FUNDAMENTALS OF HIV MEDICINE
2021 EDITION

FUNDAMENTALS OF HIV MEDICINE
2021 EDITION

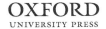

OXFORD
UNIVERSITY PRESS

Oxford University Press is a department of the University of Oxford. It furthers the University's objective of excellence in research, scholarship, and education by publishing worldwide. Oxford is a registered trade mark of Oxford University Press in the UK and certain other countries.

Published in the United States of America by Oxford University Press
198 Madison Avenue, New York, NY 10016, United States of America.

© American Academy of HIV Medicine 2021

ISSN 2752-5767 (Print)
ISSN 2752-5775 (Online)
ISBN 978–0–19–757659–5

DOI: 10.1093/med/9780197576595.001.0001

3 5 7 9 8 6 4 2

Printed by Marquis, Canada

CONTENTS

TARGET AUDIENCE

This activity has been designed to meet the educational needs of physicians, nurse practitioners, physician assistants, registered nurses, and pharmacists involved in the care of patient with HIV disease.

OVERALL LEARNING OBJECTIVES

After completing these activities, the participant should be better able to:

- Describe the evolving epidemiology of HIV disease in the US, with an emphasis on age, gender, sexuality, race/ethnicity, socioeconomic status, emerging subtypes, and viral resistance

- Implement appropriate laboratory HIV testing methods for screening and diagnosing HIV infections

- Adapt pre- and post-testing patient counseling to best meet patient needs in a variety of situations

- Provide up-to-date HIV care to a broad spectrum of infected patient populations, including pediatrics, adolescents, injection-drug users, incarcerated individuals, and an aging population

- Adjust treatment based upon the various comorbidities that are often found in HIV-infected individuals, including cardiovascular, renal, and neurologic disease

- Discuss the ethics and legal issues related to caring for HIV-infected individuals

FACULTY

LEAD EDITOR

W. David Hardy, MD, AAHIVS
Scientific and Medical Consultant Chair
Education Committee Member
Board of Directors American Academy of HIV Medicine

CO-EDITORS

Jonathan S. Appelbaum, MD, FACP, AAHIVS
Laurie L. Dozier, Jr. MD Education Director
Professor of Internal Medicine
Department of Clinical Sciences
Florida State University College of Medicine

Roberto C. Arduino, MD
Professor of Medicine
Department of Internal Medicine
Division of Infectious Diseases
McGovern Medical School
University of Texas Health Science Center at Houston

Philip Bolduc, MD
Associate Professor, Family Medicine and Community Health
University of Massachusetts Medical School
Associate Medical Director and HIV Fellowship Director
Family Health Center of Worcester

Carolyn Chu, MD, MSc
Associate Professor, Department of Family & Community Medicine
Chief Clinical Officer/PI, National Clinician Consultation Center
University of California, San Francisco

Jeffrey T. Kirchner, DO, FAAFP, AAHIVS
Medical Director Emeritus, Department of Family and Community Medicine
Physician Advisor, Department of Utilization Review and Case Management
Penn Medicine / Lancaster General Hospital

William R. Short, MD, MPH, FIDSA
Associate Professor of Medicine
Associate Professor of Obstetrics and Gynecology
Perelman School of Medicine
University of Pennsylvania

CONTRIBUTORS

Saira Ajmal, MD
Attending Physician and Clinical Assistant Professor
Department of Medicine
Advocate Christ Medical Center
University of Illinois at Chicago

Lisa Y. Armitige, MD, PhD
Assistant Medical Director, Heartland National TB Center
Associate Professor, Internal Medicine/Pediatrics/Adult ID
University of Texas Health Center at Tyler

Renata Arrington-Sanders, MD, MPH, ScM
Associate Professor
Division of Pediatrics
Division of Infectious Diseases
Johns Hopkins University

Anchalee Avihingsanon, MD, PhD
Researcher, HIV-NAT
Thai Red Cross AIDS Research Centre
Researcher, Tuberculosis Research Unit
Chulalongkorn University, Thailand

Maria Veronica Bandres, MD
Infectious Disease Fellow
Temple University Hospital

Katrina Baumgartner, MD
Lawrence General Hospital

Adam C. Bortner, MD, AAHIVS
Chief Resident
Family Medicine Residency Training Program
Family Health Centers of San Diego

Christopher M. Bositis, MD
Clinical Director, HIV and Viral Hepatitis
Greater Lawrence Family Health Center
Assistant Professor, Family Medicine
Tufts University School of Medicine

Christian Brander, PhD
ICREA Senior Research Professor
IrsiCaixa AIDS Research Institute
University of Vic, Spain

Priyanka Chakrabarti, DO
Staff Physician, Family Medicine
Partners in Primary Care

Victoria Chew, DO
Physician
Valleywise Community Health Center - McDowell Clinic

Elizabeth Y. Chiao, MD, MPH
Michael E. DeBakey VA Medical Center

Theresa Christensen, PhD
Department of Radiation Oncology
Perelman School of Medicine at the University of Pennsylvania

Eva H. Clark, MD, PhD
Assistant Professor
Division of Infectious Diseases
Baylor College of Medicine

Jennifer Cocohoba, PharmD, BCPS, AAHIVP
University of California, San Francisco, School of Pharmacy
University of California, San Francisco, Women's HIV Program

Dagan Coppock, MD
Assistant Professor
Division of Infectious Diseases
Sidney Kimmel Medical College, Thomas Jefferson University

Elizabeth H. David, MD
Associate Professor, Department of Psychiatry and Behavioral Sciences
Baylor College of Medicine
Staff Psychiatrist
Thomas Street Clinic

Abby Davids, MD, MPH, AAHIVS
HIV and Viral Hepatitis Fellowship Director
Family Medicine Residency of Idaho

Alejandro Delgado, MD
Attending Physician
Division of Infectious Diseases
Einstein Healthcare Network

Esteban A. DelPilar-Morales, MD
Attending Physician
Division of Infectious Diseases
Baystate Health/UMass Medical School

Paul W. DenOuden, MD
Physician, Site Medical Director
HIV Health Services Center
Multnomah County Health Department

Madeline B. Deutsch, MD, MPH
Associate Professor
Division of Family and Community Medicine
University of California, San Francisco

Christine M. Durand, MD
Associate Professor
Division of Medicine and Oncology
Johns Hopkins University School of Medicine

Derek M. Fine, MD
Johns Hopkins Hospital

Rajesh T. Gandhi, MD
Director, HIV Clinical Services and Education
Division of Infectious Diseases
Massachusetts General Hospital/Harvard Medical School

Deliana Garcia, MA
Director International Projects and Emerging Issues
Migrant Clinicians Network

Taylor K. Gill, PharmD, BCPS, AAHIVP
Clinical Pharmacist
Ascension Via Christi

Hannah Girard, DNP, FNP-BC, MPH
Family Nurse Practitioner
University of Massachusetts Medical School
Stanley Street Treatment and Resources (SSTAR)

Zil Garner Goldstein, FNP-BC
Associate Medical Director
Callen-Lorde Community Health Center

Dennis J. Hartigan-O'Connor, MD, PhD
Associate Professor, Department of Medical Microbiology and Immunology
Core Scientist, California National Primate Research Center
University of California, Davis

Rodrigo Hasbun, MD, MPH
Professor of Medicine
The University of Texas McGovern Medical School

Emily Heil, PharmD, MS
Associate Professor
Department of Pharmacy Practice and Science
University of Maryland School of Pharmacy

Aroonsiri (Sangarlangkarn) Howell, MD MPH
Assistant Professor
Department of Medicine
Temple University

Niyati Jakharia, MD
University of Maryland

Nikolaus Jilg, MD, PhD
Assistant in Medicine
Division of Infectious Diseases
Massachusetts General Hospital/Harvard Medical School

Boris Juelg, MD, PhD
Assistant Professor of Medicine
Division of Infectious Diseases
Massachusetts General Hospital

Angela Kapalko, PA-C, MS, AAHIVS
Education Coordinator for Advanced Practice Clinician
Students
Jonathan Lax Treatment Center
Philadelphia FIGHT Community Health Centers

Joseph S. Kass, MD, JD
Professor
Department of Neurology, Psychiatry, and Medical Ethics
Baylor College of Medicine

David E. Koren, PharmD, BCPS, AAHIVP
Clinical Pharmacist Specialist
Temple University Health System

Ramiz Kseri, MD
Assistant Professor
Clinical Sciences
Florida State University

Jonathan Lim
Johns Hopkins Medical Center

Sally Spencer-Long, MSN, ANP-BC
Adult Nurse Practitioner
Baystate Medical Center

Laszlo Madaras, MD, MPH
Chief Medical Officer, Migrant Clinicians Network
Clinical Assistant Professor of Medicine
Penn State College of Medicine

Poonam Mathur, DO, MPH
Assistant Professor
Institute of Human Virology
University of Maryland School of Medicine

Jessica A. Meisner, MD, MS, MSHP
Assistant Professor
Division of Infectious Diseases
The University of Texas Southwestern Medical Center

Steven Menez, MD
Johns Hopkins School of Medicine

Kudakwashe Mutyambizi, MD
MD Anderson Cancer Center
The University of Texas Medical School at Houston

Puja H. Nambiar, MD
Memorial Sloan Kettering Cancer Center
Weill Cornell Medical College

Thanh Thu Ngo, MD
Family Health Center of Worcester

Karin Nielsen-Saines, MD, MPH
David Geffen School of Medicine
University of California, Los Angeles

Edgar T. Overton, MD
University of Alabama School of Medicine

Bruce J. Packett, II
American Academy of HIV Medicine

Neha Sheth Pandit, PharmD
Associate Professor, Department of Pharmacy Practice and
Science
Clinical Pharmacist, THRIVE Program
University of Maryland

Ashka Patel, DO
Infectious Diseases Fellow
University of Maryland Medical Center

Manali Pednekar, MD
Memorial Hermann Health System

Lealah Pollock, MD, MS
Assistant Professor
Family and Community Medicine
University of California, San Francisco

Richard C. Prokesch, MD
Physician
Infectious Diseases Associates

Rachel A. Prosser, PhD, APRN, CNP, FAANP, AAHIVS
Hennepin County Medical Center
University of Minnesota School of Nursing
Metropolitan University School of Nursing
Centurion
RAAN
Positive Healthcare LLC

Christian B. Ramers, MD, MPH
Family Health Centers of San Diego
University of California San Diego
School of Medicine

Sarah A. Rojas, MD, MAS
Family Health Centers of San Diego

Alonso D. Pezo Salazar, MD
Infectious Diseases Fellow
The University of Texas Southwestern

Robert Shafer, MD
Professor of Medicine and Pathology
Division of Infectious Diseases
Stanford University

Jason J. Schafer, PharmD, MPH
Vice Chair and Professor
Department of Pharmacy Practice
Thomas Jefferson University

Jeffrey T. Schouten, MD
HANC Director
Office of HIV/AIDS Network Coordination
Fred Hutchinson Cancer Research Center

Claire Hutkins Seda, BA
Senior Writer and Editor
Migrant Clinicians Network

Rajagopal V. Sekhar, MD
Associate Professor of Medicine
Baylor College of Medicine

Kalpana D. Shere-Wolfe, MD
University of Maryland Medical System

Elizabeth M. Sherman, PharmD
Associate Professor, College of Pharmacy
Nova Southeastern University
Clinical Faculty, Division of Infectious Disease
Memorial Healthcare System

Daniel J. Skiest, MD
Vice Chair, Department of Medicine
Professor, Division of Infectious Diseases
Baystate Health/UMass Medical School

Benjamin Sokoloff, DO
Interim Medical Director
Cascade AIDS Project

Leah Spatafore, MD
Pediatric Resident Physician
Johns Hopkins Hospital

Gary F. Spinner, PA, MPH, AAHIVS
Medical Director, HIV/AIDS Program
Southwest Community Health Center

Rohit Talwani, MD
University of Maryland Medical Center

Erica Taylor, MD
Psychiatrist
Baylor College of Medicine
Consult-Liaison Psychiatrist
Michael E DeBakey VA Medical Center Houston

Zelalem Temesgen, MD, FIDSA
Professor of Medicine, Division of Infectious Diseases
Director, Center for Tuberculosis
Mayo Clinic

Tri Minh Trang, MD
HIV Fellow
University of Southern California

Thanh Thuy Truong, MD
Addiction Psychiatry
Department of Psychiatry and Behavioral Sciences
Baylor College of Medicine

Karen J. Vigil, MD
Associate Professor
Division of Infectious Diseases
McGovern Medical School, The University of Texas at Houston

Craig Steven Weeks, MD
Family Physician
Great Lakes Bay Health Centers
Clinical Assistant Professor
Central Michigan University

Amanda A. Westlake, MD
Physician
Division of Infectious Diseases
Baystate Medical Center/UMass Medical School

John D. Zeuli, PharmD
HIV Pharmacist
Mayo Clinic

DISCLOSURE OF CONFLICTS OF INTEREST

The Annenberg Center for Health Sciences at Eisenhower requires instructors, planners, managers and other individuals who are in a position to control the content of this activity to disclose any real or apparent conflict of interest (COI) they may have as related to the content of this activity. All identified COI are thoroughly vetted and resolved according to the Annenberg Center for Health Sciences at Eisenhower policy. The Annenberg Center for Health Sciences at Eisenhower is committed to providing its learners with high quality CME activities and related materials that promote improvements or quality in healthcare and not a specific proprietary business interest of a commercial interest.

The *faculty* reported the following financial relationships or relationships to products or devices they or their spouse/life partner have with commercial interests related to the content of this CME activity:

Name of Faculty or Presenter	Reported Financial Relationship
Saira Ajmal	Nothing to Disclose
Jonathan S. Appelbaum	Consulting Fees: Merck, ViiV Healthcare
Roberto C. Arduino	Contracted Research: ViiV Healthcare, Inc.
Lisa Y. Armitige	Nothing to Disclose
Renata Arrington-Sanders	Nothing to Disclose
Anchalee Avihingsanon	Nothing to Disclose
Maria Veronica Bandres	Nothing to Disclose
Katrina Baumgartner	Nothing to Disclose
Philip Bolduc	Nothing to Disclose
Adam C. Bortner	Nothing to Disclose
Christopher M. Bositis	Consulting Fees: Gilead
Christian Brander	Salary: Aelix Therapeutics, BCN; Contracted Research: Aelix Therapeutics, BCN; Ownership Interest: Aelix Therapeutics, BCN
Priyanka Chakrabarti	Nothing to Disclose
Victoria Chew	Nothing to Disclose
Elizabeth Y. Chiao	Nothing to Disclose
Theresa Christensen	Nothing to Disclose
Carolyn Chu	Nothing to Disclose
Eva H. Clark	Nothing to Disclose
Jennifer Cocohoba	Contracted Research: Walgreens Co.; Other: Genentech, Actelion/Janssen (Fellowship contract PI - paid to University of California San Francisco)
Dagan Coppock	Nothing to Disclose
Elizabeth H. David	Nothing to Disclose
Abby Davids	Nothing to Disclose
Alejandro Delgado	Nothing to Disclose
Esteban A. DelPilar-Morales	Nothing to Disclose
Paul W. DenOuden	Nothing to Disclose
Madeline B. Deutsch	Nothing to Disclose

Christine M. Durand	Contracted Research: Abbvie, GSK; Other: Gilead Sciences
Derek M. Fine	Consulting Fees: GSK - Drug Safety Monitoring Board
Rajesh T. Gandhi	Nothing to Disclose
Deliana Garcia	Nothing to Disclose
Taylor K. Gill	Nothing to Disclose
Hannah Girard	Nothing to Disclose
Zil Garner Goldstein	Nothing to Disclose
David Hardy	Consulting Fees: Gilead, Merck, ViiV/GSK; Contracted Research: Amgen, Gilead, Janssen, Merck, ViiV/GSK
Dennis J. Hartigan-O'Connor	Nothing to Disclose
Rodrigo Hasbun	Consulting Fees: Biofire; Contracted Research: Biofire
Emily Heil	Nothing to Disclose
Aroonsiri (Sangarlangkarn) Howell	Nothing to Disclose
Niyati Jakharia	Nothing to Disclose
Nikolaus Jilg	Nothing to Disclose
Boris Juelg	Nothing to Disclose
Angela Kapalko	Consulting Fees: ViiV Healthcare, Non-CME Fees/Commerical Interest: ViiV Healthcare, Gilead Sciences
Joseph S. Kass	Contracted Research: Biogen, Takeda, Roche/Genentech, Novartis
Jeffrey T. Kirchner	Nothing to Disclose
David E. Koren	Consulting Fees: Abbvie, Gilead, Janssen, Thera
Ramiz Kseri	Nothing to Disclose
Jonathan Lim	Nothing to Disclose
Sally Spencer-Long	Nothing to Disclose
Laszlo Madaras	Nothing to Disclose
Poonam Mathur	Nothing to Disclose
Jessica A. Meisner	Nothing to Disclose
Steven Menez	Nothing to Disclose
Kudakwashe Mutyambizi	Nothing to Disclose
Puja H. Nambiar	Nothing to Disclose
Thanh Thu Ngo	Nothing to Disclose
Karin Nielsen-Saines	Nothing to Disclose
Edgar T. Overton	Consulting Fees: ViiV Healthcare, Merck, Theratechnologies
Bruce J. Packett, II	Nothing to Disclose
Neha Sheth Pandit	Nothing to Disclose
Ashka Patel	Nothing to Disclose
Manali Pednekar	Nothing to Disclose
Lealah Pollock	Nothing to Disclose
Richard C. Prokesch	Nothing to Disclose
Rachel A. Prosser	Consulting Fees: Gilead, Contracted Research: Gilead, ViiV, GSK
Christian B. Ramers	Consulting Fees: Gilead Sciences, AbbVie, Theratechnologies, ViiV; Non-CME Fees/Commercial Interest: Gilead Sciences, AbbVie, ViiV, Merck; Contracted Research: Gilead Sciences
Sarah A. Rojas	Nothing to Disclose
Alonso D. Pezo Salazar	Nothing to Disclose
Robert Shafer	Contracted Research: Janssen Pharmaceuticals, Vela Diagnostics
Jason J. Schafer	Consulting Fees: ViiV, Merck; Contracted Research: Merck, Gilead

Jeffrey T. Schouten	Nothing to Disclose
Claire Hutkins Seda	Nothing to Disclose
Rajagopal V. Sekhar	Nothing to Disclose
Kalpana D. Shere-Wolfe	Nothing to Disclose
Elizabeth M. Sherman	Contracted Research: Gilead Sciences
William R. Short	Consulting Fees: ViiV, Non-CME Fees/Commerical Interest: ViiV, Janssen
Daniel J. Skiest	Nothing to Disclose
Benjamin Sokoloff	Nothing to Disclose
Leah Spatafore	Nothing to Disclose
Gary F. Spinner	Consulting Fees: Gilead, ViiV, Fees for Non-CME/Commerical Interest: Gilead, Ownership Interest: Gilead
Rohit Talwani	Nothing to Disclose
Erica Taylor	Nothing to Disclose
Zelalem Temesgen	Consulting Fees: ViiV Healthcare, Unrestricted Educational Grant: Gilead, ViiV, Merck
Tri Minh Trang	Nothing to Disclose
Thanh Thuy Truong	Nothing to Disclose
Karen J. Vigil	Consulting Fees: ViiV, Gilead, Napo Pharmaceuticals; Consulting Research: Merck
Craig Steven Weeks	Nothing to Disclose
Amanda A. Westlake	Nothing to Disclose
John D. Zeuli	Nothing to Disclose

The *planners and managers* reported the following financial relationships or relationships to products or devices they or their spouse/life partner have with commercial interests related to the content of this CME activity:

The Annenberg Center for Health Sciences at Eisenhower planners and managers have no conflicts to report.

The American Academy of HIV Medicine planners and managers have no conflicts to report.

The Postgraduate Institute for Medicine planners and managers have no conflicts to report.

DISCLOSURE OF UNLABELED USE

This educational activity may contain discussion of published and/or investigational uses of agents that are not indicated by the FDA. The planners of this activity do not recommend the use of any agent outside of the labeled indications.

The opinions expressed in the educational activity are those of the faculty and do not necessarily represent the views of the planners. Please refer to the official prescribing information for each product for discussion of approved indications, contraindications, and warnings.

DISCLAIMER

Participants have an implied responsibility to use the newly acquired information to enhance patient outcomes and their own professional development. The information presented in this activity is not meant to serve as a guideline for patient management. Any procedures, medications, or other courses of diagnosis or treatment discussed or suggested in this activity should not be used by clinicians without evaluation of their patient's conditions and possible contraindications and/or dangers in use, review of any applicable manufacturer's product information, and comparison with recommendations of other authorities.

1.

ENDING THE HIV EPIDEMIC
A PLAN FOR AMERICAN INITIATIVES IN THE US

Benjamin Sokoloff, Tri Minh Trang, and Thanh Thu Ngo

LEARNING OBJECTIVES

- Identify the goals of the current nationwide initiative to eliminate new HIV infections in the US

- Describe the pillars on which the initiative is built to achieve these goals

KEY POINTS

- Ending the HIV epidemic in the US is possible; the current goal is to reduce the number of new HIV infections by 75% by 2025 and by 90% by 2030.

- The four pillars of the initiative are to increase diagnosis, treatment, and prevention of HIV infection and rapid response to new clusters of HIV transmissions. These pillars are based on the strongest evidence-based science, medicine, and public health principles derived from randomized controlled clinical trials.

- The Ending the HIV Epidemic program will initially focus on 48 US counties, Puerto Rico, and Washington, DC, which have the highest rates of new infections in the US, along with seven states with the highest incidence of HIV in rural communities.

INTRODUCTION

Not only has management of persons with HIV (PWH) evolved significantly over the past three decades, but so too has the national epidemiologic plan for slowing and eventually ending the epidemic. This new chapter arrives at an auspicious time. At the time of the writing for this chapter, the United States and the world face a new global pandemic, where once again we find ourselves facing off against a novel pathogenic virus, SARS-CoV-2 and the life-threatening disease it causes, COVID-19. While COVID-19 impacts many of the same communities heavily affected by HIV, we can be grateful that, at the time of this writing, PWH do not appear

to be at higher risk for contracting SARS-CoV-2 or having more deleterious outcomes than HIV-negative persons. The US federal government throughout its history has typically responded to emerging epidemics and pandemics with legislative and executive actions with the intent of saving lives and preventing disease.

Unfortunately, new HIV infection rates have remained stubbornly high over the last decade despite many scientific and medical advances. The HIV incidence rate in 2014 was estimated to be 38,000 and the rate has remained stable since then (Centers for Disease Control and Prevention [CDC], 2020a). In addition, while the rates of new infections have declined in White men who have sex with men (MSM), they have remained stable in Black MSM and have increased in Hispanic/Latino MSM (CDC, 2020a). The CDC data from the end of 2018 also showed persistent disparities for new infections, with Blacks/African Americans making up 42% of new infections while Whites account for only 25% (CDC, 2020a). The disparities also persist in viral suppression rates between racial groups. Worse still, only 18% of persons with an indication for preexposure prophylaxis (PrEP) had a prescription for it (CDC, 2020b).

With our modern antiretroviral therapy (ART) and PrEP regimens, we should be able to suppress HIV in nearly all PWH and prevent most new infections in persons at higher risk for acquiring HIV. Using our tools of treatment as prevention (TasP) and PrEP while expanding HIV screening and focusing on those most at risk, we can see the path to zero new infections. It is clear that significant challenges remain that are preventing us from achieving this goal. And so, the Ending the HIV Epidemic (EHE) initiative was created with the bold goal of eliminating new infections in the US over the next 10 years. Mounting evidence has shown how this could be achieved, which is further cemented by the four pillars of this new program. We have come a long way from a time when HIV infection meant certain death, but we have not yet been able to stop the spread of infection on a broader scale. With this new initiative, we aspire to use the remarkable tools we have painstakingly developed to the end of this 40-year epidemic in the US.

GOALS AND TIMELINE

The EHE initiative is a 10-year plan with the goal of reducing the number of new HIV infections in the US by 75% by 2025 and by 90% by 2030, for a total of 250,000 infections averted over this time (DHHS, 2019). This translates to a reduction in the incidence of HIV infections in the US to fewer than 3,000 annually. The estimated incidence of HIV infections in the US and dependent areas in 2018 was 37,968 (CDC, 2020a). This goal, set forth by the US government, is in line with the 90-90-90 targets for ending the HIV/AIDS pandemic issued by the Joint United Nations Programme on HIV and AIDS (UNAIDS) in 2014. Based on UNAIDS-sponsored modeling, it is predicted that if 90% of persons with HIV/AIDS are diagnosed, 90% of those with a diagnosis are on ART, and 90% of those receiving ART are virally suppressed by 2020, the end of the HIV/AIDS pandemic would be achieved by 2030 (UNAIDS, 2014). At the time of this chapter's publication, 90-90-90 remains a goal attained by only a handful of countries globally. However, the EHE initiative represents the US government's ongoing commitment to eliminating HIV/AIDS as a major public health threat.

Over the 10 years of its implementation, the EHE initiative will transition through three phases. The initial phase, slated for the first 5 years, aims to target specific regions in the US—48 counties along with Puerto Rico and Washington, DC—that contributed more than 50% of all new HIV infections in the US in 2016 and 2017, as well as seven states where HIV infection remains a large burden in rural areas. Federal agencies will work with and provide support to local facilities already in place to implement the four pillars of diagnosis, treatment, prevention, and response to decrease new HIV infections by 75%. The second phase of the initiative will seek to expand on the efforts and successes achieved in phase 1 throughout the rest of the country to reach the goal of reducing the infection rate by 90% by 2030. Finally, the third phase of the initiative will focus on improving resources for individuals living with HIV who are connected to care in order to achieve viral suppression and maintain new infection rates at less than 3,000 per year (Giroir, 2020).

THE FOUR PILLARS

DIAGNOSIS

According to the latest CDC surveillance report, at the end of 2018 there were 1.2 million people living with HIV in the US. Of those, an estimated 161,800 (14%) remained undiagnosed. These individuals who are unaware of their positive HIV status are responsible for an estimated 38% of new HIV infections (CDC, 2020a). Thus, expanding HIV testing efforts to diagnose these individuals is vital not only to initiate treatment for them but also to halt further forward transmission of HIV. The first pillar of the EHE's key strategies—diagnosis—seeks to address this goal by mobilizing federal and local resources to achieve early diagnosis of all PWH. Several agencies within US Department of Health and Human Services (DHHS), including the CDC, Health Resources and Services Administration (HRSA), National Institute of Health (NIH), Indian Health Service (IHS), and Substance Abuse and Mental Health Services Administration (SAMHSA), will support community structures already in place to increase testing capabilities in both traditional settings, such as health facilities providing medical and substance abuse services, and nontraditional venues where people congregate, such as festivals, public spaces, and businesses. The overarching goal of this effort is to make HIV testing a noncontroversial, routine event for all persons in the US at least one time and repeated depending on behavioral practices.

TREATMENT

Remarkable advances in the understanding and treatment of HIV have allowed PWH taking ART to live with a stably managed chronic condition rather than a progressive, potentially life-threatening disease. Furthermore, strong evidence from the HPTN 052, PARTNER, PARTNER2, and Opposites Attract trials have repeatedly demonstrated that PWH who have consistently suppressed viral loads will not transmit the virus to their sexual partners, even by condomless sex (Bavinton et al., 2019; Cohen et al., 2011, 2016; Rodger et al., 2019). These studies provide strong support for the role of TasP. Yet, as reported by the CDC in 2018, 43% of new HIV infections come from individuals who have a known HIV diagnosis but are not receiving ART, and 20% are transmitted by HIV-positive individuals who are connected to care but have not achieved viral suppression. In 2018, 62.7% of individuals diagnosed with HIV in the US had well-suppressed viral loads. The goal of the EHE initiative is to increase this proportion to 90% by 2030. Building on the successes of clinics funded by the Ryan White HIV/AIDS Program (RWHAP), DHHS agencies seek to strengthen and expand local infrastructures while tailoring the roll-out of ART to the individual needs of each community.

PREVENTION

In 2018, there were 37,968 new HIV diagnoses in the US and dependent areas. Of those, 69% were among gay, bisexual, and other MSM; 24% among heterosexuals; and 7% among people who inject drugs (PWID). As previously discussed, Black/African American and Hispanic/Latinx individuals continue to represent a disproportionately large segment of newly HIV-positive persons (CDC, 2020a). The third pillar of the EHE initiatives aims to prevent HIV transmission by using PrEP and syringe service programs (SSPs).

PrEP significantly decreases the risk of HIV transmission via sex and injection drug use when taken daily as prescribed (Choopanya et al., 2013; Grant et al., 2010; Molina et al., 2015). However, it is estimated that fewer than 1 out of 4 of the approximately 1 million Americans at higher risk for HIV infection who are eligible for PrEP are taking it. The Ready, Set, PrEP program was created by DHHS in December 2019 as a key component of the EHE initiative to address these discrepancies. The Ready, Set, PrEP program makes PrEP available to those without prescription drug insurance coverage at no cost to them. Any individual who tests negative for HIV, has a valid PrEP prescription, and has no prescription drug insurance coverage qualifies for free PrEP medication at thousands of pharmacies nationwide. Recognizing the importance of increasing PrEP accessibility, CVS, Walgreens, and Rite Aid pharmacies have committed to dispensing free PrEP medications at their combined 21,000 locations as of March 30, 2020 (DHHS, 2019). Additionally, Gilead Sciences, the company that produces Truvada and Descovy, has committed to donating PrEP medications for up to 200,000 individuals yearly over 11 years. EHE funding will further help to expand PrEP services in local communities with particular focus on vulnerable populations such as MSM of color, women of color at higher risk for HIV, PWID, and persons between 18 and 30 years of age.

SSPs are community-based prevention programs aimed at providing comprehensive resources to PWID, including access to substance use disorder treatment, needle-exchange programs, and infectious diseases screening with linkage to care. Well-established and proven to be safe, efficacious, and cost-effective, SSPs contribute to an estimated 50% reduction in incidence of both HIV and the hepatitis C virus (HCV). In combination with medication-assisted treatment for opioid use disorder, this rate is reduced to greater than two-thirds. Thus, supporting and implementing SSPs in at-risk communities will be a powerful tool in preventing new HIV transmissions. These efforts will be spearheaded by the CDC and SAMHSA under EHE's pillar of prevention.

RESPONSE

The powerful tools that allow for rapid diagnosis and effective treatment and prevention of HIV can be wielded more successfully with thoughtful implementation of epidemiologic techniques to help guide the distribution of resources where they are most needed. The final pillar of the EHE initiative aims to strengthen communities' ability to respond quickly to new outbreaks through collaborative efforts between federal health departments and local facilities via epidemiologic trends and lab surveillance. This partnership between federal (CDC) and local public health agencies endeavors to quickly identify potential "clusters" of HIV transmission using sophisticated, real-time molecular techniques; to use epidemiologic tracing; and to offer diagnostic, therapeutic, and prophylactic interventions as appropriate.

THE TARGETED JURISDICTIONS AND FUNDING

In fiscal year (FY) 2019, DHHS allocated $33 million from the Minority HIV/AIDS Fund to be used by the phase 1–targeted jurisdictions and key stakeholders to implement initial EHE activities. Some of these activities include the launch of Ready, Set, PrEP; deployment of funds to phase 1-targeted jurisdictions and tribal communities; further support for AIDS-related treatment implementation research; and deployment of Prevention through Active Community Engagement (PACE) officers (DHHS, 2019). These officers, part of the US Public Health Service Commissioned Corps, were deployed in teams of three to work collaboratively with local leadership in Atlanta, Dallas, and Los Angeles. PACE officers have the responsibilities of assessing community needs to effectively guide and support local efforts in eliminating HIV (Giroir, 2019).

In FY20, $267 million was appropriated for EHE activities under the discretionary spending amount of $1.4 trillion. Over half of this amount (52.4%) was directed to the CDC's Division of HIV/AIDS Prevention to further expand PrEP use and develop new strategies to control clusters of new HIV outbreaks. The pillars of prevention and response took highest priority in FY20's funding package. Roughly a quarter ($63 million) of the funding was directed toward 60 RWHAPs to bolster linkage to care and overall treatment strategies (DHHS, 2020a). This was primarily provided to 39 metropolitan areas and eight states; $2.8 million was allotted to AIDS Education and Training Centers and $5 million was invested toward technical assistance and systems coordination (HRSA, 2020a).

Arguably, the most notable component of the appropriated money was used through HRSA's Primary Care HIV Prevention fund. This program was awarded $53.7 million across 195 health centers primarily located in targeted jurisdictions. It highlighted the importance of the primary care setting in achieving the goals of EHE initiative (DHHS, 2020a).

At the time of this writing, the components of FY21's budget proposal have not been confirmed and distributed. However, we note with great optimism that the proposed amount toward the EHE initiative will be more than twice that of the prior two years combined! EHE is expected to receive $716 million in FY21, with roughly half of the amount going toward the CDC and the other half going toward RWHAP health centers, a sizable increase compared to the prior fiscal year. It is also important to mention that $27 million will be dedicated to the IHS to combat the epidemic in Native American and Alaska Native communities. This component was unfortunately not appropriated in the previous fiscal year (DHHS, 2020b).

REFERENCES

Bavinton, B. R., Prestage, G. P., Jin, F., et al. Strategies used by gay male HIV serodiscordant couples to reduce the risk of HIV transmission from anal intercourse in three countries. *J Int AIDS Soc* 2019;22(4):e25277. https://doi.org/10.1002/jia2.25277

Centers for Disease Control and Prevention. Estimated HIV Incidence and Prevalence in the United States 2014–2018. HIV Surveillance Supplemental Report 2020a;25(1). https://www.cdc.gov/hiv/pdf/library/reports/surveillance/cdc-hiv-surveillance-supplemental-report-vol-25-1.pdf

Centers for Disease Control and Prevention. HIV Surveillance Report (2020b, June 8). https://www.hhs.gov/blog/2019/02/05/ending-the-hiv-epidemic-a-plan-for-america.html

Choopanya, K., Martin, M., Suntharasamai, P., et al. Antiretroviral prophylaxis for HIV infection in injecting drug users in Bangkok, Thailand (the Bangkok Tenofovir Study): a randomised, double-blind, placebo-controlled phase 3 trial. *Lancet* 2013;381(9883):2083–2090. https://doi.org/10.1016/S0140-6736(13)61127-7

Cohen, M. S., Chen, Y. Q., McCauley, M., et al. Antiretroviral therapy for the prevention of HIV-1 transmission. *N Engl J Med* 2016;375(9):830–839. https://doi.org/10.1056/NEJMoa1600693

Cohen, M. S., Chen, Y. Q., McCauley, M., et al. Prevention of HIV-1 infection with early antiretroviral therapy. *N Engl J Med* 2011;365(6):493–505. https://doi.org/10.1056/NEJMoa1105243

Department of Health and Human Services. Ending the HIV Epidemic: A Plan for America (2019, February 19). https://www.hhs.gov/blog/2019/02/05/ending-the-hiv-epidemic-a-plan-for-america.html

Department of Health Resources and Services Administration. FY 2020 Ending the HIV Epidemic Awards. (2020a, February 26). https://hab.hrsa.gov/about-ryan-white-hivaids-program/fy2020-ending-hiv-epidemic-awards

Department of Health and Human Services, Office of Infectious Disease and HIV/AIDS Policy. Ending the HIV Epidemic Funding (2020b, May 22). https://www.hiv.gov/federal-response/ending-the-hiv-epidemic/funding

Giroir, B. P. PACE announcement—Ending the HIV Epidemic (2020, July 8). https://www.hiv.gov/blog/pace-announcement

Giroir, B. P. The time is now to end the HIV epidemic. *Am J Public Health* 2020;110(1):22–24. https://doi.org/10.2105/AJPH.2019.305380

Grant, R. M., Lama, J. R., Anderson, P. L., et al. Preexposure chemoprophylaxis for HIV prevention in men who have sex with men. *N Engl J Med* 2010;363(27):2587–2599. https://doi:10.1056/NEJMoa1011205

Molina, J. M., Charreau, I., Spire, B., et al. Efficacy, safety, and effect on sexual behaviour of on-demand pre-exposure prophylaxis for HIV in men who have sex with men: an observational cohort study. *Lancet* 2015;4(9):e402–e410. https://doi.org/10.1016/S2352-3018(17)30089-9

Rodger, A. J., Cambiano, V., Bruun, T., et al. Risk of HIV transmission through condomless sex in serodifferent gay couples with the HIV-positive partner taking suppressive antiretroviral therapy (PARTNER): final results of a multicentre, prospective, observational study. *Lancet* 2019:393(10189):2428–2438. https://doi.org/10.1016/S0140-6736(19)30418-0

UNAIDS. 90-90-90: An Ambitious Treatment Target to Help End the HIV Epidemic (2014, October). https://www.unaids.org/sites/default/files/media_asset/90-90-90_en.pdf

2.

EPIDEMIOLOGY AND THE SPREAD OF HIV

Philip Bolduc, Victoria Chew, Hannah Girard, and Craig Steven Weeks

OVERVIEW OF WORLDWIDE PANDEMIC

LEARNING OBJECTIVE

- Discuss the global prevalence as well as the geographic distribution of HIV-1 and HIV-2 infections, and updates on recent shared global initiatives

WHAT'S NEW?

The World Health Organization/Joint United Nations Programme on HIV and AIDS (WHO/UNAIDS) estimates that in 2019, 38 million people worldwide were living with HIV (UNAIDS, 2020). Although the numbers of new HIV infections and AIDS-related deaths continue to decline in many regions of the world, including sub-Saharan Africa, there are still certain regions where the incidence of HIV is rising, most notably in the Eastern European and Eastern Mediterranean areas. In his foreword to the UNAIDS Global AIDS Update 2018, executive director Michel Sidibe writes, "The global AIDS response is at a precarious point—partial success in saving lives and stopping new HIV infections is giving way to complacency. At the halfway point to the 2020 targets, the pace of progress is not matching the global ambition" (Sidibe, 2018). As we approach the work yet unfinished with humility and eagerness, it is important to acknowledge improvements in the HIV care continuum. Namely, the incidence of HIV has been reduced by 40% since the peak in 1998. Since 2010 alone, the HIV incidence reported among children in 2019 has decreased by 52% (UNAIDS, 2020). The 90-90-90 initiative, which is described later in the chapter, has highlighted critical improvements and enduring deficits alike.

KEY POINTS

- UNAIDS identified several demographic subgroups at high risk for HIV infection and in danger of being left behind by the global AIDS response, including adolescent girls and young women, men who have sex with men (MSM), transgender people, people who inject drugs (PWID), prisoners, and sex workers.

- HIV occurs as types 1 and 2, with several subtypes or clades making up HIV-1. Subtype B predominates in the Western Hemisphere and Western Europe, whereas other subtypes and recombinant forms are more prevalent elsewhere. Introduction of other subtypes and recombinant strains is occurring in the Western Hemisphere and Western Europe.

Since the onset of the global epidemic, 76 million persons are estimated to have acquired HIV infection and 33 million have died of HIV/AIDS (UNAIDS, 2020). At the end of 2019, an estimated 38.0 million (31.6–44.5 million) people were living with HIV, while 1.7 million (1.2–2.2 million) people newly acquired HIV infection that year. An estimated 0.7% (0.6–0.9%) of adults aged 15 to 49 years worldwide are living with HIV, although the burden of the epidemic continues to vary considerably between countries and regions. Africa remains the most heavily burdened, with nearly 1 in every 25 adults (3.7%) living with HIV, representing more than two-thirds of the persons with HIV (PWH) globally (Figure 2.1).

Across all countries, several key demographic subgroups continue to be most impacted by the HIV/AIDS epidemic. UNAIDS has identified six populations at higher risk of acquiring HIV that are in danger of being left behind by the global AIDS response: adolescent girls and young women, men who have sex with men (MSM), transgender people, people who inject drugs (PWID), prisoners, and sex workers. The risk of acquiring HIV is 26 times higher among MSM; 29 times higher among people who inject drugs; 30 times higher for sex workers; and 13 times higher for transgender women compared to other adults in the general population (UNAIDS, 2020).

The importance of each of these populations varies by region and within countries. For example, in southern Africa, age-disparate intergenerational sexual relationships and transactional sex place adolescent girls and young women at extremely high risk for HIV; in Eastern Europe and Central Asia, most new HIV acquisitions are associated with injection drug use; and in the Latin America, the Caribbean, Western Europe, and North America, the largest proportion of new HIV diagnoses occurs among MSM. These six key populations and their sexual partners account for 47% of new HIV acquisitions globally, but with wide geographic differences: just 16% in eastern and southern Africa but 95% in Eastern Europe, central Asia, the Middle East, and North Africa (UNAIDS, 2018).

In 2014, UNAIDS launched the 90-90-90 initiative. Briefly outlined, its objectives are that 90% of persons with

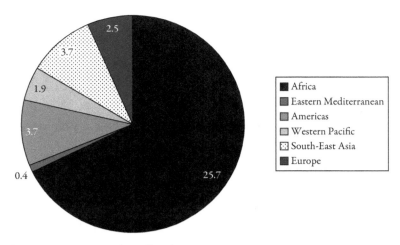

Figure 2.1 People living with HIV by WHO region, 2019 (in millions)   SOURCE: WHO estimates, 2019. Available at: https://www.who.int/gho/hiv/epidemic_status/cases_all/en/. Accessed August 17, 2020

HIV will be diagnosed, among whom 90% will be started and maintained on treatment, among whom 90% will be virally suppressed (or an overall viral suppression rate of 73%). With 75 of 170 countries reporting complete HIV testing and treatment data between 2015 and 2018, 15 were meeting the overall 73% viral suppression target. Among these, six countries accomplished each of the 90-90-90 targets, including three southern African countries, namely Botswana, Eswatini, and Namibia (Marsh et al., 2019).

In 2019, 81% of the 38 million PWH across the world knew their status (68–95%). Among them, 82% (66–97%) were accessing antiretroviral therapy (ART), and 88% (71–100%) of these persons had suppressed viral loads. Looked at another way, in 2019 67% of all PWH globally (54–79%) were on treatment and 59% (49–69%) achieved viral suppression.

Looking back, data show that we continue to close global gaps in treatment coverage, with 19 million more PWH on treatment in 2019 than in 2009. However, whereas average year-on-year increases in PWH on treatment since 2015 have been 2.0 million, an annual increase of more than 3.3 million per year will be required to meet the targets outlined for 2020. Remarkably, the viral suppression gap closed to 7.7 million people in 2018, down from over 12 million in 2015. Similarly, AIDS-related deaths dropped 60% since its peak in 2004, and AIDS-related mortality declined by 39% since 2010 (UNAIDS, 2020).

HIV DIVERSITY

There are two major types of HIV, designated HIV-1 and HIV-2. Each has a similar but distinct genome with a genetic difference of approximately 60%. The vast majority of clinical cases are caused by HIV-1, with HIV-2 representing only 1 to 2 million globally (Campbell-Yesufu & Gandhi, 2011). HIV-2 is found almost exclusively in persons from or living in West Africa and is transmitted at lower rates than HIV-1. It appears to have a longer incubation period, produce a lower plasma viral load, and lead to AIDS in fewer patients (Apetrei & Marx, 2004). HIV-1 is classified into three genetically related subtypes based on the coding sequence of the

envelope gene. Group M (Main) is the most common, and groups O (Outlier) and N (Not-M, Not-O, or New) remain rare (Apetrei & Marx, 2004). Group M has at least 11 subtypes, or clades, designated A through K.

There is limited clinical trial information on ART for HIV-2, but data do show that HIV-2 is naturally resistant to non-nucleoside reverse transcriptase inhibitors (NNRTIs) and enfuvirtide (Witvrouw et al., 2004; US Department of Health & Human Services [USDHHS], 2020). HIV-1 subtype (i.e., group) variability may eventually influence how ART is used, but at this point no data have shown any subtypes to be less sensitive to or have a greater propensity to develop resistance to current antiretroviral drugs (Gomes et al., 2002; Spira et al., 2003; Wainberg, 2004).

RECOMMENDED READING

UNAIDS. Global HIV & AIDS statistics—2020 fact sheet. http://www.unaids.org/en/resources/fact-sheet.
World Health Organization. HIV/AIDS data and statistics. http://www.who.int/hiv/data/en/.

OVERVIEW OF US EPIDEMIC

LEARNING OBJECTIVE

- Describe current demographic trends in HIV in the US, especially regarding gender, sexuality, race/ethnicity, age, injection drug use, socioeconomic status, and recent initiatives

WHAT'S NEW?

Impoverished urban areas are being defined as HIV epidemic settings. To look at the District of Columbia as an example, it estimated that 1 in every 20 adults, 1 in 7 gay or bisexual men, and 1 in 3 Black gay or bisexual men has HIV, and African Americans account for three-quarters of all persons with HIV.

KEY POINTS

- HIV incidence among young black and Latino MSM continues to increase.

- The leading mode of HIV transmission continues to be male same-sex sexual contact.

- Slowly declining incidence and more rapidly diminishing death rates continue to drive up HIV prevalence and workforce demands.

OVERALL US HIV PREVALENCE, INCIDENCE, AND DEATHS

EMPHASIS ON AREA AND KEY POPULATIONS AND PROGRAMS

According to the Centers for Disease Control and Prevention (CDC) reports on prevalence and incidence data on HIV and AIDS in the 50 US states and six dependent areas, from 2014 to 2018 the number and rate of persons living with diagnosed HIV infection increased. At year-end 2018, over 1 million (1,040,3520) adults and adolescents were living with diagnosed HIV infection, for a prevalence of 374.6 per 100,000 population (Figure 2.2). From 2014 to 2018, regionally, the rates of persons living with HIV in the Midwest, South, and West all increased, whereas the rate in the Northeast was stable. The largest percentage increase in the rate (11%) was in the Midwest. Nevertheless, at year-end 2018, prevalence remained highest in the Northeast (420.5) followed by 371.6 in the South, 260.7 in the West, and 179.8 in the Midwest. There were 37,968 new diagnoses in 2018, down from 39,782 in 2016. Among these, 69% were among gay, bisexual, and other MSM, 24% were among heterosexuals, and 7% were among PWID (CDC, 2020c).

Despite CDC and US Preventive Task Force recommendations for routine, opt-out, non–risk-factor-based HIV screening since 2006, AIDS remains disappointingly common, with 16,990 persons receiving a new AIDS diagnosis in 2018, making up 45% of the number of new HIV infections in 2018 (CDC, 2018a). New AIDS diagnoses follow a geographic and transmission trend similar to HIV diagnoses. The high rate of AIDS despite the widespread availability of

Rates per 100,000 population: Data classified using quartiles

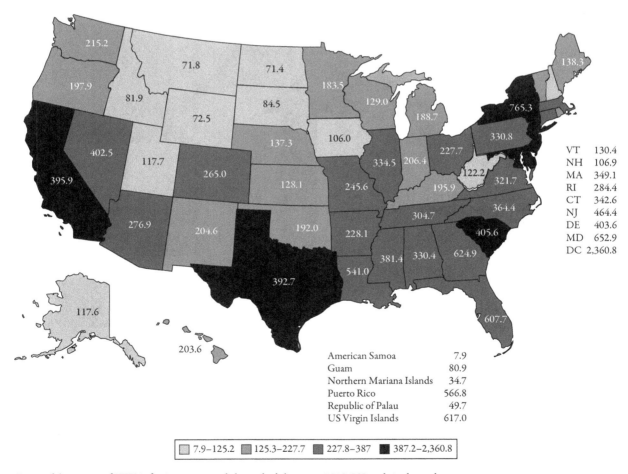

VT	130.4
NH	106.9
MA	349.1
RI	284.4
CT	342.6
NJ	464.4
DE	403.6
MD	652.9
DC	2,360.8

American Samoa	7.9
Guam	80.9
Northern Mariana Islands	34.7
Puerto Rico	566.8
Republic of Palau	49.7
US Virgin Islands	617.0

☐ 7.9–125.2　☐ 125.3–227.7　☐ 227.8–387　■ 387.2–2,360.8

Figure 2.2 Rates of diagnoses of HIV infection among adults and adolescents, 2018, US and six dependent areas　SOURCE: CDC, 2018. Available at https://www.cdc.gov/hiv/library/reports/hiv-surveillance/vol-31/content/living.html. Accessed August 17, 2020.

effective, tolerable ART highlights the need for improved HIV screening as well as care linkage, retention, and treatment for those already diagnosed with HIV (CDC, 2018a).

Death rates related to HIV continue to show a low, slow decline following the sharp drop-off with the advent of effective ART in 1996. With new infections outpacing deaths by approximately 25,000 cases each year, HIV prevalence continues to rise. Two important implications of this are that (1) more clinicians will be needed to care for the burgeoning aging HIV population and (2) more must be done to prevent HIV transmission by targeting high-risk populations with interventions of proven efficacy, such as preexposure prophylaxis (PrEP) and treatment as prevention (TasP).

THE US HIV CARE CONTINUUM

Since the USDHHS HIV/AIDS Bureau's National HIV/AIDS Strategy (NHAS) release in 2010, the HIV treatment community has focused on what is known as the HIV care continuum as the leading quality indicator in our healthcare system's response to HIV. The care continuum comprises rates of HIV diagnoses among persons estimated to have acquired HIV, care linkage, retention, and viral suppression (Figure 2.3). Although the NHAS goals (reducing new HIV diagnoses; increasing access to care and improving health outcomes for people living with HIV; reducing HIV-related health disparities) go beyond the care continuum, they nonetheless remain a fundamental indicator of progress not only for the NHAS but also for the newer Ending the HIV Epidemic initiative (see Chapter 1).

As ART has become increasingly potent, less toxic, and easier to take, the greatest challenges in suppressing what is commonly referred to as "community viral load" now exist primarily in the first three steps of the continuum. Unfortunately, little progress was made from 2010 to 2012 in these measures, and in 2012 fewer than one-third of PWH in the US were virally suppressed. However, by 2018, 86% of PWH knew their status and 65% were engaged in care, and although only 50% were retained in care, 56% had viral suppression (CDC, 2018b). On the prevention side, the number of adults prescribed PrEP increased by more than 300% from 7,972 in 2014 to 33,273 in 2015 (National HIV/AIDS Strategy: 2017 Progress Report), although even by 2018, only 18.1% of PrEP-eligible persons were prescribed it, including a disappointing 5.9% of eligible Blacks (CDC, 2018c). While these data show real progress, we still have significant work to do for the regions and groups most at risk. Providing HIV prevention, testing, and care across a variety of settings,

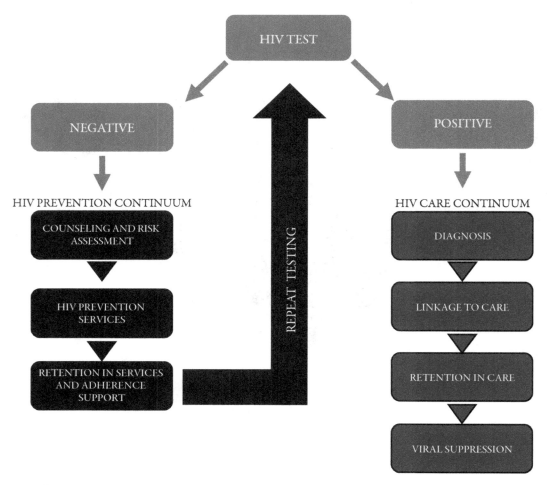

Figure 2.3 HIV testing and care continuum   Adapted from Horn et al. *J Int AIDS Soc.* 2016;19(1):21263.

particularly community health centers and other medical homes that serve affected populations with cultural competence, is critical to further improving outcomes along the care continuum.

TRANSMISSION GROUP SPECIAL CONSIDERATIONS

Though any person may acquire HIV, it is well known that the US epidemic disproportionately impacts key populations and geographic areas. As an example, Black gay and bisexual men made up 37% of new HIV diagnoses among all gay and bisexual men in 2017, more than three times their percentage of the total population (Figure 2.4). From a geographic perspective, the CDC identifies impoverished urban areas as settings of generalized epidemics. By definition, a concentrated epidemic exists when the prevalence rate is less than 1% in the general population but more than 5% in at least one high-risk subpopulation, such as is seen with HIV among MSM, PWID, and persons who exchange sex for money (sometimes referred to as commercial sex workers, or CSWs) in these areas (Denning & DiNenno, 2019).

Regrettably, we lack population-level data on CSWs given the frequently criminalized status of commercial sex work, presenting a barrier to understanding transmission dynamics and developing solutions. Similarly, important to ending the HIV epidemic is reaching out to PWID, who accounted for 9% (3,641) of the 38,739 US HIV diagnoses in 2017 (including 2,389 cases attributed to injection drug use alone and 1,252 to male-to-male sexual contact and injection drug use) (CDC, 2020a). A focus on this nexus of high-risk groups will continue to be critical to HIV work in impoverished urban areas, not all of which are located in major cities. More HIV clinicians are needed in new locations to reach underserved populations. In addition, in order to end the HIV epidemic, HIV prevention and education must expand beyond historically high-prevalence areas to newer high-incidence states and counties to reduce new infections in a way that we have not been able to do thus far.

RECOMMENDED READING

Centers for Disease Control and Prevention. HIV Surveillance Report, 2018. https://www.cdc.gov/hiv/library/reports/hiv-surveillance/vol-31/index.html

HIV AMONG COMMUNITIES OF COLOR

WHAT'S NEW?

HIV infection among Native Hawaiians/other Pacific Islanders in the US has increased.

KEY POINTS

- The prevalence of HIV among Blacks is more than three times higher than their percentage of the US population, with rates highest in the southeastern United States.

- Young Black MSM have the highest risk for HIV acquisition of any demographic group in the US.

- AIDS and AIDS-related deaths among Blacks and Hispanics are higher than population norms.

UNEQUAL BURDENS

While the annual number and rate of diagnoses of HIV infection in the United States decreased overall from 2014 to 2018, this varied widely among different subgroup populations. In Native Hawaiians/other Pacific Islanders (NHOPI), new HIV diagnoses increased 51% during this timeframe, with the majority of new cases among NHOPI MSM. In contrast, the rates of new HIV diagnoses among Asians, Blacks, Hispanics/Latinx, Whites, and persons of multiple races decreased slightly and the rate for American Indians/Alaska Natives remained stable (Figure 2.5). Although NHOPI make up less than 1% of new HIV diagnoses in the US, HIV

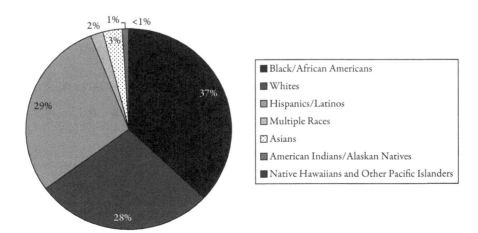

Figure 2.4 New HIV diagnoses among gay and bisexual men in the US and dependent areas by race/ethnicity, 2017   SOURCE: CDC. Diagnoses of HIV infection in the United States and dependent areas, 2017. HIV Surveillance Report 2018; 29.

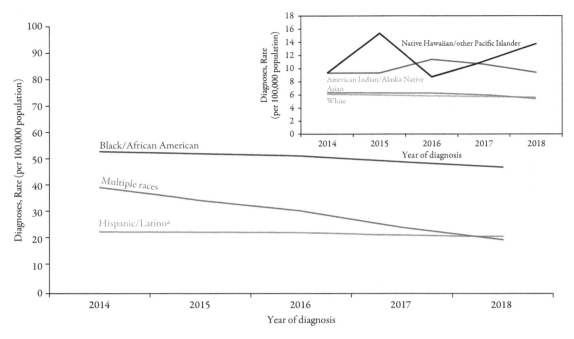

Figure 2.5 Rates of diagnoses of HIV infection among adults and adolescents by race/ethnicity, 2014–2018, United States ᵃHispanics Latinos can be of any race.
SOURCE: CDC Diagnoses of HIV infection in the United States and dependent areas, 2018. HIV Surveillance Report, 2018 (Updated); vol. 31. Available at http://www.cdc.gov/hiv/library/reports/hiv-surveillance.html. Accessed August 15, 2020.

may affect this group in ways that are not readily apparent because of their small population size (only 0.2% of the US population in 2018) and a lack of representation in clinical trials or epidemiologic analyses. In addition to societal disadvantages, including poverty and limited access to healthcare, NHOPI cultural customs, such as not discussing sex across generations, may stigmatize sexuality, especially homosexuality, and prevent NHOPI from accessing HIV prevention and care services.

However, the most critical feature to note about US epidemiologic HIV data is that Blacks continue to be the group hardest hit by HIV infections and deaths. Figure 2.6 shows how this group increased its percentage among AIDS diagnoses early in the epidemic while cases among Caucasians declined, overtaking them in 1995 before leveling off in 2000, and the number of cases among Blacks continues to far exceed all other racial groups. Blacks are vastly overrepresented among PWH compared to their percentage of the general population in 2018 (41% vs. 13%). This is also true, but to a lesser extent, for Hispanics (22% vs. 18%). These numbers for Whites, by comparison, are 29% and 60%, respectively.

The current highest-risk demographic in the US is young Black MSM who live in the South, driving the epidemic in this subgroup across the US to the extent that the CDC announced in 2016 that if current demographic trends continue, fully one-half of Black MSM (and one-quarter of Latino MSM) will be infected with HIV in their lifetime. Death rates are also heavily skewed against Blacks with HIV, with a sevenfold higher death rate than that of HIV-infected Whites. The Hispanic death rate is almost twice that of Whites, whereas other groups fare the same or better.

Regardless of how these data are examined—whether considering HIV diagnoses, AIDS, or deaths—in the US Blacks and, to a lesser extent, Hispanics shoulder a strikingly excessive burden of HIV. The 2016 National HIV/AIDS Strategy recognized this in its call to reduce racial disparities in HIV care, which should be incorporated into the mission of all local, regional, and national HIV programs. Such efforts must address the stigma, fear, discrimination, homophobia, distrust, and socioeconomic issues associated with poor access to care in these at-risk populations. The CDC and its partners are pursuing a high-impact prevention approach, increasing awareness about testing, prevention (including PrEP), and retention in care among populations disproportionately affected by HIV, particularly gay or bisexual men of color (HIV Surveillance Supplemental Report, 2018).

HIV AMONG IMMIGRANT POPULATIONS

KEY POINTS

- The percentage of new AIDS diagnoses in the United States among minority races/ethnicities continues to climb.

- HIV-2 infection, while still uncommon in the United States, may rise as more persons emigrate from West Africa.

- Different immigrant populations have widely varying rates of HIV infection, and differences within foreign and US-born racial/ethnic minorities are not fully understood.

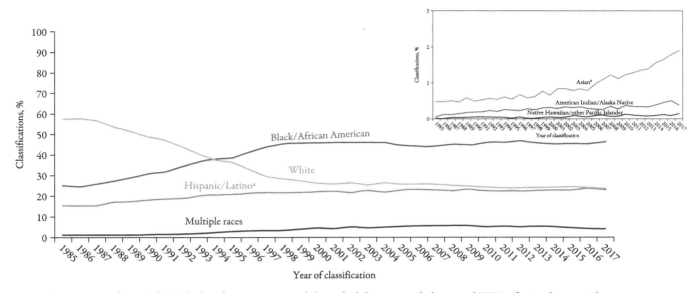

Figure 2.6 Percentages of stage 3 (AIDS) classifications among adults and adolescents with diagnosed HIV infection by race/ethnicity, 1985–2017—United States and six dependent areas   [a]Hispanics/Latinos can be of any race. [b]The Asian category includes Asian/Pacific Islander legacy cases.
SOURCE: CDC HIV/AIDS Resource Library Slide Sets. Available at http://www.cdc.gov/hiv/library/slidesets/index.html Accessed August 15, 2020.

• Immigrants, legal or not, face many barriers to engagement with the healthcare system.

For several years, the CDC has published data on the incidence and prevalence of HIV, AIDS, and HIV-related deaths among Blacks, Latinos/Hispanics, Asians, Native Americans, and Pacific Islanders. These data are summarized in Tables 2.1 and 2.2, which show the wide range of impact of HIV in these different groups and the growing overrepresentation of racial and ethnic minorities as a whole among AIDS diagnoses (72%) (Figure 2.7). However, in these data, the CDC does not separate African-born from US-born Blacks, or foreign-born versus US-born Latinos/Hispanics, making it difficult to track the HIV epidemic among these different immigrant populations. Despite this, a 2013 review found the HIV incidence among African-born versus US-born Blacks to be two-thirds higher, presentation with AIDS more frequent (30 vs. 22%), and progression to AIDS within 12 months of an HIV diagnosis more likely (45% vs. 37%), this despite the already high rates of these indicators among Blacks as a whole. Paradoxically, survival was better among African-born versus US-born Blacks (7.1 vs. 19.5 deaths per 1,000/year), possibly due to better engagement in care (Blanas et al., 2013).

Since January 4, 2010, refugees are no longer tested for HIV infection on arrival to the United States. However, since 2006, CDC guidelines have recommended universal screening for all persons 13 to 64 years of age regardless of risk factors or country of origin (Branson, 2006). Given that the chaotic and vulnerable conditions of refugee flight and refugee camps create a high risk for HIV transmission, HIV screening of

Table 2.1 ADULTS AND ADOLESCENTS LIVING WITH DIAGNOSED HIV INFECTION BY RACE/ ETHNICITY, YEAR- END 2017

RACE/ETHNICITY	NUMBER	RATE	%
American Indian/Alaskan Native	3,032	126.2	0.3
Asian	14,244	78.1	1.4
Black/African American	414,747	1,022.0	41.3
Hispanic/Latino	222,662	379.3	22
Native Hawaiian/other Pacific Islander	839	145.6	0.1
White	300,169	152.1	29.9
Multiple races	46,857	675.9	4.7
Total	1,003,782	308.7	100

SOURCE: CDC HIV/ AIDS Resource Library Slide Sets. Available at http:// www.cdc.gov/ hiv/ library/ slidesets/ index.html. Accessed August 15, 2020.

Table 2.2 DEATHS OF PERSONS WITH DIAGNOSED HIV INFECTION EVER CLASSIFIED AS STAGE 3 (AIDS) BY RACE/ ETHNICITY, YEAR- END 2017, US

RACE/ETHNICITY	NUMBER	RATE	%
American Indian/Alaskan Native	39	1.6	0.2
Asian	84	0.5	0/5
Black/African American	7049	17.4	44.1
Hispanic/Latino	2606	4.4	16.3
Native Hawaiian/other Pacific Islander	8	1.4	<1
White	5123	2.6	32.1
Multiple races	1061	15.3	6.6
Total	15,971	4.9	100

SOURCE: CDC HIV/ AIDS Resource Library Slide Sets. Available at http// www.cdc.gov/ hiv/ library/ slidesets/ index.html. Accessed August 15, 2020.

all refugees is encouraged. The CDC-recommended fourth-generation testing algorithm differentiates between HIV-1 and HIV-2, whereas older-generation HIV antibody screening tests generally do not. Therefore, if fourth-generation testing is not available, refugees or immigrants who are native to or who transited through countries with a high HIV-2 prevalence should have specific testing for HIV-2.

The CDC's 2014 surveillance case definition for HIV and AIDS applies to both variants of HIV and has specified criteria for defining HIV-2 infection. From 1988 to June 2010, 242 HIV-2 cases were reported to the CDC, but, of these, only 166 met the case definition for HIV-2. These cases were concentrated in the Northeast (66%), including 46% in New York City, occurring primarily among persons born in West Africa (81%) (CDC, 2011). During the period 2010 to 2017, use of the HIV-1/HIV-2 differentiation test increased, but the number of confirmed HIV-2 diagnoses in the US remained

less than 0.1%, consistent with previously reported findings (Peruski et al., 2020).

Data from King County, Washington, show the percentage of new HIV cases that were foreign-born rising from 23% to 34% from 2006 to 2015. The leading countries of origin were Africa (34%), Latin America (32%), and Asia (22%). Africans with HIV were more likely to be female and heterosexual, while Latin Americans and Asians were similar to US-born individuals by HIV risk factor and gender (male MSM) (Kerani et al., 2018).

Multiple factors contribute to HIV infection among immigrants. Migration within and across national borders in search of work may contribute to increased HIV risk situations. In addition, change in residence can result in loneliness, isolation, and disruption of social, familial, and sexual relationships that can lead to risk-taking behavior (Organista et al., 2004). In another study, the authors found lack of

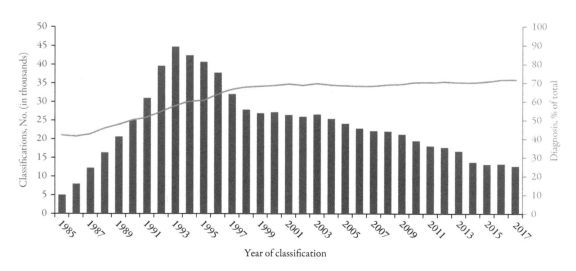

Figure 2.7 Diagnosed HIV infections classified as stage 3 (AIDS) among racial/ethnic minorities, 1985–2017, US and six dependent areas   SOURCE: CDC HIV/AIDS Resource Library Slide Sets. Available at http://www.cdc.gov/hiv/library/slidesets/index.html. Accessed August 15, 2020.

knowledge regarding HIV risk, social stigma, secrecy, and symptom-driven health-seeking behavior (as opposed to routine preventive care) as factors in delayed HIV presentation in immigrants. Furthermore, compared to US-born patients, immigrants were significantly younger; were more likely to present with indicators of more advanced HIV disease, including opportunistic infections; had lower CD4 counts; and were more likely to be hospitalized at the time of HIV diagnosis, consistent with findings specific to African-born HIV patients, as mentioned earlier (Levy et al., 2007).

RECOMMENDED READING

Blanas DA, Nichols K, Bekele M, et al. HIV/AIDS among African-born residents in the United States. *J Immigr Minor Health* 2013;15(4):718–724.

Centers for Disease Control and Prevention. HIV slide sets: HIV surveillance by race/ethnicity (through 2018). https://www.cdc.gov/hiv/library/slidesets/index.html.

HIV AMONG WOMEN, CHILDREN, AND ADOLESCENTS

WHAT'S NEW?

Nineteen percent of HIV diagnoses in 2018 in the US were among women, a figure that has remained stable since 2015. With widespread utilization of ART, transmission of HIV from mother to child has decreased to less than 1% in the United States.

KEY POINTS

- High-risk heterosexual contact remains the most common risk factor for HIV acquisition among adult women.

- The CDC recommends opt-out testing for all pregnant women in the first trimester and repeat testing in the third trimester for women at risk for infection. Adolescent HIV transmission mirrors adult patterns, with large majorities of males infected via same-sex contact and females via heterosexual contact.

WOMEN

Worldwide in 2019, women continue to account for more than half of all PWH and 48% of new infections, largely through heterosexual transmission (American Foundation for AIDS Research [amfAR], 2019). In sub-Saharan Africa, five in six new infections are among girls aged 15 to 19 years, and young women aged 15 to 24 years are twice as likely as men to be living with HIV (UNAIDS, 2020). However, in the US, women made up only 19% of HIV diagnoses in 2018, a figure that has remained stable since 2015, representing an estimated 7,190 newly diagnosed infections. This disparity is due to the preponderance of male-to-male HIV transmission in the US. Of these new diagnoses, approximately 4,336 were

stage 3 (AIDS) classifications, a number that has been declining since 1996 but remains stubbornly fixed at around one-quarter of all HIV diagnoses among women, highlighting the need to improve testing to find patients before progression to AIDS. HIV incidence among US women continues to be highest in the South, followed by the industrial states of the Northeast.

From 2014 through 2018, Black women accounted for the majority of new HIV diagnoses in US females, although the number decreased from 4,573 in 2014 to 4,114 in 2018. The seropositivity rate of these women (23 per 100,000 persons) was nearly 14 times higher than that of White females (1.7 per 100,000) and more than 4 times higher than that of Hispanic females (5.2 per 100,000). Although Black women made up only 13% of the female population, they accounted for 58% of diagnoses of HIV infection among women, which is 4.5 times the expected population-adjusted rate. Hispanic/Latino women made up 16% of the female population and accounted for 17% of diagnoses. White women were 62% of the US female population and yet accounted for only 21% of HIV diagnoses among women (CDC, 2018a).

Factors that increase a woman's risk of acquiring HIV include not knowing her partner's risk factors for HIV infection, having a lack of HIV knowledge, and having a decreased awareness of risk (CDC, 2018a). Women's relationships with their partners play a pivotal role as well: in relationships in which women are physically abused, vulnerability to HIV is increased because they may not insist on condom use due to fear of being harmed. Women with a history of sexual abuse are more likely to engage in high-risk sexual activity and to use drugs compared to women without such behaviors. This includes exchanging sexual activities for drugs and money as well as having difficulty refusing unwanted sex.

Results from the CDC's Young Men's Survey (1994–2000) found that many young Black and Latino MSM outwardly identify as heterosexual, with female spouses or partners, but also engage in same-sex encounters with other men, and that this high-risk group represents a bridge for transmitting HIV to women (Fitzpatrick et al., 2004; Millett, 2004; Valleroy et al., 2004). In addition, many poor and/or minority women lack the agency—whether economic, cultural, or otherwise—to use condoms with or to separate from abusive or unfaithful men who engage in high-risk sex with other partners or commercial sex workers. HIV prevention efforts must account for such factors to make inroads against HIV transmission in these groups.

The most common mode of transmission for women is high-risk heterosexual contact (64–92% across various groups) followed by injection drug use. These rates, current through 2018, may change with the deepening national opioid crisis and outbreaks of HIV transmission among needle-sharing networks (CDC, 2018a).

Sexual HIV transmission occurs through unprotected vaginal or anal sex, with receptive anal sex posing the highest risk and insertive vaginal sex the lowest. Oral sex is a theoretical risk if there are breaks in the oral and genital mucosa through which blood or genital secretions may pass. Similarly, sexually transmitted infections that disrupt genital mucosa

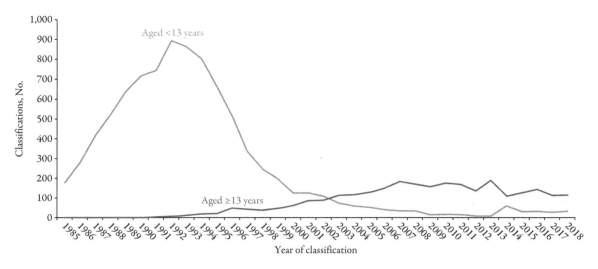

Figure 2.8 Stage 3 (AIDS) classifications among persons with perinatally acquired HIV infection, 1985–2018, US and six dependent areas   SOURCE: CDC HIV/AIDS Resource Library Slide Sets. Available at http://www.cdc.gov/hiv/library/slidesets/index.html. Accessed August 16, 2020.

and stimulate a local immune response will increase the likelihood of acquiring or transmitting HIV. Because gonorrhea and syphilis in particular have a higher rate in women of color compared to White women, this heightens their risk of HIV acquisition. Socioeconomic status also plays a role in HIV risk. In states with higher rates of poverty and limited access to healthcare, women are more likely to use drugs and exchange sex for drugs or money, factors shown to increase risk of HIV, directly or indirectly (CDC, 2018a).

CHILDREN

The reduction of perinatal HIV transmission in the United States is a major success of the antiretroviral era. Although the CDC does not publish a similar graph showing overall perinatal HIV transmission rates since the beginning of the epidemic, Figure 2.8 shows the dramatic rise and fall in perinatal AIDS diagnoses since 1985. In 1992, an estimated 952 pediatric HIV

transmissions were reported in the United States. By 2004, the number declined to 177. In 2011, there were only 53 reported perinatal infections, but this has since stabilized to around 100 infections and 50 AIDS diagnoses per year through 2017 (CDC, 2018a). The overall rate of perinatal HIV infections reported by the CDC decreased from 1.5 per 100,000 live births in 2014 to 0.9 in 2018, which meets the CDC's goal of less than one perinatal transmission per 100,000 live births (CDC, 2020b).

The recent persistence of the number of transmissions in the face of declining transmission rates is due to an increasing number of pregnancies among HIV-positive women as the powerful role of ART in preventing both horizontal and vertical transmission has been promoted among PWH. However, it bears noting that of all HIV diagnoses in children younger than age 13 years from 2010 to 2017, only 32% tested positive during their first year of life (Figure 2.9), which is closely linked to data showing that only 14% of these children's mothers were tested for HIV during their pregnancy

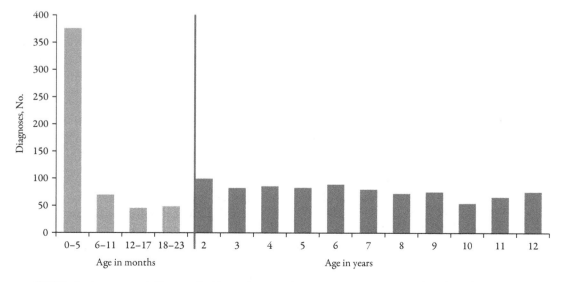

Figure 2.9 Diagnoses of HIV infection among children aged <13 years by age at diagnosis, 2010–2108, US and six dependent areas   SOURCE: CDC Diagnoses of HIV infection in the United States and dependent areas, 2018. HIV Surveillance Report, 2018 (Updated); vol. 31. Available at http://www.cdc.gov/hiv/library/reports/hiv-surveillance.html. Accessed August 15, 2020.

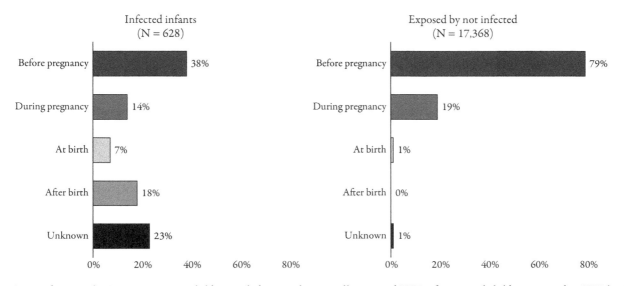

Figure 2.10 Time of maternal HIV testing among children with diagnosed perinatally acquired HIV infection and children exposed to HIV, birth years 2010–2016, US and Puerto Rico   SOURCE: CDC Diagnoses of HIV infection in the United States and dependent areas, 2018. HIV Surveillance Report, 2018 (Updated); vol. 31. Available at http://www.cdc.gov/hiv/library/reports/hiv-surveillance.html. Accessed August 15, 2020.

(Figure 2.10). Vertical transmission cannot be prevented if the mother's HIV status is not known, thus highlighting the importance of screening all pregnant women for HIV at least once during pregnancy.

As with adults, HIV disproportionately affects Black children. While accounting for 61% of diagnoses, they made up only 14% of the population of US children in 2018, whereas Hispanic (10% of HIV diagnoses, 26% of population) and White (17% of HIV diagnoses, 50% of population) children are infected far less often than their population percentages (CDC, 2018a).

ADOLESCENTS AND YOUNG ADULTS

According to 2018 CDC data, persons aged 13 to 34 account for over half of newly diagnosed HIV cases in the US. In particular, adolescents aged 13 to 24 and young adults aged 25 to 34 represented 21% and 36% of incident diagnoses, respectively. The annual number of HIV infections in 2018, compared with 2014, decreased among persons aged 13 to 24 but remained stable among all other age groups. The vast majority of these transmissions are among MSM. In the period from 2014 through 2018, diagnosis rates decreased in the 13-to-24 age group and remained stable in those aged 25 to 34; the highest rates are still observed in those aged 25 to 34 (31.5 per 100,000). These groups are particularly vulnerable, as they are least likely to be retained in care and to have a suppressed viral load (CDC, 2018a).

Transmissions remain disproportionately high among Black and Latino MSM youth. In 2018, of all adolescents and young adults aged 13 to 24 years diagnosed with HIV infection, the CDC reported that 52% were Black, again far outpacing their percentage of the general population. Hispanics/Latinos represented an additional 25% of adolescent HIV diagnoses in the same year (CDC, 2018a).

Male same-sex contact remains the predominant mode of HIV transmission in the adolescent and young adult population, accounting for 92% of new diagnoses. Heterosexual contact accounts for approximately 3%. Transmissions from injection drug use remain stable at approximately 2% (CDC, 2018a).

In 2018, females made up 15% of the HIV diagnoses in adolescents (13–19 years) and 12% in young adults (20–24 years) compared to 17% of adults older than 24 years. The mode of HIV transmission varies between sexes in this age group, as it does in adults: whereas 84% of adolescent and young adult females are infected through heterosexual contact, more than 90% of males contract HIV through male-to-male sexual contact (CDC, 2018a). Racial disparities persist among Black, Hispanic/Latino, and white adolescent and young adult females, with prevalence rates of 62%, 19%, and 13%, respectively. Perinatal transmission accounted for 41% of adolescent and young adult females living with HIV, while only 10% of cases in males with HIV were perinatally acquired. Unstable housing and employment may lead young women to engage in survival sex, leading to disproportionately high rates of HIV.

RECOMMENDED READING

Centers for Disease Control and Prevention. Adolescents and young adult surveillance. https://www.cdc.gov/hiv/pdf/library/slidesets/cdc-hiv-surveillance-adolescents-young-adults-2018.pdf

Centers for Disease Control and Prevention. HIV surveillance report: Diagnoses of HIV infection and AIDS in the United States and dependent areas. 2018. Vol. 31. https://www.cdc.gov/hiv/pdf/library/reports/surveillance/cdc-hiv-surveillance-report-2018-updated-vol-31.pdf

Centers for Disease Control and Prevention. Pediatric HIV surveillance. 2018. https://www.cdc.gov/hiv/pdf/library/slidesets/cdc-hiv-surveillance-pediatric-2018.pdf

HIV IN THE MSM AND TRANSGENDER COMMUNITIES

WHAT'S NEW?

The CDC estimated in February 2016 that, based on current trends, one in two gay Black MSM would become HIV-positive in their lifetime and that one-half of Black transgender women are already living with HIV.

KEY POINTS

- Individuals who identify as gay, bisexual, or as other MSM are the only population group in the US in which new HIV infections have steadily increased since the 1990s, with young black MSM being disproportionally affected.

- Transgender women account for the vast majority of HIV diagnoses among transgender individuals. Expanded access to PrEP is essential to help curb the spread in this at-risk population.

Since the beginning of the HIV/AIDS epidemic in the US, MSM have constituted the largest percentage of persons diagnosed with HIV/AIDS, whereas HIV transmission among women who have sex with women has been exceedingly rare. Black and Latino MSM are the only population groups in the United States in whom new infections have steadily risen from 2010 to 2018. In 2018, 82% of all HIV infections among males were attributed to male-to-male sexual contact, whereas rates of heterosexual, injection drug users, and MSM with injection drug use transmissions among men remained stable at about 9%, 5%, and 4%, respectively (CDC, 2020a). In 2018, approximately 67% of all HIV infections were attributed to MSM transmission (Figure 2.11).

The percentage of HIV cases diagnosed in the gay community differs based on race/ethnicity and age. In 2018, the estimated percentages of MSM diagnosed with HIV infection who were Black, Latino, White, and Asian were 37%, 20%, 27%, and 3%, respectively (Figure 2.12; CDC, 2018a). Native American and Pacific Islander MSM each accounted for less than 1% of new infections, and persons of mixed race 2%. Similar racial disparities exist in the adolescent and young adult population, with incidence rates of 34%, 22%, and 16%, respectively, among Black, Latino, and white MSM.

If we look at HIV transmissions among MSM as a function of age, in 2018 the largest percentage of diagnoses were in those aged 25 to 34 years (43%), followed by those aged 13 to 24 (25%), 35 to 44 (16%), 45 to 54 (11%), and more than 55 (5%). With the high prevalence of HIV in the MSM community, the cumulative risk of contracting or transmitting the virus becomes greater as these individuals age. Being unaware of one's HIV status, which is especially common among MSM of color and young MSM, increases the risk of transmitting HIV infection as well. According to CDC guidelines, MSM who are at high risk for HIV infection should be screened at least annually; this includes those who have had more than one sex partner since their last HIV test and MSM who are injection drug users. Data are insufficient to recommend more frequent screening, but "each clinician can consider the benefits of offering more frequent screening (e.g., once every 3 or 6 months) to individual MSM at increased risk for acquiring HIV infection, weighing their patients' individual risk factors, local HIV epidemiology, and local testing policies" (CDC, 2017).

Transgender individuals are one of the highest-risk groups in the United States for acquiring HIV infection, and epidemiologic data on this group are now available from the CDC. From 2009 to 2014, of the 2,351 transgender people diagnosed with HIV in the United States, 84% were transgender

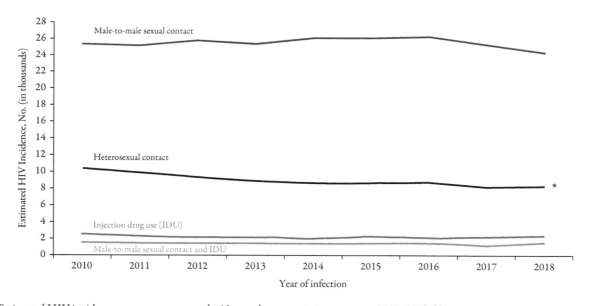

Figure 2.11 Estimated HIV incidence among persons aged ≥13 years by transmission category, 2010–2018, US SOURCE: CDC HIV/AIDS Resource Library Slide Sets. Available at https://www.cdc.gov/hiv/pdf/library/slidesets/cdc-hiv-linley-HIV-Incidence-Prevalence-2010-2018.pdf. Accessed August 12, 2020.

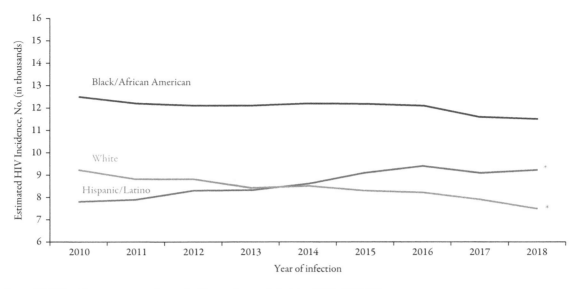

Figure 2.12 Estimated HIV incidence among males aged ≥13 years by race/ethnicity, 2010–2018, US   *Difference from 2010 estimate was deemed statistically significant (*P* < .05).
SOURCE: CDC HIV/AIDS Resource Library Slide Sets. Available at https://www.cdc.gov/hiv/pdf/library/slidesets/cdc-hiv-linley-HIV-Incidence-Prevalence-2010-2018.pdf. Accessed August 12, 2020.

women, 15% were transgender men, less than 1% had another gender identity, and half of these infected persons lived in the South. One-quarter of transgender women are estimated to have HIV; among Blacks, this figure rises to one-half (Figure 2.13).

Despite these worrisome trends, nearly two-thirds of transgender men and women in the Behavioral Risk Factor Surveillance System from 2014 to 2015 were never tested for HIV. The stigma and social rejection faced by transgender people leads to significant disparities in housing, education, employment, and access to healthcare and preventive services. While sufficient studies and firm data are lacking, it is generally observed that transgender females are often forced into survival sex, putting them at markedly increased risk for HIV acquisition. As well as social interventions like advocating for safer sexual practices and condom use, limiting number of sexual partners, using barrier protection, and advocating for stable housing and employment, modalities such as PrEP hold promise in helping to stem the tide of transmissions in

this at-risk population. This clearly represents an opportunity for improved outreach, education, and testing, as well as for addressing the many factors that put transgender people at risk for HIV infection (multiple sexual partners, condomless sex, commercial sex work, mental illness and substance abuse, homelessness, unemployment, targeted violence, and lack of family support; CDC, 2019a).

HIV AMONG OLDER ADULTS

PWH enjoy increased quality of life for longer periods of time as a result of well-tolerated and highly effective ART regimens. As such, there is a steadily increasing prevalence of HIV among all age groups (CDC, 2019b). While incidence rates among adults are generally stable, those aged 50 and older (the conventional definition of "older adult" with respect to HIV) still accounted for 17% of new HIV infections in 2018. Of the 6,640 transmissions, 4,769 (72%) were in men, mainly

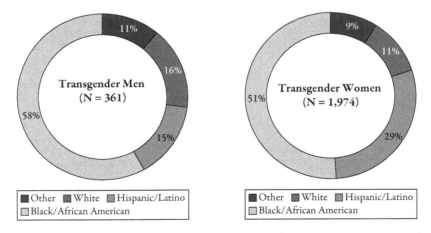

Figure 2.13 HIV diagnoses among transgender people in the US by race/ethnicity, 2009–2014. Note: Hispanics/Latinos can be of any race.   SOURCE: Clark H, et al. *AIDS Behav.* 2018;21(9):2774–2783.

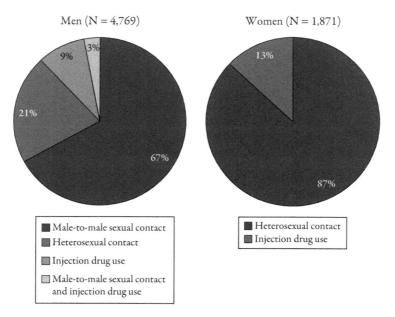

Men (N = 4,769)   Women (N = 1,871)

3%
9%
21%
67%

13%
87%

Men legend:
- Male-to-male sexual contact
- Heterosexual contact
- Injection drug use
- Male-to-male sexual contact and injection drug use

Women legend:
- Heterosexual contact
- Injection drug use

Figure 2.14 New HIV diagnoses among people aged 50 and older in the US and dependent areas by sex and transmission category, 2017 SOURCE: CDC. Diagnoses of HIV infection in the United States and dependent areas, 2017. HIV Surveillance Report 2018;29.

through male-to-male sexual contact, and 1,871 (28%) were in women, the majority of which were the result of heterosexual contact (Figure 2.14). It is important to recognize that this age group remains at significant risk of HIV acquisition and is less likely to receive guideline-based screening (US Preventive Services Task Force, 2019). A study by Adekeye et al. (2012) examining National Health Interview Survey data from 2009 demonstrated that the rate of HIV screening of individuals aged 50 and older was approximately 25%, with only half of the tests being suggested by a clinician during the encounter. This is an obvious area of opportunity for improved screening, earlier detection, linkage to care, and decreased transmission.

RECOMMENDED READING

Centers for Disease Control and Prevention. HIV among transgender people in the United States (2018). https://www.cdc.gov/hiv/group/gender/transgender/index.html

Centers for Disease Control and Prevention. HIV surveillance special report vol. 31 (2018). https://www.cdc.gov/hiv/library/reports/hiv-surveillance.html

REFERENCES

Adekeye OA, Heiman HJ, Onyeabor OS, Hyacinth HI. The new invincibles: HIV screening among older adults in the U.S. *PLoS One.* 2012;7(8):e43618. doi:10.1371/journal.pone.0043618

American Foundation for AIDS Research (amfAR). Statistics: women and HIV/AIDS. http://www.amfar.org/about-hiv-and-aids/facts-and-stats/statistics--women-and-hiv-aids

Apetrei C, Marx PA. Simian retroviral infections in human beings. *Lancet.* 2004;364(9429):137–138.

Blanas DA, Nichols K, Bekele M, Lugg A, Kerani RP, Horowitz CR. HIV/AIDS among African-born residents in the United States. *J Immigr Minor Health.* 2013;15(4):718–724. doi:10.1007/s10903-012-9691-6

Branson BM. To screen or not to screen: is that really the question? *Ann Intern Med.* 2006;145(11):857–859.

Campbell-Yesufu OT, Gandhi RT. Update on human immunodeficiency virus (HIV)-2 infection. *Clin Infect Dis.* 2011;52:780–787.

Centers for Disease Control and Prevention. HIV-2 infection surveillance—United States, 1987–2009. *MMWR Morb Mortal Wkly Rep.* 2011;60:985–988.

Centers for Disease Control and Prevention. HIV/AIDS resource library slide sets (last updated with 2018a). https://www.cdc.gov/hiv/library/slideSets/

Centers for Disease Control and Prevention. HIV and older Americans (November 12, 2019b). https://www.cdc.gov/hiv/group/age/older-americans/index.html

Centers for Disease Control and Prevention. HIV and people who inject drugs (February 6, 2020a). https://www.cdc.gov/hiv/group/hiv-idu.html

Centers for Disease Control and Prevention. HIV and transgender people (November 12, 2019a). https://www.cdc.gov/hiv/group/gender/transgender/index.html

Centers for Disease Control and Prevention. HIV and youth (May 18, 2020b). https://www.cdc.gov/hiv/group/age/youth/index.html

Centers for Disease Control and Prevention. HIV Surveillance Report (Vol 31): diagnosis of HIV infection in the United States and dependent areas, 2018 (Updated). 2020c. https://www.cdc.gov/hiv/pdf/library/reports/surveillance/cdc-hiv-surveillance-report-2018-updated-vol-31.pdf

Centers for Disease Control and Prevention. Selected National HIV Prevention and Control Outcomes. 2018b. Available at: https://www.cdc.gov/hiv/pdf/library/slidesets/cdc-hiv-prevention-and-care-outcomes-2018.pdf

Denning P, DiNenno E. Communities in crisis: is there a generalized HIV epidemic in impoverished urban areas of the United States? 2019. https://www.cdc.gov/hiv/group/poverty.html

Fitzpatrick LK, Grant L, Eure C, et al. Investigation of HIV transmission among young black men who have sex with men (MSM) in North Carolina: implications for prevention. In: *Program and Abstracts of the XV International AIDS Conference,* July 11–16, 2004; Bangkok, Thailand. Abstract C10746.

Gomes P, Diogo I, Gonca Ives MF, et al. Different pathways to nelfinavir genotypic resistance in HIV-1 subtypes B and C. In: *Program and Abstracts of the 9th Conference on Retroviruses and Opportunistic Infections,* February 24–28, 2002; Seattle, WA. Abstract 46.

Horn T, Sherwood J, Remien RH, et al. Towards an integrated primary and secondary HIV prevention continuum for the United States: a cyclical process model. *J Int AIDS Soc.* 2016;19(1):21263.

Kerani R, Bennett AB, Golden M, Castillo J, Buskin SE. Foreign-born individuals with HIV in King County, WA: a glimpse of the future of HIV? *AIDS Behav.* 2018;22(7):2181–2188. doi:10.1007/s10461-017-1914-3

Levy V, Prentiss D, Balmas G, et al. Factors in the delayed HIV presentation of immigrants in Northern California: implications for voluntary counseling and testing programs. *J Immigr Minor Health.* 2007;9(1):49–54. doi:10.1007/s10903-006-9015-9

Marsh K, Eaton JW, Mahy M, et al. Global, regional and country-level 90-90-90 estimates for 2018: assessing progress towards the 2020 target. *AIDS.* 2019;33 Suppl 3(Suppl 3):S213–S226. doi:10.1097/QAD.0000000000002355.

Millett G. Men on the "down low": more questions than answers. In: *Program and Abstracts of the 11th Conference on Retroviruses and Opportunistic Infections,* February 8–11, 2004; San Francisco, CA. Abstract 83.

National HIV/AIDS Strategy for the United States. Update to 2020. 2017 progress report. https://files.hiv.gov/s3fs-public/NHAS_Progress_Report_2017.pdf

Organista KC, Carillo H, Avala G. HIV prevention with Mexican migrants: review, critique, and recommendations. *J AIDS.* 2004;37(Suppl 4):S227–S239.

Peruski AH, Wesolowski LG, Delaney KP, et al. Trends in HIV-2 diagnoses and use of the HIV-1/HIV-2 differentiation test—United States, 2010–2017. *MMWR Morb Mortal Wkly Rep.* 2020;69:63–66. DOI: http://dx.doi.org/10.15585/mmwr.mm6903a2

Sidibe M. UNAIDS global AIDS update 2018: miles to go: closing gaps, breaking barriers, righting injustices. http://www.unaids.org/en/resources/documents/2018/global-aids-update

Spira S, Wainberg MA, Loemba H, et al. Impact of clade diversity on HIV-1 virulence, antiretroviral drug sensitivity and drug resistance. *J Antimicrob Chemother.* 2003; 51:229–240.

UNAIDS. Fact Sheet. July, 2018. https://www.react-profile.org/upload/KIT/system/uploads/UNAIDS_FactSheet_en.pdf

UNAIDS. Fact Sheet, July 2020. http://www.unaids.org/sites/default/files/media_asset/UNAIDS_FactSheet_en.pdf

US Department of Health and Human Services. Panel on Antiretroviral Guidelines for Adults and Adolescents. Guidelines for the use of antiretroviral agents in adults and adolescents living with HIV. 2020. http://www.aidsinfo.nih.gov/ContentFiles/AdultandAdolescentGL.pdf

US Preventive Services Task Force. Screening for HIV infection: US Preventive Services Task Force recommendation statement. *JAMA.* 2019;321(23):2326–2336. doi:10.1001/jama.2019.6587

Valleroy LA, MacKellar D, Behel S, Secura G. The bridge for HIV transmission to women from 15- to 29-year-old men who have sex with men in 7 US cities. In: *Program and Abstracts of the XV International AIDS Conference,* July 11–16, 2004; Bangkok, Thailand. Abstract 1367.

Wainberg MA. HIV-1 subtype distribution and the problem of drug resistance. *AIDS.* 2004;18(Suppl 3):S63–S68.

Witvrouw M, Pannecouque C, Switzer VM, et al. Susceptibility of HIV-2, SIV and SHIV to various anti-HIV-1 compounds: implications for treatment and postexposure prophylaxis. *Antivir Ther.* 2004;9:57–65.

3.

THE ORIGIN, EVOLUTION, AND EPIDEMIOLOGY OF HIV-1 AND HIV-2

Jeffrey T. Kirchner

CHAPTER GOAL

Upon completion of this chapter, the reader should be able to:
- Explain how HIV evolved from cross-species transmission of strains of simian immunodeficiency virus (SIV) to humans (viral zoonosis), spread out of Africa in the early 20th century, and eventually resulted in the global AIDS pandemic

LEARNING OBJECTIVES

- Discuss the distinct origins of HIV-1 and HIV-2 from SIVs and the multiple cross-transmission events from apes to humans

- Describe the origin of the initial HIV infections in south-central Africa, the key reasons for viral dissemination to other areas of sub-Saharan Africa, and the ultimate global spread of HIV

- Discuss the diversity of HIV, including viral groups, viral clades, and recombinant forms and their implications for future transmission of HIV, as well as treatments and vaccine developments

ORIGIN OF HIV AND ENTRY INTO HUMANS

The origin of HIV-1 can be traced to the early 1920s from southern Cameroon and then to Kinshasa in what is now the Democratic Republic of Congo (DRC). The combination of rapid population growth, changes in sexual behaviors, and the use of unsterilized needles likely contributed to the rapid spread of HIV, especially groups M and O.

KEY POINTS

- All strains of HIV-1 and HIV-2 are genetic descendants of simian immunodeficiency viruses (SIVs). Initial cross-species transmission of the virus occurred from butchering and eating of bush meat.

- HIV-1 group M ("main") and associated viral subtypes (A–L) account for approximately 95% of infections globally, with a much smaller number caused by groups N, O, and P.

- HIV-2 and its groups (A–H) are mainly limited to West Africa, but since the discovery of HIV-2 in 1986, cases have been reported in Europe and the US. Globally, HIV-2 represents approximately 3% of all HIV infections, although its prevalence appears to be declining.

- Genetic diversity of HIV, including recombination between subtypes, may continue to present challenges to the development of a globally effective vaccine.

HIV, a retrovirus and member of the lentivirus family, was identified as the cause of AIDS 2 years after the first cases were reported in 1981 (Gottlieb et al., 1981). Dr. Luc Montagnier in France and Dr. Robert Gallo in the US are both credited with identifying HIV-1 (Gallo & Montagnier, 2003). The pandemic form of HIV, also referred to as group M (for "main"), is responsible for the majority of infections globally, currently estimated to be approximately 76 million from the start of the epidemic. Since the discovery of HIV-1, followed by HIV-2 in 1986, the reasons for its emergence during the 20th century, its transmission to humans, its genetic diversity, and the pathogenesis of the virus have been the subjects of extensive research.

It was first noted in 1999, via genetic sequencing, that the chimpanzee *Pan troglodytes troglodytes* infected with SIV_{cpz} was likely the primary natural reservoir for HIV-1 (Gao et al., 1999). Later work by Keele determined that HIV-1 in humans began with cross-species transmission and recombination of two SIVs (from red-capped mangabeys [*Cercocebus torquatus*] and greater spot-nosed monkeys [*Cercopithecus nictitans*]) to chimpanzees that preyed on these animals (Keele et al., 2006). Keele and his group analyzed mitochondrial DNA and viral-specific antibody from 599 fecal samples from chimpanzees. These samples exhibited a strong and broad cross-reactive western blot profile indistinguishable from that of HIV-1 human controls. To date, serologic evidence for SIV infection has been identified in more than 45 non-human primate species (NHPS) (Peeters et al., 2014; Sharp & Hahn, 2011). The genetic diversity of these viral species is complex and includes coevolution of virus–host, cross-species transmission, and viral recombination.

Like HIV, SIV is sexually transmitted in NHPS and can be transmitted vertically. In deference to previous thinking, SIV is indeed pathogenic in most NHPS, causing CD4+ T-cell depletion (Keele et al., 2009). Chimpanzees infected with SIV have a 10- to 16-fold increased risk of death compared to those that are uninfected. Fertility and survival of offspring are also decreased in SIV-positive female chimpanzees.

WHAT'S NEW?

Researchers recently identified a new HIV subtype now called subtype L. This was based on complete genomic sequencing of three non-transmission linked cases (Yamaguchi et al., 2020). Additional strains are likely circulating in the DRC. Very strong evidence indicated that the first cross-species transmission of HIV to humans that predates emergence of group M occurred in southeast Cameroon (Sharp & Hahn, 2011). It is not known how humans acquired the zoonotic precursors of HIV-1. However, based on the recognized biology of these viruses, transmission likely arose from cutaneous or mucous membrane exposure to infected chimpanzee blood or body fluid. These exposures often occur in the context of hunting, butchering, and eating of bush meat (Sharp & Hahn, 2011).

THE SPREAD OF HIV THROUGHOUT AFRICA AND THE WORLD

A 2014 study by Faria et al. using phylogenetic analysis and "molecular clocks" (based on the assumption that retroviruses mutate over time at a constant rate) confirmed previous work by Hahn and others regarding the dissemination routes of HIV-1 in West Africa (Cohen, 2014; Faria et al., 2014; Sharp & Hahn, 2011). They have also largely determined how group M became the driver of the AIDS pandemic. It is well established that the first known infections with HIV-1 emerged from Kinshasa (formerly called Leopoldville) in the DRC in approximately 1920. Many refer to Leopoldville/Kinshasa as the cradle of the AIDS pandemic. From this area, the virus spread eastward to other communities via railway lines that carried up to 1 million passengers yearly to other areas of Africa, including the three largest population centers—Brazzaville, Mbuji-Mayi, and Lubumbashi (Cohen, 2014; Faria et al., 2014). Rivers were major travel and commerce routes and are believed to have enabled the spread of HIV geographically (Figure 3.1).

Sexual transmission is thought to be the primary mode and driver of new HIV infections and resultant dissemination of the virus. Unsterilized injections at clinics in the area

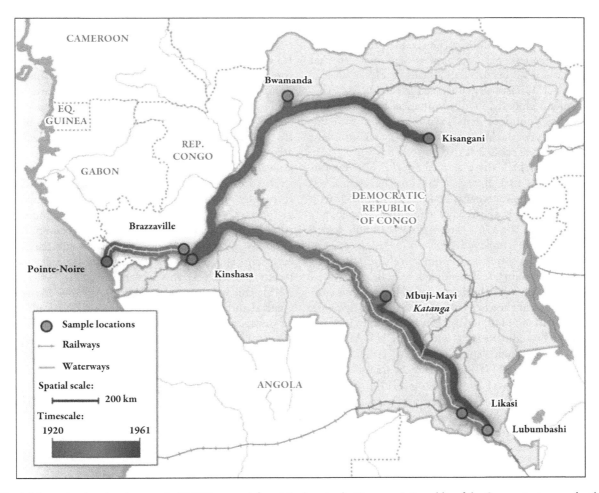

Figure 3.1 Spatial dynamics showing the spread of HIV-1 group, 1 from Kinshasa in the Democratic Republic of the Congo via rivers and railways, which were operational until about 1960   SOURCE: Faria NR, et al. *Science*. 2014;346(6205):56–61.

may have greatly contributed to the spread of HIV. According to Jacques Pepin, well-intended public health interventions by authorities in the Belgian Congo from 1921 to 1959 to treat trypanosomiasis, syphilis, yaws, malaria, and leprosy resulted in the administration of millions of injections to residents of these communities (Pepin, 2011). The majority of injections were intravenous and administered with syringes that clinicians used repeatedly without sterilizing the needles (Pepin, 2011). Consequently, thousands of these individuals may have acquired HIV iatrogenically. Data suggest similar transmission of hepatitis B and C viruses.

The epidemic histories of HIV-1 groups M and O were similar until approximately 1960, when group M infections underwent an epidemiologic transition and exponential increase, outpacing regional population growth (Faria et al., 2014). It is unknown why the growth rate of infections with HIV group M nearly tripled at approximately this time, but current explanations include virus-specific factors, population growth factors, and the widespread use of injections (Pepin, 2011; Sharp & Hahn, 2011).

Tissues samples collected from two patients in Kinshasa in 1959 and 1960 showed that HIV-1 had diversified into different subtypes much earlier than previously believed. Viral sequencing done on plasma from a sailor who died in 1959 is the oldest case of documented HIV-1 infection (Zhu et al., 1998). Worobey et al. amplified and identified HIV-1 from a lymph node specimen obtained in 1960 from a female in Kinshasa (Worobey et al., 2008). The sizable genetic difference between these two HIV specimens demonstrated that diversification of HIV-1 occurred in Kinshasa at least 20 years before the first AIDS cases were observed in the US. As HIV-1 group M spread globally, its dissemination led to population bottlenecks ("founder events") that resulted in different lineages, viral subtypes or clades, and circulating recombinant forms (CRFs) (Peeters et al., 2014).

How and when HIV first arrived in the US remains debatable. The virus first appeared in Haiti between 1960 and 1966. The probable source was Haitian professionals who returned from working in the newly independent Congo. It is estimated that during the 1960s, approximately 4,500 skilled Haitian workers were employed by the Congolese government. However, Pepin states that "a single technical assistant infected with HIV-1 subtype B went back to Haiti and stayed long enough to start a local chain of sexual transmission" (Pepin, 2011). Some authorities believe that the selling of sex to American tourists in Haiti led to HIV infection in individuals who in turn brought the virus back to the US. Although perhaps still controversial, Pepin states that "American gay and bisexual men infected Haitian male sex workers."

Work done by Gilbert et al. using HIV-1 *gag* gene sequences from five Haitian AIDS patients determined that HIV-1 subtype B definitely arrived in Haiti before it spread to the US and other Western countries (Gilbert et al., 2007). The same group of researchers noted that the most recent common ancestor of HIV-1 subtype B virus appeared in Haiti in 1966, but not in the US until 1969. Consequently, these data suggest that HIV-1 was circulating cryptically in the US for approximately 12 years before the 1981 cases of AIDS were recognized and reported (Gottlieb et al., 1981). The virus was spreading slowly among the heterosexual population before entering the higher-risk population of men who have sex with men (MSM), in which it spread much more extensively and began to be recognized clinically. The actual scientific facts will likely never be known; however, Pepin believes that the blood trade in Port-au-Prince exponentially amplified the number of HIV infections in Haiti and possibly other countries in which blood products were sold, including the US (Pepin, 2011).

HIV-1 AND HIV-2 GROUPS AND SUBTYPES AND THEIR GEOGRAPHIC DISTRIBUTIONS

HIV-1 comprises four distinct lineages that are termed groups M, N, O, and P. Each has resulted from a distinct and independent cross-species transmission event of SIVs infecting African apes. Using molecular clocks, the most recent common ancestor of group M has been dated to approximately 1920 (Sharp & Hahn, 2011). The four known HIV-1 groups share approximately 50% to 60% homology in their nucleotide sequences.

HIV-1 group M was the first lineage discovered and represents the pandemic form of HIV-1. It has a widespread global distribution and accounts for 90% to 95% of HIV-1 infections (Sharp & Hahn, 2011). The genetic diversity within HIV-1 group M is the result of subsequent evolution and spread in humans. Based on phylogenetic analysis, HIV-1 group M can be further divided into nine pure subtypes or clades (A–D, F–H, J, K, and L) and additional sub-subtypes (A1–A4 and F1–F2). The subtypes share 80% homology in their genetic sequences, meaning they differ genetically by approximately 20%. Subtypes and sub-subtypes can form additional mosaic forms through recombination of different strains inside dually or multiply infected individuals. Some recombinant forms may further achieve epidemic relevance, giving rise to known CRFs. To date, researchers have identified more than six CRFs and unique recombinant strains. Globally, subtype C, found mainly in sub-Saharan Africa, represents approximately 50% of HIV-1 infections, although recent data suggest this has increased to 75% (Faria et al., 2019). This is followed by subtype A (12%), found mainly in Central and Eastern Africa and Russia. Viral subtype B (11% of infections) is the predominant subtype in Europe, the US, and Oceania and is the most geographically dispersed subtype worldwide (Bbosa et al., 2019). Subtypes G and D respectively account for 5% and 2% of infections worldwide (Peeters et al., 2014) (Figure 3.2 and Box 3.1).

HIV-1

Group N

Group N ("N" for "non-M, non-O," or "new") was isolated in 1995 from a woman in Cameroon who had AIDS (Pepin, 2011). To date, fewer than 20 cases of group N infection have

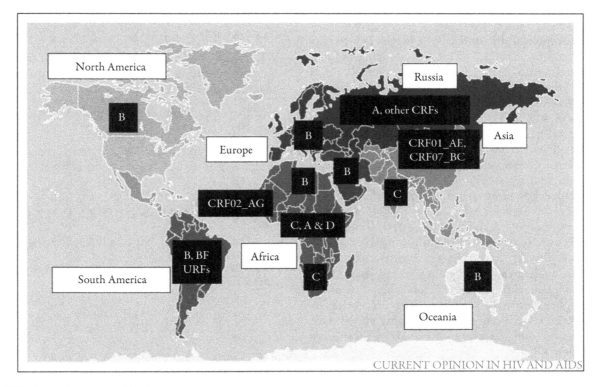

Figure 3.2 HIV subtype diversity worldwide   SOURCE: Bbosa N, et al. *Curr Opin HIV AIDS.* 2019;14:153–160.

been identified, and all except one were from Cameroon. Similar to group M, it is the result of chimpanzee-to-human transmission. The small number of infections resulting from this group and the limited genetic diversity suggest that its introduction into humans did not occur until approximately 1963 (Peeters et al., 2014).

Group O

Group O ("O" for "outlier") was first discovered in 1990 in two Cameroonians living in Belgium (De Leys, 1990) and is

Box 3.1 DISTRIBUTION OF HIV-1 SUBTYPES

Historically, the distribution of subtypes followed the geographic patterns listed here:

- *Subtype A*: Central and East Africa as well as Eastern European countries that were formerly part of the Soviet Union

- *Subtype B*: West and Central Europe, the Americas, Australia, South America, and several Southeast Asian countries (Thailand and Japan), as well as North Africa and the Middle East

- *Subtype C*: Sub-Saharan Africa, India, and Brazil

- *Subtype D*: North Africa and the Middle East

- *Subtype F*: South and Southeast Asia

- *Subtype G*: West and Central Africa

- *Subtypes H, J, and K*: Africa and the Middle East

thought to represent only approximately 1% of all HIV infections. Recent studies have determined that group O originated by cross-species transmission from western lowland gorillas (*Gorilla gorilla*) instead of chimpanzees (D'Arc et al., 2015). Like the other groups, it underwent adaptations to the human hosts. Another study found the prevalence of HIV-1 group O in Cameroon to be approximately 0.6%, indicating that the frequency of group O has been stable during the past few decades. However, the current distribution of the circulating viral strains still does not allow classification as subtypes (Villabona-Arenas et al., 2015). There are also some reports of dual infections with HIV-1 group M and group O but no recombinant forms in coinfected patients (De Oliveira et al., 2017; Ngoupo et al., 2016) Natural resistance to HIV medications, including integrase inhibitors, has not been identified. This suggests that infection with HIV-1 group O can be adequately treated in countries in which the virus circulates, but this group remains challenging in regard to diagnostic and monitoring strategies.

Group P

Group P was discovered in 2009, isolated from a Cameroonian woman living in France (Plantier et al., 2009). Despite subsequent screening for more infections caused by this group, only two cases have been identified. It is uncertain when group P virus entered the human population; it is estimated to be any time from 1845 to 1989 (Peeters et al., 2014). In addition, it remains unclear if the source was a chimpanzee or gorilla. The inability to antagonize tetherin protein (human restriction factor) may explain the limited spread of HIV-1 group P in the human population (Sauter et al., 2011).

In 1986, a morphologically similar but antigenically distinct virus was found to cause AIDS in persons living in West Africa and was termed HIV-2 (Clavel et al., 1986, 1987). It was isolated from healthy commercial sex workers in Senegal (Boswell & Rowland-Jones, 2019), This virus has only approximately 30% to 40% genetic homology with HIV-1; thus, it is considered a different virus and not another HIV-1 group (Pepin, 2011). It was determined that HIV-2 originated in sooty mangabeys (*Cercocebus atys*) with bloodborne transmission to humans, similar to HIV-1 (Chen et al., 1997; Gao et al., 1992). Molecular clock research has determined that the most common recent ancestor for HIV-2 dates to 1940 and 1945 for the first two groups—A and B (Pepin, 2011), respectively.

HIV-2 has been found mainly in Guinea-Bissau, Gambia, Senegal, Cote d'Ivoire, Mali, Nigeria, Senegal, and Sierra Leone. With widespread immigration, cases have been reported throughout Europe, the US, and other areas of the world (Campbell-Yesufu & Gandhi, 2011; Peruski et al., 2020). However, more recent data suggest that HIV-2 prevalence may be declining, at least in West Africa (Boswell & Rowland-Jones, 2019).

Since its discovery, phylogenetic analysis has identified eight different lineages of HIV-2 (groups A–H). As with HIV-1, each group represents a different host transfer of SIV from non-primate species (mangabeys) to humans. However, unlike HIV-1, only types A and B have spread to humans to any significant degree. The other groups only represent individual human cases. Of note clinically, persons infected with HIV-2 often have lower viral loads compared to those with HIV-1 (Boswell & Rowland-Jones, 2019). There is also less genital shedding in semen and cervical secretions. This likely accounts for decreased infectivity. It has also been observed that persons infected with HIV-2 have a longer asymptomatic phase and slower progression to AIDS than those with HIV-1. However, in the absence of treatment with antiretroviral agents, the progressive, albeit slower, decline in immune function and resultant disease complications will occur (Boswell & Rowland-Jones, 2019; Tzou et al., 2020).

THE FUTURE OF HIV REGIONAL AND GLOBAL GENETIC DIVERSITY

By combining historical, phylogenetic, molecular evolutionary, and epidemiologic perspectives, researchers have been able to reconstruct the history of the AIDS pandemic and many unique aspects of HIV-1 and HIV-2. It is likely that this information will be of value for HIV vaccine research and development that takes into account the genetic diversity of the virus as discussed earlier. It may also determine how strains of HIV may continue to spread and colonize new geographic regions and host populations. It also raises numerous questions:

- Given the fact that there are many other non-human primates infected with SIV, should there be concern for future zoonotic infections from cross-species transmissions?

- Will the growing prevalence of sexually transmitted infections continue to facilitate the dissemination and adaptation of HIV-1 and HIV-2?

- May there be a therapeutic role for host-restriction factors?

- Will it be possible to develop an HIV vaccine that will be effective against all HIV groups and subtypes?

RECOMMENDED READING

Pepin J. *The Origins of AIDS*. New York: Cambridge University Press; 2011.
Quammen D. *The Chimp and the River: How AIDS Emerged from an African Forest*. New York: Norton; 2015.

REFERENCES

Bbosa N, Kaleebu P, Ssemwanga D. HIV subtype diversity worldwide. *Curr Opin HIV AIDS*. 2019;14:153–160.
Boswell MT, Rowland-Jones SL. Delayed disease progression in HIV-2: The importance of TRIM5a and the retroviral capsid. *Clin Exp Immunol*. 2019;196(3):305–317. doi:10.1111/cei.13280
Campbell-Yesufu OT, Gandhi RT. Update on human immunodeficiency virus (HIV)-2 infection. *Clin Infect Dis*. 2011;52(6):780–787. doi:10.1093/cid/ciq248
Chen Z, Lucky A, Sodora DL, et al. Human immunodeficiency virus type 2 (HIV-2) seroprevalence and characterization of a distinct subtype within the range of SIV-infected sooty mangabeys. *J Virol*. 1997;71:3953–3960.
Clavel F, Guétard D, Brun-Vézinet F. Isolation of a new human retrovirus from West African patients with AIDS. *Science*. 1986;233(4761):343–346.
Clavel F, Mansinho K, Chamaret S. Human immunodeficiency virus type 2 infection associated with AIDS in West Africa. *N Engl J Med*. 1987;316:1180–1185.
Cohen J. Early AIDS virus may have ridden Africa's rails. *Science*. 2014;346:21–22.
D'Arc, M, Ayouba A, Esteban A, et al. Origin of the HIV-1 group O epidemic in western lowland gorillas. *Proc Natl Acad Sci USA*. 2015;112(11): E1343–E1352.
De Leys R. Isolation and partial characterization of an unusual HIV retrovirus from two persons of west-central Africa origin. *J Virol*. 1990;64:1207–1216.
De Oliveira F, Mourez T, Aurélia Vessiere A, et al. Multiple HIV-1/M + HIV-1/O dual infections and new HIV-1/MO inter-group recombinant forms detected in Cameroon. *Retrovirology*. 2017;14(1):1. doi:10.1186/s12977-016-0324-3
Faria NR, Rambaut A, Suchard MA, et al. The early spread and epidemic ignition of HIV-1 in human populations. *Science*. 2014;346(6205):56–61.
Faria NR, Vidal N, Lourencio J, et al. Distinct rates and patterns of spread of the major HIV-1 subtypes in Central and East Africa. *PLoS Pathog*. 2019;15(12):e1007976.
Gallo RC, Montagnier L. The discovery of HIV as the cause of AIDS. *N Engl J Med*. 2003;349:2282–2285.
Gao F, Bailes E, Robertson DL, et al. Origin of HIV-1 in the chimpanzee *Pan troglodytes troglodytes*. *Nature*. 1999;397:436–441.
Gao F, Yue L, White AT, et al. Human infection by genetically diverse SIVsm-related HIV-2 in West Africa. *Nature*. 1992;358:495–499.

Gilbert MTP, Rambaut A, Wlasiuk G, et al. The emergence of HIV/AIDS in the Americas and beyond. *Proc Natl Assoc Sci USA.* 2007;104(47):18566–18570.

Gottlieb MS, Schanker HM, Fan PT, et al. *Pneumocystis* pneumonia–Los Angeles. *MMWR.* 1981;30(21):1–3.

Keele BF, Jones JH, Terio KA, et al. Increased mortality and AIDS-like immunopathology in wild chimpanzees infected with SIV$_{cpz}$. *Nature.* 2009;460:515–519.

Keele BF, Van Heuverswyn F, Li Y, et al. Chimpanzee reservoirs for pandemic and nonpandemic HIV-1. *Science.* 2006;313(5786):523–526.

Ngoupo PA, Sadeu MB, Alain S, et al. First evidence of transmission of an HIV-1 M/O intergroup recombinant virus. *AIDS.* 2016;30(1):1–8.

Peeters M, D'Arc M, Delaporta E. The origin and diversity of human retroviruses. *AIDS Rev.* 2014;16(1):23–34.

Pepin J. *The Origins of AIDS.* New York: Cambridge University Press; 2011.

Peruski AH, Wesolowski LG, Delaney KP, et al. Trends in HIV-2 diagnosis and use of HIV-1/HIV-2 differentiation test—United States, 2010–2017. *MMWR.* 2020;69(3): 63–66.

Plantier JC, Leoz M, Dickerson JE. A new immunodeficiency virus derived from gorillas designated group "P." *Nature Med.* 2009;15:871–872.

Sauter D, Hué S, Petit S, et al. HIV-1 group P is unable to antagonize human tetherin by Vpu, Env or Nef. *Retrovirology.* 2011;8:103.

Sharp PM, Hahn BH. Origins of HIV and the AIDS pandemic. *Cold Spring Harbor Perspect Med.* 2011;1:1–22.

Tzou PL, Descamps D, Rhee SY, et al. Expanded spectrum of antiretroviral-selected mutations in human immunodeficiency virus type-2. *J Infect Dis.* 2020; 211:1962–1972.

Villabona-Arenas CJ, Domyeum J, Mouacha F, et al. HIV-1 group O infection in Cameroon from 2006–2013: prevalence, genetic diversity, evolution, and public health challenges. *Infect Genet Evol.* 2015;36:210–216.

Worobey M, Gemmel M, Teuwen DE, et al. Direct evidence of extensive diversity of HIV-1 in Kinshasa by 1960. *Nature.* 2008;455(7213):661–664.

Yamaguchi J, Vallari A, McArthur C, et al. Complete genome sequencing of GC-0018a-01 establishes HIV-1 Subtype L. *J Acquir Immune Defic Syndr.* 2020;83(3):319–322.

Zhu T, Korber BT, Nahmias AJ, et al. An African HIV-1 sequence from 1959 and implications for the origin of the epidemic. *Nature.* 1998;391(6667):594–597.

4.

MECHANISMS OF HIV TRANSMISSION

Puja H. Nambiar

CHAPTER GOALS

Upon completion of this chapter, the reader should be able to:

- Describe the relative risk of HIV transmission based on various types of sexual activity, occupational exposures, drug use, and vertical transmission

- Discuss the significance of viral load quantity and its relationship to transmission risk

- Explain the impact of co-occurring sexually transmitted diseases in HIV transmission

INTRODUCTION

With 20 years of experience demonstrating that antiretroviral therapy (ART) is highly effective in reducing the transmission of HIV, there is now clear evidence that individuals living with HIV with an undetectable viral load cannot transmit HIV sexually.

WHAT'S NEW?

- U = U campaign: Undetectable viral load equals untransmittable.

- Clinical trial data demonstrate that treatment of HIV infection is also prevention.

- It has been shown that occupational transmission is extremely rare in the United States.

KEY POINTS

- The risk of HIV transmission to a receptive partner remains higher than that to an insertive one; however, both carry a risk.

- Anything that compromises the integrity of mucous membranes, such as sexually transmitted infections, may increase the risk of transmission.

- Keeping an infected partner's viral load persistently suppressed to an undetectable level reduces the risk of transmission to an HIV-negative partner.

- Maternal transmission is a larger concern in developing countries due to lack of access to perinatal treatment with antiretroviral drugs.

SEXUAL TRANSMISSION

HIV can be transmitted through infected body fluids—blood, seminal fluid, vaginal fluid, rectal fluid, and breast milk. Sexual contact is the most common mode of HIV transmission worldwide. In the US, HIV is mainly transmitted by anal or vaginal sex and less commonly by other modes such as oral sex; mother-to-child transmission during pregnancy, birth, or breastfeeding; needle injury; blood transfusion; or organ transplants. In 2018, of the 37,968 new HIV diagnoses, 69% were due to men who have sex with men (MSM), 24% to high-risk heterosexual activity, and 7% to people who inject drugs (Centers for Disease Control and Prevention [CDC], 2020).

Acutely infected individuals, often with very high viral loads, are at the highest risk of transmitting the virus. HIV can be readily found in semen and in vaginal fluid from HIV-positive persons. There is a strong correlation between high plasma viral load and the amount of virus in genital secretions (Zhang et al., 1998). However, discordance, although rare, can exist between levels of HIV in the plasma and genital secretions. HIV-positive men on ART with undetectable virus in plasma can infrequently have detectable HIV in their seminal fluid (Zhang et al., 1998).

Unprotected anal sex has the highest risk for HIV transmission, with the receptive partner being at higher risk than the insertive partner. The person receiving the infected semen is believed to be at highest risk because of the single-cell layer of epithelium lining the rectum, which can be easily disrupted and permit entry of the virus across the rectal mucosa. The insertive partner is also at significant risk because HIV can enter the penis through the urethra; the mucosa of the nonkeratinized portions of the foreskin; or through cuts, abrasions, or open sores on the penis. Circumcision has been demonstrated to significantly reduce the risk of HIV acquisition but not of transmission (Dosekun & Fox, 2010).

Worldwide, the AIDS epidemic is being driven by new infections occurring in women of childbearing age. During unprotected vaginal intercourse, both partners are at risk of contracting HIV, although there is a higher risk of a woman contracting HIV from an infected man than a man contracting HIV from an infected woman. HIV can enter the body through the vaginal and cervical mucous membrane linings. HIV-1 replicates and persists in the vaginal epithelial dendritic cells (Pena-Cruz et al., 2018); this provides a readily understandable mechanism for transmission via the vaginal mucosa. Although the risk of men acquiring HIV through heterosexual vaginal or anal intercourse is lower, HIV is abundantly present in vaginal secretions, and the anatomic sites of potential infection in the penis are the same as those described previously for anal intercourse (Dosekun & Fox, 2010).

Sexually transmitted infections (STIs) have a significant role in HIV transmission. Genital ulcer disease (i.e., syphilis, chancroid, herpes simplex infections) and diseases causing mucosal inflammation (i.e., gonorrhea and chlamydia) have been shown to increase HIV transmission threefold. This increase is most likely due to both heightened infectivity and susceptibility. Open ulcers aid HIV entry, and inflammation recruits increased numbers of CD4+ cells that serve as targets for HIV. Early diagnosis of STIs has the potential to significantly reduce HIV incidence in general, especially if applied to high-risk populations. Another potential factor is the use of hormonal contraception in women because it may thin the vaginal mucosa, making it more susceptible to tears and trauma. However, large randomized clinical trials have provided conflicting results, and currently it is not clear whether hormonal contraception has any effect on HIV transmission.

Limiting viral replication in genital secretions is a logical approach to preventing HIV acquisition. Data from the pivotal HPTN 052 study showed dramatic reductions in HIV transmissions in serodifferent couples in which the seropositive partner was virally suppressed with ART along with monthly HIV prevention counseling and regular STI testing and treatment. This unique clinical trial showed that men and women living with HIV had a 96% reduced risk of transmitting the virus to their original linked, HIV-negative sexual partners through early initiation of ART (Cohen et al., 2011). Longer-term follow-up of the study showed a sustained, overall, 93% reduction of HIV transmission among linked couples when the HIV-positive partner was taking ART and had a suppressed viral load (Cohen et al., 2016). The results of this historic study provided the initial data to support treatment as prevention (TasP).

Taking evaluation of TasP even further, the prospective, observational PARTNER-1 (Partners of People on ART: A New Evaluation of the Risks) study, although it had limited follow-up time (median = 1.3 years per couple), showed no linked HIV transmissions with condomless anal and vaginal sex among serodifferent heterosexual and homosexual couples in which the HIV-positive partner was virologically suppressed on ART (Rodger et al., 2016). The subsequent PARTNER-2 study reported no phylogenetically linked HIV transmission in 415 couple-years of follow-up in male homosexual couples reporting condomless anal intercourse, in which the HIV-positive partners were virally suppressed and HIV-negative partners reported no use of preexposure prophylaxis (Rodger et al., 2019). An international, prospective, observational cohort study (the Opposites Attract study) examining the association between ART and viral load and HIV transmission in serodifferent male homosexual couples in Australia, Brazil, and Thailand also reported similar results (Bavinton et al., 2018). Together the PARTNER and Opposites Attract studies have reported no linked transmissions despite nearly 35,000 acts of condomless anal intercourse in HIV serodifferent male homosexual couples not using daily preexposure prophylaxis.

Developing novel approaches for the rapid detection and diagnosis of HIV infection and increasing ART coverage are the next important steps in realizing the potential public benefits of these discoveries.

TRANSMISSION IN THE HEALTHCARE SETTING

All persons working in a healthcare setting with potential for exposure to infected blood and body fluids and contaminated medical equipment or surroundings are at risk for HIV acquisition. The risk of occupational HIV transmission is low and occurs when a healthcare worker has a percutaneous injury or contact of mucous membrane or non-intact skin with HIV-infected blood, tissue, or other body fluids. The risk of HIV transmission following percutaneous and mucous membrane exposure to HIV-infected blood has been estimated to be 0.3% and 0.09%, respectively. There is virtually no risk of HIV transmission via contact of HIV-infected body fluids with intact skin (CDC, 2008a).

In addition to blood, other bodily fluids, such as cerebrospinal, synovial, amniotic, pleural, peritoneal, and pericardial fluids, are considered potentially infectious. The risk from these fluids remains unknown owing to a lack of epidemiologic studies in healthcare settings to assess the risk of HIV transmission to healthcare workers from exposure to these fluids. Although semen and cervicovaginal secretions have been shown to contain both infectious-free virus and virus-infected cells, they have not been implicated in occupational transmission from patients to healthcare workers. Feces, urine, nasal secretions, sweat, tears, sputum, vomitus, and saliva are not considered potentially infectious unless visibly bloody (Bell, 1997). The major factors influencing the possibility of transmission include the type and severity of exposure and the magnitude of viremia. A greater risk of transmission was seen with exposure to a large quantity of blood from an infected source person, deep injuries, and hollow-bore needles. The higher the titer of HIV in blood (inoculum), as seen in persons with acute HIV infection or uncontrolled HIV, the higher the transmission risk (CDC, 2008a).

Although not common, there have been several documented transmission events from healthcare workers to patients during routine medical or dental care, the most likely cause being poor adherence to infection control procedures. Furthermore, although increasingly less frequent, there have been documented cases of patient-to-patient transmission, most of which involved the use of contaminated instruments or syringes. Use of universal precautions during all healthcare procedures and encounters cannot be overemphasized. Since

1991, the CDC has investigated all cases of HIV infection reported as acquired occupationally by healthcare workers. Until now, the national HIV surveillance system recorded 58 confirmed and 150 possible cases of occupationally acquired HIV transmission among healthcare personnel. Among the 58 confirmed cases, the primary routes of exposure resulting in infection were percutaneous puncture or cut (49/58 cases), followed by mucocutaneous exposure (5), both percutaneous and mucocutaneous exposure (2), and unknown (2). The majority were in nurses (41%), followed by laboratory clinicians (35%), physicians (10%), and other health-related workers (14%). Since 1999, there has been only one case of occupationally acquired HIV (a laboratory technician who sustained a needle puncture while working with high-titer HIV cultures in 2008) (Joyce et al., 2015).

In cases in which the risk of HIV transmission can be determined, specific guidelines exist for the use of antivirals for postexposure prophylaxis (PEP). Occupational exposures require urgent medical evaluation and initiation of PEP, ideally within 2 to 6 hours after exposure. Prospective, well-controlled clinical data supporting PEP do not exist. However, by extrapolation from well-controlled animal model studies, it has been estimated that PEP reduces the risk of infection by approximately 80% and that it becomes less effective as time elapses (>72 hours). The preferred initial PEP regimen (three or more antiretroviral drugs) is tenofovir disoproxil fumarate/emtricitabine plus raltegravir (TDF/FTC + RAL) because of its ease of administration, proven potency against established HIV, and good tolerability. It is recommended to start PEP with this regimen following exposure to a source patient who is known to have HIV or for whom there is a reasonably high suspicion of having HIV. If the source person is determined to be HIV-negative, PEP can be discontinued. There is no documented transmission during the window period, and hence rapid testing would suffice. PEP is also recommended for non-occupational exposures. The recommended duration of PEP is 28 days. CDC recommendations indicate that PEP should be considered only in settings in which HIV exposure is known. Most important, based on strong animal-model data indicating time-dependent efficacy, PEP administration should not be delayed to await HIV test results but rather should be started empirically and discontinued later if tests are negative (Kuhar et al., 2013).

TRANSMISSION THROUGH THE USE OF INJECTION DRUGS

Persons who inject drugs (PWID) are at high risk of getting HIV if they use and share needles, syringes, or other drug-injection equipment previously used by someone with HIV. Sharing syringes is the second riskiest behavior for acquiring HIV. HIV survival in syringes was associated with the volume of blood remaining and the temperature of storage. Viable HIV was isolated from 50% of all syringes stored at 4 degrees Celsius for up to 42 days (Abdala et al., 2000).

In 2018, PWID accounted for 7% of new HIV diagnoses. In all regions of the US, the largest percentage of diagnosed

HIV infections among PWID was among whites, followed by African Americans and Hispanics. The prevalence of HIV remains highest among Blacks/African Americans (46%). Among women, injection drug use accounts for more than 20% of all infections.

The high-risk practices of sharing needles/syringes, engaging in risky sexual behavior, drug use, and socioeconomic factors limiting access to HIV prevention and care and substance abuse programs are some of the prevention challenges currently identified by the CDC.

The CDC is pursuing a prevention approach by distributing funds to health departments for surveillance and by supporting intervention programs such as Community PROMISE (Peers Reaching Out and Modeling Intervention Strategies); syringe service programs that provide access to sterile syringes and needles, thereby reducing transmission of HIV, hepatitis C virus, hepatitis B virus, and other blood-borne infections; and pre- and postexposure prophylaxis programs, to name a few. Providing comprehensive prevention services and medical and/or addiction treatment referrals for PWID can help increase access to healthcare and substance use treatment (CDC, 2008b).

Individuals who use recreational crystal methamphetamine are at increased risk of contracting HIV. There is no clear evidence that methamphetamine itself increases HIV transmission or acquisition, but amphetamine users, in general, report several behaviors known to be risk factors for HIV transmission, including greater numbers of sex partners, reduced use of condoms, exchange of sex for money or drugs, sex with injection drug users, and/or a history of sexually transmitted diseases. Furthermore, they are more likely to have unprotected anal or vaginal sex with partners of unknown HIV status. Individuals abusing other mind-altering drugs, such as alcohol, can also be at increased risk for HIV infection (CDC, 2007).

MOTHER-TO-CHILD TRANSMISSION

The transmission of HIV from an HIV-positive mother to her child during pregnancy, labor, delivery, or breastfeeding is referred to as perinatal transmission. Perinatal transmission of HIV is a unique setting as the infant's exposure to HIV occurs despite the presence of HIV-specific antibodies that were passively transferred from the mother while in utero. Several factors have been identified to influence the risk of perinatal HIV infection. A high maternal viral load (in the blood and the genital tract) at the time of delivery, the CD4+ T-cell count, and the clinical stage of the infection have been associated with a higher risk of perinatal HIV.

Universal perinatal HIV counseling and testing, ART for all pregnant women with HIV, scheduled cesarean delivery for women with viremia (HIV RNA > 1,000 copies/mL), infant ART, and avoidance of breastfeeding have contributed to the remarkable decline in the annual rate of perinatal transmission of HIV to less than 1% in the US. In the absence of any intervention, transmission rates can vary from 15% to 45%, and despite scaled-up prevention programs, perinatal

HIV infection continues to escalate in regions of sub-Saharan Africa (Yah & Tambo, 2019). The most common barriers and challenges were nondisclosure of HIV status, late initiation of ART treatment/adherence, screening for sexually transmitted diseases, long clinic wait times, and infant feeding methods, to name a few.

Pediatric HIV infection is associated with an accelerated course of disease and high mortality. In the absence of ART, only 65% of HIV-positive children survive until their first birthday, and less than half will reach 2 years of age. In the absence of breastfeeding and with no ART, the risk of perinatal transmission is 25%. Up to 20% more children can become infected through breastfeeding. Despite the presence of innate factors in human breast milk that display strong HIV inhibitory activity in vitro, up to 44% of HIV infections in children can be attributed to breastfeeding. The risk of acquiring HIV after a single day of breastfeeding is extremely low (0.00028 per day of breastfeeding) (Richardson et al., 2003). However, after ingesting liters of breast milk over a span of several months to years (~250 liters per year), 5% to 20% of infants born to HIV-positive women will eventually become infected with HIV in the absence of any preventive measures (WHO, UNICEF, UNFPA, and UNAIDS, 2008). Elevated levels of HIV particles (cell-free virus) and HIV-infected cells (cell-associated virus) in the breast milk of HIV-positive women are associated with an increased risk of HIV transmission during breastfeeding. Although it has been reported that a 10-fold increase in cell-free or cell-associated HIV in breast milk is associated with a 3-fold increase in transmission, it is still unclear whether cell-free virus and/or cell-associated virus are transmitted during breastfeeding. Furthermore, it is not known if the frequency of cell-free and cell-associated HIV transmission varies at different stages of lactation (i.e., colostrum, early breast milk, and mature breast milk).

REFERENCES

Abdala N, Reyes R, Carney JM, Heimer R. Survival of HIV-1 in syringes: effects of temperature during storage external icon. *Subst Use Misuse.* 2000;35(10):1369–1383.

Bavinton BR, Pinto AN, Phanuphak N, et al. Viral suppression and HIV transmission in serodiscordant male couples: an international, prospective, observational, cohort study. *Lancet HIV.* 2018;5(8):e438–e447. doi:10.1016/S2352-3018(18)30132-2

Bell DM. Occupational risk of human immunodeficiency virus infection in healthcare workers: an overview. *Am J Med.* 1997;102(5B):9–15.

Centers for Disease Control and Prevention. Methamphetamine use and risk for HIV/AIDS. January 2007. http://www.cdc.gov/hiv/resources/factsheets/meth.htm

Centers for Disease Control and Protection. HIV transmission. 2008b. https://www.cdc.gov/hiv/basics/transmission.html

Centers for Disease Control and Prevention. Recommendations for postexposure interventions to prevent infection with hepatitis B virus, hepatitis C virus, or human immunodeficiency virus, and tetanus in persons wounded during bombings and other mass-casualty events—United States, 2008a. *MMWR.* 2008;57(RR06):1–19.

Centers for Disease Control and Prevention. *HIV Surveillance Report, 2018 (Updated);* vol. 31. May 2020. http://www.cdc.gov/hiv/library/reports/hiv-surveillance.html

Cohen MS, Chen YQ, McCauley M, et al. Prevention of HIV-1 infection with early antiretroviral therapy. *N Engl J Med.* 2011;365:493–505.

Cohen MS, Chen YQ, McCauley M, et al. Final results of the HPTN 052 randomized controlled trial: antiretroviral therapy prevents HIV transmission. *N Engl J Med.* 2016;375:830–839.

Dosekun O, Fox J. An overview of the relative risks of different sexual behaviours on HIV transmission. *Curr Opin HIV AIDS.* 2010;5:291–297.

Joyce MP, Kuhar D, Brooks JT. Occupationally acquired HIV infection by healthcare personnel—United States, 1985–2013. *MMWR.* 2015;63(53):1245–1246.

Kuhar DT, Henderson DK, Struble KA, et al. Updated US Public Health Service guidelines for the management of occupational exposures to human immunodeficiency virus and recommendations for postexposure prophylaxis. *Infect Control Hosp Epidemiol.* 2013;34(11):1238.

Pena-Cruz V, Agosto LM, Akiyama H, et al. HIV replicates and persists in vaginal epithelial dendritic cells. *J Clin Invest.* 2018;128(8):3439–3444. https://doi.org/10.1172/JCI98943

Richardson BA, John-Stewart GC, Hughes JP, et al. Breast-milk infectivity in human immunodeficiency virus type 1-infected mothers. *J Infect Dis.* 2003;187:736–740.

Rodger AJ, Cambiano V, Bruun T, et al. Sexual activity without condoms and risk of HIV transmission in serodifferent couples when the HIV-positive partner is using suppressive antiretroviral therapy. *JAMA.* 2016;316(2):171–181. doi:10.1001/jama.2016.5148

Rodger AJ, Cambiano V, Bruun T, et al. Risk of HIV transmission through condomless sex in serodifferent gay couples with the HIV-positive partner taking suppressive antiretroviral therapy (PARTNER): final results of a multicentre, prospective, observational study. *Lancet.* 2019;383(10189):P2428–P2438. http://dx.doi.org/10.1016/S0140-6736(19)30418-0

WHO, UNICEF, UNFPA, and UNAIDS. *HIV Transmission Through Breastfeeding: A Review of Available Evidence: 2007 update.* Geneva: World Health Organization; 2008. http://programme.aids2018.org/Abstract/Abstract/13470

Yah CS, Tambo E. Why is mother to child transmission (MTCT) of HIV a continual threat to newborns in sub-Saharan Africa (SSA)? *J Infect Public Health.* 2019;12(2):213–223. doi:10.1016/j.jiph.2018.10.008

Zhang H, Dornadula G, Beumont M, et al. Human immunodeficiency virus type 1 in the semen of men receiving highly active antiretroviral therapy. *N Engl J Med.* 1998;339(25):1803–1809.

5.

HIV TRANSMISSION PREVENTION

Carolyn Chu, Katrina Baumgartner, and Christopher M. Bositis

INTRODUCTION

HIV prevention encompasses a vast range of approaches and tools across biomedical, behavioral, social, and structural dimensions. Recent notable developments include further implementation experience, new clinical information and medication options regarding HIV preexposure prophylaxis (PrEP), and expanded efforts with HIV treatment as prevention (TasP) through immediate initiation of antiretroviral therapy (ART). Behavioral risk reduction strategies remain critical for HIV prevention, given continued uneven access to biomedical interventions across the US and globally. Integrated HIV and substance use–related prevention and treatment programs remain somewhat underutilized and not widely implemented, although the issue continues to receive much necessary attention.

BEHAVIORAL INTERVENTIONS

LEARNING OBJECTIVE

- Provide a brief overview of behavioral factors and opportunities surrounding HIV prevention, including strategies to reduce HIV exposure risk and considerations for unique circumstances and populations

WHAT'S NEW?

Behavioral interventions continue to be refined to optimize their acceptability and effectiveness in preventing HIV and associated risk behaviors. Internet-based and mobile health platforms for delivery of prevention messaging and support offer promise as a complement or alternative to in-person prevention services. Combination interventions tailored for specific at-risk groups are as important as, if not more than, broad and undifferentiated measures for general audiences, due to varied sociocultural experiences and health disparities.

KEY POINTS

- Providers should elicit comprehensive and detailed sociobehavioral histories in a person-centered manner to identify risk areas so that appropriate and tailored prevention strategies can be shared.

- Various combinations of behavioral strategies will be effective for different populations and should be responsive to an individual's and community's needs and wishes.

Behavioral interventions to prevent HIV transmission include general educational campaigns about sexual health, substance use, and risk reduction as well as individually tailored messages. When used consistently and correctly, condoms reduce HIV transmission by over 70% (Giannou et al., 2016; Smith et al., 2015), and condom promotion/skills training remains the foundation for many sex education and HIV prevention programs. Sexual partnering practices (e.g., partner concurrency, intergenerational/age-discrepant partnering) also drive HIV risk, particularly in specific communities (Adimora et al., 2014; Anema et al., 2013). Serosorting and seropositioning—collectively termed seroadaptive strategies—are employed by some individuals at varying times. These practices utilize knowledge of an individual's HIV status, self-reported or confirmed, to inform decision-making when identifying potential partners or engaging in particular sexual practices. Although in theory such strategies should prevent transmission, each practice carries a different and uncertain level of risk due to a range of factors (Vallabhaneni et al., 2012; Wei et al., 2011).

Adolescents, younger adults, and women are at risk for HIV not only from socioeconomic and cultural factors (e.g., trafficking and violence, sexual coercion, partner substance use, economic inequalities) but also from physiologic considerations. Mucosal and immunologic features unique to the female genital tract as well as vaginal microbial dysbiosis may increase HIV susceptibility (Eastment & McClelland, 2018). For individuals of childbearing capacity, the perinatal and postpartum periods represent especially high-risk periods for HIV acquisition (Thompson et al., 2018). Therefore, behavioral interventions targeted to younger individuals—especially younger women—have involved delaying sexual debut, promoting/incentivizing condom use, ensuring routine sexually transmitted infection (STI) screening, increasing HIV-related knowledge and addressing stigma, and reducing partner concurrency and/or changes (Pettifor et al., 2013; Protogerou & Johnson, 2014). Interventions developed for youth and women have specifically utilized group-based knowledge transfer and skills training processes to support healthy decision-making, relationship building, and overall wellness.

Recently, and in part due to sustainability and dissemination/implementation challenges of in-person, group-oriented prevention activities, web-based and mobile health platforms have been explored. Using various theoretical frameworks, such interventions may be particularly acceptable to younger audiences and men who have sex with men (MSM), and some technologies offer sufficient design flexibility to deliver dynamic interventions of varying content and structure. These interventions have demonstrated efficacy with regard to reducing HIV-associated risk behaviors, delaying sexual initiation, increasing knowledge of HIV/STIs and condom self-efficacy, and increasing HIV testing (Cruess et al., 2018; Schnall et al., 2018). One systematic review characterizing the impact of digital communications technology on HIV testing among MSM and transgender women found that such interventions commonly used existing social media platforms or promotion through online peer educators, and many offered interactive features to facilitate user engagement. Testing uptake among participants exposed to digital interventions was 1.5 times higher than that of unexposed individuals, suggesting that technology-based approaches may be a useful complement to existing HIV testing efforts focused on these populations (Veronese et al., 2020).

Older adults also warrant unique consideration, as they may be less knowledgeable about current HIV-related matters, less likely to volunteer information on their sexual practices and substance use, less likely to use condoms consistently, and more likely to experience social isolation (Adekeye et al., 2012; Franconi & Guaraldi, 2018). Healthcare providers may also be less likely to inquire about these matters with older adults. Therefore, HIV prevention discussions and assessment of risk factors should still occur for older adults, and routine screening should be offered per established recommendations (US Preventive Services Task Force [USPSTF], 2019a). Timely diagnosis and treatment of HIV among older adults remains important, given the likelihood of multiple co-occurring health conditions (e.g., chronic cardiopulmonary disease, kidney disease, cognitive disorders) as well as progressive physical challenges affecting daily functioning and safety (Greene et al., 2017; Lerner et al., 2019).

Transgender individuals continue to experience some of the highest rates of HIV infection globally, and transwomen have an almost 50-fold increase in HIV prevalence (Baral et al., 2013; Caceres et al., 2011). Transgender communities face social and legal exclusion and marginalization, economic vulnerabilities, stigma/bias, and transphobia, and are at extremely high risk of experiencing violence. Transwomen who participate in transactional sex, in particular, face unique individual, interpersonal, and structural susceptibilities and challenges that confer elevated risk. Unsafe injection practices for gender-affirming therapy administration and soft-tissue filler injections, as well as substance use, may also increase risk (Poteat et al., 2017; Reback & Fletcher, 2014). Despite such disproportionate impact, HIV testing rates and PrEP use among transgender individuals remain low (Sevelius et al., 2020). Recently, prevention interventions attuned to the needs of transgender individuals have shifted from solely behavioral to combination behavioral and biomedical approaches, with the behavioral component focusing on retention in care and adherence rather than traditional outcomes such as number of sex partners and condom use (Poteat et al., 2017).

Regular HIV/STI screening remains an important cornerstone of prevention. The USPSTF recommends that all individuals aged 15 to 65 years be screened for HIV, as well as all pregnant persons; younger adolescents and older adults at increased risk of infection should also be screened (USPSTF, 2019b). Universal testing aims to (1) ensure that people with HIV (PWH) know their status, (2) identify early HIV infections reliably, (3) support safer partner disclosure, (4) encourage condom use and other risk reduction measures, and (5) assist with timely linkage to HIV care and treatment, including consideration of "rapid start" ART as soon as possible after diagnosis. In 2020, the Centers for Disease Control and Prevention (CDC) disseminated new guidance around HIV self-testing (CDC, 2021). Self-testing strategies include rapid self-testing that can be completed in any private setting and mail-in kits where specimens are processed at a laboratory with results subsequently relayed via a healthcare provider. Although follow-up testing with an instrument-based assay is generally recommended for abnormal results on currently available self-testing platforms, key advantages of self-testing include patient convenience and comfort. Data suggest self-testing is acceptable to patients, increases HIV testing rates and awareness of HIV status, may help prevent transmission to sex partners, and may also be cost-saving (Iribarren et al., 2020; MacGowan et al., 2020; Shrestha et al., 2020).

RECOMMENDED READING

Buchbinder SP, Liu AY. Virtual CROI 2020: Highlights of epidemiology, public health, and prevention research. IAS-USA. *Top Antivir Med.* 2020;28(2):439–454. https://www.iasusa.org/wp-content/uploads/2020/06/june-july2020.pdf

STRUCTURAL AND SYSTEMS-LEVEL INTERVENTIONS

LEARNING OBJECTIVES

- Briefly describe the safety of the US blood supply and new considerations that have been raised by early ART initiation (as treatment) and PrEP use among donors.

- Discuss structural/systems-level considerations and interventions that aim to decrease HIV transmission, including substance use–related practices and interventions.

WHAT'S NEW?

Substance use and HIV transmission remain inextricably linked, and the longstanding decline in HIV diagnoses among persons who inject drugs (PWID) seems to have plateaued. HIV outbreaks continue to occur among networks of PWID and have largely affected regions experiencing high poverty, unemployment, and homelessness. Systems-level advancements such as expanded harm reduction services and access to medications for substance use disorder treatment, as well as integrated substance use and HIV care and continued intensive public health efforts, remain necessary to address these overlapping epidemics.

KEY POINTS

- The US blood supply remains extremely safe, and recent policy changes regarding donor deferral practices among MSM have not been associated with an increased incidence of HIV seropositivity among donors.

- Clinicians should be able to recognize HIV transmission risks associated with both injection-related and non–injection-related substance use. Harm reduction services, substance use disorder treatment, and integrated HIV and viral hepatitis testing and care are all effective means to decrease HIV transmission.

SAFETY OF THE US BLOOD SUPPLY

The risk of transfusion-transmitted HIV is less than 1 in 1 million transfusions in the US and other developed countries (Busch et al., 2019; Zou et al., 2010). Widespread HIV-1 antibody screening began in the US in 1985, and HIV-2 antibody screening was introduced in 1992. Since 1999, donations have also been pooled for HIV-1 nucleic acid testing, facilitating more reliable detection of recently acquired HIV among donors.

In 2015, the US Food and Drug Administration (FDA) revised its guidance on donor deferral practices among MSM, changing its recommendations from indefinite deferral to a 12-month deferral since last sex (in April 2020, as part of a broader agency response to the COVID-19 pandemic, the FDA issued additional guidance changes and further reduced the recommended deferral period to 3 months) (FDA, 2020). Using data from the US Transfusion-Transmissible Infections Monitoring System, investigators compared HIV transmissions between the period before versus after the 2015 decision to establish the 12-month deferral period and found no increase in the incidence of HIV seropositivity among first-time donors (Grebe et al., 2020).

Recently, some researchers have indicated a need to revisit transfusion-related screening and monitoring practices and donor health questionnaires, citing an uncertain but potential "impact of interventions to reduce HIV through antiretroviral therapies following HIV diagnoses, and widespread availability of post-exposure and pre-exposure prophylaxis" (Custer et al., 2020). Because ART has been demonstrated to alter biomarkers of HIV infection progression and may (in rare cases) result in antibody seroreversion, current blood donation screening and testing practices may not be able to detect HIV infection in a very small subset of donors. Specifically, blood donated by individuals who started ART early after HIV acquisition could test negative for HIV-1 RNA as well as antibodies, potentially leading to transfusion-mediated transmission. PrEP use may also raise challenges for

accurate and timely HIV diagnosis (Donnell et al., 2017; Lee et al., 2020).

PREVENTION OF HIV RELATED TO SUBSTANCE USE

Injection drug use (IDU) has long been linked to HIV transmission, with risk estimates ranging from 0.63% to 2.4% per act (Baggaley et al., 2006). Of the almost 38,000 HIV diagnoses identified in the US and dependent areas in 2018, approximately 1 in 10 were among PWID (CDC, 2020a). HIV generally degrades rapidly outside the body under ambient conditions; however, studies indicate it can survive for longer periods (up to 6 weeks) within a sealed syringe (Heimer & Abdala, 2000). Higher levels of HIV present in the blood injected, larger volume of injected blood, and/or higher injection frequency can all increase risk. In addition to direct sharing of needles/syringes or equipment, various drug preparation practices (e.g., sharing water used to flush out equipment) can indirectly lead to HIV transmission. Although HIV risk has been demonstrated most clearly for intravenous drug use, any parenteral exposure—including subcutaneous and intramuscular use—to virus-containing material can potentially lead to transmission. Additionally, alcohol, stimulant, and sedative/hypnotic use have all been associated with increased HIV transmission risk by affecting decision-making and negotiation around condom use and other sex practices (Berry & Johnson, 2018; Hoenigl et al., 2016; Ickowicz et al., 2015).

Prevention of substance use–related HIV transmission remains a national public health priority. Since the 2015 HIV outbreak in Indiana, other outbreaks attributed to IDU continue to be reported in both rural and urban communities (Buchbinder & Liu, 2020). A broad, cross-sector, coordinated response should include (1) increased access to harm reduction services and naloxone; (2) improved recognition of substance use and widespread HIV/viral hepatitis education and screening practices; (3) expanded access to medications for substance use disorder treatment and HIV prevention (e.g. preexposure and postexposure prophylaxis) as well as other effective therapies for substance use; and (4) person-centered, multidisciplinary care tailored to specific community needs (Perlman & Jordan, 2018; Rich et al., 2018). Many leaders and organizations have continued to raise the visibility of structural factors and their impact on substance use; these include disparities in housing and economic opportunity, racist/aggressive policing practices and mass incarceration, and prohibitive legislation and policies (Perlman & Jordan, 2018).

Harm Reduction Approaches to IDU and HIV Prevention

Harm reduction is a concept whereby the prevention or reduction of adverse effects associated with certain behaviors is prioritized over absolute cessation of the behavior itself. Since the early 1990s, multiple harm reduction strategies—both biomedical and non-biomedical—have effectively decreased

IDU-related HIV transmission risk. Needle and syringe exchange programs, peer-based education and outreach, substance use disorder treatment, and preexposure and postexposure HIV prophylaxis have all been evaluated (Aspinall et al., 2014; CDC, 2018; MacArthur et al., 2014). In 2020, citing a 50% reduction in HIV and hepatitis C virus incidence attributable to syringe service programs (SSPs), the US Surgeon General called for policies to address the overlapping crises of drug overdoses and IDU-associated infectious disease complications, namely "state and local policies that enable implementation of comprehensive syringe services programs" (Adams, 2020). Medically supervised, safe injection facilities—also referred to as supervised injection or consumption facilities—are feasible and cost-effective and can play a uniquely meaningful role in reducing health-related harms by reducing overdose/death and linking people to medical treatment and other services (Kennedy et al., 2017).

Substance Use Screening and Expanded HIV Testing

In 2020, the USPSTF released recommendations on screening for unhealthy drug use among all adults, concluding that "screening . . . has moderate net benefit when services for accurate diagnosis of unhealthy drug use or drug use disorders, effective treatment, and appropriate care can be offered or referred" (USPSTF, 2020). For people with HIV, the overall prevalence of substance use remains fairly elevated and may be especially notable among individuals who are not virally suppressed (CDC, 2020b; Hartzler, 2017). National HIV treatment and prevention guidelines as well as many HIV professional organizations recommend assessment of substance use for all PWH as well as individuals at risk for HIV (Aberg et al., 2014; CDC, 2020b; Saag et al., 2018; US Department of Health and Human Services Panel on Antiretroviral Guidelines for Adults and Adolescents, 2019).

The CDC continues to recommend that PWID be screened for HIV at least annually. However, among one national sample of PWID, only half reported any HIV screening within the past 12 months and less than half with a new HIV diagnosis reported seeing a healthcare provider within 1 month after diagnosis (CDC, 2020b). HIV screening is not universally implemented across substance use programs, and only a small proportion offer on-site, HIV-specific services (Cohn et al., 2016). Widespread integration of HIV services within substance use programs can help complement traditional HIV testing and prevention efforts (Rich, 2018; Strathdee et al., 2012). Additionally, further efforts are needed to raise awareness and uptake of PrEP among PWID: several studies have indicated low rates of accurate PrEP knowledge as well as stigma involving providers and social networks among PWID (Bazzi et al., 2018; Biello et al., 2018).

Medical Management of Substance Use and HIV Prevention

Multiple pharmacologic therapies effectively reduce substance use and HIV transmission. However, access to—and coverage of—substance use disorder treatment remains uneven across communities and payers, with persistent disparities based on geography, socioeconomic status, and race/ethnicity (Stein et al., 2018). Provider-level barriers such as stigma and lack of prescriber comfort also contribute to high levels of unmet need with regard to substance use treatment (Haffajee et al., 2018). Multiple medications (methadone, buprenorphine, naltrexone) are available to treat opioid use disorder. For people with HIV who inject drugs, treatment of co-occurring substance use disorder can facilitate improved adherence to care and viral load suppression. One systematic review found that opioid agonist treatment increased ART coverage by over 50% and reduced ART discontinuation by approximately 20%, suggesting a positive role for integrated substance use and HIV care delivery (Low et al., 2016).

As indicated previously, non-opioid substances have also been implicated in HIV transmission. Crystal methamphetamine is a highly habit-forming stimulant that increases sexual arousal while also decreasing social inhibitions. Similar to cocaine, methamphetamine use elevates HIV risk not only through sharing equipment but also via specific sexual practices (e.g., frequently engaging in condomless and/or transactional sex, having multiple partners). Although methamphetamine use and HIV risk have been predominantly described among MSM, the population of people who use methamphetamine is varied. Novel treatment approaches are needed to address the unique complexities and challenges of its clinical management (Mimiaga et al., 2018; Substance Abuse and Mental Health Services Administration [SAMHSA], 2020).

Legal Considerations Surrounding HIV Prevention with PWID

In 2004, the World Health Organization (WHO) stated that "HIV infection [among injection drug users] is more likely to occur in legal environments where sterile injection equipment is more severely restricted" (Wodak & Cooney, 2004). In general, the US continues to have among the most severe restrictions related to syringe exchange and possession of any country. This has contributed to a broad lack of availability of SSPs, which has at times hampered HIV prevention efforts in some localities where such interventions have been critically needed to address emerging HIV outbreaks (Strathdee, 2020). As of 2018, 317 SSPs were operating in 39 states and the District of Columbia (Fernandez-Vina et al., 2020); however, only five states accounted for almost half of those programs: California, New York, New Mexico, North Carolina, and Kentucky. Although many states may now have some legal provisions explicitly authorizing SSPs, the legality of syringe possession remains ambiguous in many places, and challenges involving funding and coordination necessary to maintain such services are not insignificant. Beyond the existence of drug control laws themselves, law enforcement practices influence individual behaviors, community stigma, and the overall risk environment for PWID. One systematic review concluded that the vast majority of scientific data suggest drug criminalization has negative effects on HIV prevention and treatment (DeBeck et al., 2017).

ADDITIONAL STRUCTURAL AND SYSTEMS-LEVEL CONSIDERATIONS

Several other structural factors influence HIV risk: these represent an extensive landscape of physical, sociocultural, organizational, economic, and policy-related dynamics. Physical factors such as proximity to—and convenience of—HIV services can affect motivation to seek care. Stigma, racism, and HIV-related discrimination often influence decision-making related to testing and engagement, as well as disclosure to others. Care settings that discreetly offer co-located services and expanded access can facilitate engagement in care. Inadequate housing is a significant barrier to care and also increases HIV transmission risk (Aidala et al., 2015; Garcia et al., 2015). The intersections between behavioral/mental health and HIV have been well documented; thus, HIV providers should carefully elicit a thorough mental health history as well as screen for trauma and violence with all PWH.

Economic factors are closely intertwined with HIV: resource-limited settings are disproportionately affected by high rates of HIV, often related to deindustrialization and unemployment. Such disparities involve inequalities in poverty, gender, race, and education; economic instability; labor migration patterns; access to health resources and health literacy; local healthcare system infrastructure and funding; unmet substance use and mental health needs; drug policies and enforcement; and other factors (Zanakis et al., 2007). Despite efforts to expand testing and prevention broadly across the US, HIV diagnosis rates continue to disproportionately affect communities of color and are higher for individuals in lower socioeconomic positions (CDC, 2020b).

Health insurance status is a major determinant affecting access to primary care and preventive services. Data from the Behavioral Risk Factor Surveillance System across 2010 to 2017 demonstrated that Medicaid expansion promoted HIV testing without increasing HIV risk behavior, although there were large disparities across race/ethnicity, age, and geographic area (Gai & Marthinsen, 2019). Lack of uniform access to healthcare remains a fundamental driver of health inequity and is a critical barrier to ending the US HIV epidemic (del Rio, 2020).

The epidemiology of incarceration closely reflects that of HIV, and the complex interplay of racial and economic disparities in arrest/incarceration rates, substance use, and HIV is well described (Csete et al., 2016; Iroh et al., 2015; Wirtz et al., 2018). Incarcerated and recently released individuals generally have low rates of HIV awareness, testing, and engagement in care despite being at substantially elevated risk; one systematic review found that recent incarceration was associated with an 81% increased risk of HIV acquisition among PWID (Stone et al., 2018). Further, some analyses suggest that incarceration itself could be an important contributor to HIV transmission among networks of PWID, and the period following release represents a unique and potentially high-impact opportunity for reducing HIV transmission and adverse health outcomes, including fatal overdose (Khan et al., 2019; Stone et al., 2018). Among correctional facilities, there is considerable variation in access to and types of HIV prevention, testing, and treatment services (Valera et al., 2017). Multiple challenges unique to correctional settings include rapid turnover and transfers, lack of testing and treatment resources, limited access to condoms and harm reduction services, overcrowding and violence, low utilization of HIV preexposure and postexposure prophylaxis, variable staff training, and lack of post-release care coordination. Interventions to address such challenges have included formation of "local change teams," telemedicine/teleconsultation, and transitions programs/navigators to facilitate engagement in post-release care (Dong et al., 2017; Belenko et al., 2017).

TREATMENT AS PREVENTION: "UNDETECTABLE = UNTRANSMITTABLE"

In 2016, the Prevention Access Campaign launched its "Undetectable = Untransmittable" (U = U) campaign. This health equity initiative was based on the results of several multinational trials involving thousands of serodifferent couples (e.g. HPTN 052, PARTNER and PARTNER2, Opposites Attract). Specifically, no cases of linked sexual transmission of HIV were identified when the seropositive partner had achieved durable virologic suppression on ART. Prior to 2016, the paradigm of HIV TasP had been accepted by many in the scientific, public health, and HIV clinical provider communities; most clinical guidelines had also already removed specific $CD4^+$ thresholds for ART initiation, signaling a universal movement favoring early ART for all. Among the general population, however, ongoing stigma and skepticism have negatively affected public perception of PWH. In September 2017, the CDC officially endorsed the campaign. Goals of U = U include reducing fears of sexual transmission among PWH; broadly diminishing HIV stigma; encouraging PWH to start and remain on ART; and achieving universal access to HIV testing, treatment, and care.

Broad dissemination and scale-up of advocacy efforts and implementation of antidiscrimination policies and laws are critical achievements that can help reduce HIV-related stigma and advance universal human rights. An expert consensus statement released at the 2018 International AIDS Conference indicated that "more caution should be exercised when considering criminal prosecution, including careful appraisal of current scientific evidence on HIV-related risks and harms. This is instrumental to reduce stigma and discrimination and to avoid miscarriages of justice" (Barre-Sinoussi et al., 2018).

RECOMMENDED READING

Custer B, Quiner CA, Haaland R, et al. HIV antiretroviral therapy and prevention use in US blood donors: a new blood safety concern. *Blood.* 2020;136(11):1351–1358. doi:10.1182/blood.2020006890

Perlman D, Jordan AE. The syndemic of opioid misuse, overdose, HCV, and HIV: structural-level causes and interventions. *Current HIV/AIDS Rep.* 2018;15:96–112.

Stone J, Fraser H, Lim AG, et al. Incarceration history and risk of HIV and hepatitis C virus acquisition among people who inject drugs: a systematic review and meta-analysis. *Lancet Infect Dis.* 2018;18(12):1397–1409.

MEDICAL INTERVENTIONS FOR HIV TRANSMISSION PREVENTION

LEARNING OBJECTIVES

- Define what it means to be at high risk for HIV acquisition and identify individuals who meet these criteria

- Describe the screening, evaluation, and monitoring recommendations for PrEP, occupational postexposure prophylaxis (oPEP), and nonoccupational postexposure prophylaxis (nPEP), as well as common side effects, toxicities, and other potential risks associated with their use

- Describe three new or investigational biomedical interventions for HIV prevention and how they complement existing interventions

WHAT'S NEW?

- In 2019, the USPSTF gave a "Grade A" recommendation for tenofovir DF-based PrEP use in individuals at increased risk of HIV acquisition.

- In 2019, the FDA approved a second medication regimen (emtricitabine/tenofovir AF, or F/TAF) as PrEP for cisgender MSM and transgender women who have sex with men at higher risk of HIV acquisition, but not in any persons practicing vaginal sex.

- Interim results from the HPTN083 trial showed superiority of injectable cabotegravir as compared to daily oral emtricitabine/tenofovir DF (as PrEP) in cisgender MSM and transgender women at higher risk of HIV acquisition.

- In 2020, the European Medicines Agency (EMA) approved use of the drug-eluting dapivirine vaginal ring for women over 18 years old.

KEY POINTS

- Daily PrEP, consisting of tenofovir DF (300 mg) alone or in combination with emtricitabine (200 mg), is safe and effective for preventing HIV acquisition in a variety of at-risk groups, including MSM, transgender women, heterosexual women and men, PWID, and at-risk adolescents.

- F/TAF and event-driven PrEP may be considered for use in MSM and transgender women who have sex with men but have not yet been studied in other populations.

- Despite its effectiveness, significant disparities in PrEP use based on race, gender, geography, and risk behavior exist, threatening to exacerbate existing and similar disparities in HIV incidence.

- PEP, when taken within 72 hours of exposure, is also safe and effective for preventing HIV; PEP may be considered as a bridge to PrEP in individuals with anticipated ongoing risk exposures.

- Continued development and evaluation of novel biomedical prevention approaches are key to an effective, sustainable reduction in the number of new HIV transmissions globally.

INTRODUCTION

Biomedical interventions used to prevent HIV transmission and acquisition among individuals at risk include PrEP, oPEP, and nPEP; STI screening and treatment; voluntary medical male circumcision; prevention of perinatal HIV transmission; and TasP.

PREP

PrEP refers to the use of antiretroviral medications before HIV exposure as a means to prevent HIV acquisition in at-risk, HIV-negative individuals.

Data: Clinical Trials and Real-World Effectiveness

The FDA first approved the daily use of fixed-dose emtricitabine (FTC) 200 mg/tenofovir disoproxil fumarate (TDF) 300 mg (also known as F/TDF) as PrEP to reduce the risk of HIV through sexual acquisition in 2012. This approval was based on multiple studies showing that, when taken consistently, TDF-based PrEP is highly effective at reducing the rate of HIV acquisition in those at highest risk, including MSM, transgender women who have sex with men, PWID, and heterosexual women and men (Table 5.1). Although the point estimates of this benefit varied across different studies, with reductions in the rate of HIV transmission ranging from 44% to 75%, several common features should be highlighted:

1. It is most effective among those who are most adherent. In the iPrEx study, for example, the relative risk of HIV transmission was 92% lower among participants with detectable levels of study drug compared to those without (Grant et al., 2010), and in the Bangkok Tenofovir Study it was 70% lower (Choopanya et al., 2013).

2. It was generally well tolerated, with fewer than 10% of participants reporting serious adverse events (CDC/US Public Health Service [USPHS], 2018).

3. Infection with drug-resistant HIV in PrEP users has been rare (see discussion later in the chapter), despite historical concerns that this would limit its use.

Real-world data on the effectiveness of F/TDF as PrEP have been encouraging. Both the US Kaiser Cohort and the UK PROUD study showed substantial reductions in incident HIV infections among PrEP users compared to historical or actual controls (McCormack et al., 2016; Volk et al.,

Table 5.1 SUMMARY OF EARLY RANDOMIZED, CONTROLLED PREP TRIALS

TRIAL	STUDY POPULATION; SETTING	INTERVENTION	EFFECT–HAZARD RATIO [ESTIMATED REDUCTION IN HIV ACQUISITION] (95% CI)	REFERENCE
iPrEX	2,499 MSM and transgender women; US, South America, Thailand, South Africa	TDF/FTC	0.56 [44%] (15–63)	Grant et al., 2010
Partners PrEP	4,747 heterosexual women and men; Kenya and Uganda	TDF TDF/FTC	0.33 [67%] (0.19–0.56) 0.25 [75%] (0.13–0.45)	Baeten et al., 2012
TDF 2	1,219 heterosexual women and men; Botswana	TDF/FTC	0.38 [62%] (0.22–0.83)	Thigpen et al., 2012
Thai IDU	2,413 PWID; Thailand	TDF	0.51 [49%] (0.1–0.72)	Choopanya et al., 2013
FemPrEP	2,120 heterosexual women; Africa	TDF/FTC	0.94 [6%] (0.59–1.52)	Van Damme et al., 2012
VOICE	5,029 heterosexual women; Africa	TDF TDF/FTC	1.49 [−49%] (0.97–2.29) 1.04 [−4%] (0.73–1.49)	Marrazzo et al., 2015

2015), while data from New South Wales, Australia, and San Francisco demonstrate that rapid scale-up of PrEP in at-risk populations has coincided with population-level reductions in the number of new HIV diagnoses in these communities (Buchbinder et al., 2018; Grulich et al., 2018).

Breakthrough HIV acquisition has rarely been reported despite optimal dosing and PrEP adherence, primarily due to transmitted drug-resistant HIV (Cohen et al., 2018; Colby et al., 2018; Knox et al., 2017; Markowitz et al., 2017b; Spinelli et al., 2020; Thaden et al., 2018). Additionally, one individual acquired wild-type HIV while taking PrEP; for this case, it is thought that HIV infection progressed systemically only after PrEP discontinuation (Hoornenborg & de Bree, 2017). While such cases highlight that PrEP is not infallible, it is notable that there have been only a handful of reported cases of "PrEP failure" among extensive data supporting its efficacy, and the prevalence of multidrug-resistant HIV in individuals with unsuppressed viral load remains low overall in the US. When taken as prescribed, the vast majority of individuals on PrEP will gain protection from its use.

In 2019, the DISCOVER trial, a randomized, double-blind trial comparing emtricitabine plus tenofovir alafenamide (F/TAF) to F/TDF in 5,387 participants, was the first to lead to FDA approval of an alternative medication (F/TAF) for PrEP (Mayer et al., 2020). This trial showed non-inferiority of daily F/TAF compared to F/TDF among HIV-negative MSM and transgender women who have sex with men at high risk of sexual HIV acquisition. Results of this study cannot be generalized or widely applied, as the efficacy of F/TAF for prevention of HIV acquisition via vaginal sex or injection drug use, safety in pregnancy, and alternate or intermittent dosing has not yet been determined.

Although daily F/TDF had been the only initially approved PrEP strategy, mounting evidence now demonstrates that alternative dosing regimens are likely to be effective in certain situations. The most studied of these is often referred to as "event-driven" PrEP or "2-1-1" dosing: two pills of F/TDF taken together 2 to 24 hours prior to sexual exposure, one pill 24 hours after, and one pill 48 hours after exposure (or one pill daily until 2 sex-free days). The IPERGAY and Prévenir studies showed high rates of protection for MSM with this strategy (Molina et al., 2015, 2017, 2019), including among participants who report infrequent sex (Antoni et al., 2017). As with daily PrEP, adherence is important for the efficacy of event-driven dosing, as demonstrated by the HPTN067/ADAPT trial, where differences in adherence between daily and event-driven PrEP led to an estimated 18% efficacy reduction with the latter in the US-based cohort (Dimitrov et al., 2020). These data have led multiple national and international guidelines committees, including the International Antiviral Society—USA, to support event-driven dosing as an alternative to daily F/TDF in MSM (Saag et al., 2018).

Eligibility

Multiple guidelines on PrEP eligibility and use have been released since initial clinical trial results reporting its efficacy were first released. For the purposes of this chapter, specific recommendations are taken from the 2018 CDC/USPHS guidelines. Other guidelines of interest include those from WHO (2016, 2019); the International Antiviral Society–USA (Saag et al., 2018); and the New York State Department of Health AIDS Institute (New York State Department of Health, 2020a).

According to the CDC/USPHS guidelines, PrEP is recommended as a prevention option for adults at substantial risk of acquiring HIV, including MSM, heterosexually active women and men, and PWID (CDC/USPHS, 2018). In 2018, the FDA also approved daily F/TDF as PrEP for adolescents weighing at least 35 kg who are at increased risk of HIV acquisition. Despite a lack of data from randomized controlled trials of its efficacy among adolescents, PrEP has been shown to be an effective and important HIV prevention tool for this group (Hosek et al., 2017). It should be a component of

Table 5.2 INDICATIONS FOR PREP USE BASED ON RISK FACTORS

SEXUAL RISK FACTORS	SUBSTANCE USE RISK FACTORS
Any HIV-negative adult or adolescent weighing ≥35 kg who is not in a monogamous relationship with a recently tested, HIV-negative partner. *AND* within the last 6 months any of the following: • was diagnosed with gonorrhea or syphilis (or chlamydia if MSM or a behaviorally bisexual man [i.e., a man having sex with both men and women]) • is having condomless sex with a partner living with HIV but not on treatment or is not virally suppressed, or whose HIV status is unknown • is an MSM/bisexual man having condomless anal sex • is a heterosexual or behaviorally bisexual man or woman having condomless sex who themselves, or are involved with partner(s) who, are at increased risk of HIV (multiple or anonymous partners, partners of unknown HIV status, PWID, involved with transactional sex, transgender/MSM/bisexual male partners) • is a transgender individual with any of the above risk factors	Any HIV-negative adult or adolescent weighing ≥35 kg who injects substances. *AND* within the last 6 months: • has shared injection or drug-preparation equipment *OR* • has an injecting partner who is a PWH or has an injecting partner of unknown HIV status

Adapted from CDC/US Public Health Service (2018) and New York State Department of Health (2020a).

all HIV prevention counseling for adolescents, especially as young MSM (particularly young MSM of color) remain disproportionately affected by HIV in the US. PrEP prescribing for adolescents should always be done in the context of local regulations and laws regarding autonomy of minors and their healthcare decision-making capacity (CDC/USPHS, 2018). Importantly, the USPSTF also now recommends PrEP for those at high risk for HIV acquisition (Grade A, USPSTF, 2019a). Specific indications based on risk are listed in Table 5.2.

While CDC/USPHS guidelines do not specifically define what it means to be in a "high prevalence area or network," the majority of PrEP studies were conducted in populations in which the background HIV incidence was at least 3 per 100 person-years, and the International Antiviral Society–USA panel therefore recommends PrEP for those in which the background incidence is greater than 2% (Saag et al., 2018).

Prescribing PrEP: Baseline Assessment and Follow-Up

Prior to initiating PrEP in eligible individuals, providers should document the following:

• Absence of acute or chronic HIV

• Renal function (creatinine clearance [CrCl] $\geq$ 60 mL/min for F/TDF use; CrCl $\geq$ 30 mL/min for F/TAF)

• Hepatitis B virus (HBV) immunity or infection and vaccination status

To document absence of acute or chronic HIV, the CDC/USPHS recommends following the algorithm shown in Figure 5.1. Oral rapid HIV testing should not be used due to its lower sensitivity for detecting HIV compared to blood-based tests (CDC/USPHS, 2018), and a negative test result (preferably using combination antigen/antibody assay) should be documented within the week before PrEP initiation. For individuals who report signs or symptoms of acute HIV within the previous 4 weeks, and for those with high-risk exposures within 4 weeks prior to initiating PrEP, the most

recent testing algorithm suggests a negative antigen/antibody test alone is acceptable; others would recommend sending an HIV viral load in addition to the antigen/antibody test to confidently determine baseline HIV status (New York State Department of Health, 2020a; CDC/USPHS, 2018).

Daily F/TDF is the preferred PrEP regimen for most eligible individuals, including adolescents weighing at least 35 kg. F/TAF is an acceptable alternative for MSM and transgender women and may be preferred in people with underlying renal or bone disease. The CDC/USPHS recommends that no more than a 3-month supply of medication be prescribed at a time. Recommended follow-up and testing for PrEP toxicity and comorbid conditions are detailed in Table 5.3. While not specifically stated in the table, baseline testing for HCV is recommended and should be repeated annually in those at ongoing risk for HCV exposure (CDC/USPHS, 2018).

Concerns Related to PrEP USE

PrEP, both as daily F/TDF and F/TAF, has generally been very well tolerated in both clinical studies and real-world settings, with fewer than 10% of recipients experiencing serious adverse events (CDC, 2018; Ogbuagu et al., 2020). The most commonly reported side effects include nausea, flatulence, headache, and weight loss. Sometimes referred to as "start-up syndrome," most symptoms resolve within the first month of medication use and can usually be managed with over-the-counter medications and other supportive measures.

More serious potential PrEP toxicities include acute and/or chronic kidney injury and bone demineralization, both of which appear to be reversible with PrEP discontinuation (Mulligan et al., 2015; Solomon et al., 2014). Compared to F/TDF, F/TAF as PrEP was associated with favorable and statistically significant differences in bone mineral density and renal marker changes at 96 weeks of follow-up in the DISCOVER trial (Ogbuagu et al., 2020), supporting its use for older PrEP users and/or those with bone or renal comorbidities. However, these changes may not be clinically relevant for many PrEP users, and caution should therefore be exercised when recommending broader use of F/TAF as PrEP.

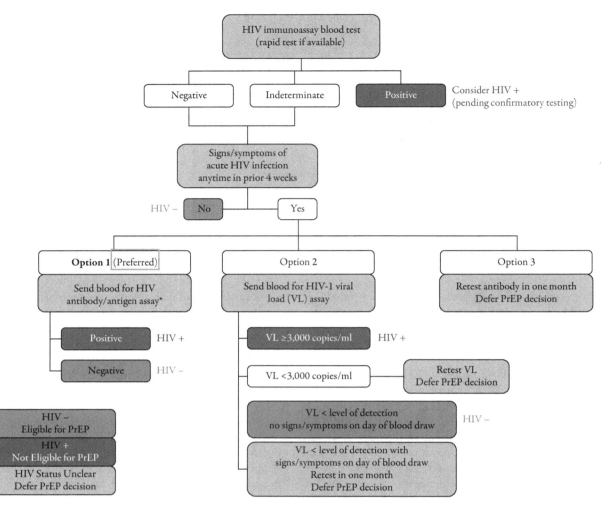

Figure 5.1 Assessment of acute/chronic HIV infection prior to PrEP initiation   SOURCE: CDC: USPHS: Preexposure prophylaxis for the prevention of HIV infection in the United States—2017 Update: a clinical practice guideline. Https://www.cdc.gov/hiv/pdf/risk/prep/cdc-hiv-prep-guidelines-2017.pdf. Published March 2018. https://www.cdc.gov/hiv/pdf/risk/prep/cdc-hiv-prep-guidelines-2017.pdf.

Table 5.3 SUMMARY GUIDELINES FOR PREP USE

	MSM	HETEROSEXUALLY ACTIVE WOMEN AND MEN	PWID
Clinically eligible if:	• Documented negative HIV test • No signs/symptoms of acute HIV infection • Renal function: CrCl ≥ 60 mL/min (F/TDF use); CrCl ≥ 30 mL/min (F/TAF) • No contraindicated medications • Documented HBV infection and vaccination status		
Prescription	• FTC/TDF (fixed-dose combination) once daily • (May use FTC/TAF once daily, or "2-1-1" event-driven dosing with FTC/TDF, as alternative for MSM or transgender women having sex with men) • No more than 3-month medication supply at a time		
Other services	• Follow-up visits at least every 3 months for HIV testing (consider early repeat HIV Ag/Ab testing after 1 month if any potential HIV exposures in the month prior to PrEP initiation), medication adherence counseling, behavioral risk reduction support, side effect assessment, and STI symptom assessment • At 3 months and every 6 months thereafter, assess renal function • Every 3 to 6 months test for gonorrhea, chlamydia, and syphilis regardless of symptoms		
	• Perform gonorrhea and chlamydia testing at all sites of exposure (including oral/rectal screening)	• Assess pregnancy intent; pregnancy test at baseline and every 3 months if potential for pregnancy	• Access to sterile needles/syringes and substance use disorder treatment services

Adapted from US Public Health Service (2019a).

For people who acquire HIV while on PrEP, there has been concern about possible development of ART resistance. Such resistance has been rarely documented to date and, with the exception of the small number of cases previously mentioned, it has been primarily observed in individuals with undiagnosed HIV at the time of PrEP initiation, underscoring the importance of evaluating for possible acute HIV before initiating PrEP (CDC/USPHS, 2018).

STI diagnoses are common among PrEP users. Whether this is due to increased frequency of screening, an increase in high-risk sexual behaviors such as condomless sex or multiple partners, or some combination thereof is not entirely clear (Baeten et al., 2012; Grant et al., 2010; Hosek et al., 2015; McCormack et al., 2016; Volk et al., 2015). Care must be taken, however, to ensure that concerns about risk compensation are not used to justify withholding PrEP from those who wish to be on it and/or might benefit from it. Rather, the focus should turn toward promoting sexual health using shared decision-making based on individual preferences and priorities, increased STI screening, and engagement in care (Marcus et al., 2019).

For people with chronic HBV as evidenced by a positive/reactive HBV surface antigen (HBsAg) test, the CDC/USPHS recommends evaluation by a clinician experienced in chronic HBV treatment. Such individuals may be given PrEP but should be counseled on the potential risk of a hepatic flare should they abruptly discontinue TDF-containing PrEP, although this has not yet been reported in HBV-positive, HIV-negative individuals (CDC/USPHS, 2018; Solomon et al., 2016). Event-driven PrEP dosing is not recommended for individuals with chronic HBV.

Individuals of childbearing capacity who wish to become pregnant or breastfeed while taking PrEP should be counseled that the vast majority of PrEP studies to date have excluded women who were or who became pregnant. However, data from the Antiviral Pregnancy Registry demonstrate no evidence of harm to fetuses exposed to F/TDF (Antiretroviral Pregnancy Registry, 2020). Further, it should be emphasized that some HIV-negative women with seropositive partners may be at increased risk for HIV acquisition during pregnancy or peri-conception. Current US guidelines recommend use of F/TDF as PrEP for women who are trying to conceive or who are pregnant when viral suppression of the seropositive partner is in question (Panel on Treatment of Pregnant Women with HIV Infection and Prevention of Perinatal Transmission, 2020). Although data are limited, use of F/TDF during lactation appears to be safe, and therefore breastfeeding is not a contraindication to its use (CDC/USPHS, 2017; US Department of Health and Human Services, 2019).

Discontinuing PrEP

PrEP should be discontinued in people who experience unacceptable side effects or toxicities, including kidney disease; are unable to adhere to the prescribed regimen or follow-up visit schedule; or change their risk status such that PrEP is no longer believed to be indicated. Individuals who acquire HIV while taking PrEP should be transitioned to ART as treatment in accordance with current HIV treatment guidelines, while awaiting genotypic testing results (CDC/USPHS, 2018).

PrEP Challenges and Disparities

Although PrEP has clearly been shown to be beneficial in the appropriate settings, questions remain. It is not clear, for example, how long PrEP can be safely prescribed. CDC/USPHS guidelines state that it should not be given for life but, rather, only during periods of highest risk of HIV acquisition; however, many PrEP-eligible individuals can be expected to remain so for extended periods (CDC/USPHS, 2018).

The role of PrEP for people in serodifferent relationships in which the partner with HIV is on suppressive ART is also not clear. It is now established that persons with HIV who maintain an undetectable viral load do not transmit HIV to their sexual partners (see earlier discussion of U = U). However, HIV-negative individuals in such relationships may have other partners of unknown status or partners who are positive but not yet on treatment. This possibility was highlighted by the fact that nearly 40% of transmissions in the HPTN052 study were unlinked (i.e., they came from someone other than their identified serodifferent partner) (Cohen et al., 2015). PrEP is likely to be beneficial for such scenarios.

The optimal strategy for initiating PrEP in some individuals with frequent, high-risk exposures is unclear and may contribute at least partly to underutilization of PrEP in PWID. When a person is identified as having a high-risk exposure within the previous 72 hours (and is not already taking PrEP consistently), current US guidelines recommend that PEP should be given for 28 days (see later in the chapter) before transitioning to PrEP, after confirming that the exposed person remains HIV-negative (CDC/USPHS, 2018). If the timing of the last exposure representing significant risk falls outside of the 72-hour window or is uncertain, and HIV cannot be confidently ruled out with immediate testing, providers should consider consultation with a PEP/PrEP-experienced provider.

Since initial FDA approval of PrEP, the number of at-risk individuals taking PrEP has increased substantially (Figure 5.2), although the number of those eligible continues to greatly exceed the number who are actually taking it.

Simultaneously, large disparities continue to exist in PrEP access and uptake in the US along lines of race, gender, geography, and risk behavior. PrEP use is greatest among white MSM and substantially lower among racial/ethnic minorities, women, and PWID (Buchbinder et al., 2018; Giler, 2017; Kuo et al., 2018; Mayer et al., 2018). In 2015, the CDC estimated that 1.1 million adults were at increased risk of HIV and met indications for PrEP, of whom 43% were Black, 24% Hispanic, and 26% white (Smith et al., 2018). This is in stark contrast to 2016 data showing that among 78,000+ people who filled PrEP prescriptions in the US, the majority (68%) were white (Figure 5.3). Regional differences were also seen: while about half of all HIV diagnoses were identified in the South, only 27% of PrEP users lived in the South (Huang et al., 2018).

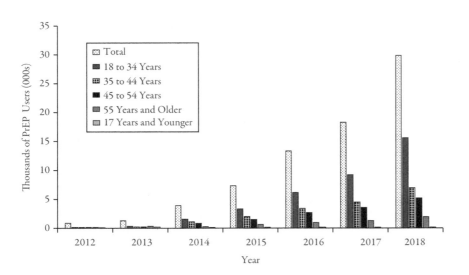

Year	Rate per 10,000 Commercially Insured Beneficiaries Prescribed PrEP
2012	0.13
2013	0.26
2014	0.76
2015	2.39
2016	4.41
2017	6.60
2018	10.56

Figure 5.2 Number of new PrEP starts by age group, 2012–2018   Adapted from Song HJ, et al. Trends in HIV Preexposure Prophylaxis Prescribing in the United States, 2012–2018. *JAMA.* 2020;324(4):395–397. doi:10.1001/jama.2020.7312

This unequal distribution of US PrEP use risks worsening disparities already seen in HIV incidence. Individual- and population-level efforts must be implemented to close these gaps while simultaneously addressing the structural racism and internalized biases that have promoted them. Increased training, especially for clinicians caring for communities of color; community-level education to promote awareness and reduce stigma; and inclusive public health campaigns all may have an impact, as would ensuring equitable access to healthcare and health insurance (Kanny et al., 2019).

Providers seeking clinical guidance on PrEP should contact local experts, if available. The National Clinician Consultation Center (nccc.ucsf.edu) also offers free teleconsultation to any

US provider through its PrEP line: (855) 448-7737 or (855) HIV-PrEP.

OPEP AND NPEP

Ethical considerations prohibit the evaluation of either oPEP or nPEP using randomized controlled trials. Data to support its use largely derive from animal models, inference from postnatal prophylaxis studies, observational studies, and one retrospective case-control study that showed an 81% reduction in the risk of HIV acquisition among healthcare workers who took zidovudine after exposure (Cardo et al., 1997; Lunding et al., 2016; Otten et al., 2000; Shih et al., 1991; Young et al., 2007).

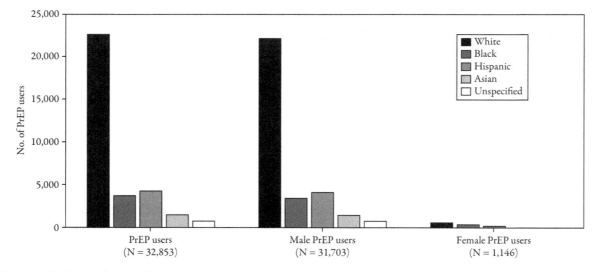

Figure 5.3 Number of PrEP users by sex and race/ethnicity, IQVIA Longitudinal Prescription Database, 2016*
*Among 32,853 (42%) persons with race/ethnicity data available, among 78,360 PrEP users identified in 2016; information on sex was missing/unknown for 4 of these 32,853 persons.
SOURCE: Huang YA, et al. MMWR. *Morb Mort Wkly Rep.* 2018;671147–1150. DOI hhtp//dx.doi.org/10.15585/mmwr.mm6741a3

oPEP

The use of ART to prevent acquisition of HIV among healthcare personnel who experience a high-risk occupational exposure was first recommended in 1990, and the US Public Health Service released its most recent oPEP guidelines in 2013 (Kuhar et al., 2013).

Risk of HIV acquisition after exposure in the healthcare setting appears to be directly related to the size of the viral inoculum, which is in turn influenced by the stage of disease of the source individual, as well as by the quantity of blood to which the worker was exposed (Kuhar et al., 2013).

Current guidelines emphasize the following:

- The HIV status of the source individual should be determined whenever possible to guide the need for initiating and/or maintaining oPEP.

- When indicated, oPEP should be started as soon as possible, preferably within 72 hours from the time of exposure.

- All oPEP regimens should include three antiretroviral medications and should generally be taken for 4 weeks (Table 5.4). The USPHS guidelines-preferred regimen is TDF plus FTC plus either raltegravir (RAL) or dolutegravir (DTG). Although USPHS PEP guidelines still include cautionary language on DTG use in pregnancy based on a 2018 safety alert regarding possible association between early pregnancy DTG exposure and neural tube defects (Zash et al., 2018), current US Department of Health and Human Services ART treatment guidelines recommend DTG as a preferred antiretroviral agent throughout pregnancy (in women with HIV), and providers should utilize an individualized approach weighing potential risks and benefits among individuals in the first trimester or trying to conceive.

- Expert consultation, with either local experts or through the national HIV Post-Exposure Prophylaxis Hotline, is recommended in certain situations (Table 5.5).

- Close follow-up services including counseling, repeat HIV testing, and drug toxicity monitoring should be provided. HIV follow-up testing should be done at 4 to 6 weeks and 3 to 4 months (if using a combination HIV antigen/antibody test) or at 6 weeks, 3 months, and 6 months if using an HIV antibody-only test (Table 5.6).

Importantly, healthcare workers who experience an occupational exposure should also be screened for HBV and hepatitis C virus (HCV). All hepatitis B–susceptible individuals should initiate the hepatitis B vaccine series, and those exposed to someone with known acute or active HBV should receive hepatitis B immune globulin as well. Currently, PEP for HCV is not recommended for occupational exposures (Moorman et al., 2020).

nPEP

The CDC's most recent nPEP guidelines were published in 2016 (Dominguez et al., 2016). In 2020, the New York State Department of Health AIDS Institute also released comprehensive, updated guidelines on the use of antiretroviral medications following nonoccupational and occupational exposures, including those involving sexual assault (New York State Department of Health, 2020b). Key points from these guidelines include the following:

Table 5.4 RECOMMENDED PEP REGIMENS: TO BE TAKEN FOR 4 WEEKS

Preferred regimen	Nucleotide reverse transcriptase inhibitor (NRTI) "backbone"	"Anchor" antiretroviral
	Emtricitabine 200 mg/Tenofovir disoproxil one tablet PO daily	Raltegravir (Isentress; RAL) 400 mg twice daily or RAL HD 1,200 mg QD, *or* dolutegravir (Tivicay; DTG) 50 mg once daily*
Alternatives	One of the following:	With one of the following:
	Tenofovir DF (Viread: TDF) \± emtricitabine (Emtriva: FTC) available as Truvada *or* Tenofovir DF (Viread: TDF)± lamivudine (Epivir; 3TC) available as Cimduo	Darunavir (Prezista; DRV) 800 mg daily + ritonavir (Norvir; RTV) 100 mg daily *or* Atazanavir (Reyataz; ATV) 300 mg daily + ritonavir (Norvir; RTV) 100 mg daily *or* Fosamprenavir (FPV; Lexiva) 1,400 mg daily + ritonavir (Norvir; RTV) 100 mg daily
	Or fixed-dose combination Stribild (EVG/COBI/FTC/TDF) once daily (elvitegravir 150 mg/cobicistat 150 mg/emtricitabine 200 mg/tenofovir disoproxil fumarate 300 mg)	

* Based on newer data and US Department of Health and Human Services recommendations, joint decision-making should be used when considering DTG for individuals who are in early pregnancy or may become pregnant.

Adapted from Kuhar (2013) and New York State Department of Health (2020b).

Table 5.5 SITUATIONS IN WHICH EXPERT CONSULTATION FOR OPEP IS RECOMMENDED

SCENARIO	COMMENTS
Delayed (i.e., later than 72 hours) exposure report	If timing of the last exposure representing significant risk falls outside of the 72-hour window or is uncertain, and HIV cannot be confidently ruled out with immediate testing
Unknown source (e.g., needle in sharps disposal container or laundry)	Use of PEP to be decided on a case-by-case basis. Consider severity of exposure and epidemiologic likelihood of HIV exposure. Do not test needles or other sharp instruments for HIV.
Known or suspected pregnancy in the exposed person	Provision of PEP should not be delayed while awaiting consultation.
Breastfeeding in the exposed person	Provision of PEP should not be delayed while awaiting consultation. It is recommended to discontinue breastfeeding for 3 months after exposure until exposed individual is confirmed to be HIV-negative
Known or suspected resistance of the source virus to antiretroviral agents	If source person's virus is known or suspected to be resistant to one or more of the drugs considered for PEP, recommend selection of drugs to which the source person's virus is unlikely to be resistant. Do not delay initiation of PEP while awaiting resistance testing results of the source person's virus.
Toxicity of the initial PEP regimen	Symptoms, if they occur, are often manageable without changing PEP regimen (e.g., antiemetic agents can be used if the exposed person develops nausea attributable to PEP medications). Counseling and support for management of side effects is important.
Serious medical illness in the exposed person	Significant underlying illness (e.g., kidney disease), or an exposed person already taking multiple medications, may increase risk of drug toxicity and drug–drug interactions.

Expert consultation can be sought with local experts or the National Clinician Consultation Center's Post Exposure Prophylaxis Hotline (PEPline) at 1-888-448-4911.

Adapted from Kuhar (2013).

- For sexual assault victims, important considerations before initiating PEP include whether or not a significant exposure occurred during the assault; whether the individual desires PEP; and knowledge of the alleged assailant's HIV status, although a lack thereof should not delay PEP initiation when warranted.

- Exposure types warranting PEP include direct contact of the vagina, penis, anus, or mouth with semen, vaginal fluids, or blood of the alleged assailant, with or without physical injury, tissue damage, or the presence of blood at the site of the assault; when broken skin or mucous membranes of the victim have been in contact with blood, semen, or vaginal fluids from the alleged assailant; and in cases of bites involving visible blood.

- Baseline HIV testing should be performed for the victim, as should a pregnancy test if indicated.

- When indicated, PEP should be initiated as soon as possible, and within 72 hours after the exposure. PEP is not recommended if it has been more than 72 hours since the exposure.

- Prophylactic treatment for gonorrhea, chlamydia, and trichomoniasis should also be offered, as should emergency contraception for individuals of childbearing capacity.

- For people with other potential nonoccupational exposures to HIV, determination of the level of risk from the exposure is critical; nPEP is generally indicated only for higher-risk exposures (Table 5.7). Other key points include the following:
  - HIV testing of the source individual should be performed when possible.
  - All exposed individuals should have the following performed at baseline: HIV testing, site-specific testing for gonorrhea and chlamydia, testing for syphilis, and pregnancy testing if indicated.
  - When indicated, PEP should be initiated as soon as possible, and within 72 hours after the exposure.
  - Person-centered risk reduction counseling should also be provided, including referrals for mental health and/or substance use care when indicated, as well as discussions of future PrEP use for individuals with anticipated ongoing risk.

- Recommended nPEP regimens include TDF plus FTC plus either RAL or DTG. See the earlier section regarding DTG use in pregnancy; guidelines currently recommend that clinicians engage in shared decision-making regarding ART selection for individuals in the first trimester or trying to conceive.

- For people who are breastfeeding at the time of potential exposure, person-centered counseling and a shared decision-making approach should be utilized, including considerations of the potential risks and benefits of continued breastfeeding (with or without PEP use) and for surveillance/follow-up testing. Current guidelines recommend

Table 5.6 RECOMMENDED MONITORING OF ADULTS AFTER EXPOSURE TO KNOWN OR SUSPECTED SOURCE WHO IS A PWH

TIME FROM EXPOSURE	RECOMMENDED SERVICES	
	COUNSELING	TESTING
Baseline	Transmission prevention (condom use; avoidance of blood/tissue donation; avoid breastfeeding if possible) Possible drug toxicities Possible drug interactions Importance of adherence	HIV antibody testing (preferably combined antigen/antibody test), even if exposed individual declines PEP Hepatitis B surface antigen (HBsAg) and surface Ab (HBsAb) Hepatitis C antibody (HCV Ab) If sexual exposure: pregnancy test, syphilis, and site-specific testing for gonorrhea and chlamydia If prescribing PEP: pregnancy test, complete blood count, liver function tests, renal function tests
48 hours (may be conducted by telephone)	Even if not taking PEP—to review additional information about exposure or the source individual if available If on PEP: Transmission prevention (condom use; avoidance of blood/tissue donation; avoid breastfeeding if possible) Possible drug toxicities Possible drug interactions Importance of adherence	
2 weeks (may be conducted by telephone)	Transmission prevention Possible drug toxicities Possible drug interactions Importance of adherence	If baseline testing abnormal or adverse effects are reported: complete blood count, liver function tests, renal function tests If sexual exposure: consider repeat STI screening
4–6 weeks	Transmission prevention	HIV Ag/Ab test, even if exposed individual declines PEP If childbearing capacity, pregnancy test If baseline testing abnormal or adverse effects are reported: complete blood count, liver function tests, renal function tests
If 4th-generation (combined antigen/antibody) HIV testing is used		
3–4 months		HIV antigen/antibody testing (if negative, HIV infection is excluded) HBsAg (unless baseline HBsAb positive/immune) HCV Ab
If 4th-generation HIV testing is not used (i.e., HIV antibody-only assay)		
12 weeks	Transmission prevention	HIV antibody testing
6 months		HIV antibody testing (if negative, HIV infection is excluded)

Adapted from Kuhar (2013), New York Department of Health (2020b).

that breastfeeding individuals with potential HIV exposure should be instructed to avoid breastfeeding for 3 months after exposure and until confirmed to be HIV-negative.

As with people who experience occupational exposures, those with nonoccupational exposures should be screened for HBV and HCV and be given appropriate treatment and follow-up as described previously.

SCREENING AND TREATMENT FOR STIS

The link between STIs and increased risk for HIV transmission/acquisition is established. This is supported by both biologic plausibility (e.g., genital tract inflammation leading to increased viral shedding in persons with HIV and increased access of HIV to subepithelial target cells) and epidemiologic synergy (Mayer & Venkatesh, 2011; Ward & Rönn, 2010). However, multiple confounders have made it difficult to estimate how much these factors contribute to increased risk, and STI treatment studies to date have failed to consistently demonstrate a reduction in HIV transmission (Mayer & Venkatesh, 2011; Ward & Rönn, 2010). The Mwanza study from Tanzania stands out as one notable exception: it demonstrated a 38% reduction in HIV incidence with syndromic STI management (Grosskurth et al., 1995). Nonetheless, the strong link argues for the importance of regular STI screening and treatment in those at risk because people who screen positive are likely to benefit from PrEP and risk reduction counseling in general. This point is highlighted by a New York City analysis demonstrating that 1 in 20 MSM with a

Table 5.7 LEVEL OF RISK BASED ON EXPOSURE TYPE FOR CONSIDERATION OF PEP

Higher-risk exposures—PEP should be recommended	• Receptive and insertive vaginal or anal intercourse with a partner living with HIV, or when the partner's HIV status is unknown • Needle sharing with a partner who is a PWH, or when the partner's HIV status is unknown • Injuries with exposure to blood or other potentially infectious fluids from a source known to be a PWH or with unknown HIV status (including needlesticks with a hollow-bore needle, human bites, and accidents)
Lower-risk exposures—require case-by-case evaluation for PEP	• Oral–vaginal contact (receptive and insertive) • Oral–anal contact (receptive and insertive) • Receptive penile–oral contact with or without ejaculation • Insertive penile–oral contact with or without ejaculation • Factors that increase risk (PEP should be offered) • Source is known to be a PWH with elevated viral load • Nonintact oral mucosa (e.g., oral lesions, gingivitis, wounds) • Blood exposure • Presence of genital ulcer disease or other sexually transmitted infections
Exposures that do *not* warrant PEP	• Kissing • Oral-to-oral contact without mucosal damage (mouth-to-mouth resuscitation) • Human bites not involving blood • Exposure to solid-bore needles or sharps not in recent contact with blood (e.g., tattoo needles, lancets) • Mutual masturbation without skin breakdown or blood exposure • Exposure to saliva not involving visible blood

Adapted from New York State Department of Health AIDS Institute (2020b).

new syphilis diagnosis were diagnosed with HIV within 1 year (Prathela et al., 2015) and Australian data showing that MSM diagnosed with rectal gonorrhea or chlamydia were two to three times more likely to be diagnosed with incident HIV in the following 12 months compared to those who were not (Cheung et al., 2016).

VOLUNTARY MEDICAL MALE CIRCUMCISION

Three large randomized trials performed in sub-Saharan Africa demonstrated that voluntary circumcision of HIV-negative men led to an approximate risk reduction for heterosexual HIV acquisition of 50% (Auvert et al., 2005; Bailey et al., 2007; Gray et al., 2007; Siegfried et al., 2009). However, this prevention benefit did not appear to extend to female partners of circumcised men with HIV (Weiss et al., 2009). Although observational data suggest that circumcision may be beneficial for MSM who practice primary insertive anal intercourse, there is currently insufficient evidence to determine whether this is the case in general for MSM (Wiysonge et al., 2011).

NEW AND INVESTIGATIONAL INTERVENTIONS FOR HIV TRANSMISSION PREVENTION

NOVEL ANTIRETROVIRALS AND DELIVERY METHODS FOR PREP

Investigation of alternative delivery methods and novel antiretrovirals for PrEP promises to further expand HIV prevention options for at-risk individuals.

Cabotegravir (CAB), a novel integrase strand transfer inhibitor, has been found to be both safe and well tolerated when delivered as an intramuscular injection every 8 weeks (Landovitz et al., 2017; Markowitz et al., 2017a). An interim analysis of HPTN083, an international, randomized, double-blind phase IIb/III trial, showed superiority of long-acting injectable CAB compared to daily oral FTC/TDF in reducing incident HIV among MSM and transgender women at high risk of HIV acquisition (Landovitz et al., 2020). While both study regimens were efficacious, injectable CAB was 66% more effective in preventing HIV acquisition. More information regarding long-acting injectable CAB will be forthcoming from this trial, as well as from HTPN084, which is evaluating long-acting injectable CAB as PrEP for cisgender women (compared to FTC/TDF) (HPTN 084, ClinicalTrials.gov.NCT03164564).

A novel antiviral, islatravir (MK-8591, a nucleoside reverse transcriptase translocation inhibitor), shows promise as a long-acting formulation with a novel mechanism of action. Islatravir was evaluated in a phase 1 trial as an implantable form of PrEP showing drug release sufficient for HIV prophylaxis for at least 1 year (Matthews et al., 2019) and will also be evaluated as a once-monthly oral form of PrEP in a phase II study (MK-8591-016, clinicaltrials.gov.NCT04003103).

MICROBICIDES

Microbicides are products applied locally to the vaginal or rectal mucosa to reduce risk of HIV and other STI acquisition. The use of microbicides or other local drug delivery devices such as vaginal rings have several potential benefits. First, they deliver high concentrations of drug to the desired tissue with minimal systemic exposure (Hendrix et al., 2013) and can thus potentially provide on-demand protection. Many products are also targeted toward women, a group disproportionately excluded from many ART and PrEP trials but who make up almost half of new HIV transmissions globally (WHO, 2016). These options may be used discreetly, represent an additional prevention option and have the potential to be coformulated with other medications such as contraceptives.

The first microbicide to receive regulatory approval for use is the dapivirine-eluting vaginal ring, approved by the EMA in 2020 based on data from the MTN-020/ASPIRE trial. This study demonstrated a 37% reduction in HIV incidence among participants who received the study ring as compared to placebo, after excluding data from two study sites with reduced rates of adherence and retention (Baeten et al., 2016). An interim analysis of its open-label extension trial provided more encouraging results: 92% of women enrolled accepted the ring, most (89%) rings were used, and HIV incidence was less than half that expected based on the infection distribution of the enrolled population (Baeten et al., 2018).

Another microbicide under investigation is TDF gel. Results of its efficacy in cisgender women have been mixed, with the greatest protection again seen in women who were most adherent (Abdool Karim et al., 2010; Dai et al., 2016; Marrazzo et al., 2015; Rees et al., 2015). Use of rectal TDF gel in MSM and transwomen is under investigation, and it has been shown to be safe and acceptable in early stage clinical trials (Cranston et al., 2017). A medicated TDF-based rectal enema (DREAM-01 trial, clinicaltrials.gov.NCT02750540) and combination topical tenofovir alafenamide/elvitegravir (TAF/EVG), as an on-demand vaginal insert (CONRAD 146 trial, clinicaltrials.gov.NCT03762772) or rectal insert (MTN-039 trial, clinicialtrials.gov.NCT04047420), are also under investigation.

VACCINES AND BROADLY NEUTRALIZING ANTIBODIES

Multiple challenges, both biomedical and social, have impeded development of an effective HIV vaccine. These include HIV diversity and pathogenesis, identification of appropriate immune correlates of protection, community preparedness and concerns about vaccine-induced positivity, and, more recently, expanded PrEP use (Hammer, 2015). With the exception of a modestly positive Thai vaccine trial, which demonstrated a 31% reduction in incident HIV among vaccine recipients, clinical trials of HIV preventive vaccines have had generally disappointing results (Table 5.8).

However, the pursuit of an effective vaccine remains important. Even with the promise of widespread ART to "end the epidemic" (as both TasP and PrEP), an effective vaccine is essential for timely, sustainable control to occur, given complexities of human behaviors and long-term funding challenges for treatment-based interventions (Fauci & Marston,

Table 5.8 SUMMARY OF HIV VACCINE EFFICACY TRIALS

TRIAL	VACCINE PRODUCT	STUDY POPULATION; SITE	RESULTS	REFERENCE
Vax 003	Recombinant gp120 (B/E)	Male and female PWID; Thailand	No efficacy	Pitisuttithum et al., 2006
Vax 004	Recombinant gp120 (B/B)	Heterosexual women and MSM; US and the Netherlands	No efficacy	Flynn et al., 2005
HVTN 502	Recombinant Ad5 (Clade B gag/pol/nef)	MSM, heterosexual women and men; North and South America, Caribbean, Australia	No efficacy	Buchbinder et al., 2008
HVTN 503	Recombinant Ad5 (Clade B gag/pol/nef)	Heterosexual women and men; South Africa	No efficacy	Gray et al., 2011
HVTN 505	6-plasmid DNA vaccine and rAd5 vector boost	MSM; US	No efficacy	Hammer et al., 2013
RV 144	ALVAC: Canarypox (gag, pol, env) \± AIDSVAX B/E recombinant gp120	Heterosexual women and men; Thailand	31% reduction in acquisition	Rerks-Ngarm et al., 2009
HVTN 702	ALVAC: Canarypox (gag, pol, env) \± AIDSVAX C recombinant gp120	Adult women and men; South Africa	No efficacy	https://www.niaid.nih.gov/news-events/experimental-hiv-vaccine-regimen-ineffective-preventing-hiv
HVTN 705	Engineered mosaic Ad26.Mos4.HIV \± clade C and mosaic gp140	Heterosexual women; sub-Saharan Africa	Ongoing	https://clinicaltrials.gov/ct2/show/NCT03060629
HVTN 706	Engineered mosaic Ad26.Mos4.HIV\ ± clade C and mosaic gp140	Cisgender MSM and transgender women; US, South America, Europe	Ongoing	https://clinicaltrials.gov/ct2/show/NCT03964415

Adapted from Rubens, 2015.

2014). The ability of a vaccine to elicit broadly neutralizing antibodies (bNAbs, antibodies that can protect against multiple pathogenic HIV strains by binding to highly conserved regions of the virus) is crucial for its success but thus far has been elusive. Use of bioinformatically developed mosaic antigens to elicit broadly protective antibody responses is a novel approach under investigation in the HIV-V-A004 trial; phase I/IIa results showed that this product produces robust immune responses in both humans and rhesus monkeys (Barouch et al., 2018; see http://www.avac.org/trial/hiv-v-a004ipcavd-009-approach).

Recent advances in the identification and understanding of bNAbs have injected new hope into HIV prevention research. One such antibody product, VRC01, targets the HIV-1 CD4 binding site and is currently under investigation in the AMP study, a collaborative HVTN 704/HPTN 085 investigation (http://ampstudy.org). 3BNC117 is another bNAb that has shown promise for further development, and in combination with 10-1074 it has been shown to be safe and well tolerated (Caskey et al., 2015; Cohen et al., 2019). These preliminary data provide optimism that BNAbs can be used as an additional PrEP strategy while awaiting development of a highly effective vaccine.

RECOMMENDED READING

Fauci AS, Marston HD. Ending AIDS: is an HIV vaccine necessary? *N Engl J Med.* 2014;370(6):495–498.

Kanny D, Jeffries WL 4th, Chapin-Bardales J, et al. Racial/ethnic disparities in HIV preexposure prophylaxis among men who have sex with men—23 urban areas, 2017. *MMWR Morb Mortal Wkly Rep.* 2019;68(37):801–806. doi:10.15585/mmwr.mm6837a2

CONCLUSION

Tremendous strides continue to be made in the vast field of HIV prevention. Although much attention has focused on ART-based interventions such as TasP and PrEP, real-world application of research findings generates important questions for clinical care delivery across varied resource landscapes, some of which remain unanswered. Ongoing disparities in access, acceptability, and consistent use of these interventions threaten to exacerbate existing disparities in HIV incidence. HIV providers can be important leaders in addressing internal biases and structural factors driving such inequities. Ultimately, a multifaceted approach including behavioral, structural, and established biomedical interventions is needed to make a significant and lasting impact on HIV globally.

REFERENCES

Abdool Karim Q, Abdool Karim SS, Frohlich JA, et al. Effectiveness and safety of tenofovir gel, an antiretroviral microbicide, for the prevention of HIV infection in women. *Science.* 2010;329(5996):1168–1174.

Aberg JA, Gallant JE, Ghanem KG, et al. Primary care guidelines for the management of persons infected with HIV: 2013 update by the HIV Medicine Association of the Infectious Diseases Society of America. *Clin Infect Dis.* 2014;58(1):e1–e34.

Adams JM. Making the case for syringe services programs. *Public Health Rep.* 2020;135(Supp 1):10S–12S.

Adekeye OA, Heiman HJ, Onyeabor OS, Hyacinth HI. The new invincibles: HIV screening among older adults in the US. *PLoS One.* 2012;7(8):e43618.

Adimora AA, Hughes JP, Wang J, et al. Characteristics of multiple and concurrent partnerships among women at high risk for HIV infection. *J AIDS.* 2014;65(1):99–106.

Aidala AA, Wilson MG, Shubert V, et al. Housing status, medical care, and health outcomes among people living with HIV/AIDS: a systematic review. *Am J Public Health.* 2015;106:e1–e23.

Anema A, Marshall BD, Stevenson B, et al. Intergenerational sex as a risk factor for HIV among young men who have sex with men: a scoping review. *Curr HIV/AIDS Rep.* 2013;10(4):398–407.

Antiretroviral Pregnancy Registry. International Interim Report for 1 January 1989–31 January 2020. http://www.apregistry.com/forms/exec-summary.pdf

Antoni G, Tremblay C, Charreau I, et al. On-demand PrEP with TDF/FTC remains highly effective among MSM with infrequent sexual intercourse: a sub-study of the ANRS IPERGAY trial. In: *Program and Abstracts of the 9th International AIDS Society Conference on HIV Science*, July 23–26, 2017, Paris, France. Abstract TUAC102.

Aspinall EJ, Nambiar D, Goldberg DJ, et al. Are needle and syringe programs associated with a reduction in HIV transmission among people who inject drugs: a systematic review and meta-analysis. *Int J Epidemiol.* 2014;43(1):235–248.

Auvert B, Taljaard D, Lagarde E, et al. Randomized, controlled intervention trial of male circumcision for reduction of HIV infection risk: the ANRS 1265 trial. *PLoS Med.* 2005;2(11):e298.

Baeten JM, Donnell D, Ndase P, et al. Antiretroviral prophylaxis for HIV prevention in heterosexual men and women. *N Engl J Med.* 2012;367:399–410.

Baeten JM, Palanee-Phillips T, Brown ER, et al. Use of a vaginal ring containing dapivirine for HIV-1 prevention in women. *N Engl J Med.* 2016;375(22):2121–2132.

Baeten J, Palanee-Phillips T, Mgodi N, et al. High uptake and reduced HIV-1 incidence in an open-label trial of the dapivirine ring. In: *Program and Abstracts of the 2018 Conference on Retroviruses and Opportunistic Infections*, March 4–7, 2018, Boston, MA. Abstract 143LB.

Baggaley R, Boily M-C, White RG, et al. Risk of HIV-1 transmission for parenteral exposure and blood transfusion: a systematic review and meta-analysis. *AIDS.* 2006;20(6):805–812.

Bailey RC, Moses S, Parker CB, et al. Male circumcision for HIV prevention in young men in Kisumu, Kenya: a randomised controlled trial. *Lancet.* 2007;369:643.

Baral SD, Poteat T, Stromdahl S, et al. Worldwide burden of HIV in transgender women: a systematic review and meta-analyses. *Lancet Infect Dis.* 2013;13(3):214–222.

Barouch DH, Thomka FL, Wegmann F et al. Evaluation of a mosaic HIV-1 vaccine in a multicentre, randomised, double-blind, placebo-controlled, phase 1/2a clinical trial (APPROACH) and in rhesus monkeys (NHP 13-19). *Lancet.* 2018;392(10143):232–243. doi:10.1016/S0140-6736(18)31364-3

Barre-Sinoussi F, Abdool Karim S, Albert J, et al. Expert consensus statement on the science of HIV in the context of criminal law. *J Int AIDS Soc.* 2018;27(7):e25161.

Bazzi AR, Biancarelli DL, Childs E, et al. Limited knowledge and mixed interest in pre-exposure prophylaxis for HIV prevention among people who inject drugs. *AIDS Patient Care STDs.* 2018;32(12):529–537.

Belenko S, Visher C, Pearson F, et al. Efficacy of structured organizational change intervention on HIV testing in correctional facilities. *AIDS Educ Prev.* 2017;29(3):241–255.

Berry MS, Johnson MW. Does being drunk or high cause HIV sexual risk behavior? A systematic review of drug administration studies. *Pharmacol Biochem Behav.* 2018;164:125–138.

Biello KM, Bazzi AT, Mimiaga MJ, et al. Perspectives on HIV pre-exposure prophylaxis (PrEP) utilization and related intervention needs among people who inject drugs. *Harm Reduction Journal.* 2018;15(1):55.

Buchbinder SP, Cohen SE, Hecht J. Getting to zero new diagnoses in San Francisco: what will it take? In: *Program and Abstracts of the 2018 Conference on Retroviruses and Opportunistic Infections,* March 4–7, 2018, Boston, MA. Abstract 87.

Buchbinder SP, Liu AY. Virtual CROI 2020: Highlights of epidemiology, public health, and prevention research. IAS-USA. *Top Antivir Med.* 2020;28(2):439–454. https://www.iasusa.org/wp-content/uploads/2020/06/june-july2020.pdf

Buchbinder SP, Mehrotra DV, Duerr A, et al. Efficacy assessment of a cell-mediated immunity HIV-1 vaccine (the Step Study): a double-blind, randomised, placebo-controlled, test-of-concept trial. *Lancet.* 2008;372(9653):1881–1893.

Busch MP, Bloch EM, Kleinman S. Prevention of transfusion-transmitted infections. *Blood.* 2019;133(17):1854–1864.

Caceres CF, Gerbase A, Lo YR, et al. *Prevention and Treatment of HIV and Other Sexually Transmitted Infections Among Men Who Have Sex with Men and Transgender People: Recommendations for a Public Health Approach.* Geneva: World Health Organization Document Production Services, 2011.

Cardo DM, Culver DH, Ciesielski CA, et al.; Centers for Disease Control and Prevention Needlestick Surveillance Group. A case control study of HIV seroconversion in health care workers after percutaneous exposure. *N Engl J Med.* 1997;337(21):1485–1490.

Caskey M, Klein F, Lorenzi JC, et al. Viraemia suppressed in HIV-1-infected humans by broadly neutralizing antibody 3BNC117. *Nature.* 2015;522(7557):487–491. doi:10.1038/nature14411

Centers for Disease Control and Prevention. HIV surveillance report. 2020a. https://www.cdc.gov/hiv/statistics/overview/index.html

Centers for Disease Control and Prevention. HIV self-testing (home testing). 2021. cdc.gov/hiv/basics/hiv-testing/hiv-self-tests.html

Centers for Disease Control and Prevention. Behavioral and clinical characteristics of persons with diagnosed HIV infection—Medical Monitoring Project, United States, 2018 cycle (June 2018–May 2019). HIV Surveillance Special Report 25. Published May 2020b. https://www.cdc.gov/hiv/library/reports/hiv-surveillance.html

Centers for Disease Control and Prevention. HIV infection risk, prevention, and testing behaviors among persons who inject drugs—National HIV Behavioral Surveillance: Injection drug use, 23 U.S. cities, 2018. HIV Surveillance Special Report 24. Published February 2020b. https://www.cdc.gov/hiv/pdf/library/reports/surveillance/cdc-hiv-surveillance-special-report-number-24.pdf

Centers for Disease Control and Prevention/US Public Health Service. Preexposure prophylaxis for the prevention of HIV infection in the United States—2017 update: a clinical practice guideline. Published March 2018. https://www.cdc.gov/hiv/pdf/risk/prep/cdc-hiv-prep-guidelines-2017.pdf

Cheung KT, Fairley CK, Read TRH, et al. HIV Incidence and predictors of incident HIV among men who have sex with men attending a sexual health clinic in Melbourne, Australia. *PLoS One.* 2016;11(5):e0156160. doi:10.1371/journal.pone.0156160

Choopanya K, Martin M, Suntharasamai P, et al. Antiretroviral prophylaxis for HIV infection in injecting drug users in Bangkok, Thailand (the Bangkok Tenofovir Study): a randomised, double-blind, placebo-controlled phase 3 trial. *Lancet.* 2013;381:2083–2090.

Clinicaltrials.gov.NCT02750540.

Clinicaltrials.gov.NCT03762772.

Clinicaltrials.gov.NCT04003103.

Clinicaltrials.gov.NCT04047420.

Cohen MS, Chen Y, McCauley M, et al. Final results of the HPTN 052 randomized controlled trial: antiretroviral therapy prevents HIV transmission. In: *Program and Abstracts of the 8th IAS Conference on HIV Pathogenesis, Treatment & Prevention,* July 19–22, 2015, Vancouver, Canada. Abstract MOAC0101LB.

Cohen SE, Sachdev D, Lee SA, et al. Acquisition of tenofovir-susceptible, emtricitabine-resistant HIV despite high adherence to daily preexposure prophylaxis: a case report. *Lancet HIV.* 2018;S2352-3018(18)30288-1. doi:10.1016/S2352-3018(18)30288-1

Cohen YZ, Butler AL, Millard K, et al. Safety, pharmacokinetics, and immunogenicity of the combination of the broadly neutralizing anti-HIV-1 antibodies 3BNC117 and 10-1074 in healthy adults: a randomized, phase 1 study. *PLoS One.* 2019;14(8):e0219142. doi:10.1371/journal.pone.0219142

Cohn A, Stanton C, Elmasry H, et al. Characteristics of US substance abuse treatment facilities offering HIV services: results from a national survey. *Psychiatr Serv.* 2016;67(6): 692–695.

Colby DJ, Kroon E, Sacdalan C, et al. Acquisition of multidrug-resistant human immunodeficiency virus type 1 infection in a patient taking preexposure prophylaxis. *Clin Infect Dis.* 2018;67(6):962–964. doi:10.1093/cid/ciy321

Cranston RD, Lama JR, Richardson BA, et al. MTN-017: a rectal phase 2 extended safety and acceptability study of tenofovir reduced-glycerin 1% gel. *Clin Infect Dis.* 2017;64(5):614–620. doi:10.1093/cid/ciw832

Cruess DG, Burnham KE, Finitsis DJ, et al. A randomized clinical trial of a brief internet-based group intervention to reduce sexual transmission risk behavior among HIV-positive gay and bisexual men. *Ann Behav Med.* 2018;52(2): 116–129.

Csete J, Kamarulzaman A, Kazatchkine M, et al. Public health and international drug policy: report of the Johns Hopkins-Lancet Commission on Drug Policy and Health. *Lancet.* 2016;387(10026):1427–1480.

Custer B, Quiner CA, Haaland R, et al. HIV antiretroviral therapy and prevention use in US blood donors: a new blood safety concern. *Blood.* 2020;136(11):1351–1358. doi:10.1182/blood.2020006890

Dai JY, Hendrix CW, Richardson BA, et al. Pharmacological measures of treatment adherence and risk of HIV infection in the VOICE study. *J Infect Dis.* 2016;213(3):335–342. doi:10.1093/infdis/jiv333

DeBeck K, Cheng T, Montaner JS, et al. HIV and the criminalization of drug use among people who inject drugs: a systematic review. *Lancet HIV.* 2017;4(8):e357–e374.

Del Rio C. How do we stop the band from playing on in the US? In: Conference on Retroviruses and Opportunistic Infections, March 8–11, 2020, Boston, MA. Abstract 61.

Dimitrov D, Moore JR, Wood D, et al. Predicted effectiveness of daily and nondaily preexposure prophylaxis for men who have sex with men based on sex and pill-taking patterns from the Human Immuno Virus Prevention Trials Network 067/ADAPT Study. *Clin Infect Dis.* 2020;71(2):249–255. doi:10.1093/cid/ciz799

Dominguez K, Smith DK, Vasavi T, et al. Updated guidelines for antiretroviral postexposure prophylaxis after sexual, injection drug use, or other non-occupational exposure to HIV—United States, 2016. US Centers for Disease Control and Prevention. Published 2016. http://stacks.cdc.gov/view/cdc/38856

Dong BJ, William MR, Bingham JT, et al. Outcomes of challenging HIV case consultations provided via teleconference by the Clinician Consultation Center to the Federal Bureau of Prisons. *J Am Pharm Assoc.* 2017;57(4):516–519.

Donnell D, Ramos E, Celum C, et al. The effect of oral preexposure prophylaxis on the progression of HIV-1 seroconversion. *AIDS.* 2017;31(14): 2007–2016.

Eastment MC, McClelland RS. Vaginal microbiota and susceptibility to HIV. *AIDS.* 2018;32(6):687–698.

Fauci AS, Marston HD. Ending AIDS: is an HIV vaccine necessary? *N Engl J Med.* 2014;370(6):495–498.

Fernandez-Vina MH, Prood NE, Herpolsheimer JD, et al. State laws governing syringe services programs and participant syringe possession, 2014–2019. *Public Health Rep.* 2020;135(Suppl):128S–137S.

Flynn NM, Forthal DN, Harro CD, et al. Placebo-controlled phase 3 trial of a recombinant glycoprotein 120 vaccine to prevent HIV-1 infection. *J Infect Dis.* 2005;191(5):654–665.

Franconi I, Guaraldi G. Pre-exposure prophylaxis for HIV infection in the older patient: what can be recommended? *Drugs Aging.* 2018;35(6):485–491.

Gai Y, Marthinsen J. Medicaid expansion, HIV testing, and HIV-related risk behaviors in the US, 2010–2017. *Am J Public Health.* 2019; 109(10): 1404–1412.

Garcia J, Parker C, Parker RG, et al. "You're really gonna kick us all out?" Sustaining safe spaces for community-based HIV prevention and control among black men who have sex with men. *PLoS One.* 2015;10(10):e0141326.

Giannou FK, Tsiara CG, Nikolopoulos GK, et al. Condom effectiveness in reducing heterosexual HIV transmission: a systematic review and meta-analysis of studies on HIV serodiscordant couples. *Expert Rev Pharmacoecon Outcomes Res.* 2016;4:489–499.

Giler RM, Magnuson D, Trevor H, et al. Changes in Truvada (TVD) for HIV pre-exposure prophylaxis (PrEP) utilization in the United States. (2012–2016). Abstract WEPEC0919. IAS 2017, July 22–26, 2017. Paris, France.

Grant RM, Lama JR, Anderson PL, et al. Preexposure chemoprophylaxis for HIV prevention in men who have sex with men. *N Engl J Med.* 2010;363:2587–2599.

Gray RH, Kigozi G, Serwadda D, et al. Male circumcision for HIV prevention in men in Rakai, Uganda: a randomised trial. *Lancet.* 2007;369:657–666.

Grebe E, Busch MP, Notari EP, et al. HIV incidence in US first-time blood donors and transfusion risk with a 12-months deferral for men who have sex with men. *Blood.* 2020;136(11):1359–1367. doi:10.1182/blood.2020007003

Greene M, Justice AC, Covinsky KE. Assessment of geriatric syndromes and physical function in people living with HIV. *Virulence.* 2017;8(5):586–598.

Grosskurth H, Mosha F, Todd J, et al. Impact of improved treatment of sexually transmitted diseases on HIV infection in rural Tanzania: randomised controlled trial. *Lancet.* 1995;346:530–536.

Grulich A, Guy RJ, Amin J, et al. Rapid reduction in HIV diagnoses after targeted PrEP introduction in NSW, Australia. In: *Program and Abstracts of the 2018 Conference on Retroviruses and Opportunistic Infections,* March 4–7, 2018, Boston, MA. Abstract 88.

Haffajee RL, Bohnert ASB, Lagisetty PA. Policy pathways to address provider workforce barriers to buprenorphine treatment. *Am J Prev Med.* 2018;54(6S3):s230–s242.

Hammer SM. Advances in preventive HIV vaccines: efficacy trial evolution. In: *ID Week 2015,* October 7–11, 2015, San Diego, CA. Oral session 0021.

Hammer SM, Sobieszczyk ME, Janes H, et al. Efficacy trial of a DNA/rAd5 HIV-1 preventive vaccine. *N Engl J Med.* 2013;369:2083–2092.

Hartzler B, Dombrowski JC, Crane HM, et al. Prevalence and predictors of substance use disorders among HIV care enrollees in the United States. *AIDS Behav.* 2017;21(4): 1138–1148.

Heimer R, Abdala N. Viability of HIV-1 in syringes: implications for interventions among injection drug users. *AIDS Reader.* 2000;10(7).

Hendrix CW, Chen BA, Guddera V, et al. MTN-001: randomized pharmacokinetic cross-over study comparing tenofovir vaginal gel and oral tablets in vaginal tissue and other compartments. *PLoS One.* 2013;8(1): e55013. doi:10.1371/journal.pone.0055013

Hoenigl M, Chaillon A, Moore DJ, et al. Clear links between starting methamphetamine and increasing sexual risk behavior: a cohort study among men who have sex with men. *J AIDS.* 2016;71(5):551–557.

Hoornenborg E, de Bree GJ. Acute infection with a wild-type HIV-1 virus in PrEP user with high TDF Levels. In: *Program and Abstracts of the 2017 Conference on Retroviruses and Opportunistic Infections,* February 13–16, 2017, Seattle, WA. Abstract 953.

Hosek SG, Landovitz RJ, Kapogiannis B, et al. Safety and feasibility of antiretroviral preexposure prophylaxis for adolescent men who have sex with men aged 15 to 17 years in the United States. *JAMA Pediatr.* November 1, 2017;171(11):1063–1071. doi: 10.1001/jamapediatrics.2017.2007.

Hosek S, Rudy B, Landowitz R, et al. An HIV pre-exposure prophylaxis (PrEP) demonstration project and safety study for young men who

have sex with men in the United States (ATN 110). In: *Program and Abstracts of the 8th IAS Conference on HIV Pathogenesis, Treatment & Prevention,* July 19–22, 2015, Vancouver, Canada. Abstract TUAC0204LB.

Huang YA, Zhu W, Smith DK, et al. Preexposure prophylaxis by race and ethnicity—United States, 2014–2016. *MMWR Morb Mortal Wkly Rep.* 2018;67:1147–1150. doi:hhtp://dx.doi.org/10.15585/mmwr.mm6741a3

Ickowicz S, Hayashi K, Dong H, et al. Benzodiazepine use as an independent risk factor for HIV infection in a Canadian setting. *Drug Alcohol Depend.* 2015;155:190–194.

Iribarren S, Lentz C, Sheinfil AZ, et al. Using an HIV self-test kit to test a partner: attitudes and preferences among high-risk populations. *AIDS Behav.* 2020 May 8. Doi: 10.1007/s10461-020-02885-3. (Online ahead of print).

Iroh PA, Mayo H, Nijhawan AE. The HIV care cascade before, during, and after incarceration: a systematic review and data synthesis. *Am J Public Health.* 2015;105(7): e5–e16.

Kanny D, Jeffries WL IV, Chapin-Bardales J, et al. Racial/Ethnic Disparities in HIV Preexposure Proplyaxis Among Men Who Have Sex with Men—23 Urban Areas, 2017. *MMWR. Morb Mortal Wkly Rep* 2019;68:801–806. DOI: http://dx.doi.org/10.15585/mmwr.mm6837a2.

Kennedy MC, Karamouzian M, Kerr T. Public health and public order outcomes associated with supervised drug consumption facilities: a systematic review. *Curr HIV/AIDS Rep.* 2017;14(5):161–183.

Khan MR, McGinnis KA, Grov C, et al. Past year and prior incarceration and HIV transmission risk among HIV-positive men who have sex with men in the US. *AIDS Care.* 2019; 31(3): 349–356.

Knox DC, Anderson PL, Harrigan R, et al. Multidrug-resistant HIV-1 infection despite preexposure prophylaxis. *N Engl J Med.* 2017;376:501–502 doi:10.1056/NEJMc1611639

Kuhar DT, Henderson DK, Struble KA, et al. Updated USPHS guidelines for the management of occupational exposures to human immunodeficiency virus and recommendations for post-exposure prophylaxis. *Infect Control Hosp Epidemiol.* 2013;34(9):875–892.

Kuo I, Agopian A, Opoku J, et al. Assessing PrEP needs among heterosexuals and people who inject drugs, Washington, DC. In: *Program and Abstracts of the 2018 Conference on Retroviruses and Opportunistic Infections,* March 4–7, 2018, Boston, MA. Abstract 1030.

Landovitz RJ, Donnell D, Clement M, et al. HPTN083 interim results: pre-exposure prophylaxis (PrEP) containing long-acting injectable cabotegravir (CAB-LA) is safe and highly effective for cisgender men and transgender women who have sex with men (MSM, TGW). *23rd International HIV Conference* (AIDS 2020: Virtual). Abstract OAXLB0101.

Landovitz R, Li S, Grinsztejn B, et al. Safety, tolerability and pharmacokinetics of long-acting injectable cabotegravir in low-risk HIV-uninfected women and men: HPTN 077. In: *Program and Abstracts of the 9th International AIDS Society Conference on HIV Science,* July 23–26, 2017, Paris, France. Abstract TUAC0106LB.

Lee SS, Anderson PL, Kwan TH, et al. Failure of pre-exposure prophylaxis with daily tenofovir/emtricitabine and the scenario of delayed HIV seroconversion. *Int J Infect Dis.* 2020;94: 41–43.

Lerner AM, Eisinger RW, Fauci AS. Comorbidities in persons with HIV: the lingering challenge. *JAMA.* 2019 [Epub ahead of print]. doi:10.1001/jama.2019.19775

Low AJ, Mburu G, Welton NJ, et al. Impact of opioid substitution therapy on antiretroviral therapy outcomes: a systematic review and meta-analysis. *Clin Infect Dis.* 2016;63(8):1094–1104.

Lunding S, Katzenstein TL, Kronborg G, et al. The Danish PEP Registry: experience with the use of post-exposure prophylaxis following blood exposure to HIV from 1999–2012. *Infect Dis (Lond).* 2016;48(3):195–200.

MacArthur GJ, van Velzen E, Palmateer N, et al. Interventions to prevent HIV and hepatitis C in people who inject drugs: a review of reviews to assess evidence of effectiveness. *Int J Drug Policy.* 2014;25(1):34–52.

MacGowan RJ, Chavez PR, Borkowf CB, et al. Effect of internet-distributed HIV self-tests on HIV diagnosis and behavioral outcomes in men who have sex with men: a randomized clinical trial. *JAMA Int Med.* 2020;180(1):117–125.

Marcus JL, Katz KA, Krakower DS, Calabrese SK. Risk compensation and clinical decision making—the case of HIV preexposure prophylaxis. *N Engl J Med.* 2019;380(6):510–512. doi:10.1056/NEJMp1810743

Markowitz M, Frank I, Grant RM, et al. Safety and tolerability of long-acting cabotegravir injections in HIV-uninfected men (ECLAIR): a multicentre, double-blind, randomised, placebo-controlled, phase 2a trial. *Lancet HIV.* 2017a;4(8):e331–e340. doi:10.1016/S2352-3018(17)30068-1

Markowitz M, Grossman H, Anderson PL, et al. Newly acquired infection with multidrug-resistant HIV-1 in a patient adherent to preexposure prophylaxis. *J Acquir Immune Defic Syndr.* 2017b;76(4):e104–e106. doi:10.1097/QAI.0000000000001534

Marrazzo JM, Gita R, Richardson BA, et al. Tenofovir-based preexposure prophylaxis for HIV infection among African women. *N Engl J Med.* 2015;372:509–518.

Matthews RP, Barrett SE, Patel M, et al. First-in-human trial of MK-8591-eluting implants demonstrates concentrations suitable for HIV prophylaxis for at least one year. *10th IAS Conference on HIV Science* (IAS 2019), July 21–24, 2019, Mexico City. Abstract TUAC0401LB.

Mayer KH, Grasso C, Levine K, et al. Increasing PrEP uptake, persistent disparities in at-risk patients in a Boston Center. In: *Program and Abstracts of the 2018 Conference on Retroviruses and Opportunistic Infections,* March 4–7, 2018, Boston, MA. Abstract 1014.

Mayer KH, Molina JM, Thompson MA, et al. Emtricitabine and tenofovir alafenamide vs. emtricitabine and tenofovir disoproxil fumarate for HIV pre-exposure prophylaxis (DISCOVER): primary results from a randomised, double-blind, multicentre, active-controlled, phase 3, non-inferiority trial. *Lancet.* 2020;396(10246):239–254. doi:10.1016/S0140-6736(20)31065-5

Mayer KH, Venkatesh KK. Interactions of HIV and other sexually transmitted diseases, and genital tract inflammation facilitating local pathogen transmission and acquisition. *Am J Reprod Immunol.* 2011;65:308–316.

McCormack S, Dunn DT, Desai M, et al. Pre-exposure prophylaxis to prevent the acquisition of HIV-1 infection (PROUD): effectiveness results from the pilot phase of a pragmatic open-label randomised trial. *Lancet.* 2016;387(10013):53–60. doi:10.1016/S0140-6736(15)00056-2

Mimiaga MJ, Pantalone DW, Biello KB, et al. A randomized controlled efficacy trial of behavioral activation for concurrent stimulant use and sexual risk for HIV acquisition among MSM: project IMPACT study protocol. *BMC Public Health.* 2018;18:914.

Molina JM, Capitant C, Charreau I, et al. On-demand PrEP with oral TDF/FTC in MSM: results of the ANRS IPERGAY trial. *N Engl J Med.* 2015;373:2237–2246.

Molina JM, Charreau I, Spire B, et al. Efficacy, safety, and effect on sexual behavior of on-demand pre-exposure prophylaxis for HIV in men who have sex with men: an observational cohort study. *Lancet.* 2017;4(9):E402–E410. doi:10.1016/S2352-3018(17)30089-9

Molina JM, Ghosn J, Algarte-Genin M, et al. Incidence of HIV infection with daily or on-demand PrEP with TDF/FTC in Paris area. Update from the ANRS Prévenir Study. *10th International AIDS Society Conference on HIV Science,* Mexico City, 2019. Abstract TUAC0202.

Moorman AC, de Perio MA, Goldschmidt R, et al. Testing and clinical management of health care personnel potentially exposed to hepatitis C virus—CDC guidance, United States, 2020. *MMWR Recomm Rep.* 2020;69(No. RR-6):1–8. doi:http://dx.doi.org/10.15585/mmwr.rr6906a1external icon

Mulligan K, Glidden DV, Anderson PL, et al. Effects of emtricitabine/tenofovir on bone mineral density in HIV-negative persons in a randomized, double-blind, placebo-controlled trial. *Clin Infect Dis.* 2015;61(4):572–580.

New York State Department of Health AIDS Institute. PrEP to prevent HIV and promote sexual health. February 2020a revision. https://www.hivguidelines.org/prep-for-prevention/

New York State Department of Health AIDS Institute. Post-exposure prophylaxis (PEP) to prevent HIV infection. June 2020b revision. https://www.hivguidelines.org/pep-for-hiv-prevention/

Ogbuagu O, Podzamczer D, Salazar L, et al. Longer-term safety of F/TAF and F/TDF for HIV PrEP: Discover Trial week-96 results. Presented at *Conference on Retroviruses and Opportunistic Infections,* March 8–11, 2020, Boston, MA. Abstract 92.

Otten RA, Smith DK, Adams DR, et al. Efficacy of postexposure prophylaxis after intravaginal exposure of pig-tailed macaques to a human-derived retrovirus (human immunodeficiency virus type 2). *J Virol.* 2000;74(20):9771–9775.

Panel on Treatment of Pregnant Women with HIV Infection and Prevention of Perinatal Transmission. Recommendations for use of antiretroviral drugs in pregnant women with HIV infection and interventions to reduce perinatal HIV transmission in the United States. 2020. https://clinicalinfo.hiv.gov/en/guidelines/perinatal/whats-new-guidelines

Perlman D, Jordan AE. The syndemic of opioid misuse, overdose, HCV, and HIV: structural-level causes and interventions. *Current HIV/AIDS Rep.* 2018;15:96–112.

Pettifor A, Bekker L-G, Hosek S, et al. Preventing HIV among young people: research priorities for the future. *J AIDS.* 2013;63(Suppl 2):S155–S160.

Pitisuttithum P, Gilbert P, Gurwith M, et al. Randomized, double-blind, placebo-controlled efficacy trial of a bivalent recombinant glycoprotein 120 HIV-1 vaccine among injection drug users in Bangkok, Thailand. *J Infect Dis.* 2006;194:1661–1671.

Poteat T, Malik M, Scheim A, Elliott A. HIV prevention among transgender populations: knowledge gaps and evidence for action. *Curr HIV/AIDS Rep.* 2017;14(4):141–152.

Prathela P, Braunstein SL, Blank S, et al. The high risk of an HIV diagnosis following a diagnosis of syphilis: a population-level analysis of New York City men. *Clin Infect Dis.* 2015;61(2):281–287.

Protogerou C, Johnson BT. Factors underlying the success of behavioral HIV-prevention interventions for adolescents: a meta-review. *AIDS Behav.* 2014;18(10):1847–1863.

Reback CJ, Fletcher JB. HIV prevalence, substance use, and sexual risk behaviors among transgender women recruited through outreach. *AIDS Behav.* 2014;18(7):1359–1367.

Rees H, Delany-Moretlwe SA, Lombard C, et al. FACTS 001 phase III trial of pericoital tenofovir 1% gel for HIV prevention in women. In: *Program and Abstracts of the 2015 Conference on Retroviruses and Opportunistic Infections,* February 2015, Seattle, WA. Abstract 26LB.

Rerks-Ngarm S, Pitisuttithum P, Nitayaphan S, et al. Vaccination with ALVAC and AIDSVAX to prevent HIV-1 infection in Thailand. *N Engl J Med.* 2009;361:2209–2220.

Rich KM, Bia J, Altice FL, et al. Integrated models of care for individuals with opioid use disorder: how do we prevent HIV and HCV? *Curr HIV/AIDS Rep.* 2018;15(3):266–275.

Rubens M, Ramamoorthy V, Saxena A, et al. HIV vaccine: recent advances, current roadblocks, and future directions. *J Immunol Res.* 2015;2015:560347.

Saag MS, Benson CA, Gandhi RT, et al. Antiretroviral drugs for treatment and prevention of HIV infection in adults: 2018 recommendations of the International Antiviral Society–USA Panel. *JAMA.* 2018;320(4):379–396. doi:10.1001/jama.2018.8431

Schnall R, Kuhns LM, Hidalgo MA, et al. Adaptation of a group-based HIV RISK reduction intervention to a mobile app for young sexual minority men. *AIDS Educ Prev.* 2018;30(6):449–462. doi:10.1521/aeap.2018.30.6.449

Sevelius JM, Poteat T, Luhur WE, et al. HIV testing and PrEP use in a national probability sample of sexually active transgender people in the United States. *J AIDS.* 2020; 84(5): 437–442.

Shih CC, Kaneshima H, Rabin L, et al. Postexposure prophylaxis with zidovudine suppresses human immunodeficiency virus type 1 infection in SCID-hu mice in a time-dependent manner. *J Infect Dis.* 1991;163(3):625–627.

Shrestha RK, Chavez PR, Noble M, et al. Estimating the costs and cost-effectiveness of HIV self-testing among men who have sex with men,

United States. *J Int AIDS Soc.* 2020;23(1):e25445. doi:10.1002/jia2.25445

Siegfried N, Muller M, Deeks JJ, et al. Male circumcision for prevention of heterosexual acquisition of HIV in men. *Cochrane Database Syst Rev.* 2009;2:CD003362. doi:10.1002/14651858.CD003362.pub2

Smith DK, Herbst JH, Zhang XJ, et al. Condom effectiveness for HIV prevention by consistency of use among men who have sex with men (MSM) in the US. *J AIDS.* 2015;68(3):337–344.

Smith DK, Van Handel M, Grey J. Estimates of adults with indications for HIV pre-exposure prophylaxis by jurisdiction, transmission risk group, and race/ethnicity, United States, 2015. *Ann Epidemiol.* 2018;28(12):850–857. doi:10.1016/j.annepidem.2018.05.003

Solomon MM, Lama JR, Glidden DV, et al. Change in renal function associated with oral FTC/TDF use for HIV pre-exposure prophylaxis. *AIDS.* 2014;28:851–859.

Solomon MM, Schechter M, Liu AY, et al. The safety of tenofovir–emtricitabine for HIV pre-exposure prophylaxis (PrEP) in individuals with active hepatitis B. *J AIDS.* 2016;71(3):281–286. doi:10.1097/QAI.0000000000000857

Song HJ, Squires P, Wilson D, et al. Trends in HIV preexposure prophylaxis prescribing in the United States, 2012–2018. *JAMA.* 2020;324(4):395–397. doi:10.1001/jama.2020.7312

Spinelli MA, Lowery B, Shuford JA, et al. Use of drug-level testing and single-genome sequencing to unravel a case of HIV seroconversion on PrEP. *Clin Infect Dis.* July 2020 [Epub ahead of print]. https://doi.org/10.1093/cid/ciaa1011

Stein BD, Dick AW, Sorbero M, el al. A population-based examination of trends and disparities in medication treatment for opioid use disorders among Medicaid enrollees. *Subst Abuse.* 2018;39(4):419–425.

Stone J, Fraser H, Lim AG, et al. Incarceration history and risk of HIV and hepatitis C virus acquisition among people who inject drugs: a systematic review and meta-analysis. *Lancet Infect Dis.* 2018;18(12):1397–1409.

Strathdee SA. Preventing HIV among people who inject drugs. In: *Conference on Retroviruses and Opportunistic Infections*, March 8-11, 2020, Boston, MA. Abstract 62.

Strathdee SA, Shoptaw S, Dyer TP, et al.; Substance Use Scientific Committee of the HIV Prevention Trials Network. Towards combination HIV prevention for injection drug users: addressing addictophobia, apathy and inattention. *Curr Opin HIV AIDS.* 2012;7(4):320–325.

Substance Abuse and Mental Health Services Administration (SAMHSA). *Treatment of Stimulant Use Disorders.* SAMHSA Publication No. PEP20-06-01-001 Rockville, MD: National Mental Health and Substance Use Policy Laboratory. Substance Abuse and Mental Health Services Administration, 2020.

Thaden JT, Gandhi M, Okochi H, et al. Seroconversion on preexposure prophylaxis: a case report with segmental hair analysis for timed adherence determination. *AIDS.* 2018;32(9):F1–F4. doi:10.1097/QAD.0000000000001825

Thigpen MC, Kebaabetswe PM, Paxton LA, et al. Antiretroviral prophylaxis for heterosexual HIV transmission in Botswana. *N Engl J Med.* 2012;367:423–434.

Thompson KA, Hughes JP, Baeten J, et al. Increased risk of HIV acquisition among women throughout pregnancy and during the postpartum period: a prospective per-coital-act analysis among women with HIV-infected partners. *J Infect Dis.* 2018; 218(1): 16–25.

US Department of Health and Human Services Panel on Antiretroviral Guidelines for Adults and Adolescents. Guidelines for the use of antiretroviral agents in adults and adolescents with HIV. Dec 2019. https://clinicalinfo.hiv.gov/en/guidelines/adult-and-adolescent-arv/whats-new-guidelines.

US Food and Drug Administration. Coronavirus (COVID-19) update: FDA provides updated guidance to address the urgent need for blood during the pandemic. 2020. https://www.fda.gov/news-events/press-announcements/coronavirus-covid-19-update-fda-provides-updated-guidance-address-urgent-need-blood-during-pandemic

US Preventive Services Task Force. Preexposure prophylaxis for the prevention of HIV Infection: US Preventive Services Task Force Recommendation Statement. *JAMA.* 2019a;321(22):2203–2213. doi:10.1001/jama.2019.6390

US Preventive Services Task Force. Screening for HIV infection: US Preventive Services Task Force Recommendation Statement. *JAMA.* 2019b;321(23):2326–2336.

US Preventive Services Task Force. Screening for unhealthy drug use: US Preventive Services Task Force Recommendation Statement. *JAMA.* 2020;323(22):2301–2309.

Valera P, Chang Y, Lian Z. HIV risk inside US prisons: a systematic review of risk reduction interventions conducted in US prisons. *AIDS Care.* 2017;29(8):943–952.

Vallabhaneni S, Li X, Vittinghoff E, et al. Seroadaptive practices: association with HIV acquisition among HIV-negative men who have sex with men. *PLoS One.* 2012;7(10):e45718.

Van Damme L, Corneli A, Ahmed K, et al. Preexposure prophylaxis for HIV infection among African women. *N Engl J Med.* 2012;367:411–422.

Veronese V, Ryan KE, Hughes C, et al. Using digital communication technology to increase HIV testing among men who have sex with men and transgender women: systematic review and meta-analysis. *J Med Internet Res.* 2020; 22(7): e14230.

Volk JE, Marcus JL, Phengrasamy T, et al. No new HIV infections with increasing use of HIV preexposure prophylaxis in a clinical practice setting. *Clin Infect Dis.* 2015;61(10):1601–1603.

Ward H, Rönn M. The contribution of STIs to the sexual transmission of HIV. *Curr Opin HIV AIDS.* 2010;5(4):305–310.

Wei C, Fisher Raymond H, Guadamuz TE, et al. Racial/ethnic differences in seroadaptive and serodisclosure behaviors among men who have sex with men. *AIDS Behav.* 2011;15(1):22–29.

Weiss HA, Hankins CA, Dickson K. Male circumcision and risk of HIV infection in women: a systematic review and meta-analysis. *Lancet Infect Dis.* 2009;9:669–677.

Wirtz AL, Yeh PT, Flath N, et al. HIV and viral hepatitis among imprisoned key populations. *Epidemiologic Rev.* 2018;40(1):12–26.

Wiysonge CS, Kongnyuy EJ, Shey M, et al. Male circumcision for prevention of homosexual acquisition of HIV in men. *Cochrane Database Syst Rev.* 2011;6.CD007496. doi:10.1002/14651858.CD007496.pub2

Wodak A, Cooney A. *Effectiveness of Sterile Needle and Syringe Programming in Reducing HIV/AIDS Among Injecting Drug Users.* Geneva: World Health Organization Document Production Services, 2004.

World Health Organization. Consolidated guidelines on the use of antiretroviral drugs for treating and preventing HIV infection. Recommendations for a public health approach—second edition, 2016. https://www.who.int/hiv/pub/arv/arv-2016/en/

World Health Organization. What's the 2+1+1? Event-driven oral preexposure prophylaxis to prevent HIV for men who have sex with men: Update to WHO's recommendation on oral PrEP. Geneva: World Health Organization, 2019 (WHO/CDS/HIV/19.8). Licence: CC BY-NC-SA 3.0 IGO.

Young TN, Arens FJ, Kennedy GE, et al. Antiretroviral post-exposure prophylaxis (PEP) for occupational HIV exposure. *Cochrane Database Sys Rev.* 2007;1:CD002835.

Zanakis SH, Alvarez C, Li V. Socio-economic determinants of HIV/AIDS pandemic and nations efficiencies. *Eur J Operational Res.* 2007;176:1811–1838.

Zash R, Holmes L, Makhema J, et al. Surveillance for neural tube defects following antiretroviral exposure from conception, the Tsepamo study (Botswana). In: *Program and Abstracts of the 22nd International AIDS Conference*, July 23–27, 2018, Amsterdam, The Netherlands. Session TUSY15.

Zou S, Dorsey KA, Notari EP, et al. Prevalence, incidence, and residual risk of human immunodeficiency virus and hepatitis C virus infections among United States blood donors since the introduction of nucleic acid testing. *Transfusion.* 2010;50(7):1495–1504.

6.

IMMUNOLOGY

Dennis J. Hartigan-O'Connor and Christian Brander

MECHANISMS OF CD4⁺ T-CELL DECLINE

LEARNING OBJECTIVE

- Describe the processes contributing to CD4⁺ T-cell decline and immune activation in untreated HIV infection

WHAT'S NEW?

Chronic inflammation in HIV disease may have its origins in translocation of microbial products across a Th17 cell-deficient mucosal barrier. Collagen deposition in lymph nodes contributes to T-cell loss by interrupting homeostasis. Sensing of intracellular pathogens, including HIV, in abortively infected cells contributes to progressive CD4⁺ T-cell loss in chronic HIV infection.

KEY POINTS

- Cytopathic infection alone is insufficient to explain CD4⁺ T-cell loss in HIV infection.

- Chronic inflammation is strongly associated with CD4⁺ T-cell loss in pathogenic lentiviral infection such as HIV but is not seen in non-pathogenic infections.

- Abortive infection of T cells leads to their elimination.

- Translocation of microbial constituents and lymph node scarring have been recognized as likely contributors to CD4⁺ T-cell decline.

The prototypic outcomes associated with HIV infection are progressive CD4⁺ T-cell decline, consequent immunodeficiency, and chronic inflammation. In untreated disease, circulating memory CD4⁺ T cells, some of which are infected, are both dividing and dying at an accelerated rate (Hellerstein et a;/, 1999). In addition, CD4⁺ T cells that reside in the gastrointestinal mucosa are important early targets of infection and are decimated early in disease (Guadalupe et al., 2003; Heise et al., 1994; Veazey et al., 1998). Although direct cytopathic infection contributes to CD4⁺ T-cell loss, many *uninfected* CD4⁺ T cells are dividing and dying in HIV disease; thus, other mechanisms must be invoked to fully explain CD4⁺ T-cell decline. The death

of infected cells is likely due to exposure to Tat, Gp120, or other toxic proteins (all of which can induce apoptosis) and/or adaptive immune clearance of HIV-infected cells (Lenardo et al., 2002). In addition, abortive infection of T cells (i.e., where cells become infected with the virus but the virus cannot complete reverse transcription and thus is not productively infected) can lead to massive cell death in the tissue. Such abortive infection drives a process known as *pyroptosis*, a form of programmed cell death that is triggered by danger signals within the abortively infected cell and that is believed to significantly contribute to the loss of CD4⁺ T cells (Ke et al., 2017). HIV can also impair CD4⁺ T-cell regeneration by destroying the immunologic niches that are required for T-cell homeostasis, by depleting essential hematopoietic progenitor cells, and by inhibiting the regenerative process through production of immune mediators (Douek et al., 2003; Grossman et al., 2002).

Chronic inflammation and immune activation have also been shown to be associated with CD4⁺ T-cell decline. For example, pathogenic lentiviral infections (such as HIV infection) and non-pathogenic infections (such as lentiviral infections of many non-human primates) are each associated with robust virus replication. Immune activation, however, is observed only in the pathogenic models, suggesting that this mechanism is directly responsible for CD4 decline and disease progression (Silvestri et al., 2003). Furthermore, chronic inflammation and CD4⁺ T-cell decline may be linked in a self-perpetuating cycle involving gut tissue. CD4⁺ Th17 cells are among those cells lost from the gastrointestinal tract in early HIV and simian immunodeficiency virus (SIV) infection (Brenchley et al., 2008; Favre et al., 2009). Th17 cells are important for maintenance of the "mucosal barrier" between gut luminal contents and circulation; when these cells are depleted, microbial constituents and even whole microbes can migrate from the gut into circulation, a process referred to as microbial translocation (Brenchley et al., 2006; Raffatellu et al., 2008). These pro-inflammatory microbial products, in particular lipopolysaccharides (LPS) from the outer membrane of gram-negative bacteria, vigorously activate the immune system, resulting in activation-induced cell death and/or altered homeostasis. This cycle is initiated early in SIV infection (Hirao et al., 2014) and appears to be an important driver of disease progression, as the presence of sufficient Th17 cells before infection can limit viral replication (Hartigan-O'Connor et al., 2012).

Two recent reports add to our understanding of the interplay between HIV and gut-homing CD4+ T cells. One showed that the frequency of a4b7hi CD4+ T cells in blood was correlated with acquisition risk in a cohort of women participating in a CAPRISA-sponsored HIV prevention study in South Africa (Sivro et al., 2018). In addition, the preinfection frequency of a4b7hi CD4+ T cells was strongly correlated with the rate of CD4+ T-cell decline following HIV infection. A second report elucidated features intrinsic to the process of naive CD4+ T-cell trafficking to gut inductive sites that facilitate viral replication in those inductive tissues (Nawaz et al., 2018). Combined stimulation with retinoic acid and the a4b7 ligand, MAdCAM, was shown to induce a distinct differentiation program in naive CD4+ T cells that leads to the generation of cells with an a4b7hi phenotype, which is supportive of viral replication.

Another increasingly recognized self-perpetuating cycle pertains to the impact of HIV-associated inflammation on lymphoid structures. The inflammatory response generated by HIV results in upregulation of certain countervailing "regulatory" responses, including production of TGF-beta, which stimulates collagen deposition (Estes et al., 2008). The scarring of the lymph nodes, which appears to be irreversible, prevents normal T-cell homeostasis and antigen presentation. The immunodeficiency that results can lead to an excess burden of a variety of microbes, including cytomegalovirus (CMV), gut microbes, and perhaps HIV itself. This microbial burden continues to the cycle by causing even more inflammation and scarring (Arthos et al., 2008).

EFFECTS OF HIV ON THE WHOLE IMMUNE SYSTEM

LEARNING OBJECTIVE

- Discuss the effects of HIV on immune cells other than CD4+ T cells

KEY POINTS

- HIV has broad effects on many immune cell types, including many cells that are not infected by the virus.

- HIV disrupts the entire lymphoid system through its effects on secondary lymphoid organs such as lymph nodes

Although HIV is tropic for CD4+ T cells, it is clear that many manifestations of HIV infection result from direct or indirect effects on other immune cell types. One example is the high death rate and turnover of CD8+ T cells, as well as numerical depletion of naive CD8+ T cells, even in the asymptomatic phase of infection (Roederer et al., 1995). HIV also has direct or indirect effects on antigen-presenting cells such as dendritic, B, and natural killer (NK) cells (Ruffin et al., 2017). One factor that likely mediates some of the effects of HIV on the broader immune system, particularly in late disease, is the destruction of lymphoid tissue architecture. In early disease,

as antigen-presenting cells are activated and initiate immune responses within lymph nodes, CD4+ T cells are retained within the nodes while activated CD8+ T cells migrate into circulation, a process that contributes to CD8+ lymphocytosis and inversion of the CD4:CD8 ratio (Bishop et al., 1990; Bujdoso et al., 1989). In later disease, there is structural damage to primary and secondary lymphoid organs resulting from fibrotic scarring (Estes et al., 2008; Samal et al., 2018). Naive T cells, including CD8+ T cells, require critical homeostatic signals and growth factors, including interleukin (IL)-7 (Link et al., 2007). Presumably, therefore, lymphoid tissue scarring is one factor that contributes to failure to fully reconstitute CD4+ and CD8+ T cells despite complete virologic suppression.

HIV-1 can also infect myeloid cells, including macrophages and dendritic cells, both of which can express CCR5. However, myeloid cells are relatively resistant to *productive* infection with HIV, as compared to CD4+ T cells (Coleman & Wu, 2009). The relative inability of SIV and HIV-2 to cause productive infection of these cells is mediated by the cellular restriction factor SAMHD1 (Hrecka et al., 2011; Laguette et al., 2011). The viral accessory protein Vpx blocks this cellular response, thus allowing infection. As HIV-1 lacks this accessory protein, it remains unclear as to how this virus might productively infect macrophages (Hrecka et al., 2011; Laguette et al., 2011; Manel et al., 2010). Surprisingly, it is now appreciated that macrophages and memory CD4+ T cells accumulate in adipose tissue during HIV infection (Damouche et al., 2017; Hsu et al., 2017; Koethe et al., 2018). Replicating virus can be recovered from these adipose tissue–resident cells, indicating that the tissue is a reservoir, though probably a minor one compared to lymphoid tissue. Antiviral effector cells, such as CD8+ T cells and NK cells, are also present in large numbers in adipose tissue. (Couturier et al., 2015, 2016; Damouche et al., 2015; Dupin et al., 2002).

Natural killer T (NKT) cells are also rapidly and selectively depleted in HIV infection (Sandberg et al., 2002; van der Vliet et al., 2002). NKT cells may be broadly divided into those that are CD4+ and those that are CD4-, with the former population secreting both Th1 and Th2 cytokines and likely providing B-cell help or carrying out immunoregulatory functions, while the latter produces mainly Th1 cytokines and has stronger cytolytic activity. The CD4+ NKT population is depleted more rapidly in HIV infection than the CD4- population but is restored more slowly after treatment with antiretroviral therapy (ART) (Li & Xu, 2008). HIV also interferes with the activation of NKT cells by downregulating expression of CD1d (a major histocompatibility complex (MHC)-related protein that presents glycolipid antigens to NKT cells) on antigen-presenting cells (Hage et al., 2005). This downregulation appears to be mediated mainly by the viral Nef protein (Cho et al., 2005).

There is continued interest in the effect of HIV and other agents of chronic infection on NK cells, particularly subsets with expanded functional capacity, including "memory" NK cells (Hwang et al., 2012; Lee et al., 2015; Lopez-Verges et al., 2011; Sun et al., 2009; Zhang et al., 2013). Such cells are considered to be innate cells with adaptive features, including more robust and rapid responses to pathogen encounter (Sun et al., 2009). Limited evidence has been presented demonstrating that HIV infection drives expansion of memory NK cells (Zhou et al., 2015). However, NK cells from SIV-infected macaques or those vaccinated with an Ad26-vectored candidate SIV/HIV vaccine can lyse targets pulsed with SIV peptides in an antigen- and NKG2-dependent fashion (Reeves et al., 2015). CMV infection, which is common in HIV-positive people, is thought to be the most important driver of memory NK cell expansion (Brodin et al., 2015; Lopez-Verges et al., 2011; Zhang et al., 2013). People coinfected with HIV and CMV may therefore present unique immunologic features.

MECHANISMS OF CHRONIC INFLAMMATION IN HIV DISEASE

LEARNING OBJECTIVE

- Discuss the mechanisms that contribute to T-cell activation and chronic inflammation in HIV disease

KEY POINTS

- Innate immune responses that result in production of type I interferons are important drivers of inflammation in early disease.

- Early depletion of CD4$^+$ T cells from the gastrointestinal mucosa likely contributes to chronic, persistent immune activation.

- CMV and other chronic infections are important contributors to T-cell activation in coinfected individuals.

It was first demonstrated more than 20 years ago that T-cell activation was associated with shorter survival in advanced HIV disease (Giorgi, 1999). One might imagine that chronic T cell activation is simply the inevitable consequence of ongoing viral replication, and that more T cell activation is indicative of more active disease. However, it is clear from studies of non-pathogenic lentiviral infections that chronic, high-level virus replication can occur without eliciting massive immune activation (Silvestri et al., 2003); indeed, in the natural hosts of SIV, the rapid reduction in immune activation appears to protect against subsequent CD4$^+$ T-cell decline and disease progression. Efforts are underway to test these factors in rare persons living with HIV and high viral loads but remarkable absence of rapid HIV disease progression (Muenchhoff et al., 2016; Palesch et al., 2018). It is now clear that HIV-associated inflammation is associated with a transformation of "immunometabolism" to greater dependence on aerobic glycolysis, which is partly dependent on mTORC1 activation (Sáez-Cirión & Sereti, 2021). This transformation can in fact be imaged using positron emission tomography (PET) scanning to reveal upregulation of the glucose transporter, GLUT1, and resultant accumulation of fluorodeoxyglucose (FDG)

tracer in persons with HIV (PWH), ranging from those with successful suppression with ART to late presenters experiencing opportunistic infection (Brust et al., 2006; Hammoud et al., 2019).

The virion itself elicits innate immune responses via activation of Toll-like receptors (TLR) 7, 8, and 9 within antigen-presenting cells. TLR engagement results in production of type-I interferons, including interferon-α (IFN-α). Indeed, a spike of IFN-α production is observed in acute HIV and SIV infection (Favre et al., 2009; Stacey et al., 2009), which doubtless shapes the ensuing adaptive immune responses. Binding of virion components to signaling molecules such as CD4 and CCR5 may also stimulate cells directly, and viral proteins such as Tat and Nef have been shown to have pro-inflammatory effects (Decrion et al., 2005), with consequences that can even affect neurogenesis and other brain functions (Fan et al., 2016). After the first 2 weeks of infection, the adaptive immune response to HIV proteins contributes to T-cell activation, although many of these activated T cells are specific for CMV and other chronic pathogens rather than HIV (Doisne et al., 2004; Papagno et al., 2004). Less appreciated is the fact that host genetics, in addition to controlling the adaptive immune response, may modulate the intensity of inflammation induced by these pro-inflammatory influences. Subjects in a Zimbabwean cohort having an IL-10 promoter mutation associated with lower inflammation experienced reductions in both mortality and CD4$^+$ T-cell loss (Erikstrup et al., 2007). Finally, lymphopenia itself can lead to T-cell activation; for example, resting T cells spontaneously become activated and proliferate when introduced into T-cell–deficient hosts (Srinivasula et al., 2011; Surh & Sprent, 2008). Thus, the progressive loss of CD4$^+$ T cells can be both a consequence and a cause of immune activation (Jones et al., 2009; King et al., 2004).

In addition to these general effects of lymphocyte depletion, the field has discovered the implications of early and profound lymphocyte depletion from the gastrointestinal mucosa (Heise et al., 1994; Veazey et al., 1998). Among the lymphocytes lost in early infection are CD4$^+$ Th17 cells (Pandiyan et al., 2016), which have an important structural role in maintaining the tight junctions between intestinal epithelial cells (Brenchley et al., 2008; Favre et al., 2009). Loss of these cells contributes to a breakdown in the physical barrier separating the gut lumen from general circulation, which allows bioactive microbial products such as LPS into the blood (Brenchley et al., 2006), while maintenance of sufficient Th17 cells is associated with reduced viral replication (Hartigan-O'Connor et al., 2012). Mucosal barrier breakdown and pro-inflammatory processes such as tryptophan catabolism, in turn, are associated with disturbance ("dysbiosis") of the gut-resident microbial community (Vujkovic-Cvijin et al., 2013, 2020). Persistent microbial dysbiosis drives further immune dysregulation and inflammation (Guillén et al., 2019), in part via loss of peroxisomal proliferator-activated receptor-α (PPARα) signaling (Crakes et al., 2019). In animal models, partial reversal of dysbiosis with *Lactobacillus plantarum* leads to recovery of the epithelium due to PPARα activation and restoration of mitochondrial structure and fatty acid β-oxidation (Crakes et al., 2019).

Occult and symptomatic opportunistic infections also contribute to chronic inflammation in HIV disease. In particular, the prevalence of CMV coinfection among PWH is at least 90% (Berry et al., 1988; Lang et al., 1989). Furthermore, CMV infection has been associated with T-cell activation in HIV-negative people (Lenkei & Andersson, 1995). Indeed, CMV-specific T cells account for nearly 10% of the circulating memory T-cell pool in seropositive individuals, suggesting that CMV replication can have a major influence on the immune system even in healthy individuals who are not immunocompromised (Sylwester et al., 2005) as well as in the growing population of elderly PWH (Margolick et al., 2018). CMV appears to have an even stronger effect on T-cell remodeling in untreated and treated HIV infection (Naeger et al., 2010). A recent pilot study tested the possibility that chronic immune activation in HIV disease could be reduced by treatment of CMV infection: 30 individuals on ART were randomized to treatment with valganciclovir or placebo (Hunt et al., 2011). A significant 20% reduction in the percentage of activated CD8[+] T cells was demonstrated in the valganciclovir group, suggesting that CMV infection (or infection with other valganciclovir-sensitive herpesviruses) is a significant contributor to T- cell activation in treated HIV- and CMV-coinfected individuals.

IMMUNOLOGIC EFFECTS OF ANTIRETROVIRAL THERAPY AND ROLE OF PERSISTENT IMMUNE DYSFUNCTION DURING THERAPY ON CLINICAL OUTCOMES

LEARNING OBJECTIVE

- Discuss the effect of ART on immune function.

KEY POINTS

- A small but clinically important subset of PWH exhibit suboptimal CD4[+] T-cell gains after treatment with ART.

- Chronic inflammation, lymphoid fibrosis, hematopoietic progenitor cell loss, and thymic dysfunction all likely contribute to failure of normal T-cell homeostasis.

- Chronic inflammation during treated disease has been associated with subsequent disease progression.

Combination ART results in complete or near-complete suppression of HIV replication. Consequently, many of the factors that cause progressive immunodeficiency are reversed. Prevention of continued CD4[+] T-cell destruction (via both direct and indirect effects) and homeostatic regeneration results in eventual restoration of CD4[+] T-cell numbers in blood and tissues. The increase in peripheral CD4[+] T-cell counts during therapy appears to be biphasic (Pakker et al., 1998). A robust increase of approximately 50

to 100 cells/mm^3 is often observed in the first several weeks following initiation of ART. Because memory cells account for most of the increase, it has long been assumed that the redistribution of cells from tissues to the periphery accounts for this rapid increase. After this early phase, CD4[+] T-cell counts increase slowly (at a rate of approximately 50 cells/mm^3 per year) until they achieve a normal range (i.e., >500 cells/mm^3; Mocroft et al., 2007). The augmented CD4[+] T-cell population includes naive cells and hence is thought to reflect true immune reconstitution. Although less well studied, CD4[+] T-cell gains also occur in tissues during effective antiviral therapy.

Although most PWH exhibit some degree of immune reconstitution during therapy, the outcome is highly variable. Some persons achieving median reference CD4[+] T-cell counts nonetheless exhibit a CD4:CD8 ratio below median because of persisting high CD8[+] T-cell counts (Gras et al., 2019). A small but clinically important subset of PWH fail to achieve normal peripheral CD4[+] T-cell counts, even after many years of therapy. These so-called immunologic nonresponders remain at relatively high risk for cancer, heart disease, liver failure, and other non-AIDS complications, but they usually achieve sufficient restoration of immune function to prevent opportunistic infections. Older persons with HIV who start ART during late-stage disease often exhibit suboptimal gains in CD4[+] T cells. In one study, approximately 40% of PWH who delayed therapy until their CD4[+] T-cell count was less than 200 cells/mm^3 failed to achieve a normal CD4[+] T-cell count after several years of viral suppression (Kelley et al., 2009). Other factors that have been associated with blunted CD4[+] T-cell gains include hepatitis C virus coinfection and high levels of T-cell activation. Historically, the use of certain nucleoside analogs (particularly the combination of stavudine and didanosine) or the use of efavirenz-based regimens (as compared to maraviroc-, raltegravir-, and protease inhibitor–based regimens) were also associated with a diminished CD4[+] T-cell response (Negredo et al., 2013).

Given its clinical importance, there is intense interest in determining the pathogenesis of immunologic failure (defined variably). In untreated disease, HIV-mediated destruction of hematopoietic stem cells, thymic tissue, lymphoid tissue, and central memory cells will all contribute to progressive CD4[+] T-cell loss. Treatment-mediated suppression of HIV replication partially restores these factors. Persistent lymph node fibrosis, thymic dysfunction, and loss of cells with stem-like properties have all been associated with CD4[+] T-cell regeneration failure and suboptimal gains during therapy (McCune, 2001; Sauce et al., 2011; Schacker et al., 2002). More recently it has been shown that immunologic nonresponders accumulate CD56[bright] NK cells with cytotoxicity against autologous activated CD4[+] T cells (Giuliani et al., 2017). Those data suggest that autoreactive NK cells, possibly linked to decreased homeostatic control by a depleted T-regulatory (T-reg) cell compartment, contribute to suboptimal immune reconstitution.

Untreated HIV infection is associated with heightened levels of immune activation. Long-term suppression of HIV replication dramatically reduces most measures of immune activation, but this effect is often incomplete, as inflammatory markers typically remain higher in treated PWH than age-matched uninfected adults (Neuhaus et al., 2010). Persistent inflammation during therapy is associated with excess risk of non-AIDS complications, including heart disease, cancer, liver disease, kidney disease, bone disease, and neurologic complications (Deeks, 2011). Persistent CMV replication may be an important cause of continued inflammation while on therapy, as higher anti-CMV IgG antibody levels are associated with increased prevalence of carotid artery lesions among women with HIV who achieve HIV suppression on ART, but not among viremic or untreated women (Gómez-Mora et al., 2017; Parrinello et al., 2012).

Persistent and possible irreversible damage to the infrastructure that supports T-cell homeostasis may account for much of the persistent immunodeficiency and inflammation often observed during therapy. Theoretically, collagen deposition and scarring of the lymphoid system during untreated disease results in a loss of the regulatory pathways (particularly those involving IL-7 and IL-27) that control T-cell regeneration and global T-cell homeostasis (Ruiz-Riol et al., 2017; Zeng et al., 2012). This disruption can result in persistently low CD4[+] T-cell counts and an inability to generate effective memory T cells in response to acute or chronic infections. Loss of lymphoid structures may also result in loss of immune surveillance and development of cancer, as well as a loss of key anti-inflammatory regulatory responses and, as a result, autoimmune-related clinical syndromes. In a self-perpetuating "vicious" cycle that persists in the absence of any HIV replication, persistent immunodeficiency results in a reduced capacity of host responses to clear pathogens. The resulting burden of these pathogens contributes to more inflammation, which in turn continues to damage the lymphoid tissues. The collective outcome is a combination of low CD4[+] T-cell counts and chronic inflammation. It is hoped that knowledge about these pathways will lead to novel interventions aimed at preventing or reversing this immunodeficient and pro-inflammatory environment.

PATHOGENESIS OF IMMUNE RECONSTITUTION INFLAMMATORY SYNDROMES (IRIS)

LEARNING OBJECTIVE

- Discuss the leading hypotheses explaining pathogenesis of IRIS, including antigen persistence and immune dysregulation

WHAT'S NEW?

The presence of a more inflammatory environment in untreated HIV disease is associated with IRIS episodes after treatment. Data on the role of T-regs in IRIS have been unclear.

KEY POINTS

- IRIS are seen most commonly in PWH initiating ART with low CD4[+] T-cell counts and preexisting opportunistic infections.

- Many IRIS symptoms are localized to sites of previous infection, suggesting the presence of persistent microbial antigens.

- Development of IRIS is associated with increased T-cell activation before initiation of treatment.

A subset of PWH who are immune-restored with ART develop inflammatory conditions known collectively as immune reconstitution inflammatory syndromes (IRIS) (Church et al., 2017). A large meta-analysis showed that 16% of PWH starting ART therapy developed an IRIS event (Muller et al., 2010). PWH most likely to be affected are those initiating ART with low CD4[+] T-cell counts and preexisting opportunistic infections (Muller et al., 2010). The symptoms of IRIS are often localized to sites of previous infection (Lawn et al., 2007), which led to the suggestion that IRIS is caused by adaptive immune responses to persistent pathogen-derived antigens (Muller et al., 2010). For example, IRIS in persons with a history of cytomegalovirus retinitis (CMVR) can manifest as inflammation of the posterior uveal tract of the eye (Nussenblatt & Lane, 1998). The most frequent clinical manifestation of cryptococcal IRIS, by contrast, is aseptic meningitis (Boulware et al., 2010).

The hypothesis that IRIS is caused by the host immune response to persistent antigen (in the form of intact organisms, dead organisms, or debris) has the appeal of simplicity, but there are surprisingly few data to support this idea. One study demonstrated that, among PWH with recent cryptococcal meningitis who were placed on ART, those developing cryptococcal IRIS had fourfold higher titers of cryptococcal antigen in serum (Boulware et al., 2010). However, in a more recent study, low cryptococcal antibody levels were associated with a significantly increased risk of developing cryptococcal IRIS (Yoon et al., 2019). Guidelines based on the Cryptococcal Optimal Antiretroviral Timing (COAT) trial (Scriven et al., 2015) recommend initial antifungal treatment followed by a minimum 5-week delay before ART (Balasko & Keynan, 2019). The approach aims to decrease the fungal burden and allow immune balance restoration prior to ART initiation. In cases of *Mycobacterium tuberculosis* or *Mycobacterium avium* complex-associated IRIS, PWH normally convert to skin test positivity, suggesting that at a minimum the disease is mediated by pathogen-specific CD4[+] T cells (French et al., 2004). Worth noting are some recent data showing that preexisting infection with *M. tuberculosis* appears to create an immune environment that influences the susceptibility of CD4[+] T cells to HIV-1 replication (He et al., 2020). In the case of CMV immune recovery uveitis, however, the presence of CMV antigens has not been demonstrated in PWH undergoing an IRIS event.

Several studies have suggested that the pretherapy inflammatory environment predicts IRIS. For example, Antonelli et al. (2010) showed that individuals who presented with an IRIS episode had a higher proportion of activated CD4+ T cells before starting ART compared with those who did not develop IRIS. These activated T cells had a Th1/Th17 skewed cytokine profile before therapy began. Furthermore, PWH with IRIS displayed higher serum IFN-γ levels near the time of their IRIS events. Another study found that understanding the importance of regulatory CD4+ T cells (T-regs) in controlling immune responses to self-antigens suggests that failure to reconstitute these anti-inflammatory cells predisposes to IRIS (Seddiki et al., 2009). However, data on this hypothesis have been inconsistent (Bourgarit et al., 2006; Hartigan-O'Connor et al., 2011). Other groups have argued that poorly regulated innate immune responses may be central to IRIS. Pretherapy and early treatment-mediated changes in various nonspecific inflammatory biomarkers (including CRP, IL-6, TNF-alpha, and D-dimers) have been associated with increased risk of IRIS and mortality during the first several months of effective ART (Barber et al., 2012; Boulware et al., 2011). In general, corticosteroids remain the only treatment for paradoxical IRIS whose use is supported by data from randomized controlled trials (Meintjes et al., 2010; Walker et al., 2018).

In summary, the pathogenesis of IRIS seems dependent on the presence of both lymphopenia and antigen-specific CD4+ T cells. These T cells may be responding to persistent pathogen-derived antigens, to self-antigens, or to unrelated foreign antigens. In these latter cases the opportunistic pathogen may be the trigger rather than the target of the pathogenic T-cell response. Lymphopenia establishes a dysregulated environment in which either the response of the antigen-specific T cells or the effect of that response on the host is exaggerated and effective control mechanisms of exuberant immune responses have been impaired throughout the period of untreated HIV infection.

MECHANISMS AND CONSEQUENCES OF VIRUS CONTROL IN "ELITE" CONTROLLERS

LEARNING OBJECTIVE

- Discuss how some individuals maintain durable control of HIV in the absence of therapy

KEY POINTS

- HIV-specific CD8+ T cells contribute to durable control of virus in HIV "elite" controllers.

- Despite the lack of readily detectable HIV RNA in plasma, "elite" controllers have higher-than-normal levels of immune activation, which may contribute to slow disease progression.

Fewer than 1% of adults with HIV who are not taking ART have no readily detectable HIV RNA in plasma. These individuals are generally referred to as "elite" controllers, although other terms have been used to define this group or similar groups of individuals who are able to suppress viral replication in the absence of ART. The term "long-term non-progressors" refers to an overlapping group of PWH who maintain healthy CD4+ T-cell counts despite HIV infection. Given that the host mechanisms that might account for virus control in these individuals could inform vaccine and cure research, there has been long-term interest in understanding their mechanisms of viral control, as well as describing the degree to which most elite controllers exhibit any evidence of disease progression.

Researchers interested in determining the mechanisms of virus control in these individuals have assessed specific candidate host factors in controllers and noncontrollers. These studies have generally been cross-sectional, making it difficult to determine if a given host response is a cause of virus control or a consequence of virus control (Deeks & Walker, 2007). Some efforts have been made to follow individuals closely during the pre-HIV infection period, both to capture information about the earliest events after infection and to study dynamic changes that may be important for eventual control (Ndhlovu et al., 2015). Confoundingly, there is reason to believe that the immune responses that bring about control of acute HIV infection are distinct from those that maintain long-term viral suppression once control of viremia has been achieved (Goulder & Deeks, 2018).

Although the mechanisms have not been conclusively defined, the collective data support a central role for potent HIV-specific CD8+ T cells and to a lesser degree CD4+ T cells in maintaining virus control. This is also supported by the fact that most genetic predictors of virus control are found on chromosome 6 in the HLA class I region that governs the antigenic specificity of CD8+ T cells (Pereyra et al., 2010). Studies in SIV-infected monkeys further support the importance of virus-specific CTL responses in virus control, although at least in the Rhesus cytomegalovirus (RhCMV)-vectored vaccine setting, their MHC class I restriction may not be universal and there may be a significant contribution of MHC class II restricted CD8+ T cells (Hansen et al., 2013a, 2013b). Similarly, the role of the Th17 cell compartment in sustaining viral replication has been highlighted in recent monkey studies and the important role of IL-17- and IL-27-producing T cells in humans has been highlighted recently (Hartigan-O'Connor et al., 2012; Ruiz-Riol et al., 2017). Other factors that have been associated with virus control include (1) strong NK cell responses (Martin et al., 2007; Sips et al., 2012), (2) prevention of apoptosis/cell death in central memory cells (van Grevenynghe et al., 2008), (3) intrinsic intracellular restriction to HIV replication mediated by p21 (Chen et al., 2011) and other as yet poorly characterized factors (O'Connell et al., 2011; Saez-Cirion et al., 2011), and (4) acquisition of a replication-deficient virus. The importance of the latter is supported by recent studies of transmitted virus in a cluster of elite controllers, showing the presence of envelope sequences with a reduced binding affinity to the CD4 receptor (Casado et al., 2018). However, care must be taken not to confuse causative, functional markers of virus control with simple correlates of controlled infection. For instance, biomarkers such as proliferative capacity of HIV-specific T cells or specific cytokine profiles may be the consequence of otherwise controlled/uncontrolled HIV infection rather than its physiologic cause (Côrtes et al., 2018; Zhang et al., 2018). Longitudinal studies, capturing PWH within days of infection and following them in the absence of treatment, may be ethically challenging but could prove highly informative in defining true causes of control in vivo.

Given that controllers are being studied as a potential model for "functional cure," the consequences of long-term, host-mediated virus control on overall health is also of interest (Migueles & Connors, 2010). HIV persists at very low levels in nearly all controllers and appears to be replicating (Hatano et al., 2009; Mens et al., 2010). Persistent virus production generates a sustained inflammatory environment (Hunt et al., 2008), which in turn might cause end-organ damage, including cardiovascular disease (Hsue et al., 2009). In addition, potential alterations in the gut microbiota of chronically infected individuals may contribute to or be the result of ongoing viral replication, even in elite controllers, and may affect the efficacy of a therapeutic HIV vaccine (Williams et al., 2015). These considerations suggest that even elite controllers might benefit from ART. Studies addressing this hypothesis are in progress.

FUTURE OF IMMUNE-BASED THERAPEUTICS IN HIV DISEASE

LEARNING OBJECTIVE

- Discuss experimental approaches to chronic inflammation in antiretroviral-treated disease

WHAT'S NEW?

Many promising immune-based therapeutics are now being tested in small clinical trials.

KEY POINTS

- Proving that HIV-associated inflammation is causally associated with disease progression will ultimately require a clinical endpoint study involving an immune-based therapy that directly affects these pathways.

- Several promising drugs are now being tested in small, pathogenesis-oriented studies.

Much of the effort of clinical investigators over the past two decades has focused on the development and optimization of combination ART for treating HIV disease. With the development of several highly effective and well-tolerated regimens for both the initial regimen and "salvage" therapy, the need for new ARTs has waned. Now that most individuals with access to ART can achieve and maintain undetectable HIV RNA levels for years, it is increasingly apparent that in order to fully restore health, other adjunctive therapies may be needed. Given the consistent observation that inflammation remains elevated despite effective therapy and that the degree of inflammation predicts disease progression, there has been a renewed effort to test existing drugs for potentially beneficial effects on inflammation in conjunction with suppressed viremia or to develop new approaches that will modify the inflammatory process (Fumaz et al., 2012; Perez-Matute et al., 2015).

A number of immune-based therapeutics have been tested in non-human primates or in human clinical trials. The results have been largely disappointing. Prednisone, hydroxyurea, cyclosporine, and mycophenolate acid have been studied in numerous clinical trials with minimal or no clinical benefit. Although there were some promising early results, all these drugs proved to be too toxic or to lack any clear efficacy, and there is hence limited interested in using nonspecific drugs that globally affect immune responses. The only exceptions to this rule are the HMB-CoA reductase inhibitors, also known simply as statins. These agents are known to have broad anti-inflammatory effects (although the mechanism for this effect remains controversial) and are safe and generally well tolerated. Pilot data in adults with HIV suggest these drugs might reduce HIV-associated T-cell activation and hence might prove to be beneficial in PWH for reasons independent of their lipid-lowering effects (Ganesan et al., 2011). At least one recent meta-analysis suggests that statins confer moderate mortality benefits in PWH (Uthman et al., 2018), although the drugs are consistently underprescribed for these individuals when compared to their HIV-uninfected counterparts (De Socio et al., 2016; Ladapo et al., 2017; van Zoest et al., 2017). A large clinical endpoint study known as REPRIEVE was started in 2015 with a current full enrollment of 7,770 PWH (Grinspoon et al., 2020). This study may prove that these drugs have unique roles in treated PWH who might not otherwise need them for lipid management.

As noted earlier, many factors contribute to persistent immune activation during therapy, including (1) irreversible breakdown of gut mucosa and subsequent microbial translocation, (2) excess CMV burden and/or enhanced immune responses to CMV (and perhaps other herpesviruses), (3) loss of immunoregulatory cells such as T-reg cells, (4) antiretroviral treatment toxicity, including generation of pro-inflammatory lipids and development of metabolic syndrome, and (5) lymphoid fibrosis, hematopoietic stem cell dysfunction, and thymic dysfunction. Many if not all of these mechanisms can be addressed therapeutically. For example, a number of drugs, including rifaximin (an antibiotic that is not absorbed systemically), sevelamer (which binds LPS/endotoxin in vivo), colostrum-related products (which bind LPS/endotoxin in the gut), chloroquine (which blocks LPS-mediated TLR signaling in myeloid cells), and mesalamine (which is an aspirin-like anti-inflammatory drug used in ulcerative colitis), have been or are being tested as means to reduce the inflammatory consequences of microbial translocation (Byakwaga et al., 2011; Gori et al., 2011; Murray et al., 2010; Piconi et al., 2011). Interventions that aim to restore certain bacterial species to the gut microbiota are also being studied, although a complete characterization of alterations in gut microbiota and related confounders is still needed before such approaches can be effective (Noguera et al., 2016; Vujkovic-Cvijin et al., 2020). Valganciclovir-mediated reduction in CMV has been shown to reduce immune activation in HIV disease (Hunt et al., 2011), and there is new optimism that letermovir may have an even greater effect (Acosta et al., 2020). Growth hormone enhances thymic function and could in theory result eventually in generation of effective immunity (Napolitano et al., 2008). The drugs pirfenidone and angiotensin-converting-enzyme (ACE) inhibitors, among other drugs, are being studied in non-human primates and humans as a means to prevent and/or reverse fibrosis. IL-7 has shown promise as a means to enhance immune function during treated disease (Levy, 2009). Although these studies will provide important insights into the mechanisms of chronic immune activation, it remains unclear how such drugs will eventually be tested in phase III clinical trials. Given the lack of a valid surrogate marker for inflammation and immunodeficiency, clinical endpoint studies will be needed. These studies are large and expensive and would be considered very high risk given the experience with the IL-2 clinical endpoint studies (Abrams et al., 2009). A relevant trial that has overcome some of these hurdles is that of tocilizumab, an IL-6 receptor blocking antibody that has the potential to interfere at a crucial point in the pro-inflammatory cascade (Fumaz et al., 2012; Rodriguez, 2014), but HIV-specific data are still lacking.

Immunomodulatory therapies may also have a contribution to make in developing a regimen that could functionally cure HIV infection, permitting durable suppression of viremia in the absence of ART. The rationale for this idea is that immunomodulators could suppress the chronic inflammation that drives HIV replication. There has been considerable interest in the potential of antibodies to $\alpha_4\beta_7$ integrin to block homing of lymphocytes to gut tissue and thus eliminate the substrate for viral growth in its most important anatomic site (Guzzo et al., 2017). A first-in-human clinical trial (Fauci, 2018) did not confirm early positive signals from SIV models; however, a more recent report demonstrated reduction in both the size and number of lymphoid aggregates in the terminal ileum (Uzzan et al., 2018). This finding is noteworthy because lymphoid aggregates are inductive sites that can support viral replication and possibly contribute to viral reservoirs. Other clinical trials have explored or will explore the immunomodulatory effects of IFN-alpha, TLR-7 agonist, TLR-9 agonist, or even vitamin D (Eckard et al., 2018; Martinsen et al., 2020; Perreau et al., 2017), some of which have shown promising results in SIV-infected non-human primate studies (Lim et al., 2018).

Given the role of chronic inflammation in heart disease and aging, it is hoped that the management of inflammation in PWH might be informed by what is happening in those other disciplines. Daily exercise; a balanced diet rich in fish, legumes, grains, and fresh vegetables (e.g., the Mediterranean diet); prevention of excess weight gain; and aggressive management of traditional risk factors such as hypertension and hyperlipidemia can all have anti-inflammatory aspects and will almost certainly contribute to successful aging in persons with HIV.

REFERENCES

Abrams D, Levy Y, Losso MH, et al. Interleukin-2 therapy in patients with HIV infection. N Engl J Med 2009;361:1548–1559.

Acosta E, Bowlin T, Brooks J, et al. Advances in the development of therapeutics for cytomegalovirus infections. J Infect Dis 2020;221:S32–S44.

Antonelli LR, Mahnke Y, Hodge JN, et al. Elevated frequencies of highly activated CD4+ T cells in HIV+ patients developing immune reconstitution inflammatory syndrome. Blood 2010;116:3818–3827.

Arthos J, Cicala C, Martinelli E, et al. HIV-1 envelope protein binds to and signals through integrin alpha4beta7, the gut mucosal homing receptor for peripheral T cells. Nat Immunol 2008;9:301–309.

Balasko A, Keynan Y. Shedding light on IRIS: from pathophysiology to treatment of cryptococcal meningitis and immune reconstitution inflammatory syndrome in HIV-infected individuals. HIV Med 2019;20:1–10.

Berry NJ, Burns DM, Wannamethee G, et al. Seroepidemiologic studies on the acquisition of antibodies to cytomegalovirus, herpes simplex virus, and human immunodeficiency virus among general hospital patients and those attending a clinic for sexually transmitted diseases. J Med Virol 1988;24:385–393.

Bishop DK, Ferguson RM, Orosz CG. Differential distribution of antigen-specific helper T cells and cytotoxic T cells after antigenic stimulation in vivo. A functional study using limiting dilution analysis. J Immunol 1990;144:1153–1160.

Boulware DR, Meya DB, Bergemann TL, et al. Clinical features and serum biomarkers in HIV immune reconstitution inflammatory syndrome after cryptococcal meningitis: a prospective cohort study. PLoS Med 2010;7:e1000384.

Bourgarit A, Carcelain G, Martinez V, et al. Explosion of tuberculin-specific Th1-responses induces immune restoration syndrome in tuberculosis and HIV co-infected patients. AIDS 2006;20:F1–F7.

Brenchley JM, Paiardini M, Knox KS, et al. Differential Th17 CD4 T-cell depletion in pathogenic and nonpathogenic lentiviral infections. Blood 2008;112:2826–2835.

Brenchley JM, Price DA, Schacker TW, et al. Microbial translocation is a cause of systemic immune activation in chronic HIV infection. Nat Med 2006;12:1365–1371.

Brodin P, Jojic V, Gao T, et al. Variation in the human immune system is largely driven by non-heritable influences. Cell 2015;160:37–47.

Brust D, Polis M, Davey R, et al. Fluorodeoxyglucose imaging in healthy subjects with HIV infection: impact of disease stage and therapy on pattern of nodal activation. AIDS 2006;20:495–503.

Bujdoso R, Young P, Hopkins, et al. Non-random migration of CD4 and CD8 T cells: changes in the CD4: CD8 ratio and interleukin 2 responsiveness of efferent lymph cells following in vivo antigen challenge. Eur J Immunol 1989;19:1779–1784.

Byakwaga H, Kelly M, Purcell DF, et al. Intensification of antiretroviral therapy with raltegravir or addition of hyperimmune bovine colostrum in HIV-infected patients with suboptimal CD4+ T-cell response: a randomized controlled trial. J Infect Dis 2011;204:1532–1540.

Casado C, Marrero-Hernández S, Márquez-Arce D, et al. Viral characteristics associated with the clinical nonprogressor phenotype are inherited by viruses from a cluster of HIV-1 elite controllers. mBio 2018;9, e02338-17.

Chen H, Li C, Huang J, et al. CD4+ T cells from elite controllers resist HIV-1 infection by selective upregulation of p21. J Clin Invest 2011;121:1549–1560.

Cho S, Knox KS, Kohli LM, et al. Impaired cell surface expression of human CD1d by the formation of an HIV-1 Nef/CD1d complex. Virology 2005;337:242–252.

Church LWP, Chopra A, Judson MA. Paradoxical reactions and the immune reconstitution inflammatory syndrome. Microbiol Spectr 2017;5(2).

Coleman CM, Wu L. HIV interactions with monocytes and dendritic cells: viral latency and reservoirs. Retrovirology 2009;6:51.

Côrtes FH, de Paula HHS, Bello G, et al. Plasmatic levels of IL-18, IP-10, and activated CD8(+) T cells are potential biomarkers to identify HIV-1 elite controllers with a true functional cure profile. Front Immunol 2018;9:1576.

Couturier J, Agarwal N, Nehete PN, et al. Infectious SIV resides in adipose tissue and induces metabolic defects in chronically infected rhesus macaques. Retrovirology 2016;13:30.

Couturier J, Suliburk JW, Brown JM. Human adipose tissue as a reservoir for memory CD4+ T cells and HIV. AIDS 2015;29:667–674.

Crakes KR, Santos Rocha C, Grishina I, et al. PPARα-targeted mitochondrial bioenergetics mediate repair of intestinal barriers at the host-microbe intersection during SIV infection. Proc Natl Acad Sci USA 2019;I16:24819–24829.

Damouche A, Lazure T, Avettand-Fenoel V, et al. Adipose tissue is a neglected viral reservoir and an inflammatory site during chronic HIV and SIV infection. PLoS Pathog 2015;11:e1005153.

Damouche A, Pourcher G, Pourcher A. High proportion of PD-1-expressing CD4(+) T cells in adipose tissue constitutes an immunomodulatory microenvironment that may support HIV persistence. Eur J Immunol 2017;47:2113–2123.

Decrion AZ, Dichamp I, Varin A, et al. HIV and inflammation. Curr HIV Res 2005;3:243–259.

Deeks SG. HIV infection, inflammation, immunosenescence, and aging. Annu Rev Med 2011;62:141–155.

Deeks SG, Walker BD. Human immunodeficiency virus controllers: mechanisms of durable virus control in the absence of antiretroviral therapy. Immunity 2007;27:406–416.

De Socio GV, Ricci E, Parruti G, et al. Statins and aspirin use in HIV-infected people: gap between European AIDS Clinical Society guidelines and clinical practice: the results from HIV-HY study. Infection 2016;44:589–597.

Doisne JM, Urrutia A, Lacabaratz-Porret C, et al. CD8+ T cells specific for EBV, cytomegalovirus, and influenza virus are activated during primary HIV infection. J Immunol 2004;173:2410–2418.

Douek D, Picker LJ, Koup RA. T cell dynamics in HIV-1 infection. Annu Rev Immunol 2003;21:265–304.

Dupin N, Buffet M, Marcelin AG, et al. HIV and antiretroviral drug distribution in plasma and fat tissue of HIV-infected patients with lipodystrophy. AIDS 2002;16:2419–2424.

Eckard AR, O'Riordan MA, Rosebush JC, et al. Vitamin D supplementation decreases immune activation and exhaustion in HIV-1-infected youth. Antivir Ther 2018;23(4):315–324.

Erikstrup C, Kallestrup P, Zinyama-Gutsire RB, et al. Reduced mortality and CD4 cell loss among carriers of the interleukin-10 -1082G allele in a Zimbabwean cohort of HIV-1-infected adults. AIDS 2007;21:2283–2291.

Estes JD, Haase AT, Schacker TW. The role of collagen deposition in depleting CD4+ T cells and limiting reconstitution in HIV-1 and SIV infections through damage to the secondary lymphoid organ niche. Semin Immunol 2008;20:181–186.

Fan Y, Gao X, Chen J, et al. HIV Tat impairs neurogenesis through functioning as a Notch ligand and activation of Notch signaling pathway. J Neurosci 2016;36:11362–11373.

Fauci AS. Durable control of HIV infections in the absence of antiretroviral therapy: opportunities and obstacles. In: AIDS 2018, Amsterdam, The Netherlands.

Favre D, Lederer S, Kanwar B, et al. Critical loss of the balance between Th17 and T regulatory cell populations in pathogenic SIV infection. PLoS Pathog 2009;5:e1000295.

French MA, Price P, Stone SF. Immune restoration disease after antiretroviral therapy. AIDS 2004;18:1615–1627.

Fumaz CR, Gonzalez-Garcia M, Borras X, et al. Psychological stress is associated with high levels of IL-6 in HIV-1 infected individuals on effective combined antiretroviral treatment. Brain Behav Immun 2012;26:568–572.

Ganesan A, Crum-Cianflone N, Higgins J, et al. High dose atorvastatin decreases cellular markers of immune activation without affecting HIV-1 RNA levels: results of a double-blind randomized placebo controlled clinical trial. J Infect Dis 2011;203:756–764.

Giorgi JV, Hultin LE, McKeating JA, et al. Shorter survival in advanced human immunodeficiency virus type 1 infection is more closely associated with T lymphocyte activation than with plasma virus burden or virus chemokine coreceptor usage. J Infect Dis 1999;179:859–870.

Giuliani E, Vassena L, Di Cesare S, et al. NK cells of HIV-1-infected patients with poor CD4(+) T-cell reconstitution despite suppressive HAART show reduced IFN-gamma production and high frequency of autoreactive CD56(bright) cells. Immunol Lett 2017;190:185–193.

Gómez-Mora E, García E, Urrea V, et al. Preserved immune functionality and high CMV-specific T-cell responses in HIV-infected individuals with poor CD4(+) T-cell immune recovery. Sci Rep 2017;7:11711.

Gori A, Rizzardini G, Van't Land B, et al. Specific prebiotics modulate gut microbiota and immune activation in HAART-naive HIV-infected adults: results of the "COPA" pilot randomized trial. Mucosal Immunol 2011;4:554–563.

Goulder P, Deeks SG. HIV control: is getting there the same as staying there? PLoS Pathog 2018;14:e1007222.

Gras L, May M, Ryder LP, et al. Determinants of restoration of CD4 and CD8 cell counts and their ratio in HIV-1-positive individuals with sustained virological suppression on antiretroviral therapy. J Acquir Immune Defic Syndr 2019;80:292–300.

Grinspoon SL, Douglas PS, Hoffman UD, et al. Leveraging a landmark trial for primary cardiovascular disease prevention in human immunodeficiency virus: introduction from the REPRIEVE coprincipal investigators. J Infect Dis 2020;222:S1–S7.

Grossman Z, Meier-Schellersheim M, Sousa AE. CD4+ T-cell depletion in HIV infection: are we closer to understanding the cause? Nat Med 2002;8:319–323.

Guadalupe M, Reay E, Sankaran S. Severe CD4+ T-cell depletion in gut lymphoid tissue during primary human immunodeficiency virus type 1 infection and substantial delay in restoration following highly active antiretroviral therapy. J Virol 2003;77:11708–11717.

Guillén Y, Noguera-Julian M, Rivera J, et al. Low nadir CD4+ T-cell counts predict gut dysbiosis in HIV-1 infection. Mucosal Immunol 2019;12:232–246.

Guzzo C, Ichikawa D, Park C, et al. Virion incorporation of integrin alpha4beta7 facilitates HIV-1 infection and intestinal homing. Sci Immunol 2017;2(11):eaam7341.

Hage CA, Kohli LL, Cho S, et al. Human immunodeficiency virus gp120 downregulates CD1d cell surface expression. Immunol Lett 2005;98:131–135.

Hammoud DA, Boulougoura A, Papadakis GZ, et al. Increased metabolic activity on 18F-fluorodeoxyglucose positron emission tomography-computed tomography in human immunodeficiency virus-associated immune reconstitution inflammatory syndrome. Clin Infect Dis 2019;68:229–238.

Hansen SG, Piatak M Jr, Ventura AB, et al. Immune clearance of highly pathogenic SIV infection. Nature 2013a;502:100–104.

Hansen SG, Sacha JB, Hughes CM, et al. Cytomegalovirus vectors violate CD8+ T cell epitope recognition paradigms. Science 2013b;340:1237874.

Hartigan-O'Connor DJ, Abel K, Van Rompay KKA, et al. SIV replication in the infected rhesus macaque is limited by the size of the pre-existing TH17 cell compartment. Sci Transl Med 2012;4:136ra169.

Hartigan-O'Connor DJ, Jacobson MA, et al. Development of cytomegalovirus (CMV) immune recovery uveitis is associated with Th17 cell depletion and poor systemic CMV-specific T cell responses. Clin Infect Dis 2011;52:409–417.

Hatano H, Delwart EL, Norris PJ, et al. Evidence for persistent low-level viremia in individuals who control human immunodeficiency virus in the absence of antiretroviral therapy. J Virol 2009;83:329–335.

He X, Eddy JJ, Jacobson KR, et al. Enhanced HIV-1 replication in CD4+ T cells derived from individuals with latent mycobacterium tuberculosis infection. J Infect Dis 2020;222(9):1550–1560.

Heise C, Miller CJ, Lackner A, et al. Primary acute simian immunodeficiency virus infection of intestinal lymphoid tissue is associated with gastrointestinal dysfunction. J Infect Dis 1994;169:1116–1120.

Hellerstein M, Hanley MB, Cesar D. Directly measured kinetics of circulating T lymphocytes in normal and HIV-1-infected humans. Nat Med 1999;5:83–89.

Hirao LA, Grishina I, Bourry O, Early mucosal sensing of SIV infection by paneth cells induces IL-1beta production and initiates gut epithelial disruption. PLoS Pathog 2014;10:e1004311.

Hrecka K, Hao C, Gierszewska M, et al. Vpx relieves inhibition of HIV-1 infection of macrophages mediated by the SAMHD1 protein. Nature 2011;474:658–661.

Hsu DC, Wegner MD, Sunyakumthorn P, et al. CD4+ cell infiltration into subcutaneous adipose tissue is not indicative of productively infected cells during acute SHIV infection. J Med Primatol 2017;46:154–157.

Hsue PY, Hunt PW, Schnell A, et al. Role of viral replication, antiretroviral therapy, and immunodeficiency in HIV-associated atherosclerosis. AIDS 2009;23:1059–1067.

Hunt PW, Brenchley J, Sinclair E. Relationship between T cell activation and CD4+ T cell count in HIV-seropositive individuals with undetectable plasma HIV RNA levels in the absence of therapy. J Infect Dis 2008;197:126–133.

Hunt PW, Martin JN, Sinclair E, et al. Valganciclovir reduces T cell activation in HIV-infected individuals with incomplete CD4+ T cell recovery on antiretroviral therapy. J Infect Dis 2011;203:1474–1483.

Hwang I, Zhang T, Scott JM, et al. Identification of human NK cells that are deficient for signaling adaptor FcRgamma and specialized for antibody-dependent immune functions. Int Immunol 2012;24:793–802.

Jones JL, Phuah CL, Cox AL, et al. IL-21 drives secondary autoimmunity in patients with multiple sclerosis, following therapeutic lymphocyte depletion with alemtuzumab (Campath-1H). J Clin Invest 2009;119:2052–2061.

Ke R, Cong ME, Li D, et al. On the death rate of abortively infected cells: estimation from simian-human immunodeficiency virus infection. J Virol 2017;91(18):e00352-17.

Kelley CF, Kitchen CM, Hunt PW, et al. Incomplete peripheral CD4(+) cell count restoration in HIV-infected patients receiving long-term antiretroviral treatment. Clin Infect Dis 2009;48:787–794.

King C, Ilic A, Koelsch K, et al. Homeostatic expansion of T cells during immune insufficiency generates autoimmunity. Cell 2004;117:265–277.

Koethe JR, McDonnell W, Kennedy A, et al. Adipose tissue is enriched for activated and late-differentiated CD8+ T cells and shows distinct CD8+ receptor usage, compared with blood in HIV-infected persons. J Acquir Immune Defic Syndr 2018;77:e14–e21.

Ladapo JA, Richards AK, DeWitt CM, et al. Disparities in the quality of cardiovascular care between HIV-infected versus HIV-uninfected adults in the United States: a cross-sectional study. J Am Heart Assoc 2017;6(11):e007107.

Laguette MJ, Abrahams Y, Prince S, et al. Sequence variants within the 3'-UTR of the COL5A1 gene alters mRNA stability: implications for musculoskeletal soft tissue injuries. Matrix Biol. 2011;30(5-6):338–345.

Lang DJ, Kovacs AA, Zaia JA, et al. Seroepidemiologic studies of cytomegalovirus and Epstein-Barr virus infections in relation to human immunodeficiency virus type 1 infection in selected recipient populations. Transfusion Safety Study Group. J Acquir Immune Defic Syndr 1989;2:540–549.

Lawn SD, Myer L, Bekker LG. Tuberculosis-associated immune reconstitution disease: incidence, risk factors and impact in an antiretroviral treatment service in South Africa. AIDS 2007;21:335–341.

Lee J, Zhang T, Hwang I, et al. Epigenetic modification and antibody-dependent expansion of memory-like NK cells in human cytomegalovirus-infected individuals. Immunity 2015;42:431–442.

Lenardo MJ, Angleman SB, Bounkeua C, et al. Cytopathic killing of peripheral blood CD4(+) T lymphocytes by human immunodeficiency virus type 1 appears necrotic rather than apoptotic and does not require env. J Virol 2002;76:5082–5093.

Lenkei R, Andersson B. High correlations of anti-CMV titers with lymphocyte activation status and CD57 antibody-binding capacity as estimated with three-color, quantitative flow cytometry in blood donors. Clin Immunol Immunopathol 1995;77:131–138.

Levy Y, Lacabaratz C, Weiss L, et al. Enhanced T cell recovery in HIV-1-infected adults through IL-7 treatment. J Clin Invest 2009;119:997–1007.

Li D, Xu XN. NKT cells in HIV-1 infection. Cell Res 2008;18:817–822.

Lim SY, Osuna CE, Hraber PT, et al. TLR7 agonists induce transient viremia and reduce the viral reservoir in SIV-infected rhesus macaques on antiretroviral therapy. Sci Transl Med 2018;10(439):eaao4521.

Link A, Vogt TK, Favre S, et al. Fibroblastic reticular cells in lymph nodes regulate the homeostasis of naive T cells. Nat Immunol 2007;8:1255–1265.

Lopez-Verges S, Milush JM, Schwartz BS, et al. Expansion of a unique CD57(+)NKG2Chi natural killer cell subset during acute human cytomegalovirus infection. Proc Natl Acad Sci USA 2011;108:14725–14732.

Manel N, Hogstad B, Wang Y, et al. A cryptic sensor for HIV-1 activates antiviral innate immunity in dendritic cells. Nature 2010;467:214–217.

Margolick JB, Bream JH, Nilles TL, et al. Relationship between T-cell responses to CMV, markers of inflammation, and frailty in HIV-uninfected and HIV-infected men in the Multicenter AIDS Cohort Study. J Infect Dis 2018;218(2):249–258.

Martin MP, Qi Y, Gao X. Innate partnership of HLA-B and KIR3DL1 subtypes against HIV-1. Nat Genet 2007;39:733–740.

Martinsen JT, Gunst JD, Højen JF, et al. The use of Toll-like receptor agonists in HIV-1 cure strategies. Front Immunol 2020;11:1112.

McCune JM. The dynamics of CD4+ T-cell depletion in HIV disease. Nature 2001;410:974–979.

Meintjes G, Wilkinson RJ, Morroni C, et al. Randomized placebo-controlled trial of prednisone for paradoxical tuberculosis-associated immune reconstitution inflammatory syndrome. AIDS 2010;24:2381–2390.

Mens H, Kearney M, Wiegand A, et al. HIV-1 continues to replicate and evolve in patients with natural control of HIV infection. J Virol 2010;84(24):12971–12981.

Migueles SA, Connors M. Long-term nonprogressive disease among untreated HIV-infected individuals: clinical implications of understanding immune control of HIV. JAMA 2010;304:194–201.

Mocroft A, Phillips AN, Gatell J, et al. Normalisation of CD4 counts in patients with HIV-1 infection and maximum virological suppression who are taking combination antiretroviral therapy: an observational cohort study. Lancet 2007;370:407–413.

Muenchhoff M, Adland E, Karimanzira O, et al. Nonprogressing HIV-infected children share fundamental immunological features of nonpathogenic SIV infection. Sci Transl Med 2016;8:358ra125.

Muller M, Wandel S, Colebunders R. Immune reconstitution inflammatory syndrome in patients starting antiretroviral therapy for HIV infection: a systematic review and meta-analysis. Lancet Infect Dis 2010;10: 251–261.

Murray SM, Down CM, Boulware DR, et al. Reduction of immune activation with chloroquine therapy during chronic HIV infection. J Virol 2010;84:12082–12086.

Naeger DM, Martin JN, Sinclair E, et al. Cytomegalovirus-specific T cells persist at very high levels during long-term antiretroviral treatment of HIV disease. PLoS One 2010;5:e8886.

Napolitano LA, Schmidt D, Gotway MB, et al. Growth hormone enhances thymic function in HIV-1-infected adults. J Clin Invest 2008;118(3):1085–1098.

Nawaz F, Goes LR, Ray JC, et al. MAdCAM costimulation through integrin-α(4)β(7) promotes HIV replication. Mucosal Immunol 2018;1:1342–1351.

Ndhlovu ZM, Kamya P, Mewalal N, et al. Magnitude and kinetics of CD8+ T cell activation during hyperacute HIV infection impact viral set point. Immunity 2015;43:591–604.

Negredo E, Massanella M, Puertas MC, et al. Early but limited effects of raltegravir intensification on CD4 T cell reconstitution in HIV-infected patients with an immunodiscordant response to antiretroviral therapy. J Antimicrob Chemother 2013;68:2358–2362.

Neuhaus J, Jacobs DR Jr, Baker JV, et al. Markers of inflammation, coagulation, and renal function are elevated in adults with HIV infection. J Infect Dis 2010;201:1788–1795.

Noguera-Julian M, Rocafort M, Guillén Y, et al. Gut microbiota linked to sexual preference and HIV infection. EBioMedicine 2016;5:135–146.

Nussenblatt RB, Lane HC. Human immunodeficiency virus disease: changing patterns of intraocular inflammation. Am J Ophthalmol 1998;125:374–382.

O'Connell KA, Rabi SA, Siliciano RF. CD4+ T cells from elite suppressors are more susceptible to HIV-1 but produce fewer virions than cells from chronic progressors. Proc Nat Acad Sci USA 2011;108:E689–E698.

Pakker NG, Notermans DW, de Boer RJ, et al. Biphasic kinetics of peripheral blood T cells after triple combination therapy in HIV-1 infection: a composite of redistribution and proliferation. Nat Med 1998;4:208–214.

Palesch D, Bosinger SE, Tharp GK, et al. Sooty mangabey genome sequence provides insight into AIDS resistance in a natural SIV host. Nature 2018;553:77–81.

Pandiyan P, Younes SA, Ribeiro SP, et al. Mucosal regulatory T cells and T helper 17 cells in HIV-associated immune activation. Front Immunol 2016;7:228.

Papagno L, Spina CA, Marchant A, et al. Immune activation and CD8(+) T-cell differentiation towards senescence in HIV-1 infection. PLoS Biol 2004;2:E20.

Parrinello CM, Sinclair E, Landay AL, et al. Cytomegalovirus immunoglobulin G antibody is associated with subclinical carotid artery disease among HIV-infected women. J Infect Dis 2012;205:1788–1796.

Pereyra F, Jia X, McLaren PJ, et al. The major genetic determinants of HIV-1 control affect HLA class I peptide presentation. Science 2010;330:1551–1557.

Perez-Matute P, Perez-Martinez L, Aguilera-Lizarraga J, et al. Maraviroc modifies gut microbiota composition in a mouse model of obesity: a plausible therapeutic option to prevent metabolic disorders in HIV-infected patients. Rev Esp Quimioter 2015;28:200–206.

Perreau M, Banga R, Pantaleo G. Targeted immune interventions for an HIV-1 cure. Trends Mol Med 2017;23:945–961.

Piconi S, Parisotto S, Rizzardini G, et al. Hydroxychloroquine drastically reduces immune activation in HIV-infected, antiretroviral therapy-treated immunologic nonresponders. Blood 2011;118:3263–3272.

Raffatellu M, Santos RL, Verhoeven DE, et al. Simian immunodeficiency virus-induced mucosal interleukin-17 deficiency promotes Salmonella dissemination from the gut. Nat Med 2008;14:421–428.

Reeves RK, Li H, Jost S, et al. Antigen-specific NK cell memory in rhesus macaques. Nat Immunol 2015;16:927–932.

Rodriguez B. AIDS 347: IL-6 blockade in treated HIV infection. 2014. ClinicalTrialsgov.

Roederer M, Dubs JG, Anderson MT, et al. CD8 naive T cell counts decrease progressively in HIV-infected adults. J Clin Invest 1995;95:2061–2066.

Ruffin N, Hani L, Seddiki N. From dendritic cells to B cells dysfunctions during HIV-1 infection: T follicular helper cells at the crossroads. Immunology 2017;151:137–145.

Ruiz-Riol M, Berdnik D, Llano A, et al. Identification of interleukin-27 (IL-27)/IL-27 receptor subunit alpha as a critical immune axis for in vivo HIV control. J Virol 2017;91(16):e00441-17.

Saez-Cirion A, Hamimi C, Bergamaschi A, et al. Restriction of HIV-1 replication in macrophages and CD4+ T cells from HIV controllers. Blood 2011;118:955–964.

Sáez-Cirión A, Sereti I. Immunometabolism and HIV-1 pathogenesis: food for thought. Nat Rev Immunol 2021;21(1):5–19.

Samal J, Kelly S, Na-Shatal A, et al. Human immunodeficiency virus infection induces lymphoid fibrosis in the BM-liver-thymus-spleen humanized mouse model. JCI Insight 2018;3(18):e120430.

Sandberg JK, Fast NM, Palacios EH, et al. Selective loss of innate CD4(+) V alpha 24 natural killer T cells in human immunodeficiency virus infection. J Virol 2002;76:7528–7534.

Sauce D, Larsen M, Fastenackels S, et al. HIV disease progression despite suppression of viral replication is associated with exhaustion of lymphopoiesis. Blood 2011;117(19):5142–5151.

Schacker TW, Nguyen PL, Beilman GJ, et al. Collagen deposition in HIV-1 infected lymphatic tissues and T cell homeostasis. J Clin Invest 2002;110:1133–1139.

Scriven JE, Rhein J, Hullsiek KH, et al. Early ART after cryptococcal meningitis is associated with cerebrospinal fluid pleocytosis and macrophage activation in a multisite randomized trial. J Infect Dis 2015;212:769–778.

Seddiki N, Sasson SC, Santner-Nanan B, et al. Proliferation of weakly suppressive regulatory CD4+ T cells is associated with over-active CD4+ T-cell responses in HIV-positive patients with mycobacterial immune restoration disease. Eur J Immunol 2009;39: 391–403.

Silvestri G, Sodora DL, Koup RA, et al. Nonpathogenic SIV infection of sooty mangabeys is characterized by limited bystander immunopathology despite chronic high-level viremia. Immunity 2003;18:441–452.

Sips M, Sciaranghella G, Diefenbach T, et al. Altered distribution of mucosal NK cells during HIV infection. Mucosal Imunol 2012;5:30–40.

Sivro A, Schuetz A, Sheward D, et al. Integrin α(4)β(7) expression on peripheral blood CD4(+) T cells predicts HIV acquisition and disease progression outcomes. Sci Transl Med 2018;10(425):eaam6354.

Srinivasula S, Lempicki RA, Adelsberger JW, et al. Differential effects of HIV viral load and CD4 count on proliferation of naive and memory CD4 and CD8 T lymphocytes. Blood 2011;118:262–270.

Stacey AR, Norris PJ, Qin L, et al. Induction of a striking systemic cytokine cascade prior to peak viremia in acute human immunodeficiency virus type 1 infection, in contrast to more modest and delayed responses in acute hepatitis B and C virus infections. J Virol 2009;83:3719–3733.

Sun JC, Beilke JN, Lanier LL. Adaptive immune features of natural killer cells. Nature 2009;457:557–561.

Surh CD, Sprent J. Homeostasis of naive and memory T cells. Immunity 2008;29:848–862.

Sylwester AW, Mitchell BL, Edgar JB, et al. Broadly targeted human cytomegalovirus-specific CD4+ and CD8+ T cells dominate the memory compartments of exposed subjects. J Exp Med 2005;202:673–685.

Uthman OA, Nduka C, Watson SI, et al. Statin use and all-cause mortality in people living with HIV: a systematic review and meta-analysis. BMC Infect Dis 2018;18:258.

Uzzan M, Tokuyama M, Rosenstein AK, et al. Anti-α4β7 therapy targets lymphoid aggregates in the gastrointestinal tract of HIV-1-infected individuals. Sci Transl Med 2018;10(461):eaau4711.

van der Vliet HJ, von Blomberg BM, Hazenberg MD, et al. Selective decrease in circulating V alpha 24+V beta 11+ NKT cells during HIV type 1 infection. J Immunol 2002;168:1490–1495.

van Grevenynghe J, Procopio FA, He Z. Transcription factor FOXO3a controls the persistence of memory CD4(+) T cells during HIV infection. Nat Med 2008;14:266–274.

van Zoest RA, van der Valk M, Wit FW, et al. Suboptimal primary and secondary cardiovascular disease prevention in HIV-positive individuals on antiretroviral therapy. Eur J Prev Cardiol 2017;24:1297–1307.

Veazey RS, DeMaria M, Chalifoux LV, et al. Gastrointestinal tract as a major site of CD4+ T cell depletion and viral replication in SIV infection. Science 1998;280:427–431.

Vujkovic-Cvijin I, Dunham RM, Iwai S, et al. Dysbiosis of the gut microbiota is associated with HIV disease progression and tryptophan catabolism. Sci Transl Med 2013;5:193ra191.

Vujkovic-Cvijin I, Sortino O, Verheij E, et al. HIV-associated gut dysbiosis is independent of sexual practice and correlates with noncommunicable diseases. Nat Commun 2020;11:2448.

Walker NF, Stek C, Wasserman S, et al. The tuberculosis-associated immune reconstitution inflammatory syndrome: recent advances in clinical and pathogenesis research. Curr Opin HIV AIDS 2018;13:512–521.

Williams WB, Liao HX, Moody MA. Diversion of HIV-1 vaccine-induced immunity by gp41-microbiota cross-reactive antibodies. Science 2015;349:aab1253.

Yoon HA, Nakouzi A, Chang CC, et al. Association between plasma antibody responses and risk for cryptococcus-associated immune reconstitution inflammatory syndrome. J Infect Dis 2019;219:420–428.

Zeng M, Southern PJ, Reilly CS, et al. Lymphoid tissue damage in HIV-1 infection depletes naive T cells and limits T cell reconstitution after antiretroviral therapy. PLoS Pathog 2012;8:e1002437.

Zhang T, Scott JM, Hwang I. Cutting edge: antibody-dependent memory-like NK cells distinguished by FcRgamma deficiency. J Immunol 2013;190:1402–1406.

Zhou J, Amran FS, Kramski M, et al An NK cell population lacking FcRgamma is expanded in chronically infected HIV patients. J Immunol 2015;194:4688–4697.

7.

HIV TESTING AND COUNSELING

Alejandro Delgado

CHAPTER GOALS

Upon completion of this chapter, the reader should be able to:

- Describe the types of HIV testing

- Prepare an overview of HIV counseling, as well as how to adapt counseling to the variety of situations or environments in which these conversations can take place

- Initiate early HIV therapy

HIV TESTING: HISTORY AND EVOLUTION

In 1985, when HIV testing first became available, the main goal of testing was for blood banks to screen the US blood supply. When it was discovered that those who simply wished to learn their HIV status were using blood donation testing sites, alternative testing sites were implemented. Because at that time no treatment was available and routes of transmission were still being investigated, opinion was divided about the value of testing. By 1987, the implications of a positive HIV serology were clear, and the US Public Health Service and the Centers for Disease Control and Prevention (CDC) issued the first set of guidelines for HIV testing and counseling (CDC, 1987). Earlier guidelines targeted those in "high-risk groups," but experience taught that a more productive approach focused on behaviors rather than membership in a particular population. Hence, the thrust of the current guidelines is that HIV screening is recommended for all persons aged 13 to 65 years, regardless of risk factors. Periodic revisions informed by the epidemiology of the pandemic extended the outreach and flexibility of testing, culminating in the "Revised Recommendations for HIV Testing of Adults, Adolescents, and Pregnant Women in Health-Care Settings" (Branson et al., 2006).

LEARNING OBJECTIVES

- List and describe the types of HIV testing.

- Present an overview of HIV counseling as well as how to adapt counseling to the variety of situations or environments in which these conversations can take place.

WHAT'S NEW?

- During the past decade, the evidence favoring the early institution of therapy for HIV has been steadily growing, showing benefits in virologic control and decreased transmission of HIV. The World Health Organization (WHO) has published data from 2017 showing that the proportion of low- to middle-income countries that have adopted the "Treat All ART initiation" has increased from 33% to 70%.

- The most recent data published in 2018 by the CDC estimate that approximately 14% of people living with HIV are unaware of their diagnosis. In certain states and among men who have sex with men (MSM), who constitute 82% of new yearly diagnoses, the percentage of people who are unaware of their HIV infection may be as high as 25%, prompting the CDC to update its HIV screening recommendations for the MSM population.

- In June 2014, the CDC revised its testing algorithm favoring the use of fourth-generation assays that are capable of early detection of HIV-1 and HIV-2 antibodies as well as the p24 antigen. This has substantially narrowed the window between initial infection and positive test results. For the first time since 1989, the CDC has eliminated the use of confirmation testing with a first-generation western blot or immunofluorescence assay, now recommending that a nucleic acid amplification test (NAAT) be used (Figure 7.1).

KEY POINTS

- HIV testing should be offered as part of routine medical care to all people. The US Preventive Services Task Force put forth recommendations in 2013 that clinicians screen all people between the ages of 15 and 65 years. Testing in younger and older persons should be offered when special circumstances deem this appropriate.

- The CDC recommends that clinicians screen asymptomatic sexually active MSM at least annually and more frequently (i.e., every 3 or 6 months) for MSM at increased risk for HIV infection.

- All persons screened for HIV should be counseled regarding risk-reduction strategies, including preexposure

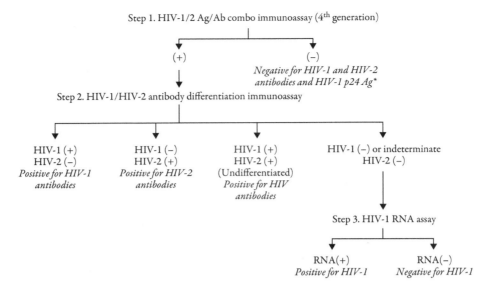

HIV Diagnostic Testing Algorithm

Step 1. HIV-1/2 Ag/Ab combo immunoassay (4th generation)

(+)

(−)
Negative for HIV-1 and HIV-2 antibodies and HIV-1 p24 Ag*

Step 2. HIV-1/HIV-2 antibody differentiation immunoassay

HIV-1 (+)
HIV-2 (−)
Positive for HIV-1 antibodies

HIV-1 (−)
HIV-2 (+)
Positive for HIV-2 antibodies

HIV-1 (+)
HIV-2 (+)
(Undifferentiated)
Positive for HIV antibodies

HIV-1 (−) or indeterminate
HIV-2 (−)

Step 3. HIV-1 RNA assay

RNA(+)
Positive for HIV-1

RNA(−)
Negative for HIV-1

(+) = Reactive (or repeatedly reactive) test result, in accordance with manufacturer's instructions
(−) = Nonreactive test result, in accordance with manufacturer's instructions
Italics = Final interpretation; No further testing indicated for the specimen
*For 3rd generation HIV-1/2 immunoassay, interpretation is 'Negative for HIV-1 and HIV-2 antibodies'.

Figure 7.1 Recommended laboratory HIV testing algorithm for serum or plasma specimens   SOURCE: Centers for Disease Control and Prevention and Association of Public Health Laboratories. Laboratory Testing for the Diagnosis of HIV Infection: Updated Recommendations. Available at http://dx.doi.org/10.15620/cdc.23447. Published June 27, 2014.

prophylaxis (PrEP) and other prevention methods, depending on test results.

- All pregnant women should be screened for HIV at the earliest instance possible.

HIV TESTING TERMINOLOGY, TYPES, AND ALGORITHM

Initially, the CDC guidelines focused on the diagnosis of HIV-1 using a sensitive antibody immunoassay with validation of those results by a more specific test such as the western blot or indirect immunofluorescence assay. By 1992, the guidelines also included testing recommendations for the diagnosis of HIV-2. In 2004, protocols for rapid antibody test results were issued with recommendations that all rapid testing be confirmed with either western blot or immunofluorescence assay. With the advent of improved immunoassays and tests, recommendations regarding HIV diagnostic testing have undergone changes.

The CDC's guidelines for laboratory testing for HIV are outlined in an algorithm (Figure 7.1). Initial testing should be done with an antigen/antibody combination immunoassay that detects both HIV-1 and HIV-2 antibodies and HIV-1 p24 antigen. If a positive result is obtained, the specimen should be tested with an antibody immunoassay that differentiates HIV-1 and HIV-2 antibodies. In the situation of a reactive antigen/antibody combination immunoassay with a nonreactive or indeterminate HIV-1/HIV-2 antibody differentiation immunoassay, the specimen should be further tested with an HIV-1 nucleic acid test. If the nucleic acid test

is reactive, then it indicates acute HIV infection if the antibody differentiation immunoassay was negative. If the antibody differentiation immunoassay was indeterminate and the nucleic acid test is reactive, this indicates confirmed infection. A negative nucleic acid test indicates a false-positive result of the initial immunoassay.

Table 7.1 enumerates the various types of HIV testing and associated terminology.

LABORATORY MARKERS FOR HIV

There is a brief period immediately after HIV infection where no laboratory markers can be detected in plasma; this is termed the *eclipse period*. After about 5 to 10 days of infection, HIV RNA can be detected by nucleic acid tests, followed by HIV-1 p24 antigen within 4 to 10 days after RNA is detected. HIV-1 p24 antigen is detected by fourth-generation immunoassays, but, as antibodies begin developing, the p24 antigens begin forming immune complexes with the antibodies and become no longer detectable. Immunoglobulin M antibodies start to be expressed about 3 to 5 days after the p24 antigen is detected, and these are detected by third- and fourth-generation immunoassays. This is followed by immunoglobulin G antibodies, which will remain throughout the course of the infection Figure 7.2 (Branson et al., 2014).

WHO SHOULD BE TESTED?

HIV testing should be undertaken in anyone who has symptoms and signs of acute or chronic HIV infection.

Table 7.1 HIV TESTING TERMINOLOGY

TEST TYPE	DESCRIPTION
Anonymous testing	No identifying information links the patient to the test sample. At the time of testing, the patient is handed a code number, and a matching code number is affixed to the sample. No institutional record of the code is kept. Results are given only verbally because no medical record is created. Treatment cannot be instituted based on this form of testing. Useful for personal informational purposes.
Confidential testing	Test is linked to patient identifiers, and access to results is available for review only by those identified within "need to know" medical standards, including local, state, and national (e.g., CDC) public health agencies.
Screening	Performing an HIV test for all persons in a defined population. For individual patients, screening is most cost-effective through an antibody-based test, the most common of which is the enzyme-linked immunosorbent assay (ELISA).
Opt-in screening	Patient approaches the provider and requests HIV testing.
Opt-out screening	Healthcare provider offers routine HIV testing to all patients unless refused by patient.
Point-of-care or rapid testing	Simplified antibody- or antibody- and antigen-based testing procedure that can give a screening-level result in approximately 20 minutes or less and that can be implemented by a trained non-healthcare individual.
Diagnostic testing	Testing prompted by the presence of clinical signs or symptoms. The term may also refer to the antigen-based confirmation of a positive ELISA. In the US, the validation test formerly used most often was the western blot analysis. New CDC guidelines now recommend using a fourth-generation HIV Ag/Ab enzyme immunoassay test or HIV RNA test for diagnostic confirmation. The validation testing may also be referred to as *confirmatory testing*.
Targeted testing	Performing an HIV test on persons perceived to be at higher risk, as defined by behavioral, clinical, or demographic characteristics. Formerly the main strategy for HIV testing, it has been supplanted by the recommendation to treat HIV screening as a routine part of medical care.

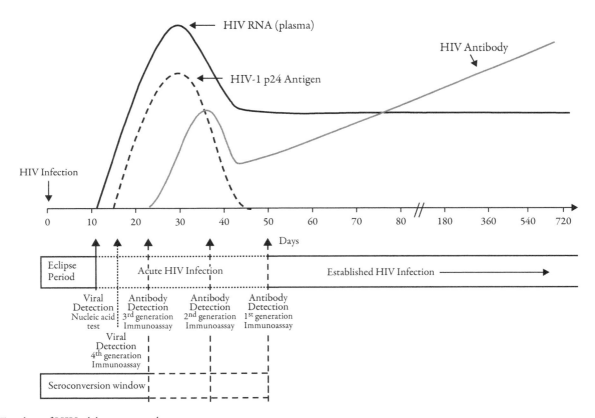

Figure 7.2 Timeline of HIV-1 laboratory markers   SOURCE: Centers for Disease Control and Prevention and Association of Public Health Laboratories. Laboratory Testing for the Diagnosis of HIV Infection: Updated Recommendations. Available at http://dx.doi.org/10.15620/cdc.23447. Published June 27, 2014. Accessed September 12, 2020.

In the healthcare setting, every individual between the ages 13 and 65 should be offered testing once in their lifetime. For higher-risk groups, repeat testing may be indicated. Healthcare providers should offer yearly testing to at-risk groups such as persons who inject drugs, people who engage in sex with an HIV-positive partner, people who exchange money for sex, MSM, or heterosexual persons who have had one more sex partner since their last HIV test. These individuals should be offered annual testing or more frequently if indicated by their risk factors.

Unless recent HIV test results are immediately available, any person whose blood or body fluid is the source of an occupational exposure for a healthcare provider should be informed of the incident and tested for HIV infection at the time the exposure occurs.

Any person seeking testing or having been diagnosed with any sexually transmitted infection (STI) should be offered HIV testing.

PRE- AND POSTTEST COUNSELING ELEMENTS

PRETEST COUNSELING

According to the CDC's 2006 recommendations for HIV testing in the healthcare setting, written consent and prevention counseling is not required. A meta-analysis of 27 published studies found that HIV counseling and testing was effective in secondary prevention but was not an effective strategy for primary prevention (Weinhardt et al., 1999). However, randomized controlled studies suggest that the quality and delivery of the counseling affects its efficacy on primary prevention. (Kamb et al., 1998; Koblin et al., 2004). As such, HIV testing in itself can offer the opportunity to refer people for prevention counseling, especially those with high-risk behaviors.

Effective pretest counseling is an interactive process of assessing risk, recognizing specific risk-inducing behaviors, and reviewing risk-reduction strategies. This may be done in a variety of ways—through written material or films or orally by a variety of trained staff. Of greatest importance is setting a nonjudgmental atmosphere, imparting accurate information in a useful format, offering an opportunity for questions, and maintaining strict confidentiality of personal information.

If deemed to be appropriate, elements of pretest counseling should include the following:

- A functional assessment of the person's decision-making capacity

- The meaning, sensitivity, and specificity of the test

- The potential ramifications of a positive test result

- A discussion about confidentiality and disclosure of test results by the healthcare providers to public health authorities and by the person to sexual and/or drug-using partners

- A frank discussion of risk-reduction behaviors

- Specific instructions about accessing treatment in the event of a positive result

POSTTEST COUNSELING

Elements of posttest counseling should include the following:

- For a negative result:
  - The validity of the negative result
  - Possible retesting if indicated
  - Reinforcement of transmission-reduction behaviors (US Department of Veterans Affairs, 2002)
  - Prevention strategies, including PrEP, condom use, safer sex practices, and clean needle and syringe services
- For a positive result (optimally given during a face-to-face meeting):
  - Review of the availability and effectiveness of treatment
  - Reinforcement of disclosure to spouse and/or sexual and/or drug-using partners
  - Reinforcement of transmission-reduction behaviors
  - An assessment of any intent to harm self or others

SPECIAL POPULATIONS AND ENVIRONMENTS

BLOOD SUPPLY SCREENING

Since 1990, all persons desiring to donate blood or plasma are required to undergo testing, as are those donating sperm for artificial insemination or tissue or organs for transplantation. The donor is notified only if the specimen tests positive. The laboratory assays used for testing blood, blood products, tissues, and organs have evolved along with those used to screen individuals (and often are the same). However, because the volume of testing is larger, pooled testing using nucleic acid tests is commonly done to improve testing and to possibly detect blood or blood products from acutely infected persons.

PERINATAL SCREENING

HIV screening should be a routine component of prenatal testing and should be performed during the first trimester or at entry into care. Retesting in the third trimester (preferably <36 weeks of gestation) is recommended for women at high risk for HIV exposure, for those who receive healthcare in high-incidence areas, and for those with signs or symptoms consistent with acute HIV infection. Women with undocumented HIV status at the time of labor or delivery should be screened with a point-of-care (POC) HIV test unless they opt out. If a mother's HIV status is unknown postpartum, POC testing of the newborn is recommended (and is legally mandated in many states) as soon as possible so that antiretroviral prophylaxis can be offered to HIV-exposed infants. The mother should be informed that the identification of

HIV antibodies in the newborn indicates that the mother is infected (Branson et al., 2006).

MSM

MSM have been identified as a population that is at high risk for HIV infection as well as STIs. Disproportionately higher rates of HIV infection are seen within the Black and Hispanic population compared to White and Asian MSM, with up to 44% being unaware of their serostatus (CDC, 2009). Due to the high-risk nature of the MSM population, the CDC recommends screening for HIV and syphilis at least annually. In addition, it is recommended to screen for urethral and rectal gonorrhea and chlamydia along with pharyngeal gonorrhea in sexually active people.

The CDC's 2015 (most current version) guidelines for sexually transmitted disease (STD) screening and treatment recommend more frequent STD screening (i.e., for syphilis, gonorrhea, and chlamydia) at 3- to 6-month intervals with MSM, including those with HIV infection, if risk behaviors persist or if they or their sexual partners have multiple partners. Evaluation for HSV-2 infection with type-specific serologic tests also can be considered if infection status is unknown in persons with previously undiagnosed genital tract infection.

TESTING SETTINGS

There are two primary models of HIV testing as per the CDC: routine testing in a standard medical setting and targeted testing in nonclinical settings. Nonclinical settings are sites where medical services are not routinely provided but select diagnostic services are offered, such as HIV testing. Examples of nonclinical settings include mobile testing units, churches, shelters, syringe services programs, and homes (CDC, 2016). The essential elements for HIV testing are the same for both a standard medical setting and a nonclinical setting. An important principle with HIV testing in a nonclinical setting is to link any person with HIV (PWH) with medical care.

HOME TESTING

Currently, there are only two home HIV tests: the Home Access HIV-1 Test System and the OraQuick In-Home HIV Test. While these tests seek to empower people and allow them to seek testing outside of healthcare settings, the limitations of oral swab testing especially should be emphasized.

The Home Access HIV-1 Test System is a home collection kit that involves pricking the finger to collect a blood sample, sending the sample to a licensed laboratory, and then calling in for results as early as the next business day. This test is anonymous. If the test is positive, a follow-up test is performed by the lab right away, and the results include the follow-up test. The manufacturer provides confidential counseling and referral for treatment. The tests conducted on the blood sample collected at home find infection later after exposure than most lab-based tests using blood from a vein but earlier than tests conducted with oral fluid.

The OraQuick In-Home HIV Test provides rapid results in the home. The testing procedure involves swabbing the gums or mucosal surface for an oral fluid sample and using a kit to test it. Results are available in 20 minutes. Those who test positive need a follow-up test. The manufacturer provides confidential counseling and referral to follow-up testing sites. Because the level of antibody in oral fluid is lower than it is in blood, oral fluid tests detect infection later after exposure than do blood tests. Up to 1 in 12 infected people may test falsely negative with this test.

STRATEGIES TO IMPROVE UPTAKE OF HIV TESTING

HIV screening should be voluntary and undertaken only with the person's knowledge and understanding. Testing is optimally undertaken with the goal of preventing newly acquired infection in those found to be negative and of providing linkage to care in those found to be positive. The knowledge imparted and self-reflection on the part of the person during testing is an essential part of the screening process. Without knowledge of risk reduction for those who are negative and linkage to care for those who are positive, screening is of little benefit to the persons being tested (CDC, 2011). The commonality of concurrent STDs in HIV practices argues against the notion that safer sex practices are promoted through knowledge of one's positive status alone. In the highly structured, technical, reimbursement-driven healthcare environment, a truly successful screening program is not one that is measured by the number of tests performed but, rather, one that takes into account that HIV screening deals with the most elemental and intimate aspects of human existence.

AREAS FOR IMPROVEMENT

Recently published data have demonstrated that, despite current recommendations by various medical organizations, including the CDC, an important percentage of at-risk individuals goes untested annually.

In a recent survey, high-risk individuals were anonymously interviewed and tested for HIV infection. Of the MSM population interviewed, 22% had a positive test result, and 8% of people who injected drugs had a positive test result. Of those who were HIV-positive, 8% of MSM and 12% of people who injected drugs were unaware of their infection. Most notably, the majority of people surveyed reported visiting a clinician but fewer than 50% were offered HIV testing.

Clearly, an opportunity for education and increased testing is still present.

ACKNOWLEDGMENT

The author would like to acknowledge the work of Hojoon You, MD, who contributed to the previous edition of this chapter.

RECOMMENDED READING

Centers for Disease Control and Prevention (CDC). 2015 sexually transmitted diseases treatment guidelines: special populations. January 25, 2017. https://www.cdc.gov/std/tg2015/specialpops.htm

Hall HI, Tang T, Espinoza L. Late diagnosis of HIV infection in metropolitan areas of the United States and Puerto Rico. *AIDS Behav.* 2016;20(5):967–972. http://www.ncbi.nlm.nih.gov/pubmed/26542730

Kelen GD, Hsieh YH, Rothman RE, et al. Improvements in the continuum of HIV care in an inner-city emergency department. *AIDS.* 2016;30(1):113–120. http://www.ncbi.nlm.nih.gov/pubmed/26731757

Truong H. Sentinel surveillance of HIV-1 transmitted drug resistance, acute infection, and recent infection. *PLoS One.* 2011;6:e25281.

Weeks BS, Alcamo EL. *AIDS: The Biological Basis.* Sudbury, MA: Jones & Bartlett; 2010.

Wejnert C, Prejean J, Hoots B, et al. Prevalence of missed opportunities for HIV testing among persons unaware of their infection. *JAMA.* 2018;319(24):2555–2557.

REFERENCES

Branson BM, Hansfield HH, Lampe MA, et al. Revised recommendations for HIV testing of adults, adolescents, and pregnant women in health-care settings. CDC MMWR Recommendations and Reports, September 22, 2006. https://www.cdc.gov/mmwr/preview/mmwrhtml/rr5514a1.htm

Branson BM, Owen SM, Wesolowski LG, et al. Laboratory testing for the diagnosis of HIV infection: updated recommendations. June 27, 2014. https://stacks.cdc.gov/view/cdc/23447

Centers for Disease Control and Prevention. Perspectives in disease prevention and health promotion public health service guidelines for counseling and antibody testing to prevent HIV infection and AIDS. August 14, 1987. https://www.cdc.gov/mmwr/preview/mmwrhtml/00015088.htm

Centers for Disease Control and Prevention. HIV infection among young black men who have sex with men: Jackson, Mississippi, 2006–2008. February 6, 2009. https://www.cdc.gov/mmwr/preview/mmwrhtml/mm5804a2.htm

Centers for Disease Control and Prevention. Vital signs: HIV prevention through care and treatment. November 29, 2011. https://www.cdc.gov/mmwr/preview/mmwrhtml/mm6047a4.htm

Centers for Disease Control and Prevention. Implementing HIV testing in nonclinical settings: a guide for HIV testing providers. March 2, 2016. https://www.cdc.gov/hiv/pdf/testing/cdc_hiv_implementing_hiv_testing_in_nonclinical_settings.pdf

Kamb ML, Fishbein M, Douglas JM, et al. Efficacy of risk-reduction counseling to prevent human immunodeficiency virus and sexually transmitted diseases. *JAMA.* 1998;280:1161–1167.

Koblin B, Chesney M, Coates T, et al. Effects of a behavioural intervention to reduce acquisition of HIV infection among men who have sex with men: the EXPLORE randomised controlled study. *Lancet.* 2004;364 (9428):41–50. https://www.ncbi.nlm.nih.gov/pubmed/15234855

US Department of Veterans Affairs. *The VA Prevention Handbook: A Guide for Clinicians.* Washington, DC: Veterans Health Administration; 2002.

Weinhardt LS, Carey MP, Johnson BT, et al. Effects of HIV counseling and testing on sexual risk behavior: a meta-analytic review of published research, 1985–1997. *Am J Public Health.* 1999;89(9):1397–1405. https://www.ncbi.nlm.nih.gov/pmc/articles/PMC1508752

8.

LABORATORY TESTING STRATEGIES, DETECTION, AND DIAGNOSIS

Alonso D. Pezo Salazar and Jessica A. Meisner

CHAPTER GOALS

Upon completion of this chapter, the reader should be able to:
- Discuss the various laboratory testing and home testing methods used for screening and diagnosis of HIV infections

- Explain how available immunoassays can be used for screening and diagnosing most early and primary HIV infections

- Discuss when virologic assays should be considered as complementary diagnostics to immunoassays for screening and confirmation of HIV-1 and HIV-2 infections

- Explain the rationale behind the HIV testing algorithm

- Describe how HIV infection can be diagnosed in newborns and children younger than age 18 months

SEROLOGIC TESTING METHODS

LEARNING OBJECTIVE

- Explain how available immunoassays can be used for screening and diagnosing most early and primary HIV infections

WHAT'S NEW?

- Fifth-generation immunoassays are approved for screening and diagnosing HIV infections in the US.

- These assays detect both antibodies to HIV-1 and HIV-2 and HIV p24 antigen and differentiate between them, thereby allowing earlier detection of acute and primary HIV infections.

KEY POINTS

- Laboratory confirmation of HIV infection is primarily through the detection of HIV antibodies and/or the p24 antigen in an individual.

- The western blot is no longer used as a confirmation test.

- The prevalence of HIV-2 is increasing in the US, so it is important to use immunoassays approved for detecting HIV-2 (as well as other non–group M HIV-1 strains).

- Using the current immunoassays and confirmatory testing, false-positive results are exceedingly rare. However, providers should use clinical judgment when interpreting test results and consider additional follow-up testing when appropriate.

- False-negative immunoassays are also exceedingly rare except for individuals who are early in their infection and have yet to produce HIV antibodies that are detectable by current assays.

- Rapid HIV tests can be useful testing options for settings such as health fairs, nonclinical locations, and other situations in which quickly receiving preliminary test results would be beneficial (e.g., pre- and/or postexposure prophylaxis).

IMMUNOLOGY BEHIND TESTING

The timelines for viremia and antibody seroconversion following initial HIV infection have been well characterized (Fiebig et al., 2003). Figure 8.1 shows the curves for viral RNA, p24 antigen, and HIV antibody development. Following HIV infection there is a seroconversion "window" that includes an "eclipse period" and an acute infection period in which an HIV infection may not be detectable by immunologic or virologic assays. Although there is no accepted laboratory definition for an acute HIV infection, a current operational definition is the detection of HIV RNA or p24 antigen in the blood before antibodies have formed (Cohen et al., 2010). In these individuals, nonserologic assays should be used or follow-up serologic testing should be performed after several weeks. In addition, it is important to understand that viral kinetics and serologic markers may not always be as accurate with non–clade B subtype infections. Additional testing may be necessary to fully understand what is occurring with regard to these markers (Hackett, 2012; Swenson et al., 2014).

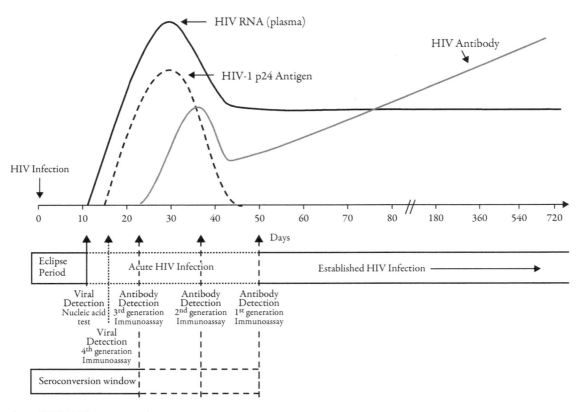

Figure 8.1 Timeline of HIV-1 laboratory markers   SOURCE: Centers for Disease Control and Prevention and Association of Public Health Laboratories. Laboratory Testing for the Diagnosis of HIV Infection: Updated Recommendations. Available at http://dx.doi.org/10.15620/cdc.23447. Published June 27, 2014. Accessed September 12, 2020.

HISTORY OF TESTING

The first enzyme immunoassay (EIA) was licensed in 1985 (Centers for Disease Control and Prevention [CDC], 1990). HIV EIAs are typically described as being from particular "generations," which helps to classify them based on technological advancements throughout the years. These advancements have shortened the detection window significantly. The first-generation EIAs used HIV lysate as an antigen to capture antibodies present in a blood sample but could only detect HIV-1. However, these had a significant number of false positives due to cellular protein contamination (Houn et al., 1987; Louie et al., 2006). The second-generation EIAs used recombinant viral proteins or peptides, which limited cellular protein contamination (Chappel et al., 2009). This generation was used to screen blood donations in the 1980s. Third-generation EIAs in the 1990s used a technique that was able to bind both immunoglobulin G (IgG) and IgM antibodies, thus even further reducing the window period.

The first western blot assay was approved in 1987; thereafter, it was recommended as a confirmatory assay for positive immunoassays (CDC, 1988). A western blot separates the individual proteins of the HIV-1 lysate into bands that allow for capturing antibodies specific to selected HIV antigens in an individual's blood or urine (Healey et al., 1992). Assays are reported positive if the bands present meet an established criterion; assays are reported as indeterminate if bands are

detected, but those detected do not meet the criteria for a positive test (CDC, 1989). Western blots are no longer used for confirmation of positive immunoassays.

EIAS

EIAs are currently the most reliable and cost-effective testing method for most individuals in the US. Screening and testing for HIV-2 infections has become more common in the US and requires the use of assays that are specifically approved to detect this virus type. HIV-2 assays are essential in locations outside the US (Hackett, 2012; Swenson et al., 2014). EIAs are still not completely reliable for screening and diagnostic testing for individuals with acute HIV infections (see the section "Virologic Assays"), in self-testing kits (see the section "HIV Self-Testing"), or for screening and diagnostic testing for infants and newborns (see the section "Alternative Algorithms for Screening and Diagnosing HIV Infections").

Antigen/antibody combination assays are also known as *fourth-generation EIAs*. These assays act as both a third-generation assay and a capture immunoassay, directly detecting the p24 antigen (Kabir et al., 2020). Thus, fourth-generation EIAs reduce the detection window period even further while maintaining the third generation's accuracy (Pandori et al., 2009; Rosenberg et al., 2015; Sickinger et al., 2004). It is important to note that fourth-generation EIAs may have a second window period in some patients, but this has not been observed in more recent testing systems that can detect IgM (Gray et al., 2018).

The fifth-generation test detects both the p24 antigen and antibodies but can separate results for HIV-1 p24 antigen, HIV-1 antibody, and HIV-2 antibody. The only fifth-generation test approved by the US Food and Drug Administration (FDA) is the Bio-Rad Bio Plex.

Current FDA-approved HIV antigen/antibody screening tests include:

- Abbott Architect HIV Ag/Ab Combo Assay
- ADVIA Centaur HIV Ag/Ab combo
- Alere Determine HIV-1/2 Ag/Ab combo
- Bio-Rad BioPlex 2200 HIV Ag-Ab
- Bio-Rad GS HIV Combo Ag/Ab EIA
- Ortho VITROS HIV Combo Test on the VITROS 3600 Immunodiagnostic System
- Roche Elecsys HIV combi PT

RAPID HIV TESTS

Rapid HIV tests detect HIV antibodies present in an oral fluid, finger-stick blood, or venipuncture whole blood/plasma sample. Fourth- and fifth-generation EIAs have shorter detection windows compared to the currently available rapid tests, but rapid tests are as accurate and test results are available in less than 30 minutes (Kabir et al., 2020). However, some data describe decreased sensitivity of HIV rapid tests in high-income countries compared to low-income countries, likely due to a larger proportion of acute infections in targeted populations (Tan et al., 2016). They show maximum potential utility in resource-limited settings, or to speed up decision-making processes by avoiding turnaround times (Setty & Hewlett, 2014). Individuals with a potential exposure and those with ongoing high risk for HIV infection who have negative rapid test results should be counseled to be retested or considered for testing that is more sensitive for detecting acute HIV infections in these situations. There are currently more than 15 rapid HIV tests approved by the FDA. Several of these rapid tests have received Clinical Laboratory Improvement Amendment (CLIA) waivers, making them available for point-of-care testing and screening in settings in which transporting specimens to a laboratory is either not possible or not practical.

Examples of CLIA waived rapid tests include:

- Chembio DPP HIV-1/2
- Chembio SURE CHECK HIV-1/2 Assay
- Clearview HIV-1/2 STAT-Pak
- Determine HIV-1/2 Ag/Ab combo test

- INSTI HIV-1/HIV-2 Antibody Test
- OraQuick ADVANCE Rapid HIV-1/2 Antibody Test
- Uni-Gold Recombigen HIV-1/2

When determining whether to use an approved rapid HIV test or EIA testing for screening and/or diagnosing HIV infections, one should consider the setting in which testing will occur, the cost, and the population being tested. Rapid tests generally cost more compared to EIA assays, especially if large numbers of tests are being performed. Rapid testing can be particularly useful for public health testing programs outside of clinical settings, such as during health fairs or at social venues where high-risk individuals may be located. Testing women who are in labor is another situation in which rapid HIV testing may be a more suitable choice compared to EIAs (Setty & Hewlett, 2014). Rapid testing platforms for point-of-care HIV RNA testing are also under development (Agutu et al., 2019; Curtis et al., 2016).

RECOMMENDED READING

Centers for Disease Control. Laboratory testing for the diagnosis of HIV infection. 2014. http://www.cdc.gov/hiv/pdf/hivtestingalgorithmrecommendation-final.pdf

Kabir MA, Zilouchian H, Caputi M, et al. Advances in HIV diagnosis and monitoring. *Crit Rev Biotech.* 2020;40(5):623–638.

Masciotra S, Luo W, Westheimer E, et al. Performance evaluation of the FDA-approved Determine HIV-1/2 Ag/Ab Combo assay using plasma and whole blood specimens. *J Clin Virol.* 2017;91:95–100.

Tan WS, Chow EPF, Fairley CK, et al. Sensitivity of HIV rapid tests compared with fourth-generation enzyme immunoassays or HIV RNA tests. *AIDS.* 2016;30(12):1951–1960.

VIROLOGIC ASSAYS

LEARNING OBJECTIVE

- Discuss when virologic assays should be considered as complementary diagnostics to immunoassays for screening and confirmation of HIV-1 and HIV-2 infections

KEY POINTS

- Virologic assays should be used in diagnosing acute HIV infections and infections in newborns and infants younger than age 18 months.

- Compared to immunoassays, virologic assays are more expensive and have an increased rate of false-positive results; virologic assays may also be falsely negative in individuals with chronic infections, undetectable viral loads, and non–clade B infections.

- To improve cost-effectiveness, several public health laboratories in the United States are pooling negative

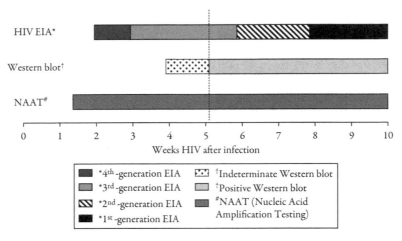

Figure 8.2 Time to detection of differences for various generations of EIAs   Modified from Branson (2007) and Patel (2010); data from Fiebig (2003) and Hecht (2011).

immunoassay samples and testing the pooled samples using a nucleic acid amplification test (NAAT). This method increases a screening program's overall accuracy by detecting individuals with acute infections who would have otherwise received a negative test result.

Virologic assays include qualitative and quantitative DNA and RNA assays as well as p24 antigen assays. Fourth- and fifth-generation antigen/antibody combination immunoassays use the HIV p24 core protein as the antigen component and thus can be considered both a serologic and a virologic assay (Stone et al., 2018). Standalone p24 antigen assays are available, although the p24 antigen rapidly becomes undetectable after antibodies develop, thereby limiting the period during which a p24 antigen assay uniquely provides diagnostic information (see Figure 8.1). Multiple p24-only tests are under investigation for a myriad of roles in HIV management and prevention, but no conclusive data are available yet (Gray et al., 2018).

Virologic assays should be considered for the following:

- Diagnosing HIV infection in newborns and infants younger than 18 months

- Diagnosing acute HIV infections in cases in which patients would likely not yet have detectable antibodies (Figure 8.2)

Because infection transmission risk correlates well with an individual's plasma viral load (Chan, 2012; Rodger et al., 2016), considerable attention has been given to detecting acute HIV infections (Cohen et al., 2010; Henn et al., 2017; Patel et al., 2010; Parekh et al., 2019). Individuals acutely infected will typically have relatively high viral loads before seroconverting and are likely unaware of their infection (Henn et al., 2017). Studies have shown that recently infected individuals are likely the source of transmission for up to 50% of all new infections (Yerly & Hirschel, 2012).

QUANTITATIVE ASSAYS FOR DETECTING HIV-1 RNA (VIRAL LOAD ASSAYS)

Several commercially available assays reliably quantify HIV-1 RNA in plasma:

- NGI UltraQual Multiplex PCR Assay for HCV, HIV-1, HIV-2, and HBV

- NucliSens HIV-1 QT (bioMérieux, Inc.)

- Procleix HIV-1/HCV Assay

- UltraQual HIV-1 RT-PCR Assay

- VERSANT HIV-1 RNA 3.0 Assay (bDNA)

- Procleix Ultrio Assay

- HIV-1 reverse transcription (RT) polymerase chain reaction (PCR) assay (manufacturer: BioLife Plasma Services, L.P.)

- Abbott RealTime HIV-1 Amplification Reagent Kit

- COBAS AmpliPrep/COBAS TaqMan HIV-1 Test

- Aptima HIV-1 Test

All of these tests quantify plasma HIV-1 RNA within a variable dynamic range. These assays detect most HIV-1 subtypes, and although they have become increasingly effective at detecting non–subtype B infections, there is some variability based on clade variations and each assay's performance characteristics. Both kPCR and RT-PCR assays are proficient at quantitation of many non–clade B strains of HIV-1 (Alvarez et al., 2015; Karasi et al., 2011; Parekh et al., 2019).

Because of the rate of false positives, these quantitative assays must be used with caution as a diagnostic test. In an acute HIV infection, plasma HIV-1 RNA levels are typically very high, whereas levels of false positives tend to be very low (Henn et al., 2017).

QUALITATIVE ASSAYS FOR DETECTING HIV-1 RNA

Currently, there is one qualitative virologic assay, frequently referred to as NAAT, approved for use as an aid in the diagnosis of HIV-1 (APTIMA; Gen-Probe, San Diego, CA). This assay can be used to assist with diagnosing an acute HIV infection and as an additional test to confirm an HIV-1 infection when an EIA or a rapid test is repeatedly reactive for HIV-1 antibodies. Qualitative assays are not commonly used because quantitative assays are the preferred detection for HIV RNA. The qualitative assays' role in point-of-care HIV management, especially in resource-limited settings, shows potential and is under investigation. Despite showing acceptable clinical accuracy, more data are required to assess its clinical utility, quality assurance, cost-effectiveness, and role in future diagnostic algorithms (Agutu et al., 2019).

HIV-2 VIROLOGIC ASSAYS

An approved HIV-2 virologic assay is not currently available in the US. Although some assays may detect a viral load, caution should be exercised when utilizing these results to monitor response to treatment because underquantification is common when viremia is detected and not all HIV-2-infected individuals will have a detectable viral load.(Campbell-Yesufu & Gandhi, 2011). A number of international laboratories use in-house (or laboratory-developed) HIV-2 viral load assays. There are two current labs in the US with HIV-2 quantitative viral loads available (New York State Department of Health and University of Washington, 2020). Reference laboratory resources are available through the CDC for public health laboratories evaluating HIV-2-reactive specimens.

RECOMMENDED READING

Chang M, Gottlieb GS, Dragavon JA, et al. Validation for clinical use of a novel HIV-2 plasma RNA viral load assay using the Abbott m2000 platform. *J Clin Virol.* 2012;55(2):128–133. doi:10.1016/j.jcv.2012.06.024

Damond F, Bernard C, Jurg Boni M, et al. An international collaboration to standardize HIV-2 viral load assays: results from the 2009 ACHIEV2E quality control study. *J Clin Microbiol.* 2011;49:3491–3497.

New York State Department of Health. HIV nucleic acid testing. Wadsworth Center website: https://www.wadsworth.org/programs/id/bloodborne-viruses/clinical-testing/hiv-2-nucleic-acid

HIV SELF-TESTING

HIV self-testing (HIVST) at home is gaining popularity as a new tool in the diagnosis of HIV, with updated 2019 guidelines from the World Health Organization (WHO) recommending it be offered as an additional approach to HIV testing services (WHO, 2019). Facility-based testing uses more sensitive assays, can provide on-site counseling, and accelerates linkage to care. However, HIVST has been shown to have high acceptability in high-risk patients from all socioeconomic strata (Figueroa et al., 2015; Krause et al., 2013; Stephenson et al., 2017) and could be very promising in low- to middle-income countries (Moshoeu et al., 2019). The processes of dissemination, adoption, and implementation remain significant hurdles, mainly due to challenges with cost, testing performance variability, risk of social harm, and linkage to care (Hurt & Powers, 2014; Johnson et al., 2014; Pai et al., 2013; Ruzagira et al., 2017; WHO, 2019).

The OraQuick In-Home HIV Test is the only HIV test approved by the FDA for home use and self-testing in the US. It tests for HIV-1/2 antibodies in the oral fluid using a swab and delivers results in 20 to 40 minutes. Main limitations are its lower sensitivity and an extended negative window of at least 3 months after exposure. Preexposure prophylaxis (PrEP) or postexposure prophylaxis (PEP) may affect results given its effect on antibody levels (CDC,2020; Kabir et al., 2020).

Despite the lower sensitivity in detecting recent HIV infection, due to the COVID-19 pandemic, CDC guidelines have added HIVST as options for PrEP monitoring when other options are not available or feasible (home specimen collection kits or self-testing via an oral swab-based test) (CDC, 2020).

RECOMMENDED READING

Figueroa C, Johnson C, Verster A, et al. Attitudes and acceptability on HIV self-testing among key populations: a literature review. *AIDS Behav.* 2015;19(11):1949–1965.

Kabir MA, Zilouchian H, Caputi M, et al. Advances in HIV diagnosis and monitoring. *Crit Rev Biotech.* 2020;40(5):623–638.

Stephenson R, Freeland R, Sullivan SP, et al. Home-based HIV testing and counseling for male couples (Project Nexus): a protocol for a randomized controlled trial. *JMIR Res Protoc.* 2017;6(5):e101.

World Health Organization. Consolidated Guidelines on HIV Testing Services for a Changing Epidemic. November 2019.

ALGORITHMS FOR SCREENING AND DIAGNOSING HIV INFECTIONS

LEARNING OBJECTIVE

- Explain the rationale behind the HIV testing algorithm

WHAT'S NEW?

Because newer serologic and virologic assays are available, new algorithms no longer use the western blot as a confirmatory assay.

KEY POINTS

- The algorithm removes the use of the western blot assay because of its limitations, particularly in confirming acute or recent HIV infections.

- The algorithm recommends using the most sensitive immunoassay (fourth-generation EIA) as a screening test, as well as following any repeatedly positive results with a different immunoassay that can discriminate between HIV-1 and HIV-2.

- Samples with a positive screening assay but negative confirmation assay should be tested using NAAT.

The current HIV testing algorithm was updated in 2014. Figure 8.3 shows the current recommended HIV testing algorithm (CDC, 2018). Key factors driving the evolution of the current algorithms are the improvement in assays for earlier detection time and availability of NAAT. In 2014, an updated testing algorithm was recommended by the CDC and the Association of Public Health Laboratories (APHL) that recommends the use of the most sensitive immunoassays for primary screening along with a confirmatory test that discriminates HIV-1 from HIV-2 after a repeatedly positive screening test (Wesolowski et al., 2017). In this algorithm, if the confirmatory test is negative, HIV NAAT should be performed. A positive NAAT would be confirmatory for an acute HIV infection.

RECOMMENDED READING

Centers for Disease Control and Prevention and Association of Public Health Laboratories. Laboratory testing for the diagnosis of HIV

infection: updated recommendations. 2014. http://dx.doi.org/10.15620/cdc. 23447

Delaney KP, Hanson DL, Masciotra S, et al. Time until emergence of HIV test reactivity following infection with HIV-1: implications for interpreting test results and retesting after exposure. *Clin Infect Dis.* 2017;64(1):53–59. doi:10.1093/cid/ciw666

Delaney KP, Wesolowski LG, Owen SM. The evolution of HIV testing continues. *Sex Transm Dis.* 2017;44(12):747–749. doi: 10.1097/OLQ.0000000000000736

Rosenberg NE, Pilcher CD, Busch MP, et al. How can we better identify early HIV infections? *Curr Opin HIV AIDS.* 2015;10(1):61–68. doi: 10.1097/COH.0000000000000121

Wesolowski LG, Parker MM, Delaney KP, et al. Highlights from the 2016 HIV diagnostics conference: the new landscape of HIV testing in laboratories, public health programs and clinical practice. *J Clin Virol.* 2017;91:63–68. doi: 10.1016/j.jcv.2017.01.009

SCREENING AND DETECTING HIV IN NEWBORNS AND CHILDREN

LEARNING OBJECTIVE

- Describe how HIV infection can be diagnosed in newborns and children younger than 18 months

WHAT'S NEW?

Virologic assays must be used for detecting HIV infection in newborns and infants younger than 18 months with perinatal and postnatal HIV exposure.

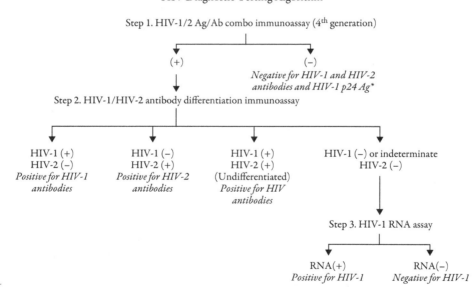

HIV Diagnostic Testing Algorithm

Step 1. HIV-1/2 Ag/Ab combo immunoassay (4th generation)

(+)   (−) *Negative for HIV-1 and HIV-2 antibodies and HIV-1 p24 Ag**

Step 2. HIV-1/HIV-2 antibody differentiation immunoassay

HIV-1 (+) / HIV-2 (−) *Positive for HIV-1 antibodies*

HIV-1 (−) / HIV-2 (+) *Positive for HIV-2 antibodies*

HIV-1 (+) / HIV-2 (+) (Undifferentiated) *Positive for HIV antibodies*

HIV-1 (−) or indeterminate / HIV-2 (−)

Step 3. HIV-1 RNA assay

RNA(+) *Positive for HIV-1*   RNA(−) *Negative for HIV-1*

(+) = Reactive (or repeatedly reactive) test result, in accordance with manufacturer's instructions
(−) = Nonreactive test result, in accordance with manufacturer's instructions
Italics = Final interpretation; No further testing indicated for the specimen
*For 3rd generation HIV-1/2 immunoassay, interpretation is 'Negative for HIV-1 and HIV-2 antibodies'.

Figure 8.3 Recommended laboratory HIV testing algorithm for serum or plasma specimens   SOURCE: Centers for Disease Control and Prevention. Updated testing algorithm for US HIV diagnosis. 2018. The 2018 Quick reference guide: Recommended laboratory HIV testing algorithm for serum or plasma specimens. January 2018. Available at: https://stacks.cdc.gov/view/cdc/50872. Accessed September 1, 2018. https://stacks.cdc.gov/view/cdc/50872.

- Maternal antibodies passed in utero are detectable in a newborn's blood using current immunoassays, so combination assays are not recommended.

- Newborn testing requires NAAT; DNA- and RNA-based assays show similar performance, so either can be used.

- HIV testing should be performed at 14 to 21 days, at 1 to 2 months, and at 4 to 6 months in all infants who are born to HIV-positive women.

- Laboratory confirmation of HIV infection requires that more than one test be positive; infections typically can be diagnosed by the age of 1 month and definitively in almost all children at age 6 months.

Maternal-to-child transmission of HIV infection can occur in utero, at the time of labor and delivery, and through breastfeeding (Kourtis et al., 2001). Because maternal antibodies passed in utero can be detected in uninfected newborns, immunoassays may be positive in uninfected newborns until 18 to 24 months of age.

When interpreting immunoassay results for an infant, it is important to consider serologic window periods after each of these potential exposure events, as well as the presence of maternal antibodies. Non-breastfed children can be considered presumptively uninfected if there are at least two negative virologic tests (at >2 weeks and >4 weeks) or one negative virologic test and one negative HIV antibody at more than 6 months, and they can be considered definitively uninfected if there are two negative virologic tests (>1 month and >4 months) or two negative serologic tests at more than 6 months (Panel on Antiretroviral Therapy and Medical Management of Children Living with HIV, 2019). Virologic assays, however, represent the gold standard for diagnostic testing of infants and children younger than 18 months (Read, 2007).

Virologic assays should be performed at birth on infants born to HIV-infected mothers who meet the following criteria: did not receive prenatal care, did not receive antepartum or intrapartum antiretroviral (ARV) drugs, received intrapartum ARV drugs only, initiated antiretroviral therapy (ART) late in pregnancy, were diagnosed with acute HIV during pregnancy, had a detectable HIV viral load close to delivery, received ARV combination drugs and did not have viral suppression (Momplaisir et al., 2015).

Additionally, testing should occur at 14 to 21 days, at 1 or 2 months of age, and at 4 to 6 months of age. Testing should also be performed for infants with higher risk of perinatal infection 2 to 4 weeks after cessation of ARV prophylaxis. Some experts also recommend serologic testing to confirm the absence of infection between 12 and 18 months. If any tests are positive, repeat testing is recommended, and the diagnosis of HIV infection can be made based on two separate positive results.

Maternal HIV antibody is present at birth; although maternal antibody fades with time, endogenous infant antibody production begins in response to an infant infection. If an infant is uninfected at birth but becomes infected through breastfeeding, HIV RNA is undetectable while the infant is uninfected but rises rapidly within the first few weeks after infection (Ciaranello et al., 2011).

While women living with HIV should be discouraged from breastfeeding, infants who are breastfed should have standard virologic testing as well as testing every 3 months throughout breastfeeding (WHO, 2010). Many experts also recommend monitoring at 4 to 6 weeks, 3 months, and 6 months after breastfeeding has stopped (Panel on Antiretroviral Therapy and Medical Management of Children Living with HIV, 2019).

Infants born to HIV-2-infected mothers should be tested with HIV-2-specific virologic assays at time points similar to those used for HIV-1 testing. HIV-2 virologic assays are not commercially available, but the National Perinatal HIV Hotline (1-888-448-8765) can provide a list of sites that perform this testing (Panel on Treatment of HIV-Infected Pregnant Women and Prevention of Perinatal Transmission, 2019).

TESTING NEWBORNS IN RESOURCE-LIMITED SETTINGS

Access to early infant diagnosis of HIV infection is improving in resource-limited settings (Ciaranello et al., 2011), but key barriers continue to exist. Virologic assays are generally more expensive than immunoassays, and additional barriers such as accurate specimen collection, transport, and laboratory processing can limit their use in these settings. However, multiple RNA and DNA PCR assays are currently being used, and the use of dried blood spots has decreased the phlebotomy requirements. Dried blood spots may be obtained through a finger or heel stick, are heat stable, are noninfectious, and can be shipped via mail or courier (Ciaranello et al., 2011).

Because breastfeeding may be recommended for children born in resource-limited settings through the age of 12 months, provided the mother and/or child is receiving ARV prophylaxis, clinical and laboratory monitoring for HIV transmission should take into consideration this ongoing exposure risk (WHO, 2010).

RECOMMENDED READING

Centers for Disease Control and Prevention and Association of Public Health Laboratories. Laboratory testing for the diagnosis of HIV infection: updated recommendations. 2014. http://stacks.cdc.gov/view/cdc/23447

Jourdain G, Mary JY, Coeur SL, et al. Risk factors for in utero or intrapartum mother-to-child transmission of human immunodeficiency virus type 1 in Thailand. *J Infect Dis.* 2007;196(11):1629–1636. http://www.ncbi.nlm.nih.gov/pubmed/18008246

King CC, Kourtis AP, Persaud D, et al. Delayed HIV detection among infants exposed to postnatal antiretroviral prophylaxis during breastfeeding. *AIDS.* 2015;29(15):1953–1961. http://www.ncbi.nlm.nih.gov/pubmed/26153671

Panel on Antiretroviral Therapy and Medical Management of Children Living with HIV. Guidelines for the use of antiretroviral agents in pediatric HIV Infection. http://aidsinfo.nih.gov/contentfiles/lvguidelines/pediatricguidelines.pdf

Panel on Treatment of Pregnant Women with HIV Infection and Prevention of Perinatal Transmission. Recommendations for the use of antiretroviral drugs in pregnant women with HIV infection and interventions to reduce perinatal HIV transmission in the United States. https://clinicalinfo.hiv.gov/sites/default/files/inline-files/PerinatalGL.pdf

Read JS. Diagnosis of HIV-1 infection in children younger than 18 months in the United States. *Pediatrics*. 2007;120(6):e1547–1562. http://www.ncbi.nlm.nih.gov/pubmed/18055670

Wessman MJ, Theilgaard Z, Katzenstein TL. Determination of HIV status of infants born to HIV-infected mothers: a review of the diagnostic methods with special focus on the applicability of p24 antigen testing in developing countries. *Scand J Infect Dis*. 2012;44(3):209–215. http://www.ncbi.nlm.nih.gov/pubmed/22074445

REFERENCES

Agutu CA, Ngetsa CJ, Price MA, et al. Systematic review of the performance and clinical utility of point of care HIV-1 RNA testing for diagnosis and care. *PLoS One*. 2019;14(6):e0218369.

Alvarez P, Martin L, Prieto L, et al. HIV-1 variability and viral load technique could lead to false positive HIV-1 detection and to erroneous viral quantification in infected specimens. *J Infect*. 2015;71(3):368–376. doi:10.1016/j.jinf.2015.05.011

Branson BM. State of the art for diagnosis of HIV infection. *Clin Infect Dis*. 2007;45(Suppl 4):S221–S225.

Campbell-Yesufu OT, Gandhi RT. Update on human immunodeficiency virus (HIV)-2 infection. *Clin Infect Dis*. 2011;52(6):780–787.

Centers for Disease Control and Prevention. Serologic testing for antibody to human immunodeficiency virus. *MMWR Morb Mortal Wkly Rep*. 1988;36:509–515.

Centers for Disease Control and Prevention. Interpretation and use of the western blot assay for serodiagnosis of human immunodeficiency virus type 1 infections. *MMWR Morb Mortal Wkly Rep*. 1989;38:1–7.

Centers for Disease Control and Prevention. Update: serologic testing for HIV-1 antibody—The United States, 1988 and 1989. *MMWR Morb Mortal Wkly Rep*. 1990;39:380–383.

Centers for Disease Control and Prevention. The 2018 quick reference guide: recommended laboratory HIV testing algorithm for serum or plasma specimens. 2018. https://stacks.cdc.gov/view/cdc/50872

Centers for Disease Control and Prevention. Information from CDC's Division of HIV/AIDS Prevention. 2020. https://www.cdc.gov/hiv/policies/dear-colleague/dcl/051520.html

Centers for Disease Control and Prevention. HIV testing—self testing. 2020. https://www.cdc.gov/hiv/testing/self-testing.html

Chan DJ. Can HIV-1 incidence be estimated from plasma viral load and sexual behavior. *Int J STD AIDS*. 2012;23(10):724–728.

Chappel RJ, Dax EM, Wilson KM. Immunoassays for the diagnosis of HIV: meeting future needs by enhancing quality of testing. *Fut Microbiol*. 2009;48:963–982.

Ciaranello AL, Park JE, Ramirez-Avila L, et al. Early infant HIV-1 diagnosis programs in resource-limited settings: opportunities for improved outcomes and more cost-effective interventions. *BMC Medicine*. 2011;9:1–15.

Cohen MS, Gay CL, Busch MP, et al. The detection of acute HIV infection. *J Infect Dis*. 2010;202:S270–S277.

Curtis KA, Rudolph DL, Morrison D, et al. Single-use, electricity-free amplification device for detection of HIV-1. *J Virol Methods*. 2016;237:132–137.

Fiebig EW, Wright DJ, Rawal BD, et al. Dynamics of HIV viremia and antibody seroconversion in plasma donors: implications for diagnosis and staging of primary HIV infection. *AIDS*. 2003;17:1871–1879.

Figueroa C, Johnson C, Verster A, et al. Attitudes and acceptability on HIV self-testing among key populations: a literature review. *AIDS Behav*. 2015;19(11):1949–1965.

Gray ER, Bain R, Varsaneux O, et al. p24 revisited: A landscape review of antigen detection for early HIV diagnosis. *AIDS*. 2018;32(15):2089–2102.

Hackett J Jr. Meeting the challenge of HIV diversity: strategies to mitigate the impact of HIV-1 genetic heterogeneity on performance of nucleic acid testing assays. *Clin Lab*. 2012;58(3–4):199–202.

Healey D, Maskill W, Howard T, et al. HIV-1 western blot: development and assessment of testing to resolve indeterminate reactivity. *AIDS*. 1992;6:629–633.

Hecht F, Wellman R, Busch M, et al. Identifying the early post-HIV antibody seroconversion period. *J Infect Dis*. 2011;204:526–533.

Henn A, Flateau C, Gallien S, et al. Primary HIV infection: clinical presentation, testing, and treatment. *Curr Infect Dis Rep*. 2017;19:37.

Houn HY, Pappas AA, Walter EM. Status of current clinical tests for human immunodeficiency virus (HIV): applications and limitations. *Ann Clin Lab Sci*. 1987;17:279–285.

Hurt CB, Powers KA. Self-testing for HIV and its impact on public health. *Sex Transm Dis*. 2014;41(1):10–12.

Johnson C, Baggaley R, Forsythe S, et al. Realizing the potential for HIV self-testing. *AIDS Behav*. 2014;18(Suppl 4):S391–S395.

Kabir MA, Zilouchian H, Caputi M, et al. Advances in HIV diagnosis and monitoring. *Crit Rev Biotech*. 2020;40(5):623–638.

Karasi JC, Dziezuk F, Quennery L, et al. High correlation between the Roche COBAS AmpliPrep/COBAS TaqMan HIV-1, v2.0 and the Abbott m2000 RealTime HIV-1 assays for quantification of viral load in HIV-1 B and non-B subtypes. *J Clin Virol*. 2011;52(3):181–186. doi: 10.1016/j.jcv.2011.07.002

Kourtis AP, Bulterys M, Nesheim SR, et al. Understanding the timing of HIV transmission from mother to infant. *JAMA*. 2001;285:709–712.

Krause K, Subklew-Sehume F, Kenyon C, et al. Acceptability of HIV self-testing: a systematic literature review. *BMC Public Health*. 2013;13:735.

Louie B, Pandori M, Wong E, et al. Use of an acute seroconversion panel to evaluate a third-generation enzyme-linked immunoassay for detection of human immunodeficiency virus-specific antibodies relative to multiple other assays. *J Clin Microbiol*. 2006;44:1856–1858.

Momplaisir FM, Brady KA, Fekete T, et al. Time of HIV diagnosis and engagement in prenatal care impact virologic outcomes of pregnant women with HIV. *PLoS One*. 2015;10(7):e0132262. http://www.ncbi.nlm.nih.gov/pubmed/26132142

Moshoeu PM, Kuupiel D, Gwala N, et al. The use of home-based HIV testing and counseling in low- and middle income countries: a scoping review. *BMC Public Health*. 2019;19:132.

New York State Department of Health. HIV nucleic acid testing. Wadsworth Center website: https://www.wadsworth.org/programs/id/bloodborne-viruses/clinical-testing/hiv-2-nucleic-acid

Pai NP, Sharma J, Shivkumar S, et al. Supervised and unsupervised self-testing for HIV in high- and low-risk populations: a systematic review. *PLoS Med*. 2013;10(4):e1001414.

Pandori MW, Hackett J Jr, Louie B, et al. Assessment of the ability of a fourth-generation immunoassay for human immunodeficiency virus (HIV) antibody and p24 antigen to detect both acute and recent HIV infections in a high-risk setting. *J Clin Microbiol*. 2009;47(8):2639–2642. doi:10.1128/JCM.00119-09

Panel on Treatment of HIV-Infected Pregnant Women and Prevention of Perinatal Transmission. Recommendations for use of antiretroviral drugs in pregnancy HIV-1 infected women for maternal health and interventions to reduce perinatal HIV transmission in the United States. 2011.

Parekh BS, Ou CY, Fonjungo PN, et al. Diagnosis of human immunodeficiency virus infection. *Clin Microbiol Rev*. 2018;32:e00064-18.

Patel P, Mackellar D, Simmons P, et al. Detecting acute human immunodeficiency virus infection using 3 different screening immunoassays and nucleic acid amplification testing for human immunodeficiency virus RNA, 2006–2008. *Arch Intern Med*. 2010;170:66–74.

Read JS; Committee on Pediatric AIDS. Diagnosis of HIV-1 infection in children younger than 18 months in the United States. *Pediatrics*. 2007;120:e1547–e1562.

Rodger AJ, Cambiano V, Bruun T, et al. Sexual activity without condoms and risk of HIV transmission in serodifferent couples when the HIV-positive partner is using suppressive antiretroviral therapy. *JAMA*. 2016;316(2):171–181.

Rosenberg NE, Pilcher CD, Busch MP, et al. How can we better identify early HIV infections. *Curr Opin HIV AIDS*. 2015;10(1):61–68. doi:10.1097/COH.0000000000000121

Ruzagira E, Baisley K, Kamali A, et al. Linkage to HIV care after home-based HIV counselling and testing in sub-Saharan Africa: a systematic review. *Trop Med Int Health*. 2017;22(7):807–821.

Setty MKHG, Hewlett IK. Point of care technologies for HIV. *AIDS Res Treat*. 2014;2014:625082.

Sickinger E, Steiler M, Kaufman B, et al. Multicenter evaluation of a new, automated enzyme-linked immunoassay for detection of human immunodeficiency virus-specific antibodies and antigen. *J Clin Microbiol*. 2004;42:21–29.

Stephenson R, Freeland R, Sullivan SP, et al. Home-based HIV testing and counseling for male couples (Project Nexus): a protocol for a randomized controlled trial. *JMIR Res Protoc*. 2017;6(5):e101.

Stone M, Bainbridge J, Sanchez AM, et al. Comparison of detection limits of fourth- and fifth-generation combination HIV antigen-antibody, p24 antigen, and viral load assays on diverse HIV isolates. *J Clin Microbiol*. 2018;56(8):e02045-17.

Swenson LC, Cobb B, Geretti AM, et al. Comparative performances of HIV-1 RNA load assays at low viral load levels: results of an international collaboration. *J Clin Microbiol*. 2014;52(2):517–523. doi:10.1128/JCM.02461-13

Tan WS, Chow EPF, Fairley CK, et al. Sensitivity of HIV rapid tests compared with fourth-generation enzyme immunoassays or HIV RNA tests. *AIDS*. 2016;30(12):1951–1960.

Wesolowski LG, Parker MM, Delaney KP, et al. Highlights from the 2016 HIV diagnostics conference: the new landscape of HIV testing in laboratories, public health programs and clinical practice. *J Clin Virol*. 2017;91:63–68. doi:10.1016/j.jcv.2017.01.009

World Health Organization. Principles and recommendations for infant feeding in the context of HIV and a summary of evidence. 2010. https://apps.who.int/iris/bitstream/handle/10665/44345/9789241599535_eng.pdf;jsessionid=15ADE7474DEDABB0968A7C34F83EF6E9?sequence=1

World Health Organization. Consolidated guidelines on HIV testing services for a changing epidemic. 2019. https://www.who.int/publications/i/item/consolidated-guidelines-on-hiv-testing-services-for-a-changing-epidemic

Yerly S, Hirschel B. Diagnosing acute HIV infection. *Expert Rev Anti Infect Ther*. 2012;10:31–41.

9.

INITIAL EVALUATION OF THE PERSON LIVING WITH HIV

HISTORY, PHYSICAL EXAMINATION, AND LABORATORY EVALUATION

Esteban A. DelPilar-Morales and Daniel J. Skiest

WHAT'S NEW?

This chapter provides additional insight into gender identity and cultural challenges that can affect the management of some people with HIV (PWH). The role of telehealth in managing PWH is covered.

LEARNING OBJECTIVES

- Describe the important details regarding the history and physical examination and appropriate laboratory evaluation for the initial evaluation of the PWH

- Discuss the challenges unique to the HIV population

KEY POINTS

- A comprehensive history, including a complete sexual and social history, is key in assessing a PWH's risks and possible barriers to treatment.

- A comprehensive physical examination and laboratory evaluation are important in order to identify any abnormal findings that may require prompt intervention and to provide a baseline for comparison with future findings.

- Awareness of a person's gender identity and cultural background will allow the healthcare provider to better understand the person's perception of their condition and is fundamental in caring for PWH.

- PWH presenting for their initial clinic visit may have early infection, asymptomatic chronic infection, or advanced HIV. Recognition of the clinical stage of infection is important so that appropriate prophylactic medications, prognosis, and counseling can be provided.

THE HIV-ORIENTED MEDICAL HISTORY

The initial office or clinic visit of a PWH, either newly diagnosed or chronically infected, has several objectives. The most obvious purpose is to obtain the information essential for current and future management. Some PWH may not feel comfortable divulging all relevant medical and social history at the first visit. The hope is that as the patient–provider relationship develops, they may feel more comfortable disclosing information at subsequent visits. The initial visit also represents an opportunity to establish a trust-based relation between patient and provider. It is important that the provider establish a nonjudgmental tone in a supportive environment. The patient–provider relationship can affect how the patient views the advice received from the provider, including beliefs about the effectiveness of the medications being prescribed (Berghoff et al., 2018). A strong patient–provider relationship has been shown to result in improved retention in care and medication adherence and is predictive of future therapeutic success (Doshi et al., 2015; Flickinger et al., 2013).

If the PWH is accompanied by another person (e.g., friend, spouse, partner, family member), the provider should not assume the accompanying person is aware of the patient's HIV diagnosis and other medical history. Prior to proceeding the provider should determine if the accompanying person is aware of the HIV diagnosis without disclosing the diagnosis. Our practice is to first ask the patient if he/she wants the accompanying person to leave the room or stay during the history. If the patient indicates they want the person to stay, the provider should then ask whether it is OK to discuss "everything" and/or "do you know why patient (name) is here today?" In most cases the person will indicate that the patient is here for HIV care; however, if it is still not clear, the provider should consider asking the person to leave the room so they can ask the patient in private, without disclosing the HIV diagnosis.

A comprehensive history that includes past medical history, social and family history, review of all medications and allergies, and review of systems and a complete physical examination should be performed at the initial visit (Tables 9.1 and 9.2). The provider should be mindful to identify possible risk factors for progression of illness and potential complications and determine if the patient has sufficient social support.

In addition to the standard history, the following items should be addressed:

Table 9.1 KEY ELEMENTS OF THE MEDICAL HISTORY AT THE INITIAL HIV VISIT

HISTORY COMPONENT	DETAILS	COMMENTS
HIV-specific history	• Date of seroconversion (if known) • Risk factors for transmission • CD4 count: nadir and pretreatment (if already on treatment) • Detailed history of previous treatment regimens as well as related adverse effects (if any) • Prior HIV resistance testing (if any) and HLA-B5701	Patients previously treated might not recall all of their past treatments, so medical records from previous providers should be obtained.
Past medical history	• Viral hepatitis: coinfection with HBV or HCV is common, can progress faster in PWH, might need treatment • Cardiovascular risk/disease: hypertension, diabetes mellitus, dyslipidemia can affect choice of ART • Other comorbidities: CKD, endocrine disorders, cerebrovascular disease, etc. • Malignancies: increased incidence in PWH, some might be indicative of AIDS • OB/GYN: prior pregnancies, present contraceptives (if any), previous Pap smears and mammography results, potential plans for future pregnancies • Tuberculosis: risk factors and potential exposures • Previous hospitalizations • Surgeries (including complications, if any) • Childhood infections	Should focus on presence of common comorbidities, particularly those that might affect choice of ART or response to it
Sexual history	• Gender identity and sexual orientation • Sexual partners: number and gender of partners • Type of sexual activities: oral, vaginal, anal, use of sex toys • Use of condoms: type and frequency • Activities associated with sex: alcohol/drug consumption, exchange for favors (money, goods, etc.) • STIs: any previous diagnosis and treatments • Partners: HIV status and other STIs	Risk of STIs varies greatly if patients are identified by gender identity and sexual orientation rather than just sex (male or female). Can identify patients who might be candidates for cervical/anal Pap smears Can help identify potential sites of testing (e.g., oral testing for chlamydia in patients who perform oral sex)
Psychiatric history	• Diagnosis and treatments • Sleep patterns: could indicate underlying depression or adverse effects of ART	Depression is frequent in PWH and if not adequately managed can significantly decrease adherence.
Medications and allergies	• List all medications currently taken (including OTCs and supplements) • Allergies and reactions	Some OTCs and supplements may interact with ART. Allergies: note reaction as well as date of first/last occurrence if known
Social history	• Employment and travel: provide insight into potential exposures and risk factors • Alcohol and tobacco use • Substance abuse: details of what type, frequency, and method of administration should be sought • Domestic violence: does the patient feel safe at home? • Hobbies and pastimes • Animal/pet exposure	Will give the provider insight into the patient's safety net and social/home support Can identify potential barriers to treatment
Family history	• First-degree family members • Any family member known to have HIV	May identify potential risk factors for heart disease Can provide information regarding support in the family if other members have HIV
Immunizations	• All vaccines with dates (if possible)	Will help determine any vaccines the patient may require
Healthcare maintenance	• Age appropriate as per guidelines • Risk factor appropriate as per guidelines	Can vary by age, gender, and exposures
Healthcare system Information	• Other healthcare providers managing the patient • Primary contact information (including emergency contacts) • Healthcare proxy and anyone authorized to access patient's information • Advance directives • Disclosure information	Patient might want restricted access to his/her information (including spouse occasionally). It is important to reinforce the confidential nature of the information provided.

Table 9.2 KEY ELEMENTS OF THE REVIEW OF SYSTEMS FOR PWH

REVIEW OF SYSTEMS

Constitutional	Intentional/unintentional weight change, fever, chills, night sweats, fatigue, malaise
Head, eyes, ears, nose, and throat (HEENT)	Hearing changes, ear pain, nasal congestion, sinus pain, hoarseness, sore throat, rhinorrhea, swallowing difficulty, oral lesion, eye pain, swelling, redness, foreign body, discharge, vision changes (floaters or blurred vision)
Cardiovascular	Chest pain, dyspnea, orthopnea, claudication, edema, palpitations
Respiratory	Cough, sputum, bloody sputum, wheezing, shortness of breath
Genitourinary	Dysmenorrhea, bleeding, dyspareunia, dysuria, urinary frequency, hematuria, urinary incontinence, urgency, flank pain, urinary flow changes, hesitancy, genital lesion
Musculoskeletal	Arthralgias, myalgias, joint swelling, joint stiffness, back pain, neck pain, injury history
Skin	Skin lesion, pruritus, hair changes, breast/skin changes, nipple discharge, rash
Neurologic	Weakness, numbness, paresthesia, loss of consciousness, syncope, dizziness, headache, coordination changes, recent falls
Psychiatric	Anxiety/panic, depression, insomnia, personality changes, delusions, rumination, suicidal ideation, homicidal ideation, hallucinations, social issues, memory changes, violence/abuse history, eating concerns
Hematologic	Bruising, bleeding, transfusion history, lymphadenopathy
Endocrine	Polyuria, polydipsia, heat or cold intolerance

- Address the emotional status of the patient.

  - What is the level of anxiety regarding the HIV diagnosis?
  - How is he or she coping with the diagnosis of HIV?
  - Does the patient have an established social support network?

- Has the patient disclosed his/her HIV status to anyone (partner, family members, or friends)?

- Which sexual partners (or needle-sharing partners) may have been exposed and are potentially at risk for HIV? Have they been notified and tested? If not, would the PWH benefit from assistance in contacting past or recent sexual or needle-sharing partners?

An important aspect of the initial clinic encounter is to determine how the PWH is coping with their HIV diagnosis (particularly if newly diagnosed) and the patient's emotional status following the diagnosis. It is also important to ask the patient if they have shared their diagnosis with anyone (e.g. friends, partner, family member, roommate) (Yu et al., 2018). Nondisclosure of HIV status may lead to lower medication adherence and increased anxiety. While some patients are fearful of the reaction of others to whom they disclose their diagnosis, we generally encourage patients to disclose their diagnosis to at least close friends and/or family members. In most cases it leads to more emotional support, less anxiety, and improved patient well-being. The provider should also ask the PWH "What fears do you have?" Often, asking and answering this question can lower the anxiety level of the patient by dispelling myths or misinformation the patient may have heard or read about (Ruffell, 2017).

THE MORE PATIENTS KNOW, THE BETTER THEY CAN CARE FOR THEMSELVES

Assessing the PWH's level of understanding of the disease process, medications, and risks is essential in the comprehensive care of the individual with HIV. Studies have demonstrated that PWH with more knowledge of their disease status do better over time. Incomplete medication knowledge has been associated with lower adherence (Miller et al., 2003; Molla et al., 2018), showing the need to ensure patients understand their condition and their medications. The level of sophistication will obviously be different depending on a person's background, level of education, health literacy, years of infection, and other factors. Lower educational level does not correlate with lower adherence (Kim et al., 2018). Any opportunity to emphasize education, understanding, and knowledge of the disease state should be fully embraced.

The provider should not assume that the patient has a thorough understanding of HIV, even in patients with long-standing infection. Open-ended questions such as the following are recommended:

"What do you know about HIV?"

"What do you think you can do to maintain your health long term?"

"How can your HIV viral load and T-cell count impact your disease?"

The provider (or team member) should explain (in simple terms, depending on the patient's level of health literacy) the significance and meaning of CD4 or T cells, HIV viral load, opportunistic infection, and risks of transmission. The "teach back" method may be useful to demonstrate the patient's level of understanding and to improve adherence to treatment in patients with chronic diseases (Ha Dinh et al., 2016).

THE PATIENT–PROVIDER RELATIONSHIP

Medical care for the PWH should be patient-centered, with the primary focus on the person's needs and preferences. The care should be sensitive to the PWH's educational, cultural, and socioeconomic background. Understanding each person in their unique circumstances not only helps establish trust but has been shown to increase adherence to treatment (Ciechanowsk et al., 2001). Previous studies have shown that PWH who feel that their HIV provider is providing personalized, patient-centered care were more likely to be adherent to treatment and to achieve an undetectable viral load (Beach et al., 2006). Ideally the patient–provider relationship will be strengthened with each encounter as the PWH gains more confidence and comfort with the provider.

SENSITIVE, RESPECTFUL, AND NONJUDGMENTAL

HIV providers frequently care for patients with a wide variety of sexual practices: patients who have been victims of abuse, people who are/have been commercial sex workers, people who have used intravenous drugs, and individuals in the gay/lesbian/transgender/bisexual/queer communities. Issues of privacy and cultural sensitivity are especially relevant in these encounters. Fostering trust—encouraging truthfulness and openness in the patient–provider relationship—requires special attention to cultivating a nonjudgmental and approachable demeanor. It is important to be sensitive to the patient's priorities, be respectful of their individuality, and be aware of their self-perception. Providers need to be aware of their own implicit biases.

CULTURAL COMPETENCY ISSUES

PWH are ethnically and culturally diverse and span the spectrum of socioeconomic status. The PWH's background may be quite different from that of the clinician providing care. Thus, it is important for the clinician to be aware of the patient's unique cultural background. Evidence shows that failing to include the cultural norms and values of target populations can act as stumbling blocks to effective communication (Uwah, 2013). The effects of cultural competency in the care of PWH were identified early in the HIV epidemic, and its impacts were notable (O'Connor, 1996). Cultural competency involves not only race identity but also sexual orientation and gender identity. At times specific groups of people can feel disenfranchised if they feel their cultural identity is not being taken into consideration (Shover et al., 2018). Cultural awareness can identify substantial economic disadvantages, pervasive childhood adversity, limited

education, and limited resources that jointly put members of a particular community at risk for the acquisition of HIV, development of depression, and addiction (Le et al., 2016). By practicing cultural humility and medicine, providers can shape patient care and strengthen the patient–provider relationship, leading to increased treatment adherence and health literacy. This highlights the importance of providers being aware of these issues, especially given the disproportionate impact of HIV/AIDS on historically underserved groups such as people of color (Mogobe et al., 2016). It is important for providers to be aware of the culture surrounding the PWH and work to minimize any barriers to treatment. As an example, some communities incorporate their religious beliefs into healthcare. Being aware of these concepts can help use that faith-based practice to promote health literacy and compliance.

LANGUAGE

PWH in the US and elsewhere originate from many regions of the world. For many patients English is not their primary language. Thus, an important issue is ensuring effective communication between the patient and the members of the healthcare team. Language-concordant care ensures that the patient and provider understand each other; it also optimizes health outcomes, advances health equity for diverse populations, and enhances trust between patient and provider (Molina & Kasper, 2019). At times, out of convenience, providers may be tempted to use family members or friends to provide language assistance. However, these strategies may be associated with a number of problems, including the translator not directly translating the provider or patient's intent, leaving out key details, etc.; it may also result in breaches of confidentiality (Bischoff & Hudelson, 2010). Providing medically trained interpreter services is vital to promoting equitable healthcare and overcoming misinterpretation and patient-perceived prejudice that can be associated with being a patient who does not speak the local language (Bischoff & Hudelson, 2010; Ngo-Metzger et al., 2009).

THE HIV-ORIENTED PHYSICAL EXAMINATION

Sir William Osler is credited with the saying, "He who knows syphilis knows medicine." The modern-day equivalent of the old adage is "He who knows HIV knows medicine," because indeed HIV infection and its sequelae can affect every organ system and can present in every clinical way possible. The HIV-oriented exam, therefore, needs to be especially comprehensive, both for the assessment of current complaints and for establishing a baseline to compare with future findings (Table 9.3). At times the physical exam can provide clues to the patient's immunologic status. As an example, erythematous candidiasis is often present at CD4$^+$ cell counts between 200 and 500 cells/µL, while pseudomembranous candidiasis often indicates more immunosuppression (≤200 cells/µL) and

Table 9.3 PHYSICAL EXAMINATION OF THE PWH

BODY ORGAN/SYSTEM	BE ESPECIALLY ATTENTIVE TO
Vital signs	Weight loss, body mass index, fat distribution, blood pressure, pulse, respiration rate, temperature Pain/tenderness
General	Body habitus, nutritional status, obvious disabilities
Skin	Rash, seborrheic dermatitis, folliculitis, moles, psoriasis, lichen planus, Kaposi's sarcoma lesions, warts, vesicular lesions, dermatophytes, molluscum contagiosum Needle marks
HEENT	Visual acuity Retinal hemorrhages and exudates (suggestive of CMV) HIV retinopathy (cotton-wool spots) Oral exam: thrush, oral hairy leukoplakia, Kaposi's lesions, gingivitis, aphthous ulcers, chancres, dentition, herpetic lesions, angular cheilitis Thyroid exam
Hemolymphatic	Regional versus generalized lymphadenopathy Splenomegaly
Cardiac	Heart sounds, murmurs, gallop
Pulmonary	Focal or generalized abnormalities
Gastrointestinal	Jaundice, hepatomegaly, splenomegaly Abdominal masses Anorectal exam (ulcers, vesicles, chancres, masses, hemorrhoids, warts) If indicated, anal Pap smear
Genitourinary	Ulcers, warts, chancres, herpetic vesicles Gender-specific exam: (1) For women: pelvic exam, cervical exam, cervical Pap smear (2) For men: testicular exam
Neurologic	Mental status, cognitive function—consider baseline HIV cognitive assessment (e.g., Montreal Cognitive Assessment test) Cranial nerves, motor strength, sensation, gait, vibratory/proprioceptive exam
Psychiatric	Depression screen should be done at baseline (PHQ-2 as a screen or other validated tools) Evidence of self-injury or self-mutilation Evidence of abuse

oral hairy leukoplakia is usually associated with a CD4 count of less than 400 cells/μL (Levy et al., 2012; Nokta, 2008). The physical exam can also provide insight into any substance use issues, particularly by noting if the person has poor personal hygiene, significant weight loss/gain, scars at injection sites on the skin, or abnormalities in the nasal mucosa associated with inhalations (Mertens et al., 2008). Other findings should be sought on physical exam that might suggest opportunistic infections, such as skin lesions suggestive of Kaposi's sarcoma or cryptococcemia or spider angiomata suggestive of chronic liver disease (hepatitis B and C) (Srivastava et al., 2015; Tappero et al., 1995).

RECOGNITION OF ACUTE AND ADVANCED HIV INFECTION

As the trend toward earlier HIV diagnosis continues (prior to any significant immune dysfunction), the majority of PWH presenting to the clinic for the initial visit will be asymptomatic or will have minor nonspecific symptoms, which the individual is typically unlikely to mention outside of a study (Robb et al., 2016). Some of these newly diagnosed patients may still have signs or symptoms of acute infection, a mononucleosis-like syndrome, which is characterized by fever, lymphadenopathy, sore throat, rash, muscle aches, diarrhea, and headache (Hoenigl et al., 2016; Niu et al., 1993) (Table 9.4). The symptoms usually resolve within 2 weeks but may persist. The presence of prolonged symptomatic illness appears to correlate with more rapid progression to AIDS (Pedersen et al., 1989). Although usually associated with later stages of HIV disease, opportunistic infections can rarely occur during transient CD4 lymphopenia and early HIV infection (Braun et al., 2015). Oral and esophageal candidiasis is the most commonly diagnosed opportunistic infection during acute HIV, but other infections, including cytomegalovirus (CMV), *Pneumocystis jirovecii* pneumonia, and cryptosporidiosis, have been reported.

Table 9.4 SIGNS AND SYMPTOMS OF ACUTE
RETROVIRAL ILLNESS

SIGNS AND SYMPTOMS	APPROXIMATE INCIDENCE (%)
Fever	48–88
Pharyngitis/sore throat	21–51
Lymphadenopathy	36–45
Rash	12–47
Oral ulcers	12–17
Myalgia/arthralgia	28–46
Diarrhea	17–35
Headache	34–44
Hepatosplenomegaly	10–15
Oral/oropharyngeal or vaginal candidiasis	10
Weight loss	21–39
Neurologic syndromes: Aseptic meningitis Peripheral neuropathy Guillain–Barré syndrome	~10

Source: Hoenigl M, et al. *Emerg Infect Dis*. 2016;22(3):532–534.

Specific symptoms and signs that suggest chronic HIV infection should prompt testing in the hopes of early diagnosis; these include the following:

- Any sexually transmitted infection
- Oral ulcers/aphthous stomatitis
- Oral hairy leukoplakia
- Oral candidiasis
- Unexplained weight loss
- Unexplained chronic fatigue
- Persistent or difficult-to-control seborrheic dermatitis
- Persistent or difficult-to-control vaginal candidiasis
- Unexplained/persistent fevers
- Herpes zoster/shingles (especially if more than one dermatome or recurrent, and especially in young people)
- Chronic diarrhea
- Persistent night sweats
- Persistent generalized lymphadenopathy
- Severe or difficult-to-control psoriasis
- Chronic or persistent herpes simplex infection of the genital tract or perianal region

Likewise, some laboratory findings may clue the clinician to the possibility of chronic HIV infection:

- Any sexually transmitted infection
- Chronic thrombocytopenia
- Leukopenia
- Anemia of chronic inflammation, especially without an alternative explanation
- Low lipid levels (low cholesterol, high-density lipoprotein [HDL], and low-density lipoprotein [LDL]), with elevated triglycerides; this has been attributed to chronic inflammatory cytokines (Grunfeld et al., 1992)
- Elevated globulin:albumin ratio, indicating polyclonal gammopathy
- Persistent or intermittent unexplained transaminitis
- Low albumin or prealbumin, especially if wasting is present
- Decreased renal function with proteinuria (HIV nephropathy)

Also, a new diagnosis of certain diseases should prompt an HIV test because their incidence is increased in individuals with HIV:

- Active tuberculosis
- Non-Hodgkin's lymphoma or Hodgkin's disease
- Cervical carcinoma in situ
- Listeriosis in an otherwise non-immunosuppressed or pregnant woman
- Extraintestinal salmonellosis
- Recurrent bacterial pneumonia
- Bacteremic pneumococcal pneumonia
- Pelvic inflammatory disease

INITIAL LABORATORY EVALUATION

A comprehensive initial laboratory evaluation should be performed at or before the first clinic visit to establish a baseline CD4 count, HIV viral load, hepatic and renal function, etc. (Table 9.5). Laboratory data should ideally be available prior to the initial interaction, but at times PWH will present for the initial evaluation without any previous records or workup aside from their positive HIV test (Aberg et al., 2014). Laboratory testing can be divided into HIV-specific testing, assessing risk factors, and routine medical care labs. The initial laboratory evaluation is fairly extensive but can be simplified thereafter, since many of the initial tests need not be repeated.

Table 9.5 INITIAL HIV LABORATORY EVALUATION

CATEGORY	TEST	FREQUENCY	COMMENTS
HIV-specific testing	HIV serology (4th-generation Ab-Ag test)	-At baseline if not available in records	-If no prior results are available and viral load is expected to be undetectable (patient on treatment), needed to establish diagnosis
	CD4 count (absolute and percentage)	-At baseline -Monitor every 3–6 months initially. -If viral load <20 copies/mL and CD4 count >300–500 for 2 years, repeat only every 12 months. If CD4 >500, CD4 monitoring is optional.	-Establishes clinical stage of HIV -Establishes risk of opportunistic complications and the need for initiation and discontinuation of opportunistic infection prophylaxis - Note: CD4 percentage should be noted as it tends to be less variable than the absolute CD4 cell count and may better assess immune function.
	HIV viral load	-At baseline -Repeat 2–8 weeks after starting ART. -Subsequently, monitor every 3–4 months. -Monitor every 6 months in adherent patients with consistent viral suppression.	-May affect selection of ART (some ART should not be used if viral load >100,000 copies/mL) -Follow-up viral load testing determines response to antiviral therapy.
	Resistance testing	-Initially -Repeat if treatment failure is noted.	-Rate of drug-resistant gene detection in developed countries is 5–15%. -Genotypic testing is preferred; phenotypic testing can be helpful in highly treatment-experienced patients with history of multiple resistance mutations. -Integrase resistance testing is generally not recommended initially–rare at baseline. Consider testing for integrase resistance if patient is failing an integrase inhibitor-based regimen.
	HLA-B5701	-At baseline, if abacavir is a consideration	-Establishes risk of abacavir hypersensitivity -If positive, abacavir contraindicated
	Tropism testing	-If CCR5 antagonist is being considered	Only use maraviroc if virus is CCR5 tropic.
	G6PD screen	-Baseline or when appropriate	-If deficient, increases risk of hemolytic anemia, particularly with the use of primaquine and dapsone
General bloodwork	CBC with differential	-Baseline and as needed thereafter	-Screen for anemia, leukopenia, lymphopenia, thrombocytopenia (incidence 30–40% in patients with advanced HIV disease) -Neutropenia could represent bone marrow suppression due to HIV or other infiltrative infections (e.g., *Mycobacterium avium*). -Anemia could indicate medication toxicity (e.g., zidovudine), viral infection (parvovirus B19), or nutritional deficiencies (iron, B12, folate). -Eosinophilia may be a clue to a parasitic infection, allergy or atopy, eosinophilic folliculitis, or drug reaction.
	Complete metabolic panel	-Baseline -Every 3–6 months thereafter	-Decreased renal function may affect selection of ART certain medications may require dosing adjustment with concomitant renal. disease -Elevated BUN/creatinine may be a sign of HIV-associated nephropathy. -Elevated transaminase and bilirubin levels may provide clues regarding possible liver pathology (e.g., viral hepatitis, drug-induced liver injury, steatohepatitis).
	Glucose and lipid profile	-Baseline -Every 6–12 months thereafter or as indicated by the risk profile	-Will help to identify any baseline metabolic abnormalities and estimate cardiovascular risk -May influence ART choice
	Vitamin D level	-Baseline -As appropriate thereafter	-Consider especially if the patient is at risk for osteopenia or osteoporosis.
	Urinalysis	-Baseline	- Assess effect of ART on kidney function (especially tenofovir). Proteinuria may be a sign of HIV nephropathy.
	Pregnancy test	-Baseline and as appropriate thereafter	-For women of childbearing age

Table 9.5 CONTINUED

CATEGORY	TEST	FREQUENCY	COMMENTS
Coinfection/ comorbidity testing	Viral hepatitis serology	-Baseline -Repeat as indicated depending on risk	-May require vaccination against hepatitis A and/or B -Identifies patients requiring further evaluation for hepatitis C infection -May influence ART selection (particularly hepatitis B)
	Tuberculosis (TB)	-Baseline and yearly thereafter	-Baseline tuberculin skin test (PPD) or IGRA is indicated in all PWH, unless there is a history of prior positive test or treatment for latent TB. -Note that a PPD result ≥5 mm induration is considered reactive in PWH. -If positive, a chest x-ray should be obtained to rule out active disease along with a careful ROS and exam to rule out extrapulmonary TB.
	STIs: Syphilis Chlamydia/ Gonorrhea	-Baseline -Annually if sexually active -More frequent testing depending on other risk factors	-Screening for trichomonas indicated in women -Test for latent syphilis. -Testing for chlamydia/gonorrhea should include pharyngeal, urine, and rectal samples, depending on sexual practices. -If positive test, treatment and counseling on preventing STIs are indicated.
	Toxoplasma	-Baseline	-If seronegative, counseling on avoidance of new infection -If seropositive, prescribe prophylaxis if CD4 count ≤100.
	Varicella and CMV	-Baseline	-To identify PWH who may require primary immunization against varicella or against herpes zoster -If CMV negative, any future blood products that should also be CMV negative for leukocyte reduced products; counseling about possibility of sexual transmission of CMV should be provided.
Other Screening	Cervical Pap smear	-Baseline -Repeat every 6–12 months	-Determines if there is HPV infection and risk for neoplastic transformation -Same frequency of testing if HPV + -Evaluate more frequently in HIV-infected women
	Anal Pap smear	-Baseline	-Consider if history of receptive anal intercourse or history of genital warts (or abnormal cervical Pap smear in women). -Optimal follow-up not yet established
	Bone density scan		-Baseline screening for osteoporosis in postmenopausal woman and men age 50 years or older -Could be considered in patients at risk (on tenofovir-based regimens)
	Age-appropriate healthcare maintenance		-Breast and colon cancer screening should follow age-appropriate guidelines. -ASCVD score should be considered to evaluate need for statin therapy. -Depression screening with repeat PHQ-2 should be considered. -Cognitive screening with MoCA -Should consider dental care as part of routine healthcare maintenance -Other risk-appropriate screening as per US Preventive Service Task Force Recommendations

DISCUSSING INITIATION OF THERAPY

In the last several years, some communities have successfully initiated "rapid initiation" programs, in which antiretroviral therapy (ART) is started immediately following diagnosis, a significant shift from previous recommendations. In the early years of the HIV epidemic, limited resources and concerns about suboptimal adherence led to a cautious approach in which PWH underwent multiple counseling sessions that could last several weeks or months before starting ART (World Health Organization [WHO], 2017). More recent data seem to support a rapid initiation (within 1 week and at times even the same day) of ART (Ford et al., 2018). This appears to improve outcomes across the HIV treatment cascade in low- and middle-income settings, including reducing loss to care. However, there is also some evidence that seems to indicate that in certain circumstances this approach could lead to an increase in loss to follow-up because of insufficient time to accept and disclose HIV status and prepare for lifelong treatment (Boyd et al., 2019; Ford et al., 2018). We agree that, when possible, ART should be started promptly, taking into consideration social and psychological aspects of committing to lifelong therapy. Contraindications such as concurrent infection with tuberculosis or cryptococcus need to be considered; if this is suspected, therapy should be delayed to lessen the likelihood of the immune reconstitution syndrome (Lawn et al., 2011).

TELEHEALTH IN HIV

The US Health Resources and Services Administration defines telehealth as the use of electronic information and telecommunications technologies to support long-distance clinical healthcare, health-related education for PWH and professionals, and public health and health administration. Many studies have supported the use of telehealth to increase convenience to PWH by decreasing travel time, improve individual satisfaction, diminish healthcare disparities, and reduce cost that will ultimately lead to improvement in clinical outcomes and quality of care (Kruse et al., 2017). Guaranteeing confidentiality, educating PWH and providers, and obtaining insurance reimbursement are some of the challenges that face the implementation of telehealth programs (Dandachi et al., 2019). During the recent COVID-19 pandemic the use of telemedicine increased and allowed providers to assess and evaluate PWH without exposing individuals or healthcare professionals to COVID-19 (Smith et al., 2020). The Centers for Medicare and Medicaid (CMS) relaxed rules and allowed providers to bill for these visits in the same manner as face-to-face visits.

Recent literature seems to indicate that telehealth programs for PWH can improve retention in care by decreasing travel time, better fitting the personal schedule, and providing more privacy; however, some worry about effective communication and examination as well as the safety of personal information (Dandachi et al., 2020). Studies of telehealth indicate that people feel relieved to avoid travel time and physical contact with the clinic itself, and most people view it positively. Many even prefer to have telehealth visits and rated it better than traditional in-clinic visits, particularly those who have difficulties with travel (more specifically, people in rural areas). Providers' concerns with the use of telehealth usually include not being able to do a physical exam, longer visit times, and inability to connect with the patient. However, in general providers feel that with the use of telehealth they are able to communicate well with patients, especially with already established PWH whom the provider knows well and with whom they have a good rapport (Dandachi et al., 2020). Barriers to telehealth include lack of access to high-speed internet service, which is common in remote areas. Technical challenges such as being comfortable with computers and computer software and new telehealth platforms can also be present (Cole et al., 2019). In general, when used appropriately, telehealth can be a useful tool for managing PWH.

RECOMMENDED READING

Aberg JA, Gallant JE, Ghanem KG, et al. Primary care guidelines for the management of persons infected with HIV: 2013 update by the HIV Medicine Association of the Infectious Disease Society of America. *Clin Infect Dis.* 2014;58:1–34.

REFERENCES

Aberg JA, Gallant JE, Ghanem KG, et al. Primary care guidelines for the management of persons infected with HIV: 2013 update by the HIV medicine association of the Infectious Diseases Society of America. *Clin Infect Dis.* 2014;58(1):e1–e34.

Beach MC, Keruly J, Moore RD. Is the quality of the patient-provider relationship associated with better adherence and health outcomes for patients with HIV? *J Gen Intern Med.* 2006;21(6):661–665.

Berghoff CR, Gratz KL, Portz KJ, et al. The role of emotional avoidance, the patient-provider relationship, and other social support in ART adherence for HIV+ individuals. *AIDS Behav.* 2018;22(3):929–938.

Bischoff A, Hudelson P. Communicating with foreign language-speaking patients: is access to professional interpreters enough? *J Travel Med.* 2010;17(1):15–20.

Boyd MA, Boffito M, Castagna A, et al. Rapid initiation of antiretroviral therapy at HIV diagnosis: definition, process, knowledge gaps. *HIV Med.* 2019;20(Suppl 1):3–11.

Braun DL, Kouyos RD, Balmer B, et al. Frequency and spectrum of unexpected clinical manifestations of primary HIV-1 infection. *Clin Infect Dis.* 2015;61(6):1013–1021.

Ciechanowski PS, Katon WJ, Russo JE, et al. The patient-provider relationship: attachment theory and adherence to treatment in diabetes. *Am J Psychiatry.* 2001;158(1):29–35.

Cole B, Pickard K, Stredler-Brown A. Report on the use of telehealth in early intervention in Colorado: strengths and challenges with telehealth as a service delivery method. *Int J Telerehabil.* 2019;11(1):33–40.

Dandachi D, Dang BN, Lucari B, et al. Exploring the attitude of patients with HIV about using telehealth for HIV care. *AIDS Patient Care STDs.* 2020;34(4):166–172.

Dandachi D, Freytag J, Giordano TP, et al. It is time to include telehealth in our measure of patient retention in HIV care. *AIDS Behav.* 2020;24(9):2463–2465.

Dandachi D, Lee C, Morgan RO, et al. Integration of telehealth services in the healthcare system: with emphasis on the experience of patients living with HIV. *J Investig Med.* 2019;67(5):815–820.

Doshi RK, Milberg J, Isenberg D, et al. High rates of retention and viral suppression in the US HIV safety net system: HIV care continuum in the Ryan White HIV/AIDS Program, 2011. *Clin Infect Dis.* 2015;60(1):117–125.

Flickinger TE, Saha S, Moore RD, et al. Higher quality communication and relationships are associated with improved patient engagement in HIV care. *J AIDS.* 2013;63(3):362–366.

Ford N, Meintjes G, Calmy A, et al. Managing advanced HIV disease in a public health approach. *Clin Infect Dis.* 2018;66(Suppl 2):S106–SS110.

Ford N, Migone C, Calmy A, et al. Benefits and risks of rapid initiation of antiretroviral therapy. *AIDS.* 2018;32(1):17–23.

Grunfeld C, Pang M, Doerrler W, et al. Lipids, lipoproteins, triglyceride clearance, and cytokines in human immunodeficiency virus infection and the acquired immunodeficiency syndrome. *J Clin Endocrinol Metab.* 1992;74(5):1045–1052.

Ha Dinh TT, Bonner A, Clark R, et al. The effectiveness of the teach-back method on adherence and self-management in health education for people with chronic disease: a systematic review. *JBI Database System Rev Implement Rep.* 2016;14(1):210–247.

Hoenigl M, Green N, Camacho M, et al. Signs or symptoms of acute HIV infection in a cohort undergoing community-based screening. *Emerg Infect Dis.* 2016;22(3):532–534.

Kim J, Lee E, Park BJ, et al. Adherence to antiretroviral therapy and factors affecting low medication adherence among incident HIV-infected individuals during 2009-2016: A nationwide study. *Sci Rep.* 2018;8(1):3133.

Kruse CS, Krowski N, Rodriguez B, et al. Telehealth and patient satisfaction: a systematic review and narrative analysis. *BMJ Open.* 2017;7(8):e016242.

Lawn SD, Torok ME, Wood R. Optimum time to start antiretroviral therapy during HIV-associated opportunistic infections. *Curr Opin Infect Dis.* 2011;24(1):34–42.

Le HN, Hipolito MM, Lambert S, et al. Culturally sensitive approaches to identification and treatment of depression among HIV-infected African American adults: a qualitative study of primary care providers' perspectives. *J Depress Anxiety.* 2016;5(2):223.

Levy TH, Jacobson DF. Dermatologic manifestations as indicators of immune status in HIV/AIDS. *J Gen Intern Med.* 2012;27(1):124.

Mertens JR, Flisher AJ, Satre DD, et al. The role of medical conditions and primary care services in 5-year substance use outcomes among chemical dependency treatment patients. *Drug Alcohol Depend.* 2008;98(1–2):45–53.

Miller LG, Liu H, Hays RD, et al. Knowledge of antiretroviral regimen dosing and adherence: a longitudinal study. *Clin Infect Dis.* 2003;36(4):514–518.

Mogobe KD, Shaibu S, Matshediso E, et al. Language and culture in health literacy for people living with HIV: perspectives of health care providers and professional care team members. *AIDS Res Treat.* 2016;2016:5015707.

Molina RL, Kasper J. The power of language-concordant care: a call to action for medical schools. *BMC Med Educ.* 2019;19(1):378.

Molla AA, Gelagay AA, Mekonnen HS, et al. Adherence to antiretroviral therapy and associated factors among HIV-positive adults attending care and treatment in University of Gondar Referral Hospital, Northwest Ethiopia. *BMC Infect Dis.* 2018;18(1):266.

Ngo-Metzger Q, Sorkin DH, Phillips RS. Healthcare experiences of limited English-proficient Asian American patients: a cross-sectional mail survey. *Patient.* 2009;2(2):113–120.

Niu MT, Stein DS, Schnittman SM. Primary human immunodeficiency virus type 1 infection: review of pathogenesis and early treatment intervention in humans and animal retrovirus infections. *J Infect Dis.* 1993;168(6):1490–1501.

Nokta M. Oral manifestations associated with HIV infection. *Curr HIV/AIDS Rep.* 2008;5(1):5–12.

O'Connor BB. Promoting cultural competence in HIV/AIDS care. *J Assoc Nurses AIDS Care.* 1996;7(Suppl 1):41–53.

Pedersen C, Lindhardt BO, Jensen BL, et al. Clinical course of primary HIV infection: consequences for subsequent course of infection. *BMJ.* 1989;299(6692):154–157.

Robb ML, Eller LA, Kibuuka H, et al. Prospective study of acute HIV-1 infection in adults in East Africa and Thailand. *N Engl J Med.* 2016;374(22):2120–2130.

Ruffell S. Stigma kills! The psychological effects of emotional abuse and discrimination towards a patient with HIV in Uganda. *BMJ Case Rep.* 2017;2017:bcr2016218024.

Shover CL, DeVost MA, Beymer MR, et al. Using sexual orientation and gender identity to monitor disparities in HIV, sexually transmitted infections, and viral hepatitis. *Am J Public Health.* 2018;108(S4):S277–S283.

Smith AC, Thomas E, Snoswell CL, et al. Telehealth for global emergencies: implications for coronavirus disease 2019 (COVID-19). *J Telemed Telecare.* 2020;26(5):309–313.

Srivastava GN, Tilak R, Yadav J, et al. Cutaneous cryptococcus: marker for disseminated infection. *BMJ Case Rep.* 2015;2015:bcr2015210898.

Tappero JW, Perkins BA, Wenger JD, et al. Cutaneous manifestations of opportunistic infections in patients infected with human immunodeficiency virus. *Clin Microbiol Rev.* 1995;8(3):440–450.

Uwah C. The role of culture in effective HIV/AIDS communication by theatre in South Africa. *SAHARA J.* 2013;10(3-4):140–149.

World Health Organization. *Guidelines for Managing Advanced HIV Disease and Rapid Initiation of Antiretroviral Therapy.* Geneva: World Health Organization; 2017.

Yu Y, Luo D, Chen X, et al. Medication adherence to antiretroviral therapy among newly treated people living with HIV. *BMC Public Health.* 2018;18(1):825.

10.

HEALTH MAINTENANCE

Ramiz Kseri

CHAPTER GOALS

Upon completion of this chapter, the reader should be able to:

- Describe tuberculosis (TB) screening indications (including exposure history) and assessment methods (including selection, interpretation, and limitations of screening tests) in people with HIV (PWH)

- Discuss the importance of routine dental care for PWH and essential information to be included in the treating physician's written referral

- Discuss the prevention of cardiovascular disease before clinical presentation among PWH

- Discuss immunization schedule for PWH

- Discuss family planning and preconception care considerations in serodiscordant and seroconcordant couples living with HIV

- Discuss the recommended frequency and specimen collection technique for cervical Pap smears in female PWH, the role of human papillomavirus (HPV) testing, and indications for specialist referral for colposcopy

HIV HEALTHCARE FLOW SHEETS FOR PRIMARY CARE

Most electronic health record (EHR) systems allow for individually designed disease-specific flow sheets. These flow sheets can be designed to address specific centers' care reporting needs. At minimum, flow sheets should include HIV-specific information such as CD4+ T-cell counts, HIV viral loads, vaccine records, and healthcare maintenance reports. HIV drug resistance test results are more difficult to enter into flow sheets. Ideally, the EHR flow sheet is designed to trigger clinical reminders regarding the need for opportunistic infection prophylaxis and vaccinations or health maintenance screening based on patients' current CD4+ T-cell counts, serologies, age, and sex (Aberg et al., 2014; Panel on Opportunistic Infections in Adults and Adolescents with HIV, 2019).

The following sections describe examples of items that should be included in HIV healthcare flow sheets. Flow sheets should be individualized to the healthcare facility's and the provider's needs.

RECOMMENDED READING

Aberg JA, Gallant JE, Ghanem KG, et al. Primary care guidelines for the management of persons infected with HIV: 2013 update by the HIV Medicine Association of the Infectious Diseases Society of America. *Clin Infect Dis.* 2014;58(1):e1–34. doi:10.1093/cid/cit665

TB SCREENING AND ASSESSMENT

LEARNING OBJECTIVE

- Describe TB screening indications (including exposure history) and assessment methods (including selection, interpretation, and limitations of screening tests) in PWH

WHAT'S NEW?

Interferon-gamma release assays (IGRAs) are an alternative to tuberculin skin tests (TSTs) for detection of *Mycobacterium tuberculosis* infection and are preferred for individuals 5 years or older who are bacillus Calmette–Guérin (BCG) vaccinated.

KEY POINTS

- Due to immunodeficiency, PWH are at increased risk for developing active TB disease and thus should be routinely screened for TB.

- PWH also frequently have other indications for TB screening, including contact with persons from areas of the world where there is a high incidence of TB and high-risk exposures in correctional and residential facilities.

- In PWH, TSTs or IGRAs should be performed at the time of initial HIV diagnosis. For persons who are initially TST or IGRA negative, testing should be repeated in those who have experienced improvement in immune function due to antiretroviral therapy (ART). Annual testing may be considered in persons with ongoing or repeated exposure to TB.

- TST responses of 5 mm or larger induration are considered positive in PWH. However, even negative TST or IGRA results may warrant preventive therapy in the setting of high-risk exposures.

- Chest radiography is indicated regardless of TST or IGRA results in PWH with recent exposure to patients with active TB or with a history of symptoms consistent with TB, as well as in any PWH with a positive test result.

HIV-associated immune compromise is associated with an increased incidence of TB among PWH, with a relative risk of 10 times that of HIV-negative persons (Horsburgh & Rubin, 2011). As with other opportunistic infections, there has been a substantial decrease in the incidence of TB among persons receiving ART. However, untreated TB is one of the few opportunistic infections transmissible to others and thus has additional public health implications for control and prevention.

PWH are at increased risk for developing active disease by reactivation of untreated latent TB infection (LTBI), at an estimated rate of 3% to 16% *per year* compared to a 5% to 10% *lifetime* risk in HIV-negative persons with no other risk factors. Once infection with *Mycobacterium tuberculosis* occurs, there can be rapid progression of newly acquired infection to disease—for example, within the first month following exposure to an infectious person. Similarly, reactivation disease may also progress rapidly, particularly in highly immunocompromised individuals. The majority of HIV-negative individuals infected with TB who develop active disease in the US were born, previously lived, or traveled for extended periods in areas where TB is endemic. Currently, 8% of individuals with active TB have underlying HIV disease. However, prior to the advent of ART, in the US, the proportion of individuals with TB who had underlying HIV was nearly 50%. TB outbreaks were identified among individuals living with HIV in US institutional settings, including healthcare facilities, correctional facilities, and homeless shelters. Although transmission in institutional settings in the US is now rare, there is substantial risk in resource-limited settings in which TB is endemic in the general population. PWH who are employees or volunteers in settings identified as high risk by local health authorities should be advised of their risk of exposure to TB and offered alternative sites of work. HIV-infected healthcare workers who intermittently work or volunteer in countries where TB is endemic should be similarly advised about their risk. The healthcare provider should help the patient assess the level of risk by evaluating factors such as the prevalence of TB in that community, the precautions against transmission that are in place, and the patient's specific duties in those settings.

PWH, especially those with CD4$^+$ T-cell counts of less than 200/μL, are more likely to present with extrapulmonary TB, miliary pulmonary disease, and disseminated TB compared to HIV-uninfected persons. PWH may have active pulmonary TB with normal chest radiographs. Similarly, patients coinfected with HIV and TB may present with negative acid-fast bacilli (AFB) sputum in up to 70% of cases (Getahun et al., 2007). In a high-incidence setting and active case-finding study of patients with culture-positive TB, up to 32% had normal chest radiographs; of those whose AFB smears were negative and who had normal chest radiographs, 8% had TB, 5% had CD4$^+$ T-cell counts of 350/μL or greater, and 10% had CD4$^+$ T-cell counts of less than 350/μL (Cain et al., 2010). Nucleic acid amplification tests such as Gene Xpert MTB/RIF are more sensitive than AFB smears, and they may identify up to 70% of smear-negative, culture-positive cases (Boehme et al., 2010).

INDICATIONS FOR LTBI SCREENING

Many indications for LTBI screening may be present concurrently in HIV-infected patients, which represent conditions with higher risk of development of TB than those without these conditions, or in situations that pose high risks of exposure or recent infection with *M. tuberculosis*. Indications for screening include the following:

- Foreign-born persons, or persons in close contact with recent immigrants or refugees, from regions with high rates of TB (i.e., Africa, Asia, Latin America, Russia, and countries of the former Soviet Union)

- Other medical conditions, such as diabetes mellitus, silicosis, chronic renal failure, being underweight (≤10% below normal), gastrectomy, injection drug use, malignancies (lymphoma, leukemia, and head and neck cancer), cardiac and renal transplantation, or use of immunosuppressive therapies (especially tumor necrosis factor-α inhibitors)

- Persons from situations with a high risk for person-to-person transmission, such as those working or residing in correctional facilities (3% of TB cases in the US), homeless shelters (6% of TB cases in the US), and other congregate settings (American Thoracic Society, Centers for Disease Control and Prevention, and Infectious Diseases Society of America, 2005)

- Close contacts of person with active TB, 30% to 40% of whom will be found to have LBTI, and 1% or 2% of whom will have active disease

- Children born to HIV-infected mothers who have TB or who are at high risk for possible LBTI (e.g., close contacts of persons with active disease)

- Persons previously treated for latent or active TB who are re-exposed to someone with active TB can become reinfected, particularly in hyperendemic settings.

SCREENING TESTS FOR
M. TUBERCULOSIS INFECTION

TST

The time-honored method for diagnosis of *M. tuberculosis* infection is the TST, which measures a polycellular delayed-type hypersensitivity response at the site of injection following the administration of purified protein derivative (PPD), an admixture of mycobacterial antigens. The preferred skin test is the intradermal, or Mantoux, method. It is administered by injecting 0.1 mL of 5 tuberculin units (TU) PPD intradermally into the dorsal or volar surface of the forearm. Tests should be read 48 to 72 hours after test administration, and the diameter of induration transverse to the long axis of the arm should be recorded in millimeters. Multiple puncture tests (i.e., tine test, Heaf test) and PPD strengths of 1 and 250 TU are not sufficiently accurate and should not be used (American Thoracic Society/Centers for Disease Control and Prevention, 2000). Induration of 5 mm or greater in PWH indicates a positive TST. TSTs require two visits to perform and confirm the results of the test and experience in intradermal placement of the test. There is some subjectivity in its interpretation, and false-positive results may occur from exposure to nontuberculous mycobacteria or prior vaccination with *M. bovis* BCG. A positive TST has been shown to be predictive of progression to active TB in PWH, who benefit from preventive therapy with a reduction in TB incidence.

IGRAs

IGRAs are blood tests that measure interferon-γ (IFN-γ) secreted by sensitized T lymphocytes after exposure to TB-specific antigens ESAT-6 and CFP-10. Two tests are currently approved by the US Food and Drug Administration (FDA) and in use for the detection of *M. tuberculosis* infection: QuantiFERON-TB Gold In-Tube (QFT-GIT) and T-SPOT TB test (T-Spot). The QFT measures the IFN-γ concentration using an enzyme-linked immunosorbent assay (ELISA), whereas the T-Spot enumerates T cells releasing IFN-γ using an ELISPOT assay. The QFT requires fresh blood to be incubated for 18 to 24 hours with plasma separation, ELISA testing, and comparison to negative and positive mitogen control antigens (phytohemagglutinin). T-Spot assays must be done on fresh blood specimens, processed within 12 hours, and incubated overnight. IGRAs require a single visit, are less subjective in interpretation than TSTs, and are more specific for detection of *M. tuberculosis* infection—that is, there is less cross-reactivity to nontuberculous mycobacteria (except *M. kansasii*, *M. szulgai*, and *M. marinum*) and BCG (Centers for Disease Control and Prevention [CDC], 2010).

Current evidence suggests that IGRAs have higher specificity (92–97%) compared to TSTs (56–95%) (NIH-CDC-HIVMA/IDSA, 2013). TSTs are more likely to identify persons with longstanding cellular immune responses to TB antigens, and IGRAs are more likely to be positive in persons with recent *M. tuberculosis* infection (Horsburgh & Rubin,

2011). For diagnosis of LTBI, the correlation between TSTs and IGRAs is poor to moderate among persons with HIV infection (Cattamanchi et al., 2011). For PWH with active TB, in one study, sensitivity was low for both QFT-GIT and TST (63% and 55%, respectively) and was inversely correlated with low CD4$^+$ T-cell counts (Raby et al., 2008). In PWH at low risk of TB exposure, false-positive tests with QFT have also been reported, suggesting the need to repeat a positive QFT test to confirm the diagnosis of LTBI when patients are at low risk of exposure (Gray et al., 2020). There have been no definitive comparisons of TSTs and IGRAs for LTBI screening of PWH in low-incidence settings.

Either TSTs or IGRAs are appropriate for TB screening among PWH in the US. Some experts have suggested using both the TST and an IGRA to screen for LTBI, but the predictive value of this approach is not clear, and use of this strategy would be more expensive and more difficult to implement. The routine use of both TSTs and IGRAs to screen for LTBI in the same patient is not recommended in the US (NIH-CDC-HIVMA/IDSA, 2020).

Testing Frequency

PWH should receive a test for LTBI at the time of initial HIV diagnosis, with repeat testing considered for those who are TST or IGRA negative initially with advanced HIV infection (CD4$^+$ T-cell counts <200/μL) and who have improvement in immune function due to ART (CD4$^+$ T-cell counts ≥200/μL). Annual testing may also be considered in those who have ongoing or repeated exposure to TB, such as individuals who travel for extended periods of time to setting where TB is hyperendemic. Intercurrent testing should be done based on recent exposure to a case of active TB, including repeat testing 8 to 12 weeks after the initial negative test for TB infection because it may take this long for the TST or IGRA to become positive following infection.

Anergy Testing

PWH are at increased risk to have impaired delayed-type hypersensitivity responses to skin test antigens due to decreased CD4$^+$ T-cell counts and, therefore, to have a compromised ability to react to TSTs (i.e., to have cutaneous anergy). Anergy testing has not been helpful in attempting to distinguish false-negative TST results due to anergy from true-negative results. Anergy testing is not recommended for routine use in PWH due to problems with test standardization and reproducibility, the variable risk for TB in the setting of anergy, and the lack of demonstrated benefit of preventive therapy in anergic PWH.

Chest Radiography and Symptom Screening in PWH

In asymptomatic persons with positive tests for LTBI, chest radiography should be done to exclude active TB. Persons with symptoms of TB, such as cough, fever, and night sweats, should be evaluated for TB regardless of IGRA or skin test results. The absence of these symptoms has a high negative predictive value for excluding active TB (Cain et al., 2010). Chest radiography should also be considered following recent exposure to a person with active TB regardless of skin test or IGRA results. PWH with pulmonary TB are more likely to exhibit atypical radiologic presentations, especially those with low CD4+ T-cell counts and, in some cases, normal chest radiographs (Palmieri et al., 2002).

Preventive Therapy

Preventive therapy is recommended following exposure to persons with active TB, regardless of initial or repeat TST results, or in persons with TST induration of 5 mm or greater and who have not been treated for active or latent TB and have no clinical evidence of active TB. Preventive therapy should be considered in persons with a history of potential exposure in high-risk settings (as listed previously) regardless of results of testing for LTBI.

For further information on evaluation and treatment of active TB disease, see Chapter 28.

RECOMMENDED READING

Centers for Disease Control and Prevention. Anergy skin testing and preventive therapy for HIV-infected persons: revised recommendations. *MMWR Morb Mortal Wkly Rep.* 1997;46(RR-15):1–12.

ACKNOWLEDGMENTS

This section is an update from the original version authored by David Cohn, MD, in the previous edition.

DENTAL CARE

LEARNING OBJECTIVE

- Discuss the importance of routine dental care for PWH and essential information to be included in the treating physician's written referral

WHAT'S NEW?

A large proportion of PWH do not receive needed dental and oral care despite the high prevalence of such disorders in this population. Referrals for dental care should include information about the patient's risk for secondary infection and bleeding, infectious status, and current medications.

KEY POINTS

- PWH are at increased risk for oral and dental problems due to immunodeficiency, salivary gland dysfunction, substance use, tobacco use, poor oral hygiene, and limited access to dental care.

- Oral cavity problems can undermine the success of ART by exacerbating existing medical, nutritional, and psychosocial problems; compromising adherence to treatment regimens; and diminishing quality of life.

- Providers should include basic oral screening in their routine clinic visits and advocate for routine dental care for patients.

- Referrals for dental care should include information about the patient's risk for secondary infection and bleeding, infectious status, and current medications.

Oral healthcare is an important component of the management of patients with HIV infection. Oral cavity problems can undermine the success of ART by exacerbating existing medical, nutritional, and psychosocial problems; compromising adherence to treatment regimens; and diminishing quality of life (New York State Department of Health AIDS Institute [NYSDOH], 2020).

Oral disease occurs disproportionately in the same individuals most affected by HIV: those of low socioeconomic status, those with limited healthcare access and use of services, and substance users whose attention to personal health and hygiene is often suboptimal (NYSDOH, 2020). They do not receive the dental care they need. In the HIV Cost and Services Utilization Study, which examined a nationally representative sample of persons in HIV care, 35% of patients had no regular source of dental care, 22% had not received dental care in more than 2 years, 25% had not received needed dental care, and 48% had no dental insurance coverage (Freed et al., 2005).

Significant proportions of PWH have HIV-related oral problems such as untreated caries (39%), gum problems (47%), missing teeth (47%), and xerostomia (dry mouth) (37%) (Freed et al., 2005). PWH with advanced immunosuppression also are at risk for serious systemic opportunistic infections and neoplasms, many of which can manifest in the oral cavity. Examples include candidiasis, hairy leukoplakia, Kaposi's sarcoma, and aphthous ulcerations (Bonito, 2001). The presence of oral candidiasis without medical explanation (e.g., recent antibiotics) is most often related to a low CD4+ T-cell number and is considered a marker for cell-mediated immunodeficiency. Deterioration of oral immunologic functions and changes in salivary flow rate and composition also aid in the development of caries and periodontal diseases, including gingivitis, which can progress to serious necrotizing gingivitis and compromise masticatory functions and nutrition (Bonito, 2001). The presence of necrotizing ulcerative periodontitis, a more aggressive form of periodontal disease, should also be considered a sign of severe immune deterioration. It is a rapidly progressing disease, and treatment should be initiated as early as possible.

Thus, oral healthcare should be an integral component of primary healthcare for PWH (NYSDOH, 2020). Providers must become familiar with oral conditions that affect PWH and include basic oral screening in routine clinic visit exams. Providers also must be aware of and advocate for oral healthcare and dental services in their communities. Finally, providers must educate patients about the importance of good oral hygiene practices and regular dental care (at least twice annually) (NYSDOH, 2020).

When considering referral to a dental specialist, the main issues of concern are the patient's risk for bleeding, risk for infection, and infectiousness. Accordingly, the following information should be provided in dental referrals:

- *Bleeding risk*: Platelet count (platelet count <60,000/mm^3 may require platelet transfusion or steroids prior to dental treatment), liver biochemical tests, history of coagulation or other bleeding disorders, history of liver disease, and current hemoglobin (to ascertain risk of anemia should significant bleeding occur)

- *Infection risk*: Total white blood cell count, absolute neutrophil count, CD4$^+$ T-cell count, history of valvular or congenital heart disease, and other medical risks for infection (e.g., active intravenous drug use posing a risk for endocarditis)

- *Antibiotic prophylaxis*: Based on the individual need of each patient, antibiotic prophylaxis may be indicated prior to dental care. The need for antibiotic prophylaxis is not based on CD4$^+$ T-cell counts, viral load, or AIDS diagnosis. Patients with severe neutropenia (neutrophil count <500/mm^3) should be premedicated with antibiotics prior to dental treatment. Otherwise, antibiotic prophylaxis is recommended based on the standard guidelines set forth by the American Heart Association (http://www.aha.org) for the prevention of bacterial endocarditis.

- *Concurrent infections*: Current HIV viral load, chronic active hepatitis B or hepatitis C infections, and contagious respiratory diseases such as active/untreated TB

All medications also should be detailed to prevent drug interactions or adverse effects if medications will be used or prescribed as part of the dental care.

RECOMMENDED READING

Freed JR, Marcus M, Freed BA, et al. Oral health findings for HIV-infected adult medical patients from the HIV Cost and Services Utilization Study. *J Am Dental Assoc.* 2005;136:1396–1405.

Greenspan JS, Greenspan D, Winkler JR. Diagnosis and management of the oral manifestations of HIV infection and AIDS. *Infect Dis Clin North Am.* 1988;2:373–385.

Integrating HIV Innovating Practices. Implementing oral healthcare into HIV primary care settings curriculum. 2013. https://careacttarget.org/library/implementing-oral-health-care-hiv-primary-care-settings-curriculum-0

Lee KC, Tami TA. Otolaryngologic manifestation of HIV disease. In: Cohen PT, Sande MA, Volberding PA, eds. *The AIDS Knowledge Base.* 3rd ed. Philadelphia, PA: Lippincott Williams & Wilkins; 1999:559–575.

IMMUNIZATIONS

LEARNING OBJECTIVE

- Discuss immunization schedule among PWH

WHAT'S NEW?

Information in this section is based on the recommendations from the Advisory Committee on Immunization Practices (ACIP), which was released in February 2020 (Freedman et al., 2020).

KEY POINTS

- Response to vaccinations is based on the CD4$^+$ T-cell count.

- Response to vaccinations is best as early as possible in the infection, or soon after immune reconstitution with ART.

- Vaccinations may need to be repeated when immune reconstitution occurs with ART, as immunosuppression can cause suboptimal response initially.

- Live virus vaccinations are not safe in PWH with a CD4$^+$ T-cell count less than 200 cells/mm^3.

CONCERN WITH IMMUNIZATIONS?

Prior to ART in the 1980s, the concern was that immunizations could inadvertently upregulate the immune system and cause elevations in HIV replication, which ultimately would accelerate the infection progression. However, it was found that this increase in HIV RNA was only transient. Also, in PWH who are on ART, immunization causes no detectable elevations in the RNA levels. The only contraindication to immunizations is a low CD4$^+$ T-cell count (<200 cells/mm^3) for live vaccinations as they can cause life-threatening disseminated infections.

HAEMOPHILUS INFLUENZA TYPE B (HIB)

Infection caused by *H. influenzae* is more common in PWH, although the annual incidence remains relatively low. In addition, only about 33% of the cases involve *H. influenzae* type B. Therefore, HIB is not recommended for routine administration to adults with HIV.

- **Bottom line:** One dose only if there is an indication (e.g., sickle cell disease, leukemia, or anatomic or functional asplenia).

HEPATITIS A VIRUS (HAV)

HAV rates in general have declined with the introduction of the vaccine in the 1990s. However, rates are increased in homeless individuals, people who inject drugs, and men who have sex with men. It is recommended to administer an HAV vaccine to all PWH regardless of CD4⁺ T-cell count.

- **Bottom line:** Two doses at least 6 months apart. A three-dose series can be administered with a combined hepatis A and hepatitis B vaccine; minimum intervals are 4 weeks between the first and second dose and 5 months between the second and third dose.

HEPATITIS B VIRUS (HBV)

There is an increased risk for PWH of acquiring HBV from injection drug use and/or condomless sex. It is recommended to administer an HBV vaccine to all PWH regardless of CD4⁺ T-cell count. Screening labs are done before and after vaccination to assess the need for the series and adequacy of response if given. Screening interpretation is as follows:

- Positive hepatitis surface antigen (HBsAg): Active infection and no indication for vaccination

- Positive antibody to hepatitis surface and core antigens (HBsAb, HBcAb): Previous infection and no need for vaccination

- Positive antibody to hepatitis surface antigen (HBsAb) with a titer of more than 10 mIU/mL: Adequately vaccinated

- **Bottom line:** Two- or three-dose series. The two-dose series is given 1 month apart. The three-dose series is given at 0, 1, and 6 months. If screening reveals a nonresponder, recommendation is to administer a four-dose series double-dose HBV vaccine at 0, 1, 2, and 6 months. If the CD4⁺ T-cell count was below 200 cells/mm³ with the initial series, waiting until immune reconstitution occurs before doing the second series is an option.

HUMAN PAPILLOMAVIRUS VIRUS (HPV)

PWH have a higher incidence of disease associated with HPV. The series is recommended for PWH who are 9 through 26 years of age; it is not recommended for older patients, although some guidelines have recommended extending the age of vaccination up to 45.

- **Bottom line:** Three-dose series given at 0, 1 to 2, and 6 months. The two-dose series should NOT be used with PWH. The series should not be given to pregnant women or continued during pregnancy. However, a pregnancy test is not required before administration. Series can be continued after the completion of pregnancy.

INFLUENZA

PWH have a higher risk of adverse outcomes with infection when compared with the general population. Recommended influenza vaccines include inactivated influenza vaccine (IIV) or recombinant influenza vaccine (RIV). Live attenuated vaccine (LAIV) is contraindicated.

- **Bottom line:** One dose annually of IIV or RIV.

MEASLES MUMPS RUBELLA (MMR)

As with influenza, PWH have a higher risk of adverse outcomes with infection when compared with the general population. It is important to remember that the MMR vaccine is a live-virus vaccine.

- **Bottom line:** Two-dose series if the CD4⁺ T-cell count is 200 cells/mm³ or greater (for at least 6 months) if born in 1957 or later. The doses are administered at least 4 weeks apart. Combination vaccination with varicella is NOT recommended. If the CD4⁺ T-cell count is less than 200 cells/mm³, both MMR and measles mumps rubella varicella (MMRV) are contraindicated. The vaccine is also contraindicated in pregnancy, which should be avoided for 28 days after vaccination.

VARICELLA VIRUS (VAR)

For PWH, primary varicella zoster virus infection is uncommon due to immunity from childhood infection. The varicella vaccine is a live-virus vaccine.

- **Bottom line:** Two doses 3 months apart. Recommended for PWH with no evidence of immunity and a CD4⁺ T-cell count of 200 cells/mm³ or greater. The vaccination is contraindicated in those with a low CD4⁺ T-cell count (<200 cells/mm³).

ZOSTER

For PWH, the incidence of zoster is 15-fold higher than among age-matched immunocompetent adults, with highest risk when the CD4⁺ T-cell count is less than 200 cells/mm³. Vaccination is intended to prevent zoster and reduce the severity of zoster if it does occur.

- **Bottom line:** Two doses of the recombinant zoster vaccine (RZV), given 2 to 6 months apart, for persons 50 years and older regardless of CD4⁺ T-cell count. RZV is preferred over the zoster vaccine live (ZVL) by the ACIP. ZVL is no longer recommended.

MENINGOCOCCUS

PWH have an increased risk of developing meningococcal disease, with the relative risk estimated at 5- to 13-fold higher than in persons without HIV. The risk in PWH appears to be higher with low CD4⁺ T-cell counts and high HIV RNA levels. Men who have sex with men are particularly at risk for meningococcal meningitis.

- **Bottom line:** For serogroups A, C, W, and Y, two doses 8 to 12 weeks apart with a booster in 5 years. Meningococcal B vaccine is recommended only in patients who are 18 years or older and who have an indication for receiving meningococcal B vaccine, such as functional or anatomic asplenia, persistent complement component deficiency, or receiving complement inhibitor. If given, the two-dose series is given 1 month apart. If the three-dose series is given, it is given at 0, 1 to 2, and 6 months.

PNEUMOCOCCUS

PWH have an increased risk of developing pneumococcal disease, with the relative risk estimated at sevenfold higher than in persons without HIV. There are two kinds of pneumococcal vaccinations available for use in the US: PCV13 and PPSV23. Recent published studies show uncertainty about the efficacy of PCV13, and in June 2019 the ACIP approved a change from its age-based recommendations to a shared clinical decision-making process.

- **Bottom line:**
  - Pneumococcal vaccine-naive: One dose of PCV13 followed by one dose of PPSV23 at least 8 weeks later. Booster of a dose of PPSV23 should be administered 5 years after the initial dose, and again after age 65.
  - Already received one dose of PPSV23 (but no dose of PCV13): One dose of PCV13 (at least 1 year after PPSV23). A booster with a dose of PPSV23 should be administered at least 5 years after the first dose of PPSV23 and at least 8 weeks after the PCV13 dose.
  - Received two prior doses of PPSV23 (but no dose of PCV13): One dose of PCV13 (at least 1 year after the last dose of PPSV23). Individuals who received the two doses of PPSV23 prior to age 65 should receive a third dose of PPSV23 after age 65 and at least 5 years after the prior dose of PPSV23 (and at least 8 weeks after the PCV13 dose).

TETANUS, DIPHTHERIA, AND PERTUSSIS (TDAP)

For PWH, an adequate immune response is usually mounted against the toxins produced from these organisms. Therefore, the recommendation for vaccination does not differ from general population.

- **Bottom line:** One dose of Tdap, followed by a Td or Tdap booster every 10 years. If previously given Td only, give one dose of Tdap. Tdap should be given in every pregnancy regardless of immunization history.

ACKNOWLEDGMENTS

We acknowledge Jean Anderson, MD, FACOG, AAHIVS. She provided the bulk of the material discussed in this section in the 2012 and 2017 editions.

REFERENCES

Aberg JA, Gallant JE, Ghanem KG, et al. Primary care guidelines for the management of persons infected with HIV: 2013 update by the HIV Medicine Association of the Infectious Diseases Society of America. *Clin Infec Dis.* 2014;28:215–222.

American Thoracic Society, Centers for Disease Control and Prevention, and Infectious Diseases Society of America. Controlling tuberculosis in the United States. *Am J Respir Crit Care Med.* 2005;172:1169–1227.

American Thoracic Society/Centers for Disease Control and Prevention. Targeted tuberculin testing and treatment of latent tuberculosis infection: joint statement of the American Thoracic Society and the Centers for Disease Control and Prevention. *Am J Respir Crit Care Med.* 2000;161:S221–S247.

Boehme CC, Nabeta P, Hillemann D, et al. Rapid molecular detection of tuberculosis and rifampin resistance. *N Engl J Med.* 2010;363(11):1005–1015.

Bonito AJ. Management of dental patients who are HIV positive. Summary, evidence report/technology assessment: number 37. AHRQ Publication No. 01-E041, March 2001. Rockville, MD: Agency for Healthcare Research and Quality. http://www.ncbi.nlm.nih.gov/books/NBK11965

Cain KP, McCarthy KD, Heilg CM, et al. An algorithm for tuberculosis screening and diagnosis in people with HIV. *N Engl J Med.* 2010;362:707–716.

Cattamanchi A, Smith R, Steingart KR, et al. Interferon-gamma release assays for the diagnosis of latent tuberculosis infection in HIV-infected individuals: a systematic review and meta-analysis. *J AIDS.* 2011;56:230–238.

Centers for Disease Control and Prevention. Updated guidelines for using interferon gamma release assays to detect *Mycobacterium tuberculosis* infection—United States, 2010. *MMWR Morb Mort Wkly Rep.* 2010;59(RR-5):1–26.

Freed JR, Marcus M, Freed BA, et al. Oral health findings for HIV-infected adult medical patients from the HIV Cost and Services Utilization Study. *J Am Dent Assoc.* 2005;136:1396–1405.

Freedman M, Kroger A, Hunter P, Ault KA. Recommended adult immunization schedule, United States, 2020. *Ann Intern Med.* 2020;172(5):337–347.

Getahun H, Harrington M, O'Brien R, et al. Diagnosis of smear-negative pulmonary tuberculosis in people with HIV infection or AIDS in resource-constrained settings: informing urgent policy changes. *Lancet.* 2007;369(9578):2042–2049.

Gray J, Reves R, Johnson S, et al. Identification of false-positive QuantiFERON-TB Gold In-Tube assays by repeat testing in PLWH at low risk of tuberculosis. *Clin Infect Dis.* 2012;54:e20–e23.

Horsburgh CR, Rubin EJ. Latent tuberculosis infection in the United States. *N Engl J Med.* 2011;364:1441–1448.

New York State Department of Health AIDS Institute. HIV and oral health: general principles. 2020. http://www.hivguidelines.org/clinical-guidelines/hiv-and-oral-health/general-principles

Palmieri F, Girardi E, Pellicelli AM, et al. Pulmonary tuberculosis in HIV-infected patients presenting with normal chest radiograph and negative sputum smear. *Infection.* 2002;30(2):68–74.

Panel on Opportunistic Infections in Adults and Adolescents with HIV. Guidelines for the prevention and treatment of opportunistic infections in adults and adolescents with HIV: recommendations from the Centers for Disease Control and Prevention, the National Institutes of Health, and the HIV Medicine Association of the Infectious Diseases Society of America. 2019. https://aidsinfo.nih.gov/contentfiles/lvguidelines/glchunk/glchunk_343.pdf

Raby E, Moyo M, Devendra A, et al. The effects of HIV on the sensitivity of a whole blood IFN-gamma release assay in Zambian adults with active tuberculosis. *PLOS One.* 2008;3(6)e2489.

11.

DIVERSITY AND HEALTH DISPARITIES

Gary F. Spinner, Renata Arrington-Sanders, Leah Spatafore, Zil Garner Goldstein, Maddie Deutsch, Angela Kapalko, Rachel A. Prosser, Abby Davids, Deliana Garcia, Claire Hutkins Seda, and Laszlo Madaras

---

CHAPTER GOALS

Upon completion of this chapter, the reader should be able to:

- Discuss the concepts of social determinants of health and racial/ethnic disparities, and how the failure to address them, leads to health inequity in HIV, COVID-19, and other diseases

- Discuss the meaning of systemic racism, and how it has contributed to, or failed to rectify, the health disparities among many persons with HIV infection (PWH)

- Discuss the diversity of PWH, the complexity of their unique cultures that are shaped by a multitude of factors, and the importance of becoming competent in developing a clinician–patient relationship across cultural differences

- Relate how a patient's values, beliefs, and judgments may create barriers to successful treatment if the HIV provider does not competently navigate the cultural differences between patient and provider, and the importance of becoming aware of one's personal biases that may hinder the patient–clinician relationship in caring for a diverse population of PWH

- Recognize the challenges in addressing racial and ethnic disparities in healthcare and in HIV

- Discuss the impact that culture, ethnicity, immigration status, sexual orientation, gender identity, religion, gender, and behavioral health problems may have on the care of PWH

- Develop and provide gender-affirming primary and HIV care and prevention for transgender persons

- Discuss limitations in HIV care and special needs among migrant populations or patients with undocumented citizenship status

---

11.1.

DIVERSITY AWARENESS

Gary F. Spinner

LEARNING OBJECTIVES

- Discuss how a patient's values, beliefs, and judgments may create barriers to successful treatment if the HIV provider does not competently navigate the cultural differences between the patient and the healthcare provider

- Recognize the challenges in addressing racial and ethnic disparities in healthcare and in HIV

- Analyze one's personal (implicit) biases regarding race, ethnicity, sexual and gender diversity, and cultural practices and understand how that bias can hinder the development of an effective patient–clinician relationship

- Discuss the impact that culture, ethnicity, immigration status, sexual orientation, gender identity, religion, gender, and behavioral health problems may have on the care of PWH

WHAT'S NEW?

- The COVID-19 pandemic does not appear to affect PWH any more than those not infected with HIV. However, the same racial and ethnic disparities that exist in the pandemic of HIV appear to hold true for COVID-19. Blacks and Latinx populations have significantly higher rates of HIV and COVID-19 infections, along with higher rates of mortality from both pandemics.

- The success of the Ryan White HIV/AIDS Program in addressing the needs of marginalized PWH has led to a significant improvement in the viral suppression rate to 87.1% for Ryan White–funded programs.

KEY POINT

- Patients with HIV come from diverse backgrounds and are often mistrustful of healthcare providers.

HIV AND COVID-19: TWO PANDEMICS, SAME RACIAL AND ETHNIC DISPARITIES

The dual pandemics of HIV, caused by the RNA virus HIV, and COVID-19, caused by the RNA virus SARS-CoV-2, share much in common beyond their viral etiologies. Both HIV and COVID-19 disproportionately affect Black and Latinx populations far more than Whites. Yet the health disparities in these two pandemics have nothing to do with any known biological differences or virus pathology. These disparities are directly related to social determinants of health, racial and ethnic health inequities, and societal policies that have either created or failed to address these unequal conditions. While PWH do not appear to be at greater risk of becoming infected with SARS-CoV-2 (Park et al., 2020), nor do they appear to have worse outcomes than HIV-uninfected people, people of color are significantly more likely to become infected with SARS-CoV-2 and have higher rates of mortality. To understand the similarities of these two pandemics is to recognize how social determinants of health create health inequity among people of color, leading to worse outcomes among those with HIV, COVID-19, and many other health conditions. The importance of knowing why racial and ethnic minorities are more likely to acquire HIV can help the HIV specialist become a more culturally competent and ultimately a better healthcare provider.

This chapter on caring for diverse populations has been updated during the COVID-19 pandemic, which is concurrent with an increase of social activism through the Black Lives Matter movement intensified by the killing of George Floyd at the hands of the Minneapolis police. The interconnection of a protest movement for racial justice and the devastation that both HIV and COVID-19 have on persons of color will be explored, contextualizing the health disparities of both pandemics and how social determinants of health adversely impact the health and well-being of people of color. According to the World Health Organization, "Social determinants of health (SDH) are the conditions in which people are born, grow, work, live, and age, and the wider set of forces and systems shaping the conditions of daily life. These forces and systems include economic policies and systems, development agendas, social norms, social policies and political systems" (World Health Organization, 2020).

Blacks, Latinxs, and Native Americans all experience significant health disparities in the US. A health disparity is "a particular type of health difference that is closely linked with social, economic, and/or environmental disadvantage" (Health.gov, 2020). Health disparities adversely affect groups of people who have systematically experienced greater obstacles to healthcare based on their racial or ethnic group; religion; socioeconomic status; gender; age; mental health;

cognitive, sensory, or physical disability; sexual orientation or gender identity; geographic location; or other characteristics historically linked to discrimination or exclusion (US Department of Health and Human Services (DHHS, 2020). While unequal access to healthcare can be one determinant of less-than-equal health outcomes, the disparities go far beyond access to care. For example, even with equal access to healthcare in the Veterans Health Administration, there were mortality disparities for Black veterans with stage 4 chronic kidney disease, colon cancer, diabetes, HIV, rectal cancer, and stroke; for Native American and Alaska Native veterans undergoing noncardiac major surgery; and for Latinx veterans with HIV (Peterson et al., 2018).

What follows are examples of the racial and ethnic disparities for HIV and for COVID-19, and why it is important for HIV specialists to have a sound understanding of these disparities and how they affect clinical outcomes. Healthcare providers' attitudes, biases, and beliefs will also be addressed, as it is important for the HIV specialist to recognize how racial and ethnic biases, whether conscious or unconscious, can have a profound impact on the health outcomes of patients.

HIV: RACIAL AND ETHNIC DISPARITIES

Black and Latinx populations account for a vastly disproportionate percentage of PWH. According to data from the US Centers for Disease Control and Prevention (CDC, 2020b), while Blacks account for only 13.4% of the US population, they made up 42% of all newly diagnosed PWH in the US in 2018. Latinxs account for 18.5% of the US population but represented 28% of HIV incidence in 2018. Black men and women have higher rates of some sexually transmitted infections (STIs) than other racial/ethnic groups, increasing their risk for HIV acquisition and transmission (CDC, 2020b). The lifetime risk of acquiring HIV is six times higher for Black men, and nearly three times higher for Latino men, than for Whites. Black women have a 14 times higher lifetime risk of HIV and Latina women have a 3 times higher lifetime risk of acquiring HIV as compared with Whites. Among men who have sex with men (MSM), one of every two black MSM has a lifetime risk of HIV acquisition, compared with 1 in 6 Latino MSM and 1 in 11 White MSM (CDC, 2016).

In every category, comparing viral suppression between Whites and Blacks, Whites are more likely to be virally suppressed (Crepaz et al., 2018). While 56% of whites were suppressed, only 41% of Blacks were suppressed, and this held true by gender, by age, among MSM, and among people who inject drugs.

Preexposure prophylaxis (PrEP) is 99% effective in the prevention of HIV when taken optimally, yet while Blacks and Latino MSM have the highest risk of acquiring HIV, PrEP is far more likely to be offered to Whites (Kanny et al., 2019). This disparity between White and Black MSM persisted among those who had health insurance and had a usual source of healthcare.

In summary, Blacks and Latinxs have higher rates of HIV transmission, have a higher risk of infection, are less likely to be virally suppressed when on antiviral therapy, and are less likely to be offered HIV prevention with PrEP than Whites.

COVID-19: RACIAL AND ETHNIC DISPARITIES

Like HIV, COVID-19 disproportionately affects people of color, who are more likely to become infected with COVID-19 than Whites and more likely to have severe disease and death.

A *New York Times* analysis of CDC data looking at the characteristics of 640,000 persons with COVID-19 found that Latinxs and Blacks in the US were three times more likely to have COVID-19 and twice as likely to die from this disease (Oppel et al., 2020).

Although the CDC data are incomplete, missing racial and ethnic data for many patients, a study analyzing data through mid-April 2020 (Millett, 2020b) from counties in which there are disproportionately more Blacks residing, found that 97% of predominantly Black counties had at least one COVID-19 case compared to 80% of other counties. They also found that 49% of Black counties had at least one COVID-19 death compared with 28% in all other non-majority-Black counties. The predominantly Black counties tended to have lower rates of insurance, higher rates of unemployment, crowded housing, poor air quality, and reduced ability to practice social distancing. In addition, employed persons in predominantly Black counties were more likely to be classified as essential workers, to use public transportation, and to have jobs that did not allow working from home. When using the same methodology to look at Latinx-majority counties, a similar outcome of disproportionately high COVID-19 cases and deaths was found.

In a safety-net hospital in Chicago (Parra-Rodriguez & Stroger, 2020), 53% of Latinxs and 44% of Blacks had severe COVID-19 disease compared with 22% of Whites. A CDC analysis (Wortham et al., 2020) found that almost one-third of U.S. non-Whites who die with COVID-19 are younger than 65, more than twice the proportion in Whites, according to analysis of over 10,000 deaths in 15 states and New York City. These data also showed that twice as many Latinxs under age 65 died from COVID-19 as compared to Whites. The authors of this study speculated that non-Whites were more likely to have jobs that precluded social distancing.

In California, where Latinxs represent 39% of the state population, they accounted for 46% of all COVID-19 deaths as of July 2020. Latinxs also accounted for a disproportionate share of COVID-19 deaths in Florida and Arizona through July 2020 (Thebault & Fowers, 2020).

Native Americans have also been impacted disproportionately by COVID-19. While CDC data on race and ethnicity for COVID-19 have been incomplete and problematic, a *New York Times* article (Conger et al., 2020) found that in New Mexico, Native Americans accounted for nearly 40% of virus cases even though they make up 9% of the population. In the Phoenix, Arizona, area, Native Americans were infected at four times the rate of Whites. "The disparities we see there with COVID-19 are aligned with those that we see for hospitalizations and deaths due to influenza and other respiratory viruses," said Allison Barlow, director of the Center for American Indian Health at Johns Hopkins University.

"Native Americans—particularly those living on reservations—are more prone to contract the virus because of crowded housing conditions that make social distancing difficult," she said, along with years of underfunded health systems, food and water insecurity, and other factors that contribute to underlying health conditions that can make the illness more severe once contracted.

Among the social factors most likely contributing to the increased morbidity and mortality of COVID-19 in racial and ethnic minorities are poverty, high density and crowded housing, employment that precludes working from home, and the higher likelihood of being employed as essential services workers. Other factors include reliance on public transportation; overrepresentation in jails, prisons, homeless shelters, and detention centers, where social distancing is not possible; living in multigenerational households where it is difficult to protect older family members; not having sick leave (which increases the likelihood that someone keeps working while ill); lack of health insurance; distrust of the healthcare system; and racism, stigma, and systemic inequities (CDC, 2020a).

COVID-19 AND HIV AND THEIR LINK TO SYSTEMIC RACISM

Health equity (DHHS definition) is the attainment of the highest level of health for all people. It requires valuing everyone equally, with focused and ongoing societal efforts to address avoidable inequalities, historical and contemporary injustices, and the elimination of health and health care disparities (DHHS, 2020).

The significant health disparities experienced by people of color are examples of health inequity. The unequal adverse health impact of HIV and COVID-19 holds true for other health conditions as well, including certain cancers, respiratory diseases, diabetes, hypertension, and other conditions, along with worse healthcare outcomes for most of these conditions. Infant mortality for Black infants is 2.5 times higher than for White infants (CDC, 2016). A Black man's life expectancy is nearly 5 years shorter than a White man's (CDC, 2017), and he is 30% more likely to die from heart disease, twice as likely to be diagnosed with diabetes, twice as likely to have a stroke, and 40% more likely to have hypertension but 10% less likely to have it under control (Graham, 2015).

The Black Lives Matter movement taking place at the time of this writing is not only about Blacks being more than 2.5 times as likely to be killed while in the hands of the police (Roper, 2020) or incarcerated at 5.1 times the rate for Whites (Nellis, 2016) but also about these health inequities, among other issues making up systemic racial injustice.

To truly understand the racial and ethnic disparities of the pandemics of HIV and COVID-19, one must recognize the pandemic of racism. According to Ibram Kendi (2019), a scholar of race and discriminatory policy in America, "Racism is a marriage of racist policies and racist ideas that produces and normalizes racial inequities, and that racial inequity is when two or more racial groups are not standing on approximately equal footing. A racist policy is any measure that produces or sustains racial inequity between racial groups."

The social conditions that lead to adverse health conditions (including poverty, lack of access to healthcare, lower-wage employment, segregated and overcrowded housing, and educational disadvantages, among many other inequities) are systemic problems related either to policies that have created these disadvantages or to a lack of appropriate policies to address and eliminate these disadvantages.

Systemic racism, also known as institutional racism (Wikipedia, 2020), is a form of racism that is embedded as normal practice within society or an organization that can lead to such issues as discrimination in employment, housing, healthcare, political power, criminal justice, education, among other issues.

Systemic racism must be recognized for causing many of the social inequities that people of color experience. Crowded, high-density housing; low-wage essential service jobs that preclude working from home; and reliance on public transportation are linked to COVID-19. There are a multitude of programs and policies that can be traced back to racial and ethnic discrimination. For example, the practice of banks denying housing loans to Blacks, or charging them higher rates of interest with stricter repayment terms, has led to fewer Blacks than Whites owning homes. Historically, the Federal Housing Administration's refusal to insure mortgages in Black neighborhoods, and their requirement of developers receiving subsidized loans to build subdivisions that specifically exclude Blacks, are systemically racist policies that created segregated and more densely populated housing and denied Blacks of one of the most common ways to build personal wealth, home ownership (Rothstein, 2017).

Another example of systemic racism relates to unemployment benefits for workers laid off due to COVID-19. Almost a quarter of Black workers live in the South, where 52% of all new HIV infections currently occur, and where race has long played a role in limiting safety-net programs. During the COVID-19 pandemic, the US unemployment rate has skyrocketed, but the unemployment insurance program is state controlled, and many Southern states have excluded from unemployment programs many of the jobs that are more likely to employ Blacks and Latinxs. The average high-school-educated White is twice as likely to receive unemployment benefits as the average high-school-educated Black (Nichols & Simms, 2012), and Blacks receive lower rates of compensation than Whites, according to Kathryn Edwards of the Rand Corporation (Badger et al., 2020).

Despite the significant progress in treating PWH, there continues to be approximately 38,000 new HIV infections each year. While people of color are far more likely to acquire HIV, and PrEP is 99% effective in preventing infection when taken optimally, people of color are less likely to be offered it. "Ending the HIV Epidemic: A Plan for America" was the Trump administration's effort to address some of the geographic disparities where people are at greatest risk of acquiring HIV. It targets the 48 counties along with 7 rural communities with greatest risk for HIV (Health Resources and Services Administration, 2020). However, the social determinants of health faced by people of color threaten to undermine the plan's intended progress. A modeling study of HIV incidence (Nosyk et al., 2020) suggests the goal of ending the HIV epidemic is unlikely to be met due to many barriers, including lack of access to healthcare, proposed cutbacks to and/or outright elimination of the Affordable Care Act, and failure to expand Medicaid in many of the Southern states. Millett et al. pointed out at the AIDS 2020 conference that income inequality, poverty, and the degree of Black/White segregation, housing instability, and homelessness are associated with HIV in certain communities where poverty, vacant housing, unemployment, and isolation are most prevalent (Millett et al., 2020a).

WHAT NEEDS TO BE DONE?

The Ryan White HIV/AIDS Program has been a hugely successful program, with significantly better outcomes in Ryan White–funded clinics compared with other HIV clinics in the US. Serving over half a million patients with HIV, 73.6% of whom are racial and ethnic minorities and 62.8% of whom are living below the federal poverty level, the highest measure of HIV treatment success—viral suppression—was 87.1% for Ryan White–funded clinics compared with the national average of 62.7% (Cheever, 2019; Hall et al., 2015). Ryan White clinics are funded to address barriers many patients face, such as transportation, primary medical care, food bank services, housing, linguistic services, child care services, emergency financial services, substance use treatment services, case management, and a host of other services. Through the Ryan White clinics' efforts to address these barriers, the level of health equity for patients served by this program is raised. The program's success can be attributed to its intent to specifically address the racial and ethnic disparities impacting people of color, as well as other marginalized groups.

PROVIDING CULTURALLY COMPETENT CARE

It is not uncommon for healthcare providers to harbor false beliefs about biological differences between Blacks and Whites. One study of medical students and residents found that half of those surveyed believed one or more false statements about biological differences between Blacks and Whites, including the belief that Blacks do not feel pain the same way that Whites do or that skin is thicker in Blacks than Whites (Hoffman et al., 2016). These prejudices alienate patients, who rightfully perceive the racism and implicit bias that their healthcare providers harbor.

Provider bias, and sometimes overt racism, can lead to longer waiting times for people of color as compared with Whites, taking patient concerns less seriously, doing a less thorough workup of problems, and recommending different treatment options based on a perceived lack of patient adherence, along with many other differences in the treatment of some racial and/or ethnic groups. A systematic review of 15 peer-reviewed studies to identify implicit racial and ethnic bias among healthcare providers found that in 14 of those 15 studies, most healthcare providers demonstrated implicit bias through more favorable attitudes toward Whites and negative attitudes toward Blacks and Latinxs (Hall et al., 2015). Four studies found that healthcare providers saw Blacks as less cooperative, less compliant, and less responsive to medical advice. Several studies found that healthcare providers associated poor adherence and noncompliance with Latinx patients, and two studies found moderate amounts of bias against darker-skinned patients than lighter-skinned patients.

Even healthcare providers who see themselves as providing equitable care may unknowingly be interacting with their patients of color differently and less effectively than with their White patients. Clearly, our system of medical education needs to more actively address issues of race and ethnicity in the training of physicians, nurses, and other healthcare workers. Unless we acknowledge and change our individual racist and ethnic biases and work to implement health and social policies that eliminate racism and ethnic bias, we will continue to perpetuate the health disparities we see with HIV, COVID-19, and a multitude of other health conditions. What follows in this chapter are further examples of the diversity of patients with HIV and how we can elevate our awareness and appreciation of those who entrust us with their healthcare.

RETENTION IN CARE

Retaining patients in care requires culturally competent staff at all levels of an organization. It could be easy for the busy HIV specialist to focus more intensely on the complex medical aspects of HIV medicine and relegate the issues of diversity and cultural competence to "soft areas" that are less important than learning resistance mutations or developing expertise in the use of the latest antiviral drugs. However, to do so runs the risk of failing to adequately comprehend how patients' behaviors, beliefs, and the characteristics of their unique social, ethnic, racial, religious, gender identity, sexual orientation, or country of origin may affect their engagement with the healthcare system. Failing to understand the important cultural context within which patients interact with the healthcare system often leads to poor patient adherence with treatment, misunderstandings about the treatment plan, or, worse, loss of retention in care. To successfully treat patients and to achieve the treatment goals, we need to do our best to understand the unique context of our diverse group of patients and to provide care that acknowledges the cultural values that may impact their acceptance of treatment.

An analysis (Skarbinski et al., 2015) estimated that PWH who were out of care were responsible for 61% of new HIV infections in the US. Furthermore, a statewide study from North Carolina that analyzed patients with acute HIV infection found that most transmission events (77%) were attributable to partners with previously diagnosed infection, of whom only 23% were reportedly in care and taking antiviral medication within the time that transmission was likely to have occurred (Cope et al., 2015). This is compelling evidence that the system of HIV care in the US is failing to treat and retain many PWH. There are likely many reasons for lack of success in patient retention, but it underscores the crucial need to improve the ways healthcare providers interact with patients in order to keep them engaged in care and adherent with their antiviral medications. Developing competence in understanding the attributes of a diverse patient population is challenging, but failure to do so will allow greater numbers of PWH to lose contact with care. The greater challenge in becoming culturally competent is for healthcare providers to develop awareness of their own values, beliefs, and attitudes and what biases may be inherent in their own culture.

DIVERSITY OF PATIENTS

Medical providers caring for PWH are likely caring for a population of patients from racial or ethnic groups different from their own. In the US, PWH are disproportionately Black and Latinx and, regardless of race or ethnicity, are often affected by poverty, drug or alcohol abuse, mental health problems, lack of employment, lack of permanent housing, histories of incarceration, inadequate education, and sexual preferences different from those of the general population. Some patients may be immigrants or refugees whose language and cultural differences may cause barriers to acceptance of healthcare services from a system of care culturally different from their own. Understanding how patients' spiritual and religious values may impact their healthcare decisions is important when caring for a diverse group of patients. However, in our attempt to develop cultural understanding of their diversity, it is critical to avoid stereotyping patients, which also creates barriers to acceptance of treatment. The values, beliefs, and judgments of patients may differ from ours, and unless we can withhold judgment of a patient's circumstances, a trusting relationship may never develop.

IMPORTANCE OF TRUST

Trust is a critically important component of a successful patient–clinician relationship. Without trust, patients are less likely to adhere to a treatment plan. Patients who do not trust their healthcare provider or the healthcare system will be less likely to take prescribed medications, keep scheduled appointments, or accept clinicians' advice.

Mistrust by certain racial and ethnic minorities in the US is common. A telephone survey by the Kaiser Family Foundation (James, 1999) found that one-third of Blacks and one-third of Latinxs reported experiencing unfair treatment by the healthcare system; figures for White were less than half those numbers. Blacks were used without their informed consent in medical experimentation by the US Public Health Service from 1932 to 1972 in the notorious Tuskegee syphilis

study, which created a legacy of mistrust (Skarbinski et al., 2015). Mistrust has led to conspiracy theories about the origins of HIV. In 2005, a national telephone survey of 500 Blacks (Bogart & Thorburn, 2005) found that 53% agreed that "there is a cure for AIDS, but it is being withheld from the poor," 27% agreed that "AIDS was produced in a government laboratory," and 16% agreed that "AIDS was created by the government to control the Black population."

DISPARITIES IN HEALTHCARE

The HIV epidemic in the US is characterized by significant racial and ethnic disparities. In 2018, the distribution of new diagnoses of HIV by race/ethnicity was 26% for Whites, 26% for Latinx/Latino, 42% for Blacks, 2% for Asians, 1% for Native Americans/Alaska Natives, 2% for those of multiple races, and less than 1% for Native Hawaiian/Other Pacific Islanders (CDC, 2019). For many patients, the route of HIV transmission carries significant stigma. Among Black men, of whom 80% contracted the disease by male-to-male sexual contact, being gay or bisexual carries a stigma that is prevalent both in the general population and within the Black community. Stigma creates barriers that keep many men from being tested for HIV or connecting to care once identified as being PWH. To understand the effect of stigma and to develop nonjudgmental ways to communicate effectively with patients, we must first acknowledge that patients may enter their relationship with a healthcare provider assuming the healthcare provider harbors the same biases as the general population. Becoming culturally competent requires clinicians to develop strategies with each patient to allay the patient's fear of disapproval by the healthcare provider as well as to provide reassurance that the patient's personal health information will be protected and kept confidential.

With significant racial and ethnic disparities concerning who is living with HIV, the need to provide culturally appropriate care is evident. Failing to adequately understand a patient's culture—best defined as the unique set of beliefs, characteristics, and behaviors formed by the communities in which a patient resides—can create a barrier between the patient and the healthcare provider. A lack of trust by the patient may prevent successful treatment. Mistrust of healthcare providers occurs particularly if patients believe they will receive unequal treatment. Many studies across all disease states have documented the unequal treatment provided to Blacks and Latinxs. According to the Institute of Medicine (Smedley, 2003), racial and ethnic minorities often receive a lower quality of healthcare services even when insurance status and income are the same as those for non-minorities. Black and Latinx patients have a higher risk of acute myocardial infarction and rehospitalization and death from acute coronary syndrome but are less likely than Whites to receive angiography or other coronary interventions (Graham, 2015).

Healthcare clinicians need to understand what objections a patient may have to the recommended treatment in an effort to help the patient understand potential consequences that may occur without treatment. Clinicians need to take the time to ask patients open-ended questions. Asking questions such as "What are your concerns about taking this medication?" allows patients to express their concerns and gives the healthcare provider the opportunity to address them.

BIAS IN HEALTHCARE

Cultural competence requires taking time to learn what cultural barriers might exist. Healthcare providers who are ethnocentric only view a patient's culture from their own culture's perspective and risk losing patients' trust. Healthcare providers are not immune to the biases that exist in the general population. Weisse et al. (2001) found that White males were twice as likely to be prescribed analgesics for pain as Black males, whereas female physicians prescribed higher doses for Blacks than for Whites. A study examining how the patient's race affects physicians' perceptions found that physicians rated Black patients as less intelligent, less educated, more likely to abuse drugs and alcohol, and less likely to adhere to treatment even when considering the patient's income and education (van Ryn & Burke, 2000). In a systematic review of 15 studies that looked at racial and ethnic biases, all but one study showed that racial and ethnic bias by healthcare providers existed (Hall et al., 2015). These studies show how racism and personal bias can lead to unequal care.

Bias can be either overt (explicit) or covert (implicit). Derogatory comments made by either providers or office staff about particular "types" of patients are an example of bias. Judgmental comments about how frequently certain patients develop STIs, use the emergency room, look for pain medications, and have too many uncared-for children are examples of overt bias and stereotyping. Such comments, in addition to being highly unprofessional and judgmental, may reinforce among medical staff involved in patient care that bias and judgment are an acceptable form of professional conduct. Negative comments about a patient, especially if overheard by other patients, can transmit the message to patients that they may be the topic of unwanted conversation. Healthcare organizations need to make certain that staff at all levels and functions within the institution become culturally competent. Recognizing the cultural differences that might exist between a patient and a healthcare provider is an essential step to welcoming each patient with acceptance and understanding. Only by attempting to recognize and to understand these differences can a healthcare provider comprehend what may be needed to best inspire patient trust in the provider, the institution, and the plan of treatment.

WOMEN AND HIV

There are 18 million women worldwide living with HIV, and in the US 19% of PWH are women (UN AIDS, 2015). Most women diagnosed with HIV (75%) acquire the virus through heterosexual sex (CDC, 2017). Black women are disproportionately HIV positive: 58% of US women living with HIV are Black (CDC, 2017). Women living with HIV experience intimate partner violence at twice the national average (Gruskin et al., 2014). The 2014 meta-analysis by Gruskin et al. showed that 55% of women with HIV in the US have experienced trauma and violence. Women and transgender women living with HIV who have experienced trauma and violence had a fourfold higher likelihood of nonadherence to their antiretroviral therapy (ART) regimen (Machtinger et al., 2012). HIV providers should inquire about a history of violence and abuse and should refer the patient to appropriate crisis and domestic violence services as needed. Healthcare providers should understand that many women who are victims of domestic abuse feel powerless and trapped because of economic dependency, primary responsibility for children, and fear of homelessness. Many women may be slow or unwilling to seek help. A careful mental health and depression screening should be done, and referral to appropriate mental health services should be made when indicated.

SEXUAL AND GENDER MINORITY PATIENTS

Many lesbian, gay, bisexual, transgender and queer (LGBTQ+) patients do not feel welcome by their healthcare providers. Many do not seek medical care because they have had bad experiences with healthcare providers (National LGBT Health Education Center, 2015). One recent study of Black MSM found that 29% experienced racial and sexual stigma from their healthcare providers, and 48% reported mistrust of the healthcare system (Eaton et al., 2015). If patients feel uncomfortable speaking about their sexual orientation, they are far more likely to withhold important information. Ways to help LGBTQ+ patients feel more welcome include using gender-neutral pronouns, allowing LGBTQ+ patients to be called by their preferred name (even if their legal name may be different), and training staff to have a nonjudgmental attitude. Learning and using the language that patients use may make patients feel more comfortable. For example, patients may use the terms "top" or "bottom" to describe insertive or receptive anal sex. Asking patients about the gender(s) of their partner(s) is an appropriate way to learn patients' sexual orientation. Avoidance of words that imply a patient has a relationship with someone of the opposite sex is also important. "Do you have a partner?" or "Are you in a relationship?" is a more appropriate question than "Do you have a husband/wife?" Patients who feel accepted by their healthcare provider are more likely to return for care. Conversely, those who perceive disapproval of their lifestyle, sexual orientation, or practices will feel uncomfortable and are much less likely to return.

BEHAVIORAL HEALTH PROBLEMS

The HIV Costs and Services Utilization Study found that nearly 50% of adults treated for HIV have symptoms of a psychiatric disorder, a prevalence that is four to eight times higher than in the general population (Bing et al., 2001). In the general population, there is a 10- to 20-year reduction in life expectancy in people with severe mental health disorders (Chang et al., 2011). Mental illness caries a risk of mortality greater than that of smoking (Chesney et al., 2014).

Identifying patients with mental illness or addiction is crucial in caring for PWH. A careful history followed by referral to mental health services as needed is important because patients with mental illness have been reported to have lower levels of adherence (Paterson & Swindells, 2000). Stigma about mental health diagnoses may keep many patients from accessing mental health services. On-site behavioral health services increase the likelihood that patients will connect to treatment. Many patients with substance abuse problems may experience a sense of rejection when they reveal that they have chemical dependency or are participating in a substance abuse treatment program. They may assume that mentioning pain will be perceived as drug seeking by their healthcare provider—a common stereotype of healthcare providers. Cultural competence requires communicating with patients openly and without judgment. It requires efforts to develop trust and to help reduce the stigma that most drug users have about their chemical dependency.

LANGUAGE AND COMMUNICATION

Language comprehension and communication are essential to patient understanding and, ultimately, to good adherence. Many PWH speak languages other than English. Language barriers can interfere with the success of treatment. Exit interviews of emergency room patients found that Spanish-speaking patients were less likely to understand their discharge instructions or carry out follow-up plans (Crane, 1997).

Hiring bilingual and bicultural staff is important in a culturally competent organization when there are significant numbers of patients in the local population who speak a particular language. The culturally competent clinical practice needs to make use of professional interpreter services for patients who do not speak the language of the healthcare provider. The use of family members or friends may inhibit patient honesty when asked to discuss personal information. Telephone interpreter services, although costly, are a necessary tool when on-site interpretation is unavailable. This is especially important for immigrant populations, for whom linguistic barriers, often combined with significant cultural differences, may greatly impede the delivery of healthcare. Patients who used the interpreter services received significantly more recommended preventive services, made more office visits, and had more prescriptions written and filled (Jacobs et al., 2004).

RELIGION AND SPIRITUALITY

A 2014 Gallup survey found that 81% of Americans identify with a particular religion (Newport, 2014). Patients turn to religion in times of illness, and this often influences the way people perceive and cope with their situation. Many PWH have strong religious affiliations (Cotton, 2006). A patient's faith may sometimes conflict with medical advice, which can lead to a lack of adherence to treatment. It is important to ask patients about their spiritual beliefs and how those beliefs may affect their perception of illness and acceptance of treatment.

CREATING A CULTURALLY COMPETENT, PATIENT-CENTERED HIV PRACTICE

Racial and ethnic diversity in healthcare leadership and staff is a priority in building culturally competent healthcare organizations. Including community members and consumer representatives on governing boards, as is done at Federally Qualified Health Centers (FQHCs), can help hold an organization accountable for providing culturally competent care to a diverse patient population. Providing materials that are linguistically appropriate to the population being served at a literacy level appropriate to the level of most patients is important.

Changing the model of care from the traditional physician-centered practice to a model that places the patient in the center of the relationship—the patient-centered medical home (PCMH) model—can improve the quality of care. This model relies on reorganizing care to ensure that it is comprehensive, with integrated physical and mental health services. Care that is patient centered supports patients' efforts to manage their own care to whatever degree they may choose. It is coordinated so that there is a smoother transition across levels of care, such as primary care, hospital care, and specialty care. Services are accessible, with after-hours access to a healthcare provider, along with flexible office hours. Last, there is a focus on quality and safety, using evidence-based standards and data for performance improvement (Agency for Healthcare Research and Quality, 2015). Culturally and linguistically appropriate services are offered. In one study, retention in care for PWH was improved with the PCMH model (Sitapati et al., 2012).

Patients want healthcare providers who communicate with them and who are empathic. Better healthcare outcomes have been associated with providers with whom patients can share their feelings and thoughts. Patients of empathic and communicative healthcare providers are far more likely to comply with their treatment plans (Sitapati et al., 2012).

The patient-centered approach incorporates cultural competency interventions in order to better address the racial, ethnic, and cultural differences between provider and patient, and it offers training to providers and to all staff who interact with patients in order to make them more culturally competent. Healthcare provider training to improve providers' knowledge and attitudes about diverse populations is essential to creating a culturally competent system of care.

Perhaps most important, aspiring culturally competent healthcare providers must raise their awareness of their own cultural beliefs, values, and attitudes and any biases that may be inherent in them. Consciousness of one's own cultural biases and an honest attempt to transcend them will allow the HIV provider to communicate effectively, with empathy, and without prejudgment, facilitating an improved and mutually satisfying relationship with each patient.

11.2.

ADOLESCENT HIV CARE

Leah Spatafore and Renata Arrington-Sanders

LEARNING OBJECTIVE

- Describe the developmental, cognitive, social, and environmental factors that may affect treatment adherence and secondary prevention in adolescents

WHAT'S NEW?

Worldwide, adolescent women represent the majority of new HIV cases. In the US, rates of infection have increased among young MSM of color.

KEY POINTS

- Adolescents are at risk for HIV through sexual behaviors; most adolescents acquire HIV through condomless sex.

- Adolescents in late puberty per Sexual Maturity Rating (SMR) staging (Stage 4 or 5) can be managed according to adult/adolescent guidelines; prepubescent and early pubescent adolescents (per SMR staging Stage 1–3) can be managed according to pediatric guidelines.

- Psychosocial factors that could affect adherence should be addressed before initiating treatment.

- Sexual risk behaviors in adolescents living with HIV should be given special attention.

The period of adolescence (defined as ages 12–24 years) is a critical time of physical, social, emotional, and cognitive growth and development (Sanders, 2013). However, adolescents are the most uninsured and underinsured age group in the US and the least likely group to use primary care and other outpatient medical services (Kaiser Foundation, 2007). Those with specific health and social problems, as well as those with particular difficulty obtaining appropriate medical care and other services, are at heightened risk for HIV acquisition. These groups include gender and sexual minority adolescents who identify as gay, lesbian, bisexual, or transgender; youth with unstable housing; injection drug users; individuals who have a mental illness; and those who have been sexually or physically abused, are incarcerated, or are in foster care.

Health disparities occur as a result of an individual's interaction with socioenvironmental factors at the interpersonal (e.g., family and social/sexual networks), intermediate structural (e.g., community, social institutions, culture, social norms, and values), and macrostructural (e.g., socioeconomic conditions) levels (McLeroy et al., 1988) that contribute to high rates of HIV. For example, young Black men who have sex with men and bisexual men and other MSM were disproportionately impacted by HIV in the US between 2010 and 2017 (CDC, 2020b) and accounted for the majority of new HIV transmissions in their age group (CDC, 2020b). Worldwide, adolescent females disproportionately account for new HIV transmissions (UNICEF). Such high rates do not result from increased individual behavior but rather from the complex interrelationship of multiple social identities—such as race, ethnicity, gender, socioeconomic status, and sexual orientation—that intersect at the individual's experience and reflect larger social-structural inequities experienced on the macro level (Bowleg, 2013; Crenshaw, 1991; Haltikis et al., 2013).

Approximately 1 million adults living in the US are transgender (i.e., a person who has a gender identity that differs from the sex they were assigned at birth; Meerwijk & Sevelius, 2017). From 2009 to 2014, 2,351 transgender people were diagnosed with HIV in the US, and a meta-analysis estimates that 14% of transgender women in the US are living with HIV (Becasen et al., 2019). More than one-third (36.3%) of these women were adolescents and young adults less than 24 years old (Clark et al., 2017). This represents a 34-fold increased odds of HIV infection compared to that of all reproductive-age adults (Baral et al., 2013). Transwomen of color are particularly affected. Data from the meta-analysis referred to previously report that rates of HIV are as high as 44% among Black transgender women (Becasen et al., 2019). Higher rates of HIV are attributed to experiences of stigma, discrimination, negative healthcare encounters, lack of familial support, limited healthcare and housing access, and a high incidence of mental health diagnoses. These factors contribute to increased drug and alcohol abuse, sex work, incarceration, homelessness, and attempted suicide.

Adolescents with HIV from perinatal transmission are another group of adolescents and young adults living with HIV. Given there is near-universal maternal screening and treatment in most high-income countries, this population is small; however, the same cannot be said for low-resource countries, in which perinatal transmission continues to be an ongoing concern. Adolescents infected via perinatal transmission share many common issues with those who acquired HIV behaviorally—namely stigma, sexuality, disclosure, unplanned pregnancy, nonadherence, and substance misuse and abuse. However, this population generally is on more complicated ART regimens based on the development of resistance mutations during childhood.

The same socio-ecologic factors (discrimination, isolation, microaggressions, and minority stress) that contribute to HIV risk predispose youth to comorbidities (high rates of mental health and substance use disorders) and medical nonadherence in their HIV treatment and management. Differences in the treatment cascade of care by age have been hypothesized as an explanation for the increase in HIV infections by at-risk youth nationally (Zanoni & Mayer, 2014). Less than half (40%) of those aged 13 to 29 years are aware of their HIV status, and best estimates suggest that only 62% of those are connected to care within their first year of diagnosis (Zanoni & Mayer, 2014). Other studies have suggested that adolescents have much lower linkage rates, ranging from 29% to 73% successfully linked within the first year of diagnosis (Craw et al., 2008; Torian et al., 2008). The CDC and the US Preventive Services Task Force recommend routine HIV screening for all youth (Branson et al., 2006; Moyer, 2013). Annual screening is recommended based on risk, and gay and bisexual youth should be screened every 3 to 6 months (CDC MMWR, 2017). Venue-based and social networking testing is another effective strategy to reach high-risk youth and increase the identification and linkage of youth into care (Barnes et al., 2010; Boyer et al., 2013; Straub et al., 2011). Once diagnosed with HIV, special efforts to improve engagement in care are often necessary to maximize youth accessing care.

DEVELOPMENTAL ISSUES

Adolescents face the same barriers to treatment adherence as adults, but they have additional challenges due to their developmental stage and legal circumstances. Social stigma, fear of alienation from peer groups, medication side effects, lack of transportation, dependence on parents or other caregivers, growing autonomy, and "feeling fine" are major contributors to nonadherence (Futterman, 2005; Radcliff et al., 2010).

MEDICAL MANAGEMENT

Currently, most adolescents acquire HIV through sexual transmission and are unaware of their diagnosis, making them excellent candidates for prevention counseling, linkage to and engagement in care, and initiation of ART (DHHS, 2020). Adolescents often experience high viral loads at diagnosis (mean HIV viral load in a cohort of adolescents from 15 HIV sites was 94,398 copies/mL [Ellen et al., 2014]) and multiclass resistance at diagnosis. Multiclass resistance suggests a transmission dynamic that includes older partners who have been on medications (Agwu et al., 2012). Data extrapolated

from the START and TEMPRANO trials favor initiating ART in all individuals who are able and willing to commit to treatment, understand the benefits and risks of therapy, and understand the importance of adherence (DHHS, 2020). The course of disease in youth is similar to that in adults, and they generally should be treated according to the same guidelines (DHHS, 2020).

The newest guidelines recommend ART for all individuals with HIV, regardless of CD4$^+$ T-cell count and age. Therapy should be initiated as soon as possible, and deferred treatment should be determined on a case-by-case basis. Recent guidelines for adolescents and young adults include data on the efficacy and feasibility of immediate ART and recommendations for certain populations. Earlier initiation of ART has been associated with reduced morbidity and mortality associated with HIV.

Concerns have been raised about some of the regimens in patients who acquired infection from perinatal transmission. Initial data from the Tsepamo study raised concerns about dolutegravir (DTG)-based regimens predisposing newborns of women on this medication to neural tube defects (NTDs). However, data presented at AIDS 2020 by Dr. Rebecca Zash, who reviewed 39,200 births surveyed from March 2019 to April 2020, found that newborns of mothers who were on DTG at the time of conception were not significantly more likely to have NTDs compared with newborns of mothers taking non-DTG ARTs (HIV.gov). In the ADVANCE trial, presented at AIDS 2020, weight gain was more common among study participants on the DTG-based regimens compared to the efavirenz-based regimen. Providers should be aware of side effects that can occur with regimens (HIV.gov).

SEXUAL RISK

The high rate of HIV in adolescents is multifactorial. Data have suggested that many adolescents do not have more sexual partners but that risk results from multiple psychosocial factors that predispose youth to HIV. Sexual networks, which include a partner who is living with HIV, are more common among adolescents living in higher-density, lower-income areas characterized by violence and limited access to care. Adolescents with HIV infection exist in communities with high rates of unintended pregnancy (Nachman et al., 2009), STIs (Trent et al., 2007), and condomless sex (Clum et al., 2009; Weiner et al., 2007). This, combined with rates of screening for STIs in HIV clinics that lag rates of non-HIV clinics, can promote high rates of STI and transmission of HIV (Berry et al., 2015). Additionally, condom negotiation is often not always a simple task for some adolescents. In one sample, females with HIV had lower self-efficacy overall (B = −0.15, p = 0.01), to discuss safe sex with one's partner (B = −0.14, p = 0.01), and to refuse sex without a condom (B = −0.21, p = 0.01), and lower self-efficacy was related to condomless vaginal and anal intercourse episodes (Boone et al., 2015). In young men, some have suggested that alcohol and other substances may be a key contributor to condomless sex with HIV-negative or unknown-status partners (Bruce et al., 2013). Other studies suggest a complicated relationship with psychological stress, substance use, and mental health that contributes to condomless sex (Nugent et al., 2010). Disclosure is complicated by HIV stigma and fear of rejection personally with partners and publicly (Toska et al., 2015).

There is a need to regularly address the risk for pregnancy, acquiring STIs, and the secondary transmission of HIV to sexual partners. The CDC recommends screening for STIs in women younger than 25 years because of the high rates of STIs in this age range. In young MSM, screening for STIs is recommended from extragenital body sites because oropharyngeal, rectal, and urethral infections are commonly present in this population (Workowski & Bolan, 2015). The CDC provides complete screening guidelines for youth living with HIV, and clinic-based motivational interviewing can improve condom use (Chen et al., 2011; Naar-King et al., 2006). The CDC also recommends PrEP for persons at high risk for HIV acquisition. PrEP is recommended for adolescents with an HIV-positive partner; for those with a high number of sexual partners (more than one partner in the last 6 months); for HIV-negative gay or bisexual men who report inconsistent condom use or STI diagnosis in the last 6 months; for heterosexual adolescents with inconsistent condom use or a recent diagnosis of gonorrhea or syphilis, living in a high-prevalence area or network, or engaging in sex with high-risk partners; for adolescents who inject drugs or have a partner who injects drugs; and for adolescents who have engaged in exchange of sex for goods, money, housing, or service (CDC, 2017). PrEP is approved for use in adolescents and young adults weighing 35 kg or more.

A client-centered approach that includes culturally grounded risk reduction and addresses not only the client's individual risk but also the complicating contextual factors that impact risk is most helpful. For example, to be effective, providers will also need to also address key social factors that may contribute to risk, including discrimination, housing, employment, food insecurity, mental health, and substance use. Personalized cognitive counseling (PCC) and Many Men, Many Voices (MMMV) are two evidence-based interventions that have been suggested to address the needs of vulnerable, at-risk communities. PCC uses an individual approach focusing on their last sexual risk behavior, while MMMV attempts to address the intersecting factors and identities impacting adolescents.

SUBSTANCE ABUSE

According to the 2017 National Youth Risk Behavior Survey (YRBS), approximately 40% of youth described ever having sex, with 29% of high school students reporting that they were currently sexually active. Among youth who described being currently sexually active, 19% drank alcohol or used drugs prior to their last sexual intercourse. Substance use predisposes adolescents to other high-risk sexual behaviors like inadequate condom use, and, for adolescents with HIV infection, substance use can interfere with clinical care. In a large AIDS Treatment Network (ATN) study of 1,712 youth, 61% of males and 45% of females scored 2 or higher on the CRAFT screening tool (Fernandez et al., 2015). Daily or weekly use of cannabis was 33% for males and 19% for females. Daily or weekly use of alcohol was 27% for males and 12% for females. Substance use prior to and during sex was commonly described. The regular assessment of substance abuse with appropriate counseling and referral is a key requirement in care.

MENTAL HEALTH

In the ATN study of 1,712 youth, 21% had a positive screen for depression and 15% for anxiety. Fifteen percent of the cohort had reported seriously considering suicide, and 14% were prescribed psychotropics. Seventy percent of the cohort recalled seeing a mental health provider while in care, and 38% of men and 42% of women reported currently wanting to receive mental health services (data presented at the October 2011 ATN meeting). These data suggest that regular screening and referral for mental health disorders is crucial. Stigma is another common concern for youth living with and at risk for HIV (Arrington-Sanders et al., 2020; Dowshen et al., 2009; Swendeman et al., 2006) and can relate to HIV status, sexual identity, or racial/ethnic minority status. Stigma can lead to feelings of marginalization and mistrust; engagement in risky behaviors, including condomless sex and nonadherence to medications; and delay in HIV testing care. Providers will need to approach adolescents with HIV infection using an intersectionality lens to be effective, acknowledging all identities (e.g., race/ethnicity, gender identity, socioeconomic status).

MEDICATION ADHERENCE

Youth living with HIV are at risk for nonadherence because of the aforementioned psychosocial, developmental, and cognitive factors. Several studies have documented nonadherence in youth living with HIV (Belzer et al., 1999, Belzer & Olson, 2008; Reisner et al., 2009). Rates of adherence to HIV medications during the past 30 days range from 28% to 70% (Reisner et al., 2009). Barriers include medical, psychological, and logistical issues. Medical barriers include an AIDS diagnosis (Martinez et al., 2012; Murphey et al., 2003), a difficult ART regimen (Buchanan et al., 2012), the absence of symptoms, and an unwelcoming medical environment (Philbin et al., 2014). Psychological barriers include depression, anxiety (Tanney et al., 2012; Wagner et al., 2011), stigma associated with the diagnosis or transmission history (Rao et al., 2007), and lack of social support (Williams et al., 2006). In addition, behavioral problems impact 50% of youth living with HIV (Bing, 2001). Positive self-efficacy and outcome expectancy were associated with better adherence, and logistical barriers such as lack of housing, insurance, and transportation were associated with poorer adherence (Rudy et al., 2008). A comprehensive, multidisciplinary healthcare team is required to serve the medical, logistical, and psychosocial needs of adolescents with HIV. Individually tailored interventions that address social and psychological factors (e.g., substance use, lack of insurance despite universal access to care, and lack of social support) and structural barriers (e.g., housing and insurance instability) will need to be developed in order to better meet the needs of youth living with HIV. Attention to potential barriers to adherence prior to treatment initiation is likely to improve outcomes.

COVID-19

In late 2019, a new pathogen, SARS-CoV2, spread across the globe, killing hundreds of thousands of people. Older adults experience the highest rates of SARS-CoV2, but adolescents and young adults, aged 15 to 25 years, account for up to 20.5% of new COVID-19 infections in some US locales, despite data suggesting that youth have lower COVID-19 testing rates (CDC, 2020a). Black and Latinx adolescents and emerging adults, aged 18 to 29, disproportionately account for 35.6% of COVID-related age-specific deaths (CDC, 2020a). The same social determinants of health that predispose communities to COVID-19 illness contribute to high rates of HIV in adolescents at risk for HIV. These include concomitant comorbidities, adverse social determinants of health, structural racism, access to testing centers, population density, inadequate housing, and poor access to healthy foods. Newer data have emerged about an illness specific to children and adolescents—multisystem inflammatory syndrome in children (MIS-C)—associated with COVID-19.

Adolescents with HIV should follow COVID-19 prevention, testing, and treatment guidelines from the CDC, including use of facial coverings/masks, social distancing at 6 feet, washing hands, cleaning and disinfecting surfaces frequently, and limiting travel. Further guidance suggests that they should maintain an adequate supply of medications to ensure there will be no barriers to medication access during the pandemic. It is important for providers to consider when in-person visits, including laboratory visits, are necessary pending the patient's clinical status and needs. When possible, they should use telemedicine visits, assist youth in using electronic hardware for appointments (e.g., webcams, virtual platforms), and adjust schedules to meet the needs of adolescents with HIV (Armbruster et al., 2020). It will be important to ensure that adolescents keep up to date on immunizations, including pneumococcal and influenza immunizations, and are provided necessary care for manifestations of mental health and substance use issues, which may increase during the COVID-19 pandemic. These additional comorbidities are prevalent in adolescents with HIV, so it is vital that providers address these topics and refer patients to appropriate mental health and substance use providers when necessary and continue to use a multidisciplinary team to support these patients.

CARE MODELS

Based on the high rates of psychosocial problems reviewed previously, developmentally based care models that utilize multidisciplinary care teams are preferable. When a multidisciplinary model is not available, it becomes imperative to facilitate the management of complex youth with behavioral problems by close communication among physicians, nurses, social workers or case managers, and behavioral health providers. Avoiding potentially catastrophic health outcomes, including rapid HIV progression, multiclass drug resistance, depression and suicide, chronic homelessness, prolonged incarceration, drug addiction, and secondary transmission of HIV, will likely require intensive attention to psychosocial issues. At times, a temporary approach of delaying early ART initiation may improve outcomes by allowing time to focus on developmental and social barriers.

TRANSITION TO ADULT CARE

Finally, clinicians must plan for the transition of adolescents with HIV into adult care. In a joint statement, the American Academy of Pediatrics, the American Academy of Family Physicians, the American College of Physicians, and the American Society of Internal Medicine affirmed that all adults, including those with special medical needs, benefit from care by doctors who are trained in adult medicine (Cohen et al., 2002). They recommended that an identified healthcare provider be responsible for the transition, that a portable medical summary be maintained, and that a written transition plan be developed with the patient and family by age 14 years. In addition to these recommendations, Valenzuela et al. (2011) recommended the following:

- Optimizing provider communication between adolescent and adult clinics

- Identifying adult care providers willing to care for adolescents and young adults

- Addressing patient and family resistance to transition of care caused by lack of information, concerns about stigma or risk of disclosure, and differences in practice styles

- Helping youth develop life skills, including counseling them on the importance of appropriate use of a primary care provider, managing appointments, symptom recognition and reporting, and self-efficacy

- Identifying an optimal clinic model based on specific needs

- Implementing ongoing evaluation to measure the success of a selected model

- Engaging adult and adolescent care providers in regular multidisciplinary case conferences

- Implementing interventions that may improve outcomes, such as support groups and mental health consultation

- Incorporating a family planning component into clinical care

- Educating HIV care teams and staff about transitioning

The National Health Alliance also has resources that organize transition into "Six Core Elements." These resources can effectively be used in any clinical setting (https://www.gottransition.org/six-core-elements/). Guidance from Straub (2018) identifies additional key components of transition, including formal, written transition policies; staff training in adolescent development, life skills, and self-care plans for adolescents with HIV; tailored programs that target resources toward adolescents with HIV; and integrative patient registries that can be shared across pediatric and adult clinics.

SUMMARY

Adolescents or youth who are living with HIV may have multiple developmental, cognitive, social, contextual, and environmental challenges that impact their identification, linkage, and engagement with care. Attention to the factors noted previously will likely improve the care, treatment, and adherence of youth living with HIV and potentially will prevent them from "falling through the cracks."

11.3.

HIV AND TRANSGENDER POPULATIONS

Zil Garner Goldstein and Madeline B. Deutsch

LEARNING OBJECTIVE

- Equip providers with the knowledge and skill to develop and provide gender-affirming primary and HIV care and prevention for transgender persons

WHAT'S NEW?

It is increasingly recognized that the development of transgender-specific programs and interventions and avoiding grouping transgender people with MSM populations results in improved care and prevention outcomes. Biomedical interactions between hormones and antiretroviral medications (ARVs) are unlikely, but transgender people may have poorer HIV outcomes or adherence to PrEP due to the stigma and discrimination experienced by this population.

KEY POINTS

- Transgender people have a range of identities and sexual orientations as well as transition-related goals; each transgender patient should be approached as an individual.

- Transgender people and programs should not be aggregated with MSM; programs and materials should be developed specifically for transgender populations using a culturally grounded approach.

- Gender-affirming hormone therapy with estrogens and androgen blockers is generally safe and compatible with ART regimens.

- Hormone therapy and other gender-affirming interventions improve HIV outcomes and reduce risk.

- Transgender patients require ongoing primary and preventive care, as do cisgender patients; it is important to tailor transgender primary care based on each patient's hormonal status and organ inventory.

- Providers should maintain a high index of suspicion for injected silicone and other fillers and related morbidity.

EPIDEMIOLOGY, DEMOGRAPHICS, AND TERMINOLOGY

"Transgender" is an umbrella term used to describe persons whose gender identity and/or expression of gender is different from the sex they were assigned at birth. Some transgender persons may seek only gender-affirming hormone therapy (HT), whereas others may seek surgical interventions such as genital reassignment surgery or other procedures on the face, breast, or body. Still other transgender persons may present with a more complex gender identity; some may choose to seek HT or surgical treatments but continue to live part or full time in their birth gender, whereas others may assume a fluid gender expression that is not categorizable in either polar gender (Deutsch et al., 2015a). Some transgender people may choose to not pursue any gender-affirming medical or surgical treatments. A 2015 national survey of transgender people found that 30% of respondents identified as genderqueer or nonbinary; that is, neither male nor female (James et al., 2016). Table 11.1 presents a description of selected terminology and identities. The sexual orientations of transgender persons also lie on a spectrum; in the same 2015 survey, 15% identified as heterosexual, 16% as gay or lesbian, 21% as queer, and 32% as bi/pansexual. In most cases, transgender persons define their sexual orientation based on their affirmed gender. For example, a transgender man who has sex with men would identify as gay. However, this also varies across cultural and linguistic lines, and the most effective method for determining the sexual history and health of a patient is to ask, "What are the gender(s) of people you have sex with? Are any of them transgender people? What kind of genitals do they have? A penis? A vagina?" "What kind of genitals are involved in the sex you have?" (Deutsch, 2018). Allowing transgender persons to define their own identity and experience and viewing them as individuals rather than as a stereotype will enhance the patient–provider relationship and may serve to improve adherence with ART and other care (Melendez & Pinto, 2009).

The World Professional Association for Transgender Health's *Standards of Care for the Health of Transsexual, Transgender and Gender Non-Conforming People*, seventh version (SOCv7; Coleman et al., 2012) states,

> Gender nonconformity refers to the extent to which a person's gender identity, role, or expression differs

Table 11.1. SELECTED TERMINOLOGY AND IDENTITIES

TERM	DESCRIPTION
Transgender	Umbrella term for gender-nonconforming persons; more "modern" and inclusive term, preferred by many
Transsexual	Older, more clinical term, some use this to identify those seeking medical or surgical treatment
Trans	Colloquial term increasingly used in place of "transgender," especially among younger populations
Non-binary	Describes a range of gender identities that are neither male nor female
Travestí	Term used by some Latina/Spanish-speaking transgender women
Gay	Term used by some Latina/Spanish-speaking transgender women with complex gender/sexual identities
Transgender woman/ transfeminine person	Person with a female or feminine-spectrum non-binary gender identity who was assigned male birth sex
Transgender man/ transmasculine person	Person with a male or masculine-spectrum gender identity who was assigned female birth sex

Note: People may use pronouns and/or names that differ from those listed on legal identity documents. Some may use gender-neutral "they/them" pronouns.

from the cultural norms prescribed for people of a particular sex. . . . Gender dysphoria refers to discomfort or distress that is caused by a discrepancy between a person's gender identity and that person's sex assigned at birth (and the associated gender role and/or primary and secondary sex characteristics).

SOCv7 further states,

Transsexual, transgender, and gender nonconforming individuals are not inherently disordered. Rather, the distress of gender dysphoria, when present, is the concern that might be diagnosable and for which various treatment options are available. The existence of a diagnosis for such dysphoria often facilitates access to healthcare and can guide further research into effective treatments. Research is leading to new diagnostic nomenclatures, and terms are changing in both the DSM [Diagnostic and Statistical Manual of Mental Disorders] . . . and the ICD [International Classification of Disease].

In order to access covered medical and surgical procedures, transgender people are generally given a billable diagnosis. Historically this has been "Gender Dysphoria," described in both the DSM-5 and the ICD-10 as a state of distress caused by mismatch between gender identity and birth-assigned sex. The need for a diagnosis to access care, including ongoing routine care when dysphoria is absent after gender transition has occurred, has historically forced all transgender people to carry a mental health diagnosis. The World Health Organization has recently announced that the ICD-11 will include a new diagnosis of "gender incongruence" that will be moved from the

mental health section to a new section on sexual health (Gander, 2018).

Epidemiologic surveillance in transgender populations has been limited due to inconsistencies in the collection of gender identity data. Incomplete or inconsistent identification of transgender populations represents a significant structural determinant of the health disparities seen in transgender populations. Best practice for the measurement of gender identity data involves the use of at least two questions, such as gender identity and birth assigned sex (Cahill & Makadron, 2013; Cahill & Makadron, 2014; Deutsch et al., 2013), or some other combination of questions that allow differentiation of all transgender and gender nonbinary people, including those who identify as "male" or "female," from cisgender people, which records both the current gender identity and the birth assigned sex (Cahill & Makadron, 2013; Cahill & Makadron 2014; Deutsch et al., 2013). This method has been found to identify twice as many transgender people as a "one-step" method in which a single "sex/gender" question is asked (Tate et al., 2012). A population-based statewide telephone survey in Massachusetts found a prevalence of 0.5% (Conron et al., 2012). The current estimate of the proportion of the transgender population by the UCLA Williams Institute recently doubled from 0.3% to 0.6% (Flores et al., 2016).

A 2019 meta-analysis found an HIV prevalence of 14.3% among transgender women living in the US (Becasen et al., 2019). This striking rate is driven by interactions between structural, personal, behavioral, and biological risks unique to transgender women. Structural factors include a lack of legal recognition or protections that often result in survival sex work. Personal factors include the higher rates of mood disorders seen in transgender populations as a result of ongoing discrimination as well as drive for gender affirmation; the model of gender affirmation describes the relationship between denial of gender affirmation (through lack of access to medical interventions or legal rights such as the ability to change one's name and gender on identity documents) and high-risk sexual behavior (Sevelius, 2013). Increasing gender affirmation through HT and surgery has been shown to have a positive effect on viral load suppression (Sevelius et al., 2019). Other behavioral factors include increased rates of condomless sex with primary male partners and anecdotes of increased earnings from sex work when no condom is used. Biological factors have not been explored in depth, but they could include changes to the anal epithelium in the presence of feminizing hormones, reduced erectile function resulting in impaired condom effectiveness, and unknowns such as HIV transmission through receptive vaginal sex in those who have undergone vaginoplasty (Poteat et al., 2015).

Transgender women have lower rates of virologic suppression (81% vs. 87% national overall average) in 2018 Ryan White HIV/AIDS Program monitoring data (HRSA, 2019). A study of HIV indicators comparing transgender women to cisgender male and female controls found significant differences between transgender women and cisgender men in rates of ART adherence (78.4% vs. 87.4%, $p = 0.0143$ for 100% last-3-day adherence) and virologic suppression (50.8% vs. 61.4%, $p = 0.0127$) but no difference in these measures when compared to cisgender women (Mizuno et al., 2015). Another study found that a high rate of adherence to HT regimens was associated with a positive odds ratio of 34.5 ($p = 0.002$) for reported high ART adherence, though there was no effect on the rate of undetectable viral load. Satisfaction with current gender expression was also associated with higher reported adherence (odds ratio 2.56, $p = 0.03$) but not with undetectable viral load (Sevelius et al., 2014b). Other factors associated with viral load suppression are having a primary care provider who manages both hormone therapy and HIV, stable housing, employment, longer time since HIV diagnosis, and achieving gender affirmation as desired (Bukowski et al., 2018; Jin, 2019; Sevelius et al., 2019; Sabino et al., 2021).

Few data exist on HIV risks and prevalence among transgender men, although some data suggest an increased risk (Green et al., 2015). A 2010 San Francisco study found that 61% of transgender men engaged in sex with other men, with 51% participating in vaginal receptive sex and 39% participating in anal receptive sex. Transgender men have reported feeling that HIV testing was less accessible to them than cisgender male controls (43.5% vs. 56.9%, $p = 0.04$) (Sevelius et al., 2014a).

INITIATING HT

Gender-affirming HT has been found to have a number of benefits on quality of life and on symptoms of depression, anxiety, and poor social functioning (Colton et al., 2011; Gómez-Gil et al., 2012). SOCv7 defines hormonal and surgical treatment as medically necessary and states that it is unethical to deny surgical care solely on the basis of HIV or hepatitis B or C serostatus. SOCv7 departs from prior practices that uniformly required a mental health referral "letter" prior to initiating gender-affirming HT. There are no minimums with regard to time spent in psychotherapy prior to HT, and it is also stated that primary care providers with adequate skill and experience may make their own determination of readiness for initiation of HT. This "informed consent" pathway destigmatizes and depathologizes transgender identities, and it overcomes several perceived or actual barriers to accessing HT; a rigorous mental health screening process may neither be available (lack of resources or lack of trained/willing providers) nor culturally applicable (language barriers and cultural differences between Western-oriented psychotherapy and persons of Latinx, African, Aboriginal, or Asian background) (Deutsch, 2012). It is also appropriate to offer physician-supervised HT to those patients who may otherwise turn to unprescribed sources of hormones (internet and street purchase) or who have already fully adjusted and socially transitioned to the affirmed (new) gender. A 2009 study of transgender women in New York City found that 10% receiving physician-supervised HT were also obtaining hormones from other sources and that patients were frequently taking two or three concomitant hormone regimens. This same study reported as barriers to accessing physician-supervised HT a lack of a knowledgeable provider (32%), lack of a transgender-friendly provider (30%), cost (29%), location (18%), and language (13%) (Sanchez et al., 2009). It is important that transgender persons have reasonable and realistic expectations about what HT and other treatments can and cannot do. Effectiveness of treatment relates to the age at initiation and the overall health state of the individual, as well as genetic factors. Once gender-affirming HT has begun, there should be continued monitoring for underlying psychosocial factors or mental health conditions, with interventions provided as indicated.

FEMINIZING HORMONE REGIMENS

Feminizing HT involves testosterone blockade in combination with estrogen replacement and the possible use of a progestogen. The most commonly used testosterone blocker in the US is spironolactone, a potassium-sparing diuretic taken in divided doses of 50 to 300 mg twice daily. Caution must be used with patients on angiotensin-converting enzyme (ACE) inhibitors or those with impaired renal function. Concomitant use of ARVs that may affect renal function, such as tenofovir, is a theoretical risk; however, no case reports exist of spironolactone causing or worsening renal function in these patients. Fosamprenavir and amprenavir are the only ARVs known to have interactions with estrogens that result in lower ARV drug levels, but these ARVs are rarely used. Side effects of spironolactone are mainly orthostatic hypotension and polyuria, both of which tend to resolve after several weeks. Routine monitoring of potassium and renal function (baseline, every 3 months for the first year, and then every 6 months) is reasonable. Creatinine levels should be compared to the male normal range. In patients with contraindications to spironolactone, 5-α-reductase inhibitors such as finasteride

5 mg daily or dutasteride 0.5 mg daily may be used. Some transgender women, especially those whose only opportunity for income is sustenance sex work, prefer to retain erectile function and may choose to avoid or use lower doses of testosterone blockers (Hembree et al., 2017).

Estrogen treatment may be via an oral, transdermal, or injectable route. The transdermal route of estradiol (50- to 200-µg patch changed one or two times per week) has been studied extensively and is very safe with respect to risk of thromboembolic disease: a 2008 meta-analysis of vascular thrombotic events (VTEs) in postmenopausal HT found a relative risk of VTEs in users of transdermal estradiol of 1.1 versus nonuser controls. This same review found a two- to threefold increased risk of VTEs among users of any type of oral estrogen in the first year of treatment only; however, this increase translates to only an additional 1.5 VTEs per 1,000 woman-years (Canonico et al., 2008). A subsequent 2019 review found the incidence of VTE to be 2.3 events per 1,000 patient years (Khan et al., 2019). The transdermal route also delivers fairly constant and physiologic serum estradiol levels, which helps minimize common estrogenic symptoms such as migraine, weight gain, or mood swings; however, transdermal preparations tend to be expensive, may irritate the skin, and are not always included in HIV formularies. Oral 17β-estradiol in divided doses of 2 to 4 mg twice daily also delivers a constant and physiologic dose and is well tolerated. Some providers recommend administering oral estradiol sublingually to minimize first-pass metabolism and effects on clotting factors. Prior studies reporting 20- to 40-fold increases in VTE risk in transgender women involved the use of high-dose, highly thrombogenic synthetic ethinyl estradiol, which is no longer used in cross-sex treatment, and did not control for tobacco use (Asscheman, 1989 et al; van Kesteren et al., 1997). More recent outcome studies of patients using 17β-estradiol have mixed findings, with one cohort of Dutch transgender women using only transdermal estradiol showing no increased risk of VTE and a US cohort of transgender enrollees in a managed healthcare plan using estrogen therapy showing a 3.2-fold increased risk (Asscheman et al., 2011; Nash et al., 2018).

Many patients may arrive at clinic requesting, or even demanding, injectable estrogens. Although estradiol valerate 20 to 40 mg intramuscular and estradiol cypionate 2.5 to 5 mg twice monthly have been used historically, these routes may deliver supraphysiologic estrogen levels that can vary widely over the injection cycle. Almost no data exist on the short- or long-term effects of this route, although anecdotally it is well tolerated. This route may be useful in a harm-reduction setting in which there is concern that a patient may turn to unprescribed hormone sources if an injected medication is not prescribed. This route may also be useful in patients who have low psychosocial functioning, poor medication adherence, or high pill burden, or to provide an opportunity to bundle HIV-related and other care with frequent hormone injection visits (Ickovics, 2008). Fluctuation of levels may be minimized by dividing the dose into weekly injections and, if needed, titrating peak and trough serum estradiol levels to manage any estrogenic side effects. Furthermore, changes in the hormonal milieu can lead to changes in the balance of Th1–Th2 T-lymphocyte function and theoretical alterations in cellular immunity, furthering the argument in favor of constant and physiologic dosing of estrogen.

Interactions between estrogen HT and ARVs are complex and inconsistent. Three small studies have investigated possible drug–drug interactions between PrEP and feminizing HT. Tenofovir/emtricitabine (TDF/FTC) does not affect the levels of feminizing HT, and both masculinizing and feminizing HT reduce serum and target tissue TDF concentrations (Cottrell et al., 2018; Hiransuthikul et al., 2018). While a sub-analysis of the iPrex study showed that there was no significant increase in risk for HIV transmission among transgender women with serum levels equivalent to taking TDF/FTC five or more times per week, subsequent data suggest that achieving this concentration of serum TDF may require better adherence than was previously thought (Deutsch et al., 2015b). These data also suggest that "PrEP on demand" requires further study in transgender populations before it can be recommended as an effective prevention strategy to transgender people on HT.

Data from contraceptive studies are mixed with regard to findings that protease inhibitors (PIs) and nonnucleoside reverse transcriptase inhibitors (NNRTIs) may cause changes in serum estrogen and progesterone levels (Kearney & Mathias, 2009; Marrazzo et al., 2015). However, should a patient previously on a stable HT regimen begin to experience symptoms of estrogen excess (migraines, weight gain, and mood swings) or deficiency (hot flashes) after a change in ART regimens, it is reasonable to check serum estradiol levels and/or adjust HT dosages empirically. In addition to the previously mentioned tests, monitoring of transgender women using HT should include baseline fasting glucose and lipid profiles, with subsequent monitoring as clinically indicated.

Progestogens have been suggested to enhance breast development and feminization of the body contours, and they may play a role in improving libido and mood. Patients may have a wide range of emotional responses to progestogens, with some patients preferring its effects and others feeling worse. It is reasonable to attempt a trial of oral micronized progesterone 100 to 200 mg every night at bedtime or, if unavailable, medroxyprogesterone acetate 5 to 10 mg orally at bedtime in patients who request this medication, including those with limited breast development or for those experiencing unpleasant mood or libido changes. However, regardless of estrogens used, there is an increase in thrombogenicity with the addition of medroxyprogesterone acetate, and a lesser increase with the use of other progestogens (Scarabin, 2018).

MASCULINIZING HORMONE REGIMENS

Female-to-male treatment primarily involves testosterone administration. Routes include intramuscular testosterone cypionate or enanthate at 25 to 100 mg once a week or transdermal routes such as patches (2–8 mg/d) or gels and creams (20–50 mg/d). Testosterone undecanoate is available in both an intramuscular injection formulation that is given every 10 weeks after two monthly loading doses and as a twice-daily oral regimen. Intranasal testosterone cypionate is also available but must be administered three times daily. Long-acting implantable testosterone pellets are also available; however, insertion involves a minor in-office procedure, and maintaining cisgender male range testosterone levels often requires placement of new pellets every 2 to 4 months. An oral testosterone undecanoate preparation was recently approved for use in the US. This medication requires a dosing up-titration and is administered twice daily. A Food and Drug Administration (FDA) "black box" warning has been placed on this medication regarding a risk of hypertension; notably, the effect size of the increase in blood pressure when seen is small (Swerdloff et al., 2020). Recently, many providers have begun using the subcutaneous route with testosterone cypionate and enanthate, which is less painful and traumatic and has been found to be noninferior (Olson et al., 2014). Dosing can be adjusted to 100 to 200 mg every 2 weeks; however, this may result in wide fluctuations in hormone levels. This treatment is well tolerated, with a minimum of side effects in most cases. Dose is titrated to cessation of menses and progression of virilization. HIV providers familiar with administering testosterone to cisgender men with low testosterone levels should be aware that transgender men in general will require higher and more frequent dosing since they require complete replacement rather than supplementation. Prior concerns about hepatic injury are currently unfounded with the use of nonoral, nonsynthetic androgens. Monitoring should include baseline and periodic (every 6–12 months) fasting serum lipids, glucose, and hematocrit. Due to the lack of menstruation and the hematopoietic influence of testosterone, hematocrit should be compared to male normal ranges. Because testosterone administration alone is not a reliable contraceptive, even in the setting of prolonged amenorrhea, transgender men who are sexually active with someone who has a penis and testes should be counseled on contraceptive use and the teratogenic risks of unplanned pregnancy while using testosterone. The effects of testosterone on the vagino-cervical mucosa with regard to HIV transmission risk are unknown, though transgender men using testosterone do tend to have higher rates of atrophic vaginitis and inadequate specimens on cervical Pap sampling (Peitzmeier et al., 2014). Primary human papillomavirus (HPV) screening via self-swab is a viable alternative for transmasculine patients who are uncomfortable with a pelvic exam. This method of screening is preferred by transmasculine people and increases cervical cancer screening rates in the clinical setting but is less sensitive than traditional provider-collected specimens (Reisner et al., 2017). However, increases in screening rates lead to the detection of more high-risk HPV infection than screening fewer individuals with a more sensitive test (Goldstein et al., 2019). Conversely, since many high-risk HPV infections do not result in cervical dysplasia requiring intervention, high-risk HPV-only screening may result in overdetection and unnecessary downstream testing such as colposcopy, which can be particularly of concern in those transgender men and transmasculine people for whom pelvic examinations are traumatic (Deutsch et al., 2020).

SURGICAL CONSIDERATIONS

SOCv7 requires a readiness and capacity to provide informed consent by a mental health provider prior to most gender-affirming surgical procedures. Common surgical procedures and recommendations from SOCv7 for referral to surgery are listed in Table 11.2. Expanded insurance coverage for gender-affirming surgeries is available under the Affordable Care Act, and in some states, Medicaid has made such procedures available to patients with lower levels of psychosocial functioning and health literacy. Providers should consider additional and ongoing assessments of such perioperative essentials as housing, social support, transportation, and ability for self-care, and they should provide resources and support to address identified needs or gaps (Deutsch, 2016). Patients may also present with a history of any number of surgical procedures. In some cases, the surgery may have been performed in another state or even overseas; as such, local primary care providers may be called upon to provide postoperative care. Most surgeons are willing to work with local physicians and when contacted may ask for photographs to be transmitted by email. For those patients with a complex wound care issue and remote surgeon, referral to a local wound care center may be a reasonable alternative approach.

More than 90% of vaginoplasties are performed using a penile-inversion technique; the erectile tissue is removed and a "neovagina" is created by inverting the penile skin into a pocket created in the pelvis. A clitoris is created using the glans penis, and labia are created with scrotal and possibly urethral skin. The neovagina requires lifelong periodic dilation and/or sexual activity to maintain depth and girth, and an artificial lubricant is required for penetration. Diseases of the neovagina are usually a result of remaining or recurrent granulation tissue (which may be cauterized using silver nitrate) or mixed-skin flora or sebum and debris conditions resulting from a deep inverted pocket of keratinized skin. Candida infections are uncommon, and the pH would not be expected to be acidic as in a natal vagina (Weyers et al., 2009). Although it is not possible to perform a Pap smear on a neovagina, providers should maintain a reasonable index of

Table 11.2. COMMON SURGICAL PROCEDURES

FEMINIZING	MASCULINIZING
Vaginoplasty	Mastectomy (male chest reconstruction, "top surgery")
Orchiectomy	Hysterectomy ± oophorectomy
Augmentation mammoplasty	Metoidioplasty (removal of clitoral hood and ligaments)
Rhinoplasty	Phalloplasty
Jaw/mandible contouring	
Reduction thyrocondroplasty (Adam's apple reduction)	
Forehead reconstruction/ hairline advancement	

suspicion for occult penile conditions such as Bowen's disease. A small minority of transgender patients receive a vaginoplasty in which a self-lubricating vagina is created using a segment of sigmoid colon. These patients must be monitored for possible malignancy or inflammatory bowel disease of the neovagina. Due to the anatomic differences of the surgically constructed neovagina, an anoscope may facilitate improved visualization and better patient tolerance compared to a vaginal speculum. The prostate is not removed during the vaginoplasty procedure; examination of the prostate in a patient who undergone vaginoplasty may be more effective when performed endovaginally. The risk of transmission of HIV via penile–neovaginal receptive sex in transgender women is unknown. Care of transgender women with a history of silicone or saline implant breast augmentation is identical to that of non-transgender persons.

PRIMARY CARE

Transgender persons require the same general primary and preventive care considerations as do non-transgender persons. However, it is important to take an inventory of organs on a patient-by-patient basis. For example, transgender women will retain their prostate after vaginoplasty, and some transgender men may have a hysterectomy but retain their ovaries or cervix. All organ screening should be based on a combination of age and risk factors, maintaining sensitivity to the patient's anxiety, which may be provoked due to examinations and studies on organs related to the birth sex. Screening for breast cancer in transgender women has not been studied; case series exist showing a possible increased risk above that of non-transgender men but lower risk than that of non-transgender women (Brown et al., 2015; Gooren et al., 2013). Some experts recommend that after 5 to 10 years of HT, patients should be considered for breast cancer screening, as are their age-matched non-transgender peers. Overall, providers should attribute HT as the etiology of any new health condition only after other more common causes have been excluded. Solid, long-term health outcome data are lacking. The largest population-based study on mortality outcomes to date is a retrospective series in the Netherlands of more than 2,000 transgender men and women. In this study, overall mortality among transgender women was increased by 51% in comparison to that of the general Dutch population; however, besides a 64% increase in risk of death due to cardiovascular disease, most of this increase was due to HIV, suicide, and substance abuse, and the study did not control for tobacco use. Transgender men did not have an increased overall mortality compared to the general population, but they had a 25-fold increased mortality relating to substance abuse (Asscheman et al., 2011).

HIV CARE AND PREVENTION CONSIDERATIONS

HIV prevention, care, and research programs have historically grouped transgender women with MSM. This linkage fails to recognize the significant behavioral and social differences between these two groups, not the least of which is that transgender women are not men (Poteat et al., 2015). Other than the possible negative impact of estrogens on amprenavir and fosamprenavir, and theoretical renal interaction between tenofovir and spironolactone, there are no clear biomedical differences in the prevention or management of HIV in transgender persons (El-Ibiary et al., 2008). The most important considerations are ensuring that programs and clinic settings are culturally appropriate; electronic medical record systems should have the capacity to record and display preferred name and pronoun, social marketing and recruitment materials should include imaging and messaging appropriate for transgender populations, waiting rooms should have transgender-oriented pamphlets and wall art, and clinic bathroom policies should be inclusive and clearly posted. Providers and clinic staff should have adequate cultural fluency and sensitivity (Sevelius et al., 2014a).

HIV PrEP in transgender women has not been studied in depth. The only published study to date of PrEP in transgender women is a subgroup analysis of the iPrEx trial that found no efficacy on an intention-to-treat basis. However, none of the transgender women who seroconverted had detectible drug levels at the time of HIV detection. Hormone use was associated with lower drug levels overall, as well as lower likelihood of having therapeutic drug levels, but the relationship between specific drug levels and HIV risk was identical between MSM and transgender women. It remains to be determined if reduced drug levels in transgender women using hormones are due to a direct interaction or to other confounders, such as increased pill burden or personal fear of interaction between hormones and ARVs (Deutsch et al., 2015b).

SILICONE

The use of injected silicone and other soft tissue fillers ("pumping") has become an increasingly prevalent practice, particularly among transgender women of color and sex workers. Unscrupulous practitioners, medical assistants, or laypersons will inject up to 1 liter or more of medical- or industrial-grade silicone, lubricant oil, insulating caulk, tire sealant, and other chemicals with the intent of bringing drastic and rapid changes to the physique (Silva-Santisteban, 2013). Most patients are unaware of exactly what is being injected, and the colloquial "silicone" may refer to any one of a number of injected fillers. In addition to the risks associated with the injected material, risks of acute bacterial infections and sepsis as well as transmission of HIV and hepatitis are high under these uncontrolled operating conditions. Some patients may have a sterile systemic inflammatory response mimicking sepsis or suffer embolization syndromes. The free filler substances could serve as an immunoadjuvant that precipitates an immune reconstitution inflammatory syndrome (IRIS) (Alvarez et al., 2016). Long-term risks include chronic pain and disfigurement as the injected material migrates and calcifies. It is particularly important to assess for injected fillers when using parenteral hormone regimens as the location of fillers may affect available injection sites, and the effects of fillers on transdermal estrogens are unknown.

This procedure is sought due to a variety of factors; in addition to peer pressure and a lack of understanding of the risks, more complex factors of survival are at play. Patients engaging in survival sex work may believe that they need to obtain a hyperfeminine figure in order to be competitive—and therefore pay for food and rent. Others may place a priority on erectile function and avoid HT, using silicone as their sole method of body feminization. Still others may live in neighborhoods in which they do not feel safe being identified as a transgender person, and they believe that silicone will assist them in blending in as a non-transgender person (Clark et al., 2008).

Treatment of silicone-related morbidities is limited and mostly supportive. Two case reports describe improved symptoms with subcutaneous etanercept 25 mg twice weekly; however, the applicability of etanercept when chemicals other than silicone are used, as well as its safety in PWH, is unclear (Desai et al., 2006; Pasternack et al., 2005; Rapaport, 2005).

An additional concern is subcutaneous or intramuscular medications used in PWH, such as penicillin and enfuvirtide, and how these injections may be affected by or complicate pre-existing soft tissue fillers. One case report described the safe and successful use of subcutaneous enfuvirtide in a patient with extensive migratory silicone material under ultrasound guidance (Gabrielli et al., 2010).

SUMMARY

Most of the special considerations in the care of transgender people living with HIV relate to provider and staff cultural competency, the tone and content of messaging, using the correct name and pronoun, and avoiding categorizing transgender women together with MSM. Gender affirmation through hormone and surgical treatment improves quality of life and, when bundled with HIV care or prevention efforts, may have synergistic benefits. More study is needed to evaluate the role of PrEP in transgender communities.

11.4.

CARE OF HOMELESS PWH

Angela Kapalko

LEARNING OBJECTIVE

- Describe special considerations affecting the medical management of homeless or displaced individuals

WHAT'S NEW?

- Thirteen single-pill combination regimens for HIV treatment are currently available; this should enhance adherence and reduce pill burden and complexity.

- Innovative programs for linkage and retention in care are operational.

- Opioid reversal (naloxone) programs are lifesaving.

- Needle exchange programs are essential in preventing clusters of HIV and hepatitis infections in injection drug users.

KEY POINTS

- HIV and homelessness are overlapping epidemics.

- Poverty, mental illness, substance use, and discrimination are barriers to care for both.

- Establishing mutual trust is paramount.

- Linkage to care and retention in care require enhanced teamwork.

Homelessness and HIV are two overlapping epidemics that each lead to worse health outcomes. They share many of the same risk factors of poverty, mental illness, substance use, racism, homophobia, stigmatization, and other forms of discrimination. Linkage to care and retention in care are challenging and are best met through the establishment of a trusting relationship, outreach, case management, partnering with supportive housing programs, and client-centered innovative local programs to reduce the barriers to care.

The federal government estimates that there are approximately 567,715 people who are homeless on any given night in January 2019 (HUD Continuum of Care Homeless Assistance Program, 2019). Advocates point to 2 to 3 million persons experiencing homelessness annually (National Law Center on Homelessness and Poverty, 2015). The HIV prevalence among homeless populations exceeds national averages. It is estimated that 3.4% of homeless people are HIV positive, compared to less than 0.5% nationally (National Coalition for the Homeless, 2009). In certain areas, the HIV prevalence among homeless people is much higher. In San Francisco, 20% of new HIV transmissions occur in people are currently homeless (San Francisco Department of Public Heath, 2019). It has also been estimated that one-third to one-half of people with advanced HIV are either homeless or at imminent risk of homelessness. Rising costs of housing, diminishing stock of single-room occupancies and public housing, and low wages make it nearly impossible to maintain stable housing in many cities.

Obtaining information about housing status and stability should be a routine part of obtaining a psychosocial history for PWH. Questions phrased in the vein of "What is your living situation?" are readily understood and are preferable to "Are you homeless?" A follow-up question on the stability of current living arrangements can also give insight into a patient's housing status. If the patient is marginally housed or homeless, knowing how to contact the patient is extremely important. Be aware of any contact phone numbers, as well as places they usually visit, including any agencies that they use, case managers, and food lines and stores that they frequent. This will allow one to contact them in case of abnormal lab results, important appointments, and if they are lost to follow-up. Some social service agencies provide free voice mail, which can be a confidential way for the patient to receive messages. Free cellphones are available for low-income individuals. Text messages relaying appointment reminders and motivating messages have been shown to increase attendance at appointments. In Kenya, text messages significantly improved adherence and viral suppression (Lester et al., 2010). In the era of electronic health records, patient portals grant patients more access to their health records and healthcare providers; however, having access to a smartphone or a computer is key and could be a limiting factor for many people experiencing homelessness. Health status is poorer in homeless populations than in the general population. A systematic review that included 152 studies representing 139,757 patients found that worse housing status was independently associated with worse outcomes among PWH (Aidala et al., 2016). The issue of tuberculosis (TB) exposure and transmission is a serious problem for homeless PWH, and TB transmission in shelters is well documented (McElroy et al., 2003). Aggressive screening for TB is recommended. Louse-borne and rat-borne infections are probably underrecognized given that the seroprevalence of rickettsial and other related infections is as high as 50% in homeless populations studied both in the US and in Europe (Brouqui et al., 2005). Body lice can transmit a variety of bacterial infections, including relapsing fever caused by *Borrelia recurrentis*, trench fever caused by *Bartonella quintana*, epidemic typhus caused by *Rickettsia prowazekii*, and bacillary angiomatosis caused by *Bartonella henselae* and *B. quintana*. Bacillary angiomatosis occurs in severely immunosuppressed PWH; infestation with body lice is an important factor in transmission of *Bartonella*, the causative organism (Foucault, 2006). Recently, widespread outbreaks of hepatitis A among congregate living conditions, both within and outside shelters, have been occurring throughout the US. In February 2019, the CDC and the Advisory Committee on Immunization Practices (ACIP) updated its recommendations for hepatitis A vaccination to include people experiencing homelessness (Doshani et al., 2019).

PREVENTION, MORTALITY, AND MORBIDITY

Homelessness remains an important risk factor for HIV transmission (Golden et al., 2018; San Francisco Department of Public Health, 2019). Current prevention strategies including postexposure prophylaxis and PrEP have not been well studied in homeless populations, but indications are positive that these would be effective and acceptable (Doblecki-Lewis et al., 2016). Although PrEP is effective if taken, in a survey among young adults experiencing homelessness, only 29% had knowledge of PrEP, even though 84% were eligible for it based on risk (Santa Maria, 2018). The success of efforts to eliminate transmission by reducing community viral loads will almost certainly pivot on the ability to reach and ensure adherence in homeless and multiply diagnosed populations.

Although death rates for HIV have steadily declined since their peak in 1995, homeless people experience excess mortality compared to the general population. Among the homeless in Boston, the mortality rate was 9-fold higher in 25- to 44-year-olds and 4.5-fold higher in 45- to 64-year-olds. One-third of the deaths were due to drug overdoses (Baggett et al., 2013). In a population-based incidence-density case-control study in San Francisco, people who were homeless at time of their HIV diagnosis had a 27-fold higher odds of death compared with those with housing (Spinelli et al., 2019). An analysis assessing the differences in causes of death among housed and homeless people diagnosed with HIV in San Francisco between 2002 and 2016 included 4,158 individuals. Compared to those reported as housed at death, those who were homeless were more likely to be younger, to be Black, to have a history of injection drug use, to be female or transgender, and to live below the poverty level and were less likely to have been prescribed ART. Additionally, deaths due to mental disorders related to substance use were higher in the individuals experiencing homelessness (Hessol et al., 2019). Studies suggest that

substance use treatment, opiate reversal programs, treatment of hepatitis B and C, cancer screening, and supportive housing may be lifesaving in homeless HIV-infected persons.

Harm reduction measures such as needle exchange programs and naloxone distribution programs can also be lifesaving. In May 2015, the CDC (2015) reported that in a rural county in Indiana, 135 persons were diagnosed with HIV in a community of 4,200. The cases were linked to syringe-sharing partners injecting oxymorphone. Coinfection with the hepatitis C virus (HCV) was found in 114 patients. A public health emergency was declared, and a needle exchange program was authorized by the governor. Needle exchange programs are important for reducing the spread of HIV and HCV, as well as for linking persons to substance use programs and methadone treatment. In a report on more than 10,000 opioid reversals, the CDC (2012) stated that making training in the use and distribution of naloxone available to opioid drug users is a strategy that reduces overdose deaths. Opioid reversal programs using naloxone have been credited with saving numerous lives. Patients who are prescribed opioids or who use them or are on methadone or buprenorphine should have access to naloxone and training on how to use it. With access to naloxone increasing across the country and the rate of opioid-related overdoses continuing, providing naloxone discussion and training to all PWH during medical or social service visits should be considered.

Clearly, team-based care is essential to address the multiple needs of homeless patients. Randomized controlled trials have shown that HIV-infected homeless people randomized to intensive case management linked to housing were more likely to obtain permanent housing and achieve an undetectable viral load than those who received usual hospital discharge planning (Buchanan et al., 2009). San Francisco has a respite unit with medical and social services. Homeless patients can have their medications administered, wound care provided, and follow-up appointments tracked. They also may be able to transition into permanent housing. Results from the Seattle Eastlake "wet housing" project showed that heavy alcohol users who were admitted and allowed to drink in the housing significantly decreased their heavy drinking days, reduced their daily intake from 21 to 11 drinks per day, had a major decrease in withdrawal tremors, and saved the city $4 million in the first year (Collins et al., 2012). Street medicine and mobile healthcare programs such as the Homeless Outreach Team (SF HOT) and HIV Homeless Outreach Mobile Engagement (HHOME) in San Francisco assertively provide continuity to patients who would otherwise be lost from the healthcare system aside from high-cost acute services. Ironically, cities with budget deficits may find that providing more care and housing can save money. Failure to do so can result in disastrous increases in HIV infection and morbidity and mortality, as has happened as a result of the austerity measures in Athens, Greece (Sypsa et al., 2015). Case management programs can coordinate the comprehensive wraparound services that complex patients need; administrators can accompany these patients to important appointments and find them in the field when necessary. Nevertheless, in recognition of the large disparities that continue to exist for homeless PWH, the Health Resources and Services Administration (HRSA) has initiated a multisite demonstration project called Building a Medical Home for Multiply Diagnosed HIV-Positive Homeless Populations that will evaluate and disseminate information on best practices in caring for this population (Phillips et al., 2018).

Recent research has demonstrated the pervasive occurrence of chronic pain in this population (Miaskowski et al., 2011) and the complexity of managing pain in these patients (Hansen et al., 2011). The National Health Care for the Homeless Clinicians Network has developed a useful guideline for care of homeless patients with chronic pain (Wismer et al., 2011). Efforts to develop innovative and comprehensive programs to manage pain and co-occurring mental health and chemical dependency in this population are under way in San Francisco and other locations.

With the availability of electronic medical records, quality improvement programs can track measures such as missed appointments, loss to follow-up, detectable viral loads, show-up rates for new patients, or various healthcare maintenance measures, including Pap smears, mammograms, and colorectal cancer screening. Causes for poor performance can be studied locally, and solutions can be tested with quality improvement methods.

HIV TREATMENT

Although homeless people may face challenges to adherence and compliance that housed individuals may not face, homelessness should not be a limiting factor in the decision to prescribe ART. With more recent guidelines nationally and internationally recommending ART regardless of CD4+ T-cell count, thoughtfulness around factors that could impact an individual experiencing homelessness need to be discussed at all points in an individual's care. In a prospective study conducted among the San Francisco-based Shelter, Health and Drug Outcomes Among Women (SHADOW) study, data from 120 PWH were analyzed to determine independent associations between factors common in low-income women and unsuppressed viral loads. An unsuppressed viral load was detected in 60% during the study period of 3 years and 19% were unsuppressed at all visits. Having an unsuppressed viral load increased by more than 10% for every 10 nights sleeping on the street or spent in a shelter, and odds were over three-fold higher for women who were recently incarcerated (Riley et al., 2019). Linkage to care and ART directly from incarceration could help with viral suppression, even if it is not long lasting. A study of PWH injection drug users on ART in Miami showed that homeless subjects had higher rates of anxiety and perceived stress but similar rates of depression as housed subjects. In the study, depression was significantly related to lower adherence, although housing status was not. Sixty-three percent of homeless subjects reported 100% adherence. This study showed that depression is a potent predictor of nonadherence, suggesting that HIV-infected homeless individuals should be screened and treated for depression (Waldrop-Valverde et al., 2005).

Strategies to improve adherence in homeless people are similar to those recommended for general populations. There are several additional strategies, including building on existing routines, such as those related to shelter, meals, or even drug-using routines. To assist patients, providers must ask about and understand these routines when prescribing and providing adherence counseling.

We recommend single-pill combination regimens, if possible, to prevent running out of part of the regimen and to ease pill burden. In choosing an ART regimen, there are some special considerations, such as whether medications should be taken on an empty stomach or have particular food restrictions, requirements for dose timing that may be difficult to maintain, and food times and types that may not be under a person's control. Large numbers of pill bottles or weekly pill boxes are recognizable and difficult to conceal in a shelter setting; as a result, stigmatization, discrimination, or theft of medications may occur. Medication bottles can be kept by a case manager or program director, and small pill boxes that can be refilled frequently may be useful in these cases. Currently, there are 13 single-pill combination regimens. A long-acting injectable combination therapy of cabotegravir and rilpivirine is on the horizon, and while it has not been studied specifically in people who experience homelessness, the idea of needing a injection only every month or every other month for HIV could be very appealing and assist with adherence. Unboosted integrase inhibitor–based regimens currently top the 2020 DHHS treatment guidelines. Coformulated bictegravir, emtricitabine, and tenofovir alafenamide (Biktarvy) can be taken with or without food, has a high genetic barrier to resistance (which is helpful if adherence is a concern), and has a favorable side effect profile. The coformulated tablet of dolutegravir, lamivudine, and abacavir (Triumeq) is another option with no food requirements; however, the patient must be HLA B5701 negative before starting. With one less medication, dolutegravir and lamivudine (Dovato) has come onto the list of single-tablet options. Patients who are new to starting Dovato need to not be coinfected with hepatitis B and have an HIV RNA of more than 500,000 copies/mL. Other single-tablet regimens are available and would need more consideration when prescribing. Coformulated efavirenz-based regimens (Atripla, Symfi, and Symfi Lo) may cause sedation and decreased awareness of one's environment and may affect street safety or worsen underlying psychiatric problems. Rilpivirine-based regimens (Complera, Odefsey, Juluca) lack the central nervous system side effects of efavirenz but must be taken with a 500-calorie meal (see Complera/Odefsey website for sample meals) because nutritional supplements are not adequate. Furthermore, proton pump inhibitors (PPIs) cannot be used, and Complera and Odefesy are less effective as an initial treatment regimen in those with a baseline viral load greater than 100,000 copies/mL. Juluca, which is a two-drug single tablet combination of rilpivirine and dolutegravir, is only indicated for patients who already have an HIV RNA of less than 50 copies/mL and have no resistance to the components. Coformulated doravirine, lamivudine, and tenofovir DF (Delstrigo) is the newest triple single-tablet regimen with no food requirement and a low side effect profile. Since it does have tenofovir disoproxil fumarate (DF), it is only indicated for patients with creatinine clearance of greater than 60 mL/min. Lastly, any of the coformulated regimens that include cobicistat, a pharmacokinetic booster, like emtricitabine, cobicistat, tenofovir, and elvitegravir (Stribild or Genvoya) or darunavir, cobicistat, emtricitabine, and tenofovir AF (Symtuza), are recommended to be taken with food. Cobicistat is a CYP3A inhibitor, and there are multiple drug interactions; it is also an inhibitor of several of the transporter systems, so monitoring drug interactions is important.

THE MODEL OF CARE

There are more than 100 healthcare for the homeless programs throughout the US. Linking with a local program or getting advice from a national healthcare for the homeless organization is helpful to HIV providers working with homeless people. Shelter staff are also key resource providers in education and prevention efforts as well as support. Providing housing, particularly supportive housing targeted to formerly homeless people, is a critical health service function.

Homeless PWH have a high prevalence of mental health disorders, especially depression, which is associated with poorer adherence to medications. Histories of both physical and sexual assault are common, especially among homeless women and transgender individuals. In one study, 32% of women and 38% of transgender persons reported a history of either sexual or physical assault in the previous year. It has also been reported that Black women with a history of childhood abuse have an increased risk of being homeless and using crack cocaine (Wechsberg et al., 2003).

Building a trusting relationship and providing a nonjudgmental medical home in which patients can feel that they are valued as individuals is of utmost importance. The healthcare team should be able to recognize and treat posttraumatic stress disorder, depression, and other psychiatric disorders. A harm reduction approach is recommended. An effective program will also need to coordinate services with local jails and prisons because incarceration is more common among the homeless and those living with HIV. Many homeless people are devoted to their pets and will not take care of their own health needs unless their pets are safe. Some cities have a special arrangement with the local humane society or have special services for pets.

In San Francisco, the Positive Health Access to Services and Treatment (PHAST) team works to encourage testing in the inpatient setting, emergency room, and urgent care and primary care clinics. The PHAST team provides easy linkage to care and actively works with new PWH or people who have fallen out of care, meeting them in the emergency room or in their inpatient room. PHAST works to stabilize patients, navigate them through often complex healthcare and benefits systems, and work on their barriers as defined by the patients. Patients are followed closely to link them to and retain them in care. The key is not giving up on the patients; it may take a long time for them to fully engage. The San Francisco Department of Public Health's Linkage, Navigation, Integration, and Comprehensive Services (LINCS) program takes referrals for all San Francisco clients who would benefit from connecting or reconnecting with services. LINCS has outreach workers who search for both newly diagnosed patients and patients lost to follow-up.

11.5.

INCARCERATED POPULATIONS

Rachel A. Prosser

LEARNING OBJECTIVE

- Discuss the provision of HIV care and release planning in the context of correctional facilities

WHAT'S NEW?

In light of the 2020 DHHS ART guidelines, which recommend treating everyone who is HIV positive with ART irrespective of CD4[+] T-cell count, correctional facilities may need to reevaluate and prioritize their ARV formulary list. The splitting of coformulated tablets into their respective components and generic drug preferences may become more common practice as part of efforts to treat more HIV-infected inmates while being fiscally prudent. Caution is urged that correctional facilities do not stray from the DHHS-recommended regimens for treatment-naive individuals.

KEY POINTS

- The US has the highest incarceration rate in the world.

- Persons of color are disproportionately incarcerated.

- Rates of HIV infection and AIDS diagnoses are 5 and 2.5 times higher, respectively, in state and federal correctional facilities compared to the general public.

- Correctional facilities pose unique barriers to ART adherence.

- Strategies for successful release planning may include having an appointment with an HIV provider soon after release and working with case managers/social workers to obtain medical coverage and referrals to community HIV organizations.

According to US Department of Justice statistics, approximately 6,937,600 offenders were under the supervision of correctional systems at the end of 2012. Of these individuals, 4,781,300 were supervised via probation or parole systems. The remaining individuals were living in jails or state or federal prisons. The number of individuals incarcerated in the US has been declining slowly since 2009. At the end of 2012, 1 in every 35 adults in the US was under some form of correctional observation. This is the lowest rate observed since 1997.

The risk factors associated with acquiring HIV infection and having an interaction with the criminal justice system are similar. In 2014, approximately half of federal inmates and 16% of state inmates were serving time for drug-related offenses. Black, non-Hispanic males have a 3.8 to 10.5 times higher rate of incarceration compared to their White, non-Hispanic counterparts. Similarly, Black, non-Hispanic females have a 1.6 to 4.1 times higher rate of incarceration compared to White, non-Hispanic females. In 2014, women accounted for approximately 7% of the total prison population. White women make up 50% and Black women 21% of all incarcerated women. An estimated 7.3% of Black men between the ages of 30 and 34 years were in a state or federal correctional facility (Guerino et al., 2011).

HIV EPIDEMIOLOGY IN CORRECTIONAL FACILITIES

Within state and federal correctional systems, HIV infection prevalence is five times higher than that in the general population. Rates of confirmed AIDS cases in prisons are approximately 2.5 times greater than those of nonincarcerated populations (Maruschak, 2009; Spaulding et al., 2002). Results from studies conducted with HIV-infected inmates demonstrated that being Black or Hispanic, being an MSM, having a history of injection drug use, having an STI, and having a psychiatric condition were all positive predictors of HIV infection (Beckwith et al., 2010).

The prevalence of HCV coinfection among HIV-infected inmates varies greatly depending on region. Rates of HIV/HCV coinfection in correctional settings have been estimated to be as high as 65% to 70% (Weinbaum et al., 2005).

PROBLEMS WITH HIV PREVENTION IN PRISONS

Although risk behaviors such as tattooing, drug use, and sex are forbidden in correctional facilities, these activities are common. Condoms are not available and are deemed contraband in most facilities. Not surprisingly, clean needles are not provided, and needle exchange programs do not exist. Thus, prevention programs cannot provide the materials necessary to prevent the spread of STIs and other illnesses. Fortunately, to date, the actual transmission rate of HIV within correctional facilities is thought to be relatively low, and it is believed to be lower in comparison to that in the general public. However, the true rate of HIV acquisition among inmates is difficult to ascertain because routine HIV testing on entry and exit from correctional facilities is poorly documented. Effective treatment of HIV will further decrease the risk of HIV transmission in correctional settings.

BARRIERS TO HIV TREATMENT IN CORRECTIONAL FACILITIES

Policies governing the provision of care and access to medical testing vary across prisons and jails. For example, some state prisons require HIV testing, whereas some merely recommend it. The CDC (2009) has recommended routine opt-out testing of inmates. In 2005, only 33% of state and federal prisons were performing routine mandatory HIV testing (Hammett et al., 2007). Not surprisingly, routine opt-out testing strategies yield greater numbers of screening and subsequent HIV diagnoses. Jails, as opposed to prisons, typically have an extremely rapid turnover rate, making routine or opt-out HIV screening and follow-up difficult to implement. According to Minton and Sabol (2009), the average weekly turnover rate in jails was 66.5% in 2008.

Facilities may or may not meet national standards; they may or may not have access to HIV specialists and to specialty tests, such as coreceptor tropism assays, integrase inhibitor resistance testing, HLA-B*5701 screening and testing, or resistance genotypes (Bernard et al., 2006).

Similar to the nonincarcerated population, there are many reasons for nonadherence to ART among inmates, but some are unique to correctional facilities. Movement between facilities, being in segregation, and lockdowns (when officials forbid any departures from the cells of certain wings or halls by inmates for periods of time) can cause disruptions in adherence. Facilities not receiving medications in a timely manner or inmates not being alerted to pick up their medications can serve as barriers to adherence. Inmates cannot always keep their own medication ("keep on person" [KOP]), and some are required to pick up medication daily at the pharmacy or infirmary (DOT). Confidentiality can be a major concern, for example, when picking up medications or going for DOT. Sometimes the exposure of HIV status can have severe consequences in prisons. Getting medications on schedule and meeting food requirements can be difficult. Inmates may be required to attend programs or report for jobs that interfere with the timely ingestion of medication, especially in DOT situations. Meals are served at specific times that may not coincide with the timing for a particular medication. Taking efavirenz at bedtime may not be possible. DOT regimens do not encourage autonomy on the part of the patient. Facilities that require DOT could consider allowing the more real-life KOP system for a specified time before discharge.

Additional barriers unique to correctional facilities stem from limited budgets and the costs of HIV care. Some facilities may have guidelines or restrictions on when providers can initiate ART. Many correctional facilities have formulary restrictions that appear to be cost-effective. Less expensive ART options often result in more pills daily, twice-daily dosing schedules, and greater side effects (all well-documented correlates of nonadherence). Costs incurred as a result of the need for additional medications to counter common ART side effects are difficult to capture and often not included in cost analyses.

ART USE IN CORRECTIONAL FACILITIES

Providers should include the inmate's length of stay and future transfers in the decision-making process for initiating ART. Often, inmates who are released from prison and violate parole will be brought to a jail and then transferred to prison or brought directly back to prison. This movement often results in missed doses of ART. Note that the selection of ART regimens with a higher barrier to resistance will likely provide greater success for persons unable to fill ART prescriptions and for persons who will be in and out of correctional facilities. In the spirit of cost savings, selection of more durable regimens may prevent the development of drug-resistant HIV. Subsequently, avoiding the development of drug-resistant HIV may save on future lab costs and also costs associated with adding agents to effectively treat drug-resistant strains of HIV. Anecdotally, inmates have reported efavirenz-containing regimens as having "street value" in correctional facilities: the drug can be ground up and huffed or snorted for hallucinogenic effects.

RELEASE PLANNING

A key to success of many programs is collaboration among stakeholders—for example, correctional systems, academic institutions, and medical centers in the community (Braithwaite et al., 1996). A multitude of resources are available for persons living with HIV. It would behoove individuals working with discharge planning and reentry to the community of HIV-positive inmates to become familiar with the resources available. In some communities, housing and food supplies are available to persons based solely on their HIV diagnosis.

Additional considerations for successful release to the community are scheduling appointments with an HIV provider soon after release and assisting inmates with their linkage to HIV care. Some facilities provide inmates 1 week of medication and a 30-day prescription at time of release. Without some type of healthcare coverage in place, however, many inmates are unable to fill the prescriptions. In fact, only approximately 20% of released inmates fill their ART prescription within 30 days of release (Baillargeon et al., 2009).

11.6.

RURAL POPULATIONS AND HIV

Abby Davids

LEARNING OBJECTIVE

- Describe obstacles to and best practices for optimal HIV care for PWH in rural settings

WHAT'S NEW?

PWH in rural areas face unique challenges. The 2014 HIV outbreak in rural Indiana illustrates the need for expanded HIV prevention, testing, and care services targeted to the needs of rural populations.

KEY POINTS

- The HIV epidemic in the US has begun to shift to more rural areas.

- Rural residence creates barriers for HIV care and is a risk factor for lower HIV testing overall, later HIV diagnosis, and increased HIV-related mortality.

- The increasing rurality of the US opioid epidemic highlights additional challenges and needs for both HIV and HCV care in rural areas.

Although the HIV epidemic in the US began in large cities, it has since moved to more rural areas (Schafer et al., 2017). The southern US currently has the highest incidence and prevalence of HIV in the country; although only 37% of the US population lives in the South, the region accounts for approximately 46% of all HIV transmissions and 52% of new transmissions (CDC, 2020c). Some non-urban counties in the South now have a higher HIV prevalence than many large US cities (CDC, 2011). Racial disparities in the burden of HIV transmissions, particularly among Black populations, are amplified in the South as well (CDC, 2015).

Rural/non-urban residence creates several barriers to engagement in the HIV continuum of care. HIV testing rates are lower in rural areas; in one study, the rate of lifetime HIV testing was 66% for non-urban participants versus 88% for urban participants (Wallace, 2011). MSM in rural areas are less likely to be tested for HIV than those in urban areas, as are undocumented migrant and seasonal farmworkers in rural areas (Fernandez, 2005; Goldenberg et al., 2014). Rural providers may not offer HIV testing routinely as well; in one study, primary care providers in North Carolina were only 10% adherent to CDC HIV testing guidelines, despite being aware of the recommendations (White et al., 2015).

Access to care also remains a challenge for PWH in rural areas. Many rural residents travel to urban areas for their medical care, citing lack of local provider expertise as one reason for this. In 2013, 95% of non-urban counties in the US lacked a Ryan White HIV medical provider, compared to 69% of urban counties (Vyavaharkar et al., 2013). In 2017, of the 2000 organizations funded by the Ryan White program, only 6% were located in rural areas (Klein, 2020). Additionally, PWH in rural areas were less likely to have regular outpatient visits with their HIV care provider than PWH in urban areas, and they were less likely to take ART. PWH in rural areas were also less likely to be prescribed newer ARVs than those living in urban areas (Schafer et al., 2017). In one study from the US Veterans Administration, PWH in rural areas had more advanced HIV infection at diagnosis than those in urban areas, and the mortality hazard ratio for rural PWH versus urban PWH was 1.34 (Ohl et al., 2010). Additional barriers to care for PWH in rural areas include stigma, lack of support services, and transportation difficulties.

Rural areas are also less likely than urban areas to have harm reduction programs in place to reduce one of the root causes of HIV transmission. The 2014 outbreak of HIV in rural Scott County, Indiana, showcases the potential for rapid progression of HIV and HCV through communities affected by the opioid epidemic. Currently in the US, new opioid injectors reside primarily in non-urban areas, and opioid users who switch from oral formulations to injection use engage in injection practices with greater risk of HIV and HCV transmission. The CDC estimates that the counties at greatest risk for an HIV outbreak associated with injection drug use are mostly rural, and this, combined with high rates of poverty and lower educational attainment, makes rural areas particularly vulnerable. HCV similarly affects non-urban populations disproportionately, and many of the areas with highest rates of acute HCV in the US are in rural Appalachian states (Schranz et al., 2018).

Clearly, to provide state-of-the-art healthcare to the large rural population of PWH, programs are needed to address barriers to care and stigma that PWH in rural areas face. Strategies that keep in mind the social determinants of health and the importance of involving local community members have proven to be most successful (Schafer et al., 2017). These include:

- Community engagement: involving community members in research and programming, such as lay health advisor interventions

- Leveraging existing data sources: agreement on a universal definition of "rurality" in order to study and understand populations in rural areas more fully

- Human resource capacity development: addressing the shortage of HIV care providers in rural areas and conducting needs assessments of rural primary care providers to better understand knowledge gaps and training needs

- Innovative service delivery: consideration of non-clinic-based locations to deliver HIV prevention and testing, such as emergency departments or pharmacies; use of tele-health to reach remote patients; use of teleconferencing to connect specialists in urban areas with primary care providers in rural areas; and optimizing the use of technology, including text messaging and app-based services

Resources for rural HIV care are available through the National Rural Health Association and the Rural Health Information Hub; the latter includes an HIV/AIDS Prevention and Treatment Toolkit (available at https://www.ruralhealthinfo. org/toolkits/hiv-aids). A web resource is available to locate nearby federally funded community health centers (DHHS; available at http://findahealthcenter.hrsa.gov/Search_HCC.aspx).

11.7.

CARE OF MIGRANT AND IMMIGRANT PERSONS WITH HIV

Deliana Garcia, Claire Hutkins Seda, and Laszlo Madaras

LEARNING OBJECTIVE

- Discuss the important distinction between migrants and immigrants

- Discuss the differences in HIV risk, presentation, and comorbidities among immigrants from different regions of the world

- Discuss the impact of stigma on healthcare-seeking behavior, treatment adherence, and safe practices

WHAT'S NEW?

- Migration or human movement as an overlay to other social determinants of health requires a careful assessment of the person beyond ethnicity and language preference.

KEY POINTS

- The complex combination of population characteristics and barriers to care requires a careful consideration of each person's circumstances when considering HIV risk, testing, treatment adherence, and perceived or experienced stigma.

- Research in these populations is challenging due to a myriad of factors, including recruitment issues, ethical challenges, and subgroup differentiation.

- A distinction between premigration transmission and postmigration transmission appears when considering migrants from the Americas versus those from the African continent.

- The prevalence and incidence of HIV in Hispanics and African Americans in the US are higher than those of Whites, and these populations have less access to care and treatment than do Whites.

- Among immigrant populations living with HIV, the prevalence and presentation of opportunistic infections or coinfections differ from those of US-born PWH.

Migrants (those in the US for a time-limited stay, usually to engage in remunerated activity like farm work) and newly arrived immigrants (those who wish to resettle permanently in the US) are largely Latinx from Mexico and Central America. A smaller percentage are from Africa and Asia (Radford, 2019). Some migrants and recent immigrants live and work in the US without authorization, although it is unclear how many. A crucial characteristic of these target populations is their geographic instability and high mobility. Migrants, by definition, move frequently for work purposes, family reunification, or pursuit of safe haven, contributing to an unstable and stressful lifestyle (IOM, 2020).

A natural consequence of such mobility is that migrants face many barriers to accessing care. Mobility is just one negative social determinant of health (SDH), a condition in which people are born, raised, and work. Some SDHs include a person's employment and working conditions, income and social status, social support and connectedness, environment and housing, access to healthcare and literacy, and gender issues (O'Laughlin, 2018). The discrepancies attributable to these categories shape individual health status and outcomes through their impact on intermediary determinants such as living conditions, psychosocial circumstances, behavioral and/or biological factors, and the health system itself (WHO, 2019). In addition to mobility, migrants and new immigrants face numerous negative SDHs that overlap and amplify each other. They frequently work in labor-based occupations with high risk for injury and illness (Levy et al., 2007). Low income, a lack of strong networks in the receiving communities, and considerable social and cultural isolation (frequently the result of language barriers, economic limitations, cultural differences, and fear over immigration status) are common SDHs among migrants and new immigrants. These SDHs limit migrants' and new immigrants' access to HIV health education, testing, and treatment. They also limit migrants' and new immigrants' participation in data collection and surveys.

As a result, developing an accurate picture of the HIV epidemic among migrants and immigrants to the US has been hampered by a lack of national data. The CDC only recently began tracking country of origin for PWH, and currently there are few national publications on the topic. Most published reports on HIV and immigrant populations are based on studies at the county, city, and state levels. An example is a report from a study conducted through the San Mateo County Health Department in California. Immigrants within the study population presented with lower CD4+ T-cell counts and were more likely to have an opportunistic infection and be hospitalized at the time of HIV diagnosis. Immigration status was significantly associated with delayed presentation, although the study did not separate out newly arrived immigrants and long-term immigrants (Levy et al., 2007). Historically, such local epidemiologic studies have been the predominant method for assessing need and planning services for immigrant populations.

A 2018 review of published literature since 2015 on known HIV outcomes among migrants from low- and middle-income countries living in high-income countries suggests that a high proportion of migrants acquire HIV after migration and are disproportionally affected by HIV (Ross et al., 2018). Migrants from Latin America and the Caribbean have the highest rates of postmigration infection and migrants from Africa have the lowest.

Research in these populations is challenging as migrants living with HIV are difficult to identify and monitor. The combination of factors such as stigma along with increased risk behaviors and reluctance to use condoms or seek testing increases the risk of migrants acquiring HIV infection (Ross et al., 2018). High levels of mobility are predictive of poor engagement in HIV care and ART disruption (Ross et al., 2018). Reliance on the community for daily survival may negatively affect care seeking and adherence if the migrant living with HIV fears ostracism from the social group. Studies of sexual practices among male migrants note riskier behaviors such as sex with casual female partners and sex workers, condomless anal and vaginal intercourse, and substance use, likely while transiting or in the receiving country. For example, in Mexico after MSM the greatest risk for HIV transmission is among those who have migrated to the US or had a partner who migrated (Hirsch et al., 2002, 2007). Poor HIV outcomes are primarily driven by stigma and limited access to care (Ross et al., 2018). Additionally, there is limited evidence on appropriate interventions for migrants living with HIV.

Among immigrants, the picture is slightly clearer, although the available data do not segment newly arrived immigrants from those who may have lived in the US for many years. HIV was diagnosed in 191,697 persons in the US between 2007 and 2010, with 16.2% among those born outside the US. Nearly half of those diagnosed with HIV for whom a specific country or region of birth outside of the US was known were from Central America and Mexico. A little more than 20% were from the Caribbean and approximately 15% were from Africa. California, Florida, New York, and Texas reported the highest numbers of persons born outside the US diagnosed with HIV. They are also the states with the highest overall case rates. Slightly more than 73% persons born outside the US living with HIV were male. The racial breakdown for PWH born outside the US was as follows: 3.3% were White, 10% were Black, 42.2% were Hispanic, and 64.3% were Asian. Thirty-nine percent of persons born outside the US were infected through heterosexual contact versus 27.2% for US-born persons (Prosser et al., 2012).

Migrants and newly arrived immigrants living with HIV are vulnerable to numerous comorbidities. TB is the most common presenting comorbidity among migrant and immigrant PWH. In regions of the world where TB is endemic, the *Mycobacterium tuberculosis* can persist for years in a person who has been exposed yet not developed active disease. TB infection can progress from latent to active disease if the PWH has a suppressed CD4+ count, and it can involve every organ system. Extrapulmonary TB should be considered if the person presents with fatigue, weakness, weight loss, and fever but without an active productive cough. ART may be more toxic in persons with chronic hepatitis, and the prevalence of HBV infection in Asian immigrants may complicate attempts to treat HIV. Opportunistic infections not usually seen in US-born persons may present in immigrant PWH, reflecting the epidemiology of their country of origin. Examples include *Penicillium marnefii* in persons of Southeast Asian origin and a variety of parasitic diseases in persons of African descent.

Immigrants and migrants face significant barriers to accessing medical care, including for diagnosis and treatment of HIV and comorbidities. Efforts to reduce these barriers should include legislation that will support and enhance the public health system, improved access to HIV services, better epidemiologic data on immigrants to the US with HIV, and enhanced training and support for healthcare providers who serve immigrant populations. Often crucial to success in working with migrant and immigrant populations is using a team approach involving interpreters, social workers, and case managers; hiring culturally appropriate staff; including peer navigators and community health workers; networking with local community-based organizations working with the impacted populations; Ryan White program and 340B Pharmacy access; and legal services. The CDC has a useful website dedicated to immigrant and refugee health issues (http://www.cdc.gov/immigrantrefugeehealth).

REFERENCES

Agency for Healthcare Research and Quality. Defining the PCMH. 2015. https://www.pcmh.ahrq.gov/page/defining-pcmh

Aberg JA, et al. Primary care guidelines for the management of persons infected with HIV: 2013 update by the HIV medicine association of the Infectious Diseases Society of America. *Clin Infect Dis.* 2014;58(1):e1.

Agwu AL, Bethel J, Hightow-Weidman LB, et al. Substantial multi-class transmitted drug resistance and drug-relevant polymorphisms among treatment-naive behaviorally HIV-infected youth. *AIDS Patient Care STDS.* 2012;26(4):193–196.

Aidala AA, Wilson MG, Shubert V, et al. Housing status, medical care, and health outcomes among people living with HIV/AIDS: a systematic review. *Am J Public Health.* 2016;106:e1–e23. http://doi.org/10.2105/AJPH.2015.302905.

Alvarez H, Marino A, Garcia-Rodriquez JF, et al. Immune reconstitution inflammatory syndrome in an HIV-infected patient using subcutaneous silicone fillers. *AIDS.* 2016;30(16):2561–2563.

Armbruster M, Fields EL, Campbell N, et al. Addressing Health Inequities Exacerbated by COVID-19 Among Youth With HIV: Expanding Our Toolkit. 2020. *J Adolesc Health.* 2020;67(2):290–295.

Arrington-Sanders R, Hailey-Fair K, Wirtz AL, Morgan A, Brooks D, Castillo M, Trexler C, Kwait J, Dowshen N, Galai N, Beyrer C, Celentano D. Role of Structural Marginalization, HIV Stigma, and Mistrust on HIV Prevention and Treatment Among Young Black Latinx Men Who Have Sex with Men and Transgender Women: Perspectives from Youth Service Providers. *AIDS Patient Care STDS.* 2020;34:7–15.

Asscheman H, Giltay EJ, Megens JAJ, et al. A long-term follow-up study of mortality in transsexuals receiving treatment with cross-sex hormones. *Eur J Endocrinol.* 2011;164(4):635–642.

Asscheman H, Gooren LJG, Eklund PLE. Mortality and morbidity in transsexual patients with cross-gender hormone treatment. *Metabolism.* 1989;38(9):869–873.

Badger E, Parlapiano A, Bui Q. Black workers will hurt the most if Congress doesn't extend jobless benefits. *New York Times,* August 7, 2020.

Baggett TP, Hwang SW, O'Connell JJ, et al. Mortality among homeless adults in Boston: shifts in causes of death over a 15-year period. *JAMA Intern Med.* 2013;173:189–195.

Baillargeon J, Giordano T, Rich J, et al. Accessing antiretroviral therapy following release from prison. *JAMA.* 2009;301(8):848–857.

Baral SD, Poteat T, Strömdahl S, et al. Worldwide burden of HIV in transgender women: a systematic review and meta-analysis. *Lancet Infect Dis.* 2013;(3):214–222.

Barnes W, D'Angelo L, Yamazaki M, et al. Identification of HIV-infected 12–24-year-old men and women in 15 cities through venue-based testing. *Arch Pediatr Adolesc Med.* 2010;164:273–276.

Becasen JS, Denard CL, Mullins MM, et al. Estimating the Prevalence of HIV and Sexual Behaviors Among the US Transgender Population: A Systematic Review and Meta-Analysis, 2006–2017. *Am J Public Health.* 2019;(1)e1–e8.

Beckwith C, Zaller N, Fu J, et al. Opportunities to diagnose, treat, and prevent HIV in the criminal justice system. *J AIDS.* 2010;55(suppl 1):S49–S55.

Belzer ME, Fuchs DN, Luftman GS, et al. Antiretroviral adherence issues among HIV-positive adolescents and young adults. *J Adolesc Health.* November 1999;25(5):3316–3319.

Bernard K, Sueker J, Colton E, et al. Provider perspectives about the standard of HIV care in correctional settings and comparison to the community standard of care: how do we measure up? *Infect Dis Corrections Rep.* 2006;9(3):1–6.

Berry SA, Ghanem KG, Mathews WC, et al. Brief report: gonorrhea and chlamydia testing increasing but still lagging in HIV clinics in the United States. *J AIDS.* 2015;70(3):275–279.

Bing EG, Burnam A, Longshore D, et al. Psychiatric disorders and drug use among HIV-infected adults in the US. *Arch Gen Psychiatry.* 2001;58:721–728.

Bogart LM, Thorburn S. Are HIV/AIDS conspiracy beliefs a barrier to HIV prevention among African-Americans? *J AIDS.* 2005;38(2):213–218.

Boone MR, Cherenack EM, Wilson PA, et al. Self-efficacy for sexual risk reduction and partner HIV status as correlates of sexual risk behavior among HIV-positive adolescent girls and women. *AIDS Patient Care STDS.* 2015;29(6):346–353.

Bowleg L. "Once you've blended the cake, you can't take the parts back to the main ingredients": black gay and bisexual men's descriptions and experiences of intersectionality. *Sex Roles.* 2013;68(11–12):754–767.

Boyer CB, Hightow-Weidman L, Bether J, et al. An assessment of the feasibility and acceptability of a friendship-based social network recruitment strategy to screen at-risk African American and Hispanic/Latina young women for HIV infection. *JAMA Pediatr.* 2013; (3):289–296.

Braithwaite R, Hammett T, Mayberry R. *Prisons and AIDS: a public health challenge.* San Francisco: Jossey-Bass; 1996.

Branson B, Handsfield H, Lampe M, et al. Revised recommendations for HIV testing of adults, adolescents, and pregnant women in health-care settings. *MMWR.* 2006;55(RR14):1–17.

Brouqui P, Stein A, Dupont HT, et al. Ectoparasitism and vector-borne diseases in 930 homeless people from Marseilles. *Medicine (Baltimore).* January 2005;84(1):61–68.

Brown GR, Jones KT. Incidence of breast cancer in a cohort of 5,135 transgender veterans. *Breast Cancer Res Treat.* 2015;149(1):191–198. http://doi.org/10.1007/s10549-014-3213-2.

Bruce D, Kahana S, Harper G, et al. Alcohol use predicts sexual risk behavior with HIV-negative or partners of unknown status among young HIV-positive men who have sex with men. *AIDS Care.* 2013;25(5):559–565.

Buchanan AL, Montepiedra G, Sirois PA, et al. Barriers to medication adherence in HIV-infected children and youth based on self- and caregiver report. *Pediatrics.* 2012;129:e1244–e1251.

Buchanan DB, Kee R, Sadowski LS, et al. The health impact of supportive housing for HIV-positive homeless patients: a randomized controlled trial. *Am J Public Health.* 2009;99(6):S675–S680.

Bukowski LA, Chandler CJ, Creasy SL, et al. Identifying barriers and facilitators to HIV diagnosis and viral suppression among black transgender women in the United States. *J Acquir Immune Defic Syndr.* 2018;79(4):413–420.

Cahill S, Makadon H. Sexual orientation and gender identity data collection in clinical settings and in electronic health records: a key to ending LGBT health disparities. *LGBT Health.* 2013. http://online.liebertpub.com/doi/abs/10.1089/lgbt.2013.0001.

Cahill S, Makadon HJ. Sexual orientation and gender identity data collection update: US Government takes steps to promote sexual orientation and gender identity data collection through meaningful use guidelines. *LGBT Health.* 2014. http://doi.org/10.1089/lgbt.2014.0033.

Canonico M, Plu-Bureau G, Lowe G, et al. Hormone replacement therapy and risk of venous thromboembolism in postmenopausal women: systematic review and meta-analysis. *BMJ.* 2008;336(7655):1227.

Centers for Disease Control and Prevention. Health equity considerations and racial and ethnic minority groups. 2020a. https://www.cdc.gov/coronavirus/2019-ncov/need-extra-precautions/racial-ethnic-minorities.html

Centers for Disease Control and Prevention. HIV and African Americans, 2018. May 2020b. https://www.cdc.gov/hiv/group/racialethnic/africanamericans/index.html

Centers for Disease Control and Prevention. HIV surveillance report, 2018 (updated); vol. 31. May 2020c. http://www.cdc.gov/hiv/library/reports/hiv-surveillance.html

Chang CK, Hayes RD, Perera G, et al. Life expectancy at birth for people with serious mental illness and other major disorders from a secondary mental healthcare case register in London. *PLoS One.* 2011;10:1371.

Cheever L. HRSA announced highest HIV viral suppression rate in new Ryan White HIV/AIDS Program client-level data report. December 2019. https://www.hiv.gov/blog/hrsa-announces-highest-hiv-viral-suppression-rate-new-ryan-white-hivaids-program-client-level-0

Chen X, Murphy DA, Naar-King S, et al. A clinic-based motivational intervention improves condom use among subgroups of youth living with HIV. *J Adolescent Health.* 2011;49:193–198.

Chesney E, Goodwin GM, Fazel S. Risks all-cause and suicide mortality in mental disorders: a meta-review. *World Psychiatry.* 2014;13(2):153–160.

Clark H, Babu AS, Wiewel EW, Opoku J, Crepaz N. Diagnosed HIV infection in transgender adults and adolescents: results from the national HIV surveillance system, 2009–2014. *AIDS Behav.* 2017;21(9):2774–2783.

Clark RF, Cantrell FL, Pacal A, et al. Subcutaneous silicone injection leading to multi-system organ failure. *Clin Toxicol.* 2008;46(9):834–837. http://doi.org/10.1080/15563650701850025.

Clum G, Chung S, Ellen J. Mediators of HIV related stigma and risk behavior in HIV infected young women. *AIDS Care.* 2009;21:1455–1462.

Cohen D, Farley T, Taylor S, et al. When and where do youths have sex? The potential role of adult supervision. *Pediatrics.* 2002;110:1–6.

Coleman E, Bockting W, Botzer M, et al. Standards of care for the health of transsexual, transgender, and gender-nonconforming people, version 7. *Intl J Transgenderism*. 2012;13(4):165–232.

Colton Meier SL, Fitzgerald KM, Pardo ST, et al. The effects of hormonal gender affirmation treatment on mental health in female-to-male transsexuals. *J Gay Lesbian Mental Health*. 2011;15(3):281–299.

Conron KJ, Scott G, Stowell GS, et al. Transgender health in Massachusetts: results from a household probability sample of adults. *Am J Public Health*. 2012;102(1):118–122.

Conger K, Gebeloff R, Oppel Jr. RA. Native Americans feel devastated by the virus yet overlooked in the data. *New York Times*, July 31, 2020.

Cope AB, Power KA, Kuruc JD, et al. Ongoing HIV transmission and the HIV care continuum in North Carolina. *PLoS One*. 2015;10(6):e0127950.

Cotton S. Puchalski CM, Sherman SN, et al. Spirituality and religion in patients with HIV/AIDS. *Gen Intern Med*. 2006;12(21, suppl 5):S5–S13.

Cottrell ML, Prince HM, Maffuid K, et al. Altered TDF/FTC pharmacology in a transgender female cohort: implications for PrEP. TUPDX0106. http://programme.aids2018.org/Abstract/Abstract/11225.

Crane JA. Patient comprehension of doctor–patient communication on discharge from the emergency department. *Emerg Med*. 1997;15(1):1–7.

Craw JA, Gardner LI, Marks G, et al. Brief strengths-based case management promotes entry into HIV medical care: results of the antiretroviral treatment access study-II. *J AIDS*. 2008;(5):597–606.

Crenshaw K. Mapping the margins: Intersectionality, identity politics, and violence against women of color. *Stanford Law Rev*. 1991;43:1241–1299.

Crepaz N, Dong X, Wang X, et al. Racial and Crane JA. Patient comprehension of doctor–patient communication on discharge from the emergency department. *Emerg Med*. 1997;15(1):1–7.

Department of Health of Human Services (DHHS). Panel on Antiretroviral Guidelines for Adults and Adolescents. Guidelines for the Use of Antiretroviral Agents in Adults and Adolescents with HIV. Department of Health and Human Services. 2020. https://clinicalinfo.hiv.gov/sites/default/files/inline-files/AdultandAdolescentGL.pdf

Desai AM, Browning J, Rosen T. Etanercept therapy for silicone granuloma. *J Drugs Dermatol*. 2006;5(9):894–896.

Deutsch MB. Use of the informed consent model in the provision of cross-sex hormone therapy: a survey of the practices of selected clinics. *Intl J Transgenderism*. 2012;13(3):140–146. http://doi.org/10.1080/15532739.2011.675233.

Deutsch MB, Green J, Keatley J, et al. (2013). Electronic medical records and the transgender patient: Recommendations from the World Professional Association for Transgender Health EMR Working Group. *J Am Med Informat Assoc*. 2012, 001472. Available at http://doi.org/10.1136/amiajnl-2012-001472.

Deutsch MB, Bhakri V, Kubicek K. Effects of cross-sex hormone treatment on transgender women and men. *Obstet Gynecol*. 2015a;125(3):605–610.

Deutsch MB, Glidden DV, Sevelius J, et al. HIV pre-exposure prophylaxis in transgender women: a subgroup analysis of the iPrEx trial. *Lancet HIV*. 2015b. http://doi.org/10.1016/S2352-3018(15)00206-4.

Deutsch MB. *J Health Care Poor Underserved*. 2016;27(2):386–391.

Deutsch MB. Pre-Exposure Prophylaxis in Trans Populations: Providing Gender-Affirming Prevention for Trans People at High Risk of Acquiring HIV. *LGBT Health*. 2018 Oct;5(7):387–390.

Deutsch MB, Reisner SL, Peitzmeier S, et al. Recent penile sexual contact is associated with an increased odds of high-risk cervical human papilloavirus infection in transgender men. *Sex Transm Dis*. 2020;47(1):48–53.

Doblecki-Lewis S, Lester L, Schwartz B, et al. HIV risk and awareness and interest in pre-exposure and post-exposure prophylaxis among sheltered women in Miami. *Intl J STD AIDS*. 2016;27(10):873–881. http://doi.org/10.1177/0956462415601304

Doshani M, Weng M, Moore KL, Romero JR, Nelson NP. Recommendations of the Advisory Committee on Immunization Practices for Use of Hepatitis A Vaccine for Persons Experiencing Homelessness. *MMWR Morb Mortal Wkly Rep*. 2019;68:153–156.

Dowshen N, Binns HJ, Garofalo R. Experiences of HIV-related stigma among young men who have sex with men. *AIDS Patient Care and STDs*. 2009;23:371–376.

Eaton LA, Driffin DD, Kegler C, et al. The role of stigma and medical mistrust in the routine healthcare engagement of black men who have sex with men. *Am J Public Health*. 2015;105(2):75–82.

El-Ibiary SY, Cocohoba JM. Effects of HIV antiretrovirals on the pharmacokinetics of hormonal contraceptives. *Eur J Contraception Reproduc Health Care*. 2008;13(2):123–132. http://doi.org/10.1080/13625180701829952.

Ellen JM, Kapogiannis B, Fortenberry JD, et al. HIV viral load levels and CD4$^{\+}$ cell counts of youth in 14 cities. *AIDS*. 2014;28(8):1213–1219.

Evron S, Glezerman M, Harow E, et al. Human immunodeficiency virus: anesthetic and obstetric considerations. *Anesth Analg*. 2004;98(2):503–511.

Fernández MI, Collazo JB, Bowen GS, et al. Predictors of HIV testing and intention to test among Hispanic farmworkers in South Florida. *J Rural Health*. 2005;21:56–64.

Fernández MI, Huszti HC, Wilson PA, et al. Profiles of Risk Among HIV-Infected Youth in Clinic Settings. *AIDS Behav*. 2015;19(5):918–930.

Flores AR, Herman JL, Gates GJ, et al. How many adults identify as transgender in the United States? The Williams Institute. June 2016. https://williamsinstitute.law.ucla.edu/wp-content/uploads/How-Many-Adults-Identify-as-Transgender-in-the-United-States.pdf.

Futterman D. HIV in adolescents and young adults: half of all new infections in the United States. *Top HIV Med*. August–September 2005;13(3):101–105.

Gabrielli E, Ferraioli G, Ferraris L, et al. Enfuvirtide administration in HIV-positive transgender patient with soft tissue augmentation: US evaluation. *New Microbiologica*. 2010;33:263–265.

Gander K. Being transgender is not a mental illness, World Health Organizations says. Newsweek. June 19, 2018. https://www.newsweek.com/being-transgender-not-mental-illness-world-health-organization-says-983869.

Golden MR, Lechtenberg R, Glick SN, et al. Outbreak of Human Immunodeficiency Virus Infection Among Heterosexual Persons Who Are Living Homeless and Inject Drugs — Seattle, Washington, 2018. *MMWR Morb Mortal Wkly Rep*. 2019;68:344–349.

Goldenberg T, McDougal SJ, Sullivan PS, et al. Preferences for a mobile HIV prevention app for men who have sex with men. *JMIR Mhealth Uhealth*. 2014;2:e47.

Goldstein ND, LeVasseur MT, Tran NK, et al. Modeling HPV vaccination scale-up among uban young men who have sex with men in the context of HIV. *Vaccine*. 2019;37(29):3883–3891.

Gómez-Gil E, Zubiaurre-Elorza L, Esteva I, et al. Hormone-treated transsexuals report less social distress, anxiety and depression. *Psychoneuroendocrinology*. 2012;37(5):662–670.

Gooren LJ, van Trotsenburg MAA, Giltay EJ, et al. Breast cancer development in transsexual subjects receiving cross-sex hormone treatment. *J Sexual Med*. 2013;10(12):3129–3134. http://doi.org/10.1111/jsm.12319.

Gordon MR, Smale A, Lyman R. US will accept more refugees as crisis grows. *New York Times*, September 20, 2015.

Graham G. Disparities in cardiovascular disease risk in the United States. *Curr Cardiol Rev*. 2015;11(3):238–245.

Green, N, Hoenigl, M, Morris, S, et al. Risk behavior and sexually transmitted infections among transgender women and men undergoing community-based screening for acute and early HIV infection in San Diego. *Medicine*. 2015;94(41):e1830.

Gruskin S, Safreed-Harmon K, Moore CL, et al. HIV and gender-based violence: welcome policies and programmes, but is the research keeping up? *Reprod Health Matters*. 2014;22(44):174–184.

Guerino P, Harrison P, Sabol W. Prisoners in 2010. US Department of Justice, Bureau of Justice Statistics. 2011. http://www.bjs.gov

Hall WJ, Chapman MV, Lee KM, et al. Implicit racial/ethnic bias among health care professionals and its influence on health care outcomes: a systematic review. *Am J Public Health*. 2015;105(12):e60–e76.

Hammet T, Kennedy S, Kuck S. National survey of infectious diseases in correctional facilities: HIV and sexually transmitted diseases. US Department of Justice. 2007. https://www.ncjrs.gov/pdffiles1/nij/grants/217736.pdf

Hansen L, Penko J, Guzman D, et al. Aberrant behaviors with prescription opioids and problem drug use history in a community-based cohort of HIV-infected individuals. *J Pain Symptom Management*. 2011;42(6):893–902.

Health Resources and Services Administration. Ending the HIV Epidemic: A Plan for America. February 2020. https://www.hrsa.gov/ending-hiv-epidemic

HealthyPeople.gov. Healthy People 2020. The Secretary's Advisory Committee on National Health Promotion and Disease Prevention Objectives for 2020. Phase I report: Recommendations for the framework and format of Healthy People 2020. Section IV: Advisory Committee findings and recommendations [cited 2010 January 6]. http://www.healthypeople.gov/sites/default/files/PhaseI_0.pdf

Hembree WC, Cohen-Kettenis P, Gooren L, et al. Endocrine treatment of gender-dysphoric/gender-incongruent persons: An endocrine society clinical practice guideline. *Endocr Pract*. 2017;23(12):1437.

Hessol NA, Eng M, Vu A, et al. A longitudinal study assessing differences in causes of death among housed and homeless people diagnosed with HIV in San Francisco. *BMC Public Health*. 2019;19:1440. https://doi.org/10.1186/s12889-019-7817-7

Hiransuthikul A, Himmad K, Kerr S, et al. Drug-drug interactions between the use of feminizing hormone therapy and pre-exposure prophylaxis among transgender women: the iFACT study. TUPDX0107LB. http://programme.aids2018.org/Abstract/Abstract/13177.

Hirsch J, Higgins J, Bentley M, et al. The social constructions of sexuality: marital infidelity and sexually transmitted disease: HIV risk in a Mexican migrant community. *Am J Public Health*. 2002;92(8):1227–1237.

Hirsch J, Meneses S, Thompson B, et al. The inevitability of infidelity: sexual reputation, social geographies, and marital HIV risk in rural Mexico. *Am J Public Health*. 2007;97(6):986–996.

Hoffman KM, Trawalter S, Axt JR, Oliver MN. Racial bias in pain assessment and treatment recommendations, and false beliefs about biological differences between blacks and whites. *Proc Natl Acad Sci U S A*. 2016;113(16):4296–4301.

Ickovics JR. "Bundling" HIV prevention: Integrating services to promote synergistic gain. *Prevent Med*. 2008;46(3):222–225. http://doi.org/10.1016/j.ypmed.2007.09.006.

Institutional racism—Wikipediaen.wikipedia.org › wiki › Institutional_racism. https://en.wikipedia.org/wiki/Institutional_racism

International Organization for Migration. Key migration terms. 2020. https://www.iom.int/key-migration-terms

Jacobs EA, Shepard D, Suaya JA, et al. Overcoming language barriers in healthcare: costs and benefits of interpreter services. *Am J Public Health*. 2004;94(5):866–869.

James C. Race, ethnicity and medical care: a survey of public perceptions and experiences. Kaiser Family Foundation, September 1999.

James, SE, Herman, JL, Rankin, S, et al. The Report of the 2015 U.S. Transgender Survey. 2016. Washington, DC: National Center for Transgender Equality.

Jin H, Restar A, Biello K, et al. Burden of HIV among young transgender women: factors associated with HIV infection and HIV treatment engagement. *AIDS Care*. 2019;31(1):125–130.

Kaiser Family Foundation. *Key Facts: Race, Ethnicity, and Medical Care*. Menlo Park, CA: Kaiser Family Foundation; 2007.

Kanny D, Jeffries 4th WL, Chapin-Bardales J, et al. Racial/ethnic disparities in HIV preexposure prophylaxis among men who have sex with men—23 urban areas, 2017. *Morb Mortal Wkly Rep*. 2019;68(37):801–806.

Kearney BP, Mathias A. Lack of effect of tenofovir disoproxil fumarate on pharmacokinetics of hormonal contraceptives. *Pharmacotherapy*. 2009;29(8):924–929. http://doi.org/10.1592/phco.29.8.924.

Kendi IX. *How to be antiracist*. Penguin Random House, LLC; 2019.

Khan J, Schmidt RL, Spittal MJ, et al. Venous thrombotic risk in transgender women undergoing estrogen therapy: A systematic review and metaanalysis. *Clin Chem*. 2019;65(1):57–66.

Lester RT, Ritvo P, Mills E, et al. Effects of a mobile phone short message service on antiretroviral treatment adherence in Kenya (WelTel Kenya1): a randomized trial. *Lancet*. 2010;376:1838–1845.

Levy V, Prentiss D, Balmas G, et al. Factors in the delayed HIV presentation of immigrants in northern California: implications for voluntary counseling and testing programs. *J Immigrant Minority Health*. 2007;9:49–54. https://doi.org/10.1007/s10903-006-9015-9

Machtinger EL, Haberer JE, Wilson TC et al. Recent Trauma is Associated with Antiretroviral Failure and HIV Transmission Risk Behavior Among HIV-Positive Women and Female-Identified Transgenders. *AIDS Behav*. 2012;16:2160–2170.

Marrazzo JM, Ramjee G, Richardson BA, et al. Tenofovir-based pre-exposure prophylaxis for HIV infection among African women. *N Engl J Med*. 2015;372(6):509–518. http://doi.org/10.1056/NEJMoa1402269.

Maruschak L. HIV in prisons, 2007–08. US Department of Justice, Bureau of Justice Statistics. 2009. http://www.bjs.gov/content/pub/pdf/hivp08.pdf

Martinez J, Harper G, Carleton RA, et al. The impact of stigma on medication adherence among HIV-positive adolescent and young adult females and the moderating effects of coping and satisfaction with healthcare. *AIDS Patient Care STDS*. 2012;26:108–115.

Massachusetts Department of Public Health (MDPH). HIV/AIDS Fact sheet: persons born outside the US.

McElroy PD, Southwick KL, Fortenberry ER, et al. Outbreak of tuberculosis among homeless persons coinfected with human immunodeficiency virus. *Clin Infect Dis*. 2003;36(10):1305–1312.

Meerwijk EL, Sevelius JM. Transgender population size in United States: a meta-regression of population-based probability samples. *Am J Public Health*. 2017;107(2):e1–e8.

Melendez RM, Pinto RM. HIV prevention and primary care for transgender women in a community-based clinic. *J Assoc Nurses AIDS Care*. 2009;20(5):387–397.

Miaskowski C, Penko JM, Guzman D, et al. Occurrence and characteristics of chronic pain in a community-based cohort of indigent adults living with HIV infection. *J Pain*. 2011;12(9):1004–1016.

Millett G. Casualties on the road to ending HIV: context matters in addressing HIV disparities. Prime Session 1. 40 Year HIV Pandemic, July 7, 2020a. AIDS2020.org Virtual IAS Conference, July 4–10, 2020.

Millett G, Jones AT, Benkeser D, et al. Assessing differential impacts of Covid-19 on Black communities. *Ann Epidemiol*. 2020b;47:37–44.

Minton T, Sabol W. Jail inmates at midyear 2008—Statistical tables. US Department of Justice, Bureau of Justice Statistics. 2009. Available at http://bjs.ojp.usdoj.gov/content/pub/pdf/jim08st.pdf.

Mizuno Y, Frazier EL, Huang P, et al. Characteristics of transgender women living with HIV receiving medical care in the United States. *LGBT Health*. 2015;2(3):228034.

Murphy DA, Sarr M, Durako SJ, et al. Barriers to HAART adherence among HIV-infected adolescents. *Arch Pediatr Adolesc Med*. 2003;157:249–255.

Moyer VA; US Preventive Services Task Force. Screening for HIV: US Preventive Services Task Force recommendation statement. *Ann Intern Med*. July 2, 2013;159(1):51–60.

Naar-King S, Wright K, Parsons JT, et al. Health choices: Motivational enhancement therapy for health risk behaviors in HIV-positive youth. *AIDS Educ Prevent*. 2006;18:1–11.

Nachman SA, Cheroff M, Gona P, et al. Incidence of noninfectious conditions in perinatally HIV-infected children and adolescents in the HAART era. *Arch Pediatr Adolesc Med*. 2009;163:164–171.

Nash GD, Flanders WD, Baird TC, et al. Cross-sex hormones and acute cardiovascular events in transgender persons: a cohort study. *Ann Intern Med.* August 21, 2018;169(4):205–213. doi: 10.7326/M17-2785. Epub July 10, 2018.

National Coalition for the Homeless, 2009, July. HIV/AIDS and Homelessness. https://www.nationalhomeless.org/factsheets/hiv.html.

National LGBT Health Education Center. Providing welcoming services and care for LGBT people. 2015. http://www.lgbthealtheducation.org/wp-content/uploads/Learning-Guide.pdf

National Law Center on Homelessness and Poverty. Homelessness in America: Overview of data and causes. January 2015. http://www.nlchp.org/documents/Homeless_Stats_Fact_Sheet.

Nellis A. The color of justice: racial and ethnic disparity in state prisons. The Sentencing Project. June 14, 2016. https://www.sentencingproject.org/publications/color-of-justice-racial-and-ethnic-disparity-in-state-prisons/

Newport F. Three-quarters of Americans identify as Christian. Gallup.com. December 2014.

Nichols A, Simms M. Racial and ethnic differences in receipt of unemployment insurance benefits during the great recession. Urban Institute. June 2012. https://www.urban.org/sites/default/files/publication/25541/412596-Racial-and-Ethnic-Differences-in-Receipt-of-Unemployment-Insurance-Benefits-During-the-Great-Recession.PDF

Nosyk B, Zang X, Krebs E, et.al. Ending the HIV epidemic in the USA: an economic modeling study in six cities. *Lancet HIV.* 2020;7(7):e491–e503.

Nugent NR, Brown LK, Belzer M, et al. Youth living with HIV and problem substance use: elevated distress is associated with nonadherence and sexual risk. *J Int Assoc Phys AIDS Care.* 2010;9(2):113–115.

Ohl M, Tate J, Duggal M, et al. Rural residence is associated with delayed care entry and increased mortality among veterans with human immunodeficiency virus infection. *Medicare Care.* 2010;48:1064–1070.

Olson J, Schrager SM, Clark LF, et al. Subcutaneous testosterone: An effective delivery mechanism for masculinizing young transgender men. *LGBT Health.* 2014. http://doi.org/10.1089/lgbt.2014.0018.

O'Laughlin B. Structural reform and the politics of inequality in global public health. *Development and Change.* 2018;47(4):686–711. doi:10.1111/dech.12251

Oppel Jr. RA, Gebeloff R, Lai R, et al. The fullest look yet at the racial inequity of coronavirus. *New York Times*, July 5, 2020. https://www.nytimes.com/interactive/2020/07/05/us/coronavirus-latinos-african-americans-cdc-data.html

Park LS, Rentsch CT, Sigel K, et al. COVID-19 in the largest U.S. cohort. Presented at: 23rd International AIDS Conference. 2020. Virtual.

Parra-Rodriguez L, Stroger Jr JH. Racial and ethnic disparities in COVID-19 admissions in a safety-net health system in Chicago. International AIDS Society Cirtual 2020 Covid-19 Conference, July 10–11, 2020. https://www.natap.org/2020/COVID/072920_04.htm

Pasternack FR, Fox LP, Engler DE. Silicone granulomas treated with etanercept. *Arch Dermatol.* 2005;141(1):13.

Paterson DL Swindells S. Adherence to protease inhibitor therapy and outcomes in patients with HIV infection. *Ann Intern Med.* 2000;133:21–30.

Peitzmeier SM, Reisner SL, Harigopal P, et al. Female-to-male patients have high prevalence of unsatisfactory Paps compared to non-transgender females: Implications for cervical cancer screening. *J Gen Intern Med.* May 2014;29(5):778–784.

Peterson K, Anderson J, Boundy E, et al. Mortality disparities in racial/ethnic minority groups in the Veterans Health Administration: an evidence review and map. *Am J Public Health.* 2018;108(3):e1–e10.

Philbin MM, Tanner AE, Duval A, et al. Linking HIV-positive adolescents to care in 15 different clinics across the United States: creating solutions to address structural barriers for linkage to care. *AIDS Care.* January 2014;26(1):12–19.

Phillips HJ, Tinsley MJ, Rajabiun S. Building a Medical Home for HIV-Positive, Multiply Diagnosed Homeless Populations. *Am J Public Health.* 2018;108(Suppl 7):S518. doi:10.2105/AJPH.2018.304863

Prosser AT, Tang T, Hall HI. HIV in persons born outside the United States 2007—2010. *JAMA.* 2012;308(6):601–607.

Poteat T, Wirtz AL, Radix A, et al. HIV risk and preventive interventions in transgender women sex workers. *Lancet.* 2015;385(9964):274–286. http://doi.org/10.1016/S0140-6736(14)60833-3.

Radcliff J, Doty N, Hawkins LA, et al. Stigma and sexual risk in HIV-positive African American young men who have sex with men. *AIDS Patient Care STD.* 2010;24:493–499.

Radford J. Key findings about U.S. immigrants. Pew Research Center. 2019 https://www.pewresearch.org/fact-tank/2019/06/17/key-findings-about-u-s-immigrants/

Rao D, Kekwaletswe TC, Hosek S, et al. Stigma and social barriers to medication adherence with urban youth living with HIV. *AIDS Care.* 2007;19:28–33.

Rapaport MJ. Silicone granulomas treated with etanercept. *Arch Dermatol.* 2005;141(9):1171. http://doi.org/10.1001/archderm.141.9.1171-a.

Reisner SL, Deutsch MB, Peitzmeier SM, et al. Comparing self- and provider-collected swabbing for HPV DNA testing in female-to-male transgender adult patients: a mixed-methods biobehavioral study protocol. *BMC Infect Dis.* 2017;17(1):444.

Reisner SL, Mimiaga MJ, Bland S, et al. HIV risk and social networks among male-to-female transgender sex workers in Boston, Massachusetts. *J Assoc Nurses AIDS Care.* 2009 Sep-Oct;20(5):373–386.

Riley ED, Vittinghoff E, Koss CA, et al. Housing First: Unsuppressed Viral Load Among Women Living with HIV in San Francisco. *AIDS Behav.* 2019;23:2326–2336. https://doi.org/10.1007/s10461-019-02601-w

Rose D, Collins M, Kelban R. Complications of surgery in HIV-infected patients. *AIDS.* 1998;12:2243–2251.

Roper W. Black Americans 2.5x more likely than Whites to be killed by police. Statista.com. June 2, 2020. https://www.statista.com/chart/21872/map-of-police-violence-against-black-americans

Ross J, Cunningham CO, Hanna DJ, HIV outcomes among migrants from low- and middle-income countries living in high-income countries: a review of recent evidence. *Curr Opin Infect Dis.* 2018;31(1):25–32. doi:10.1097/QCO.0000000000000415

Rothstein R. *The color of law: a forgotten history of how our government segregated America.* Liveright; 2017.

Rudy BJ, Murphy DA, Harris DR, et al. Patient-related risks for nonadherence to antiretroviral therapy among HIV-infected youth in the United States: a study of prevalence and interactions. *AIDS Patient Care STD.* 2008;23:1–10.

Sanchez NF, Sanchez JP, Danoff A. Health care utilization, barriers to care, and hormone usage among male-to-female transgender persons in New York City. *Am J Public Health.* 2009;99(4):713.

Sanders RA. Adolescent psychosocial, social, and cognitive development. *Pediatr Rev.* August 2013;34(8):354–358; quiz 358–359.

San Francisco Department of Public Health Population Health Division (SFDPH). (2019, September) HIV Epidemiology Annual Report 2018. https://www.sfdph.org/dph/files/reports/RptsHIVAIDS/HIV-Epidemiology-Annual-Report-2018.pdf.

Scarabin PY. Progestogens and venous thromboembolism in menopausal women: an updated oral versus transdermal estrogen meta-analysis. *Climacteric.* 2018;21(4):341–345.

Schafer KR, Albrecht H, Dillingham R, et al. The Continuum of HIV Care in Rural Communities in the United States and Canada: What Is Known and Future Research Directions. *J Acquir Immune Defic Syndr.* 2017;75(1):35–44.

Schranz AJ, Barrett J, Hurt CB, Malvestutto C, Miller WC. Challenges Facing a Rural Opioid Epidemic: Treatment and Prevention of HIV and Hepatitis C. *Curr HIV/AIDS Rep.* 2018;15(3):245–254.

Sevelius JM. Gender affirmation: a framework for conceptualizing risk behavior among transgender women of color. *Sex Roles.* 2013;68(11–12):675–689.

Sevelius JM, Patouhas E, Keatley JG, et al. Barriers and facilitators to engagement and retention-in-care among transgender women living with human immunodeficiency virus. *Ann Behav Med.* 2014a;47(1):5–16.

Sevelius JM, Saberi P, Johnson MO. Correlates of antiretroviral adherence and viral load among transgender women living with HIV. *AIDS Care*. August 2014b;26(8):976–982.

Sevelius J, Chakravarty D, Neilands TB, et al. Evidence for the Model of Gender Affirmation: The Role of Gender Affirmation and Healthcare Empowerment in Viral Suppression Among Transgender Women of Color Living with HIV. HRSA SPNS Transgender Women of Color Study Group. *AIDS Behav*. 2019 doi:10.1007/s10461-019-02544-2. Online ahead of print.

Sitapati AM, Limneos J, Bonet-Vázquez M, et al. Retention: building a patient-centered medical home in HIV primary care through PUFF (patients unable to follow-up found). *J Health Care Poor Underserved*. 2012;23(3 suppl):81–95.

Skarbinski J, Rosenberg E, Paz-Bailey G, et al. Human immunodeficiency virus transmission at each step of the care continuum in the United States. *JAMA Intern Med*. 2015;175(4):596–597.

Smedley D, Stith A, Nelson A (Eds.). *Unequal Treatment—Confronting Racial and Ethnic Disparities in Healthcare*. Washington, DC: 2003. Institute of Medicine, The National Academies Press.

Spaulding A, Stephenson B, Macalino G, et al. Human immunodeficiency virus in correctional facilities. *Clin Infect Dis*. 2002;35:305–312.

Spinelli MA, Hessol, NA, et al. Homelessness at diagnosis is associated with death among people with HIV in a population-based study of a US city. *AIDS*. 2019;33:1789–1794.

Straub DM, Arrington-Sanders R, Harris DR, et al. Correlates of HIV testing history among urban youth recruited through venue-based testing in 15 US cities. *Sex Transm Dis*. August 2011;38(8):691–696.

Sabino TE, Avelino-Silva VI, Cavalcantte C, et al. Adherence to antiretroviral treatment and quality of life among transgender women living with HIV/AIDS in Sao Paulo, Brazil. *AIDS Care*. 2021;33(1):33–38.

Swendeman D, Rotherman-Borus MJ, Comulada S, et al. Predictors of HIV-related stigma among young people living with HIV. *Health Psychology*. 2006;25:501–509.

Swerdloff RS, Wang C, White WB, et al. A new oral testosterone undecanoate formulation restores testosterone to normal concentrations in hypogonadal men. *J Clin Endocrinol Metab*. 2020;105(8):2515–2531.

Sypsa V, Paraskevis D, Malliori M, et al. Homelessness and other risk factors for HIV infection in the current outbreak among injection drug users in Athens, Greece. *Am J Public Health*. January 2015;105(1):196–204.

Tanney MR, Naar-King S, MacDonnell K. Depression and stigma in high-risk youth living with HIV: a multi-site study. *J Pediatr Health Care*. 2012;26:300–305.

Tate CC, Ledbetter JN, Youssef CP. A two-question method for assessing gender categories in the social and medical sciences. *J Sex Research*. 2012;50,1–10.

Thebault R, Fowers A. Pandemic's weight falls on Hispanics and Native Americans as deaths pass 150,000. *Washington Post*, July 31, 2020.

Torian LV, Wiewel EW, Liu K, et al. Risk factors for delayed initiation of medical care after diagnosis of human immunodeficiency virus. *Arch Intern Med*. 2008;(11):1181–1187.

Toska E, Cluver LD, Hodes R, et al. Sex and secrecy: how HIV-status disclosure affects safe sex among HIV-positive adolescents. *AIDS Care*. December 2015;27(Suppl 1):47–58.

Trent M, Chung SE, Ellen JM, et al. New sexually transmitted infections among adolescent girls infected with HIV. *Sex Transmitted Infect*. 2007;83:468–469.

UNAIDS. How AIDS changed everything—MDG6: 15 years, 15 lessons of hope from the AIDS response. July 2015. UNAIDS Secretariat, Geneva, Switzerland. https://issuu.com/unaids/docs/mdg6_executivesummary_en

US Department of Health and Human Services. Office of Minority Health. HHS action plan to reduce racial and ethnic health disparities: a nation free of disparities in health and health care. 2010. https://www.minorityhealth.hhs.gov/npa/files/Plans/HHS/HHS_Plan_complete.pdf

Valenzuela JM, Buchanan CL, Radcliffe J, et al. Transition to adult services among behaviorally infected adolescents with HIV: a qualitative study. *J Pediatr Psychol*. March 2011;36(2):134–140.

van Kesteren PJ, Asscheman H, Megens JA, et al. Mortality and morbidity in transsexual subjects treated with cross-sex hormones. *Clin Endocrinol*. 1997;47(3):337–342.

van Ryn M, Burke J. The effect of patient race and socioeconomic status on physicians' perceptions of patients. *Social Sci Med*. 2000;50:813–828.

Vyavaharkar M, Glover S, Leonhirth D, et al. HIV in Rural America: Prevalence and Service Availability. A Technical Report by the South Carolina Rural Health Research Center. 2013.

Wagner GJ, Goggin K, Remien RH, et al. A closer look at depression and its relationship to HIV antiretroviral adherence. *Ann Behav Med*. 2011;42:352–360.

Waldrop-Valverde D, Valverde E. Homelessness and psychological distress as contributors to antiretroviral nonadherence in HIV-positive injecting drug users. *AIDS Patient Care STD*. May 2005;19(5):326–334.

Wechsberg WM, Lam WK, Zule W, et al. Violence, homelessness, and HIV risk among crack-using African-American women. *Subst Use Misuse*. February–May 2003;38(3–6):669–700.

Weinbaum C, Sabin K, Santibanez S. Hepatitis B, hepatitis C, and HIV in correctional populations: a review of epidemiology and prevention. *AIDS*. 2005;19(Suppl 3):S41–S46.

Weiner LS, Battles HR, Wood LV. A longitudinal study of adolescents with perinatally or transfusion acquired HIV infection: sexual knowledge, risk reduction self efficacy and sexual behavior. *AIDS Behav*. 2007;11:471–478.

Weisse CS, Sorum PC, Sanders KN, et al. Do gender and race affect decisions about pain management? *J Gen Intern Med*. 2001;16(4):211–217.

Weyers S, Verstraelen H, Gerris J, et al. Microflora of the penile skin-lined neovagina of transsexual women. *BMC Microbiol*. 2009;9(1):102. http://doi.org/10.1186/1471-2180-9-102.

White BL, Walsh J, Rayasam S, et al. What makes me screen for HIV? Perceived barriers and facilitators to conducting recommended routine HIV testing among primary care physicians in the Southeastern United States. *J Int Assoc Provid AIDS Care*. 2015;14:127–135.

Williams PL, Storm D, Montepiedra G, et al. Predictors of adherence to antiretroviral medications in children and adolescents with HIV infection. *Pediatrics*. 2006;118:e1745–e1757.

Wismer B, Amann T, Diaz R, et al., eds. *Adapting Your Practice: Recommendations for the Care of Homeless Adults with Chronic Non-malignant Pain*. Nashville, TN: Health Care for the Homeless Clinicians' Network, National Health Care for the Homeless Council; 2011:119.

Workowski K, Bolan G. Sexually transmitted diseases treatment guidelines, 2015. *MMWR Recomm Rep*. 2015;65(3).

World Health Organization. TB and HIV and other comorbidities. 2019.

World Health Organization. Social determinants of health. 2020. https://www.who.int/social_determinants/en/

Wortham JM, Lee JT, Althomsons S, et al. Characteristics of persons who died with COVID-19—United States, February 12–May 18, 2020. *Morb Mortal Wkly Rep*. 2020;69(28):923–929.

Zanoni BC, Mayer KH. The adolescent and young adult HIV cascade of care in the United States: exaggerated health disparities. *AIDS Patient Care STD*. 2014;28(3):128–135.

12.

COMPLEMENTARY AND ALTERNATIVE MEDICINE/INTEGRATIVE MEDICINE APPROACHES

Ashka Patel and Kalpana D. Shere-Wolfe

LEARNING OBJECTIVES

- Discuss the fundamentals and practice of complementary and integrative medicine as it pertains to care for persons with HIV (PWH)

- Describe the established and evolving science of natural products, mind–body practices, and traditional medical systems

WHAT'S NEW?

This edition contains updated information on the effects of micronutrient supplementation on CD4+ T-cell counts and HIV disease progression as well as fish oil supplementation. In addition, herb–drug interactions are reviewed, with new data presented on interactions with newer antiretroviral medications.

KEY POINTS

- Complementary and alternative medicine (CAM) use is common in PWH. Physicians caring for PWH should be aware of the high prevalence of CAM use and the failure of most patients to disclose CAM use. Physicians need to routinely ask about CAM use, particularly herbal medicines and supplements.

- Nutritional supplementation with micronutrients—vitamins A, B, C, and E, zinc, and selenium—has been shown to improve markers of HIV progression and, in some studies, to also affect mortality.

- Natural health products (herbs, vitamins, and supplements) have the potential for significant drug interactions, which may lower the efficacy or increase the adverse effects of antiretroviral therapy (ART).

- Fish oil supplementation remains controversial. The American Heart Association does not recommend fish oil for primary prevention, but there is evidence of its use in secondary prevention of cardiovascular disease and in hypertriglyceridemia.

- Evidence suggests gut microbiota changes in PWH, but, currently, the routine use of probiotics is not recommended in PWH.

- Some data suggest that stress, anxiety, and depression can affect HIV progression. Mind–body practices such as meditation, mindfulness, yoga, and tai chi can reduce stress, improve blood pressure, and improve quality of life. In addition, they may affect adverse health behaviors. The effects of these practices on CD4+ T-cell counts and disease progression are currently under investigation.

- Acupuncture may be of benefit in patients with musculoskeletal pain and sleep issues.

WHAT IS CAM AND INTEGRATIVE MEDICINE?

CAM is a group of diverse medical and healthcare systems, practices, and products that are not currently considered part of conventional medicine. Although the terms *complementary* and *alternative* are used simultaneous and interchangeably, they refer to different entities. If a non-mainstream practice is used together with conventional medicine, it is considered "complementary." If a non-mainstream practice is used in place of conventional medicine, it is considered "alternative." True alternative medicine is uncommon in developed countries but may be commonly found in resource-limited settings. Most people who use non-mainstream approaches use them along with conventional treatments (see the National Center for Complementary and Integrative Health [NCCIH] website at https://nccih.nih.gov). Integrative medicine, the increasingly more common term in use, refers to the use of CAM modalities with conventional medicine in an evidence-based integrated manner with emphasis on the importance of the relationship between practitioner and patient. Cornerstones of integrative medicine—nutrition, stress management, and exercise/movement—overlap those of conventional medicine but vary in their emphasis and approach.

Complementary and integrative health approaches encompass three broad areas: natural products, mind and body practices, and traditional medical systems. Natural products are herbs or botanicals, vitamins and minerals, and probiotics. They are widely marketed and available and typically are sold as dietary supplements. Mind and body practices include a large and diverse group of techniques typically administered by trained practitioners. They include yoga, chiropractic and osteopathic manipulation, meditation, massage therapy, acupuncture, relaxation techniques (e.g., breathing exercises, guided imagery, and progressive muscle relaxation), tai chi, qi gong, healing touch, movement therapies, and hypnotherapy. Traditional medical systems include various types of healers, Ayurvedic medicine, Chinese medicine, homeopathy, and naturopathy. The research on these various modalities varies widely. Although there are many studies on certain herbal products, acupuncture, yoga, spinal manipulation, and meditation, there have been fewer studies on other practices. Moreover, studies using these modalities in PWH are limited.

USE OF CAM BY PWH

Historically, CAM was popular among PWH prior to the development of ART, and it remains popular. This is true in the US, Canada, Australia, many European countries, Asia, and Africa. Now that effective treatment options exist for PWH and the life expectancy of these patients parallels that of people without HIV, CAM therapies are being sought for general wellness, mood disorders, stress reduction, and reduction of medication-associated side effects, as well as for boosting the immune system (Lorenc & Robinson, 2013; Thompson et al., 2012). Importantly, one of the key reasons why CAM is being used by patients is because it enables them to have a more active role in their healthcare as well as a sense of control. CAM use is a way to shift the focus away or "demedicalize" HIV management and focus on sense of wellness and normalcy (Littlewood & Vanable, 2011). Factors that contribute to the increasingly popular concept of wellness include good nutrition, exercise, physical relaxation, and mental ease.

Reports of CAM use vary due to differences in study populations and definitions of CAM and CAM therapies. CAM is used by approximately 30% to 60% of PWH; however, when restricted to practitioner-based CAM, the prevalence is approximately 15% or 16% (Bahall, 2017; Dhalla et al., 2006; Greene et al., 1999; Halpin et al., 2018; Josephs et al., 2007; Kelso-Chichetto et al., 2016; London et al., 2003; Lorenc & Robinson, 2013; Standish et al., 2001; Visser & Grierson, 2002). CAM use is predicted by higher levels of education, men who have sex with men, female gender, longer disease duration, symptom severity and time on ART, and financial resources (Agnoletto et al., 2006; Halpin et al., 2018; Littlewood & Vanable, 2008; Lorenc & Robinson, 2013). Vitamins, herbs, and supplements are most common, followed by prayer, meditation, and spiritual approaches. In developing countries and areas with poor access to conventional HIV treatment, traditional culture-based systems are widely used. In general, patients have a high level of satisfaction with CAM modalities, with 50% to 70% reporting improvement in malaise, various symptoms, and quality of life (Agnoletto et al., 2003; Duggan et al., 2001).

There are insufficient data regarding adherence and CAM use (Kelso-Chichetto et al., 2016; Owen-Smith et al., 2007).

In general, most studies have found that CAM users do not have decreased adherence to conventional medication, nor do they reject conventional ART. Rather, they use CAM in an integrated manner with their conventional HIV care (Littlewood & Vanable, 2008, 2014; Liu et al., 2009; Milan et al., 2008).

PHYSICIAN ATTITUDES TOWARD CAM

There are limited data on physician attitudes toward CAM. In one study of 89 HIV care providers, 63% believed that CAM and integrative medicine therapies may be helpful for PWH, and 36% had personally used one (Wynia et al., 1999). A national survey of infectious disease physicians demonstrated that they are familiar with various CAM modalities, including vitamin and mineral supplementation, massage, acupuncture, chiropractic, yoga, and herbal medicine. They most recommended vitamin and mineral supplementation (80%) and massage (62%). Data regarding clinical efficacy, drug interactions, and safety appear to be important factors that influence infectious disease physicians' use of these modalities for their patients (Shere-Wolfe et al., 2013).

PATIENT DISCLOSURE REGARDING CAM USE

Studies have shown that the majority of physicians do not ask their patients about CAM use and that patients may not disclose CAM use for various reasons unless asked directly (Patel et al., 2017; Wahner-Roedler et al., 2014; Wynia et al., 1999). CAM use disclosure rates vary across studies from 38% to 90% (Littlewood & Vanable, 2008). It is important that clinicians caring for PWH ask about CAM use to identify any potential drug interactions and safety issues.

Discussing CAM use is important, especially with respect to natural products. Concerns regarding drug interaction are paramount; however, also important are issues related to contamination of natural products. One study found that 21% of Ayurvedic medicines purchased via the internet contained detectable levels of lead, mercury, and arsenic (Saper et al., 2008). Similarly, Chinese herbal medicines may have microbial and heavy metal contamination (Ting et al., 2013). Heavy metal toxicity and testing may be considered in patients with new symptoms after initiating Chinese or Ayurvedic medicine. Other safety issues include side effects from taking extremely large doses of vitamins. High doses of vitamin A can cause liver and bone damage as well as increase the risk of birth defects. High-dose vitamin C intake apparently increases the risk of kidney stones. High doses of zinc (>75 mg/day) have been linked to copper deficiency.

Questions such as "Are you taking any vitamins, supplements, or herbs?" can be asked immediately after inquiring about conventional medications and compliance. For foreign patients, asking "Are you taking any natural medicines from your country?" may elicit information that might not otherwise be offered. A brief statement such as "This is important as many natural products can interfere with your HIV medication" or "I want to make sure what you are using is safe. Even simple things like vitamins can hurt you if you take too much" can help elicit information and foster a partnership relationship. With increasing use of electronic medical records, this information can be included and tracked easily. It is important to ask in a nonjudgmental manner that allows the patient to feel comfortable with disclosure. Many patients may not be well informed about the products they are using. It may be helpful to direct patients to the National Institutes of Health's Medline Plus website for free, easy-to-understand, evidence-based information about many herbal products.

NATURAL HEALTH PRODUCTS TO CONSIDER FOR USE IN PWH

NUTRITIONAL SUPPLEMENTATION

Micronutrients (vitamin and minerals) are important for human development, disease prevention, and well-being. They are not produced in the body and must be derived from the diet. Vitamins A, D, E, C, and B, as well as zinc, iron, and selenium, play an important role in immunity. PWH have been found to have various micronutrient deficiencies that are prevalent before symptomatic disease and occur in patients who are ART-naive as well as those taking ART (Baum et al., 1995; Beach et al., 1992; Hepburn et al., 2004; Remacha et al., 2003). Micronutrient supplementation has been shown to improve markers of HIV progression (cluster of differentiation T-lymphocyte cell count [CD4+] and viral load) and mortality in both early (Baum et al., 2013) and late stages of HIV (Filteau et al., 2015; Jiamton et al., 2003; Kaiser et al., 2006; Range et al., 2006) as well as in pregnant women (Fawzi et al., 2004). However, there are very limited and conflicting reports regarding whether micronutrient supplementation increases HIV shedding (Jiamton et al., 2005; McClelland et al., 2004; Sudfeld et al., 2014).

The effects of multivitamins (vitamins A, B, C, and E) on the health status of pregnant PWH in Tanzania were studied. A double-blind, randomized controlled trial found a significantly lower rate of progression to World Health Organization (WHO) stage 4 AIDS and a significantly lower death rate in the multivitamin group compared to the placebo group. Multivitamin use also resulted in significantly higher CD4+ T-cell counts and significantly lower viral loads (Fawzi et al., 2004).

A retrospective cohort study of 67,707 patients in Tanzania demonstrated the effectiveness of routine supplementation with vitamin B complex, vitamin C, and vitamin E in PWH. Among the 48,207 ART-naive patients, supplementation reduced the risk of mortality, incidence of tuberculosis, and meeting ART eligibility. Among 46,077 ART-experienced patients, supplementation reduced the risk of mortality, incidence of tuberculosis, and immunologic failure. The benefits of multivitamin supplementation were greatest in the first year of ART (Sudfeld et al., 2019).

Zinc deficiency is common in adult PWH and is independently associated with disease progression (Baum et al., 1997, 2003; Beach et al., 1992; Falutz et al., 1988; Graham et al., 1991; Jones et al., 2006). In a randomized, double-blind,

placebo-controlled trial of 231 PWH with low plasma zinc levels, zinc supplementation at 12 to 15 mg of elemental zinc for 18 months resulted in a fourfold decrease in the likelihood of immunologic failure, defined as a decrease in CD4+ T-cell count to 200 cells/mm³, compared to placebo. Viral load was not affected by zinc supplementation. Zinc supplementation also significantly reduced diarrhea compared with placebo. Respiratory diseases and HIV-related mortality were not affected by supplementation. Zinc testing and supplementation should be considered in PWH with a high prevalence of zinc deficiency, such as drug users, children, men who have sex with men, and populations in developing countries (Baum et al., 2010).

Zinc deficiency has also been studied in PWH with liver disease secondary to concomitant hepatitis C (HCV) infection or alcohol use disorder. In Russia, a cross-sectional study of 204 ART-naive patients with HIV/HCV coinfections complicated with heavy drinking noted that the prevalence of advanced liver fibrosis was not associated with zinc deficiency (Barocas et al., 2019).

Similarly, a double-blinded placebo-controlled randomized clinical trial of 254 PWH who were ART-naive and had past-30-day heavy alcohol consumption was conducted in Russia to assess if zinc gluconate supplementation (15 mg for men and 12 mg for women) taken daily for 18 months could change the Veterans Aging Cohort Study (VACS) Index score (a higher VACS Index score indicates higher mortality risk). The study concluded that zinc supplementation did not change the score at 18 months. Also, there was no change in the secondary outcomes, which included a change in CD4+ T-cell count, an assessment of cardiovascular risk based on the Reynolds Risk Score, and changes in inflammatory or microbial translocation biomarkers at 18 months (Freiberg et al., 2020).

Another single nutrient that has been studied in the HIV population is selenium. A systematic review of randomized controlled trials comparing selenium with placebo and reporting outcomes of its effect on viral load and CD4+ T-cell count concluded that daily supplementation with 200 micrograms of selenium can delay CD4+ T-cell count decline in PWH, but there were no quantifiable data showing that it suppresses or reduces viral load (Muzembo et al., 2019).

Pregnant PWH with selenium deficiency were noted to have an eightfold higher risk for preterm delivery ($p = 0.03$) (Okunade et al., 2018). However, selenium supplementation should be used with caution in primiparous women not receiving ART because at least one study has shown increased HIV-1 RNA detection in the breast milk of these women with selenium supplementation (Sudfeld et al., 2014).

Vitamin D deficiency is also common among PWH, although estimates range widely from 10% to 88% (Sherwood et al., 2012; Zhang et al., 2017). The wide range of estimates is likely due to differences in demographics, location, climate/season, and definitions. Etiology of vitamin D deficiency in PWH is likely multifactorial too. It includes both traditional risk factors such as dietary deficiency, darker skin, obesity, chronic kidney disease, lack of sun exposure, malabsorption, etc. and HIV-related factors such as ART regimens, especially those with efavirenz, which has been shown to interfere with vitamin D metabolism. Vitamin D plays an important role in osteoporosis, cardiovascular disease (CVD), and the immune system (Eckard & McComsey, 2014). Some but not all data from randomized controlled trials in the general population demonstrate that vitamin D supplementation improves bone mineral density and decreases fractures (Bischoff-Ferrari et al., 2005; Dawson-Hughes et al., 1997; Jackson et al., 2006). The degree to which vitamin D deficiency contributes to osteopenia and osteoporosis, CVD, and disease progression in PWH is unknown. The Endocrine Society recommends that at-risk persons be screened, including all persons receiving ART. The European AIDS Clinical Society also recommends screening for vitamin D deficiency in persons with the risk factors mentioned earlier in the paragraph, those with a history of low bone mineral density and/or fracture, or those with a high risk for fracture (Holick et al., 2011; EACS Online, 2019).

A trial demonstrated that for adolescents and young adults ($n = 214$) ages 16 to 24 years on a regimen containing tenofovir disoproxil fumarate (TDF), monthly vitamin D supplementation (50,000 IU) improved vitamin D levels and lumbar spine bone mineral density regardless of baseline vitamin D status (Havens et al., 2018). In adults 25 to 47 years of age, supplementation with high-dose vitamin D3 (4,000 IU) and calcium carbonate (1,000 mg) with ART initiation (efavirenz, emtricitabine, and tenofovir) increased 25-(OH) D levels and attenuated increases in bone turnover markers and bone loss at the hip and lumbar spine by approximately 50% at 48 weeks (Overton et al., 2015). Lastly, a prospective, open-label, multicenter trial of 167 participants who were virologically suppressed, age 60 years or older, and on a TDF-containing regimen showed that bone mineral density improved when the TDF-containing regimen was switched to a elvitegravir, cobicistat, emtricitabine, and tenofovir alafenamide–based regimen (Maggiolo et al., 2019).

Vitamin D deficiency may also play a role in risk for tuberculosis (TB) in PWH. In a diverse cohort of adults with advanced HIV infection in high-burden TB countries. Vitamin D deficiency at ART initiation was found to be independently associated with an increased risk of incident TB in the next 96 weeks (Tenforde et al., 2017). Also, in Lima, Peru, a nested case–control study, systemic review, and individual-participant data meta-analysis showed that vitamin D predicts TB disease in a dose-dependent manner and that the risk of TB disease is the highest among PWH with severe vitamin D deficiency (Aibana et al., 2019).

Studies show mixed results regarding the role of vitamin D deficiency and CD4+ T-cell count recovery. One trial of vitamin D supplementation in children living with HIV on ART did not show an effect on CD4+ T-cell count (Ezeamama et al., 2016; Kakalia et al., 2011; Sudfield et al., 2012). In another double-blinded, randomized, placebo-controlled trial in Ethiopia, daily supplementation with 5,000 IU of vitamin D3 and phenylbutyrate in treatment-naive PWH was shown to improve vitamin D3 status but did not reduce viral load, restore T-cell counts, or improve body mass index or middle-upper-arm circumference (Ashenafi et al., 2019).

Hence, given the data in the general population supporting the use of vitamin D and calcium supplementation to decrease the risk of fractures and improve bone mineral density and the increasing number of studies in PWH, especially those on efavirenz (EFV)- and TDF-containing regimens, that show improvement in bone mineral density, it seems reasonable to screen high-risk PWH and provide supplementation to minimize HIV-related complications of osteoporosis and potentially affect immune function and disease progression. However, individuals on integrase strand transfer inhibitor (INSTI)-containing regimens should be counseled on the drug interactions between INSTIs and divalent minerals and the risk of potential treatment failure. They should be advised to take multivitamins/minerals either 2 hours before or 6 hours after INSTIs.

More recently, a systematic review of the effects of vitamin D, selenium, or zinc supplementation was conducted. Twenty-four single-supplement trials involving 5,948 participants were included in the review. Seven vitamin D trials showed no harmful or beneficial effects of vitamin D supplementation on HIV progression. Six selenium trials found that selenium supplementation increased CD4+ T-cell counts, the risk of diarrhea, and the hospital admission rate for HIV-related conditions. Eleven zinc trials showed a potential benefit of supplementation on diarrhea and immune function (Kayode & Anaba, 2020). Thus, it is recommended that each PWH be evaluated on an individual basis taking into account all the risks and benefits.

FISH OILS

Data show that CVD mortality for PWH has increased significantly from 1999 to 2013 (Feinstein et al., 2016). The use of fish oils for cardioprotection is controversial, and there are to date no studies looking at the use of omega-3 fatty acids for CVD in PWH. A meta-analysis of randomized trials of omega-3 fatty acid supplements involving approximately 78,000 participants in 10 trials with a history of coronary heart disease (CHD), stroke, or diabetes found no evidence that fish oils have cardioprotective effects (Aung et al., 2018). Similarly, a randomized placebo-controlled trial of 24,871 patients that showed supplementation with marine omega-3 fatty acids did not result in a lower incidence of major cardiovascular events or cancer than placebo (Manson et al., 2019). However, an updated meta-analysis of 13 trials concluded that marine omega-3 supplementation lowers the risk for myocardial infarction, CHD death, total CHD, CVD death, and total CVD (Hu et al., 2019). Hence, the use of fish oils as primary prevention of CVD remains controversial and is not currently recommended by the American Heart Association (Feinstein et al., 2019).

There is evidence that inflammation and oxidative stress is important in the pathogenesis of CVD, which is particularly important in PWH. Nonetheless, a randomized parallel, placebo-controlled trial in Brazil of PWH on ART did not show any effect of 3 g of fish oils on high-sensitivity C-reactive protein (hs-CRP), fibrinogen, factor VIII, interleukin (IL)-6, IL 1-beta, or tumor necrosis factor (TNF)-alpha (Oliveira et al., 2015). In another randomized parallel controlled clinical trial, 70 PWH in Mexico were given 2.4 g of omega-3 fatty acids compared to a placebo. A reduction in markers for oxidative stress such as nitric oxide catabolites, lipoperoxides, or glutathione could not be shown in the treatment arm (Amador-Licona et al., 2015). Lastly, in a randomized, controlled, double-blinded clinical trial of 37 PWH between the ages of 40 and 70 who were given fish oil 1.6 g/day for 12 weeks or a placebo, there were no significant differences between the treatment and control groups on any measures of inflammation or immunosenescence in both CD4[+] and CD[+] 8 T-cell counts (Swanson et al., 2018).

Omega-3 fatty acid supplementation has also been studied for depression in the general population with mixed results. Some studies have suggested that EPA may be more beneficial than DHA and that omega-3 fatty acids may best be used in addition to antidepressant medication rather than in place of it (Grosso et al., 2015). A randomized placebo-controlled trial of 100 PWH assigned to omega-3 fatty acids (720 mg EPA and 480 mg DHA daily) versus a placebo control group showed a reduction of depression scores in the patients in the treatment group over time (Ravi et al., 2016).

Fish oils appear to be beneficial for the treatment of hypertriglyceridemia. In a multicenter randomized trial, patients with CVD or diabetes or other risk factors on a statin therapy with a fasting triglyceride (TG) level of 135 to 499 mg/dL and a low-density-lipoprotein cholesterol level of 41 to 100 mg/dL were given 4 g of icosapent ethyl or placebo. Results showed that the risk of ischemic events, including cardiovascular death, was lower among those who received icosapent ethyl compared to placebo (Bhatt et al., 2019). Fish oils are relatively safe and do not have significant drug interactions with ART. In 100 PWH receiving ART with hypertriglyceridemia, fish oils at doses of approximately 6 g/day significantly reduced TG concentrations with no significant effect of fish oils on CD4[+] T-cell counts, immune function, or lopinavir trough concentrations (Gerber et al., 2008). This result was confirmed in another randomized controlled trial of 48 PWH on ART as well as fenofibrate (Peters et al., 2012). Fish oils alone have also been shown to decrease TG levels without adverse effects on immune parameters or antiretroviral pharmacokinetics (De Truchis et al., 2005). In a study of PWH on combination ART with elevated fasting TG levels, the use of 3 g of fish oils combined with diet counseling and exercise resulted in a decrease in TG levels of 25% at 4 weeks versus a 2.8% increase in the control group (Wohl et al., 2005). Additionally, a meta-analysis of nine clinical studies comprising 578 PWH revealed that omega-3 fatty acids significantly reduced TG levels while increasing levels of high-density-lipoprotein cholesterol (Fogacci et al., 2020).

Doses greater than 3 g/day should be used with caution in patients with bleeding disorders or on anticoagulants. Unlike other supplements, fish oils are also available in prescription form such as Lovaza for use in hypertriglyceridemia. It is reasonable that fish oils—either as supplements or as fatty fish twice a week (salmon, mackerel, herring, lake trout, sardines, and albacore tuna)—be considered in PWH with hypertriglyceridemia and possibly those with CVD, especially if they are not medically optimized.

PROBIOTICS

The intestinal microbiota serves to preserve the intestinal barrier, to provide resistance to pathogenic colonization, and to stimulate the development of gut-associated lymphoid tissue. The gut microbiota is changed in PWH compared to the uninfected healthy population (Dillon et al., 2014; Dinh et al., 2015; Lozupone et al., 2013; Mutlu et al., 2014; Vujkovic-Cvijin et al., 2013). However, currently, probiotics cannot be recommended for PWH. They do deserve further investigation, particularly as immunomodulators.

INTERACTION OF NATURAL HEALTH PRODUCTS WITH ART

Concurrent use of natural health products with ART is common among PWH. Of all the CAM modalities, herbal supplements have the greatest potential for adverse effects due to potential drug–drug interactions. The following considerations add to the complexity and unpredictability of these interactions (MacDonald et al., 2009):

1. Many herbal remedies are complex products made of many different phytochemicals, some of which may not be fully characterized and standardized.

2. Some natural health products induce and inhibit gastrointestinal and hepatic enzymes simultaneously.

3. Many ART medications are substrates, inhibitors, or inducers of the drug-metabolizing enzymes (CYP family) and drug transporters (P-glycoprotein [P-gp]).

4. In vitro experiments may not predict in vivo effects due to various effects of intestinal enzymes, colonic microflora, and other factors.

5. Because of variations in extraction methods, constituents, and plant type/part, results from one study are not generalizable to other brands and formulation of natural health products.

For these reasons, it is difficult to state that any natural health product is free from the possibility of potential drug–drug interactions. Most ART drug–drug interactions occur through the cytochrome P450 pathway and through drug transporters, which includes the P-gp efflux drug transporter (Brooks et al., 2017).

The major isoform responsible for protease inhibitor (PI) metabolism is CYP3A4, and are substrates of P-gp. Non-nucleoside reverse transcriptase inhibitors (NNRTIs) are metabolized by CYP3A4 and CYP2B6. PIs inhibit CYP3A4, whereas most NNRTIs induce CYP3A4. INSTIs (dolutegravir and raltegravir) neither induce nor inhibit CYP3A4. Conversely, nucleoside reverse transcriptase inhibitors (NRTI) and raltegravir are not inducers, inhibitors, or substrates of CYPs; therefore, they have fewer drug–drug interactions.

Thus, any medications, supplements, or herbs that interfere with CYP, P-gp, or uridine diphosphate glucuronosyltransferase (UGT) have the potential to result in changes in concentration of HIV and non-HIV drugs. ART–herbal interactions are bidirectional, and ART may affect the concentrations, efficacy, and side/adverse effects of herbal medicines (Ladenheim et al., 2008; Lamorde et al., 2012).

GUIDE FOR NATURAL HEALTH PRODUCT–DRUG INTERACTION

Some commonly used CAM products, such as cod liver oil and flax/flaxseed oil, have no known interactions with ART medications. Kava kava (*Piper methysticum*), black cohosh (*Cimicifuga racemose*), valerian (*Valeriana officinalis*), bitter orange (*Citrus aurantium*), saw palmetto (*Serenoa repens*), and Siberian ginseng (*Eleutheroccus senticosus*) have not been found to interact with CYP3A4. Therefore, it is unlikely that clinically significant pharmacokinetic interactions would occur with PIs or NNRTIs, but they may affect other ART regimens (Lee et al., 2006). Potential CAM products that interact with antiretroviral medications can be viewed in Table 12.1.

1. Red yeast rice extract (RYRE) is sometimes used by patients to lower cholesterol. It is made by fermenting a type of yeast called *Monascus purpureus* over red rice. RYRE contains several compounds, known as monacolins, that block the production of cholesterol. One of these, monacolin K, has the same structure as the drugs lovastatin and mevinolin (Ma et al., 2000). Lovastatin is exclusively metabolized by CYP3A4 and is contraindicated in patients taking PIs. Red yeast rice was marketed in the United States as the dietary supplement Cholestin. The US Food and Drug Administration banned it in 1998. However, RYREs are still available, and some of them still contain lovastatin. Patients should be cautioned to avoid RYRE if they are on PIs or statins.

2. St. John's wort (*Hypericum perforatum*) is an herbal product used for depression. It is known to be an inducer of CYP3A4 and P-gp. It also contains constituents that can affect other CYPs, including CYP2D6. It has been shown to alter levels of nevirapine, rilpivirine, and indinavir (de Maat et al., 2001; Hafner et al., 2010; Piscitelli et al., 2000). St. John's wort should be avoided by patients on ART.

Table 12.1 POTENTIAL CAM PRODUCTS THAT INTERACT WITH ANTIRETROVIRAL MEDICATIONS

LIKELY SAFE	USE CAUTION BASED ON IN VITRO AND CASE REPORTS	AVOID	TO BE DETERMINED	ADJUST TIMING OF SUPPLEMENT
Cod liver oil	Ginseng	Red yeast rice extract	Evening primrose	Calcium carbonate
Flaxseed oil/flaxseed	Gingko	St. John's wort	Echinacea	Ferrous fumarate
Fish oils	Cat's claw		Cranberry	Multivitamins
Vitamin C	Goldenseal		Cancer bush	Other minerals—magnesium, zinc, copper, chromium, selenium
Aloe vera	Garlic		Goji	
	African potato		Green tea	
	Milk thistle		Harpagophyton	
	Echinacea		Horse chestnut	
	Piperine		Horsetail	
	Bitter orange		Moringa	
	Sweet orange		Saw palmetto	
	Borage		Milk thistle	
	Grapefruit		Red vine	
			Spirulina	
			Valerian	
			Wintergreen	

3. Echinacea (*Echinacea angustifolia, E. purpurea*) is commonly used for viral infections and immunologic boosting. *E. purpurea* has been shown to induce CYP3A4 metabolism of darunavir but with no effect on overall darunavir and ritonavir pharmacokinetics (Molto et al., 2011). Echinacea was also not found to affect etravirine concentrations (Molto et al., 2012b) or the pharmacokinetics of lopinavir/ritonavir (Penzak et al., 2010).

4. Garlic is often taken to prevent heart disease, high cholesterol, and high blood pressure and to boost the immune system. However, garlic may induce intestinal CYP3A4 or P-gp (Berginc et al., 2010). In one study, garlic markedly reduced the concentration of saquinavir, although the results suggested that it affected the bioavailability of saquinavir rather than its systemic clearance (Piscitelli et al., 2002). In single-dose pharmacokinetic (PK) studies, garlic extract did not affect the area under the curve (AUC) or the maximum concentration recorded (C_{max}) of ritonavir or saquinavir (Gallicano et al., 2003; Jacek et al., 2004). Garlic should be avoided by patients on ART.

5. Milk thistle (*Silybum marianum*) inhibits CYP3A4 and P-gp activity in vitro but has not been shown to significantly affect darunavir–ritonavir concentrations in one study (Molto et al., 2012b) or indinavir pharmacokinetics in three separate PK studies (DiCenzo et al., 2003; Mills et al., 2005; Piscitelli et al., 2002).

6. Ginseng (*Panax ginseng*) may induce CYP3A4 activity in the liver and gastrointestinal tract. Two multidose PK studies showed no effect of ginseng on lopinavir/ritonavir or indinavir levels (Andrade et al., 2008; Calderón et al., 2014). One case of a PWH on raltegravir + lopinavir/ritonavir therapy who developed liver failure after starting ginseng has been reported (Mateo-Carrasco et al., 2012).

7. *Ginkgo biloba* was not found to significantly alter raltegravir or lopinavir/ritonavir pharmacokinetics in healthy volunteers (Blonk, 2012; Robertson et al., 2008), but it was reported to potentially affect the efficacy of efavirenz (Naccarato et al., 2012; Wiegman et al., 2009).

8. Cat's claw (*Uncaria guianensis, U. tomentosa*), which is used for a wide variety of ailments, including inflammatory and infectious diseases, may increase atazanavir, ritonavir, and saquinavir levels due to CYP3A4 inhibition (Galera et al., 2008).

9. Goldenseal (*Hydrastis canadensis*) has potent CYP3A4 inhibition properties but was not shown to affect indinavir levels (Sandhu et al., 2003). Patients taking goldenseal should be monitored for increased toxicity of CYP3A4 substrate drugs.

10. Fish oil in combination with lopinavir/ritonavir showed no significant decrease in ART level (Gerber et al., 2008).

11. Vitamin C decreased the AUC of indinavir by 15% and C_{max} by 23% in healthy volunteers. However, other studies in healthy individuals found no difference in CYP3A4 activity (Jalloh et al., 2016; Slain et al., 2005; van Heeswijk et al., 2005).

12. Two popular African herbs, African potato (*Hypoxis hemerocallidea*) and cancer bush (*Lessertia frutescens*), have been shown to inhibit CY3A4 and P-gp in vitro (Awortwe et al., 2014). African potato (*H. hemerocallidea, H. obtuse*) was studied in two PK studies and was found to have no significant effect on AUC or C_{max} with efavirenz and lopinavir/ritonavir (Gwaza et al., 2013). Cancer bush can reduce the absorption and bioavailability of antiretrovirals, so patients should be monitored for plasma concentration and viral load (Bordes et al., 2020).

13. Evening primrose inhibits CYP3A4 and CYP2D6. There is one case report of evening primrose increasing lopinavir levels (Beukel et al., 2008).

14. Calcium carbonate and ferrous fumarate significantly decrease serum levels of dolutegravir; chelation is suspected as the mechanism (Song et al., 2015). Patients on INSTI-based regimens taking calcium, magnesium, iron, zinc, copper, chromium, or selenium should be educated on this interaction and counseled to take the INSTI 2 hours before or 6 hours after the calcium or iron supplement (Brooks et al., 2017).

15. Multivitamin supplementation decreased dolutegravir levels in healthy volunteers (Patel et al., 2011).

16. Black pepper contains the active alkaloid piperine, which is often combined with turmeric to increase absorption. It has been shown to inhibit CYP3A4, P-gp, and UGT isoforms. Nevirapine levels increased significantly in individuals receiving 20 mg of piperine daily. Piperine may induce and/or inhibit other ART medications as well (Kasibhatta & Naidu, 2007).

17. Grapefruit (*Citrus pardis, C. maxima*) is also known to inhibit CYP3A4 and P-gp. There is a risk of increasing the absorption and bioavailability of certain antiretrovirals. Need to be cautious with PIs, NNRTIs, elvitegravir, bictegravir, dolutegravir, and maraviroc and bioavailability with citrus. Bordes et al., 2020).

18. Horse chestnut (*Aesculus hippocastanum*) inhibits CYP3A4 and P-gp. It interacts with NNRTIs, elvitegravir, abacavir, tenofovir, indinavir, raltegravir, PIs, efavirenz, dolutegravir, bictegravir, and maraviroc (Bordes et al., 2020).

19. Horsetail (*Equisetum arvense*) inhibits CYP1A2 and CYP2D6. It can increase viral load. It interacts with lamivudine, zidovudine, efavirenz, emtricitabine, and tenofovir (Bordes et al., 2020).

20. Moringa (*Moringa oleifera*) inhibits CYP3A4, 1A2, and 2D6 and interacts with nevirapine and efavirenz (Bordes et al., 2020).

21. Red vine (*Vitis vinifera*) inhibits CYP2C9, 2D6, and 3A4 and interacts with PIs, NNRTIs, dolutegravir, elvitegravir, bictegravir, and maraviroc (Bordes et al., 2020).

22. Spirulina (*Arthrospira platensis*) inhibits CYP2C9 and interacts with etravirine (Bordes et al., 2020).

23. Sweet orange (*Citrus sinensis*) inhibits the OATP1A2 transporter, allowing intestinal absorption of substrate drugs for 4 hours. It interacts with saquinavir, lopinavir, and darunavir (Bordes et al., 2020).

24. Wintergreen causes renal toxicity and interacts with tenofovir (Bordes et al., 2020).

Lack of high-quality studies in humans and lack of standardization of herbal formulations, among other factors, limit our knowledge on ART and herbal interactions. Other than a few herbal products such as St. John's wort, there is no simple guide to which natural health product and antiretroviral combinations clearly have significant clinical interactions. In vitro testing may be helpful for identifying products to screen, but it is limited in its clinical extrapolation. Therefore, caution is advised and consultation with a pharmacist regarding any natural health product and antiretroviral interaction is warranted. Resources for information on natural health products for both clinicians and patients are listed in Table 12.2. Particularly useful for clinicians is the Natural Medicines Database website (formerly known as Natural Standard and Natural Medicine Comprehensive Database), which has an extensive database on herbal medicines with in-depth information as well as a drug interaction checker. The database is available through subscription and is usually also available through most academic libraries or applications for smartphones. ART–herbal interactions can also be checked at http://www.hiv-druginteractions.org. The NCCIH also has concise evidence-based information on common herbs and links for information on herb–drug interactions.

HERBAL MEDICINES FOR HIV TREATMENT

In a meta-analysis of 12 randomized controlled trials involving 881 patients with AIDS, traditional Chinese medicine (TCM) interventions were associated with significantly reduced plasma viral load compared with placebo ($p = 0.04$). Patients receiving TCM interventions had significantly higher CD4$^+$ T-cell counts compared with the placebo group ($p = 0.002$) as well as improved clinical symptoms ($p < 0.00001$). Additionally, TCM interventions were significantly more likely to result in improved clinical symptoms ($p < 0.00001$). TCM interventions conferred a similar risk of adverse events compared with control interventions ($p = 0.29$). Nonetheless, the reductions in plasma viral load significantly favored conventional Western medical therapy alone over integrated traditional Chinese and Western medical therapy ($p = 0.004$) (Deng et al., 2014).

MIND–BODY APPROACHES

Mind and body practices include a large and diverse group of procedures or techniques typically administered by trained practitioners or teachers rather than by physicians. They include yoga, chiropractic and osteopathic manipulation, meditation, massage therapy, acupuncture, relaxation techniques (e.g., breathing exercises, guided imagery, and progressive muscle relaxation), tai chi, qi gong, healing touch, and hypnotherapy. Central to these modalities is the elicitation of the relaxation response.

RELAXATION RESPONSE

The relaxation response can be described as a state of deep rest that changes the short- and long-term physical and emotional responses to stress (e.g., decreases in heart rate, blood pressure, rate of breathing, and muscle tension)—it is the opposite of the fight-or-flight response (Benson et al., 1974). Preliminary studies suggest that this response can affect gene expression related to energy metabolism, inflammatory response, and stress as well affect telomere length, which is associated with premature mortality and predicts a variety of health risks and diseases (Bhasin et al., 2013; Buric et al., 2017; Epel et al., 2004; Lavretsky et al., 2013). The clinical implications of these changes at the level of gene expression and telomeres are currently unknown.

STRESS, DEPRESSION, AND HIV PROGRESSION

HIV infection presents many stresses and challenges—mental, emotional, and physical—that vary from the time

Table 12.2 INTERNET RESOURCES FOR NATURAL HEALTH PRODUCTS INFORMATION AND NATURAL HEALTH PRODUCT–DRUG INTERACTIONS

RESOURCE	WEBSITE
Natural Medicines	http://www.naturalmedicines.therapeuticresearch.com
National Center for Complementary and Integrative Health	https://nccih.nih.gov/health/herbsataglance.htm
HIV–Drug Interaction	http://www.hiv-druginteractions.org
National Institutes of Health, Office of Dietary Supplements Dietary Supplement Label Database	http://www.dsld.nlm.nih.gov/dsld/index.jsp
National Institutes of Health, Office of Dietary Supplements	https://ods.od.nih.gov
National Institutes of Health, MedlinePlus Herbs and Supplements Directory	https://nlm.nih.gov/medlineplus/druginfo/herb_All.html
Consumer Lab	http://www.consumerlab.com

of diagnosis to coping with drug adherence and medication-related side effects, aging issues, and dealing with the loss of infected loved ones. Not surprisingly, PWH have a higher incidence of depression and anxiety than the uninfected population (Pence et al., 2006; Whetten et al., 2008). Psychosocial variables and stress can affect measurable factors such as CD4$^+$ T-cell counts and viral loads in a variety of ways, including drug adherence, immune function, and health behaviors.

Stress has been shown in prospective human observational studies, animal studies, and laboratory experiments to be associated with depression, CVD, and progression of HIV. This effect is generally thought to be mediated by negative affective states such as anxiety and depression, behavioral patterns (adherence, substance abuse, etc.), and stress-elicited endocrine responses mediated by the hypothalamic–pituitary–adrenocortical axis and the sympathetic–adrenal–medullary system (Cohen et al., 2007). In PWH, some studies have shown that stress may be associated with reductions in natural killer cell and cytotoxic T-lymphocyte phenotypes (Leserman et al., 1997).

Results from studies prior to 2000 were inconsistent with respect to the effect of stress and depression on HIV progression. However, several studies after 2000 have suggested a link between stress and HIV progression (Leserman, 2008). Among 96 asymptomatic, gay PWH not on ART at baseline who were followed every 6 months for up to 9 years, each additional moderately severe stress event increased the risk of progression to AIDS by 50% and of developing an AIDS-related clinical condition by 2.5-fold after controlling for demographics, baseline CD4$^+$ T cells and viral load, and ARVs (Leserman et al., 2002). In a study of 177 men and women living with HIV, baseline depression and hopelessness predicted the slope of CD4$^+$ T cells and viral load. High cumulative depression and avoidant coping were associated with approximately twice the rate of CD4$^+$ T-cell decline and greater increases in viral load (Ironson et al., 2005).

MEDITATIVE PRACTICES

Meditation is a practice of concentrated focus on a sound, object, visualization, the breath, movement, or attention itself in order to increase awareness of the present moment, reduce stress, promote relaxation, and enhance personal and spiritual growth. Examples include mantra meditation and mindfulness meditation. Yoga, tai chi, and qi gong are forms of breath-coordinated movement meditations.

Research suggests that meditative practices may reduce blood pressure, symptoms of irritable bowel syndrome, anxiety and depression, and insomnia (https://www.nccih.nih.gov/health/meditation-in-depth). In 2017, the American Heart Association issued a scientific statement on meditation and CVD risk reduction stating that overall, studies on meditation suggest a possible benefit on cardiovascular risk and may be considered as adjunctive therapy for cardiovascular risk reduction (Levine et al., 2017).

YOGA

Several yoga studies in the general population show possible benefits for stress management, mental/emotional health, sleep, and healthy lifestyle behaviors (https://www.nccih.nih.gov/health/yoga-what-you-need-to-know). In one large analysis of approximately 35,000 US adults, yoga users reported high rates of health behavior outcomes such as motivation to exercise (~60%), eat healthier (~40%), cut back or stop drinking alcohol (12%), and cut back or stop smoking cigarettes (25%). More than 80% perceived reduced stress as a result of practicing yoga (Stussman et al., 2015).

Well-designed studies of yoga in the PWH are sparse. One prospective controlled study of yoga in PWH with CVD risk factors showed that 20 weeks of supervised yoga was effective in significantly reducing resting systolic and diastolic blood pressure by an average of 5/3 mmHg, reductions similar to those achieved with the Dietary Approaches to Stop Hypertension (DASH) diet. Studies suggest that a 10-mmHg reduction in systolic blood pressure and a 5-mmHg reduction in diastolic blood pressure predict a 40% to 50% lower risk of death from coronary artery disease (CAD). Extrapolating from these data in HIV-uninfected adults, yoga intervention would theoretically translate into a decreased risk of death from CAD by 20% to 25% in PWH. Yoga did not affect body weight, fat mass, pro-atherogeneic lipids, glucose tolerance, or immune or virologic status (Cade et al., 2010).

A 1-month yoga program was found to improve depression, anxiety, and CD4$^+$ T-cell counts in 22 PWH on ART compared to 22 control persons (Naoroibam et al., 2016). Mantra meditation (repetition of a word or phrase) was found to be effective in reducing anger, improving quality of life, and improving spiritual well-being in a randomized controlled study of PWH (Bormann et al., 2006). Recent meta-analyses of yoga studies in the HIV population demonstrated significant effects on stress, anxiety, and positive affect (Dunne et al., 2019; Ramirez-Garcia et al., 2019).

MINDFULNESS-BASED STRESS REDUCTION

Mindfulness-based stress reduction (MBSR) is a technique that uses cultivation of nonjudgmental awareness in the present moment. It is usually taught as an 8-week structured program. MBSR has been shown to decrease the side effects of ART and alleviate symptoms. In one randomized wait-list controlled study of 76 PWH with ART-related side effects, MBSR was found to significantly reduce the frequency of symptoms and distress related to symptoms (Duncan et al., 2012). In another randomized controlled trial of 117 PWH, MBSR was found to result in a reduction in avoidance, higher positive affect, and improvement in depression at 6 months (Gayner et al., 2012). A recent trial in 72 PWH aged 14 to 22 years old showed significantly higher levels of mindfulness, problem-solving coping, and life satisfaction as well as lower aggression; participants were more likely to have or to maintain reductions in viral load at 3 months (Webb et al., 2018).

Few studies have examined the effect of MBSR on CD4$^+$ T-cell count. One small randomized controlled short-term study of a diverse group of PWH suggested that MBSR could buffer CD4+ T-cell decline (Creswell et al., 2009). In a later randomized controlled trial of 40 long-term diagnosed and treated PWH, mindfulness-based cognitive therapy (which combined elements of MBSR and cognitive-behavioral therapy), patients were found to have decreased stress, anxiety, and depression and also a significantly increased CD4+ T-cell count at week 20 compared to placebo ($p < 0.001$), with no change in viral load (Gonzalez-Garcia et al., 2014). In contrast, a recent randomized, controlled trial of MBSR in PWH with CD4+ T-cell counts of more than $350/mm^3$ who were not on ART did not show benefit of MBSR with respect to CD4+ T-cell counts, CRP, IL-6, viral load, or D-dimer (Hecht et al., 2018).

TAI CHI

In the general population, studies suggest that tai chi may improve balance and stability in older people and those with Parkinson's disease; reduce pain from knee osteoarthritis, fibromyalgia, and back pain; and promote quality of life and mood in people with heart failure and cancer (https://www.nccih.nih.gov/health/meditation-in-depth). Data specific to PWH are limited. In a small study of 38 PWH randomized to tai chi, exercise, and control groups, both tai chi and exercise were found to improve physiologic parameters, functional outcomes, and quality of life. These patients were also noted to have improved social interactions (Galantino et al., 2005).

In a large group of 252 PWH, those randomized to three 10-week stress management approaches—cognitive-behavioral relaxation training, focused tai chi training, and spiritual growth—were compared to a wait-listed control group. Both the cognitive-behavioral relaxation and tai chi groups used less emotion-focused coping and had augmented lymphocyte proliferative function. Moreover, the tai chi group had an increase in quality of life, related mainly to an increase in emotional well-being (McCain et al., 2008).

Meditative practices can increase quality of life; reduce stress, anxiety, and depression; and affect health-related behaviors. These practices have not been shown to have harmful side effects, and they should be considered for interested patients with stress, depression, anxiety, and adverse health behaviors. These practices may also be considered for patients who are unwilling to utilize psychological counseling, support, or cognitive-behavioral therapy. Many meditative practices are available. Which one is best depends on patient preference, which may be influenced by cultural factors, convenience, and finances. The practice most likely to be effective is the one that the patient is most likely to do.

ACUPUNCTURE

Pain is a frequently reported symptom in PWH (Vogl et al., 1999). Pain may be secondary to peripheral neuropathy or to musculoskeletal issues. Results from several studies suggest that acupuncture may help with chronic pain syndromes related to low back pain, neck pain, and osteoarthritis/knee pain (Hinman et al., 2014; Linde et al., 2009; Manheimer et al., 2010; Vickers et al., 2012; Witt et al., 2006). Acupuncture may also help reduce the frequency of tension headaches and prevent migraine headaches. Clinical practice guidelines issued by the American Pain Society and the American College of Physicians in 2007 recommended acupuncture as one of several nonpharmacologic approaches that physicians should consider when patients with chronic low back pain do not respond to practices such as remaining active, applying heat, and taking pain-relieving medications (Chou et al., 2007).

Few studies have examined the effect of acupuncture in PWH. A large multicenter, modified double-blind, randomized, placebo-controlled study comparing acupuncture and sham acupuncture for symptomatic treatment of HIV-related neuropathy revealed a modest decrease in average pain scores in both groups but no significant improvement with acupuncture (Shlay et al., 1998). In another small study of 23 PWH with sleep disturbances at least three times per week, patients received acupuncture two evenings a week for 5 weeks. Both sleep time and sleep quality were reported as improved (Phillips & Skelton, 2001). A recent meta-analysis of interventions for HIV-related neuropathic pain showed only a marginal benefit of acupuncture for this indication (Amaniti et al., 2019).

Although studies of acupuncture in PWH are limited, it seems reasonable to consider acupuncture in patients with musculoskeletal pain and perhaps those with sleep disturbances, especially in those who are either reluctant to take or intolerant of conventional medications.

EXERCISE

Substantial evidence indicates that regular physical activity contributes to the primary and secondary prevention of several chronic diseases, such as CVD, osteoporosis, and diabetes, and is associated with a reduced risk of premature death (Warburton et al., 2006). Moreover, studies have shown that in PWH, exercise can improve strength, endurance, time to fatigue, and body composition; increase quality of life and sense of well-being; mitigate excessive bone loss; and decrease depression and anxiety (Dudgeon et al., 2004; MacArthur et al., 1993; Perazzo et al., 2018; Rigsby et al., 1992; Stringer et al., 1998). It may also preserve or improve cognition in people living with HIV (Quigley et al., 2019). Given the increased risk of CVD, muscle wasting, and bone disease, it makes sense that some form of physical activity be encouraged for capable PWH. Physicians have an important role in educating and encouraging exercise as a measure for well-being and disease prevention.

MANUAL THERAPIES

Manual CAM therapies include massage, shiatsu, reiki, therapeutic touch, acupressure, and chiropractic manipulation. Manual modalities are often used by patients for their purported effects of increasing circulation, pain alleviation, relaxation, and stimulation of immune function (Power et al., 2002). One small randomized controlled trial showed that massage therapy combined with stress management resulted in a decrease in medical care usage and an increase in health perceptions in PWH (Birk et al., 2000). A Cochrane review of massage in PWH showed that there appears to be a positive effect on the quality of life of affected individuals, particularly when massage is combined with other interventions such as meditation and stress management (Hillier et al., 2010).

TRADITIONAL MEDICINE

It is beyond the scope of this chapter to review the major traditional medical systems of India, China, and Africa. These systems are broad and complex, and they often combine different therapeutic modalities discussed previously in this chapter, such as a combination of herbal remedies and mind–body practices. Reasons for the use of these traditional systems by PWH stem from cultural beliefs, economic considerations, and limited accessibility to ART. Data from well-designed clinical trials regarding the efficacy and safety of these systems are sparse.

Traditional Indian medicine consisting of Ayurveda, Unani medicine, Siddha medicine, homeopathy, and naturopathy is used by two-thirds of the Indian population—especially in rural areas—for both primary care needs and HIV (Fritts et al., 2008).

Similarly, in Africa, a large portion of the population uses herbs for primary healthcare, HIV, and HIV-related health problems (Calitz et al., 2014). Although there is increasing study of herbal medicines and their potential for drug interactions in vitro, clinical trials are lacking.

TCM has probably been the most studied of the traditional systems, with data showing potential efficacy of TCM herbs for HIV and HIV-associated conditions. To date, no data exist to support the use of these systems as primary treatment for HIV. Some data exist on efficacy, especially of TCM on endpoints such as CD4[+] T cells and viral load; however, they have been inferior to ART. There may be a role for these systems in the management of symptoms, HIV-associated conditions, and delaying of HIV progression in those not on ART, but more data are needed with respect to their efficacy and herb–drug interactions.

Other aspects of traditional medical systems excluding herbal medicines, such as spiritual and healing practices and attitudes toward sickness and death (provided they do not harm), should be acknowledged and respected by physicians.

SUMMARY

Complementary, integrative, and alternative modalities are widely used by PWH. True alternative medicine for HIV is rare in developed countries but widespread in resource-limited areas. Physicians caring for PWH need to be aware of the prevalence of complementary therapies among their patients, the potential for herbal–drug interactions, and the potential toxicities of herbal medicines.

Physicians can also play an important role in fostering partnerships with their patients who use CAM modalities by using nonjudgmental and open communication about their benefits and risks. Some natural health products, such as fish oils and multivitamins, should be considered for use in PWH. Strategies to delay HIV progression using micronutrients, probiotics, and traditional natural products in PWH with high CD4[+] T-cell counts deserve further research, particularly in resource-limited settings in which access to ART is limited. Many mind–body techniques are useful for reducing stress, anxiety, and depression—all of which may affect HIV disease progression. These techniques may be especially useful in patients with adverse health behaviors who are unwilling to undergo formal therapy. They should also be considered in resource-limited settings as a self-empowering, low-cost means of coping with the emotional and physical challenges associated with HIV.

Treatment of HIV remains complex and multifactorial. Complementary and integrative modalities with low potential for adverse effects, such as mind–body techniques and certain natural products, should be considered in the balanced approach to dealing with the multidimensional aspects of HIV disease. The use of such practices will likely increase in the future. Therefore, it behooves physicians caring for these patients to understand the range of available options, their potential interactions with standard therapeutic regimens, and the ongoing data regarding their potential efficacy and safety.

RECOMMENDED READING

Baum, M. K., Campa, A., Lai, S., et al. (2013). Effect of micronutrient supplementation on disease progression in asymptomatic, antiretroviral-naive, HIV-infected adults in Botswana: a randomized clinical trial. JAMA, 310(20), 2154–2163.

Bhasin, M. K., Dusek, J. A., Chang, B., et al. (2013). Relaxation response induces temporal transcriptome changes in energy metabolism, insulin secretion and inflammatory pathways. PLoS One, 8(5), e62817. doi:10.1371/journal.pone.0062817

Brooks, K. M., George, J. M., & Kumar, P. (2017). Drug interactions in HIV treatment: complementary and alternative medicines and over-the-counter products. Expert Rev Clin Pharmacol, 10(1), 59–79.

Buric, I., Farias, M., Jong, J., et al. (2017). What is the molecular signature of mind–body interventions? A systematic review of gene expression changes induced by meditation and related practices. Front Immunol, 8, 670.

Cade, W., Reeds, D. N., Mondy, K. E., et al. (2010). Yoga lifestyle intervention reduces blood pressure in HIV-infected adults with cardiovascular disease risk factors. HIV Med, 11(6), 379–388.

Dinh, D. M., Volpe, G. E., Duffalo, C., et al. (2015). Intestinal microbiota, microbial translocation, and systemic inflammation in chronic HIV infection. J Infect Dis, 211(1), 19–27. doi:10.1093/infdis/jiu409

Halpin, S. N., Carruth, E. C., Rai, R. P., et al. (2018). Complementary and alternative medicine among persons living with HIV in the era of combined antiretroviral treatment. AIDS Behav, 22(3), 848–852.

Havens, P. L., Stephensen, C. B., Van Loan, M. D., et al. (2017). Vitamin D3 supplementation increases spine bone mineral density in adolescents and young adults with human immunodeficiency virus infection being treated with tenofovir disoproxil fumarate: a randomized, placebo-controlled trial. Clin Infect Dis, 66(2), 220–228.

Jalloh, M. A., Gregory, P. J., Hein, D., et al. (2017). Dietary supplement interactions with antiretrovirals: a systematic review. Int J STD AIDS, 28(1), 4–15. doi:10.1177/0956462416671087

Jiménez-Nácher, I., Alvarez, E., Morello, J., et al. (2011). Approaches for understanding and predicting drug interactions in human immunodeficiency virus-infected patients. Expert Opin Drug Metabol Toxicol, 7(4), 457–477.

Klatt, N. R., Canary, L. A., Sun, X., et al. (2013). Probiotic/prebiotic supplementation of antiretrovirals improves gastrointestinal immunity in SIV-infected macaques. J Clin Invest, 123(2), 903–907. doi:10.1172/JCI66227

Lavretsky, H., Epel, E., Siddarth, P., et al. (2013). A pilot study of yogic meditation for family dementia caregivers with depressive symptoms: effects on mental health, cognition, and telomerase activity. Int J Geriatr Psychiatry, 28(1), 57–65.

Saper, R. B., Phillips, R. S., Sehgal, A., et al. (2008). Lead, mercury, and arsenic in US-and Indian-manufactured Ayurvedic medicines sold via the Internet. JAMA, 300(8), 915–923.

REFERENCES

Agnoletto, V., Chiaffarino, F., Nasta, P., et al. (2003). Reasons for complementary therapies and characteristics of users among HIV-infected people. Int J STD AIDS, 14(7), 482–486. doi:10.1258/095646203322025803

Agnoletto, V., Chiaffarino, F., Nasta, P., et al. (2006). Use of complementary and alternative medicine in HIV-infected subjects. Complement Ther Med, 14(3), 193–199.

Aibana, O., Huang, C. C., Aboud, S., et al. (2019). Vitamin D status and risk of incident tuberculosis disease: a nested case-control study, systematic review, and individual-participant data meta-analysis. PLoS Med, 16(9), e1002907.

Amador-Licona, N., Díaz-Murillo, T. A., Gabriel-Ortiz, G., et al. (2016). Omega 3 fatty acids supplementation and oxidative stress in HIV-seropositive patients. A clinical trial. PloS One, 11(3), e0151637.

Amaniti, A., Sardeli, C., Fyntanidou, V., et al. (2019). Pharmacologic and non-pharmacologic interventions for HIV-neuropathy pain. A systematic review and a meta-analysis. Medicina, 55, 762.

Andrade, A. S., Hendrix, C., Parsons, T. L., et al. (2008). Pharmacokinetic and metabolic effects of American ginseng (Panax quinquefolius) in healthy volunteers receiving the HIV protease inhibitor indinavir. BMC Complement Altern Med, 8, 50-6882-8-50. doi:10.1186/1472-6882-8-50

Ashenafi, S., Amogne, W., Kassa, E., et al. (2019). Daily nutritional supplementation with vitamin D(3) and phenylbutyrate to treatment-naive HIV patients tested in a randomized placebo-controlled trial. Nutrients, 11(1), 133.

Aung, T., Halsey, J., Kromhout, D., et al. (2018). Associations of omega-3 fatty acid supplement use with cardiovascular disease risks: meta-analysis of 10 trials involving 77,917 individuals. JAMA Cardiol, 3(3), 225–234.

Awortwe, C., Bouic, P. J., Masimirembwa, C. M., et al. (2014). Inhibition of major drug metabolizing CYPs by common herbal medicines used by HIV/AIDS patients in Africa—Implications for herb-drug interactions. Drug Metab Lett, 7(2), 83–95. doi:DML-EPUB-58874

Bahall, M. (2017). Prevalence, patterns, and perceived value of complementary and alternative medicine among HIV patients: a descriptive study. BMC Complement Altern Med, 17(1), 422.

Barocas, J. A., So-Armah, K., Cheng, D. M., et al. (2019). Zinc deficiency and advanced liver fibrosis among HIV and hepatitis C co-infected anti-retroviral naive persons with alcohol use in Russia. PLoS One, 14(6), e0218852.

Baum, M. K., Campa, A., Lai, S. (2003). Zinc status in human immunodeficiency virus type 1 infection and illicit drug use. Clin Infect Dis, 37(Suppl 2), S117–S123. doi:CID30489

Baum, M. K., Campa, A., Lai, S., et al. (2013). Effect of micronutrient supplementation on disease progression in asymptomatic, antiretroviral-naive, HIV-infected adults in Botswana: a randomized clinical trial. JAMA, 310(20), 2154–2163.

Baum, M. K., Lai, S., Sales, S., et al. (2010). Randomized, controlled clinical trial of zinc supplementation to prevent immunological failure in HIV-infected adults. Clin Infect Dis, 50(12), 1653–1660. doi:10.1086/652864

Baum, M. K., Shor-Posner, G., Lai, S., et al. (1997). High risk of HIV-related mortality is associated with selenium deficiency. J AIDS, 15(5), 370–374.

Baum, M. K., Shor-Posner, G., Lu, Y., et al. (1995). Micronutrients and HIV disease progression. AIDS, 9(9), 1051–1056.

Beach, R. S., Mantero-Atienza, E., Shor-Posner, G., et al. (1992). Specific nutrient abnormalities in asymptomatic HIV-1 infection. AIDS, 6(7), 701–708.

Benson, H., Beary, J. F., & Carol, M. P. (1974). The relaxation response. Psychiatry, 37(1), 37–46.

Berginc, K., Trdan, T., Trontelj, J., et al. (2010). HIV protease inhibitors: garlic supplements and first-pass intestinal metabolism impact on the therapeutic efficacy. Biopharm Drug Dispos, 31(8–9), 495–505.

Beukel van den Bout-van den, C. J., Bosch, M. E., Burger, D. M., et al. (2008). Toxic lopinavir concentrations in an HIV-1 infected patient taking herbal medications. AIDS (London), 22(10), 1243–1244. doi:10.1097/QAD.0b013e32830261f4

Bhasin, M. K., Dusek, J. A., Chang, B., et al. (2013). Relaxation response induces temporal transcriptome changes in energy metabolism, insulin secretion and inflammatory pathways. PLoS One, 8(5), e62817. doi:10.1371/journal.pone.0062817

Bhatt, D. L., Steg, P. G., & Miller, M. (2019). Cardiovascular risk reduction with icosapent ethyl. Reply. N Engl J Med, 380(17), 1678.

Birk, T. J., McGrady, A., MacArthur, R. D., et al. (2000). The effects of massage therapy alone and in combination with other complementary therapies on immune system measures and quality of life in human immunodeficiency virus. J Altern Complement Med, 6(5), 405–414.

Bischoff-Ferrari, H. A., Willett, W. C., Wong, J. B., et al. (2005). Fracture prevention with vitamin D supplementation: a meta-analysis of randomized controlled trials. JAMA, 293(18), 2257–2264.

Blonk, M., Colbers, A., Poirters, A., et al. (2012). Effect of ginkgo biloba on the pharmacokinetics of raltegravir in healthy volunteers. Antimicrob Agents Chemother, 56(10), 5070–5075. doi:10.1128/AAC.00672-12

Bordes, C., Leguelinel-Blache, G., Lavigne, J.-P., et al. (2020). Interactions between antiretroviral therapy and complementary and alternative medicine: a narrative review. Clin Microbiol Infect, 26(9), 1161–1170. doi:10.1016/j.cmi.2020.04.019

Bormann, J. E., Gifford, A. L., Shively, M., et al. (2006). Effects of spiritual mantram repetition on HIV outcomes: a randomized controlled trial. J Behav Med, 29(4), 359–376.

Brooks, K. M., George, J. M., & Kumar, P. (2017). Drug interactions in HIV treatment: complementary and alternative medicines and over-the-counter products. Exp Rev Clin Pharmacol, 10(1), 59–79.

Buric, I., Farias, M., Jong, J., et al. (2017). What is the molecular signature of mind–body interventions? A systematic review of gene expression changes induced by meditation and related practices. Front Immunol, 8, 670.

Cade, W., Reeds, D. N., Mondy, K. E., et al. (2010). Yoga lifestyle intervention reduces blood pressure in HIV-infected adults with cardiovascular disease risk factors. HIV Med, 11(6), 379–388.

Calderón, M. M., Chairez, C. L., Gordon, L. A., et al. (2014). Influence of Panax ginseng on the steady state pharmacokinetic profile of lopinavir–ritonavir in healthy volunteers. Pharmacotherapy, 34(11), 1151–1158.

Calitz, C., Steenekamp, J. H., Steyn, J. D., et al. (2014). Impact of traditional African medicine on drug metabolism and transport. Exp Opin Drug Metab Toxicol, 10(7), 991–1003.

Chou, R., Qaseem, A., Snow, V., et al. (2007). Diagnosis and treatment of low back pain: a joint clinical practice guideline from the American College of Physicians and the American Pain Society. Ann Intern Med, 147(7), 478–491.

Creswell, J. D., Myers, H. F., Cole, S. W., et al. (2009). Mindfulness meditation training effects on CD4+ T cell T lymphocytes in HIV-1 infected adults: a small randomized controlled trial. Brain Behav Immun, 23(2), 184–188.

Dawson-Hughes, B., Harris, S. S., Krall, E. A., et al. (1997). Effect of calcium and vitamin D supplementation on bone density in men and women 65 years of age or older. N Engl J Med, 337(10), 670–676.

de Maat, M. M., Hoetelmans, R. M., Mathôt, R. A., et al. (2001). Drug interaction between St. John's wort and nevirapine. AIDS, 15(3), 420–421.

Deng, X., Jiang, M., Zhao, X., et al. (2014). Efficacy and safety of traditional Chinese medicine for the treatment of acquired immunodeficiency syndrome: a systematic review. J Tradit Chin Med, 34(1):1–9.

De Truchis, P., Kirstetter, M., Perier, A., et al. (2005). Treatment of hypertriglyceridemia in PWH under HAART, by (n-3) polyunsaturated fatty acids: a double-blind randomized prospective trial in 122 patients [Abstract 39]. Paper presented at the 12th Conference on Retroviruses and Opportunistic Infections, Boston, February 22–25.

Dhalla, S., Chan, K. J., Montaner, J. S., et al. (2006). Complementary and alternative medicine use in British Columbia—A survey of HIV positive people on antiretroviral therapy. Complement Ther Clin Pract, 12(4), 242–248.

DiCenzo, R., Shelton, M., Jordan, K., et al. (2003). Coadministration of milk thistle and indinavir in healthy subjects. Pharmacotherapy, 23(7), 866–870.

Dillon, S., Lee, E., Kotter, C., et al. (2014). An altered intestinal mucosal microbiome in HIV-1 infection is associated with mucosal and systemic immune activation and endotoxemia. Mucosal Immunol, 7(4), 983–994.

Dinh, D. M., Volpe, G. E., Duffalo, C., et al. (2015). Intestinal microbiota, microbial translocation, and systemic inflammation in chronic HIV infection. J Infect Dis, 211(1), 19–27. doi:10.1093/infdis/jiu409

Dudgeon, W. D., Phillips, K. D., Bopp, C. M., et al. (2004). Physiological and psychological effects of exercise interventions in HIV disease. AIDS Patient Care STDs, 18(2), 81–98.

Duggan, J., Peterson, W. S., Schutz, M., et al. (2001). Use of complementary and alternative therapies in PWH. AIDS Patient Care STDs, 15(3), 159–167.

Duncan, L. G., Moskowitz, J. T., Neilands, T. B., et al. (2012). Mindfulness-based stress reduction for HIV treatment side effects: a randomized, wait-list controlled trial. J Pain Symptom Manage, 43(2), 161–171.

Dunne, E. M., Balletto, B. L., Donahue, M. L., et al. (2019). The benefits of yoga for PWH: a systematic review and meta-analysis. Complement Ther Clin Pract, 34, 157–164. doi:10.1016/j.ctcp.2018.11.009

Eckard, A. R., & McComsey, G. A. (2014). Vitamin D deficiency and altered bone mineral metabolism in HIV-infected individuals. Curr HIV/AIDS Rep, 11(3), 263–270.

Epel, E. S., Blackburn, E. H., Lin, J., et al. (2004). Accelerated telomere shortening in response to life stress. Proc Natl Acad Sci USA, 101(49), 17312–17315. doi:0407162101

Ezeamama, A. E., Guwatudde, D., Wang, M., et al. (2016). Vitamin-D deficiency impairs CD4 T-cell count recovery rate in HIV-positive adults on highly active antiretroviral therapy: a longitudinal study. Clin Nutr, 35(5), 1110–1117.

Falutz, J., Tsoukas, C., & Gold, P. (1988). Zinc as a cofactor in human immunodeficiency virus-induced immunosuppression. JAMA, 259(19), 2850–2851.

Fawzi, W. W., Msamanga, G. I., Spiegelman, D., et al. (2004). A randomized trial of multivitamin supplements and HIV disease progression and mortality. N Engl J Med, 351(1), 23–32.

Feinstein, M. J., Bahiru, E., Achenbach, C., et al. (2016). Patterns of cardiovascular mortality for HIV-infected adults in the United States: 1999–2013. Am J Cardiol, 117(2), 214–220.

Feinstein, M. J., Hsue, P. Y., Benjamin, L. A., et al. (2019). Characteristics, prevention, and management of cardiovascular disease in people living with HIV: a scientific statement from the American Heart Association. Circulation, 140(2), e98–e124.

Filteau, S., PrayGod, G., Kasonka, L., et al.; NUSTART (Nutritional Support for Africans Starting Antiretroviral Therapy) Study Team (2015). Effects on mortality of a nutritional intervention for malnourished HIV-infected adults referred for antiretroviral therapy: a randomised controlled trial. BMC Med, 13, 17-014-0253-8. doi:10.1186/s12916-014-0253-8

Fogacci, F., Strocchi, E., Veronesi, M., et al. (2020). Effect of omega-3 polyunsaturated fatty acids treatment on lipid pattern of HIV patients: a meta-analysis of randomized clinical trials. Mar Drugs, 18(6):292. doi:10.3390/md18060292

Freiberg, M. S., Cheng, D. M., Gnatienko, N., et al. (2020). Effect of zinc supplementation vs placebo on mortality risk and HIV disease progression among HIV-positive adults with heavy alcohol use: a randomized clinical trial. JAMA Netw Open, 3(5), e204330.

Fritts, M., Crawford, C. C., Quibell, D., et al. (2008). Traditional Indian medicine and homeopathy for HIV/AIDS: a review of the literature. AIDS Res Ther, 5, 25-6405-5-25. doi:10.1186/1742-6405-5-25

Galantino, M. L., Shepard, K., Krafft, L., et al. (2005). The effect of group aerobic exercise and t'ai chi on functional outcomes and quality of life for persons living with acquired immunodeficiency syndrome. J Altern Complement Med, 11(6), 1085–1092.

Galera, R. L., Pascuet, E. R., Mur, J. E., et al. (2008). Interaction between cat's claw and protease inhibitors atazanavir, ritonavir and saquinavir. Eur J Clin Pharmacol, 64(12), 1235–1236.

Gallicano, K., Foster, B., & Choudhri, S. (2003). Effect of short-term administration of garlic supplements on single-dose ritonavir pharmacokinetics in healthy volunteers. Br J Clin Pharmacol, 55(2), 199–202.

Gayner, B., Esplen, M. J., DeRoche, P., et al. (2012). A randomized controlled trial of mindfulness-based stress reduction to manage affective symptoms and improve quality of life in gay men living with HIV. J Behav Med, 35(3), 272–285.

Gerber, J. G., Kitch, D. W., Fichtenbaum, C. J., et al. (2008). Fish oil and fenofibrate for the treatment of hypertriglyceridemia in HIV-infected subjects on antiretroviral therapy: results of ACTG A5186. J AIDS, 47(4), 459–466. doi:10.1097/QAI.0b013e31815bace2

Gonzalez-Garcia, M., Ferrer, M. J., Borras, X., et al. (2014). Effectiveness of mindfulness-based cognitive therapy on the quality of life, emotional status, and CD4+ T cell count of patients aging with HIV infection. AIDS Behav, 18(4), 676–685.

Graham, N. M., Sorensen, D., Odaka, N., et al. (1991). Relationship of serum copper and zinc levels to HIV-1 seropositivity and progression to AIDS. J AIDS, 4(10), 976–980.

Greene, K. B., Berger, J., Reeves, C., et al. (1999). Most frequently used alternative and complementary therapies and activities by participants in the AMCOA study. J Assoc Nurses AIDS Care, 10(3), 60–73.

Grosso, G., Micek, A., Marventano, S., et al. (2016). Dietary n-3 PUFA, fish consumption and depression: a systematic review and meta-analysis of observational studies. J Affect Disord, 205, 269–281.

Gruppo italiano per lo studio della sopravvivenza nell'infarto miocardico. (1999). Dietary supplementation with n-3 polyunsaturated fatty acids and vitamin E after myocardial infarction: results of the GISSI-prevenzione trial. Lancet, 354(9177), 447–455. doi:S0140673699070725

Gwaza, L., Aweeka, F., Greenblatt, R., et al. (2013). Co-administration of a commonly used Zimbabwean herbal treatment (African potato) does not alter the pharmacokinetics of lopinavir/ritonavir. Int J Infect Dis, 17(10), e857–e861.

Hafner, V., Jager, M., Matthee, A. K., et al. (2010). Effect of simultaneous induction and inhibition of CYP3A by St. John's wort and ritonavir on CYP3A activity. Clin Pharmacol Ther, 8(2), 191–196.

Halpin, S. N., Carruth, E. C., Rai, R. P., et al. (2018). Complementary and alternative medicine among persons living with HIV in the era of combined antiretroviral treatment. AIDS Behav, 22(3), 848–852.

Havens, P. L., Stephensen, C. B., Van Loan, M. D., et al. (2017). Vitamin D3 supplementation increases spine bone mineral density in adolescents and young adults with human immunodeficiency virus infection being treated with tenofovir disoproxil fumarate: a randomized, placebo-controlled trial. Clin Infect Dis, 66(2), 220–228.

Hecht, F. M., Moskowitz, J. T., Moran, P., et al. (2018). A randomized, controlled trial of mindfulness-based stress reduction in HIV infection. Brain Behav Immun, 73, 331–339. doi:S0889-1591(18)30190-9

Hepburn, M. J., Dyal, K., Runser, L. A., et al. (2004). Low serum vitamin B$_{12}$ levels in an outpatient HIV-infected population. Int J STD AIDS, 15(2), 127–133. doi:10.1258/095646204322764334

Hillier, S. L., Louw, Q., Morris, L., et al. (2010). Massage therapy for people with HIV/AIDS. Cochrane Database Syst Rev, 1, CD007502.

Hinman, R. S., McCrory, P., Pirotta, M., et al. (2014). Acupuncture for chronic knee pain: a randomized clinical trial. JAMA, 312(13), 1313–1322.

Holick, M. F., Binkley, N. C., Bischoff-Ferrari, H. A., et al. (2011). Evaluation, treatment, and prevention of vitamin D deficiency: an Endocrine Society clinical practice guideline. J Clin Endocrin Metab, 96(7), 1911–1930.

Hu, Y., Hu, F. B., Manson, J. E. (2019). Marine omega-3 supplementation and cardiovascular disease: an updated meta-analysis of 13 randomized controlled trials involving 127,477 participants. J Am Heart Assoc, 8(19), e013543. doi:10.1161/JAHA.119.013543

Ironson, G., O'Cleirigh, C., Fletcher, M. A., et al. (2005). Psychosocial factors predict CD4$^+$ T cell and viral load change in men and women with human immunodeficiency virus in the era of highly active antiretroviral treatment. Psychosom Med, 67(6), 1013–1021. doi:67/6/1013

Jacek H., Rentsch, K. M., Steinert, H. C., et al. (2004). No effect of garlic extract on saquinavir kinetics and hepatic CYP3A4 function measured by the erythromycin breath test. Clin Pharmacol Ther, 75(2), P80. doi:10.1016/j.clpt.2003.11.304

Jackson, R. D., LaCroix, A. Z., Gass, M., et al. (2006). Calcium plus vitamin D supplementation and the risk of fractures. N Engl J Med, 354(7), 669–683.

Jalloh, M. A., Gregory, P. J., Hein, D., et al. (2017). Dietary supplement interactions with antiretrovirals: a systematic review. Int J STD AIDS, 28(1), 4–15. doi:10.1177/0956462416671087

Jiamton, S., Chaisilwattana, P., & Pepin, J. (2005). A randomized placebo-controlled trial of the impact of multiple micronutrient supplementation on HIV-1 genital shedding among Thai subjects. J AIDS, 37(1), 1216–1218.

Jiamton, S., Pepin, J., Suttent, R., et al. (2003). A randomized trial of the impact of multiple micronutrient supplementation on mortality among HIV-infected individuals living in Bangkok. AIDS, 17(17), 2461–2469.

Jones, C. Y., Tang, A. M., Forrester, J. E., et al. (2006). Micronutrient levels and HIV disease status in PWH on highly active antiretroviral therapy in the nutrition for healthy living cohort. J AIDS, 43(4), 475–482. doi:10.1097/01.qai.0000243096.27029.fe

Josephs, J., Fleishman, J., Gaist, P., et al. (2007). Use of complementary and alternative medicines among a multistate, multisite cohort of PWH. HIV Med, 8(5), 300–305.

Kaiser, J. D., Campa, A. M., Ondercin, J. P., et al. (2006). Micronutrient supplementation increases CD4$^+$ T cell count in HIV-infected individuals on highly active antiretroviral therapy: a prospective, double-blinded, placebo-controlled trial. J AIDS, 42(5), 523–528. doi:10.1097/01.qai.0000230529.25083.42

Kakalia, S., Sochett, E. B., Stephens, D., et al. (2011). Vitamin D supplementation and CD4 count in children infected with human immunodeficiency virus. J Pediatr, 159(6), 951–957.

Kasibhatta, R., & Naidu, M. (2007). Influence of piperine on the pharmacokinetics of nevirapine under fasting conditions. Drugs in R & D, 8(6), 383–391.

Kayode, I., & Anaba, U. (2020). Effect of vitamin D, selenium, or zinc supplementation in human immunodeficiency virus: a systematic review. AIDS Rev, 22, 1–10.

Kelso-Chichetto, N. E., Okafor, C. N., Harman, J. S., et al. (2016). Complementary and alternative medicine use for HIV management in the state of Florida: medical monitoring project. J Altern Complement Med, 22(11), 880–886.

Ladenheim, D., Horn, O., Werneke, U., et al. (2008). Potential health risks of complementary alternative medicines in HIV patients. HIV Med, 9(8), 653–659.

Lamorde, M., Byakika-Kibwika, P., & Merry, C. (2012). Pharmacokinetic interactions between antiretroviral drugs and herbal medicines. Br J Hosp Med, 73(3), 132–136.

Lavretsky, H., Epel, E., Siddarth, P., et al. (2013). A pilot study of yogic meditation for family dementia caregivers with depressive symptoms: effects on mental health, cognition, and telomerase activity. Int J Geriatr Psychiatry, 28(1), 57–65.

Lee, L. S., Andrade, A. S., & Flexner, C. (2006). Interactions between natural health products and antiretroviral drugs: pharmacokinetic and pharmacodynamic effects. Clin Infect Dis, 43(8), 1052–1059. doi:CID39658

Leserman, J. (2008). Role of depression, stress, and trauma in HIV disease progression. Psychosom Med, 70(5), 539–545. doi:10.1097/PSY.0b013e3181777a5f

Leserman, J., Petitto, J., Gu, H., et al. (2002). Progression to AIDS, a clinical AIDS condition and mortality: psychosocial and physiological predictors. Psychol Med, 32(06), 1059–1073.

Leserman, J., Petitto, J. M., Perkins, D. O., et al. (1997). Severe stress, depressive symptoms, and changes in lymphocyte subsets in human immunodeficiency virus-infected men: a 2-year follow-up study. Arch Gen Psychiatry, 54(3), 279–285.

Levine, G. N., Lange, R. A., Bairey-Merz, C. N., et al. (2017). Meditation and cardiovascular risk reduction: a scientific statement from the American Heart Association. J Am Heart Assoc, 6(10), e002218.

Linde, K., Allais, G., Brinkhaus, B., et al. (2009). Acupuncture for tension-type headache. Cochrane Database Syst Rev, 1, CD007587.

Littlewood, R. A., & Vanable, P. A. (2008). Complementary and alternative medicine use among HIV-positive people: research synthesis and implications for HIV care. AIDS Care, 20(8), 1002–1018.

Littlewood, R. A., & Vanable, P. A. (2011). A global perspective on complementary and alternative medicine use among PWH in the era of antiretroviral treatment. Curr HIV/AIDS Rep, 8(4), 257–268.

Littlewood, R. A., & Vanable, P. A. (2014). The relationship between CAM use and adherence to antiretroviral therapies among persons living with HIV. Health Psychol, 33(7), 660.

Liu, C., Yang, Y., Gange, S. J., et al. (2009). Disclosure of complementary and alternative medicine use to health care providers among HIV-infected women. AIDS Patient Care STDs, 23(11), 965–971.

London, A. S., Foote-Ardah, C. E., Fleishman, J. A., et al. (2003). Use of alternative therapists among people in care for HIV in the United States. Am J Public Health, 93(6), 980–987.

Lorenc, A., & Robinson, N. (2013). A review of the use of complementary and alternative medicine and HIV: issues for patient care. AIDS Patient Care STDs, 27(9), 503–510.

Lozupone, C. A., Li, M., Campbell, T. B., et al. (2013). Alterations in the gut microbiota associated with HIV-1 infection. Cell Host Microbe, 14(3), 329–339.

Ma, J., Li, Y., Ye, Q., et al. (2000). Constituents of red yeast rice, a traditional Chinese food and medicine. J Agric Food Chem, 48(11), 5220–5225.

MacArthur, R. D., Levine, S. D., & Birk, T. J. (1993). Supervised exercise training improves cardiopulmonary fitness in HIV-infected persons. Med Sci Sports Exer, 25(6), 684–688.

MacDonald, L., Murty, M., & Foster, B. C. (2009). Antiviral drug disposition and natural health products: risk of therapeutic alteration and resistance. Expert Opin Drug Metab Toxicol, 5(6), 563–578. doi:10.1517/17425250902942302

Maggiolo, F., Rizzardini, G., Raffi, F., et al. (2019). Bone mineral density in virologically suppressed people aged 60 years or older with HIV-1 switching from a regimen containing tenofovir disoproxil fumarate to an elvitegravir, cobicistat, emtricitabine, and tenofovir alafenamide single-tablet regimen: a multicentre, open-label, phase 3b, randomised trial. Lancet HIV, 6(10), e655–e666.

Manheimer, E., Cheng, K., Linde, K., et al. (2010). Acupuncture for peripheral joint osteoarthritis. Cochrane Database Syst Rev, 1, CD001977.

Manson, J. E., Cook, N. R., Lee, I. M., et al. (2019). Marine n-3 fatty acids and prevention of cardiovascular disease and cancer. N Engl J Med, 380(1), 23–32.

Mateo-Carrasco, H., Gálvez-Contreras, M. C., Fernández-Ginés, F. D., et al. (2012). A potential drug–herbal interaction between ginkgo biloba and efavirenz. J Int Assoc Physicians AIDS Care, 11(2), 98–100. doi:10.1177/1545109711435364

McCain, N. L., Gray, D. P., Elswick Jr, R., et al. (2008). A randomized clinical trial of alternative stress management interventions in persons with HIV infection. J Consult Clin Psychol, 76(3), 431.

McClelland, R. S., Baeten, J. M., Overbaugh, J., et al. (2004). Micronutrient supplementation increases genital tract shedding of HIV-1 in women: results of a randomized trial. J AIDS, 37(5), 1657–1663.

Milan, F. B., Arnsten, J. H., Klein, R. S., et al. (2008). Use of complementary and alternative medicine in inner-city persons with or at risk for HIV infection. AIDS Patient Care STDs, 22(10), 811–816.

Mills, E., Wilson, K., Clarke, M., et al. (2005). Milk thistle and indinavir: a randomized controlled pharmacokinetics study and meta-analysis. Eur J Clin Pharmacol, 61(1), 1–7.

Molto, J., Valle, M., Miranda, C., et al. (2011). Herb–drug interaction between Echinacea purpurea and darunavir–ritonavir in PWH. Antimicrob Agents Chemother, 55(1), 326–330. doi:10.1128/AAC.01082-10

Molto, J., Valle, M., Miranda, C., et al. (2012a). Effect of milk thistle on the pharmacokinetics of darunavir–ritonavir in PWH. Antimicrob Agents Chemother, 56(6), 2837–2841. doi:10.1128/AAC.00025-12

Molto, J., Valle, M., Miranda, C., et al. (2012b). Herb–drug interaction between Echinacea purpurea and etravirine in PWH. Antimicrob Agents Chemother, 56(10), 5328–5331. doi:10.1128/AAC.00025-12

Mutlu, E. A., Keshavarzian, A., Losurdo, J., et al. (2014). A compositional look at the human gastrointestinal microbiome and immune activation parameters in HIV-infected subjects. PLoS Pathog, 10(2), e1003829.

Muzembo, B. A., Ngatu, N. R., Januka, K., et al. (2019). Selenium supplementation in HIV-infected individuals: a systematic review of randomized controlled trials. Clin Nutr ESPEN, 34, 1–7.

Naoroibam, R., Metri, K. G., Bhargav, H., et al. (2016). Effect of integrated yoga (IY) on psychological states and CD4 counts of HIV-1 infected patients: a randomized controlled pilot study. Int J Yoga, 9(1), 57–61. doi:10.4103/0973-6131.171723

Okunade, K. S., Olowoselu, O. F., Osanyin, G. E., et al. (2018). Selenium deficiency and pregnancy outcome in pregnant women with HIV in Lagos, Nigeria. Int J Gynaecol Obstet, 142(2), 207–213.

Oliveira, J. M., Rondó, P. H., Yudkin, J. S., et al. (2014). Effects of fish oil on lipid profile and other metabolic outcomes in PWH on antiretroviral therapy: a randomized placebo-controlled trial. Int J STD AIDS, 25(2), 96–104.

ORIGIN Trial Investigators. (2008). Rationale, design, and baseline characteristics for a large international trial of cardiovascular disease prevention in people with dysglycemia: the ORIGIN trial (Outcome Reduction with an Initial Glargine Intervention). Am Heart J, 155(1), 26–32.

Overton, E. T., Chan, E. S., Brown, T. T., et al. (2015). Vitamin D and calcium attenuate bone loss with antiretroviral therapy initiation: a randomized trial. Ann Intern Med, 162(12), 815–824.

Owen-Smith, A., Diclemente, R., & Wingood, G. (2007). Complementary and alternative medicine use decreases adherence to HAART in HIV-positive women. AIDS Care, 19(5), 589–593.

Patel, P., Song, I., Borland, J., et al. (2011). Pharmacokinetics of the HIV integrase inhibitor S/GSK1349572 co-administered with acid-reducing agents and multivitamins in healthy volunteers. J Antimicrob Chemother, 66(7), 1567–1572. doi:10.1093/jac/dkr139

Patel, S. J., Kemper, K. J., & Kitzmiller, J. P. (2017). Physician perspectives on education, training, and implementation of complementary and alternative medicine. Adv Med Educ Practice, 8, 499.

Pence, B. W., Miller, W. C., Whetten, K., et al. (2006). Prevalence of DSM-IV-defined mood, anxiety, and substance use disorders in an HIV clinic in the southeastern United States. J AIDS, 42(3), 298–306. doi:10.1097/01.qai.0000219773.82055.aa

Penzak, S. R., Robertson, S. M., Hunt, J. D., et al. (2010). Echinacea purpurea significantly induces cytochrome P450 3A activity but does not alter lopinavir–ritonavir exposure in healthy subjects. Pharmacotherapy, 30(8), 797–805. doi:10.1592/phco.30.8.797

Perazzo, J. D., Webel, A. R., Alam, S. K., et al. (2018). Relationships between physical activity and bone density in people living with HIV: results from the SATURN-HIV study. J Assoc Nurses AIDS Care, 29(4), 528–537.

Peters, B. S., Wierzbicki, A. S., Moyle, G., et al. (2012). The effect of a 12-week course of omega-3 polyunsaturated fatty acids on lipid parameters in hypertriglyceridemic adult PWH undergoing HAART: a randomized, placebo-controlled pilot trial. Clin Ther, 34(1), 67–76.

Phillips, K. D., & Skelton, W. D. (2001). Effects of individualized acupuncture on sleep quality in HIV disease. J Assoc Nurses AIDS Care, 12(1), 27–39.

Piscitelli, S. C., Burstein, A. H., Chaitt, D., et al. (2000). Indinavir concentrations and St. John's wort. Lancet, 355(9203), 547–548.

Piscitelli, S. C., Burstein, A. H., Welden, N., et al. (2002). The effect of garlic supplements on the pharmacokinetics of saquinavir. Clin Infect Dis, 34(2), 234–238. doi:CID010586

Piscitelli, S. C., Formentini, E., Burstein, A. H., et al. (2002). Effect of milk thistle on the pharmacokinetics of indinavir in healthy volunteers. Pharmacotherapy, 22(5), 551–556.

Power, R., Gore-Felton, C., Vosvick, M., et al. (2002). HIV: effectiveness of complementary and alternative medicine. Prim Care, 29(2), 361–378.

Quigley, A., O'Brien, K., & Parker, K. (2019). Exercise and cognitive function in people living with HIV: a scoping review. Disabil Rehabil, 41(12), 1384–1395.

Ramirez-Garcia, M. P., Gagnon, M. P., Colson, S., et al. (2019). Mind-body practices for people living with HIV: a systematic scoping review. BMC Complement Altern Med, 19(1), 125.

Range, N., Changalucha, J., Krarup, H., et al. (2006). The effect of multivitamin/mineral supplementation on mortality during treatment of pulmonary tuberculosis: a randomised two-by-two factorial trial in Mwanza, Tanzania. Br J Nutr, 95(4), 762–770.

Ravi, S., Khalili, H., Abbasian, L., et al. (2016). Effect of omega-3 fatty acids on depressive symptoms in HIV-positive individuals: a randomized, placebo-controlled clinical trial. Ann Pharmacother, 50(10), 797–807.

Remacha, A. F., Cadafalch, J., Sarda, P., et al. (2003). Vitamin B-12 metabolism in PWH in the age of highly antiretroviral therapy: role of homocysteine in assessing vitamin B-12 status. Am J Clin Nutr, 77(2), 420–424.

Rigsby, L. W., Dishman, R., Jackson, A. W., et al. (1992). Effects of exercise training on men seropositive for the human immunodeficiency virus-1. Med Sci Sports Exercise, 24(1), 6–12.

Robertson, S. M., Davey, R. T., Voell, J., et al. (2008). Effect of Ginkgo biloba extract on lopinavir, midazolam and fexofenadine pharmacokinetics in healthy subjects. Curr Med Res Opin, 24(2), 591–599. doi:10.1185/030079908X260871

Sandhu, R. S., Prescilla, R. P., Simonelli, T. M., et al. (2003). Influence of goldenseal root on the pharmacokinetics of indinavir. J Clin Pharmacol, 43(11), 1283–1288.

Saper, R. B., Phillips, R. S., Sehgal, A., et al. (2008). Lead, mercury, and arsenic in US- and Indian-manufactured Ayurvedic medicines sold via the Internet. JAMA, 300(8), 915–923.

Shere-Wolfe, K. D., Tilburt, J. C., D'Adamo, C., et al. (2013). Infectious diseases physicians' attitudes and practices related to complementary and integrative medicine: results of a national survey. Evid Based Complement Altern Med, 2013, Article ID 294381.

Sherwood, J. E., Mesner, O. C., Weintrob, A. C., et al. (2012). Vitamin D deficiency and its association with low bone mineral density, HIV-related factors, hospitalization, and death in a predominantly black HIV-infected cohort. Clin Infect Dis, 55(12), 1727–1736.

Shlay, J. C., Chaloner, K., Max, M. B., et al. (1998). Acupuncture and amitriptyline for pain due to HIV-related peripheral neuropathy: a randomized controlled trial. JAMA, 280(18), 1590–1595.

Slain, D., Amsden, J. R., Khakoo, R. A., et al. (2005). Effect of high-dose vitamin C on the steady-state pharmacokinetics of the protease inhibitor indinavir in healthy volunteers. Pharmacotherapy, 25(2), 165–170.

Song, I., Borland, J., Arya, N., et al. (2015). Pharmacokinetics of dolutegravir when administered with mineral supplements in healthy adult subjects. J Clin Pharmacol, 55(5), 490–496. doi:10.1002/jcph.439

Standish, L., Greene, K., Bain, S., et al. (2001). Alternative medicine use in HIV-positive men and women: demographics, utilization patterns and health status. AIDS Care, 13(2), 197–208.

Stringer, W. W., Berezovskaya, M., O'Brien, W. A., et al. (1998). The effect of exercise training on aerobic fitness, immune indices, and quality of life in HIV patients. Med Sci Sports Exercise, 30(1), 11–16.

Stussman, B. J., Black, L. I., Barnes, P. M., et al. (2015). Wellness-related use of common complementary health approaches among adults: United States, 2012. Natl Health Stat Rep, 85, 1–12.

Sudfeld, C. R., Aboud, S., Kupka, R., et al. (2014). Effect of selenium supplementation on HIV-1 RNA detection in breast milk of Tanzanian women. Nutrition, 30(9), 1081–1084.

Sudfeld, C. R., Buchanan, A., Ulenga, N., et al. (2019). Effectiveness of a multivitamin supplementation program among HIV-infected adults in Tanzania. AIDS, 33(1):93–100.

Sudfeld, C. R., Wang, M., Aboud, S., et al. (2012). Vitamin D and HIV progression among Tanzanian adults initiating antiretroviral therapy. PloS One, 7(6), e40036.

Swanson, B., Keithley, J., Baum, L., et al. (2018). Effects of fish oil on HIV-related inflammation and markers of immunosenescence: a randomized clinical trial. J Altern Complement Med, 24(7):709–716. doi:10.1089/acm.2017.0222

Tenforde, M. W., Yadav, A., Dowdy, D. W., et al. (2017). Vitamin A and D deficiencies associated with incident tuberculosis in PWH initiating antiretroviral therapy in multinational case-cohort study. J AIDS, 75(3), e71–e79.

Thompson, M. A., Aberg, J. A., Hoy, J. F., et al. (2012). Antiretroviral treatment of adult HIV infection: 2012 recommendations of the International Antiviral Society–USA panel. JAMA, 308(4), 387–402.

Ting, A., Chow, Y., & Tan, W. (2013). Microbial and heavy metal contamination in commonly consumed traditional Chinese herbal medicines. J Tradit Chin Med, 33(1), 119–124.

van Heeswijk, R. P., Cooper, C. L., Foster, B. C., et al. (2005). Effect of high-dose vitamin C on hepatic cytochrome P450 3A4 activity. Pharmacotherapy, 25(12), 1725–1728.

Vickers, A. J., Cronin, A. M., Maschino, A. C., et al. (2012). Acupuncture for chronic pain: individual patient data meta-analysis. Arch Intern Med, 172(19), 1444–1453.

Visser, R. D., & Grierson, J. (2002). Use of alternative therapies by PWH in Australia. AIDS Care, 14(5), 599–606.

Vogl, D., Rosenfeld, B., Breitbart, W., et al. (1999). Symptom prevalence, characteristics, and distress in AIDS outpatients. J Pain Symptom Manage, 18(4), 253–262.

Vujkovic-Cvijin, I., Dunham, R. M., Iwai, S., et al. (2013). Dysbiosis of the gut microbiota is associated with HIV disease progression and tryptophan catabolism. Sci Transl Med, 5(193), 193ra91. doi:10.1126/scitranslmed.3006438

Wahner-Roedler, D. L., Lee, M. C., Chon, T. Y., et al. (2014). Physicians' attitudes toward complementary and alternative medicine and their knowledge of specific therapies: 8-year follow-up at an academic medical center. Complement Ther Clin Practice, 20(1), 54–60.

Warburton, D. E., Nicol, C. W., & Bredin, S. S. (2006). Health benefits of physical activity: the evidence. Can Med Assoc J, 174(6), 801–809. doi:174/6/801

Webb, L., Perry-Parrish, C., Ellen, J., & Sibinga, E. (2018). Mindfulness instruction for HIV-infected youth: a randomized controlled trial. AIDS Care, 30(6), 688–695.

Whetten, K., Reif, S., Whetten, R., et al. (2008). Trauma, mental health, distrust, and stigma among HIV-positive persons: implications for effective care. Psychosom Med, 70(5), 531–538. doi:10.1097/PSY.0b013e31817749dc

Wiegman, D. J., Brinkman, K., & Franssen, E. J. (2009). Interaction of Ginkgo biloba with efavirenz. AIDS, 23(9), 1184–1185.

Witt, C. M., Jena, S., Brinkhaus, B., et al. (2006). Acupuncture for patients with chronic neck pain. Pain, 125(1), 98–106.

Wohl, D. A., Tien, H. C., Busby, M., et al. (2005). Randomized study of the safety and efficacy of fish oil (omega-3 fatty acid) supplementation with dietary and exercise counseling for the treatment of antiretroviral therapy-associated hypertriglyceridemia. Clin Infect Dis, 41(10), 1498–1504. doi:CID37106

Wynia, M. K., Eisenberg, D. M., & Wilson, I. B. (1999). Physician–patient communication about complementary and alternative medical therapies: a survey of physicians caring for patients with human immunodeficiency virus infection. J Altern Complement Med, 5(5), 447–456.

Zhang, L., Tin, A., Brown, T. T., et al. (2017). Vitamin D deficiency and metabolism in HIV-infected and HIV-uninfected men in the multicenter AIDS cohort study. AIDS Res Hum Retroviruses, 33(3), 261–270. doi:10.1089/AID.2016.0144

13.

HIV CARE COORDINATION

Amanda A. Westlake, Sally Spencer-Long, and Daniel J. Skiest

IMPORTANCE OF AN INTERDISCIPLINARY APPROACH TO HIV PATIENT CARE

LEARNING OBJECTIVE

Describe the importance of an interdisciplinary team approach to the optimal management of PWH

WHAT'S NEW?

- An interdisciplinary team is an essential comprehensive care strategy to approaching the HIV continuum of care—to help diagnose, link, engage, and successfully treat PWH who increasingly have other chronic illnesses. The interdisciplinary HIV team can effectively address the full range of medical, psychosocial, and behavioral comorbidities.

KEY POINTS

- As PWH are surviving longer there is an increased prevalence of non–HIV-related comorbidities, which has resulted in an increasing need for chronic disease management.

- The barriers to each of the steps in the HIV continuum of care need to be identified, anticipated, and addressed. Often, addressing these barriers entails medical, psychosocial, and other specialized services.

- Coordination of care using a patient-centered interdisciplinary team model of care, which usually involves multiple clinicians and healthcare team members working together to meet the needs of the patient, can be an effective strategy for initial and continued engagement in care, especially for complicated patients and/or those with few resources.

Currently available antiretroviral therapies (ART) have higher efficacy, are associated with better adherence, and have lower side effect profiles compared to ART available in previous decades. This has led to prolonged survival, approaching that of the general population (Samji et al., 2014; Wada et al., 2014). This prolonged survival, coupled with the fact that the US incidence of HIV has decreased only moderately over the past decade (Centers for Disease Control and Prevention [CDC], 2020), has resulted in an increased number of PWH needing complex medical care.

In 2018, over half of PWH were age 50 or older (CDC, 2020). HIV accentuates the complications of aging, manifested by the earlier onset of cardiovascular disease, cognitive impairment, certain types of cancer, and diabetes in PWH relative to their HIV-negative peers. As a result of both factors (increased age of PWH and increased risk of certain comorbidities), PWH often require chronic disease management in addition to the treatment of HIV infection (Chu & Selwyn, 2011). Thus, care for PWH is often provided by clinicians with expertise in general medicine, behavioral health, and substance abuse treatment, in addition to HIV medicine and infectious diseases.

The HIV epidemic disproportionately affects people of color, those with less education, lower income, lack of adequate insurance, lack of permanent housing, and a history of incarceration. Black men who have sex with men (MSM) have the highest rates of new infection (CDC, 2020). Ongoing stigma discourages HIV testing and may result in late presentations to care with more advanced disease. There may be real or perceived personal, cultural, or system-based barriers to care (Bauman et al., 2013; CDC, 2011; Irvine et al., 2014; Scanlon & Vreeman, 2013), which in some individuals can result in lower levels of continued engagement and suboptimal viral suppression (Gardner et al., 2011; White House Office of National AIDS Policy, 2014).

The social determinants of health play an important role in caring for PWH. Many PWH are facing the day-to-day struggles of poverty—unstable housing, lack of transportation, inadequate medical insurance—which can impact their engagement in HIV care. These individuals are also likely to have more difficulty navigating the increasingly complicated US healthcare system, resulting in fragmented care or disengagement. If not addressed, these issues may result in lower levels of continued engagement.

The goals of HIV clinical care are to suppress viral replication, decrease HIV-related morbidities, improve immune status, prolong survival, improve quality of life, and decrease HIV transmission (US Department of Health and Human Services, 2020b). The key steps needed to achieve these goals have been described as the HIV continuum of care and include timely diagnosis, linkage to and subsequent retention in care, and finally initiation and continuation of ART (CDC Fact Sheets, 2019). The steps in the HIV continuum are the basis of the recent US plan "Ending the HIV Epidemic: A Plan for America," which includes the goal to decrease HIV incidence by 90% by 2030 (US Department of Health and Human Services, 2020a) (Figure 13.1).

The first step in the HIV continuum of care is the timely diagnosis of HIV infection. This requires a combination of targeted community outreach to increase testing in high-risk populations as well as routine HIV screening in the general population (US Preventive Services Task Force, 2019). The next step is (prompt) linkage to care, followed by engagement in care, and retention of the patient in care while ART is initiated. A growing body of literature supports prolonged benefits (increased likelihood of viral suppression and retention in care) with same-day or rapid (within 14 days of diagnosis) ART initiation (Ford et al., 2018). Once ART is initiated—and potentially for decades to follow—the patient needs to be effectively followed and supported in care to ensure durable virologic suppression. There are barriers to success at each step in the continuum that need to be identified, anticipated, and addressed by clinicians and others providing care. The goals in the HIV continuum are cost-effective (Gopalappa et al., 2012), but achieving them can be challenging and often requires input and expertise from multiple providers and allied health workers, often as an interdisciplinary HIV care team working together to address potential barriers, including depression, substance abuse, lack of housing, and lack of medical insurance (Dombrowski et al., 2015).

The following are illustrative case examples of the types of complex comorbidities and chronic conditions that currently characterize the care of PWH:

1. A 35-year-old man recently released from jail, where he was diagnosed with HIV. His CD4 count is 50 cells/mm^3 and he is currently homeless and opioid-dependent.

This patient has several immediate needs: ART, stable housing, substance abuse treatment, and opportunistic infection prophylaxis. The priorities of the patient and the HIV provider may not be in the same order; the patient may feel that treatment of opioid use disorder and housing take precedence, while the provider prioritizes ART initiation. To effectively meet his needs and provide appropriate medical care, the treating clinician will likely require the assistance of multiple HIV team members, including a case manager, financial counselor, recovery coach, and social worker and a provider who treats opioid use disorder. Ensuring access to medication-assisted treatment for opioid use disorder is critical, as those who are treated with methadone or buprenorphine have a two-fold increase in ART adherence and a corresponding 48% increase in viral suppression (MacArthur et al., 2012).

2. An obese 55-year-old woman who has a history of major depression and prior inconsistent medication adherence, which led to virologic failure. She is currently taking ART and has an undetectable viral load.

This patient stopped seeing her therapist and psychiatrist 1 year ago because she felt she no longer required mental health treatment. However, she was recently divorced, lost her job (and thus her health insurance), and is not accepting of her new diagnosis of type 2 diabetes mellitus. Although this patient's HIV is currently controlled, the HIV provider is concerned about her recent major life events leading to a depressive episode, which may impact medication adherence, and thought this may have caused the decreased efficacy of her first HIV

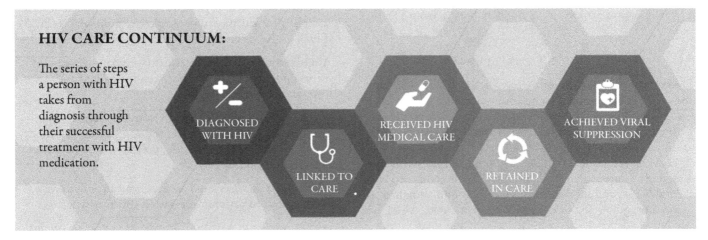

HIV CARE CONTINUUM:

The series of steps a person with HIV takes from diagnosis through their successful treatment with HIV medication.

DIAGNOSED WITH HIV

LINKED TO CARE

RECEIVED HIV MEDICAL CARE

RETAINED IN CARE

ACHIEVED VIRAL SUPPRESSION

Figure 13.1 The HIV care continuum. SOURCE: Centers for Disease Control and Prevention. HIV.Care.Continuum/HIV.gov. Available at: https://files.hiv.gov/s3fs-public/care-continuum-banner-v1.jpg

regimen. This patient will need several issues addressed simultaneously, including treatment of her depression, applying for Medicaid and AIDS Drug Assistance Program (ADAP), and treatment of her obesity and diabetes. She would benefit from prompt referrals to behavioral health for treatment of her depression (both therapist and psychiatrist), to a case manager and financial counselor for assistance with ADAP and Medicaid, and to a nutritionist and endocrinologist for treatment of coexisting medical problems.

3. A perinatally infected 24-year-old woman who has a history of intermittent viral suppression. She is in an abusive relationship with her boyfriend. She presents with vaginal bleeding after an episode of domestic violence and is found to have a positive urine pregnancy test.

This patient presents unique challenges to the provision of optimal care, including obstetrical needs, mental health concerns, and safe housing, and she may require additional efforts to retain in care. A social worker would be helpful to work with the patient to identify housing that would be both safe and supportive (e.g., family shelter) and to provide guidance with implementation of a restraining order to prevent future harmful events. The case manager could assist with linkage to a primary care provider and with transportation needs required to keep appointments for continued engagement in care. A high priority would be arranging prenatal visits as well as primary care and specialist evaluations (e.g., high-risk obstetrician and infectious diseases). Clinicians would need to request assistance from behavioral health specialists to provide ongoing support for the current pregnancy, situational stress/depression, posttraumatic stress, and acceptance of her HIV disease, which will involve life-long engagement in care to maintain optimal health.

RECOMMENDED READING

National Center for HIV/AIDS. Viral hepatitis, STD, and TB prevention 2017. Accessed August 29, 2018.
Saag MS, Gandhi RT, Hoy JF, et al. Antiretroviral drugs for treatment and prevention of HIV infection in adults: 2020 Recommendations of the International Antiviral Society—USA Panel. *JAMA*. Published online October 14, 2020. doi:10.1001/jama.2020.17025

INTERDISCIPLINARY TEAM CARE

Due to the complexities of caring for the PWH, including the often concomitant diagnoses of substance use disorder and mental illness, coordinated, patient-centered care is optimally delivered in an ambulatory, chronic disease model by an interdisciplinary (multidisciplinary) team (Gallant et al., 2011; Mugavero et al., 2011, Ojikutu et al., 2014). In this integrated HIV care model, HIV primary care is combined with mental health and substance abuse services into a single coordinated program. The integrated HIV care model, which has been used effectively to meet the medical and social needs of PWH for decades (largely via Ryan White funding; see later discussion), is essentially a patient-centered medical home. In fact, it has been suggested that the HIV integrated care model can be used as a template for primary care clinic medical homes (Beane et al., 2014). In the integrated or coordinated care model, the goal is to treat the *patient* rather than the *disease*. Team members work together with the patient to clarify goals of care. This leads to improved outcomes by engaging various healthcare workers to work together to help the patient navigate through the complex healthcare system (Bauman et al., 2013; Boyd & Lucas, 2014; Chu & Selwyn, 2011).

Studies have demonstrated that shared and coordinated patient care among different disciplines can increase the efficiency of care without duplication of services among multiple healthcare service providers (Gallant et al., 2011; Horberg et al., 2012). A recent study of PWH on Medicaid and with chronic health problems (asthma, chronic obstructive pulmonary disease, diabetes, congestive heart failure) and psychiatric illness and/or substance use disorders found that patients in a medical home model of care had more efficient care, which resulted in substantial cost savings, compared to patients not cared for in a medical home model (Crits-Christoph et al., 2018).

ROLES OF HIV PATIENT CARE TEAM

A comprehensive HIV care team will typically have a physician, nurse, case manager (often a nurse), advanced practitioner, mental health provider, social worker, nutritionist, health educator, clinical pharmacist, substance abuse treatment counselor, and financial counselor (Gallant et al., 2011; Horberg et al., 2012). The makeup of a particular HIV care team will be specific to the needs of the local patients served and the resources available. Some teams may not have all of the listed positions, and some members of a care team may undertake tasks not traditionally part of their job description. In many cases the roles may overlap (Table 13.1).

- Physicians and advanced practitioners diagnose, treat, refer to other specialists, and often lead the interdisciplinary care team.

- Public health workers, nurses, and health educators offer initial HIV screening; provide HIV prevention education, including information on preexposure prophylaxis (PrEP) if HIV negative; and link PWH to an HIV provider.

- Administrative staff and case managers arrange appointments and serve as liaisons between the patient and healthcare providers.

- Social workers and financial advisors link patients to available community resources (housing, disability, food assistance, etc.) and assist with applications for healthcare insurance, including ADAP.

- Clinical pharmacists and health educators provide assistance with medication information and adherence.

- Nursing staff and nutritionists provide education on nutrition, adherence, and healthy lifestyles.

Table 13.1 DIFFERENT ROLES OF HIV PATIENT CARE TEAM

	ROLES	RESPONSIBILITIES	POTENTIALLY INVOLVED PERSONNEL
Diagnosis (prevention)	Community outreach	Offer HIV screening Link patients to primary care (offer preexposure prophylaxis [PrEP] if HIV negative)	Public health worker Researcher Nurse Health educator
Linkage to care	Patient navigation	Arrange appointments Function as a liaison between patient and the healthcare provider	Administrative staff Nurse Case manager
Linkage to care Prescribing ART	Insurance/social support	Link patients to available community resources Apply for medical insurance, including ADAP Advocate for patient's needs	Social worker Financial advisor Case manager Advocacy group liaison
Engagement/retention	Retention/engagement	Outreach to out-of-care patients Outreach to public health and community-based organizations Gather patient data on retention	Administrative staff Nurse Case manager Public health worker
Engagement/retention	Mental health	Provide counseling Provide mental health treatment Provide psychosocial support	Social worker Psychologist Psychiatrist Substance abuse counselor
Prescribing ART Viral suppression	Medical care	Provide medical management Refer to appropriate specialist(s) Educate on medication adherence	HIV specialist or primary care clinician Pharmacist/local pharmacy worker Nurse
Viral suppression	Patient education	Provide education on nutrition, adherence, drug interaction, healthy lifestyle, etc.	Nurse Adherence counselor Nutritionist Health educator Pharmacist HIV specialist or primary care clinician
Linkage Engagement/retention Prescribing ART Viral suppression	Population health management	Gather data on each step of HIV continuum of care Conduct quality improvement Measure patient outcomes Evaluate projects/programs	Electronic medical record provider Administrative staff Data support staff Researcher HIV specialist or primary care clinician Public health worker
All stages of care	Team lead	Provide system-based coordination Develop infrastructure	Any team member Commonly done by a clinician

- Psychiatrists, therapist/counselors, and substance abuse counselors respectively provide mental health assessment and treatment, psychosocial support, and treatment of addiction (including substance use disorder).

A team leader is usually designated (physician or advanced practitioner). The team leader should facilitate communication among various team members to support the goal of quality care for patients. Ongoing communication (via electronic health records [EHR], meetings, phone consultation) between the interdisciplinary team and the patient is essential to ensure collaborative and patient-centered care (Gallant et al., 2011; Nancarrow et al., 2013). Regular meetings to discuss the needs of patients and to reassess team members' roles are important. The complexity of the patient's medical and psychosocial needs can often be overwhelming, and learning the

patient's priorities and making partnered decisions with the patient can help interdisciplinary coordination of care among healthcare professionals and the patient (Gallant et al., 2011; Mugavero et al., 2011). There are limited data on standardized ways of measuring interdisciplinary team care (Boyd & Lucas, 2014). However, periodic internal review of the interdisciplinary members' responsibilities and infrastructure can help improve and consolidate responsibilities, avoid duplication of tasks, and augment the efficiency and effectiveness of the team. One survey indicated that patients who received care in an interdisciplinary HIV care model had high levels of satisfaction (Vachirasudlekha et al., 2014).

Numerous factors result in the need for more resources to manage PWH, including the higher rates of homelessness, substance abuse, and mental illness. Providing comprehensive care for these patients often requires referrals to other healthcare providers, financial counselors, social workers, and ancillary services. Depending on the model and scope of HIV care, the referrals may occur within the same interdisciplinary HIV team, to another provider in the same institution, or to someone outside the system. Effective referrals can be initiated through a structured referral process utilizing established referral sources.

While there is no one approach that will work for all HIV providers or delivery models with regard to appropriate referrals, certain practices may be widely applicable. Initially, an assessment of the patient's referral needs should be performed and objectives for the referral should be clearly defined. Ideally, providers from different disciplines should work together to meet the identified patient healthcare needs. In the interdisciplinary team-based approach, decisions regarding referrals and patient care are shared. In collaborative arrangements, decision-making responsibilities are shared and ownership of changes in care may shift depending on the level of expertise required at a given time.

It is helpful for team members to become familiar with the various agencies in their community, especially those that maintain a core group of professionals committed to the care of PWH. This encourages further support and involvement in the patient's progress. Referral of patients to on-site providers is preferred, but referrals off-site may be necessary. This can present its own set of challenges, especially regarding transportation, communication, and reimbursement. In some cases, if resources allow, the case manager may accompany the patient to ensure the patient attends the appointment and any recommendations are understood by the patient and are carried out. Clear two-way communication between the HIV provider and the specialist is important for the goals of care to be met. The specialist should clearly identify the questions and objectives of the referring provider and the patient and should clearly state the plan of care, which should be readily accessible. A shared EHR can help to alleviate the communication issue. However, direct communication between the referring provider and the specialist, as well as with other team members, is optimal.

Responsibility for the implementation and follow-up of recommended changes in the plan of care should be clearly outlined. Making one team member responsible for tracking the status of referrals helps ensure their completion. Frequent and timely communication between the referring organization and the referral providers can decrease gaps in care and ensure continuity of quality care.

QUALITY IMPROVEMENT

The goal of the HIV care is to optimize patient health, decrease HIV transmission, and end the AIDS epidemic. A clear vision with focused efforts to improve clinical outcomes and quality can help to develop, improve, and sustain effective patient care practices (Gallant et al., 2011; Mugavero et al., 2011). An up-to-date and available patient registry with relevant clinical and retention data can help monitor and measure patient care outcomes. Examples of relevant clinical and retention data include adherence, missed appointments,

recent contact information and outreach, detectable viral load, status of ART, and evidence of failing or failed care (e.g., development of antiretroviral resistance, new opportunistic infections, onset or worsening of comorbid conditions, or clinical decline).

In a resource-limited setting, targeted data collection may be beneficial instead of attempting to obtain all data at once. For example, it may be beneficial to prioritize and focus resources to high-risk and vulnerable patients, such as those who have been out of care for more than 6 months or have a detectable viral load. A patient registry with clinical and laboratory data can also support the measurement of and improve patient outcomes by strategizing quality-improvement projects. Examples include annual influenza vaccination among patients with HIV and appropriate sexually transmitted disease screening.

FUNDING FOR HIV CARE – THE RYAN WHITE HIV/AIDS PROGRAM

The Ryan White HIV/AIDS Program is an important component of HIV patient care (HRSA HIV/AIDS, 2021; Sood et al., 2014). This federal program, which began in 1991, funds healthcare and services to PWH. Program funding is distributed among Parts A through F. Part A provides emergency assistance to eligible areas that are most severely affected by HIV/AIDS. Part B provides grants to all 50 states and US territories or associated jurisdictions. Part C provides outpatient-based comprehensive primary healthcare for PWH. Part D provides family-centered care for women, infants, children, and youth with HIV/AIDS. Part F provides funds for a variety of programs, such as health information technology, social media, and outreach programs. The program also funds dental care, special projects, training programs, and minority AIDS initiatives.

The Ryan White Program funds cities, states, and local community-based organizations to provide HIV care and treatment services to more than half a million people each year and assists approximately 52% of all people diagnosed with HIV in the United States. In fiscal year 2018, the Ryan White Program provided $2.34 billion in funding (HRSA, 2021). The program is known for its "wrap-around" services to patients with HIV. However, coverage and requirements of Ryan White–funded programs may vary state to state, and grantees of the program should review eligibility and criteria for renewal (including required data collection and conformance with standards of care) (HRSA, 2021). The Ryan White Program is always the "payer of last resort."

An important component of the Ryan White Program (under Part B) is ADAP, which provides medications approved by the US Food and Drug Administration to low-income people living with HIV who have limited or no health coverage from private insurance, Medicaid, or Medicare. ADAP funds may also be used to purchase health insurance for eligible clients and for services that enhance access to, adherence to, and monitoring of drug treatments. Different states have varied eligibility criteria and renewal processes, including documentation of income status (15 states established income eligibility at 200% or less of the federal poverty level), diagnosis of

HIV, opportunistic infections, chronic medical conditions, and/or other service needs (HRSA ADAP, 2021).

Several studies have demonstrated better clinical outcomes for patients receiving care at Ryan White–funded clinics versus nonfunded clinics. Wrap-around clinical and case management services provided by Ryan White Programs result in increased retention in care and consequently in increased viral suppression (Kay et al., 2018). Assistance with necessities such as food and transportation (utilized by one in three patients served by the Ryan White Program) and housing (utilized by one in five patients) is a key component of support for people with HIV with incomes at or below the poverty level. In a study of 8,000 people with HIV, nearly 75% of patients receiving care at Ryan White–funded facilities achieved viral suppression despite a greater likelihood of poverty and unstable housing. Further, patients with incomes at or below the poverty level were more likely to achieve viral suppression if they received care at a Ryan White–funded facility (Weiser et al., 2015).

Ryan White programs ensure access to ART among uninsured and underinsured PWH and are thus associated with increased viral suppression among those groups. In an analysis of over 18,000 patients in which 41% had Ryan White assistance, patients whose private or Medicaid coverage was supplemented by the Ryan White program were both more likely to be prescribed ART and to sustain viral suppression than those without Ryan White supplementation (Bradley et al., 2016). A recent study of over 3,000 MSM enrolled in the Miami-Dade County Ryan White Program demonstrated that nearly 85% of the men achieved sustained viral suppression (Sheehan et al., 2020). In this study, one of the factors associated with increased odds of sustained viral suppression was having an HIV physician who serves a larger volume of Ryan White clients. The central role of the medical case manager as part of the multidisciplinary Ryan White team was identified as one reason the rate of viral suppression was higher than expected.

RECOMMENDED READING

Gardner LI, Giordano TP, Marks G, et al. Enhanced personal contact with HIV patients improves retention in primary care: a randomized trial in six US HIV clinics. *Clin Infect Dis.* 2014;59(5):725–734.

Henry Kaiser Family Foundation. Total federal HIV/AIDS grant funding. 2014. Available at http://kff.org/hivaids/state-indicator/total-federal-grant-funding. Accessed August 2, 2018.

Joint United Nations Programme on HIV/AIDS (UNAIDS). 90-90-90: an ambitious treatment target to help end the AIDS epidemic. 2014. Available at https://new.pancap.org/pc/pcc/media/pancap_document/90-90-90_Targets.pdf. Accessed November 29, 2015.

Newhouse RP, Spring B. Interdisciplinary evidence-based practice: moving from silos to synergy. *Nurs Outlook.* 2010;58(6):309–317.

Shah M, Risher K, Berry SA, et al. The epidemiologic and economic impact of improving HIV testing, linkage, and retention in care in the United States. *Clin Infect Dis.* 2016;62(2):220–229.

REFERENCES

Bauman LJ, Braunstein S, Calderon Y, et al. Barriers and facilitators of linkage to HIV primary care in New York City. *J AIDS.* 2013;64(1):S20–S26.Beane SN, Culyba RJ, DeMayo M, Armstrong W. Exploring the medical home in Ryan White HIV care settings: a pilot study. *J Assoc Nurses AIDS Care.* May–June 2014;25(3):191–202.

Boyd CM, Lucas GM. Patient-centered care for people living with multi-morbidity. *Curr Opin HIV AIDS.* 2014;9(4):419–427.

Bradley H, Viall AH, Wortley PM, et al. Ryan White HIV/AIDS program assistance and HIV treatment outcomes. *Clin Infect Dis.* January 1, 2016;62(1):90–98.

Centers for Disease Control and Prevention. HIV.Care.Continuum/HIV. gov. Available at: https://files.hiv.gov/s3fs-public/care-continuum-banner-v1.jpg.

Centers for Disease Control and Prevention (CDC). HIV surveillance—United States, 1981–2008. *MMWR Recomm Rep.* 2011;60(21):689–693.

Centers for Disease Control and Prevention (CDC). HIV Surveillance Report, 2018 (Updated). Published May 2020. Available at http://www.cdc.gov/hiv/library/reports/hiv-surveillance.html. Accessed July 26, 2020.

Centers for Disease Control and Prevention (CDC), Division of HIV/AIDS Prevention. Understanding the HIV care continuum. 2019. Available at https://www.cdc.gov/hiv/pdf/library/factsheets/cdc-hiv-care-continuum.pdf. Accessed January 21, 2021.

Chu C, Selwyn PA. An epidemic in evolution: the need for new models of HIV care in the chronic disease era. *J Urban Health.* 2011;88(3):556–566.

Crits-Christoph P, Gallop R, Noll E, et al. Impact of a medical home model on costs and utilization among comorbid HIV-positive Medicaid patients. *Am J Manag Care.* 2018;24:368–375.

Dombrowski JC, Simoni JM, Katz DA, et al. Barriers to HIV care and treatment among participants in a public health HIV care relinkage program. *AIDS Patient Care STDs.* 2015;29:279–287.

Ford N, Migone C, Calmy A, et al. Benefits and risks of rapid initiation of antiretroviral therapy. *AIDS.* 2018;32(1):17–23.

Gallant JE, Adimora AA, Carmichael JK, et al. Essential components of effective HIV care: a policy paper of the HIV Medicine Association of the Infectious Diseases Society of America and the Ryan White Medical Providers Coalition. *Clin Infect Dis.* 2011;53:1043–1050.

Gardner EM, McLees MP, Steiner JF, et al. The spectrum of engagement in HIV care and its relevance to test-and-treat strategies for prevention of HIV infection. *Clin Infect Dis.* 2011;52(6):793–800.

Gopalappa C, Farnham PG, Hutchinson A, et al. Cost effectiveness of the national HIV/AIDS strategy goal of increasing linkage to care for HIV-infected persons. *J AIDS.* 2012;66(1):99–105.

Health Resources and Services Administration (HRSA). The Ryan White HIV/AIDS program. Available at http://hab.hrsa.gov/abouthab/aboutprogram.html. Accessed January 20, 2021.

Health Resources and Services Administration (HRSA). The Ryan White HIV/AIDS program. Part B: AIDS Drub Assistance Program> Available at https://hab.hrsa.gov/about-ryan-white-hivaids-program/part-b-aids-drug-assistance-program. Accessed January 20, 2021.

Horberg MA, Hurley LB, Towner WJ, et al. Determination of optimized multidisciplinary care team for maximal antiretroviral therapy adherence. *J AIDS.* 2012;60(2):183–190.

Irvine MK, Chamberlin SA, Robbins RS, et al. Improvements in HIV care engagement and viral load suppression following enrollment in a comprehensive HIV care coordination program. *Clin Infect Dis.* 2014;60:298–310.

Kay ES, Batey DS, Mugavero MJ. The Ryan White HIV/AIDS Program: Supplementary Service Provision Post-Affordable Care Act [published correction appears in AIDS Patient Care STDS. 2019 Aug;33(8):379–380]. *AIDS Patient Care STDs.* 2018;32(7):265–271. doi:10.1089/apc.2018.0032

MacArthur GJ, Minozzi S, Martin N, et al. Opiate substitution treatment and HIV transmission in people who inject drugs: systematic review and meta-analysis. *BMJ.* 2012;345:e5945.

Mugavero MJ, Norton WE, Saag MS. Health care system and policy factors influencing engagement in HIV medical care: piecing together the fragments of a fractured health care delivery system. *Clin Infect Dis.* 2011;52(Suppl 2):S238–S246.

Nancarrow SA, Booth A, Ariss S, et al. Ten principles of good interdisciplinary team work. *Hum Resour Health*. 2013;11:19.

Ojikutu B, Holman J, Kunches L, et al. Interdisciplinary HIV care in a changing healthcare environment in the USA. *AIDS Care*. 2014;26(6):731–735.Samji H, Cescon A, Hogg RS, et al. Closing the gap: increases in life expectancy among treated HIV-positive individuals in the United States and Canada. *PLoS One*. 2014;8(12):e81355.

Scanlon ML, Vreeman RC. Current strategies for improving access and adherence to antiretroviral therapies in resource-limited settings. *HIV AIDS (Auckl)*. 2013;5:1–17.

Sheehan DM, Dawit R, Gbadamosi SO, et al. Sustained HIV viral suppression among men who have sex with men in the Miami-Dade County Ryan White Program: the effect of demographic, psychosocial, provider and neighborhood factors. *BMC Public Health*. 2020;20(1). doi:10.1186/s12889-020-8442-1

Sood N, Juday T, Vanderpuye-Orgle J, et al. HIV care providers emphasize the importance of the Ryan White program for access to quality of care. *Health Affairs*. 2014;33(3):394–400.

US Department of Health and Human Services. *About ending the HIV epidemic: plan for America*. 2020a. Available at https://www.hiv.gov/federal-response/ending-the-hiv-epidemic/overview. Accessed August 30, 2020.

US Department of Health and Human Services. Panel on antiretroviral guidelines for adults and adolescents: guidelines for the use of antiretroviral agents in HIV-1-infected adults and adolescents. 2020b. Available at https://clinicalinfo.hiv.gov/en/guidelines/adult-and-adolescent-arv/whats-new-guidelines. Accessed October 4, 2020.

US Preventive Services Task Force, Owens DK, Davidson KW, Krist AH, et al. Screening for HIV infection: US Preventive Services Task Force Recommendation Statement. *JAMA*. June 18, 2019 18;321(23):2326–2336.

Wada N, Jacobson LP, Cohen M, et al. Cause-specific mortality among HIV-infected individuals, by CD4+ cell count at HAART initiation, compared with HIV-uninfected individuals. *AIDS*. 2014;28:257–265.

Weiser J, Beer L, Frazier E, et al. Service delivery and patient outcomes in Ryan White HIV/AIDS program-funded and nonfunded health care facilities in the United States. *JAMA Intern Med*. 2015;175(10):1650–1659.

White House Office of National AIDS Policy. *National HIV/AIDS strategy: update of 2014 federal actions to achieve national goals and improve outcomes along the HIV care continuum*. Washington, DC: White House Office of National AIDS Policy, 2014.

Vachirasudlekha B, Cha A, Berkowitz L, et al. Interdisciplinary HIV care—patient perceptions. *Int J Health Care Qual Assur*. 2014;27(5): 405–413.

14.

THE PHARMACIST'S ROLE IN HIV CARE

Jennifer Cocohoba

INTRODUCTION

HIV, a chronic disease, requires a multidisciplinary approach to ensure that all aspects of a patient's health are addressed. Medications are essential tools used for prevention, treatment, and the management of comorbid conditions. Pharmacists play an important role in all of these because they facilitate access to medications and ensure accurate dispensing. Pharmacist specialists have also become essential members of the healthcare team because their expertise extends beyond dispensing. When included on the healthcare team, HIV pharmacist expertise can be utilized to improve the selection, safety, efficacy, and overall quality of medication therapy.

LEARNING OBJECTIVES

- Describe common settings in which HIV pharmacists practice.

- List three potential ways in which pharmacists can contribute to the care of people with HIV (PWH).

WHAT'S NEW?

- Data and experience continue to accumulate on the innovative and meaningful ways that pharmacists contribute to improved HIV health outcomes along the care continuum and how pharmacists can help increase access to timely HIV-related services, including testing and preexposure prophylaxis (PrEP). Systematic interventions such as antiretroviral stewardship programs involving clinical pharmacists can also prevent and address hospital medication errors as well as contribute to cost savings.

KEY POINTS

- HIV pharmacists are a diverse group of providers who work to improve the health of PWH via medication therapy management, quality assurance practices, research, and other avenues.

- HIV pharmacists may be particularly skilled at managing complex antiretroviral drug–drug interactions, recommending therapies for people with complex antiretroviral therapy (ART) resistance patterns, and providing education and support with regard to adherence.

- If practicing with a physician under a collaborative drug therapy management agreement, an HIV pharmacist may be able to provide more direct disease state management (e.g., prescribing and ordering lab tests), including PrEP, HIV treatment, and associated conditions.

THE HIV CLINICAL PHARMACIST SPECIALIST

Medications for HIV have become more convenient but not less complex. Approximately half of PWH in the US are over the age of 50, and a large proportion of them take five or more medications (Okoli et al., 2020). For this reason, having a clinical pharmacist as a part of the healthcare team can greatly enhance HIV care. HIV-specialized clinical pharmacists typically receive advanced training in HIV during postdoctorate residencies, infectious diseases fellowship programs, or HIV-specific fellowship programs, although some acquire their HIV knowledge through practice-based experience and intense self-study. Certification programs such as the American Academy of HIV Medicine's HIV Pharmacist (AAHIVP) certification program and the HIV Pharmacotherapy Continuing Education Program offered through the University of Buffalo can help distinguish pharmacists who are well versed in many aspects of HIV pharmacotherapy (McLaughlin et al., 2018). Many HIV pharmacists also pursue Board of Pharmacy Specialties certification in infectious diseases (BCIDP) or ambulatory care (BCACP) due to the wide knowledge base, roles, and responsibilities that can be associated with caring for PWH.

SETTINGS IN WHICH HIV PHARMACISTS PROVIDE PATIENT CARE

PWH encounter many different pharmacists who contribute to their care across the spectrum of their disease and medical visits. For patients who are acutely ill, the first setting in which they may interact with an HIV-specialized pharmacist is in the hospital. In many health systems, the infectious diseases (ID) team oversees consultative care for PWH, and HIV/ID pharmacists on these multidisciplinary teams contribute skills and knowledge to enhance HIV care. For example, the current paradigm of "test and treat" has increased the number of patients diagnosed with HIV and immediately initiated on ART during a hospital stay, but HIV pharmacotherapy is riddled with complex drug–drug interactions and requires close monitoring to dose adjust for renal insufficiency or hepatic dysfunction. HIV pharmacists on inpatient clinical services assist the team in selecting appropriate ART and opportunistic infection regimens, screen for complex drug–drug interactions, assist in ordering and interpreting resistance testing or therapeutic drug monitoring assays (if indicated), provide discharge counseling for patients initiating new ART, and can help coordinate benefit coverage for any antiretroviral therapies prescribed during an inpatient hospital stay (Durham et al., 2017).

Patients in a clinic may interact with HIV-specialized pharmacists who work as part of an interdisciplinary ambulatory care team. These HIV clinical pharmacists have a wide range of duties commensurate with their experience and level of expertise. Responsibilities can include dispensing medications in a clinic-associated pharmacy; reviewing patient charts to ensure optimal pharmacotherapy; providing one-on-one patient education; consulting with patients and medical providers regarding medication-related problems, adherence, or resistance testing results; initiating and managing ART or PrEP; ordering lab tests; and initiating, adjusting, or discontinuing medications for opportunistic infections and other concomitant disease states.

ART is typically dispensed by a community pharmacist. Nearly all PWH will interact with community pharmacists at some point; in fact, the community pharmacist may be the healthcare provider with whom a healthy PWH interacts most frequently. In larger metropolitan areas, pharmacists and staff who are knowledgeable about HIV disease may frequently be found at pharmacies that specialize in HIV care. These HIV-focused pharmacies may belong to large retail chains, may be independently owned, or may be integrated within a larger health system (Gilbert & Gerzenshtein, 2016). The pharmacy may elect to undergo an accreditation process to be officially recognized as a specialty pharmacy, although this designation tends to indicate expertise in many disease states and not just HIV alone. Patient education and counseling, provision of reminder devices and adherence aids, managing the practical aspects of synchronizing and coordinating medication refills, facilitating procurement of antiretrovirals, and working with patients to address medication-related financial barriers (e.g., copay fees) are just a few of the activities conducted by HIV community pharmacists. As a testament to some of the less tangible but positive impact of community pharmacies, a large demonstration project by the Centers for Disease Control and Prevention (CDC) found a 12.9% improvement in retention in care when medical clinics partnered with community pharmacies in a patient-centered medical home model (Byrd et al., 2019).

PHARMACIST CONTRIBUTIONS TO HIV CARE: A SAMPLE OF SPECIFIC SKILLS

Pharmacists make ideal treatment facilitators due to their extensive training in comprehensive medication therapy management (MTM). The goal of MTM is for a pharmacist to optimize a patient's treatment through identification, resolution, and prevention of medication-related problems (American Pharmacists Association and the National Association of Chain Drug Stores Foundation, 2008). This definition of MTM is intentionally broad so that it may accommodate the wide variety of activities a pharmacist may perform to optimize a patient's therapy. For example, during a medication therapy review, a pharmacist may discover dangerous drug–drug interactions and poor patient adherence. The pharmacist may work closely with the patient and their medical provider to create an action plan that addresses these issues. This section presents a sample of some of the evidence supporting the positive impact pharmacists have when caring for PWH.

AMELIORATING ANTIRETROVIRAL ERRORS

HIV-specialized pharmacists play an important role in preventing and ameliorating medication errors. Published literature suggests that PWH are at high risk of incurring medication errors when hospitalized and that these errors—including incorrect antiretroviral regimens, incorrect dosing strategies, incorrect scheduling, or drug–drug interactions—may occur at various points during their hospital stay (Li & Foisy, 2014).

Pharmacist-led antiretroviral stewardship programs have resulted in reduced ART medication errors in hospitalized persons with HIV. A joint statement endorsed by the American Academy of HIV Medicine, the HIV Medicine Association, and the Infectious Disease Society of America recommends inclusion of a clinical pharmacist on interdisciplinary antiretroviral stewardship teams and highlights the contributions of pharmacists in improving antiretroviral use in hospitalized patients (Koren et al., 2020). One hospital found that 45% of their 334 inpatients with HIV had at least one medication error occur during their stay, and 31% of these patients still had uncorrected errors at the time of discharge (Zucker et al., 2016). After 1 year, a prospective audit and feedback strategy was employed and the proportion of admissions with errors dropped to 31%, although 31% still had uncorrected errors at discharge. During the second year, prospective review plus intervention was implemented. The proportion of medication errors remained stable at 37%, but the rate of uncorrected errors at discharge dropped to 12%. A Texas antiretroviral stewardship program implemented pharmacist education, a pharmacist-led ART checklist, and modifications to the hospital order-entry and verification system to support prospective audit and feedback; this combination of interventions significantly reduced the number of ART-related errors from 208 to 24 (Shea et al., 2018). An antiretroviral stewardship program implemented in Philadelphia found that of 567 hospital admissions involving persons with HIV, 43% required at least one stewardship intervention and the cost savings associated with the program was estimated at $263,428 over a 1-year period (DePuy et al., 2019). Finally, errors of omission can greatly impact the health of hospitalized patients. A small study of 139 patients found that hospital pharmacist intervention improved the rates of appropriate opportunistic infection prophylaxis from 58% to 93% (Schatz et al., 2016).

IDENTIFYING AND MANAGING DRUG–DRUG INTERACTIONS AND POLYPHARMACY

Many antiretroviral agents strongly induce or inhibit the cytochrome P450 system, particularly the 3A4 isoform. Because approximately 60% of the most commonly prescribed drugs are also metabolized via cytochrome P450 3A4, pharmacists are trained to carefully review a patient's medication list to identify adverse drug interactions that may result in excess toxicity or subtherapeutic levels of the object drug or that may result in alterations in the HIV drug concentrations. Pharmacists provide management strategies for known interactions. For important theoretical interactions, pharmacists may suggest using therapeutic drug monitoring and can help interpret the levels garnered from these tests. In a single-center study, 248 persons with HIV were referred to a clinical pharmacist for medication review (McNicholl et al., 2017). Patients were taking an average of 11.6 ± 5.7 medications in addition to their ART. The pharmacist identified medications that were potentially inappropriate (as defined by Beers Criteria) in 63% of the cohort, uncovered contraindicated drug interaction pairs in 20 patients, and was able to de-prescribe at least one medication for 69% of patients in this study (Fick et al., 2019).

SUPPORTING ADHERENCE AND PROVIDING PATIENT EDUCATION

In every setting, HIV pharmacists strive to support patient adherence to antiretrovirals by addressing system-related and patient-related barriers to taking medications. One very basic barrier PWH may face is difficulty adhering to medications because they cannot afford them. Pharmacists can provide patients with information and resources regarding pharmaceutical company–run patient assistance programs and state-run AIDS drug assistance programs to help them afford their regimens. In the modern era of broad utilization management practices, pharmacists and their technicians can play a critical role in selecting antiretroviral regimens that adhere to insurance formulary guidelines, providing clinical justification for prior authorizations, and managing those submissions so that patients do not have lapses in therapy.

Pharmacists have access to a wealth of reminder devices and tools that may improve medication adherence (Mahtani et al., 2011; Saberi & Johnson, 2011). Some pharmacies offer specialized unit-dose packaging in plastic "bubble packs" or on medication cards ("blister packs") to help patients remember to take their doses. Pharmacists can train patients on how to use weekly medication boxes. Some community and clinic pharmacists may offer text messaging or may work with patients to set up cellphone alarms to serve as automated medication reminders. Pharmacies may offer a variety of other adherence-enhancing services, such as online management of medications, automatic prescription refills, telephone refill reminders, and home mailing or courier medication delivery.

Pharmacist services also include patient counseling to enhance adherence. HIV clinical pharmacists make ideal treatment advocates because they are knowledgeable about ART and may help bridge the gap between patients and their clinic providers. They offer personalized patient education regarding HIV as a chronic disease, HIV treatment and opportunistic infection prophylaxis, and management of adverse effects. Using evidence-based counseling techniques such as motivational interviewing, pharmacists may help assess a patient's readiness to initiate ART and can help motivate the patient toward that goal (D'Antonio, 2010; Krummenacher et al., 2011). Although these topics may be discussed during the treating clinician's visit rather than during a pharmacist visit, this type of education often takes up more time than allowed in a brief clinic visit, which is typically focused on acute medical problems. A visit with a pharmacist provides additional time for complementary education and serves as an extension of the provider's care.

Pharmacists may package all of these services into structured adherence programs that span the range of patient assessment, education, and counseling; offering reminder devices; dispensing medications; and providing continuity in the refill process. Although no two pharmacist-run adherence programs are exactly alike, many studies have illustrated their benefits with regard to patient outcomes. A study of 10,801 PWH conducted at Kaiser Permanente in California compared different clinic team structures to determine the optimal combination of clinicians that would increase adherence (Horberg et al., 2012). For patients starting a new ART regimen, the largest adherence increases at 12 months were attributable to multidisciplinary teams composed of a clinical pharmacist, a social worker/benefits coordinator, and a non–HIV-specialized primary care provider (8.1% increase in mean adherence; 95% confidence interval [CI], 2.7–13.5%). Kaiser Permanente also conducted an ecological study to assess the effects of its HIV clinical pharmacists on adherence, healthcare utilization, and HIV outcomes (Horberg et al., 2007). Refill adherence at 24 months was significantly higher for patients seen by an HIV clinical pharmacist (76.7% vs. 68.9%, $p = 0.02$). Odds of having a suppressed viral load or increase in CD4$^+$ T-cell count were modestly better for patients seen by HIV pharmacists. However, these point estimates in laboratory changes did not achieve statistical significance and varied based on other factors (such as provider panel size) and patient factors (such as duration of [known] HIV infection). Rathbun et al. (2005) conducted a small randomized controlled clinical trial testing the effect of a pharmacist-run clinic adherence program on adherence and viral load. The intervention consisted of patient education, monitoring, and provision of adherence reminder devices. Patients were counseled at a clinic visit prior to starting ART. After initiation, they were contacted via telephone within 1 week and seen at a clinic visit after 2 weeks. Patients could be followed in additional clinic visits as necessary for the 12-week duration of the study. At week 28, adherence, as recorded by electronic drug monitors (74% vs. 51%), proportion of patients with viral suppression of less than 50 copies/mL (63% vs. 53%), and median CD4$^+$ T-cell count increases (142 vs. 97 cells) were all higher in the clinic pharmacist intervention group, although the point estimates did not achieve statistical significance. Apart from this unique randomized controlled trial, most of the published research evaluating the impact of HIV pharmacists in clinic settings used quasi-experimental before-and-after study designs. These studies, which examine pharmacist-run adherence programs situated within community clinics, hospital clinics, and academic medical center clinics, found improvements in CD4$^+$ T-cell counts, increased rates of viral suppression, fewer acute medical visits, and increased adherence for patients who interact with an HIV clinical pharmacist (Saberi et al., 2012). Future research should also focus on cost savings associated with pharmacist adherence support; a small study provided a cost-avoidance estimate of $49,702 for 16 PWH who completed a 6-month pharmacist-led adherence program (Dilworth et al., 2018).

Community pharmacies may also have an important impact on antiretroviral adherence. A California Medicaid pilot program examined 10 community pharmacies that provided MTM and various adherence-related services for 1,353 PWH (Hirsch et al., 2009, 2011; Rosenquist et al., 2010). At 3 years, people with HIV filling their ART at the pilot pharmacies ($n = 2,234$) demonstrated higher medication possession ratios (69.4% vs. 47.3%, $p < 0.001$) and higher odds of having optimal adherence (odds ratio, 2.74; 95% CI, 2.44–3.10) compared to those filling ART at traditional pharmacies, after controlling for age, gender, and ethnicity (Hirsch et al., 2009, 2011). Costs at the end of the first year of the program were approximately $1,014 per patient. In a study of community pharmacies that partnered with medical clinics to create a patient-centered medical home model, ART adherence did not substantially change for the group of 765 persons with HIV after the model was implemented, although rates of viral suppression improved from 75% before implementation to 86% after implementation ($p < 0.001$) (Byrd et al., 2020). These studies suggest the potential for improvement in adherence and HIV viral suppression when patients use HIV-knowledgeable community pharmacies.

TESTING FOR HIV INFECTION

HIV testing is a service that is emerging predominantly in community pharmacies, although pharmacists in other settings are often included as members of multidisciplinary testing teams (Sherman et al., 2014). These models of care typically employ point-of-care "rapid" HIV tests, counseling, and linkage to confirmatory testing and/or care. In general, pharmacy-based testing appears to be acceptable to both patients and pharmacists (Amesty et al., 2015; Darin et al., 2015). In 2011 the CDC facilitated the development of an HIV testing model for adoption in community pharmacies (Weidle et al., 2014). A total of 1,540 point-of-care HIV tests were administered across 21 sites, with pre- and post-test counseling requiring 3 to 4 minutes and patients waiting an average of 23 minutes for their test results. The average cost per person tested ranged from $32.17 to $47.21 (Lecher et al., 2015). This demonstration project resulted in the inclusion of testing in retail pharmacies as one of the CDC's effective interventions for enhancing diagnosis of HIV. A statewide HIV testing program implemented in pharmacies in Virginia also found that HIV testing in pharmacies was a successful way to connect with "hard-to-reach" populations (Collins et al., 2018). Of the 3,630 tests conducted over a 2-year period, 46% of clients reported that they had either never been tested before or were unsure whether they had received an HIV test. Collectively, these studies as well as others demonstrate the importance of pharmacies serving as HIV testing sites and pharmacists as key personnel identifying new HIV infections.

EXPANDING PATIENT CARE VIA COLLABORATIVE PRACTICE AGREEMENTS

In the US, most states have legislation that allows for pharmacists to engage in collaborative practice; however, the requirements and regulations vary from state to state. In some states, pharmacists may enhance the care of PWH via collaborative drug therapy management (CDTM) agreements. The specifics of any CDTM agreement depend on the collaborating physician and the qualifications and experience of the pharmacist.

The American College of Clinical Pharmacy defines a CDTM agreement as

> a collaborative practice agreement between one or more physicians and pharmacists wherein qualified pharmacists working within the context of a defined protocol are permitted to assume professional responsibility for performing patient assessments; ordering drug therapy-related laboratory tests; administering drugs; and selecting, initiating, monitoring, continuing, and adjusting drug regimens. (Hammond et al., 2003, p. 1210)

The American Society of Health Systems Pharmacists published a statement on pharmacist involvement in HIV care that attempts to summarize the scope of practice for an HIV pharmacist (Schafer et al., 2016). Collaborative protocols with physicians may allow pharmacists to select and initiate ART or opportunistic infection prophylaxis, draw and interpret pertinent labs that monitor efficacy or toxicity of the regimen, simplify regimens using fixed-dose combination tablets, and manage common antiretroviral-related side effects such as nausea and diarrhea. Knowledgeable pharmacists may order, interpret, and change a patient's ART based on resistance tests. Ma et al. (2010) conducted a before-and-after comparison of clinical outcomes for patients consulting with an HIV clinical pharmacist in a drug optimization clinic. Pharmacists reviewed patient medication histories and resistance tests, simplified or adjusted their ART regimens, and provided adherence training and education. After the pharmacist intervention, refill adherence was improved (89% vs. 81%, $p = 0.003$), a higher proportion of patients achieved undetectable viral loads (96% vs. 63%, $p < 0.001$), and a higher proportion of patients had increased absolute CD4$^+$ T-cell counts (491 vs. 423 cells/mm^3 at visit, $p < 0.001$).

In addition to managing ART, some protocols allow pharmacists to assess and adjust medication therapy for

HIV-related comorbidities such as depression, diabetes, hypertension, hepatitis C, or dyslipidemia. One retrospective cohort study found that an interdisciplinary primary care team that included an HIV pharmacist produced significantly improved outcomes in lipid management and smoking cessation for patients with HIV and diabetes, hypertension, or hyperlipidemia ($n = 96$) compared to a control group ($n = 50$) that was managed by an individual healthcare provider (Cope et al., 2015). The interdisciplinary team achieved a cost savings of approximately $3,000 per patient.

A collaborative, interdisciplinary practice coupled with good communication between providers can serve as an excellent model for enhancing HIV care and extend the provider's ability to reach the greatest number of patients. The roles, responsibilities, and impact of HIV pharmacists in clinical practice are likely to expand in the future as the profession advocates for all pharmacists to be recognized as healthcare providers under US federal law.

ENHANCING PREVENTION EFFORTS WITH PREP

An emerging opportunity to utilize CDTM agreements is in the provision of PrEP. Recent studies have highlighted gaps in access to PrEP (Huang et al., 2018). Some of these gaps may be related to clinician familiarity or time to discuss or manage PrEP, or lack of access to healthcare for certain populations who might benefit from PrEP. Community pharmacists may offer unique access to some of these patient populations. CDTM agreements would allow pharmacists to screen for clinical appropriateness, prescribe PrEP under protocol, draw and review monitoring labs, assess and support adherence, and refill as appropriate. The critical need to expand access to HIV prevention therapies has led to some states, such as California and Colorado, passing laws to widen pharmacist scope of practice to furnish preexposure and postexposure prophylaxis under statewide protocols. These types of laws provide an alternative pathway for pharmacists to provide HIV prevention therapies when establishing an individual pharmacist–physician CDTM agreement may be challenging.

Various studies have confirmed patients' acceptability of pharmacists screening them for PrEP indications and for pharmacy-run PrEP programs (Crawford et al., 2020; Zhu et al., 2020). The One-Step-PrEP program in Seattle, Washington, is an example of a pharmacy-run PrEP program operating under a CDTA (Tung et al., 2018). Over a 3-year period from 2015 to 2018, 714 patients sought out this pharmacy-based PrEP service. Of those, 695 persons initiated PrEP and most of these patients (98%) did not have to pay for their PrEP medication. An impressive retention of 75% was achieved over the first 3 years of operation. This study demonstrates that pharmacy-based PrEP services are feasible and desired and remain a promising avenue for pharmacists to contribute to the public health goal of preventing new infections.

A novel avenue for pharmacists to enhance prevention efforts is to facilitate rapid ART initiation. A pharmacist was the first point of contact for persons newly diagnosed with HIV for a pharmacist-driven rapid ART program at a Ryan White–funded clinic in Rhode Island in 2019 (Brotherton et al., 2020). During the visit, the pharmacist assessed ART readiness, provided education, screened for drug interactions, facilitated ART access, recommended patient-specific ART to the triage physician for initiation, and called the client 2 weeks after initiation. A retrospective analysis of the program found significantly reduced time from intake to ART start (16 vs. 0 days, $p < 0.001$) and reduced time to viral suppression (81 vs. 34 days, $p = 0.001$). Programs such as this one hold great potential to rapidly reduce viral loads and potentially impact HIV transmissions.

PHARMACISTS: UNLIMITED POTENTIAL

The benefit of having an HIV clinical pharmacist extends beyond direct patient services. Pharmacists are becoming increasingly important members of HIV hospital or clinic quality improvement teams. Performance measures often involve chart abstraction and generation of reports to benchmark rates of ART, viral suppression, opportunistic infection prophylaxis, and adherence. HIV pharmacists have the clinical background and skills to assess these and other key indicators quickly, accurately, and thoroughly. Pharmacists can also offer valuable insight for "plan–do–study–act" projects designed to improve any below-target performance measures.

Finally, an increasing number of trained HIV clinical pharmacist scientists are making a strong impact on HIV-related research. A solid understanding of study design, drug therapy monitoring, and pharmacotherapy makes HIV clinical pharmacists ideal study coordinators or project managers for research studies being conducted within clinical settings. Advanced training through master's degree programs and complementary PhD programs also places HIV clinical pharmacists in an optimal position to serve as principal investigators on research studies regarding pharmacokinetics, pharmacodynamics, investigational drugs, adherence, drug resistance, or provision of health services. As pharmacists become further trained in clinical research methods, they will continue to contribute valuable information to the body of HIV care knowledge.

CONCLUSION

HIV clinical pharmacists are a diverse group of healthcare practitioners with specialized skills and knowledge. Whether they are engaged in direct patient care, quality assurance, research, or a combination of these, they strive to benefit people with HIV through their efforts. Although not all clinics or hospitals have available resources or funding to house an HIV-specialized pharmacist, collaborations with HIV-focused community pharmacists can ensure that patients have access to this valuable healthcare team member and that they receive the highest-quality medication care possible.

RECOMMENDED READING

Durham SH, Badowski ME, Liedtke MD, et al. Acute care management of the HIV-infected patient: a report from the HIV Practice and Research Network of the American College of Clinical Pharmacy. *Pharmacotherapy*. 2017;37:611–629.

Hill LA, Ballard C, Cachay ER. The role of the clinical pharmacist in the management of people living with HIV in the modern antiretroviral era. *AIDS Rev*. 2019;21(4):195–210.

Koren DE, Scarsi KK, Farmer EK, et al. A call to action: the role of antiretroviral stewardship in inpatient practice. A joint policy paper of the Infectious Diseases Society of America, HIV Medicine Association, and American Academy of HIV Medicine. *Clin Infect Dis*. 2020;70(11):2241–2246.

Schafer JJ, Cocohoba JM, Sherman EM, et al. (Eds.). *HIV Pharmacotherapy: The Pharmacist's Role in Care and Treatment*. Bethesda, MD: American Society of Health-System Pharmacists; 2018.

REFERENCES

American Pharmacists Association and National Association of Chain Drug Stores Foundation. Medication therapy management in pharmacy practice: core elements of an MTM service model (version 2.0). *J Am Pharm Assoc*. 2008;48(3):341–353.

Amesty S, Crawford ND, Nandi V, et al. Evaluation of pharmacy-based HIV testing in a high-risk New York City community. *AIDS Patient Care STDS*. 2015;29(8):437–444. doi:10.1089/apc.2015.0017.

Brotherton AL, Shah RB, Garland J, et al. Pharmacist-driven rapid ART reduces time to virologic suppression in Rhode Island. Conference on Retroviruses and Opportunistic Infections. Boston, MA, March 8–11, 2020. Abstract 498.

Byrd KK, Hardnett F, Clay PG, et al.; Patient-Centered HIV Care Model Team. Retention in HIV care among participants in the patient-centered HIV care model: a collaboration between community-based pharmacists and primary medical providers. *AIDS Patient Care STDS*. 2019;33(2):58–66.

Byrd KK, Hou JG, Bush T, et al. Adherence and viral suppression among participants of the patient-centered human immunodeficiency virus (HIV) care model project: a collaboration between community-based pharmacists and HIV clinical providers. *Clin Infect Dis*. 2020;70(5):789–797.

Collins B, Bronson H, Elamin F, et al. The "no wrong door" approach to HIV testing: results from a statewide retail pharmacy-based HIV testing program in Virginia, 2014–2016. *Public Health Rep*. 2018;133(2 suppl):34S–42S.

Cope R, Berkowitz L, Arcebido R, et al. Evaluating the effects of an interdisciplinary practice model with pharmacist collaboration on HIV patient co-morbidities. *AIDS Patient Care STDS*. 2015;29(8):445–453.

Crawford ND, Albarran T, Chamberlain A, et al. Willingness to discuss and screen for pre-exposure prophylaxis in pharmacies among men who have sex with men. *J Pharm Pract*. 2020:897190020904590.

D'Antonio N. Including motivational interviewing skills in the PharmD curriculum. *Am J Pharm Educ*. 2010;74(8):152d.

Darin KM, Scarsi KK, Klepser DG, et al. Consumer interest in community pharmacy HIV screening services. *J Am Pharm Assoc*. 2015;55(1):67–72.

DePuy AM, Samuel R, Mohrien KM, et al. Impact of an antiretroviral stewardship team on the care of patients with human immunodeficiency virus infection admitted on an academic medical center. Open Forum Infect Dis. 2019;6(7): ofz290.

Dilworth TJ, Klein PW, Mercier RC, et al. Clinical and economic effects of a pharmacist-administered antiretroviral therapy adherence clinic for patients living with HIV. *J Manag Care Pharm*. 2018;24(2):165–172.

Fick DM, Semla TP, Steinman M, et al. American Geriatrics Society 2019 updated AGS Beers Criteria for potentially inappropriate medication use in older adults. *J Am Geriatr Soc*. 2019;67(4):674–694.

Gilbert EM, Gerzenshtein L. Integration of outpatient infectious diseases clinic pharmacy services and specialty pharmacy services for patients with HIV infection. *Am J Health Syst Pharm*. 2016;73(11):757–763.

Hammond RW, Schwartz AH, Campbell MJ, et al. Collaborative drug therapy management by pharmacists—2003. *Pharmacotherapy*. 2003;23(9):1210–1225.

Hirsch JD, Gonzales M, Rosenquist A, et al. Antiretroviral therapy adherence, medication use, and health care costs during 3 years of a community pharmacy medication therapy management program for Medi-Cal beneficiaries with HIV/AIDS. *J Manag Care Pharm*. 2011;17(3):213–223.

Hirsch JD, Rosenquist A, Best B, et al. Evaluation of the first year of a pilot program in community pharmacy: HIV/AIDS medication therapy management for Medi-Cal beneficiaries. *J Manag Care Pharm*. 2009;15(1):32–41.

Horberg MA, Hurley LB, Silverberg MJ, et al. Effect of clinical pharmacists on utilization of and clinical response to antiretroviral therapy. *J AIDS*. 2007;44(5):531–539.

Horberg MA, Hurley LB, Towner WJ, et al. Determination of optimized multidisciplinary care team for maximal antiretroviral therapy adherence. *J AIDS*. 2012;60(2):183–190.

Huang YA, Zhu W, Smith DK, et al. HIV preexposure prophylaxis, by race and ethnicity—United States, 2014–2016. *MMWR Morb Mortal Wkly Rep*. 2018;67:1147–1150.

Koren DE, Scarsi KK, Farmer EK, et al. A call to action: the role of antiretroviral stewardship in inpatient practice. A joint policy paper of the Infectious Diseases Society of America, HIV Medicine Association, and American Academy of HIV Medicine. *Clin Infect Dis*. 2020;70(11):2241–2246.

Krummenacher I, Cavassini M, Bugnon O, et al. An interdisciplinary HIV-adherence program combining motivational interviewing and electronic antiretroviral drug monitoring. *AIDS Care*. 2011;23(5):550–561.

Lecher SL, Shrestha RK, Botts LW, et al. Cost analysis of a novel HIV testing strategy in community pharmacies and retail clinics. *J Am Pharm Assoc*. 2015;55(5):488–492.

Li EH, Foisy MM. Antiretroviral and medication errors in hospitalized HIV-positive patients. *Ann Pharmacother*. 2014;48(8):998–1010.

Ma A, Chen DM, Chau FM, et al. Improving adherence and clinical outcomes through an HIV pharmacist's interventions. *AIDS Care*. 2010;22(10):1189–1194.

Mahtani KR, Heneghan CJ, Glasziou PP, et al. Reminder packaging for improving adherence to self-administered long-term medications. *Cochrane Database System Rev*. 2011;9:CD005025.

McLaughlin M, Gordon LA, Kleyn TJ, et al. Assessment of the benefits of and barriers to HIV pharmacist credentialing. *J Am Pharm Assoc*. 2018;58(2):168–173.

McNicholl IR, Gandhi M, Hare CB, et al. A pharmacist-led program to evaluate and reduce polypharmacy and potentially inappropriate prescribing in older HIV-positive patients. *Pharmacotherapy*. 2017;37(12):1498–1506.

Okoli C, de los Rios P, Eremin A, et al. Relationship between polypharmacy and quality of life among people in 24 countries living with HIV. *Prev Chronic Dis*. 2020;17:190359.

Rathbun RC, Farmer KC, Stephens JR, et al. Impact of an adherence clinic on behavioral outcomes and virologic response in the treatment of HIV infection: a prospective, randomized, controlled pilot study. *Clin Ther*. 2005;27(2):199–209.

Rosenquist A, Bes BM, Miller TA, et al. Medication therapy management services in community pharmacy: a pilot programme in HIV specialty pharmacies. *J Eval Clin Pract*. 2010;16(6):1142–1146.

Saberi P, Dong BJ, Johnson MO, et al. The impact of HIV clinical pharmacists on HIV treatment outcomes: a systematic review. *Patient Prefer Adherence*. 2012;6:297–322.

Saberi P, Johnson MO. Technology-based self-care methods of improving antiretroviral adherence: a systematic review. *PLoS One*. 2011;6(11):e27533.

Schafer JJ, Gill TK, Sherman EM, et al. ASHP guidelines on pharmacist involvement in HIV care. *Am J Health Syst Pharm.* 2016;73:468–494. http://www.ajhp.org/content/73/7/468

Schatz K, Guffey W, Maccia M, et al. Pharmacists' impact on opportunistic infection prophylaxis in patients with HIV/AIDS. *J Hosp Infect.* 2016;94(4):389–392.

Shea KM, Hobbs AL, Shumake JD, et al. Impact of an antiretroviral stewardship strategy on medication error rates. *Am J Health Syst Pharm.* 2018;75(12):876–885.

Sherman EM, Elrod S, Allen D, et al. Pharmacist testers in multidisciplinary health care team expand HIV point-of-care testing program. *J Pharm Pract.* 2014;27(6):578–581.

Tung EL, Thomas A, Eichner A, et al. Implementation of a community pharmacy-based pre-exposure prophylaxis service: a novel model for pre-exposure prophylaxis care. *Sex Health.* 2018;15(6):556–561.

Weidle PJ, Lecher S, Botts LW, et al. HIV testing in community pharmacies and retail clinics: a model to expand access to screening for HIV infection. *J Am Pharm Assoc.* 2014;54(5):486–492.

Zhu V, Tran D, Banjo O, et al. Patient perception of community pharmacists prescribing pre-exposure prophylaxis for HIV prevention. *J Am Pharm Assoc.* 2020;60(6):781–788.

Zucker J, Mittal J, Jen SP, et al. Impact of stewardship interventions on antiretroviral medication errors in an urban medical center: a 3-year, multiphase study. *Pharmacotherapy.* 2016;36(3):245–251.

15.

PALLIATIVE CARE AND END-OF-LIFE SUPPORT

Paul W. DenOuden

CHAPTER GOAL

Upon completion of this chapter, the reader should be able to:

- Discuss both hospice and palliative care options in the context of end-stage HIV and determine when each option may be most appropriate

- Know when each option may be most appropriate

- Optimally counsel and educate persons with HIV (PWH) and their families in an effective, professional, and sensitive manner

- Be identify with common end-of-life symptoms and how to effectively treat them

KEY POINTS

- Palliative care can be accessed at any stage of illness to alleviate ongoing or severe symptoms even in the absence of a terminal illness.

- Hospice care involves an interdisciplinary approach to diagnosing and managing suffering and addressing the physical, psychosocial, and spiritual needs of PWH and their families at the end of life.

- Hospice care should be considered when no further interventions or treatments can cure or prolong the life of a terminally ill PWH with an estimated life expectancy of 6 months or less.

- Making the decision for hospice care is often challenging for the PWH, family, and clinicians alike.

CARING FOR THE TERMINALLY ILL PWH

In the early years of the HIV epidemic, before the introduction of antiretroviral therapy (ART), caring for the terminally ill PWH was a regular and inevitable part of HIV care, as the disease would progressively advance to terminal stages without effective ART. Most HIV-treating clinicians were dealing with terminal illness on a daily basis, and, in dealing with multiple opportunistic infections and AIDS-related

malignancies, there would come a point when the focus changed to palliative/hospice care. Many US cities had multiple AIDS hospices for terminally ill PWH. As ART evolved and became increasingly successful, and especially from the late 1990s onward as death rates plummeted, many hospices closed or changed their focus to skilled nursing, and the daily focus of clinicians became much more geared toward ongoing care of stable PWH. However, given the still significant death rates and changing dynamics of causes of mortality in HIV, it is still important for HIV clinicians to be comfortable with and fluent in caring for PWH with terminal illnesses. The number of end-stage opportunistic infections has decreased, whereas the number of PWH with more common malignancies, end-stage liver disease, cardiovascular disease, and age-related comorbidities has increased.

Keeping focus on maintaining a close provider–individual relationship in the transition to terminal illness is essential; providers not only have a responsibility to the PWH to journey with them through chronic illness to recovery, stabilization, or death but also have a responsibility to themselves to do so. By caring for the dying and attempting to provide PWH with "good" deaths, physicians may feel a greater sense of professional satisfaction. Providing good end-of-life care makes physicians better communicators, helping them to better understand and treat suffering while offering them a deeper understanding of the nature of life (Block, 2001; Cherny et al., 1996).

It is important to reassure PWH that they will not be abandoned when hospice care has begun. PWH and their families usually prefer their primary physicians to stay in contact until death, even if the main tasks of palliative care are taken on by another clinician (Han & Arnold, 2005). Maintaining contact throughout the dying process is most likely the best policy, within reasonable bounds of previous clinical involvement (Quill & Cassel, 1995).

Of note, despite years of pushing for increased HIV screening, a significant proportion of PWH (about 30% in the US) are still initially diagnosed with HIV late in the stage of illness (Xia et al., 2015). These individuals would have been considered to have end-stage illness in the pre-ART era and may have quickly transitioned to palliative/hospice care. In our current extremely effective ART era, virtually all of these PWH with advanced-stage disease can be successfully treated and often return to normal functioning and a good long-term prognosis. Many healthcare providers who do not primarily work in the HIV field may not realize this, and the issues and goals of quick improvement versus hospice/palliative interventions get blurred. This may be especially true in resource-poor settings where ART is not as immediately available. These situations are a particularly important time to have an HIV specialist with knowledge of effective ART and outcomes be involved in care from the beginning to help PWH, their family, and other healthcare providers be in alignment with realistic goals.

HOSPICE CARE

DEFINITION OF HOSPICE CARE

Hospice care is defined as a comprehensive system of care for persons with limited life expectancy. This system is flexible and can take place either at home or in an inpatient care facility (hospital or nursing home). Hospice care works from a bio-psychosocial model rather than a disease model, and it focuses on comfort, dignity, and personal growth at life's end. This encompasses biomedical, psychosocial, and spiritual aspects of the dying experience, emphasizing quality of life and healing or strengthening of interpersonal relationships rather than prolonging the dying process at any cost. A quality hospice program comprises an interdisciplinary team of experts that deals with all aspects of the dying process (Emanuel et al., 2005).

Often, people interchange the terms "palliative care" and "hospice care." *Palliative care* is used to address suffering at any stage of illness, from diagnosis to recovery or death. *Hospice* is a formal structured environment for delivering quality palliative care at the end of life.

INDICATIONS FOR HOSPICE CARE

In the early days of the HIV epidemic in the US, death was common and survival unusual. Advances in ART and treatment of AIDS-related illnesses have resulted in dramatic increases in the life expectancy of PWH. Unfortunately, several end-stage conditions remain very difficult to treat in PWH with extensive antiretroviral resistance or in PWH who refuse or cannot tolerate medications. It may be appropriate in these circumstances to discuss end-stage options. In this way, hospice care can focus on comfort and quality of life rather than on treatments with uncomfortable side effects and no further benefit.

One study found that the cause of death of PWH in the ART era is increasingly likely to be a chronic medical condition such as hepatic failure or malignancies, with opportunistic infections (OIs) declining in importance (Sansone & Frengley, 2000). Crum et al. (2006) found that 80% of pre-ART deaths were related to AIDS-defining conditions. This declined to 65% in the early post-ART era and reduced further to 56% in the late post-ART era (Crum et al., 2006).

Since the advent of ART, the biology of HIV has shifted, requiring both PWH and healthcare providers to consider the cumulative impact of chronic HIV infection and the long-term side effects of treatment. With longer life spans,

people with HIV have become prone to diseases of aging—such as heart disease, cancer, diabetes, and osteoporosis—and to progressive conditions such as chronic viral hepatitis (Highleyman, 2005). Chronic viral hepatitis can lead to end-stage liver damage as PWH coinfected with HIV and hepatitis B virus and/or hepatitis C virus live longer. Cardiovascular disease is seen with increasing frequency, due to both the chronic inflammatory nature of persistent HIV viral infection and sometimes increased long-term metabolic toxicities from certain ART regimens.

These changes in end-stage disease have resulted in changes in the approach that caregivers take to the PWH they care for and, thus, in how physicians and other clinicians discuss end-of-life options with PWH as they reach the terminal phases of disease. However, it is important to keep in mind that AIDS-defining conditions may still appear, especially toward the end of life, and prevention and treatment of OIs will still have a role in the end-of-life care (Welch & Morse, 2002).

ADVANTAGES OF HOSPICE CARE

Hospice and palliative care represent an interdisciplinary approach to the diagnosis and management of suffering. *Suffering* is a multidimensional disorder of consciousness that includes physical, psychosocial, and spiritual elements. The unit of care in palliative care is the individual–caregiver dyad, with the needs of the family and loved ones being addressed along with the needs of the PWH (Emanuel et al., 2005). Given that there is still stigma associated with HIV and that, for many reasons, families are sometimes alienated from PWH, special care needs to be taken with family dynamics issues that often come to the fore in hospice care with this population. As the usefulness of medical treatments diminishes, the effectiveness of psychosocial and spiritual interventions increases (Peterson et al., 1996).

When a PWH becomes progressively weaker and debilitated despite maximal treatment, it is time to consider hospice care. Early hospice evaluation with clear goals can provide great comfort to PWH and their loved ones. Palliative care clinicians are experts in pain and symptom management and can usually improve the PWH's level of comfort. If symptoms do not respond to conventional medical therapy, addressing psychological and spiritual suffering may benefit the individual. Alternative and complementary therapies may be used, including relaxation, music therapy, meditation, herbal therapy, and acupuncture (Chesney & Folkman, 1994; O'Neill & Alexander, 1997).

It takes time to prepare for a good death, and the earlier a hospice referral is made, the more likely the individual will be able to benefit. Unfortunately, the average length of stay in hospice is only 2 weeks, which may be an indication of missed opportunities for referral.

Understanding, reconciliation, acceptance, and, for many, spiritual growth at the end of life may provide great comfort. Table 15.1 lists many of the practical issues involved in the care of dying persons (Cherny et al., 1996), which encompasses much more than strictly medical issues.

Table 15.1 PRACTICAL ISSUES TO BE ADDRESSED IN THE CARE OF DYING PWH

ISSUE	SPECIFICS TO BE ADDRESSED
Communication	With individual With family With other participating caregivers
Symptom control	Physical Psychological Existential
Evaluation of family well-being	Coping Resources
Evaluation of therapeutic plan	Primary therapies Supportive pharmacotherapies Hydration and nutrition
Contingency planning	Crisis planning Addressing do-not-resuscitate orders
Ongoing care planning	Home/inpatient Home care backup Observation 24-hour availability of clinician with decision-making authority

Adapted from Cherny et al. *Hematol Oncol Clin North Am.* 1996;10:261–286, with permission from Elsevier.

Many people with terminal illnesses prefer to die at home if possible, and individuals and their families may want to consider end-of-life care at home using an interdisciplinary care management approach. Home hospice services can be cost-effective and can enhance quality of life for terminally ill PWH with HIV (Huba et al., 1998). Home hospice care usually requires stable housing and willing family, partners, or friends to help with the dying process at home. Sometimes this can be challenging to accomplish for many social reasons, even if an individual is interested in pursuing home hospice.

DIFFICULTIES OF HOSPICE IN THE ART ERA

With the use of ART, death is less common and often less anticipated. Poor outcome is sometimes related to nonadherence, and feelings of guilt and other emotional responses can become a major issue for the PWH and the caregiver. People dying of HIV tend to be younger and often suffer from depression and other mental health issues that need evaluation and treatment.

Several issues can lead to difficult deaths, including the biology of HIV disease, provider and system barriers to accepting hospice care, family issues, and the individual's values and choices. PWH can experience dramatic improvement even when close to death; however, deaths from comorbid conditions such as hepatitis and cancer are often more abrupt, unpredictable, and devastating (Karascz et al., 2003).

Many PWH and providers may be very reluctant to abandon research and experimental treatment options even in the late stages of disease. There is evidence that even PWH with severe immunosuppression, very low CD4 T-cell counts, high viral loads, and/or symptomatic HIV can still derive significant benefit from ART (Highleyman, 2005). This further complicates the choice to seek hospice care. Many people arrive at the end of life with limited assets. Although hospice can find community support and provide services not covered by ordinary government and private insurance, most insurance coverage of hospice care, following the lead of Medicare rules, generally prohibits curative options for those seeking coverage for hospice and palliative care at the end of life (Scala-Foley et al., 2004).

PWH may face very difficult decisions in choosing to stop ART, both for symptom control and psychological reasons, because so many have been conditioned to stay fully adherent and never stop ART and the complications with hospice coverage make it more difficult to decide how they and their physicians should best face this challenge (Karascz et al., 2003). Individuals with advanced HIV frequently do not fit the cancer model on which hospice often rests. For these PWH, an insurance program that requires cessation of ART or that will not cover other treatments is often problematic and may result in difficulty in planning and decision-making. Generally, ART is not covered under the Medicare hospice benefit.

PALLIATIVE CARE

Palliative care is often a major part of hospice care, but it can and should be used for any suffering persons even if they are not actively in hospice. Palliative care has been defined by the World Health Organization (WHO, 1990) as

> the active total care of patients whose disease is not responsive to curative treatment. Control of pain, of other symptoms, and of psychological, social, and spiritual problems, is paramount. The goal of palliative care is to achieve the best quality of life for patients and their families.

The subset of palliative care tailored to the terminally ill and associated with hospice care is more accurately termed "end-of-life care." Many end-stage symptoms can be successfully treated in a palliative care setting, making the end of life as comfortable as possible for terminally ill hospice PWH. Common and distressing symptoms in terminally ill people can often be successfully managed.

The use of non-oral routes of medication delivery can be helpful in a palliative setting for other symptom management in addition to pain control. Examples of non-oral administration include rectal administration (prochlorperazine suppositories for nausea and diazepam suppositories for agitation), sublingual administration (lorazepam for hiccups or agitation), or subcutaneous/intramuscular administration (clonazepam or haloperidol for acute agitation) (Enck, 2002; Woodruff, 1999).

The following sections describe several common symptoms to be aware of and focus on when providing palliative care to a PWH.

PAIN

A common fear of PWH at end of life is that of pain. There are many medication approaches to pain control, and a common treatment model is given by the WHO in its report on cancer pain relief and palliative care (WHO, 1990). There is a large body of palliative care literature and many protocols available on how to effectively manage pain at end of life, which should be reviewed if this is not a routine part of the provider's work, and tailored to each unique situation.

In the terminal phase of disease, oral medications become more difficult for people to take, and alternative routes such as the transdermal approach have been shown to be safe and effective in PWH (Newshan & Lefkowitz, 2001). Another widely used route for effective pain medication delivery is continuous subcutaneous infusion, which is common in the hospice setting and has many potential advantages, including ease of administration/access, decreased infection-site complications, less volume overload, and lower cost (Herndon & Fike, 2001). Other modalities of pain control in addition to classic opiates are important to remember to optimize effective pain management for people (Table 15.2).

SEIZURES

In persons whose terminal AIDS condition involves intracerebral masses or central nervous system (CNS) infections such as toxoplasmosis or CNS lymphoma, seizures can be a frequent symptom requiring management. There are several common antiepileptic drugs, and because no one drug has shown superiority over the others, they are often used interchangeably, with substitution as needed for lack of effectiveness or side effects (Krouwer et al., 2000). Adding or increasing corticosteroids to treat related peritumoral edema may be indicated if seizures are occurring with a therapeutic antiepileptic drug level (Krouwer et al., 2000).

Table 15.2 MODALITIES OF PAIN CONTROL

OPIATES	NEUROPATHIC PAIN MEDICATIONS	ADJUVANT TREATMENTS
Codeine	Carbamazepine	Acetaminophen
Fentanyl	Duloxetine	Acupuncture
Hydromorphone	Gabapentin	Benzodiazepines
Methadone	Pregabalin	Cannabinoids
Morphine	Tricyclics	Corticosteroids
Oxycodone	Valproic acid	Focal radiation
Oxymorphone		Lidocaine (topical)
		Muscle relaxants
		Nonsteroidal anti-inflammatories (NSAIDs)
		Massage therapy
		Guided imagery
		Music therapy

Depression, Fatigue, and Sleep Disturbance

Depression, fatigue, and sleep disturbance are all common and interrelated symptoms that can be addressed effectively in palliative care. Because fatigue and sleep difficulties are common manifestations of depression, effective standard antidepressant treatment (e.g., with a selective serotonin reuptake inhibitor [SSRI] or other appropriate psychopharmaceuticals) may need to be instituted (see Chapter 33 on psychiatric complications). Psychostimulants (e.g., methylphenidate or dextroamphetamine) have been studied in the palliative care setting and have been found to be effective in treating depression, opioid-induced sedation, and fatigue. Often dosed in the morning and early afternoon, psychostimulants may improve the cognition, neuropsychological function, and energy of terminally ill PWH and allow for better quality of life and interaction with loved ones during the final days of life (Dein & George, 2002).

DELIRIUM

Another related CNS symptom that many individuals in hospice experience is delirium, which is defined as a transient disorder of cognition and attention, often accompanied by disruption of the normal sleep–wake cycle (Enck, 2002). The causes of delirium are broad and include metabolic disturbances; acute infection and fever; brain metastases; hypoxia; and side effects of drugs frequently used in palliation, such as opiates and corticosteroids (Enck, 2002; Woodruff, 1999).

Management should be directed at the suspected cause; for example, if hypoxia is suspected, empiric oxygen can be administered via cannula/mask, and if a drug side effect is implicated, nonessential medications can be discontinued or the opioid changed (Woodruff, 1999). Sedation may be necessary to alleviate severe agitation, and neuroleptics, most commonly haloperidol (which can be given orally, intravenously, or intramuscularly as needed), are effective and can be titrated individually (Woodruff, 1999). In the last few days of life, an agitated delirium often termed "terminal restlessness" occurs in some individuals (Woodruff, 1999). Benzodiazepines are commonly used in this situation because they specifically aid in relieving myoclonus, seizure activity, and restlessness. There are many options with varying half-lives and many possible routes of delivery, such as diazepam rectal suppository, sublingual lorazepam, and subcutaneous clonazepam.

PRURITUS

Pruritus is common and may be a symptom of dry skin, may be due to underlying organ dysfunction or tumor, or may be induced by opioid use (Krajnik & Zylicz, 2001; WHO, 1998). Directed treatment often includes topical steroid creams and emollients for dry skin (WHO, 1998). Systemic antihistamines, corticosteroids, and even SSRIs have been found to be of benefit (Krajnik & Zylicz, 2001; WHO, 1998). Nursing care for the skin can include colloidal oatmeal soap baths and warm compresses for comfort.

DRY MOUTH

Dry mouth or oral mucosa breakdown has many etiologies, and symptom relief can be quite helpful for personal comfort. Often in advanced HIV infections contribute to this problem, and treatment is related to the specific cause—for example, antifungals for oral candidiasis or antivirals for herpes simplex ulcers. Mouthwashes, hydration techniques such as use of ice chips or popsicles, and oral hygiene using mouth swabs called toothettes can also lessen discomfort (WHO, 1998). Painful aphthous ulcers can be aided by the topical corticosteroid Orabase and local analgesic agents (WHO, 1998), such as viscous lidocaine; use of thalidomide has also been shown to be effective in PWH (Woodruff, 1999).

HICCUPS

Hiccups can be difficult and multifactorial in nature. Promoting gastric emptying with metoclopramide can help (Kinzbrunner et al., 2002). Treating esophagitis, a common cause of hiccups in advanced HIV (Albrecht & Stellbrink, 1994), can be accomplished with antifungals and antacids as appropriate. Symptomatic treatment often includes chlorpromazine or baclofen trials to calm the CNS response (Kinzbrunner et al., 2002).

DYSPNEA

Dyspnea is a common end-of-life symptom and can be an unpleasant sensation causing much anxiety to the PWH, which often exacerbates the breathlessness. As with other symptoms, the causes are highly variable, and treatment is always directed to the root cause when known. For example, diuretics may be helpful in cases of heart failure or fluid overload, and significant pleural effusions can be drained for symptom relief. If bronchospasm is noted, inhaled bronchodilators can be used, often in nebulized form with a mask if the PWH is unable to use a metered-dose inhaler; systemic corticosteroids can also cause effective bronchodilation. Oxygen therapy is of benefit if the PWH is hypoxic (e.g., pulse oximeter saturation <90%) and can be titrated for comfort via either nasal prongs or face mask.

Many PWH may remain dyspneic even with oxygen use and other interventions, and the use of morphine may be indicated for the relief of continued respiratory symptoms rather than solely for pain control because morphine has been shown to decrease the respiratory rate and sensation of air hunger. Morphine also has the benefit of administration via the oral, subcutaneous, intravenous, intramuscular, rectal, or even nebulized route. The anxiety that accompanies and often worsens dyspnea can be managed using any of the benzodiazepines via any appropriate route and timing schedule (Enck, 2002; Woodruff, 1999).

The final stages of the dying process are variable but commonly involve irregular or Cheyne–Stokes respirations and difficulty in clearing upper airway secretions. The sounds made by these retained secretions during respiration in this phase, often referred to as "death rattle" or "tracheal secretions," may be quite disturbing to family and caregivers of the terminally ill PWH. Standard measures to reduce this potentially disquieting sound include positioning, decreasing parenteral hydration, and gentle suctioning, as well as antisecretory drug therapy. Several anticholinergic drugs have been reported to be successful, including scopolamine, atropine, and hyoscyamine (Wildiers & Menten, 2002).

NAUSEA

Intractable nausea is common in end-stage HIV (Karus et al., 2005), and often the source of the nausea is elusive. The many possible causes of discomfort, including both side effects from therapies and direct effects of OIs, make therapies difficult to generalize (Karus et al., 2005; Reiter & Kudler, 1996). The most effective method is to begin with a phenothiazine such as prochlorperazine or trimethobenzamide, increase the dose to the highest tolerable level, and then add another agent of a different class such as ondansetron. Many other classes of medications are effective, including butyrophenones, benzodiazepines, benzamides, and cannabinoids. However, simultaneous use of three or four agents may be needed to provide adequate relief (Reiter & Kudler, 1996).

REFERENCES

Albrecht H, Stellbrink HJ. Hiccups in people with AIDS. *J Acquir Immune Defic Syndr.* 1994;7(7):735.

Block SD. Perspectives on care at the close of life. Psychological considerations, growth, and transcendence at the end of life: the art of the possible. *JAMA.* 2001;285:2898–2905.

Cherny NI, Coyle N, Foley KM. Guidelines in the care of the dying cancer patient. *Hematol Oncol Clin North Am.* 1996;10:261–286.

Chesney MA, Folkman S. Psychological impact of HIV disease and implications for intervention. *Psychiatr Clin North Am.* 1994;17:163–182.

Crum NF, Riffenburgh RH, Wegner S, et al. Comparisons of causes of death and mortality rates among HIV-infected persons: analysis of the pre-, early, and late HAART (highly active antiretroviral therapy) eras. *J AIDS.* 2006;41:194–200.

Dein S, George R. A place for psychostimulants in palliative care? *J Palliat Care.* 2002; 18:196–199.

Emanuel LL, Ferris FD, von Gunten CF, Von Roenn J. *EPEC-O: Education in Palliative and End-of-Life Care—Oncology.* Chicago: The EPEC Project; 2005.

Enck RE. *The Medical Care of Terminally Ill Patients.* 2nd ed. Baltimore: Johns Hopkins University Press; 2002.

Han PK, Arnold RM. Palliative care services, patient abandonment, and the scope of physicians' responsibilities in end-of-life care. *J Palliat Med.* 2005;8:1238–1245.

Herndon CM, Fike DS. Continuous subcutaneous infusion practices of United States hospices. *J Pain Symptom Manage.* 2001;22:1027–1034.

Highleyman L. Mortality trends: toward a new definition of AIDS? *BETA.* 2005;17:18–28.

Huba GJ, Cherin DA, Melchior LA. Retention of clients in service under two models of home health care for HIV. *Home Health Care Serv Q.* 1998;17:17–26.

Karascz A, Dyche L, Selwyn P. Physicians' experiences of caring for late-stage HIV patients in the post-HAART era: challenges and adaptations. *Soc Sci Med.* 2003;57:1609–1620.

Karus D, Raveis DH, Alexander C, et al. Patient reports of symptoms and their treatment at three palliative care projects servicing individuals with HIV. *J Pain Symptom Manage.* 2005;30:408–417.

Kinzbrunner BM, Weinreb NJ, Policzer JS (Eds.). *Twenty Common Problems in End-of-Life Care*. New York: McGraw-Hill; 2002.

Krajnik M, Zylicz Z. Understanding pruritus in systemic disease. *J Pain Symptom Manage*. 2001;21:151–168.

Krouwer HG, Pallagi JL, Graves NM. Management of seizures in brain tumor patients at the end of life. *J Palliat Med*. 2000;3:465–475.

Newshan G, Lefkowitz M. Transdermal fentanyl for chronic pain in AIDS: a pilot study. *J Pain Symptom Manage*. 2001;21:69–77.

O'Neill JF, Alexander CS. Palliative medicine and HIV. *Prim Care*. 1997;24:607–615.

Peterson JL, Folkman S, Bakeman R. Stress, coping, HIV status, psychosocial resources, and depressive mood in African American gay, bisexual, and heterosexual men. *Am J Community Psychol*. 1996;24:461–487.

Quill TE, Cassel CK. Nonabandonment: a central obligation for physicians. *Ann Intern Med*. 1995;122:368–374.

Reiter GS, Kudler NR. Palliative care and HIV. Part II: systemic manifestations and late-stage issues. *AIDS Clin Care*. 1996;8:27–30, 33, 36.

Sansone GR, Frengley JD. Impact of HAART on causes of death of persons with late-stage AIDS. *J Urban Health*. 2000;77:166–175.

Scala-Foley MA, Caruso JT, Archer D, et al. Medicare's hospice benefits: when cure is no longer the goal, Medicare will cover palliative care. *Am J Nurs*. 2004;104:66–67.

Welch K, Morse A. The clinical profile of end-stage AIDS in the era of highly active antiretroviral therapy. *AIDS Patient Care STDS*. 2002;16:75–81.

Wildiers H, Menten J. Death rattle: prevalence, prevention and treatment. *J Pain Symptom Manage*. 2002;23:310–317.

Woodruff R. *Palliative Medicine: Symptomatic and Supportive Care for Patients with Advanced Cancer and AIDS*. Oxford: Oxford University Press; 1999.

World Health Organization. Cancer pain relief and palliative care. Report of a WHO expert committee. *World Health Organ Tech Rep Ser*. 1990;804:1–75.

World Health Organization. *Symptom Relief in Terminal Illness*. Geneva: World Health Organization; 1998.

Xia Q, Kobrak P, Wiewel E, et al. The high proportion of late HIV diagnoses in the USA is likely to stay: findings from a mathematical model. *AIDS Care*. 2015;27(2):206–212. doi:10.1080/09540121.2014.958430

16.

VIROLOGY AND NATURAL HISTORY OF HIV

Poonam Mathur

CHAPTER GOALS

Upon completion of this chapter, the reader should be able to:

- Demonstrate and apply knowledge of the established and evolving science of HIV virology, both in the cell and in the host

- Describe how HIV virology informs treatment aimed at various stages of the viral life cycle

HIV STRUCTURE AND LIFE CYCLE

LEARNING OBJECTIVE

- Discuss basic HIV virology and its relevance to current and potential drug targets

WHAT'S NEW?

Expanded discussion of viral classification, entry, and production is presented.

KEY POINTS

- HIV is a member of the lentivirus subfamily of retroviruses.

- The HIV life cycle can be divided into two phases: (1) virus entry, reverse transcription, entry into the nucleus, and integration of double-stranded DNA (the provirus) and (2) regulation of production of viral proteins and new infectious virions.

- HIV enters the cell via the CD4 receptor and chemokine coreceptors, primarily CCR5 and CXCR4.

- The viral genome is transcribed from RNA to DNA by reverse transcriptase and integrated into the host genome by integrase.

- The HIV genome encodes 15 proteins comprising three categories: structural, regulatory, and accessory.

- After budding from the host cell, the virus matures into its infectious form through cleavage of viral precursor proteins by protease.

VIRAL CLASSIFICATION

HIV is a member of the lentivirus subfamily of retroviruses, differing from HTLV-1 and HTLV-2, which are oncoviruses. Two distinct groups of HIV lentiviruses are pathogenic in humans: HIV-1 and HIV-2. Both are transmitted sexually and known to cause immunodeficiency disease. HIV-2 is less pathogenic and is epidemiologically distinct from HIV-1, as it was first isolated from persons with HIV (PWH) in West Africa. Subsequent discussion will focus on HIV-1 infection and pathogenesis.

HIV-1 is subclassified into three groups: M (major), O (outlier), and N (non-M, non-O) (Simon et al., 1998). The vast majority of HIV-1 infections belong to group M. Group M has at least nine known genetically distinct subtypes (or clades): A, B, C, D, F, G, H, J, and K. Subtype A remains the most prevalent strain in parts of East Africa, Russia, and the former Soviet Union; subtype B in Europe and the Americas; and subtype C in Southern Africa and India (Bbosa et al., 2019). Occasionally, genetic material from different clades of HIV-1 may recombine within the same host to form hybrid viruses, called *circulating recombinant forms* or *CRFs* (Salminen et al., 1997). Ninety inter-subtype recombinants have been shown to be recurrent among circulating HIV-1, and recent studies based on nearly full-length genome sequencing have highlighted the growing importance of recombinant variants and subtype C viruses (Bbosa et al., 2019). For a current listing of these CRFs, see https://www.hiv.lanl.gov/content/sequence/HIV/CRFs/CRFs.html (Song et al., 2018).

VIRAL STRUCTURE

HIV-1 is an RNA virus, and its basic genomic structure is typical of other retroviruses. The integrated form of HIV is known as the *provirus*, which is flanked at both ends by a repeated sequence known as the *long terminal repeats* (LTRs). The genes of HIV are located in the central region of the proviral DNA and encode 15 distinct proteins divided into three classes: structural proteins (Gag, Pol, and Env), regulatory proteins (Tat and Rev), and accessory proteins (Vpu, Vpr, Vif, and Nef) (Klimkait et al., 1990; Willey et al., 1992). In the mature HIV-1 virion, the inner capsid contains two molecules of single-stranded RNA and key enzymes necessary for infection: reverse transcriptase, integrase, protease, and accessory proteins (Figure 16.1). The capsid is surrounded by structural

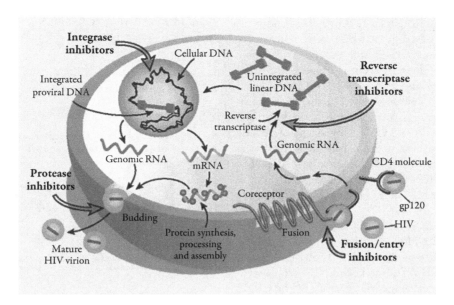

Figure 16.1 HIV life cycle and drug targets.   SOURCE: Reproduced from Fauci 2003 with permission from Macmillan Publishers Ltd: *Nat Med*, copyright 2003.

matrix protein, itself contained within the viral envelope. Composed of a phospholipid bilayer derived from the host cell, the envelope contains trimers of the viral glycoproteins gp120 and gp41. The exposed surfaces of gp120 exhibit a high level of variability, limiting the humoral immune response to circulating virus (Tilton & Doms, 2010).

VIRAL ENTRY

The viral envelope contains the necessary proteins for cell fusion and viral entry, initiating infection of the host cell.

HIV gains access to its target cells via multiple interactions of viral proteins with receptors on the cell membrane (Figure 16.2). The viral glycoprotein gp120 binds with high affinity to the CD4 receptor, which normally functions as a coreceptor in the activation of helper T cells. CD4 binding induces a conformational change in gp120, exposing its binding sites for coreceptors (either CCR5 or CXCR4) on the host cell surface. Binding of gp120 to the coreceptor exposes the fusion domain of the viral glycoprotein gp41. Then, glycoprotein gp41 inserts its hydrophobic peptide into the target cell membrane, forming a pore through which the

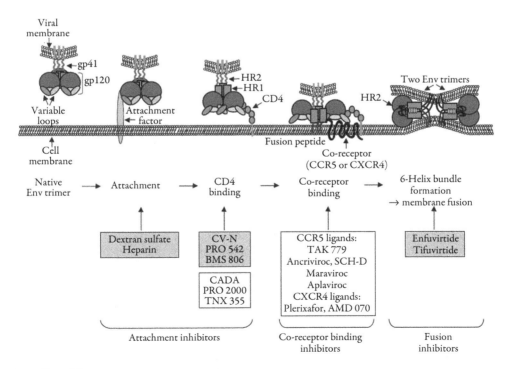

Figure 16.2 HIV entry into cells and drug targets.   SOURCE: Reeves J, et al. *Drugs*. 2005;65(13);1747–1766 with permission from Springer Nature.

viral capsid enters (Tavasolli, 2011). This process is known as *fusion*. Gp41 is a target of drugs that bind to this glycoprotein and prevent formation of the fusion pore.

Viral strains vary in their coreceptor usage. Those that bind the chemokine receptors CCR5 or CXCR4 are classified as R5-tropic or X4-tropic, respectively. During HIV transmission and early infection, R5-tropic strains predominate. Individuals who do not express CCR5, by virtue of genetic mutation, are highly resistant to HIV infection (Reiche et al., 2007). Mutant alleles in the CCR5 gene have also been shown to prevent HIV infection by creating a partially nonfunctional coreceptor for HIV entry (Liu et al., 1996; Samson et al., 1996).

Drugs that target CCR5 and bind to the coreceptor alter its interaction with gp120. However, these drugs can only be used in PWH whose virus is R5-tropic. Through evolution within the host, some HIV strains become X4-tropic, rendering them resistant to these agents. Deletion of the CCR5 gene through stem cell transplantation or gene therapy has been a proposed mechanism for curing HIV (Deeks et al., 2012). There have been three cases reported to achieve sustained HIV remission through stem cell transplantation from CCR5-Δ32 mutation homozygous donor cells, and efforts to modify CCR5 receptors to maintain HIV-1 remission in the absence of ART are ongoing (Gupta et al., 2019).

REVERSE TRANSCRIPTION AND INTEGRATION

After fusion, viral disassembly (which is distinct from and not merely the reverse of viral assembly) occurs before reverse transcription can take place. In order for HIV-1 to fully establish infection in a susceptible cell, the RNA must undergo reverse transcription into double-stranded DNA and integrate into the host genome (Tekeste et al., 2015). Reverse transcription starts when the viral RNA is released into the host cell cytoplasm, shedding associated proteins in a process known as *uncoating*. The viral enzyme reverse transcriptase (RT) then produces double-stranded DNA from the viral RNA template. RT is a heterodimer composed of a larger, functional subunit (p66) and a smaller, structural subunit (p51). At this stage, the host's natural antiviral immunity is activated, and the enzyme APOBEC3G, found in CD4+ T cells and macrophages, terminates the elongating viral DNA by causing hypermutations. However, HIV has the protein Vif, which binds APOBEC3G and leads to its degradation, overriding the host's natural immunity and allowing propagation of viral DNA (Table 16.1) (Tavasolli, 2011).

The newly synthesized viral DNA then integrates into the host DNA. Integration is a vital step in the sustained life of the virus and its progeny; integrase (IN)-negative HIV mutants do not integrate and therefore do not produce infectious virions (Wiskerchen & Muesing, 1995). Integration is catalyzed by IN, in conjunction with the nuclear localization factor Vpr, to form the preintegration complex. Once in the nucleus, a critical interaction between integrase and the host protein LEDGF/p75 directs this complex to the host DNA (Tavasolli, 2011), and IN mediates strand transfer, linking

Table 16.1 VIRAL ACCESSORY AND REGULATORY PROTEIN FUNCTIONS

GENE	FUNCTION
Tat	Transcriptional transactivator
Rev	Allows unspliced viral genomes to leave the nucleus
Nef	Downregulates CD4 receptor and major histocompatibility complex (MHC) class I, alters T-cell activation, aids viral infectivity
Vif	Counters the host restriction factor APOBEC3G
Vpr	Facilitates the nuclear localization of the viral genome
Vpr	Downregulates CD4 receptor, increases viral release

Adapted from Miller MD, et al. *Trends Microbiol.* August 1994;2(8):294–298.

viral and host DNA through covalent bonds. Coopting host cell proteins, HIV relies on the cell's normal DNA repair mechanism to complete integration.

The newest class of antiretroviral medications endorsed by the US Department of Health and Human Services are integrase strand transfer inhibitors (INSTIs), which block the penultimate step of integration by preventing strand transfer to the host DNA. Also, since it has been demonstrated in vitro that the RT–IN interaction is biologically significant for reverse transcription (Tekeste et al., 2015), the interaction between these two enzymes has been a target for development of two-drug combination therapy, which has demonstrated viral suppression and a safety profile consistent with current antiretroviral therapy (ART) regimens (Llibre et al., 2018).

VIRUS PRODUCTION

Once integrated into the host DNA, the viral genome can remain latent or undergo active expression. Active expression is dependent on cellular and viral factors that activate viral promotors, including coinfection with other agents, production of inflammatory cytokines, and cellular activation (Honda et al., 1998). In active infection, viral DNA is first transcribed into mRNA. Some of the early mRNAs produced are 2 kb in size and serve as viral regulatory proteins. These mRNAs can be detected by Southern blot analysis (Kim et al., 1989) or even polymerase chain reaction (PCR) within 6 hours of infection (Klotman et al., 1991). Many of the same transcription factors involved in CD4+ T-cell activation also bind to the HIV LTR, promoting expression of the viral genome (Pereira et al., 2000). The resulting mRNA is spliced, processed, and ultimately translated into viral proteins by the host cell machinery. In a positive feedback loop, the viral protein Tat (trans-activator) promotes further viral transcription by facilitating elongation of nascent viral transcripts (Kao et al., 1987).

The viral protein Gag mediates assembly of progeny virions by packaging genomic RNA within virus particles. Finally, HIV protease catalyzes the cleavage of the gag-pol precursor polyprotein (p55), yielding the structural proteins that form the mature virion. Assembly of mature virus occurs at the cell membrane, and these virus particles exit the cell in a process known as *viral budding*. Budding occurs in areas called *lipid rafts*, located in the cell membrane, composed of high concentrations of cholesterol, sphingolipids, and glycolipids (Liao et al., 2001). HIV-1 generation time in vivo is 2 days, and the half-life of infected CD4$^+$ T cells is 0.7 days (Markowitz et al., 2003). The ubiquitin proteasome system (UPS), which is a major protein degradation mechanism for eukaryotic cellular processes, may also play a critical role in in regulation of proteasomal degradation of viral and cellular counterparts during the HIV-1 life cycle, ultimately resulting in a contest for host or virus survival. However, the coordination and significance of viral protein degradation at different stages of the life cycle remains elusive and warrants further investigation (Rojas & Park, 2019).

RECOMMENDED READING

Fauci AS. HIV and AIDS: 20 years of science. *Nat Med.* 2003;9(7): 834–843.
Greene WC, Peterlin BM. Molecular insights into HIV biology. http://hivinsite.ucsf.edu/InSite?page=kb-02-01-01
Moore JP, Kitchen SG, Pugach P, et al. The CCR5 and CXCR4 coreceptors: central to understanding the transmission and pathogenesis of human immunodeficiency virus type 1 infection. *AIDS Res Hum Retroviruses.* 2004;20(1):111–126.
Reeves JD, Piefer AJ. Emerging drug targets for antiretroviral therapy. *Drugs.* 2005;65(13):1747–1766.

HIV NATURAL HISTORY

LEARNING OBJECTIVE

- Discuss the course of HIV infection and its dynamics in the host over time

WHAT'S NEW?

Overview of establishment of the viral reservoir

Overview of the current status of latency reversal agents and their mechanisms of action

KEY POINTS

- In mucosal transmission, HIV crosses the epithelial barrier and establishes an expanding infection at the site of entry.

- During acute infection, HIV disseminates to lymphatic tissue throughout the body.

- The rate of fall in plasma viremia with ART reflects the kinetics of different types of infected host cells.

- HIV exhibits remarkable levels of diversity, both globally and within a single host.

- HIV establishes latent infection in a subset of host cells, allowing it to persist despite ART.

ESTABLISHMENT OF INFECTION

In sexual transmission, HIV must first breach the epithelial barrier of the genital or rectal mucosa. This may occur via physical breaks in the epithelium related to trauma or sexually transmitted infections, particularly herpes simplex virus. However, HIV can also cross intact mucosa via specialized dendritic cells in the genital tract or transcytosis in the gastrointestinal tract (Morrow et al., 2008). Upon crossing the epithelial barrier, the virus encounters multiple potential target cells. The major cellular receptor for fusion and entry of HIV is CD4$^+$ T cells, whose critical role in HIV infection was identified in 1984 (Dalgleish et al., 1984; Klatzmann et al., 1984). Initial infection is propagated by dendritic cells (especially the Langerhans cells), components of the innate immune system, which deliver HIV to CD4$^+$ T cells; or the virus may directly infect local CD4$^+$ T cells without the aid of dendritic cells. The initial proliferation of HIV represents a genetic bottleneck in which a large viral inoculum gives rise to a small founder population of infected cells. In heterosexual transmission, infection results from a single viral genotype in 80% of cases, with preference for the CCR5 coreceptor (Haase, 2010).

The *eclipse phase* refers to the period after mucosal exposure, when the virus remains undetectable in plasma, and lasts approximately 10 days. Once a founder viral population is established at the portal of entry, it must expand locally by rapid migration to regional lymph nodes and dissemination to distant draining lymph nodes via the bloodstream. In a chain reaction of cell-to-cell signaling, termed the *virologic synapse* (Piguet & Steinman, 2007), dendritic and Langerhans cell-type T cells' exposure to HIV induces the recruitment of more plasmacytoid dendritic cells and ultimately more CD4$^+$ T cells (Haase, 2010). Therefore, in addition to the role that lymphoid tissue (in particular dendritic cells) plays in the initiation of HIV infection, it also is responsible for the dissemination of HIV infection. These early events may be altered to prevent infection, and they figure prominently in research on microbicides, preexposure and postexposure prophylaxis, and preventive vaccines.

ACUTE INFECTION

Once infection is established in draining lymph nodes, activated CD4$^+$ T lymphocytes become the predominant source of viral replication. Immune activation increases the pool of susceptible activated CD4$^+$ T cells, creating a positive feedback loop. An exponential increase in plasma viremia ensues, and PWH may develop symptoms of the acute retroviral syndrome. HIV disseminates and infects other lymphatic tissues throughout the body. The CD4$^+$ T-cell count in peripheral blood declines markedly, thought to occur through several proposed mechanisms: increased destruction of cells by direct infection by HIV, activation of apoptosis, increased lymphocyte turnover, decreased production by reduced thymic output, and redistribution of cells from peripheral blood to lymphoid tissue. A profound depletion of CD4$^+$ T cells also occurs in the gut-associated lymphatic tissue (GALT), causing permanent damage.

The events in acute infection have long-term consequences for the patient. Activation of CD4$^+$ T cells and HIV RNA replication causes fibrosis to occur in the lymphoid architecture, leading to incomplete immune reconstitution after initiation of ART (Brenchley et al., 2004). Damage to the gastrointestinal epithelium and mucosal immune response allows an increase in microbial translocation (Haase, 2010), which may serve as a stimulus to systemic immune activation, magnifying the positive feedback loop for the virus. Over time, microbial translocation likely contributes to chronic immune activation and progression to AIDS. Finally, a reservoir of latently infected cells is established, which later prevents viral eradication with ART. Important reservoir sites include the GALT and peripheral lymphoid tissues. In the rare cases in which HIV is diagnosed during primary infection, immediate ART may have potential to attenuate, although not reverse, these changes.

The establishment of the HIV reservoir and viral latency is widely discussed as the barrier to curing HIV (Castro-Gonzalez et al., 2018). Current therapies do not completely eliminate the reservoir after it has been established, since infected cells harbor replication-competent proviruses that are transcriptionally inactive and thus are not utilizing the replication enzymes that are targets for ART.

VIRAL KINETICS AND LATENCY

Plasma HIV RNA levels reflect a dynamic interplay between the infection of susceptible cells and the destruction of infected cells. With initiation of ART, susceptible host cells are protected from infection. Consequently, the rate of decline in the viral load following initiation of ART reflects the kinetics of the death of HIV-infected cells (Figure 16.3) (Palmer et al., 2011).

Viral decay occurs in four distinct phases. The viral load declines dramatically in the first phase of 7 to 10 days, reflecting clearance of activated CD4$^+$ T cells ($t_{1/2}$ = 1 or 2 days), with roughly 90% of the decrease in plasma HIV occurring

in these first weeks of therapy (Markowitz et al., 2003). The second phase, characterized by a more gradual decline in viral load and an average viral half-life of 14 days (Andrade et al., 2013), correlates with the intermediate half-lives of partially activated CD4$^+$ T cells, macrophages, and possibly dendritic cells. In the third phase, plasma HIV continues to decline, although at levels detectable only by ultrasensitive assays. This phase may represent decay of latently infected resting CD4$^+$ T cells that are producing HIV, but HIV RNA levels are unobserved since they have fallen below the limit of detection (Andrade et al., 2013). The fourth phase occurs 4 to 5 years after ART initiation and finally stabilizes at very low levels (<1–5 copies/mL) (Siliciano et al., 2003). Research has focused on the resting memory CD4$^+$ T cell as the source of viral replication during these latter stages. Despite fully suppressive ART, the proportion of resting CD4$^+$ T cells that are latently infected shows minimal decline over time, yielding an estimated half-life of 44 months (Siliciano et al., 2003). By this estimate, HIV eradication would require more than 70 years of uninterrupted ART.

Since HIV latency is the chief obstacle to eradicating HIV, increasing attention has turned to the mechanisms that maintain latent infection. In latent infection, proviral DNA is integrated into the host genome but remains in a transcriptionally silent, but inducible, state. Latently infected cells serve as a reservoir for virus that can reactivate and drive HIV viral loads to pretreatment levels if ART is interrupted (Rouzine et al., 2015). In rhesus macaque models, simian immunodeficiency virus (SIV) established latency in reservoir cells as early as 3 days after infection, before viremia was detected (Whitney et al., 2014). Different biological processes, such as host transcription factors, histone deacetylase-mediated epigenetic silencing, and cytokines, have been shown to play a role in HIV latency. The host transcription factors (NF-κB, NFAT, and P-TEFβ) and the viral protein tat promote expression of proviral DNA, but they are present at low levels in resting CD4$^+$ T cells, thus maintaining latency. Histone deacetylation and DNA methylation at the HIV LTR alter the local

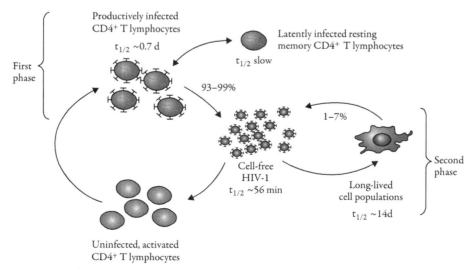

Figure 16.3 Rates of clearance of different cell populations and viral turnover.   SOURCE: Simon V et al. *Nat Rev Microbiol.* 2003;1(3):181–190.

chromatin environment, denying access to the machinery of transcription (Palmer et al., 2011). Establishment of the reservoir is also facilitated by cell-to-cell transmission of HIV, rather than cell-free transmission, which is more efficient and does not expose virus particles to the challenges of surviving in the extracellular environment (Pedro et al., 2019).

Therapies that promote expression of the proviral genome or activate resting CD4$^+$ T cells have the potential to speed decay of the latent reservoir. Two recent studies demonstrated robust and persistent latency reversal in mice and SIV models in multiple tissues and peripheral blood by activating the noncanonical NF-κB pathway (Nixon et al., 2020) and by interleukin-15 stimulation combined with depletion of CD8$^+$ T cells (McBrien et al., 2020). Further investigations on latency reversal agents are reviewed in more detail in Chapter 6.

VIRAL DIVERSITY

During untreated infection, HIV replicates at an extraordinary rate, with roughly 10 billion new virions produced each day. Reverse transcriptase, in contrast to DNA polymerases, lacks proofreading activity (Taylor et al., 2008). As a result, frequent mutations occur in the daughter viral genome, potentially altering the structure and function of viral proteins. HIV recombination is another means of viral diversity and occurs when one person is coinfected with two strains of the virus that replicate within the cell (Taylor et al., 2008). The rapid rate of production, combined with frequent mutations and recombination, leads to the production of diverse quasi-species. Strikingly, the genetic diversity observed in a single individual after 6 years of HIV infection is roughly equivalent to that observed worldwide in influenza A virus within a given year (Korber et al., 2001). However, the genetic diversity that occurs in acute infection occurs at a much higher rate than in chronic infection. The high number of replication cycles also allows for selection of resistant variants, due to either drug pressure or the immune system. Emergence of drug resistance mutations is governed by selection forces and drift (Maldarelli et al., 2013).

Viral diversity presents a unique challenge for producing an HIV vaccine. Historically, vaccines have prevented infection by stimulating antibody or cell-mediated immunity in susceptible PWH. Both HIV and SIV have been shown to escape from these host immune responses by virtue of their extreme diversity. An effective HIV vaccine may need to elicit broad immune responses that protect against multiple quasi-species and possibly other HIV subtypes. An international phase 3 study known as Mosaico (NCT03964415) was started in 2019 to investigate an experimental HIV vaccine that targets more strains of HIV than any other vaccine produced, and in vitro results indicate lasting immune response for at least 2 years after vaccine administration (Mega, 2019). The vaccine trial is ongoing, and results are pending.

The impact of viral diversity is well known to clinicians engaged in the treatment of HIV. The administration of multiple agents, initially called drug cocktails but now known as combination therapy, is required to suppress viral replication to levels at which drug-resistant strains are unlikely to emerge—in other words, viral diversity underpins the importance of strict adherence to HIV therapy. Similarly, the continuous evolution of HIV has required resistance testing in clinical practice and the continued development of antiretrovirals with novel therapeutic mechanisms.

RECOMMENDED READING

Finzi D, Blankson J, Siliciano JD, et al. Latent infection of CD4+ T cells provides a mechanism for lifelong persistence of HIV-1, even in patients on effective combination therapy. *Nat Med.* 1999;5(5):512–517.

Harris RS, Liddament MT. Retroviral restriction by APOBEC proteins. *Nat Rev Immunol.* 2004;4(11):868–877.

Mehandru S, Tenner-Racz K, Racz P, et al. The gastrointestinal tract is critical to the pathogenesis of acute HIV infection. *J Allergy Clin Immunol.* 2005;116(2):419–422.

Persaud D, Zhou Y, Siliciano JM, et al. Latency in human immunodeficiency virus type 1 infection: no easy answers. *J Virol.* 2003;77(3):1659–1665.

Simon V, Ho DD. HIV-1 dynamics in vivo: implications for therapy. *Nat Rev Microbiol.* 2003;1(3):181–190.

ACKNOWLEDGMENT

This chapter was based on previous additions written by Schuyler Livingston, Martin Markowitz, William Wright, Benjamin Young, and Bruce L. Gilliam.

REFERENCES

Andrade A, Rosenkranz S, Cillo A, et al. Three distinct phases of HIV-1 RNA decay in treatment-naïve patients receiving raltegravir-based antiretroviral therapy: ACTG A5248. *J Infect Dis.* 2013;208(6):884–891.

Bbosa N, Kaleebu P, Sswemwanga D. HIV subtype diversity worldwide. *HIV AIDS.* 2019;14(3):153–160.

Brenchley JM, Schacker TW, Ruff LE, et al. CD4+ T cell depletion during all stages of HIV disease occurs predominantly in the gastrointestinal tract. *J Exp Med.* 2004;200(6):749–759.

Castro-Gonzalez S, Colomer-Lluch M, Serra-Moreno R. Barriers for HIV cure: the latent reservoir. *AIDS Res Hum Retroviruses.* 2018;34(9):739–759.

Dalgleish AG, Beverly PC, Clapham PR, et al. The CD4(T4) antigen is an essential component of the receptor for the AIDS retrovirus. *Nature.* 1984;312:763–767.

Deeks SG, Autran B, Berkhout B, et al.; International AIDS Society Scientific Working Group on HIV Cure. Towards an HIV cure: a global scientific strategy. *Nat Rev Immunol.* 2012;12:607–614.

Gupta RK, Abdul-Jawad S, McCoy LE, et al. HIV-1 remission following CCR5Δ32/Δ32 haematopoietic stem-cell transplantation. *Nature.* 2019;568(7751):244–248.

Haase A. Targeting early infection to prevent HIV-1 mucosal transmission. *Nature.* 2010;464:217–223.

Honda Y, Rogers L, Nakata K, et al. Type I interferon induces inhibitory 16-kD CCAAT/enhancer binding protein (C/EBP) beta, repressing the HIV-1 long terminal repeat in macrophages: pulmonary tuberculosis alters C/EBP expression, enhancing HIV-1 replication. *J Exp Med.* 1998;188:1255–1265.

Kao SY, Calman AF, Luciw PA, et al. Anti-termination of transcription within the long terminal repeat of HIV-1 by tat gene product. *Nature*. 1987;330(6147):489–493.

Kim SY, Byrn R, Groopman J, et al. Temporal aspects of DNA and RNA synthesis during human immunodeficiency virus infection: evidence for differential gene expression. *J Virol*. 1989;63:3708–3713.

Klatzmann D, Champagne E, Chamaret S, et al. T-lymphocyte T4 molecule behaves as receptor for human retrovirus LAV. *Nature*. 1984;312:767–768.

Klimkait T, Strebel K, Hoggan MD, et al. The human immunodeficiency virus type 1-specific protein vpu is required for efficient virus maturation and release. *J Virol*. 1990;64(2):621–629.

Klotman ME, Kim S, Buchbinder A, et al. Kinetics of expression of multiply spliced RNA in early human immunodeficiency virus type 1 infection of lymphocytes and monocytes. *Proc Natl Acad Sci USA*. 1991;88:5011–5015.

Korber B, Gaschen B, Yusim K, et al. Evolutionary and immunological implications of contemporary HIV-1 variation. *Br Med Bull*. 2001;58:19–42.

Liao Z, Cimakasky LM, Hampton R, et al. Lipid rafts and HIV pathogenesis: host membrane cholesterol is required for infection by HIV type 1. *AIDS Res Hum Retroviruses*. 2001;17:1009–1019.

Liu R, Paxton W, Choe S, et al. Homozygous defect in HIV-1 coreceptor accounts for resistance of some multiply-exposed individuals to HIV-1 infection. *Cell*. 1996;86:367–377.

Llibre J, Chien-Ching H, Brinson C, et al. Efficacy, safety, and tolerability of dolutegravir-rilpivirine for the maintenance of virological suppression in adults with HIV-1: phase 3, randomised, non-inferiority SWORD-1 and SWORD-2 studies. *Lancet*. 2018;391(10123):839–849.

Maldarelli F, Kearney M, Palmer S, et al. HIV populations are large and accumulate high genetic diversity in a nonlinear fashion. *J Virol*. 2013;87(18):10313–10323.

Markowitz M, Louie M, Hurley A, et al. A novel antiviral intervention results in more accurate assessment of human immunodeficiency virus type 1 replication dynamics and T-cell decay in vivo. *J Virol*. 2003;77:5037–5038.

McBrien JB, Mavigner M, Franchitti L, et al. Robust and persistent reactivation of SIV and HIV by N-803 and depletion of CD8+ cells. *Nature*. 2020;578(7793):154–159.

Mega ER. Mosaic HIV vaccine to be tested in thousands of people across the world. *Nature*. 2019;572:165–166.

Miller MD, Feinberg MB, Greene WC. The HIV-1 nef gene acts as a positive viral infectivity factor. *Trends Microbiol*. 1994;2(8):294–298.

Morrow G, Vachot L, Vagenas P, et al. Current concepts of HIV transmission. *Curr Infect Dis Rep*. 2008;10(2):133–139.

Nixon CC, Mavigner M, Sampey GC, et al. Systemic HIV and SIV latency reversal via non-canonical NF-κB signaling in vivo. *Nature*. 2020;578(7793):160–165.

Palmer S, Josefsson L, Coffin JM. HIV reservoirs and the possibility of a cure for HIV infection. *J Intern Med*. 2011;270(6):550–560. doi:10.1111/j.1365-2796.2011.02457.x

Pedro K, Henderson A, Agosto L. Mechanisms of HIV-1 cell-to-cell transmission and the establishment of the latent reservoir. *Virus Res*. 2019;265:115–121.

Pereira LA, Bentley K, Peeters A, et al. A compilation of cellular transcription factor interactions with the HIV-1 LTV promoter. *Nucleic Acids Res*. 2000;28(3):663–668.

Piguet V, Steinman RM. The interaction of HIV with dendritic cells: outcomes and pathways. *Trends Immunol*. 2007;28:503–510.

Reeves JD, Piefer AJ. Emerging drug targets for antiretroviral therapy. *Drugs*. 2005;65:1747–1766. 10.2165/00003495-200565130-00002

Reiche EM, Bonametti AM, Voltarelli JC, et al. Genetic polymorphisms in the chemokine and chemokine receptors: impact on clinical course and therapy of the human immunodeficiency virus type 1 infection (HIV-1). *Curr Med Chem*. 2007;14:1325–1334.

Rojas V, Park I-W. Role of the ubiquitin proteasome system (UPS) in the HIV-1 life cycle. *Int J Mol Sci*. 2019;20(12):2984.

Rouzine I, Weinberger A, Weinberger L. An evolutionary role for HIV latency in enhancing viral transmission. *Cell*. 2015;160(5):1002–1012.

Salminen MO, Carr JK, Robertson DL, et al. Evolution and probably transmission of intersubtype recombinant human immunodeficiency virus type 1 in a Zambian couple. *J Virol*. 1997;71(4)2647–2655.

Samson M, Libert F, Doranz B, et al. Resistance to HIV-1 infection in Caucasian individuals bearing mutant alleles of the CCR-5 chemokine receptor gene. *Nature*. 1996;382:722–725.

Siliciano JD, Kaidas J, Finzi D, et al. Long-term follow-up studies confirm the stability of the latent reservoir for HIV-1 in resting CD4+ T cells. *Nat Med*. 2003;9(6):727–728. doi:10.1038/nm880

Simon F, Mauclere P, Roques P, et al. Identification of a new human immunodeficiency virus type 1 distinct from group M and group O. *Nat Med*. 1998;4(9):1032–1037.

Song H, Giorgi E, Ganusov V, et al. Tracking HIV-1 recombination to resolve its contribution to HIV-1 evolution in natural infection. *Nat Commun*. 2018;9:1928.

Tavasolli A. Targeting the protein-protein interactions of the HIV lifecycle. *Chem Soc Rev*. 2011;40(3):1337–1346.

Taylor B, Sobieszczyk M, McCutchan F, et al. The challenge of HIV-1 subtype diversity. *N Engl J Med*. 2008;358(15):1590–1602.

Tekeste SS, Wilkonson TA, Weiner EM, et al. Interaction between reverse transcriptase and integrase is required for reverse transcription during HIV-1 replication. *J Virol*. 2015;89(23):12058–12069.

Tilton JC, Doms RW. Entry inhibitors in the treatment of HIV-1 infection. *Antiviral Res*. 2010;85(1):91–100. doi:10.1016/j.antiviral.2009.07.022

Whitney JB, Hill AL, Sanisetty S, et al. Rapid seeding of the viral reservoir prior to SIV viraemia in rhesus monkeys. *Nature*. 2014;512:74–77.

Willey RL, Maldarelli F, Martin MA, et al. Human immunodeficiency virus type 1 Vpu protein regulates the formation of intracellular gp160-CD4 complexes. *J Virol*. 1992;66(1):226–234.

Wiskerchen M, Muesing MA. Human immunodeficiency virus type 1 integrase: effects of mutations on viral ability to integrate, direct viral gene expression from unintegrated viral DNA templates, and sustain viral propagation in primary cells. *J Virol*. 1995;69:376–386.

17.

SCIENTIFIC BASIS OF ANTIRETROVIRAL THERAPY

David E. Koren, Neha Sheth Pandit, and Emily Heil

CHAPTER GOALS

Upon completion of this chapter, the reader should be able to:

- Describe the classes of antiretroviral (ARV) agents and their mechanisms of action

- Discuss the clinical trials underpinning new trends in antiretroviral therapy (ART)

- Explain the basic principles of applied pharmacokinetics, pharmacodynamics, and pharmacogenomics of ARV agents

- Recognize the benefits of coformulated ART regimens versus the need for tailored ARV dosing

- Enumerate key principles of clinical trial design and expanded-access programs

---

CLASSES AND MECHANISMS OF ANTIRETROVIRAL AGENTS

LEARNING OBJECTIVE

- Describe the mechanisms of action of the traditional and newer ARV classes

WHAT'S NEW?

Fostemsavir, a CD4 attachment inhibitor, is a new oral medication that inhibits initial viral entry into the CD4$^+$ T cell and is not affected by viral tropism.

KEY POINTS

- There are five major categories of antiretroviral agents: inhibitors of viral entry, two types of HIV-1 reverse transcriptase inhibitors, inhibitors of HIV-1 protease, and inhibitors of HIV-1 integrase.

- Combination ART is recommended for all people with HIV (PWH).

INTRODUCTION

Conventional terminology refers to individual antiretroviral agents as ARVs, whereas a combination of ARVs taken to control HIV infection is known as antiretroviral therapy, or ART. As recommended by the US Department of Health and Human Services (DHHS, 2020) since 2012 and as further validated by the Start (Insight Start Group, 2015) and Temprano (Temprano ANRS 12136 Study Group, 2015) trials, ART is indicated for all PWH without regard to CD4$^+$ T-cell count. There have been 33 unique US Food and Drug Administration (FDA)-approved agents to treat HIV, targeting five major steps in the HIV replication cycle (Figure 17.1). Classes of ARVs can be divided into nucleoside/nucleotide reverse transcriptase inhibitors (NRTIs/NtRTIs), nonnucleoside reverse transcriptase inhibitors (NNRTIs), protease inhibitors (PIs), entry inhibitors (comprising an attachment inhibitor [AI], a fusion inhibitor [FI], a C-C chemokine receptor type 5 coreceptor antagonist [CCR5], and a postattachment inhibitor), and integrase strand transfer inhibitors (INSTIs). The primary goal of ART is to achieve viral suppression (DHHS, 2020).

NRTIS/NTRTIS

NRTIs inhibit the HIV-encoded reverse transcriptase enzyme in the host cell cytoplasm. This blocks the conversion of single-stranded viral RNA to double-stranded DNA, ultimately preventing incorporation of HIV genetic material into the host double-stranded DNA. NRTIs are nucleoside and nucleotide analogs; when reverse transcriptase incorporates them into the growing DNA, chain elongation is terminated. NRTIs must first be activated in the cell through three phosphorylation steps before they can become active chain terminators; NtRTIs require only two phosphorylation steps. NRTIs are poor substrates for human nuclear DNA polymerase alpha, but some NRTIs can be utilized by human mitochondrial DNA polymerase gamma and thus can cause toxicity. This class of antiretrovirals include the nucleosides abacavir (ABC), emtricitabine (FTC), lamivudine (3TC), and zidovudine (AZT) and the nucleotides tenofovir disoproxil fumarate (TDF) and tenofovir alafenamide (TAF) as well as three older NRTIs (didanosine [DDI], deoxycytidine, and stavudine [D4T]), which are no longer used clinically.

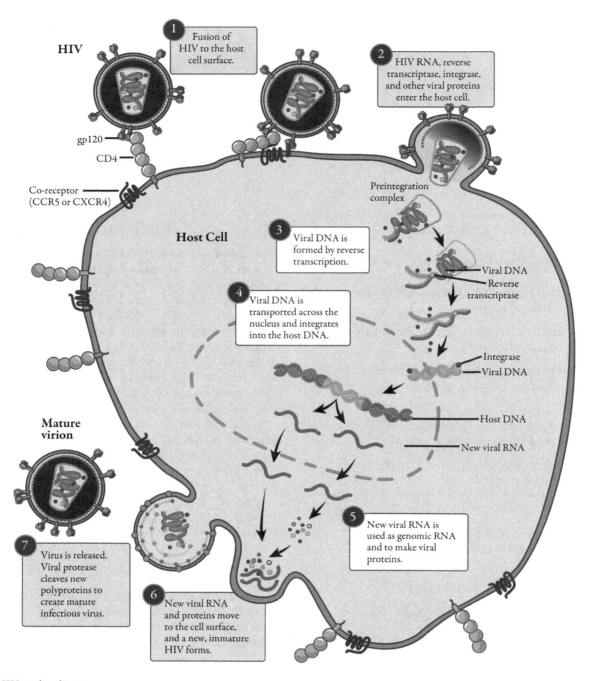

HIV

① Fusion of HIV to the host cell surface.

② HIV RNA, reverse transcriptase, integrase, and other viral proteins enter the host cell.

gp120

CD4

Co-receptor (CCR5 or CXCR4)

Preintegration complex

Host Cell

③ Viral DNA is formed by reverse transcription.

Viral DNA

Reverse transcriptase

④ Viral DNA is transported across the nucleus and integrates into the host DNA.

Integrase

Viral DNA

Host DNA

New viral RNA

Mature virion

⑤ New viral RNA is used as genomic RNA and to make viral proteins.

⑦ Virus is released. Viral protease cleaves new polyproteins to create mature infectious virus.

⑥ New viral RNA and proteins move to the cell surface, and a new, immature HIV forms.

Figure 17.1 HIV viral replication. SOURCE: NIH. Available at: https://www.niaid.nih.gov/diseases-conditions/hiv-replication-cycle

NNRTIS

NNRTIs also inhibit reverse transcriptase in the cytoplasm of the host cell. They act at the same point in the HIV-1 replication cycle as do the NtRTIs, but NNRTIs bind the reverse transcriptase adjacent to the active site, causing structural alterations in the enzyme that sterically prevent it from adding any new nucleosides to the growing DNA chain. Because of this different mechanism of action, the viral mutations that encode for resistance to NNRTIs are different from those that encode for resistance to NtRTIs. Doravirine, efavirenz (EFV), etravirine, nevirapine, and rilpivirine (RPV) make up the clinically relevant, FDA-approved NNRTIs.

PIS

PIs act when a nearly mature virion is budding from the surface of the infected host cell. These compounds bind HIV-1 protease, preventing it from cleaving the gag precursor polyprotein, an essential process for HIV core maturation. Thus, the viruses that bud from the cell have immature cores, rendering them defective and unable to infect further host cells. First-line PI regimens that include a pharmacologically boosted PI characteristically are associated with no to very low rates of treatment-emergent drug resistance at the time of virologic failure. While there are nine currently FDA-approved PIs, only two, atazanavir (ATV) and darunavir (DRV), are recommended in the DHHS Guidelines (DHHS, 2020) in certain clinical situations. The remaining seven (saquinavir; ritonavir [RTV]; indinavir; low-dose, RTV-boosted lopinavir [LPV/r], nelfinavir; fosamprenavir; and tipranavir) are no longer recommended in the DHHS guidelines.

ENTRY INHIBITORS

HIV entry inhibitors are a diverse class with different mechanisms of action. Fostemsavir, the most recently FDA-approved agent, is an attachment inhibitor; it binds to the HIV envelope protein gp120 and prevents viral attachment. Enfuvirtide (T-20), a fusion inhibitor, binds to the HIV envelope protein gp41, preventing virus envelope–cell membrane fusion. Chemokine coreceptor inhibitors act by binding to the CCR5 coreceptor, resulting in allosteric changes that prevent HIV binding and attachment. The only FDA-approved coreceptor inhibitor is maraviroc, a CCR5 coreceptor antagonist, which requires the testing of viral coreceptor tropism or utilization. Patients who harbor virus partially or fully using the alternative coreceptor CXCR4 should not be prescribed maraviroc. Ibalizumab, a monoclonal antibody characterized as a postattachment inhibitor, sterically inhibits post-CD4 receptor binding through attachment to domain 2 of the CD4 receptor of T cells.

INSTIS

Integrase inhibitors inhibit the viral enzyme integrase, which is responsible for inserting HIV proviral DNA into the host cell's DNA. There are four FDA-approved integrase inhibitors: raltegravir (RAL), elvitegravir (EVG), dolutegravir (DTG), and bictegravir (BIC). Regimens that include an INSTI are associated with the most rapid viral load declines of all ARVs and greater CD4+ T-cell increases than NNRTI- or PI-based regimens. An additional integrase inhibitor, cabotegravir (CAB), is likely to receive FDA approval in 2021.

KEY CHARACTERISTICS AND FINDINGS OF RECENT CLINICAL TRIALS OF US DHHS-RECOMMENDED REGIMENS

BIC-BASED REGIMENS

BIC is the fourth FDA-approved INSTI and is available only in a fixed-dose single-tablet regimen with the NtRTI TAF and the NRTI FTC. BIC/TAF/FTC is a regimen recommended by the DHHS for most PWH. BIC is generally very well tolerated and adverse drug reactions are uncommon. Characteristic adverse effects are diarrhea, nausea, and headache.

BIC is dosed once daily and has no dietary requirements. As with all INSTIs, oral absorption of BIC is affected by divalent cations, and so dose separation between BIC and products containing divalent cations (aluminum, magnesium, iron, and calcium) is recommended. Alternatively, iron- and calcium-containing supplements can be taken with BIC together with food (as with DTG). BIC causes reversible inhibition of renal tubular transporters, resulting in decreased tubular excretion of creatinine. This has the effect of increasing serum creatinine levels without impairment of glomerular filtration, also as seen with DTG. Increases were seen in clinical trials after 4 weeks and remained stable through week 48.

Two phase 3 clinical trials evaluated BIC-containing treatments (with either TAF/FTC or ABC/3TC) for initial therapy in adults. GS-380-1489 was a multicenter, randomized, double-blind noninferiority study comparing once-daily BIC/TAF/FTC versus DTG/ABC/3TC in 631 patients. The primary endpoint at week 48 demonstrated noninferiority between the two regimens with regard to viral suppression (<50 copies/mL) (Gallant et al., 2017).

GS-380-1490 was a similarly designed multicenter, randomized, double-blind noninferiority study comparing once-daily BIC/TAF/FTC versus DTG ± TAF/FTC in 657 treatment-naive adults. Overall, the two regimens performed very similarly at week 48, demonstrating noninferiority between the two regimens with regard to viral suppression (<50 copies/mL) (Sax et al., 2017). These studies suggest that BIC, dosed as part of a single-tablet regimen, is a potent available treatment option for persons initiating therapy.

No treatment-emergent resistance mutations resulted in either clinical trial. BIC retains in vitro activity against some viral strains resistant to other INSTIs (namely RAL and EVG), although cross-resistance is possible in isolates harboring a resistance mutation at integrase gene codon 118 or with multiple integrase resistance mutations in combination.

DTG-BASED REGIMENS

DTG is an INSTI commercially available as a standalone product (Tivicay); a fixed-dose three-drug regimen with the two NRTIs, ABC and 3TC (Triumeq); a fixed-dose, two-drug regimen with 3TC (Dovato); and a fixed-dose combination with the NNRTI RPV (Juluca). DTG + TDF/FTC or TAF/FTC, DTG/ABC/3TC, and DTG/3TC are DHHS-recommended preferred initial treatment regimens (the latter depending on certain patient characteristics to meet eligibility for treatment). DTG is generally very well tolerated, and adverse drug reactions are uncommon, including diarrhea, nausea, and headache.

DTG has multiple dosing recommendations in adults: once daily in INSTI-naive patients or in those who are INSTI-experienced without associated resistance substitutions, and twice daily in patients who are INSTI-experienced with associated INSTI-resistance substitution or who are receiving concurrent cytochrome P450-3A4 inducers (e.g., carbamazepine or rifampin). DTG has no dietary requirements. Oral absorption of INSTIs is affected by divalent cations. Dose separation between DTG and products containing divalent cations (aluminum, magnesium, iron, and calcium) is recommended. Alternatively, iron- and calcium-containing supplements can be taken with DTG together with food. To reduce the risk of ABC hypersensitivity reaction, DTG/ABC/3TC should be administered only to individuals who test negative for the HLA B-5701 allele. DTG causes reversible inhibition of the renal tubular transporter, resulting in decreased tubular excretion of creatinine. This has the effect of increasing serum creatinine levels without impairment of glomerular filtration.

Six phase 3 clinical trials evaluated DTG-containing treatments (with either TDF/FTC or ABC/3TC or in a two-drug combination with 3TC) for initial therapy in adults. The SINGLE study was a randomized, double-blind, 144-week study that compared DTG + TDF/FTC to single-tablet EFV/TDF/FTC in approximately 800 treatment-naive adults (Pappa et al., 2014; Walmsley et al., 2013). The primary endpoint demonstrated statistical superiority of DTG + TDF/FTC, with the difference driven by discontinuations due to EFV-related side effects rather than differing rates of viral suppression between on-treatment groups. The superiority of the DTG study arm was maintained through 144 weeks of follow-up.

SPRING-2 was a randomized double-blind study comparing DTG to twice-daily RAL, paired with either NRTI backbone ABC/3TC or TDF/FTC in approximately 800 treatment-naive patients (Raffi et al., 2013). Overall, the two study arms performed similarly, with approximately 3% discontinuation due to treatment-related adverse effects and rare treatment-emergent drug resistance (none in the DTG arm), demonstrating noninferiority between the two INSTIs.

FLAMINGO was an open-label clinical trial comparing DTG to DRV/r (again with TDF/FTC or ABC/3TC) in treatment-naive adults (Clotet et al., 2014; Molina et al., 2014). The 48- and 96-week results demonstrated the superiority of DTG to DRV/r. The difference between the two study arms was driven by a combination of more frequent virologic and tolerability discontinuations in the DRV/r arm. Changes in fasting lipid levels were lower among subjects in the DTG arm.

ARIA was the first fully powered all-women's phase 3 clinical trial comparing DTG/ABC/3TC to RTV-boosted ATV + TDF/FTC in 499 women (Orrell et al., 2017). After 48 weeks, DTG/ABC/3TC met a predetermined statistical noninferiority endpoint of viral suppression of less than 50 copies/mL compared to the RTV-boosted PI arm. Fewer patients receiving DTG reported drug-related adverse effects than with ATV/r (83 [33%] vs. 121 [41%]). Additionally, fewer patients receiving the INSTI-based regimen experienced adverse effects that led to discontinuation (10 [4%] vs. 17 [7%]).

Challenging the dogma of requiring three medications from two classes for an initial ART regimen, the GEMINI 1 and 2 trials determined the efficacy of a two-drug therapy among treatment-naive patients. These two identically designed, multicenter, double-blind, randomized, noninferiority phase 3 trials evaluated efficacy and safety of a once-daily two-drug regimen comprising DTG + 3TC compared to DTG + TDF/FTC in ART-naive patients (Cahn et al., 2019). At week 48, 90% and 93% of patients receiving a two-drug regimen across GEMINI 1 and 2 respectively reached the primary endpoint of an HIV-1 RNA less than 50 copies per mL per intention-to-treat analysis; per-protocol results were 92% and 94%, and noninferiority was met compared to a three-drug regimen. No emergence of INSTI or NRTI

resistance-conferring mutations were detected in any patient meeting virologic withdrawal criteria (<1% of participants overall) through week 96 (Cahn et al., 2020). Of note, inclusion criteria for these studies consisted of initial viral loads greater than 1,000 but less than 500,000 copies/mL and excluded patients coinfected with hepatitis B or with known ARV resistance mutations.

TANGO was an open-label, multicenter phase 3 study that evaluated the efficacy and safety of a switch to DTG/3TC in adults living with suppressed HIV-1 on a three- or four-drug TAF-based regimen (van Wyk et al., 2020). At week 48, only one participant in the DTG/3TC group (0.3%) and two participants in the TAF-based regimen group (0.5%) had HIV RNA of more than or equal to 50 copies/mL, demonstrating noninferiority. Zero participants in the DTG/3TC group and one in the TAF-based regimen group met confirmed virologic withdrawal criteria. Post hoc analysis described that all seven participants (4/322 in the DTG/3TC group and 3/321 in the TAF-based regimen group) who had preexisting archived M184V/I mutations (all mixtures with wild-type) maintained an HIV-1 RNA of less than 50 copies/mL at all on-treatment timepoints through week 48. Of note, a higher proportion of adverse events resulting in study withdrawal occurred in patients receiving DTG/3TC (3.5%, vs. 0.5% in TAF group). Weight gain was reported more frequently in patients receiving TAF; however, adjusted mean weight increase was only 0.8 kg in both groups ($p = 0.863$). A statistically significant difference was seen in the DTG/3TC group with respect to improved lipid parameters.

Treatment-emergent resistance to DTG in treatment-naive clinical trials is exceptionally rare, with only one case reported with no corresponding decrease in DTG susceptibility (ViiV Healthcare, Tivicay package insert, 2018). Moreover, resistance to NRTI components to initial therapy has not been reported in phase 3 clinical trials. DTG retains activity against some viral strains resistant to RAL and EVG, although cross-resistance is possible in isolates harboring resistance mutations at integrase gene codon 148 (in combination with at least two other integrase inhibitor-resistance mutations).

A final reflection on recent DTG trials concerns perinatal outcomes. In 2018, an interim analysis of the Tsepamo surveillance trial of birth outcomes in Botswana was released after four cases of neural tube defects were seen in infants from HIV-positive mothers who had received DTG prior to and through conception and pregnancy (Zash et al., 2017). Follow-up data published in 2019 analyzing 119,033 deliveries reported that among the 1,683 deliveries in which the mother was taking DTG-based ART at conception, 5 neural tube defects were found (0.30% of deliveries), compared with 15 defects among 14,792 (0.10%) infants born to mothers taking any non-DTG ART at conception (Zash et al., 2019). Study investigators stated that although the prevalence of neural tube defects was three times higher with DTG than with non-DTG ARVs, this represented only approximately two excess defects per 1,000 exposures. A more recent analysis from the AIDS 2020 conference contained 39,200 additional births surveyed from March 2019 to April 2020 and reported that newborns of mothers who were on DTG at the time of conception were not significantly more likely to have neural tube defects (0.19%) compared with newborns of mothers taking non-DTG ARVs (0.12%), an evolution of data showing extinguishing of this initially concerning signal. As of August 2020, US guidelines list DTG as an alternative rather than a preferred treatment option in an individual trying to conceive, but as a preferred agent in women who are already pregnant and presumed to be beyond the window of early organogenesis. Ultimately, given the changing nature of these recommendations, providers are recommended to check current DHHS or World Health Organization (WHO) guidance when starting DTG in women of childbearing age.

RAL-BASED REGIMENS

RAL was the first FDA-approved INSTI (2007). The combination of RAL with TDF/FTC is a DHHS-recommended initial regimen. RAL is generally very well tolerated, and adverse drug reactions are uncommon. Characteristic adverse effects are diarrhea, nausea, and headache.

Depending on formulation, RAL can be dosed once or twice daily and has no dietary restrictions. RAL is metabolized by glucuronidation and has no interaction with CYP3A4 substrates. Oral absorption of RAL is decreased by divalent cations; coadministration with aluminum- or magnesium-containing antacids is not recommended.

STARTMRK was a 240-week, randomized, double-blind, placebo-controlled study comparing RAL + TDF/FTC compared to EFV/TDF/FTC in 566 ART-naive individuals (DeJesus et al., 2012). At the primary endpoint of 48 weeks, RAL + TDF/FTC was noninferior to EFV/TDF/FTC. The 4- and 5-year analysis showed virologic and immunologic superiority of RAL, with the virologic differences driven by EFV/TDF/FTC discontinuations due to adverse effects (Rockstroh et al., 2013).

ACTG A5257 was a large randomized open-label trial of more than 1,800 treatment-naive subjects comparing twice-daily RAL with once-daily ATV/r or once-daily DRV/r, each administered with TDF/FTC (Lennox et al., 2014). At week 96, the RAL group was statistically superior to both once-daily PI regimens. Although the regimens had similar virologic suppression rates, there were differences in discontinuations due to side effects and toxicity. Of note, participants receiving RAL had less change in fasting lipid levels and less decrease in bone mineral density compared to both boosted PI arms.

SPRING-2 was a double-blind study that randomized treatment-naive subjects to receive RAL or DTG and was discussed previously (Raffi et al., 2013). Over 96 weeks of follow-up, the two study arms performed nearly identically, demonstrating noninferiority of the two INSTIs.

The phase 3 ONCEMRK trial was a randomized, double-blind, active controlled trial comparing RAL 400 mg twice daily versus RAL 1,200 mg daily, dosed as two 600-mg tablets (plus TDF/FTC) in approximately 800 treatment-naive patients. Noninferiority was met at week 48 using a snapshot analysis, including in patients with pretreatment viral loads greater than 100,000 copies/mL (Cahn et al., 2018).

Resistance to RAL is characterized by mutations at codons 143, 148, and 155 in the viral integrase gene. Resistance to RAL typically confers cross-resistance to EVG and much less commonly to DTG. Despite a lower genetic barrier to resistance in RAL compared to DTG or BIC, treatment-emergent resistance to RAL is uncommon. In the STARTMRK and SPRING-2 studies, in individuals initiating ART with RAL + TDF/3TC, INSTI resistance was detected after virologic failure in 4 of 281 (STARTMRK; 240-week data) and 1 of 411 (SPRING-2; 96-week data) treated individuals. No INSTI resistance emerged after the first 48 weeks of treatment.

OTHER RECENTLY FDA-APPROVED ARVS

Fostemsavir (Rukobia) is the prodrug of temsavir, a first-in-class investigational oral HIV-1 attachment inhibitor that binds directly to the viral envelope glycoprotein 120 (gp120), affecting the conformational change required for attachment and entry of the virus into the CD4 cell. FTR is an attractive treatment option for participants known to have multidrug-resistant HIV-1 infection as it has no in vitro cross-resistance with other classes of ARVs, contains a favorable drug–drug interaction profile, and can be used regardless of HIV-1 CCR5 coreceptor tropism. The BRIGHTE trial is an ongoing phase 3 trial that enrolled 371 adult patients with a known history of multidrug-resistant HIV-1 infection who had failure of their current ARV regimen and had exhausted at least four to six classes of ARVs (Kozal et al., 2020). Patients were assigned to one of two study arms. The first arm consisted of patients who had at least one or two fully active ARVs and were randomly assigned to receive FTR versus placebo + failing regimen the first 8 days to be followed with open-label FTR combined with optimized background therapy (most commonly used agents were DTG, DRV, and tenofovir) on day 9. The second arm had no fully active ARVs and received open-label FTR (600 mg twice daily) and optimized background therapy from day 1. The primary endpoint was defined as change in $\log_{10}$ level of HIV-1 RNA from day 1 through day 8 and was demonstrated to be statistically significant in the FTR groups (0.79 $\log_{10}$ decline). At week 48, the percentage of patients with an HIV-1 RNA level of less than 40 and less than 200 copies/mL was 62% and 84%, respectively. Adverse events and complications were associated with advanced AIDS (7% discontinuation rate associated with infections) and other drug-related events such as nausea and diarrhea. Virologic failure was seen in 18% of participants in the randomized group versus 46% in nonrandomized group and was associated with gp120 amino acid substitutions.

In 2018, the first single-tablet regimen containing a PI was approved by the FDA based on the results of the AMBER (treatment-naive) and EMERALD (treatment-experienced) clinical trials (Orkin et al., 2020b and 2018, respectively). The combination comprises TAF, FTC, DRV, and COBI (Symtuza) and is an alternative agent in the DHHS guidelines for initial ART but is one of the preferred regimens for rapid ART initiation if the results of genotyping and HBV and HLA-B5701 status are yet unknown.

WHAT'S ON THE HORIZON?

In March 2020, two studies were published in the *New England Journal of Medicine* evaluating the use of combination injectable long-active CAB (an INSTI) and RPV (an NNRTI) (Cabenuva) after oral induction for initial treatment of HIV-1 (FLAIR) and maintenance of suppression (ATLAS). The common focus of these studies was to evaluate the use of a long-acting injectable regimen to improve the overall ARV side-effect profile, decrease the burden of daily regimens, and improve engagement with care.

FLAIR was a phase 3 randomized open-label trial enrolling 629 adults with HIV-1 infection who had not previously received ART (Orkin et al., 2020a). Participants were given 20 weeks of daily oral induction therapy with DTG/ABC/3TC and at 16 weeks (once HIV-1 RNA levels were <50 copies/mL) were randomly assigned to continue oral therapy or switch to oral CAB + RPV for 1 month followed by monthly injections of the same agents. The primary endpoint at 48 weeks was the percentage of participants with HIV-1 RNA of 50 or more copies/mL. At week 48, an HIV-1 RNA level of 50 copies/mL or higher was found in six participants (2.1%) in the long-acting-therapy arm and in seven participants (2.5%) in the oral-therapy arm, meeting noninferiority criteria. The most common side effect was injection-site reaction (86% of participants). Virologic failure was seen in four participants in the long-acting therapy arm, with possible correlations to body mass index of more than 30, integrase polymorphisms, and low drug concentrations. Despite the reported adverse reactions, satisfaction scores were higher in the long-acting-therapy group.

ATLAS was a randomized, multicenter, parallel-group, open-label trial of long-acting CAB and RPV switch therapy compared to current oral therapy in virologically suppressed (<50 copies/mL) PWH (Swindells et al., 2020). Participants were randomized to continue their current therapy or switch to the long-acting-therapy regimen dosed every 4 weeks. At week 48 an HIV-1 RNA level less than 50 copies/mL was found in 92.5% of participants in the long-acting arm and 95.5% in the oral-therapy arm, meeting criteria for noninferiority. Injection-site reactions occurred in 83% of participants in the long-acting-therapy group, causing study withdrawal for four participants (1%). At week 44, participants in the long-acting-therapy group reported greater treatment satisfaction. Per the HIV Treatment Satisfaction Questionnaire assessment, 97% of participants in the long-acting-therapy group selected the injectable regimen over the daily oral therapy as their preferred HIV treatment.

Although Cabenuva was approved in Canada 2020, the FDA issued a complete response letter without approval, citing concerns for chemistry manufacturing and controls, while simultaneously noting no reported safety issues or changes in the safety profile. (ViiV Healthcare, 2019). Approval is thought to be likely in 2021.

RECOMMENDED READING

Cahn P, Madero J, Arribas J, et al. Dolutegravir plus lamivudine versus dolutegravir plus tenofovir disoproxil fumarate and emtricitabine in antiretroviral-naïve adults with HIV-1 infection (GEMINI-1 and GEMINI-2): week 48 results from two multicentre, double-blind, randomised, non-inferiority, phase 3 trials. *Lancet.* 2019;393:143–155.

Kozal M, Aberg, J, Pialoux G, et al. Fostemsavir in adults with multidrug-resistant HIV-1 infection. *N Engl J Med.* 2020;382:1232–1243.

Orkin C, Arasteh K, Gorgolas M, et al. Long-acting cabotegravir and rilpivirine after oral induction for HIV-i Infection. *N Engl J Med.* 2020a;382:1124–1135.

Swindells S, Andrade-Villanueva J, Richmond GJ, et al. Long-acting cabotegravir and rilpivirine for maintenance of HIV-1 suppression. *N Engl J Med.* 2020;382:1112–1123.

Van Wyk J, Ajana F, Bisshop F, et al. Efficacy and safety of switching to dolutegravir/lamivudine fixed-dose 2-drug regimen vs continuing a tenofovir alafenamide–based 3- or 4-drug regimen for maintenance of virologic suppression in adults living with human immunodeficiency virus type 1: phase 3, randomized, noninferiority TANGO study. *Clin Infect Dis.* 2020;71(8)L1920–1929. doi:10.1093/cid/ciz1243

Zash R, Holmes L, Diseko M, et al. Neural-tube defects and antiretroviral treatment regimens in Botswana. *N Engl J Med.* 2019;381:827–840.

PHARMACOKINETICS, PHARMACODYNAMICS, AND PHARMACOGENOMICS

LEARNING OBJECTIVES

- Describe the basic pharmacokinetic properties of classes of ARV agents

- Explain the benefits and shortcomings of using RTV or COBI for pharmacokinetic enhancement of PIs and/or INSTIs

- Review the potential role for therapeutic drug monitoring (TDM) for ARV agents

- Demonstrate how pharmacogenomics are applied in the clinical management of PWH

KEY POINTS

- Pharmacokinetics and local drug exposure can differ significantly within anatomic sanctuary sites compared with the systemic compartment.

- High variability in interpatient ARV concentrations is common, which makes population ARV pharmacokinetics difficult to interpret.

- Suboptimal ARV concentrations can result in drug resistance and virologic failure.

- TDM can be considered in certain cases.

- Pharmacogenomic testing for the HLA-B*5701 haplotype reduces the risk of ABC hypersensitivity reaction and is recommended prior to the initiation of ABC-containing therapy.

INTRODUCTION

The science of *pharmacokinetics* studies the amount of drug in various compartments of the body and attempts to explain the effect that the body has on the drug through the assessment of multiple factors known as **ADME**: (1) **A**bsorption or bioavailability of the drug, (2) **D**istribution of the drug throughout body compartments, (3) **M**etabolism of the drug, and (4) **E**limination or excretion of the drug from the body. Clinical pharmacokinetics is the application of these pharmacokinetic principles to the therapeutic management of a drug in a patient with the goal of enhancing efficacy while minimizing toxicity.

In contrast, *pharmacodynamics* examines the relationship between the drug concentration and response or the impact that the drug has on the body, which may have an intended or unintended pharmacologic effect. It also attempts to describe how drugs may interact with each other and display an additive, synergistic/multiplying, or antagonistic effect. An example is the combination of AZT and ganciclovir causing additive bone marrow toxicity resulting in neutropenia. The combination of AZT and D4T is antagonistic as both drugs compete for the same site of action on the viral reverse transcriptase target. Similarly, FTC and lamivudine should not be used together as they are unlikely to have additive antiviral activity due to similar chemical structures (DHHS, 2020).

Finally, *pharmacogenomics* is the practice of using host or viral genetic variation to individualize therapeutic decisions.

PHARMACOKINETICS

Absorption

Medication absorption highly depends on the route of administration. Oral formulations of ARV medications have varying degrees of bioavailability that affect a patient's serum ARV concentration. Currently, only AZT and ibalizumab are available in an intravenous formulation, and enfuvirtide is the only ARV available for subcutaneous injection. Ibalizumab, a humanized monoclonal antibody, was approved as an intravenous infusion given every 14 days for heavily treatment-experienced patients (Emu et al., 2017). Long-acting injectable formulations of RPV and an investigational INSTI, CAB, have been evaluated for intramuscular administration and shown to be noninferior to continued oral ARV in virologically suppressed adults (Swindells et al., 2020). For the solid dosage forms, absorption first requires the dissolution of the tablet or capsule, allowing the drug to be absorbed through the gastrointestinal tract and then into the systemic circulation, from which it will be distributed to its site of action.

Drug absorption is a function of ionization and aqueous solubility, which can be impacted by factors such as gastric pH, gastric mobility (emptying), absorptive capacity, biliary function, gastrointestinal enzymes, splanchnic blood flow, CYP enzyme expression in the gut, and transporters, such as P-glycoprotein. Absorption can be further affected under different patient conditions, such as use of nasogastric or percutaneous endoscopic gastrostomy tubes (G-tube) for medication administration, or when liquid formulations of medications are required, such as for pediatric patients or patients who have difficulty swallowing solid dosage forms. Many ARVs are available in oral solutions or suspensions to facilitate administration in these circumstances. The bioavailability of many ARV medications can be significantly compromised by manipulation of the dosage form, such as crushing tablets or opening up the contents of capsules (Bastiaans et al., 2014). For example, administration of crushed lopinavir/RTV tablets significantly decreased the exposure of both components, with a decrease in area under the plasma drug concentration–time curve (AUC) of 45% and 47%, respectively, compared to swallowing the tablets whole (Best et al., 2011). Additionally, certain medications like BIC and RPV are insoluble in water, so crushing these medications to mix in water for administration via G-tube could compromise drug concentrations (Biktarvy et al., 2019; Edurant et al., 2019).

Food can impact the bioavailability and rates of absorption for certain medications because food increases the pH in the stomach and delays gastric emptying to the small intestine, which serves as the site of absorption for many medications. For example, the relative bioavailability and maximum plasma drug concentration (C_{max}) of EFV are increased after a high-fat meal, and it is recommended that the drug be taken on an empty stomach (Sustiva, 2019). The solubility of a drug and surface area for absorption can be affected by gastric bypass procedures, which may impact the absorption of ART (Smith et al., 2011). In addition, the AUC and trough concentrations of INSTIs can be significantly reduced when coadministered with polyvalent cation products such as iron and calcium supplements or antacids containing aluminum, magnesium, or calcium. INSTIs should be given at least 2 hours before polyvalent cations under fasting conditions or at the same time if administered with food (DHHS, 2020).

Some ARVs require an acidic environment for solubility to occur, and acid-reducing agents may impact the dissolution of these drugs. ATV is a PI whose absorption is dependent on a highly acidic environment. Up to 40 mg by mouth twice daily of famotidine with boosted and unboosted ATV was found to decrease ATV AUC by approximately 20% (Wang et al., 2011). A pharmacokinetic study of boosted ATV and omeprazole 20 mg reported a 42% reduction in ATV AUC and a 46% reduction in ATV trough concentration (C_{trough}) compared with boosted ATV alone (Zhu et al., 2011). An increased gastric pH by acid-reducing agents such as proton pump inhibitors does not cause changes in absorption with other PIs such as DRV/RTV (DHHS, 2020). Increased gastric pH will also decrease RPV absorption, leading to suboptimal concentrations. RPV 150 mg was given with omeprazole 20 mg to 16 HIV-negative patients, resulting in an AUC and C_{max} decrease of 40%. Based on this study, proton pump inhibitors are contraindicated with RPV, and H_2 antagonists should be taken 12 hours before or 4 hours after RPV ingestion (Crauwels et al., 2008).

Distribution

After ARVs are absorbed into the bloodstream, they distribute into the interstitial and intracellular fluids depending on the individual physiochemical properties (pK, molecular weight/size, and lipophilicity) of each drug (Minuesa et al., 2011). Many of the ARVs circulate in the bloodstream reversibly bound to plasma proteins. Albumin primarily binds acidic drugs, and α_1 acid glycoprotein primarily binds basic drugs. Only free, or unbound, drug is pharmacologically active, and the greater the free fraction of the drug, the better it distributes into tissues or compartments. A decrease in plasma protein binding may be seen in patients with cirrhosis or cancer (Morse et al., 2006). Unbound drug can enter cells or tissues primarily through carrier-mediated transport mechanisms, although some drugs can pass through via transcellular diffusion (Griffin et al., 2011).

The individual distribution characteristics of ARV compounds are under extensive investigation because each ARV drug may differ in its ability to penetrate into "sanctuary sites" throughout the body. These are areas where HIV can undergo compartmentalized viral replication with the potential to select resistant viral mutations due to suboptimal ARV drug concentrations within these sites, such as the male and female genital tract and/or the central nervous system (CNS; Pomerantz, 2002; Tseng et al., 2014). Drug distribution to the male and female genital tracts is influenced by many factors, including hormonal changes, inflammation, concomitant sexually transmitted infections, and drug factors such as protein binding and lipophilicity (Trezza & Kashuba, 2014). Consequently, understanding drug distribution in the genital tract is essential for selecting agents for preexposure prophylaxis.

Metabolism

Many ARV drugs, including CCR5 inhibitors, NNRTIs, and PIs, are metabolized by CYP enzymes, which are located in the smooth endoplasmic reticulum in cells throughout the body, primarily the liver and intestines. Inhibition of gut CYP3A4 enzymes leads to increased bioavailability of these agents, whereas inhibition of liver CYP3A4 metabolism results in delayed elimination and a prolonged elimination half-life. RTV, an early protease inhibitor, is a highly potent CYP3A4 inhibitor, and coadministration of a subtherapeutic dose (~100 mg) of RTV is sufficient to enhance (or "boost") the pharmacokinetic profile of all but one (nelfinavir) of the currently licensed PIs (Larson et al., 2014). COBI, a similarly potent inhibitor of CYP3A enzymes, is approved by the FDA to provide pharmacokinetic enhancement to PIs such as ATV and DRV and the INSTI EVG. Due to its selective inhibition of CYP3A enzymes, cobicistat has less potential for off-target drug interactions compared to RTV. Unlike RTV, COBI has no anti-HIV activity; it is also more soluble than RTV, facilitating the development of coformulated products (Larson et al., 2014; Shah et al., 2013).

Pharmacokinetic enhancement of PI and INSTI concentrations with RTV or COBI, although increasing the risk of interactions with other agents, has several benefits, including:

- Higher C_{trough} levels, reducing the risk of selection for drug-resistant viral quasi-species

- Higher plasma levels throughout the day, minimizing or eliminating:
  - food requirements
  - the significance of interactions with other agents that induce the metabolism of PIs and INSTIs
  - the effects of interpatient variations in drug levels due to factors such as gender, smoking, alcohol consumption, or liver disease
- Increased plasma half-life, resulting in reduced dosing frequency and pill burden
- Increased levels of "forgiveness" with missed or late doses, potentially delaying/preventing the development of viral mutations

P-glycoprotein (P-gp) is a cellular protein pump involved in transporting molecules in and out of the cell. P-gp is found extensively in the intestine, and its action is important in drug exposure and bioavailability. PIs are known to be substrates for P-gp. Overexpression of P-gp by certain individuals may result in lower intracellular concentrations of some PIs and thus decreased overall drug exposure (Sankatsing et al., 2004). RTV is a potent inhibitor of P-gp, whereas COBI is a weak P-gp substrate and inhibitor that does not lead to clinically relevant interactions (Larson et al., 2014; Shah et al., 2013).

Excretion

ARVs are eliminated from the body either unchanged by the process of excretion or converted to metabolites that may be more readily excreted. The kidney is the most important organ for the elimination of drugs and their metabolites, whereas the liver is the principal organ responsible for drug metabolism and biliary excretion (Verbeeck & Musuamba, 2009). Renal and hepatic diseases are progressive illnesses that may occur as comorbidities in PWH. Chronic kidney disease is a condition marked by deteriorating kidney function and subsequent decreases in medication elimination. NRTIs are primarily eliminated via the kidney, with the exception of ABC. If there is a decrease in the glomerular filtration rate (GFR) in chronic kidney disease, it may be necessary to decrease the NRTI dose or increase the dosing frequency interval to prevent high systemic drug concentrations that may lead to adverse drug reactions.

It is important for the clinician to routinely check kidney function at least every 6 months (DHHS, 2020). The National Kidney Foundation Kidney Disease Outcomes Quality Initiative recommends the use of kidney function–estimating equations of either Cockcroft–Gault or the Modification of Diet in Renal Disease (MDRD) for the routine estimation of GFR. Note that most FDA medication package insert dosage guidelines for renal impairment are based on only the Cockcroft–Gault estimating equation. Guidelines for renal dosage adjustments of ARV agents are provided in all prescribing information in addition to DHHS guidelines (DHHS, 2020).

PHARMACODYNAMICS AND TDM

The need to maintain adequate drug concentrations that are effective in controlling HIV replication and preventing resistance has resulted in considerable interest in the relationship between ARV drug exposure, virologic response, and drug-related toxicity. The ideal ARV dosing strategy ensures the highest probability of success at maintaining viral suppression with the lowest possible dose. This relationship can be examined through TDM. A retrospective study of 1,807 samples found that the majority of concentrations for ARVs are above the upper therapeutic threshold and could likely benefit from dose optimization using TDM (Cattaneo et al., 2014). Currently, the only ARV approved at the lowest efficacious dose was RPV, but postapproval dose reduction has been seen ARVs such as AZT, DDI, D4T, and EFV. Other medications shown to be efficacious but not yet approved at lower doses include lopinavir, ATV, DVR, and RAL (Crawford et al., 2012).

DTG has predictable pharmacokinetics, with minimal intersubject variability and a defined exposure–response relationship (Cottrell et al., 2013). Early studies showed that DTG toxicities occurred at dosing ranges used for evaluation (Boffito et al., 2020). A study of 43 PWH over the age of 60 showed a significantly higher C_{min} of DTG compared to controls, with many PWH presenting with toxicities of DTG (Elliot et al., 2019). Despite this, the use of TDM for routine ART management has not been standard of care in most situations due to a lack of several key elements, including large prospective studies showing improved outcomes, established therapeutic concentration ranges for ARV agents, and laboratories that reliably perform ARV concentrations. These factors, plus intrapatient variability in drug concentrations, challenge the use of ARV TDM in clinical practice (DHHS, 2020; Pretorius et al., 2011).

Nevertheless, TDM of ARVs could be considered for patients who may have compromised ADME or in populations where pharmacokinetic studies are limited. For example, absorption may be disrupted in patients with drug interactions or impairment of gastrointestinal, hepatic, and renal function. TDM of ARVs may be beneficial in pregnant, pediatric, obese, or elderly patients (Cattaneo et al., 2020; DHHS, 2020). Metabolism may be affected in patients on concurrent CYP P450-interacting ARVs, and excretion may be compromised, leading to toxicities for patients with hepatic or renal impairment (Cattaneo et al., 2020; DHHS, 2020). For patients who are experiencing virologic rebound, adherence to their treatment regimen should be thoroughly evaluated prior to TDM as noncompliance is the most common cause for treatment failure.

PIs

All PIs are CYP3A4 substrates and most are CYP3A inhibitors; thus, there is a risk of drug interactions with commonly used medications that may be substrates of, induce, or inhibit the same CYP enzymes. The most common example of this type of interaction is the boosting effect of RTV or COBI on other PIs or the INSTI EVG, but many medications used for comorbidities common in PWH also have CYP3A4-based interactions. In addition, boosting can potentiate the toxicity of the target drug. A retrospective analysis of 240 PWH on boosted and unboosted ATV found a direct correlation between ATV plasma concentrations and the incidence and severity of hyperbilirubinemia, percentage increase in triglycerides, and incidence of nephrolithiasis. These toxicities and increased plasma concentrations were seen mostly in the boosted ATV group, and the study suggested that concentrations greater than 800 ng/mL were likely the cause (Gervasoni et al., 2015).

NNRTIs

Like PIs, NNRTIs are substrates of the CYP3A4 enzyme; unlike PIs, however, most NNRTIs are CYP3A4 inducers, not inhibitors, and thus NNRTIs are also at high risk for drug interactions. Whereas PIs have a high genetic barrier to resistance, single-point mutations such as K103N or Y181C can cause complete virologic resistance to first-generation NNRTIs. Second-generation NNRTIs such as etravirine and RPV (and, later, doravirine) have a higher genetic barrier to resistance (Usach et al., 2013) and maintain activity against K103N virus. As one might expect, the risk of virologic failure with EFV-based ART was associated with low EFV plasma levels in one small study (Marzolini et al., 2001). In a larger study, however, trough levels and AUC_{24} of nevirapine and EFV were not significantly predictive of virologic failure, although for EFV there was an association between these parameters and virologic failure (Van Leth et al., 2006). An analysis of etravirine from the DUET trials failed to show any relationship between its pharmacokinetics and efficacy or toxicities (Kakuda et al., 2010). These studies suggest that when reliably taken at prescribed doses, NNRTIs retain full activity, with resistance occurring more due to improper adherence than pharmacokinetic issues. RPV is currently being studied as a long-acting subcutaneous injection that could be given at least every 4 and perhaps every 8 weeks. The plasma RPV concentrations seen in the long-acting studies have been similar to those seen with oral RPV use (Williams et al., 2015).

EFV-induced CNS toxicities have been correlated with elevated plasma concentrations (Marzolini et al., 2001). Through the use of TDM and dose adjustment, elevated plasma EFV concentrations were reduced to the recommended therapeutic range while maintaining undetectable viral loads (Mello et al., 2011). Although subjects in this trial were stable on long-term EFV, a significant improvement in anxiety scores and a trend toward lower stress scores were noted with the reduction in concentrations. EFV 400 mg was also compared to the standard 600-mg dose, and it was found that the lower 400-mg dose was noninferior to the standard 600-mg dose for virologic suppression and was associated with fewer EFV-related adverse events (ENCORE1 Study Group, 2015). A fixed-dose combination tablet including EFV 400 mg has FDA approval to help minimize toxicities (Symfi Lo, 2019).

INSTIs

RAL, DTG, and BIC are metabolized by UGT1A1, whereas EVG acts similarly to a PI as a substrate of CYP3A4 requiring pharmacokinetic enhancing, with the attendant potential for drug interactions. BIC is a minor substrate of CYP3A4, so coadministration of potent inducers of CYP3A, P-gp, or UGT1A1 should be avoided (Biktarvy et al., 2019).

A study that evaluated RAL 800 mg once daily compared to 400 mg twice daily, both given with FTC/TDF, in treatment-naive individuals found that although patients in both groups had similar AUCs, a sixfold decrease was seen in C_{trough} in the 800-mg group (Rizk et al., 2012). Even with the decrease in C_{trough}, similar response rates were seen in both groups with a baseline viral load of 100,000 copies/mL or less. However, the once-daily dosing arm was statistically inferior to the standard twice-daily dosing arm in those patients with a baseline viral load of more than 100,000 copies/mL and a CD4$^+$ T-cell count of 200 mm^3 or less (Eron et al., 2011).

A different study comparing RAL 1,200 mg once daily to 400 mg twice daily, both in combination with FTC/TDF, in ART-naive patients found that the once-daily option was noninferior to twice-daily dosing. RAL HD 600-mg tablets are available and have FDA approval for a total 1,200-mg dosage taken orally once daily (Deeks, 2017). A final feature seen with INSTIs has been a rapid decline in HIV viral load after initiation. DTG 50 mg daily was shown to achieve a 2.5-log decrease in HIV RNA after 10 days of therapy (Lalezari et al., 2009), and similar results were seen with the use of EVG, which resulted in a decrease of greater than 1 log in HIV RNA after once- and twice-daily dosing (DeJesus et al., 2006).

CNS Effectiveness of ARVs

The CNS is reached by considerable blood flow, but two anatomic barriers, the blood–brain barrier and the blood–cerebrospinal fluid (CSF) barrier, prevent the free passage of drugs into the brain (Calcagno et al., 2014). The CNS HIV Antiretroviral Therapy Effects Research (CHARTER) study group developed the CNS penetration-effectiveness (CPE) ranking scheme of CNS effectiveness of ARVs based partly on the physiochemical properties of the drug, such as lipophilicity, protein binding, and efflux substrate, that affect penetration into the CNS (Letendre et al., 2008). Regimens with higher CPE scores were proposed to have greater effectiveness in controlling HIV replication in the CSF. However, the use of CPE rankings to affect the course and severity of HIV-associated neurocognitive disorder has not been demonstrated consistently (Caniglia et al., 2014; Ellis et al., 2014; Mukerji et al., 2018; Santos et al., 2019).

PHARMACOGENOMICS

Pharmacogenomics refers to the concept of using information about genetic variation to identify the most effective or well-tolerated ARV medications for an individual patient. Pharmacogenomic applications can be broadly categorized into the following areas: (1) ARV susceptibility, (2) explaining pharmacokinetic or pharmacodynamic variability, and (3) predicting adverse drug reactions. An example of the first category is genotypic resistance testing, which uses viral, not host, genetic markers to predict susceptibility to ARV medications. It is recommended prior to the initiation of treatment

and in response to treatment failure. An example of the third category is seen with EFV, which is associated with characteristic neuropsychological side effects correlating with plasma levels. Its metabolism is variable, with higher levels associated with genetic polymorphisms of cytochrome CYP2B6 (Rotger et al., 2007). In one clinical trial from Japan, individuals harboring the CYP2B6*6 or -*26 allele successfully maintained plasma EFV levels despite dose reduction (Gatanaga et al., 2007).

Perhaps the best example, however, of using pharmacogenomic biomarkers to predict adverse drug reactions is the association between the HLA-B*5701 allele and ABC hypersensitivity. Without genetic screening, approximately 5% to 8% of individuals exposed to ABC develop a hypersensitivity reaction (HSR), which can be fatal upon drug rechallenge. Genetic screening identified the HLA-B*5701 allele as a predictor of HSR; subsequently, the PREDICT study (Mallal et al., 2008) randomized 1,956 predominantly White individuals who were treated with ABC-containing ART. The use of HLA genetic screening dramatically reduced clinically suspected HSR from 7.8% to 3.4%. Skin patch test immunologically confirmed HSR was reduced from 2.7% to 0%. In a large, racially diverse group of North American patients, HLA-B*5701 screening resulted in 0.8% of individuals having clinically suspected HSR and no immunologically confirmed cases (Young et al., 2008). HLA-B*5701 allele screening is now recommended prior to the use of ABC by multiple national treatment guidelines (DHHS, 2020).

SUMMARY

Understanding the basic principles of applied clinical pharmacokinetics, pharmacodynamics, and pharmacogenomics can help the clinician gain insight into contemporary HIV pharmacotherapy and improve therapeutic responses. This information can be used to improve ART for the individual patient by gaining a fundamental working knowledge of concepts that contribute to the occurrence of drug–drug interactions, adverse drug reactions, poor adherence, decreased efficacy, and the selection of viral resistance. These factors, alone or in combination, can lead to treatment failure of ART and subsequent progression of HIV disease.

ARV DOSING AND COFORMULATIONS

LEARNING OBJECTIVES

- Describe food requirements, typical dosing, and modified dosing according to weight and renal and hepatic clearance for FDA-approved ARV therapies.

- Identify coformulations used in HIV therapy.

WHAT'S NEW?

Safety data with regard to TAF and FTC expanded certain FDA dosing recommendations in the setting of renal dysfunction.

KEY POINTS

- The selection of an ARV dose should take into consideration the drug concentration that inhibits viral replication and the concentration that causes toxicity.

- Current ARV agents are dosed either once or twice daily without need for exact 24- or 12-hour dosing.

- Multiple factors affect drug exposures, including renal and/or hepatic insufficiency, ARV food requirements, and drug interactions.

- Coformulated medications reduce pill burden and improve adherence to ART.

The selection of an appropriate ARV dosage is based on the amount of drug needed to inhibit viral replication and the ability to physiologically obtain these concentrations without causing significant toxicities. Ideally, the maximum concentration should not cause adverse events, and the minimum drug concentrations at the end of a dosing interval should be in excess of the target concentration needed to inhibit viral replication.

Many ARV agents are metabolized by the liver and/or eliminated by the kidney; thus, changes in hepatic or renal function can cause drug accumulation. This increases the potential for adverse drug events and might necessitate dose changes. A single-arm, open-label study by Eron et al. (2019) dosed EVG/COBI/TAF/FTC daily in patients with severe renal dysfunction (with estimated creatinine clearances <15 mL/min) and in patients on intermittent hemodialysis; no significant adverse effects were seen. From these data, the FDA expanded dosing recommendations among several tablets that include these agents. However, in situations in which renal and/or hepatic impairment requires dosage modifications, the use of certain fixed-dose single-tablet regimens (STRs; e.g., Atripla, Biktarvy, Complera, Delstrigo, Dovato, Genvoya, Odefsey, Stribild, and Triumeq) may not be possible; these situations may require the use of individual agents, when available, with the proper dosage adjustment for each agent. As of 2020, there are 22 coformulations licensed for use in HIV therapy in the US (Table 17.1).

Table 17.1 APPROVED COMBINATION ARV FORMULATIONS

MEDICATIONS IN FORMULATION	ABBREVIATION	TRADE NAME	APPROVAL DATE
Abacavir and lamivudine	ABC/3TC	Epzicom	8/2/2004
Abacavir, dolutegravir, and lamivudine	ABC/DTG/3TC	Triumeq	8/22/2014
Abacavir/lamivudine and zidovudine	ABC/3TC/ZDV	Trizivir	11/14/2000
Atazanavir and cobicistat	ATV/Cobi	Evotaz	1/29/2015
Bictegravir, emtricitabine, and tenofovir alafenamide	BIC/FTC/TDF	Biktarvy	2/7/2018
Darunavir and cobicistat	DRV/Cobi	Prezcobix	1/29/2015
Darunavir, cobicistat, emtricitabine, and tenofovir alafenamide	DRV/Cobi/FTC/TAF	Symtuza	7/17/2018
Dolutegravir and lamivudine	DTF/3TC	Dovato	4/18/2019
Dolutegravir and rilpivirine	DTG/RPV	Juluca	11/21/2017
Doravirine, lamivudine, and tenofovir disoproxil fumarate	DOR/3TC/TDF	Delstrigo	8/30/2018
Efavirenz, emtricitabine, and tenofovir disoproxil fumarate	EFV/FTC/TDF	Atripla	7/12/2006
Efavirenz, lamivudine, and tenofovir disoproxil fumarate	EFV/3TC/TDF	Symfi	3/22/2018
Efavirenz, lamivudine, and tenofovir disoproxil fumarate	EFV/3TC/TDF	Symfi Lo	2/4/2019
Elvitegravir, cobicistat, emtricitabine, and tenofovir alafenamide	EVG/Cobi/FTC/TAF	Genvoya	11/5/2015
Elvitegravir, cobicistat, emtricitabine, and tenofovir disoproxil fumarate	EVG/Cobi/FTC/TDF	Stribild	8/27/2012
Emtricitabine, rilpivirine, and tenofovir alafenamide	FTC/RPV/TAF	Odefsey	3/1/2016
Emtricitabine, rilpivirine, and tenofovir disoproxil fumarate	FTC/RPV/TDF	Complera	8/10/2011
Emtricitabine and tenofovir alafenamide	FTC/TAF	Descovy	4/4/2016
Emtricitabine and tenofovir disoproxil fumarate	FTC/TDF	Truvada	8/2/2004
Lamivudine and tenofovir disoproxil fumarate	3TC/TDF	Cimduo	2/28/2018
Lamivudine and zidovudine	3TC/ZDV	Combivir	9/27/1997
Lopinavir and ritonavir	LPV/r	Kaletra	9/15/2000

Adapted from https://hivinfo.nih.gov/understanding-hiv/fact-sheets/fda-approved-hiv-medicines.

Counseling patients on optimal dosing and adherence is critical to the success of ART. Evidence-based guidelines for improving adherence are available and include recommendations for the routine collection of self-reported adherence data and the use of pharmacy refill data adherence monitoring (International Advisory Panel on HIV Care Continuum Optimization, 2015). Nearly all ARVs currently prescribed are dosed either once or twice daily. Note that this does not imply, nor require, that patients take their medications exactly every 24 or 12 hours; rather, they may aim to take their medications within a more generous time window.

Many ARVs should be taken with food for optimal absorption. Some medications require an acidic stomach environment and may have negative drug interactions with acid-lowering agents such as proton pump inhibitors (e.g., ATV and RPV). Others require dietary fat for optimal absorption (e.g., RPV). Counseling about and patient adherence to dietary restrictions are important elements for optimal response to ART. The adult and adolescent DHHS guidelines list the standard dose, food requirements, and dosage adjustments in renal and/or hepatic impairment for the FDA-approved ARVs (DHHS, 2020).

Coformulated ARVs have been used for the treatment of HIV since 1997. The rationale for coformulation is to decrease pill burden, thereby facilitating treatment adherence while decreasing risk of selective nonadherence or supply chain gaps. A meta-analysis comparing STRs to multitablet ARV regimens (MTRs) concluded that STRs were associated with statistically significantly higher adherence compared to patients on MTRs of any frequency (odds ratio [OR], 2.37; 95% confidence interval [CI], 1.68–3.35; $p < 0.001$; four studies), twice-daily MTR (OR, 2.53; 95% CI, 1.13–5.66; $p = 0.02$; two studies), and once-daily MTR (OR, 1.81; 95% CI, 1.15–2.84; $p = 0.01$; two studies) (Clay et al., 2015). The relative risk (RR) for 48-week viral load suppression was improved with STRs (RR, 1.09; 95% CI, 1.04–1.15; $p = 0.0003$; three studies), whereas RR of grade 3 to 4 laboratory abnormalities was lower among patients on STRs (RR, 0.68; 95% CI, 0.49–0.94; $p = 0.02$; two studies).

RECOMMENDED READING

Cattaneo D, Baldelli S, Cozzi V, et al. Impact of therapeutic drug monitoring of antiretroviral drugs in routine clinical management of people living with HIV: a narrative review. *Ther Drug Monit.* 2020;42(1):64–74. doi:10.1097/FTD.0000000000000684

Clay PG, Nag S, Graham CM, et al. Meta-analysis of studies comparing single and multi-tablet fixed dose combination HIV treatment regimens. *Medicine.* 2015;94(42):e1677.

CLINICAL TRIALS DESIGN AND ACCESS PROGRAMS

LEARNING OBJECTIVE

- Describe the differences between phase 1, 2, 3, and 4 research clinical trials and expanded-access programs.

WHAT'S NEW?

The Right-to-Try Pathway is an expanded-access program external to the FDA for patients with life-threatening diseases or conditions who are unable to enroll in a clinical trial and who have exhausted all other treatment options.

KEY POINTS

- Phase 1 studies are the earliest clinical trials, focusing mainly on safety and pharmacokinetics.

- Phase 2 studies further evaluate safety and begin to evaluate efficacy and dosing. Dose selection is done in early phase 2.

- Phase 3 studies focus on safety and efficacy in the target population.

- Phase 4 studies, sometimes referred to as *postmarketing trials*, occur after FDA approval and study the use of the drug in different patient populations and its long-term safety.

- Expanded-access programs make a drug available to patients who are in particular need before the drug becomes available commercially. These programs are generally not established until after phase 3 studies have been fully enrolled.

PHASES OF CLINICAL TRIALS

In general, there are four phases to drug development, which are guided by procedures described in the US Code of Federal Regulations 21 CFR 314.126 (FDA, 2020b):

- Phase 1 is the most preliminary clinical work in small numbers of human subjects and helps to determine safety/toxicity (FDA, 2020a). Phase 1 studies usually start as single-dose studies and then progress to multiple-dose studies, mainly using healthy volunteers. They evaluate a range of aspects, such as pharmacokinetics (including drug bioavailability), dosing interval, food effects, tolerability, and toxicity in order to define the maximum tolerated dose, sentinel adverse effects, and target-organ toxicity.

- Phase 2 studies further evaluate toxicity and the effectiveness of the drug for a particular indication in a larger number of patients who have the disease or condition under study, and they potentially establish dosage (FDA, 2020a). This is usually the initial assessment of activity or proof-of-concept study. It includes several doses and a short course of monotherapy or functional monotherapy. It may include randomized dosing and control or may be dose-escalating. Phase 2 studies also collect data on pharmacokinetics, dose response, tolerability, and toxicity. In HIV, these studies are usually divided into phase 2a and phase 2b:

    Phase 2a trials are generally conducted in a small number of HIV-infected patients and usually are of short duration.

Phase 2b trials usually involve longer-term dosing, almost always involve combination with other agents, and have a control arm. Longer-term tolerability, toxicity, and effectiveness are important outcomes.

- Phase 3 studies are primarily geared toward large cohort efficacy and, along with the accumulated weight of safety and toxicity studies, form the basis for submission to and approval by the FDA (FDA, 2020a). Phase 3 studies are typically large, randomized studies that provide the core information for submission and regulatory approval. They frequently include blinded therapy. For ARVs, the endpoint for the most part has traditionally been some measurement of HIV-1 RNA response.

- Phase 4 studies are postmarketing or postapproval trials and may be mandated by the FDA to further determine long-term toxicities or may serve as vehicles for expanded indications or dosing changes (DHHS, 2005).

EXPANDED-ACCESS PROGRAMS

Expanded-access programs are often created for patients in particular need to make a drug available before it is licensed. These programs are an outgrowth of the expedited review process for HIV drugs and are usually limited in the number of patients enrolled and the duration of availability. Typically, expanded-access programs are established after phase 3 studies have been fully enrolled and before drug approval. They are subject to FDA oversight (FDA, 2020a, 2020c; US Code, 2020), although considerably less so than are registrational trials. Due to the number of treatment options available today, expanded-access programs are much less common than in the past.

There are five mechanisms for expanded access.

Emergency Investigational New Drug

For an emergency investigational new drug (E-IND), a physician, on behalf of the patient, contacts the FDA and/or pharmaceutical manufacturer. In this type of emergency situation, a written submission is not needed; however, the FDA expects the physician to submit an IND application as soon as possible (FDA, 2020a).

Open-Label Protocol

Open-label protocol is designed to account for the time between the completion of a clinical trial and the FDA approval of an investigational drug. This allows for the continuation of treatment and the end of a phase 3 study. Compliance with the patient safeguard processes must also be demonstrated (FDA, 2020a).

Treatment Investigational New Drug

The treatment investigational new drug (T-IND) allows patients, most of whom are very ill, access to investigational drugs when there are no alternative therapies. These are sometimes referred to as "compassionate use" studies and are used to collect safety data in very ill patients who use the new therapy (FDA, 2020a).

Parallel Track

This mechanism has been developed to expand availability of INDs to patients with AIDS or other related diseases. Patients in a parallel track study, or a study that is being run in parallel with controlled clinical studies for a particular investigational agent, are those who would not otherwise have access to the treatment because of geographic location or because they do not meet the specific entry criteria for the original study. Only patients who cannot enroll in the available original trial and who are not eligible for marketing standard treatment may enroll in these studies (FDA, 2020c).

In 2009, the FDA issued two new rules related to expanded access. The first rule, titled "Expanded Access to Investigational Drugs for Treatment Use," clarifies the criteria for access to investigational drugs, enumerates the requirements for access submissions, establishes safeguards to protect patients from adverse side effects, and implements mechanisms for maintaining meaningful data about treatment use and results. Per the rule, those who may be granted access to investigational drugs include individuals with a serious or immediately life-threatening disease and for whom there is no comparable satisfactory alternative therapy; intermediate-size patient populations comprising individuals who are ineligible to participate in clinical trials or whose disease is so rare that a drug is not being developed; and larger populations under a treatment protocol or in a trial conducted as part of an IND application.

The expanded-access rule specifies that pharmaceutical companies are responsible for submitting IND safety reports (and annual reports when the protocol continues for 1 year or more) and for providing treating physicians with necessary information to maximize the benefits and minimize the risks of treatment. Physicians who administer the treatments, who are considered "investigators" for purposes of this rule, must report adverse drug events to the sponsor, ensure that informed consent requirements are met, and maintain accurate case histories and drug disposition records.

The second rule, titled "Charging for Investigational Drugs Under an Investigational New Drug Application," amends the existing rules concerning when drug manufacturers may charge patients for investigational drugs. This rule specifies that a company that wishes to charge a clinical trial participant for a drug must show that the drug may provide a significant advantage over other available treatments (as demonstrated by the trial), that the data from the trial are essential to demonstrating the drug's safety and efficacy, and that charging participants is essential because the cost of the drug is "extraordinary to the sponsor" (FDA, 2020c).

Right-to-Try

The Trickett Wendler, Frank Mongiello, Jordan McLinn, and Matthew Bellina Right-to-Try Act of 2017 created a new expanded-access pathway for certain investigational agents that have not yet been approved by the FDA. This pathway exists for patients who (1) have a life-threatening disease or condition, (2) have exhausted all approved treatment options for the disease or condition and are unable to participate in a clinical trial, and (3) have given informed consent. A patient's physician may work with a company developing a post-phase 1 drug to access it without involvement of the FDA. Medications must be continuously under clinical trial in order to be eligible for Right-to-Try; if the investigational process is placed on a clinical hold, the drug is ineligible (FDA, 2020d).

RECOMMENDED READING

Food and Drug Administration. Expanded access to investigational drugs for treatment use. Title 21 CFR Parts 312 and 316. 2020c. https://www.accessdata.fda.gov/scripts/cdrh/cfdocs/cfCFR/CFRSearch.cfm?CFRPart=312&showFR=1&subpartNode=21:5.0.1.1.3.9

Food and Drug Administration. Expanded access to investigational drugs for treatment use—Questions and answers: guidance for industry. 2016. https://www.fda.gov/regulatory-information/search-fda-guidance-documents/expanded-access-investigational-drugs-treatment-use-questions-and-answers

REFERENCES

Bastiaans DET, Cressey TR, Vromans H, et al. The role of formulation on the pharmacokinetics of antiretroviral drugs. *Expert Opin Drug Metab Toxicol.* 2014;10(7):1019–1037. doi:10.1517/17425255.2014.925879

Best BM, Capparelli EV, Diep H, et al. Pharmacokinetics of lopinavir/ritonavir crushed versus whole tablets in children. *J AIDS.* 2011;58(4):385–391. doi:10.1097/QAI.0b013e318232b057

Biktarvy [package insert]. Foster City, CA. Gilead, 2019.

Boffito M, Waters L, Cahn P, et al. Perspectives on the barrier to resistance for dolutegravir + lamivudine, a two-drug antiretroviral therapy for HIV-1 infection. *AIDS Res Human Retroviruses.* 2020;36(1):13–18. doi:10.1089/AID.2019.0171

Cahn P, Madero J, Arribas J, et al. Dolutegravir plus lamivudine versus dolutegravir plus tenofovir disoproxil fumarate and emtricitabine in antiretroviral-naïve adults with HIV-1 infection (GEMINI-1 and GEMINI-2): week 48 results from two multicentre, double-blind, randomised, non-inferiority, phase 3 trials. *Lancet.* 2019;393:143–155.

Cahn P, Madero JS, Arribas JR, et al. Durable efficacy of dolutegravir plus lamivudine in antiretroviral treatment-naïve adults with HIV-1 infection: 96-week results from the GEMINI-1 AND GEMINI-2 randomized clinical trials. *J AIDS.* 2020;83(3):310–318. doi:10.1097/QAI.0000000000002275

Cahn P, Sax PE, Squires K, et al.; ONCEMRK Study Group. Raltegravir 1200 mg once daily vs 400 mg twice daily, with emtricitabine and tenofovir disoproxil fumarate, for previously untreated HIV-1 infection: week 96 results from ONCEMRK, a randomized, double-blind, noninferiority trial. *J AIDS.* 2018;78(5):589–598. doi:10.1097/QAI.0000000000001723

Calcagno A, Di Perri G, Bonora S. Pharmacokinetics and pharmacodynamics of antiretrovirals in the central nervous system. *Clin Pharmacokinet.* 2014;53(10):891–906. doi:10.1007/s40262-014-0171-0

Caniglia EC, Cain LE, Justice A, et al. Antiretroviral penetration into the CNS and incidence of AIDS-defining neurologic conditions. *Neurology.* 2014;83(2):134–141. doi:10.1212/WNL.0000000000000564

Cattaneo D, Baldelli S, Castoldi S, et al. Is it time to revise antiretrovirals dosing? A pharmacokinetic viewpoint. *AIDS.* 2014;28(16):2477–2479. doi:10.1097/qad.0000000000000440

Cattaneo D, Baldelli S, Cozzi V, et al. Impact of therapeutic drug monitoring of antiretroviral drugs in routine clinical management of people living with HIV: a narrative review. *Ther Drug Monit.* 2020;42(1):64–74. doi:10.1097/FTD.0000000000000684

Clay PG, Nag S, Graham CM, et al. Meta-analysis of studies comparing single and multi-tablet fixed dose combination HIV treatment regimens. *Medicine.* 2015;94(42):e1677. doi:10.1097/MD.0000000000001677

Clotet B, Feinberg J, van Lunzen J, et al.; the ING114915 Study Team. Once-daily dolutegravir versus darunavir plus ritonavir in antiretroviral-naïve adults with HIV-1 infection (FLAMINGO): 48 week results from the randomised open-label phase 3b study. *Lancet.* 2014;383(9936):2222–2231. [Erratum in *Lancet.* 2015;385(9987):2576.]

Cottrell ML, Hadzic T, Kashuba ADM. Clinical pharmacokinetic, pharmacodynamic, and drug interaction profile of the integrase inhibitor dolutegravir. *Clin Pharmacokinet.* 2013;52(11):981–994. doi:10.1007/s40262-013-0093-2

Crauwels HM, van Heeswijk RP, Kestens D, et al. The pharmacokinetic interaction between omeprazole and TMC 278, an investigational NNRTI [Abstract P239]. Presented at the 9th International Congress on Drug Therapy in HIV Infection, Glasgow, Scotland, November 2008.

Crawford KW, Ripin DHB, Levin AD, et al. Optimising the manufacture, formulation, and dose of antiretroviral drugs for more cost-effective delivery in resource-limited settings: a consensus statement. *Lancet Infect Dis.* 2012;12(7):550–560. doi:10.1016/S1473-3099(12)70134-2

Deeks ED. Raltegravir once-daily tablet: a review in HIV-1 infection. *Drugs.* 2017;77(16):1789–1795. doi:10.1007/s40265-017-0827-9

DeJesus E, Berger D, Markowitz M, et al. Antiviral activity, pharmacokinetics, and dose response of the HIV-1 integrase inhibitor GS-9137 (JTK-303) in treatment-naïve and treatment-experienced patients. *J AIDS.* 2006;43(1):1–5. doi:10.1097/01.qai.0000233308.82860.2f

DeJesus E, Rockstroh JK, Lennox JL, et al. Efficacy of raltegravir versus efavirenz when combined with tenofovir/emtricitabine in treatment-naïve HIV-1-infected patients: week-192 overall and subgroup analyses from STARTMRK. *HIV Clin Trials.* 2012;13(4):228–232.

Department of Health and Human Services. Information on clinical trials and human research studies: glossary. 2005. http://www.clinical-trials.gov/ct/gui/info/glossary#phasel

Department of Health and Human Services. Panel on Antiretroviral Guidelines for Adults and Adolescents. Guidelines for the use of antiretroviral agents in adults and adolescents. 2020. https://clinicalinfo.hiv.gov/en/guidelines/adult-and-adolescent-arv/whats-new-guidelines

Edurant [package insert]. Titusville, NJ. Janssen Therapeutics, 2019.

Elliot ER, Wang X, Singh S, et al. Increased dolutegravir peak concentrations in people living with human immunodeficiency virus aged 60 and over, and analysis of sleep quality and cognition. *Clin Infect Dis.* 2019;68(1):87–95. doi:10.1093/cid/ciy426

Ellis RJ, Letendre S, Vaida F, et al. Randomized trial of central nervous system-targeted antiretrovirals for HIV-associated neurocognitive disorder. *Clin Infect Dis.* 2014;58(7):1015–1022. doi:10.1093/cid/cit921

Emu B, Fessel WJ, Schrader S, et al. Forty-eight-week safety and efficacy on-treatment analysis of ibalizumab in patients with multi-drug resistant HIV-1. *Open Forum Infect Dis.* 2017;4(Suppl 1):S38–S39. doi:10.1093/ofid/ofx162.093

ENCORE1 Study Group. Efficacy and safety of efavirenz 400 mg daily versus 600 mg daily: 96-week data from the randomized, double-blind, placebo-controlled, non-inferiority ENCORE1 study. *Lancet Infect Dis.* 2015;15(7):793–802. doi:10.1016/S1473-3099(15)70060-5

Eron JJ, Lelievre JD, Kalayjian, et al. Safety of elvitegravir, cobicistat, emtricitabine, and tenofovir alafenamide in HIV-1-infected adults with end-stage renal disease on chronic haemodialysis: an open-label, single-arm, multicenter, phase 3b trial. *Lancet HIV*. 2019;6(1):e15–e24. doi:10.1016/S2352-3018(18)30296-0

Eron JJ, Rockstroh JK, Reynes J, et al. Raltegravir once daily or twice daily in previously untreated patients with HIV-1: a randomised, active-controlled, phase 3 non-inferiority trial. *Lancet Infect Dis*. 2011;11(12):907–915. doi:10.1016/S1473-3099(11)70196-7

Food and Drug Administration. Information sheets: Guidance for Institutional Review Boards (IRBs), Clinical Investigators, and Sponsors. https://www.fda.gov/science-research/guidance-documents-including-information-sheets-and-notices/information-sheet-guidance-institutional-review-boards-irbs-clinical-investigators-and-sponsors

Food and Drug Administration. 21 CFR 312.21. Investigational new drug application. In: Food and Drugs. 2020a. https://www.accessdata.fda.gov/scripts/cdrh/cfdocs/cfcfr/CFRSearch.cfm?fr=312.21

Food and Drug Administration. 21 CFR 314.126. Applications for FDA approval to market a new drug. In: Food and Drugs. 2020b. https://www.accessdata.fda.gov/scripts/cdrh/cfdocs/cfCFR/CFRSearch.cfm?fr=314.126

Food and Drug Administration. Charging for investigational drugs under an investigational new drug application. 2009a. https://www.fda.gov/regulatory-information/search-fda-guidance-documents/charging-investigational-drugs-under-ind-questions-and-answers

Food and Drug Administration. Expanded access to investigational drugs for treatment use. Title 21 CFR Parts 312 and 316. 2020c. https://www.accessdata.fda.gov/scripts/cdrh/cfdocs/cfCFR/CFRSearch.cfm?CFRPart=312&showFR=1&subpartNode=21:5.0.1.1.3.9

Food and Drug Administration. Right to try. 2020d. https://www.fda.gov/patients/learn-about-expanded-access-and-other-treatment-options/right-try

Gallant J, Lazzarin A, Mills A, et al. Bictegravir, emtricitabine, and tenofovir alafenamide versus dolutegravir, abacavir, and lamivudine for initial treatment of HIV-1 infection (GS-US-380–1489): a double-blind, multicenter, phase 3, randomized controlled noninferiority trial. *Lancet*. 2017;390(10107):2063–2072.

Gatanaga H, Hayashida T, Tsuchiya K, et al. Successful efavirenz dose reduction in HIV type 1-infected individuals with cytochrome P450 2B6*6 and *26. *Clin Infect Dis*. 2007;45(9):1230–1237. doi:10.1086/522175

Gervasoni C, Meraviglia P, Minisci D, et al. Metabolic and kidney disorders correlate with high atazanavir concentrations in HIV-infected patients: is it time to revise atazanavir dosage? *PLoS One*. 2015;10(4):1–12. doi:10.1371/journal.pone.0123670

Griffin L, Annaert P, Brouwer KL. Influence of drug transport proteins on the pharmacokinetics and drug interactions of HIV protease inhibitors. *J Pharm Sci*. 2011;100(9):3636–3654. doi:10.1002/jps.22655

Insight Start Study Group. Initiation of antiretroviral therapy in early asymptomatic HIV Infection. *N Eng J Med*. 2015;373(9):795–807. doi:10.1056/NEJMoa1506816

International Advisory Panel on HIV Care Continuum Optimization. IAPAC guidelines for optimizing the HIV care continuum for adults and adolescents. *J Int Assoc Provid AIDS Care*. 2015;14(Suppl 1):S3–S34. doi:10.1177/2325957415613442

Kakuda TN, Wade JR, Snoeck E, et al. Pharmacokinetics and pharmacodynamics of the non-nucleoside reverse-transcriptase inhibitor etravirine in treatment-experienced HIV-1-infected patients. *Clin Pharmacol Ther*. 2010;88(5):695–703. doi:10.1038/clpt.2010.181

Kozal M, Aberg J, Pialoux G, et al. Fostemsavir in adults with multidrug-resistant HIV-1 infection. *N Engl J Med*. 2020;382:1232–1243.

Lalezari J, Sloan L, DeJesus E, et al. Potent antiviral activity of S/GSK1349572, a next generation integrase inhibitor (INI) in INI-naïve HIV-1-infected patients: ING111521 protocol [Abstract TUAB105]. Presented at the 5th Conference on HIV Pathogenesis, Treatment and Prevention; Cape Town, South Africa, July 19–22, 2009.

Larson KB, Wang K, Delille C, et al. Pharmacokinetic enhancers in HIV therapeutics. *Clin Pharmacokinet*. 2014;53(10):865–872. doi:10.1007/s40262-014-0167-9

Lennox JL, Landovitz RJ, Ribaudo HJ, et al. Efficacy and tolerability of 3 nonnucleoside reverse transcriptase inhibitor-sparing

antiretroviral regimens for treatment-naïve volunteers infected with HIV-1: a randomized, controlled equivalence trial. *Ann Intern Med*. 2014;161(7):461–471.

Letendre S, Marquie-Beck J, Capparelli E, et al. Validation of the CNS penetration-effectiveness rank for quantifying antiretroviral penetration into the central nervous system. *Arch Neurol*. 2008;65(1):65–70. doi:10.1001/archneurol.2007.31

Mallal S, Phillips E, Carosi G, et al. HLA-B*5701 screening for hypersensitivity to abacavir. *N Engl J Med*. 2008;358(6):568–579. doi:10.1056/NEJMoa0706135

Marzolini C, Telenti A, Decosterd LA, et al. Efavirenz plasma levels can predict treatment failure and central nervous system side effects in HIV-1-infected patients. *AIDS*. 2001;15(1):71–75. doi:10.1097/00002030-200101050-00011

Mello AF, Buclin T, Decosterd LA, et al. Successful efavirenz dose reduction guided by therapeutic drug monitoring. *Antivir Ther*. 2011;16(2):189–197. doi:10.3851/IMP1742

Minuesa G, Huber-Ruano I, Pastor-Anglada M, et al. Drug uptake transporters in antiretroviral therapy. *Pharmacol Ther*. 2011;132(3):268–279. doi:10.1016/j.pharmthera.2011.06.007

Molina JM, Clotet B, van Lunzen J, et al. Once-daily dolutegravir is superior to once-daily darunavir/ritonavir in treatment-naïve HIV-1-positive individuals: 96 week results from FLAMINGO. *J Int AIDS Soc*. 2014;17(4 Suppl 3):19490.

Morse GD, Catanzaro LM, Acosta EP. Clinical pharmacodynamics of HIV-1 protease inhibitors: use of inhibitory quotients to optimise pharmacotherapy. *Lancet Infect Dis*. 2006;6(4):215–225. doi:10.1016/S1473-3099(06)70436-4

Mukerji SS, Misra V, Lorenz DR, et al. Impact of antiretroviral regimens on cerebrospinal fluid viral escape in a prospective multicohort study of antiretroviral therapy-experienced human immunodeficiency virus-1-infected adults in the United States. *Clin Infect Dis*. 2018;67(8):1182–1190. doi:10.1093/cid/ciy267

Orrell C, Hagins DP, Belonosova E, et al. Fixed-dose combination dolutegravir, abacavir, and lamivudine versus ritonavir-boosted atazanavir plus tenofovir disoproxil fumarate and emtricitabine in previously untreated women with HIV-1 infection (ARIA): week 48 results from a randomized, open-label, noninferiority, phase 3b study. *Lancet HIV*. 2017;4(12):e536–e546.

Orkin C, Arasteh K, Hernandez-Mora MG, et al. Long-acting cabotegravir and rilpivirine after oral induction for HIV-1 infection. *N Engl J Med*. 2020a;382(12):1124–1135. doi:10.1056/NEJMoa1909512

Orkin C, Eron JJ, Rockstroh J, et al.; AMBER Study Group. Week 96 results of a phase 3 trial of darunavir/cobicistat/emtricitabine/tenofovir alafenamide in treatment-naive HIV-1 patients. *AIDS*. 2020b;34(5):707–718. doi:10.1097/QAD.0000000000002463.

Orkin C, Molina JM, Negredo E, et al.; EMERALD study group. Efficacy and safety of switching from boosted protease inhibitors plus emtricitabine and tenofovir disoproxil fumarate regimens to single-tablet darunavir, cobicistat, emtricitabine, and tenofovir alafenamide at 48 weeks in adults with virologically suppressed HIV-1 (EMERALD): a phase 3, randomised, non-inferiority trial. *Lancet HIV*. 2018;5(1):e23–e34. doi:10.1016/S2352-3018(17)30179-0

Pappa K, Baumgarten A, Felizarta F, et al. Dolutegravir (DTG) plus abacavir/lamivudine once daily superior to tenofovir/emtricitabine/efavirenz in treatment-naïve HIV subjects: 144-week results from SINGLE (ING114467). Paper presented at the Interscience Conference on Antimicrobial Agents and Chemotherapy (ICAAC), Washington, DC, 2014.

Pomerantz RJ. Reservoirs of human immunodeficiency virus type 1: the main obstacles to viral eradication. *Clin Infect Dis*. 2002;34(1):91–97. doi:10.1086/338256

Pretorius E, Klinker H, Rosenkranz B. The role of therapeutic drug monitoring in the management of patients with human immunodeficiency virus infection. *Ther Drug Monit*. 2011;33:265–274.

Raffi F, Jaeger H, Quiros-Roldan E, et al. Once-daily dolutegravir versus twice-daily raltegravir in antiretroviral-naïve adults with HIV-1 infection (SPRING-2 study): 96 week results from a randomised, double-blind, noninferiority trial. *Lancet Infect Dis.* 2013;13(11):927–935.

Rizk ML, Hang Y, Luo WL, et al. Pharmacokinetics and pharmacodynamics of once-daily versus twice-daily raltegravir in treatment-naïve HIV-infected patients. *Antimicrob Agents Chemother.* 2012;56(6):3101–3106. doi:10.1128/AAC.06417-11

Rockstroh JK, DeJesus E, Lennox JL, et al. Durable efficacy and safety of raltegravir versus efavirenz when combined with tenofovir/emtricitabine in treatment-naïve HIV-1-infected patients: final 5-year results from STARTMRK. *J AIDS.* 2013;63(1):77–85.

Rotger M, Tegude H, Colombo S, et al. Predictive value of known and novel alleles of CYP2B6 for efavirenz plasma concentrations in HIV-infected individuals. *Clin Pharmacol Ther.* 2007;81(4):557–6. doi:10.1038/sj.clpt.6100072

Sankatsing SUC, Beijnen JH, Schinkel AH, et al. P glycoprotein in human immunodeficiency virus type 1 infection and therapy. *Antimicrob Agents Chemother.* 2004;48(4):1073–1081. doi:10.1128/aac.48.4.1073-1081.2004

Santos GMA, Locatelli I, Métral M, et al. Cross-sectional and cumulative longitudinal central nervous system penetration effectiveness scores are not associated with neurocognitive impairment in a well treated aging human immunodeficiency virus-positive population in Switzerland. *Open Forum Infect Dis.* 2019;6(7):ofz277. https://doi.org/10.1093/ofid/ofz277

Sax PE, Pozniak A, Montes ML, et al. Coformulated bictegravir, emtricitabine, and tenofovir alafenamide versus dolutegravir with emtricitabine and tenofovir alafenamide, for initial treatment of HIV-1 infection (GS-US-380-1490): a randomized, double-blind, multicenter, phase 3, noninferiority trial. *Lancet.* 2017;390(10107):2073–2082.

Shah BM, Schafer JJ, Priano J, et al. Cobicistat: a new boost for the treatment of human immunodeficiency virus infection. *Pharmacotherapy.* 2013;33(10):1107–1116. doi:10.1002/phar.1237

Smith A, Henrisksen B, Cohen A. Pharmacokinetic considerations in Roux-en-Y gastric bypass patients. *Am J Health Syst Pharm.* 2011;68(23):2241–2247. doi:10.2146/ajhp100630

Sustiva [package insert]. Princeton, NJ: Bristol-Myers Squibb; 2019.

Swindells S, Andrade-Villanueva J, Richmond GJ, et al. Long-acting cabotegravir and rilpivirine for maintenance of HIV-1 suppression. *N Engl J Med.* 2020;382(12):1112–1123. doi:10.1056/NEJMoa1904398

Symfi Lo [package insert]. Morgantown, WV: Mylan; 2019.

Temprano ANRS 12136 Study Group. A trial of early antiretrovirals and isoniazid preventive therapy in Africa. *N Engl J Med.* 2015;373(9):808–822. doi:10.1056/NEJMoa1507198

Trezza CR, Kashuba AD. Pharmacokinetics of antiretrovirals in genital secretions and anatomic sites of HIV transmission: implications for HIV prevention. *Clin Pharmacokinet.* 2014;5(7)3:611–624. doi:10.1007/s40262-014-0148-z

Tseng A, Seet J, Phillips EJ. The evolution of three decades of antiretroviral therapy: challenges, triumphs and the promise of the future. *Br J Clin Pharmacol.* 2014;79(2):182–194. doi:10.1111/bcp.12403

Usach I, Melis V, Peris JE. Non-nucleoside reverse transcriptase inhibitors: a review on pharmacokinetics, pharmacodynamics, safety and tolerability. *J Int AIDS Soc.* 2013;16(1):1–14. doi:10.7448/IAS.16.1.18567

US Code. 21 USC 360bbb. General provisions relating to drugs and devices: expanded access to unapproved therapies and diagnostics. In: Food and Drugs: Drugs and Devices. January 24, 2002. https://uscode.house.gov/view.xhtml?edition=prelim&req=granuleid%3AUSC-prelim-title21-chapter9-subchapter5-partE&num=0

Van Leth F, Kappelhoff BS, Johnson D, et al. Pharmacokinetic parameters of nevirapine and efavirenz in relation to antiretroviral efficacy. *AIDS Res Hum Retroviruses.* 2006;22(3):232–239. doi:10.1089/aid.2006.22.232

van Wyk J, Ajana F, Bisshop F, et al. Efficacy and safety of switching to dolutegravir/lamivudine fixed-dose two-drug regimen versus continuing a tenofovir alafenamide-based three- or four-drug regimen for maintenance of virologic suppression in adults with HIV-1: phase 3, randomized, non-inferiority TANGO Study. *Clin Infect Dis.* 2020;71(8):1920–1929.

Verbeeck RK, Musuamba FT. Pharmacokinetics and dosage adjustment in patients with renal dysfunction. *Eur J Clin Pharmacol.* 2009;65(8):757–773. doi:10.1007/s00228-009-0678-8

ViiV Healthcare. Tivicay package insert. September 2018. https://www.gsksource.com/pharma/content/dam/GlaxoSmithKline/US/en/Prescribing_Information/Tivicay/pdf/TIVICAY-PI-PIL.PDF#page=1

ViiV Healthcare. ViiV Healthcare receives complete response letter from US FDA for use of investigational cabotegravir and rilpivirine long-acting regimen in the treatment of HIV. December 21, 2019. https://viivhealthcare.com/en-gb/media/press-releases/2019/december/complete-response-letter-from-us-fda/

Walmsley SL, Antela A, Clumeck N, et al. Dolutegravir plus abacavir–lamivudine for the treatment of HIV-1 infection. *N Engl J Med.* 2013;369(19):1807–1818.

Wang X, Boffito M, Zhang J, et al. Effects of the H2-receptor antagonist famotidine on the pharmacokinetics of atazanavir-ritonavir with or without tenofovir in HIV-infected patients. *AIDS Patient Care STDs.* 2011;25(9):509–515. doi:10.1089/apc.2011.0113

Williams PE, Crauwels HM, Basstanie ED. Formulation and pharmacology of long-acting rilpivirine. *Curr Opin HIV AIDS.* 2015;10(4):239–245. doi:10.1097/COH.0000000000000164

Young B, Squires K, Patel P, et al. First large, multicenter, open-label study utilizing HLA-B*5701 screening for abacavir hypersensitivity in North America. *AIDS.* 2008;22(13):1673–1681. doi:10.1097/QAD.0b013e32830719aa

Zash R, Holmes L, Diseko M, et al. Neural-tube defects and antiretroviral treatment regimens in Botswana. *N Engl J Med* 2019;381:827–840.

Zash R, Jacobson D, Mayondi GDM, et al. Dolutegravir/tenofovir/emtricitabine (DTG/TDF/FTC) started in pregnancy is as safe as efavirenz/tenofovir/emtricitabine (EFV/TDF/FTC) in nationwide birth outcomes surveillance in Botswana. 9th IAS, Paris, France, 2017.

Zhu L, Persson A, Mahnke L, et al. Effect of low-dose omeprazole (20 mg daily) on the pharmacokinetics of multiple dose atazanavir with ritonavir in health subjects. *J Clin Pharmacol.* 2011;51(3):368–377. doi:10.1177/0091270010367651

18.

PRESCRIBING ANTIRETROVIRAL THERAPY

*Poonam Mathur, Maria Veronica Bandres, Saira Ajmal, Zelalem Temesgen,
and David E. Koren*

CHAPTER GOALS

Upon completion of this chapter, the reader should be able to:

- Enumerate the goals of antiretroviral treatment (ART) and rationale for treatment of all persons with HIV (PWH) as soon as possible

- List the US Department of Health and Human Services (DHHS) panel's recommended initial HIV treatments

- Describe important criteria in selecting an initial treatment regimen

- Identify when ART should be switched and how to do so

OVERVIEW OF ART

WHAT'S NEW?

- DHHS guidelines recommend starting ART immediately or as soon as possible after the diagnosis of HIV is made.

- HIV integrase inhibitors are the standard of care for initial therapy, with all five DHHS recommended initial treatment regimens pairing an integrase strand transfer inhibitor (INSTI) with tenofovir (TFV) or abacavir (ABC) and emtricitabine (FTC) or lamivudine (3TC) for most PWH. Additional recommendations for certain clinical situations exist, including protease inhibitor (PI)-based or nonnucleoside reverse transcriptase inhibitors (NNRTI)-based and nucleoside reverse transcriptase inhibitors (NRTI)-sparing regimens.

- Bictegravir (BIC), dolutegravir (DTG), or boosted darunavir (DRV/r) paired with TFV/FTC can be used for rapid ART initiation before initial lab results are available.

- The DTG + 3TC fixed-dose two-drug regimen was approved for initial treatment except for individuals with HIV RNA of more than 500,000 copies/mL, those

with coinfection with hepatitis B virus (HBV), or those in whom ART is to be started before the results of HIV genotypic resistance testing or HBV testing are available.

- 3TC can be used as a single NRTI with DRV/r if ABC, tenofovir alafenamide (TAF), or tenofovir disoproxil fumarate (TDF) cannot be used.

KEY POINTS

- Uncontrolled HIV replication is associated with inflammation, accelerated aging, and a higher rate of comorbid illnesses, effects that have been shown to be reduced by earlier initiation of ART.

- Studies demonstrate improved clinical outcomes with treatment initiation at $CD4^+$ cell counts greater than $500/mm^3$, and treatment is now recommended for all PWH regardless of $CD4^+$ cell count.

- Treatment of HIV with ART is highly effective at preventing HIV-1 transmission.

- ART regimen selection considers what is best suited for the patient to ensure adherence and long-term durability with regard to medication tolerability and toxicities, resistance, and patient comorbidities.

INTRODUCTION

Great strides have been made in ART since the introduction of zidovudine in 1987 and combination therapy in 1996. ART has reduced both HIV-associated and non-HIV-associated morbidity and mortality, making HIV a chronic disease that can be managed with potent and simple medication regimens, affording PWH a low risk of AIDS-related complications; few, if any, significant side effects from medications; and near-normal life expectancy (Samji et al., 2013). In addition, treatment with ART has been shown to reduce HIV transmission. However, in 2018 only 65% of PWH in the US had suppressed viral loads (HIV.gov, 2020) due to undiagnosed infections or difficulty linking PWH to and retaining them in care.

Paramount to the success of ART is the patient's willingness and commitment to adhere to lifelong therapy. In the past, acute and long-term adverse effects associated with ART limited adherence to therapy, often leading to treatment failure. However, current combinations are associated with less toxicity, reduced pill burden, and improved potency, allowing many PWH to achieve the greater than 95% adherence required for stable, long-term viral suppression. Nevertheless, PWH continue to face several factors that can have a significant impact on ART success, including access to and the cost of long-term ART, particularly in resource-limited areas; drug interactions; comorbid medical conditions such as hepatitis B and C, tuberculosis, cardiovascular and renal disease, diabetes, osteoporosis or osteopenia, psychological disorders, and chemical dependency; and other social, economic, geographic, racial, and gender identity factors that disproportionately impact PWH. Recognizing and addressing the individual barriers to adherence for each patient prior to ART initiation can have a dramatic effect on long-term treatment outcomes.

As reviewed in the last chapter, there are 33 US Food and Drug Administration (FDA)-approved individual antiretroviral drugs (ARVs) classified in seven categories based on their mechanism of action, plus two pharmacokinetic boosters. A panel of leading HIV specialists, convened by the DHHS, has been developing and updating recommendations for use of ARV agents in PWH since the early days of the ART era. These guidelines and those published by the International Antiviral Society–USA (IAS-USA) (Saag et al., 2018) are similar and are periodically updated to reflect the release of new medications and HIV treatment in special populations. The guidelines also address patient readiness for therapy, barriers to adherence, and comorbid conditions, as well as providing information on dosing and drug interactions. At the time of this writing, the most recent DHHS guidelines released on December 18, 2019, included key updates to several sections, including changes in recommendations for initial regimens for the ARV-naive patient and when to start treatment (DHHS, 2020).

CURRENT TREATMENT GUIDELINES: WHEN TO START

Both DHHS and IAS-USA guidelines recommend starting ART immediately or as soon as possible after the diagnosis of HIV is made, with an intent to improve the uptake of ART and linkage to care, decrease the time to virologic suppression, and reduce HIV transmission (DHHS, 2020; Saag et al., 2018). This guidance reflects data from the START trial supporting treatment in all PWH regardless of CD4+ T-cell count in order to reduce the morbidity and mortality associated with HIV infection (Lundgren et al., 2015). START and HPTN-052 (first in 2011, again in 2020) also demonstrated the power of ART-driven viral suppression to prevent HIV transmission (Cohen et al., 2011, 2020), a phenomenon known as "treatment as prevention," or TasP.

In some cases, ART may initially be deferred due to psychosocial factors, but these cases should be the exception, and ART should be started as soon as psychosocial factors have stabilized and the patient is ready for treatment. The following conditions should be considered urgent and discourage deferral of treatment initiation: pregnancy; CD4+ T-cell count less than 200 cells/mm³; AIDS-defining malignancies, opportunistic infections, and conditions such as HIV-associated dementia; HIV-associated nephropathy; coinfection with HBV or hepatitis C virus (HCV); and acute or early HIV infection. Whether for acute or chronic HIV infection, DHHS guidelines also recommend not waiting for resistance test results in newly diagnosed PWH as long as an ARV with a high genetic barrier to resistance such as BIC, DTG, or DRV/r is chosen (DHHS, 2020).

Same-day HIV testing and ART initiation (e.g., "rapid start") is supported by randomized clinical trials conducted in South Africa (Rosen et al., 2016), Haiti (Koenig et al., 2017), and Lesotho (Labhardt et al., 2018). Additionally, clinic-based observational cohort studies in San Francisco (Rapid ART Program for Individuals with an HIV Diagnosis, or RAPID) and Atlanta (Rapid Entry and ART in Clinic for HIV, or REACH) demonstrated a significant decrease in time to viral suppression and time to initial provider appointment with immediate ART initiation (Coffey et al., 2019; Colasanti et al., 2018; Pilcher et al., 2017). These studies provide evidence that same-day HIV diagnosis and ART initiation is feasible and may be beneficial, whether in a resource-rich setting with a multidisciplinary support system or in more resource-limited settings. Additionally, since persons recently infected with HIV often have very high viral loads during the first several weeks and are therefore at increased risk of infecting other persons, coupling early diagnosis with rapid ART initiation has great potential to reduce HIV transmission.

The combination of data showing both personal and public health benefits of universal ART for PWH creates a powerful impetus to improve all facets of the HIV care continuum discussed in the chapter on HIV epidemiology (Chapter 2)—that is, to diagnose all PWH and assist them in linkage, engagement, and retention in healthcare that provides fully suppressive ART and comprehensive care for HIV comorbidities. High ART potency and low pill and side effect/toxicity burdens make this more feasible now than ever before, even to the point of starting treatment at the time of diagnosis for many patients.

CURRENT TREATMENT GUIDELINES: WHAT TO START

Selection of an Initial ART Regimen

Currently, there are 33 different ARV agents comprising seven different mechanisms of action aimed at providing maximal viral suppression when used in combination (DHHS, 2020; Saag et al., 2018). The available classes of agents and pharmacokinetic (PK) enhancers were reviewed extensively in the preceding chapter. Regimens that do not require boosting are favored in order to reduce the potential for drug interactions (Saag et al., 2018). Since 1996, effective combination ART regimens have been defined as a three-drug combination consisting of two NRTIs (NRTI backbone) with an NNRTI, PI, or INSTI with or without an added PK enhancer. Such regimens have resulted in favorable virologic and immunologic outcomes in most patients in clinical trials as well as in clinical practice, particularly as pill burdens and toxicities decreased over the years.

Per the latest DHHS HIV treatment guidelines from December 2019, five different INSTI-based regimens are recommended as initial therapy for most people with HIV, based on efficacy and toxicity, as evidenced from published reports of randomized, prospective clinical trials with an adequate sample size and adequate duration. Boosted DRV/TFV/FTC or 3TC, which had previously been one of the preferred regimens for initial therapy, is now relegated to the category of "Recommended Initial Regimens in Certain Clinical Situations" based on evidence of better outcomes with INSTI-based regimens due to more adverse drug events with DRV-based regimens.

The previous guidelines recommended against the use of DTG during the first trimester of pregnancy and in those of childbearing potential who are trying to conceive or who are sexually active and not using effective contraception due to preliminary data from Botswana suggesting an increased risk of neural tube defects (0.9%) (Zash et al., 2018). Updated results showed that the prevalence is lower than reported in the preliminary data (0.3%) but still higher than in infants who were exposed to ART that did not contain DTG (0.1%) (Raesima et al., 2019; Zash et al., 2019). It is not yet known if this is a class effect, and the DHHS recommendation for individuals of childbearing potential still favors raltegravir (RAL) over DTG. If a patient becomes pregnant on DTG or is already pregnant before ART initiation, DTG is preferred.

Perhaps the most novel change in the most recent version of the DHHS guidelines is the recommendation of the single-tablet regimen (STR) DTG + 3TC as an initial ART regimen based on the GEMINI trials, as reviewed in the preceding chapter (Cahn et al., 2018), with some caveats related to patient selection. In general, however, when selecting an ART regimen, providers must consider comorbid conditions, past and present resistance test results, patient readiness and barriers to adherence such as cost and convenience (e.g., pill burden and dosing frequency), pregnancy state or potential among women of childbearing age, and the potential for drug interactions. A summary of patient and regimen-specific factors to consider when selecting an ARV regimen is provided in Table 18.1, and the five DHHS-recommended initial HIV regimens are shown in Box 18.1.

choosing between Recommended NRTI Backbones

The NRTI combinations of TDF or TAF with FTC (TDF/FTC or TAF/FTC) or ABC/3TC represent the nucleoside backbone in each of the recommended and alternative regimens. All of these NRTI combinations are available as coformulated, fixed-dose tablets and as components of coformulated STRs. Choosing between the NRTI pairs is directed mainly by differences between TDF, TAF, and ABC. TAF, an oral prodrug of TFV, is available in several coformulated preparations (TAF/FTC, EVG/cobi/TAF/FTC, RPV/TAF/FTC, DRV/cobi/TAF/FTC, BIC/TAF/FTC).

In two clinical studies, ACTG 5202 and ASSERT, regimens with ABC/3TC were shown to have an inferior virologic response compared with regimens containing TDF/FTC. ACTG 5202 compared the efficacy and safety of ABC/3TC to that of TDF/FTC when each was used in combination with either efavirenz (EFV) or ritonavir (RTV)-boosted atazanavir (ATV/r); differences in virologic efficacy were noted in those with a baseline HIV RNA level greater than 100,000 copies/mL (Sax et al., 2009). The ASSERT study compared ABC/3TC to TDF/FTC, with each also receiving EFV. The proportion of participants with HIV RNA less than 50 copies/mL was lower among ABC/3TC-treated participants (Post et al., 2010). However, other studies have documented virologic equivalence between ABC/3TC and TDF/FTC. The HEAT study compared ABC/3TC to TDF/FTC, each in combination with RTV-boosted lopinavir (LPV/r); there was no difference in virologic efficacy, including in patients with a baseline HIV RNA greater than 100,000 copies/mL (Smith et al., 2009). Similarly, ABC/3TC has shown comparable virologic efficacy to TDF/FTC when used in combination with DTG (Walmsley et al., 2013).

Table 18.1 FACTORS FOR CONSIDERATION IN ART REGIMEN SELECTION

PATIENT CHARACTERISTICS	COMORBIDITIES	REGIMEN-SPECIFIC CONSIDERATIONS
Pretreatment HIV RNA level	Cardiovascular disease, hyperlipidemia, renal disease, osteoporosis, psychiatric illness, neurologic disease, drug abuse requiring opioid replacement therapy	Regimen's genetic barrier to resistance
Pretreatment CD4$^+$T cells	Pregnancy or pregnancy potential	Potential adverse effects of medications
HIV genotypic drug resistance	Coinfections: hepatitis C, hepatitis B, tuberculosis	Drug interactions
HLA-B*5701 status		Convenience—pill burden, dosing frequency, availability of fixed-dose combination products, food requirement
Patient's anticipated compliance		Cost
Patient's preference		Timing of initiation

Adapted from Adult Panel on Antiretroviral Guidelines for Adults and Adolescents. Guidelines for the Use of Antiretroviral Agents in Adults and Adolescents with HIV. Department of Health and Human Services. Available at https://clinicalinfo.hiv.gov/sites/default/files/inline-files/AdultandAdolescentGL.pdf

Box 18.1 RECOMMENDED INITIAL ART REGIMENS

INSTI-Based Regimens (in Alphabetical Order)

Bictegravir/emtricitabine/tenofovir alafenamide (BIC/FTC/TAF)[b] (A1)

Dolutegravir/abacavir/lamivudine (DTG/ABC/3TC)[a,b]—if HLA-B*5701 negative (A1)

Dolutegravir + tenofovir/emtricitabine (DTG + TDF/FTC or TAF/FTC)[a,c,d] (A1)

Raltegravir + tenofovir/emtricitabine (RAL + TDF/FTC or TAF/FTC)[a,c,d] (BII/BIII)

Dolutegravir/lamivudine (DTG/3TC)—if HIV RNA <500,000 copies/mL, no HBV coinfection, and able to wait for HIV genotypic resistance testing for reverse transcriptase/HBV testing (A1)

[a] Lamivudine (3TC) may be interchanged with emtricitabine (FTC) or vice versa.
[b] Single-pill, once-daily regimen.
[c] Fixed-dose coformulated product for nucleoside backbone.
[d] TAF and TDF are two forms of tenofovir approved by the FDA. TAF has better bone and kidney toxicity markers than TDF, while TDF is associated with lower lipid levels. Safety, cost, and access are among the factors to consider when choosing between these drugs.

Adapted from Adult Panel on Antiretroviral Guidelines for Adults and Adolescents. Guidelines for the Use of Antiretroviral Agents in Adults and Adolescents with HIV. Department of Health and Human Services. Available at https://clinicalinfo. hiv.gov/sites/default/files/inline-files/AdultandAdolescentGL.pdf

The serious and potentially fatal ABC hypersensitivity reaction was reviewed in the preceding chapter, but it bears repeating the need to check HLA-B*5701 status first and avoid this drug in patients who are positive (ViiV Healthcare et al., 2013). ABC has also been associated with myocardial infarction (MI) in some observational studies but not in others (Monforte et al., 2013; Palella et al., 2015; Sabin et al., 2014; Worm et al., 2010; Young et al., 2015). However, more recent literature suggests a correlation (Dorjee et al., 2017), and in the HIV treatment community a consensus has emerged that ABC should be avoided in patients at increased cardiac risk.

TDF has been associated with renal impairment and reduced bone mineral density, which may be exacerbated when TDF is used in regimens containing PIs or elvitegravir (EVG) boosted with RTV or cobicistat (cobi) (Mocroft et al., 2015, McComsey et al., 2011). TAF is an oral prodrug of TFV that has been designed to achieve higher active metabolite concentrations inside peripheral blood CD4 and mononuclear cells; it may therefore be administered at lower doses than TDF with comparable antiviral efficacy but less renal and bone mineral adverse effects. The approval of TAF and the two TAF-containing regimens—EVG 150 mg/cobi 150 mg/FTC 200 mg/TAF 10 mg (EVG/cobi/ FTC/TAF) and rilpivirine (RPV) 25 mg/TAF 25mg/FTC 200 mg (RPV/FTC/TAF)—was supported by 48-week data from two pivotal phase 3 studies. In the first, EVG/c/ TAF/FTC was found to be noninferior to EVG 150 mg/ cobi150 mg/FTC 200 mg/TDF 300 mg (EVG/cobi/FTC/ TDF) among treatment-naive adult patients. The safety and efficacy of FTC/TAF were also demonstrated in one switch study of virologically suppressed patients randomized to continue FTC/TDF or switch to TAF/FTC (Gallant et al., 2016; Pozniak et al., 2016). Bioequivalence studies also demonstrated that standalone TAF/FTC achieved the same drug levels of TFV in target cells as with EVG/cobi/FTC// TDF. Similar studies also demonstrated that RPV/TAF/ FTC achieved similar drug levels of FTC and TFV in the blood as with EVG/cobi/FTC/TAF, and similar drug levels of RPV as standalone RPV. TAF/FTC is now included as a component of several recommended regimens and offers clinicians an additional NRTI backbone option. Two doses of TAF have been approved: 25 and 10 mg. The 10-mg dose is intended for use in combination with RTV or cobi; otherwise, the 25-mg dose of TAF is recommended.

Choosing Between third drug options

The choice of the third drug in an initial ARV regimen lies between an INSTI, NNRTI, or PI and is based on consideration of the regimen's likely efficacy, genetic barrier to resistance, adverse effects, convenience, comorbidities, and drug interactions. Based on these considerations, the following observations have been noted (complementing and reinforcing data presented in the preceding chapter):

- The efficacy and safety of DTG-based regimens with either ABC/3TC or FTC/TDF have been evaluated in three clinical trials (SPRING-2, SINGLE, and FLAMINGO), where they were found to be noninferior or superior to other INSTI-, NNRTI-, or PI-based regimens. Thus, DTG/ABC/3TC and DTG + FTC/TDF are among recommended first-line ART regimens (Clotet et al., 2014; Raffi et al., 2013; Walmsley et al., 2013).

- Recently, the two-drug regimen of DTG/3TC has been added as well, based on 96-week data from the GEMINI 1 and GEMINI 2 trials, which showed that the efficacy of the two-drug regimen was similar to the three-drug regimen of DTG + FTC/TDF (in patients with HIV RNA <500,000 copies/mL, no HBV coinfection, if HIV genotypic resistance testing for reverse transcriptase (RT) and HBV is available).

- The efficacy and safety of RAL (with either FTC/TDF or ABC/3TC) have been evaluated in a number of clinical trials, in which it was shown to be superior to EFV-, ATV/r-, and DRV/r-based regimens and noninferior to

DTG-based regimens (Lennox et al., 2009, 2014; Raffi et al., 2013).

- The fixed-dose combination EVG/cobi/FTC/TDF was evaluated in two randomized clinical trials and found to be noninferior to EFV/FTC/TDF or ATV/r + FTC/TDF (Rockstroh et al., 2013; Zolopa et al., 2013).

- BIC is available as part of a single-tablet, once-daily regimen that includes TAF and FTC (BIC/FTC/TAF). The efficacy of BIC in ART-naive adults was compared to DTG plus two NRTIs in two large, phase 3, randomized, double-blinded clinical trials (Gallant et al., 2017; Sax et al., 2017). The proportion of participants with plasma HIV RNA less than 50 copies/mL at week 48 in the BIC arms was noninferior to that noted in the DTG arms in both trials (89% vs. 93% and 92.4% vs. 93%, respectively).

- Clinical studies of DRV/r + FTC/TDF have shown it to be noninferior to RAL and superior to LPV/r. Compared to DTG-based regimens in the FLAMINGO study, DRV/r was inferior to DTG, with adverse events being the primary driver for this difference (Clotet et al., 2014).

- Historically, EFV, particularly the single-tablet regimen EFV/FTC/TDF (Atripla), played a central role in the preferred first-line ARV regimen category. This was based on its demonstrated superiority or noninferiority to all the regimens against which it was compared. However, more recent studies have shown superiority of DTG, RAL, and RPV (the latter in patients with baseline HIV RNA <100,000 copies/mL and CD4 cell count >200 cells/mm³) to EFV; these results were primarily driven by differences in adverse events. Concern regarding EFV-related adverse events was further enhanced by a possible association with suicidality observed in one analysis of four clinical trials (Mollan et al., 2014). Thus, EFVFTC/TDF has been relegated to the alternative "Recommended Initial Regimens in Certain Clinical Situations" category.

- Previously, ATV/r + FTC/TDF was among the preferred first-line ARV regimens based on its virologic efficacy, which is equivalent to that of a number of comparator regimens, including EFV/FTC/TDF, EFV + ABC/3TC, LPV/r + FTC/TDF, and EVG/cobi/FTC/TDF. However, a more recent study, ACTG 5257, compared ATV/r with DRV/r or RAL, each in combination with FTC/TDF. On-treatment virologic efficacy was comparable among the three groups; however, more adverse events and treatment discontinuations were noted among patients on ATV/r compared to the other two groups (Lennox et al., 2015). Thus, ATV/r has been relegated to the "Recommended Initial Regimens in Certain Clinical Situations" category.

- Data suggest greater weight gain with certain INSTI-based regimens, particularly when paired with TAF, compared to other ARV drugs (Bhagwat et al., 2018; Bourgi et al., 2020; Sax et al., 2020; Venter et al., 2019).

RECOMMENDED INITIAL REGIMENS IN CERTAIN CLINICAL SITUATIONS

The DHHS guidelines provide an evidence-based menu for selecting an initial ART regimen, and the vast majority of patients will be eligible for one of the five recommended initial regimens. However, it remains the responsibility of clinicians to select the regimen most suited to the clinical scenario at hand. Other ART regimens listed as alternatives in Tables 6a and 7 of the DHHS guidelines are effective but may have some potential disadvantages (e.g., pill burden, dosing, schedule, toxicity profile, baseline HIV RNA levels or CD4 cell count restrictions) compared to preferred regimens for most people, or they may have fewer supporting data from randomized clinical trials. However, there may be situations in which these agents might be preferred for an individual patient. These alternative regimens are categorized as INSTI-, NNRTI-, and PI-based regimens and regimens when ABC, TAF, and TDF cannot be used; these regimens and clinical scenarios that might prompt their use are shown here in Tables 18.2, 18.3, and 18.4. Additionally, comments are made here on the new NNRTI doravirine (DOR):

- DOR is available as either a single agent (Pifeltro) or as part of an STR (DOR/TDF/3TC, Delstrigo), which was shown to be noninferior to EFV/FTC/TDF (Orkin et al., 2019).

- DOR was also compared to DRV/r, each with either ABC/3TC or FTC/TDF, and found to be noninferior (Molina et al., 2018).

- DOR/TDF/3TC and DOR + FTC/TDF or FTC/TAF are classified as "Recommended Initial Regimens in Certain Clinical Situations."

WHEN TO SWITCH OR SIMPLIFY ART

Because PWH must take ARVs for life, side effects and toxicities must be addressed to avoid metabolic complications and adherence problems that can lead to virologic failure. With the advent of newer agents with improved toxicity profiles, easier dosing schedules, and fewer pills, providers are often confronted with the question of whether to change individual agents or whole regimens. Although the optimal time for changing therapy remains undetermined, most studies have investigated changes in therapy for PWH who have been controlled on an ART regimen for at least 6 months. The main goal of switching therapy is to maintain viral suppression without jeopardizing the availability of future treatment options. According to the IAS-USA and DHHS, the following are some reasons to consider changing therapy (DHHS, 2020; Saag et al., 2018):

1. Reduce pill burden or dosing frequency

2. Reduce short- or long-term toxicity and enhance tolerability

3. Change food or fluid requirements

Table 18.2 ALTERNATIVE ART REGIMENS

INSTI-BASED REGIMENS	NNRTI-BASED REGIMENS	PI-BASED REGIMENS	WHEN ABC, TAF, AND TDF CANNOT BE USED
Elvitegravir/cobisistat/tenofovir/emtricitabine (EVG/c/TDF/FTC or TAF/FTC)[d] (B1)	Efavirenz/tenofovir/emtricitabine (EFV/TDF/FTC)[b,c] (EFV 400 mg or 600 mg with TDF/3TC) (B1)	Cobicistat-boosted atazanavir (ATV/c) + tenofovir/emtricitabine (TDF/FTC)[a,c]—only if pretreatment estimated CrCl ≥70 mL/min (B1)	DTG/3TC—if HIV RNA <500,000 copies/mL, no HBV coinfection, and able to wait for HIV genotypic resistance testing for reverse transcriptase/HBV testing (A1)
	Rilpivirine/tenofovir/emtricitabine (RPV/TDF/FTC)[a,b]—if pretreatment HIV RNA <100,000 copies/mL and CD4+ T-cell count >200 cells/mm³ (B1)	Ritonavir-boosted atazanavir (ATV/r) + tenofovir/emtricitabine (TDF/FTC)[a,c] (B1)	DRV/r plus RAL twice daily—if pretreatment HIV RNA <100,000 copies/mL and CD4+ T-cell count >200 cells/mm (C1)
		Cobicistat-boosted darunavir (DRV/c) or ritonavir-boosted darunavir (DRV/r) + abacavir/lamivudine (ABC/3TC)[a,c]—if HLA-B*5701 negative (BII)	DRV/r + 3TC (C1)
		Cobicistat-boosted darunavir (DRV/c) + tenofovir/emtricitabine (TDF/FTC)[a,c] (A1)	

[a] Lamivudine (3TC) may be interchanged with emtricitabine (FTC) or vice versa.

[b] Single-pill, once-daily regimen.

[c] Fixed-dose coformulated product for nucleoside backbone.

[d] TAF and TDF are two forms of tenofovir approved by the FDA. TAF has fewer bone and kidney toxicities than TDF, while TDF is associated with lower lipid levels. Safety, cost, and access are among the factors to consider when choosing between these drugs.

Adapted from Adult Panel on Antiretroviral Guidelines for Adults and Adolescents. Guidelines for the Use of Antiretroviral Agents in Adults and Adolescents with HIV. Department of Health and Human Services. Available at https://clinicalinfo.hiv.gov/sites/default/files/inline-files/AdultandAdolescentGL.pdf

4. Minimize drug interactions

5. Optimize ART regimen for pregnancy or in case of pregnancy

6. Reduce cost

Switching to a simplified, less toxic regimen in PWH with an extensive treatment history remains complex. Simply changing one agent may not be possible, and a complete review of the patient's treatment history, resistance testing, treatment tolerance, and drug interactions should be conducted prior to designing a new regimen. In general, two approaches to changing therapy in virally suppressed PWH have been changing one agent to another either within the same class or in another class (DHHS, 2020). Within-class simplification can decrease toxicity, dosing frequency, and pill burden, especially when coformulated agents are used. For example, a regimen that includes the NRTI zidovudine could be changed to a regimen that includes TFV or ABC, reducing side effects and dosing frequency (DHHS, 2020). Another example of a within-class change is switching from TDF to TAF for decreased long-term bone and renal effects (Gallant et al., 2016). However, the long-term adverse effects of the NRTIs TFV, ABC, and 3TC should be noted. In a 2013

Table 18.3 BASELINE CONDITIONS

SCENARIO	RECOMMENDED ACTION
Low CD4+ T-cell count (<200 cells/mm³)	Do not use RPV or DRV/r plus RAL.
Pretreatment HIV RNA >100,000 copies/mL	Do not use RPV, ABC/3TC with EFV or ATV/r, or DRV/r plus RAL.
Pretreatment HIV RNA >500,000 copies/mL	Do not use RPV-based regimens, ABC/3TC with ATV/r, DRV/r + RAL, or DTG/3TC.
ARV to be started before HIV drug resistance results are available	Recommended regimens: BIC/TAF/FTC, DTG + (TAF or TDF) + (3TC or FTC), (DRV/r or DRV/c) + (TAF or TDF) + (3TC or FTC). Avoid ABC, NNTRI-based regimen, and DTG/3TC.

Adapted from Adult Panel on Antiretroviral Guidelines for Adults and Adolescents. Guidelines for the Use of Antiretroviral Agents in Adults and Adolescents with HIV. Department of Health and Human Services. Available at https://clinicalinfo.hiv.gov/sites/default/files/inline-files/AdultandAdolescentGL.pdf

Table 18.4 CONCOMITANT MEDICAL CONDITIONS

SCENARIO	RECOMMENDED ACTION
Cardiac disease	Consider avoiding ABC, LPV/r, and DRV/r.
Chronic kidney disease	Avoid TDF with a PK enhancer, in particular: ▪ EVG/cobi/FTC//TDF ▪ ATV/cobi with TDF ▪ DRV/cobi with TDF Avoid ATV. TAF may be used if CrCl >30 mL/min or if on chronic hemodialysis.[b] ABC may be used if HLA-B*5701 negative. Options when ABC, TAF, or TDF cannot be used: DTC/3TC, DRV/r + 3TC, DRV/r + RAL.
HIV-associated dementia	Avoid EFV because its psychiatric effects may cloud the clinical picture. Favor use of DRV- or DTG-based regimens due to the possibility of increased central nervous system penetration.
Osteoporosis	Avoid TDF.
Hyperlipidemia	EFV, ABC, PIRTV or PI/cobi, and EVG/cobi have been associated with increases in lipid levels. TDF lowers lipid levels, so switching from TDF to TAF is associated with increased lipid levels.
Psychiatric illness	Consider avoiding EFV and RPV. They can exacerbate psychiatric symptoms and may be associated with suicidality.
HBV coinfection	Use FTC/TDF or 3TC/TDF. If TDF use is contraindicated, recommend use of FTC or 3TC with entecavir.
Tuberculosis	If rifampin is used, EFV/FTC/TDF is the recommended regimen, although DTG 50 mg twice daily has been shown to be effective. If a PI/r-based ART regimen is used, rifabutin is the rifamycin of choice in the tuberculosis regimen, but it requires dose adjustment.
Gastroesophageal reflux disease requiring proton pump inhibitors	Avoid ATV or RPV.
Situations when neither tenofovir nor abacavir can be used	DTG/3TC (no HBV coinfection, no history of resistance, and HIV RNA <500,000 copies/mL) DRV/r plus RAL (treatment-naive) LPV/r plus 3TC (treatment-naive) DTG/RPV (virally suppressed with no previous virologic failure)

[a] Lamivudine (3TC) may be interchanged with emtricitabine (FTC) or vice versa.

[b] Only studied with EVG/cobi/FTC/TAF.

Adapted from Adult Panel on Antiretroviral Guidelines for Adults and Adolescents. Guidelines for the Use of Antiretroviral Agents in Adults and Adolescents with HIV. Department of Health and Human Services. Available at https://clinicalinfo.hiv.gov/sites/default/files/inline-files/AdultandAdolescentGL.pdf

population-based study of approximately 100 patients, these NRTIs were shown to inhibit telomerase activity, leading to accelerated shortening of telomere length in mononuclear cells (TFV was found to be the most potent inhibitor). This study suggests that even the NRTIs commonly in use today are a potential contributor to HIV-associated accelerated aging, and switching PWH off NRTI-based regimens may become a higher priority in the future (Leeansyah et al., 2013).

Similar to NRTIs, within-class simplification of NNRTIs can reduce toxicities and adverse side effects. For example, switching from EFV to RPV (Hagins et al., 2018) or DOR (Johnson et al., 2019) demonstrated noninferior efficacy for maintaining virologic suppression for 96 weeks and 48 weeks, respectively, and both RPV and DOR possess a superior neuropsychiatric profile when compared to EFV as shown in previous studies (Orkin et al., 2019; van Lunzen et al., 2016).

The majority of studies investigating class switches have evaluated the replacement of a PI with an alternative class, such as an NNRTI or INSTI. This can be done to reduce toxicity or drug interactions or to change to a simpler, once-daily coformulated combination. Although this is generally successful in PWH without resistance, it can lead to virologic failure in PWH with previous underlying resistance. This was seen in the SWITCHMRK 1 and 2 studies, where PWH randomized to change from boosted LPV to RAL had improved serum lipid concentrations but also had a higher virologic failure rate than those who remained on LPV/RTV, leading to study termination at 24 weeks (Eron et al., 2010). Therefore, DHHS recommends a careful review of the drug-resistance profile and consultation with a clinician who has expertise in HIV drug resistance before ART changes are made in persons with a history of treatment failure and drug resistance (DHHS, 2020).

One recent development in HIV treatment is that there are now two two-drug ART regimens shown to be effective for PWH who are virologically suppressed (DTG/RPV or

DTG/3TC) or treatment-naive (DTG/3TC) who have no prior evidence of resistance to either drug in the combination. Both DTG/3TC studies were discussed in the preceding chapter, showing noninferiority with this regimen in switches (TANGO) and naive (GEMINI) patients. For DTG/RPV, in the SWORD 1 and SWORD 2 studies 1,024 participants with viral suppression for at least 1 year with no history of virologic failure or significant drug resistance mutations were randomized to remain on their ART or switch to DTG/RPV, either at the start of the study (early switch) or at week 52 (late switch). At week 100, 89% of the early-switch arm and 93% of the late-switch arm had maintained fewer than 50 HIV RNA copies per milliliter (Aboud et al., 2019). One caveat to note about these two-drug approaches, however, is that neither one has adequate anti-HBV activity, so they are not recommended for persons coinfected with HBV or whose HBV status is unknown (DHHS, 2020).

In the aforementioned switch studies, ART changes were made in PWH who were virologically suppressed. If regimen switching is prompted by virologic failure or suboptimal viral load reduction, HIV drug-resistance testing must be performed to guide selection of active ART drugs. For PWH with virologic failure while on an INSTI, genotype testing specifically for INSTI resistance should be performed, in addition to the standard genotyping performed on the protease and reverse transcription regions of the genome. Genotyping should be done while the patient is either on ART or within 4 weeks of discontinuation before the dominant strain may revert to wild-type virus and important mutations fade into the CD4$^+$ archive. The addition of phenotypic testing to genotypic testing traditionally was recommended for PWH with complex resistance patterns, although over time the sophistication and reliability of algorithmic genotype interpretations such as the Stanford Drug Resistance Database have largely obviated the need for phenotypic testing. The new attachment inhibitor fostemsavir is now an option for patients expected to have incomplete activity from an optimized background regimen, helping 62% and 84% of such patients achieve HIV-1 RNA counts of less than 40 and less than 200 copies/mL, respectively, at 48 weeks (Kozal et al., 2020).

If switching to an ABC-based regimen, HLA-B*5701 allele testing must be done to reduce the risk of a hypersensitivity reaction. When switching regimens for someone with HBV coinfection, a drug regimen effective for both HIV and HBV should be used; typically this means using TFV, but if that is not possible, the patient should receive entecavir in addition to their HIV ART regimen.

After switching regimens, PWH should be evaluated closely to ensure that no new side effects have emerged, and a repeat viral load 4 to 8 weeks after a regimen switch should be obtained to ensure the patient is virally suppressed. If preexisting laboratory abnormalities were attributed to the previous ART regimen (e.g., hyperlipidemia assumed to be from PIs), these laboratory values should be rechecked 3 months after switching regimens (DHHS, 2020).

SUMMARY

The DHHS, IAS-USA, World Health Organization, European AIDS Clinical Society, and British HIV Association guidelines now recommend treatment of all PWH, regardless of the CD4$^+$ count. Currently, the critical issues in ART are focused on optimizing regimens for the individual patient. Barriers to adherence and addressing those factors remain paramount, and resolution prior to treatment initiation is important to achieve treatment success. Once the patient is ready for therapy, the key issues are tailoring medication regimens for the patient's medical comorbidities, medication toxicities, and lifestyle. Switching to newer agents must be done prudently, with careful consideration of the patient's resistance history and comorbidities. Just as there has been enormous progress in the past, we will continue to witness significant change in the future as we seek to find the optimal treatments for PWH.

RECOMMENDED READING

Department of Health and Human Services, Panel on Antiretroviral Guidelines for Adults and Adolescents. Guidelines for the use of antiretroviral agents in HIV-1-infected adults and adolescents. December 18, 2019. https://www.aidsinfo.nih.gov/ContentFiles/AdultandAdolescentGL.pdf

Saag M, Benson C, Gandhi R, et al. Antiretroviral drugs for treatment and prevention of HIV infection in adults: 2018 recommendations of the International Antiviral Society-USA Panel. *JAMA.* 2018;320(4):379–396.

REFERENCES

Aboud M, Orkin C, Podzamczer D, et al. Efficacy and safety of dolutegravir-rilpivirine for maintenance of virological suppression in adults with HIV-1: 100-week data from the randomised, open-label, phase 3 SWORD-1 and SWORD-2 studies. *Lancet HIV.* 2019;6(9):e576–e587.

Bhagwat P, Ofotokun I, McComsey GA, et al. Changes in waist circumference in HIV-infected individuals initiating a raltegravir or protease inhibitor regimen: effects of sex and race. *Open Forum Infect Dis.* 2018;5(11):ofy201.

Bourgi K, Rebeiro PF, Turner M, et al. Greater weight gain in treatment naive persons starting dolutegravir-based antiretroviral therapy. *Clin Infect Dis.* 2020;70(7):1267–1274.

Cahn P, Sierra Madero JS, Arribas JR, et al. Dolutegravir plus lamivudine versus dolutegravir plus tenofovir disoproxil fumarate and emtricitabine in antiretroviral-naïve adults with HIV-1 infection (GEMINI-1 and GEMINI-2): week 48 results from two multicenter, double-blind, randomized, non-inferiority, phase 3 trials. *Lancet.* 2018;393(10167):143–155. doi:10.1016/S0140-6736(18)32462-0

Clotet B, Feinberg J, van Lunzen J, et al. Once-daily dolutegravir versus darunavir plus ritonavir in antiretroviral-naive adults with HIV-1 infection (FLAMINGO): 48 week results from the randomised open-label phase 3b study. *Lancet.* 2014;383(9936):2222–2231.

Coffey S, Bacchetti P, Sachdev D, et al. RAPID antiretroviral therapy: high virologic suppression rates with immediate antiretroviral therapy initiation in a vulnerable urban clinic population. *AIDS.* 2019;33(5):825–832.

Cohen MS, Chen YQ, McCauley M, et al. Prevention of HIV-1 infection with early antiretroviral therapy. *N Engl J Med.* 2011;365:493–505.

Cohen MS, Gamble T, McCauley M. Prevention of HIV transmission and the HPTN 052 study. *Annu Rev Med.* 2020;71:347–360. doi:10.1146/annurev-med-110918-034551

Colasanti J, Sumitani J, Mehta CC, et al. Implementation of a rapid entry program decreases time to viral suppression among vulnerable persons living with HIV in the Southern United States. *Open Forum Infect Dis.* 2018;5(6):ofy104.

Department of Health and Human Services. Guidelines for the use of antiretroviral agents in adults and adolescents with HIV. 2020. https://clinicalinfo.hiv.gov/en/guidelines/adult-and-adolescent-arv/whats-new-guidelines

Dorjee K, Baxi SM, Reingold AL, et al. Risk of cardiovascular events from current, recent, and cumulative exposure to abacavir among persons living with HIV who were receiving antiretroviral therapy in the United States: a cohort study. *BMC Infect Dis.* 2017;17(1):708. doi:10.1186/s12879-017-2808-8

Eron JJ, Young B, Cooper DA, et al.; the SWITCHMRK 1 and 2 investigators. Switch to a raltegravir-based regimen versus continuation of a lopinavir–ritonavir-based regimen in stable HIV-infected patients with suppressed viremia (SWITCHMRK 1 and 2): two multicentre, double-blind, randomized controlled trials. *Lancet.* 2010;375:396–407.

Gallant JE, Daar ES, Raffi F, et al. Efficacy and safety of tenofovir alafenamide versus tenofovir disoproxil fumarate given as fixed-dose combinations containing emtricitabine as backbones for treatment of HIV-1 infection in virologically suppressed adults: a randomised, double-blind, active-controlled phase 3 trial. *Lancet HIV.* 2016;3(4):e158–e165.

Gallant J, Lazzarin A, Mills A, et al. Bictegravir, emtricitabine, and tenofovir alafenamide versus dolutegravir, abacavir, and lamivudine for initial treatment of HIV-1 infection (GS-US-380-1489): a double-blind, multicentre, phase 3, randomised controlled non-inferiority trial. *Lancet.* 2017;390(10107):2063–2072.

Hagins D, Orkin C, Daar ES, et al. Switching to coformulated rilpivirine (RPV), emtricitabine (FTC) and tenofovir alafenamide from either RPV, FTC and tenofovir disoproxil fumarate (TDF) or efavirenz, FTC and TDF: 96-week results from two randomized clinical trials. *HIV Med.* 2018;19(10):724–733.

HIV.gov. Overview: data and trends: US statistics. 2020. https://www.hiv.gov/hiv-basics/overview/data-and-trends/statistics

Johnson M, Kumar P, Molina JM, et al. Switching to doravirine/lamivudine/tenofovir disoproxil fumarate (DOR/3TC/TDF) maintains HIV-1 virologic suppression through 48 weeks: results of the DRIVE-SHIFT trial. *J AIDS.* 2019;81(4):463–472.

Koenig SP, Dorvil N, Devieux JG, et al. Same-day HIV testing with initiation of antiretroviral therapy versus standard care for persons living with HIV: a randomized unblinded trial. *PLoS Med.* 2017;14(7):e1002357.

Kozal M, Aberg, J, Pialoux G, et al. Fostemsavir in adults with multidrug-resistant HIV-1 infection. *N Engl J Med.* 2020;382:1232–1243.

Labhardt ND, Ringera I, Lejone TI, et al. Effect of offering same-day ART vs usual health facility referral during home-based HIV testing on linkage to care and viral suppression among adults with HIV in Lesotho: the CASCADE randomized clinical trial. *JAMA.* 2018;319(11):1103–1112.

Leeansyah E, Cameron P, Solomon A, et al. Inhibition of telomerase activity by human immunodeficiency virus (HIV) nucleos(t)ide reverse transcriptase inhibitors: a potential factor contributing to HIV-associated accelerated aging. *J Infect Dis.* 2013;207:1157–1165.

Lennox JL, DeJesus E, Lazzarin A, et al. Safety and efficacy of raltegravir-based versus efavirenz-based combination therapy in treatment-naïve patients with HIV-1 infection: a multicentre, double-blind randomised controlled trial. *Lancet.* 2009;374(9692):796–806.

Lennox JF, Landovitz RJ, Ribaudo HJ. Three nonnucleoside reverse transcriptase inhibitor-sparing antiretroviral regimens for treatment-naïve volunteers infected with HIV-1. *Ann Intern Med.* 2015;162(6):461–462.

Lundgren J, Babiker A, Gordin F, et al.; Insight Start Study Group. Initiation of antiretroviral therapy in early asymptomatic HIV infection. *N Engl J Med.* 2015;373(9):795–807.

McComsey GA, Kitch D, Daar ES, et al. Bone mineral density and fractures in antiretroviral-naive persons randomized to receive abacavir-lamivudine or tenofovir disoproxil fumarate-emtricitabine along with efavirenz or atazanavir-ritonavir: AIDS Clinical Trials Group A5224s, a substudy of ACTG A5202. *J Infect Dis.* 2011;203(12):1791–1801.

Mocroft A, Lundgren JD, Ross M, et al. Exposure to antiretrovirals (ARVs) and development of chronic kidney disease (CKD) [Abstract 142]. Presented at the 2015 Conference on Retroviruses and Opportunistic Infections, Seattle, WA, February 23–24, 2015.

Molina JM, Squires K, Sax PE, et al. Doravirine versus ritonavir-boosted darunavir in antiretroviral-naive adults with HIV-1 (DRIVE-FORWARD): 48-week results of a randomised, double-blind, phase 3, non-inferiority trial. *Lancet HIV.* 2018;5(5):e211–e220.

Mollan KR, Smurzynski M, Eron JJ, et al. Association between efavirenz as initial therapy for HIV-1 infection and increased risk for suicidal ideation or attempted or completed suicide: an analysis of trial data. *Ann Intern Med.* 2014;161(1):1–10.

Monforte AD, Reiss P, Ryom L, et al. Atazanavir is not associated with an increased risk of cardio- or cerebrovascular disease events. *AIDS.* 2013;27(3):407–415.

Orkin C, Squires KE, Molina JM, et al. Doravirine/lamivudine/tenofovir disoproxil fumarate is non-inferior to efavirenz/emtricitabine/tenofovir disoproxil fumarate in treatment-naive adults with human immunodeficiency virus-1 infection: week 48 results of the DRIVE-AHEAD trial. *Clin Infect Dis.* 2019;68(4):535–544.

Palella F, Althoff KN, Moore R, et al. NA-ACCORD: recent abacavir use and risk of MI [Abstract 749 LB]. Presented at the 2015 Conference on Retroviruses and Opportunistic Infections, Seattle, WA, February 23–26, 2015.

Pilcher CD, Ospina-Norvell C, Dasgupta A, et al. The effect of same-day observed initiation of antiretroviral therapy on HIV viral load and treatment outcomes in a U.S. public health setting. *J AIDS.* 2017;74(1):44–51.

Post FA, Moyle GJ, Stellbrink HJ, et al. Randomized comparison of renal effects, efficacy, and safety with once-daily abacavir/lamivudine versus tenofovir/emtricitabine, administered with efavirenz, in antiretroviral-naive, HIV-1-infected adults: 48-week results from the ASSERT study. *J AIDS.* 2010;55(1):49–45.

Pozniak A, Arribas JR, Gathe J, et al. Switching to tenofovir alafenamide, coformulated with elvitegravir, cobicistat, and emtricitabine, in HIV-infected patients with renal impairment: 48-week results from a single-arm, multicenter, open-label phase 3 study. *J AIDS.* 2016;71(5):530–537.

Raesima MM, Ogbuabo CM, Thomas V, et al. Dolutegravir use at conception—additional surveillance data from Botswana. *N Engl J Med.* 2019;381(9):885–887.

Raffi F, Jaeger H, Quiros-Roldan E, et al. Once-daily dolutegravir versus twice-daily raltegravir in antiretroviral-naive adults with HIV-1 infection (SPRING-2 study): 96 week results from a randomised, double-blind, non-inferiority trial. *Lancet Infect Dis.* 2013;13(11):927–935.

Rockstroh J, DeJesus E, Henry K, et al. A randomized, double-blind comparison of coformulated elvitegravir/cobicistat/emtricitabine/tenofovir DF vs. ritonavir-boosted atazanavir plus coformulated emtricitabine and tenofovir DF for initial treatment of HIV-1 infection: analysis of week 96 results. *J AIDS.* 2013;62(5):483–486.

Rosen S, Maskew M, Fox MP, et al. Initiating antiretroviral therapy for HIV at a patient's first clinic visit: the RapIT randomized controlled trial. *PLoS Med.* 2016;13(5):e1002015.

Saag M, Benson C, Gandhi R, et al. Antiretroviral drugs for treatment and prevention of HIV infection in adults: 2018 recommendations of the International Antiviral Society-USA Panel. *JAMA.* 2018;320(4):379–396.

Sabin C, Reiss P, Ryom L, et al. Is there continued evidence for an association between abacavir and myocardial infarction risk? [Abstract 747]. Presented at the 21st Conference on Retroviruses and Opportunistic Infections, Boston, MA, 2014.

Samji H, Cescon A, Hogg RS, et al.; North American AIDS Cohort Collaboration on Research and Design (NA-ACCORD) of IeDEA. Closing the gap: increases in life expectancy among treated

HIV-positive individuals in the United States and Canada. *PLoS One*. 2013;8(12):e81355. doi:10.1371/journal.pone.0081355

Sax PE, Erlandson KM, Lake JE, et al. Weight gain following initiation of antiretroviral therapy: risk factors in randomized comparative clinical trials. *Clin Infect Dis*. 2020;71(6):1379–1389.

Sax PE, Pozniak A, Montes ML, et al. Coformulated bictegravir, emtricitabine, and tenofovir alafenamide versus dolutegravir with emtricitabine and tenofovir alafenamide, for initial treatment of HIV-1 infection (GS-US-380-1490): a randomised, double-blind, multicentre, phase 3, non-inferiority trial. *Lancet*. 2017;390(10107):2073–2082.

Sax P, Tierney C, Collier A, et al. Abacavir–lamivudine versus tenofovir–emtricitabine for initial HIV-1 therapy. *N Engl J Med*. 2009;361(23):2230–2240.

Smith KY, Patel P, Fine D, et al. Randomized, double-blind, placebo-matched, multicenter trial of abacavir/lamivudine or tenofovir/emtricitabine with lopinavir/ritonavir for initial HIV treatment. *AIDS*. 2009;23(12):1547–1556.

van Lunzen J, Antinori A, Cohen CJ, et al. Rilpivirine vs. efavirenz-based single-tablet regimens in treatment-naive adults: week 96 efficacy and safety from a randomized phase 3b study. *AIDS*. 2016;30(2):251–259.

Venter WDF, Moorhouse M, Sokhela S, et al. Dolutegravir plus two different prodrugs of tenofovir to treat HIV. *N Engl J Med*. 2019;381(9):803–815.

ViiV Healthcare. Ziagen (abacavir) US prescribing information. 2013. http://www.accessdata.fda.gov/drugsatfda_docs/label/2012/020977s025,020978s029lbl.pdf

Walmsley SL, Antela A, Clumeck N, et al. Dolutegravir plus abacavir–lamivudine for the treatment of HIV-1 infection. *N Engl J Med*. 2013;369(19):1807–1818.

Worm SW, Sabin C, Weber R, et al.; DAD Study Group. Risk of myocardial infarction in patients with HIV infection exposed to specific individual antiretroviral drugs from 3 major drug classes. *J Infect Dis*. 2010;201:318–330.

Young J, Xiao Y, Moodier EE, et al. Effect of cumulating exposure to abacavir on the risk of cardiovascular disease events in patients from the Swiss HIV cohort study. *J AIDS*. 2015;69(4):413–421.

Zash R, Holmes L, Diseko M, et al. Neural-tube defects and antiretroviral treatment regimens in Botswana. *N Engl J Med*. 2019;381(9):827–840.

Zash R, Makhema J, Shapiro RL. Neural-tube defects with dolutegravir treatment from the time of conception. *N Engl J Med*. 2018;379(10):979–981.

Zolopa A, Sax P, DeJesus E, et al. A randomized double-blind comparison of coformulated elvitegravir/cobicistat/emtricitabine/tenofovir disoproxil fumarate versus favirenz/emtricitabine/tenofovir disoproxil fumarate for initial treatment of HIV-1 infection: analysis of week 96 results. *J AIDS*. 2013;63:96–100.

19.

THE HIV RESERVOIR AND CURE AND REMISSION STRATEGIES

Rajesh T. Gandhi, Boris Juelg, Nikolaus Jilg, Niyati Jakharia, and Rohit Talwani

---

CHAPTER GOALS

Upon completion of this chapter, the reader should be able to:

- Identify key hurdles for HIV eradication strategies and explain approaches that might overcome these challenges

- Discuss new antiretroviral drugs (ARVs) in development

- Discuss current research on preventive and therapeutic vaccines and immunomodulatory and genetic agents

---

INTRODUCTION

Currently available ARVs consistently achieve durable suppression of HIV but are not able to eliminate the latent reservoir of infection or significantly modulate host immune responses in a manner that improves clinical outcomes. In this chapter, we will discuss new ARVs in development and various strategies targeting immune dysregulation and T-cell homeostasis. We also update the status of clinical research evaluating immunomodulators and vaccines.

WHAT'S NEW?

Novel strategies to promote HIV latency reversal and approaches to boost HIV-specific immunity are being evaluated in clinical trials aimed at eradicating HIV. A new generation of broadly neutralizing antibodies has demonstrated potency at suppressing HIV-1 viremia in clinical trials and may play a role in immunotherapy and prevention. Latency-reversing agents (e.g., histone deacetylase inhibitors) and gene therapy strategies using autologous CD4$^+$ T cells and hematopoietic stem cells continue to be evaluated in trials.

KEY POINTS

- HIV-1 persists quiescently in cellular reservoirs not detected by the immune system due to the lack of active viral replication; these reservoirs represent the biggest obstacle to cure approaches.

- Reversal of HIV-1 latency and induction of virus expression by a variety of interventions may render infected cells susceptible to immune recognition and active clearance.

- Strategies to boost immune responses via active or passive immunization, immunomodulation, or gene therapy are being evaluated with the aim of achieving HIV-1 control without antiretroviral therapy (ART), if not viral eradication.

WHY SHOULD WE TRY TO CURE HIV?

Although current ART is highly effective at controlling HIV-1 replication, it does not eradicate or cure the infection. There are several compelling reasons for trying to cure HIV-1. First, despite efforts to expand access to treatment, many people with HIV (PWH) worldwide are not receiving ART, which leads to ongoing transmission of the virus. Second, because current ART does not eradicate HIV-1, PWH must take ART for many decades, which may eventuate in difficulties with adherence, substantial cost, and the potential for long-term side effects. Third, PWH have increased rates of cardiovascular disease, liver disease, neurocognitive disorders, and other noninfectious complications that may be driven by elevated levels of inflammation that persist despite suppressive ART. Fourth, many PWH treated with ART alone do not achieve immune restoration despite viral suppression; in a large trial of HIV-positive adults achieving virologic suppression for 3 years with CD4$^+$ T-cell counts of 200 cells/mL or less, these patients had significantly greater mortality compared to those with CD4$^+$ T-cell counts of more than 200 cells/mL (adjusted hazard ratio, 2.6) (Engsig et al., 2014). Given significant evidence that CD4$^+$ T-cell counts have been correlated with normal life expectancy (ART Collaboration Cohort et al., 2008; Lewden et al., 2007), attention has turned to strategies to control chronic immune activation and loss of normal T-cell homeostasis seen in HIV. Finally, HIV-1 infection continues to be associated with stigma and social isolation, which adversely affects quality of life. Given these limitations of current ART, there is a concerted effort to find a cure for HIV-1.

While complete viral eradication, or a "sterilizing cure," is the ultimate goal, the concept of a "functional cure" or "HIV-1 remission" has been introduced, which includes strategies aimed at achieving host control of the virus without the need for ART. Several clinical observations within the past few years have fueled the belief that one or the other of these types of "cure" might be possible. Certainly, the most compelling example is that of the "Berlin patient." This man with HIV-1 and virologic suppression on ART received, as treatment for acute myelogenous leukemia, allogeneic hematopoietic stem cell transplants from a donor who carried a homozygous deletion in CCR5 (CCR5Δ32/Δ32), the coreceptor for HIV-1, thereby making his new CD4$^+$ T cells resistant to infection (Hutter et al., 2009). Following discontinuation of ART, no HIV-1 RNA has been detected in the Berlin patient's peripheral blood; moreover, multiple attempts to detect HIV-1 RNA or proviral DNA in cellular reservoirs and other tissue compartments have been negative (Yukl et al., 2013).

These findings were replicated in the "London patient" who underwent a similar allogeneic stem cell transplant with cells that did not express CCR5; following the transplant, no replication-competent virus in blood, cerebrospinal fluid, intestinal tissue, or lymphoid tissue was detected at 30 months following ART discontinuation (Gupta et al., 2020). Because of the risk of stem cell transplantation, however, this intensive approach is not appropriate in PWH who do not have a hematologic malignancy.

Another notable "proof of concept" came from studies of early initiation of ART during acute HIV-1 infection. The VISCONTI study identified 14 PWH whose viremia remained controlled for years after the interruption of ART that had been initiated during primary infection (Saez-Cirion et al., 2013). Furthermore, the CHAMP (Control of HIV After Antiretroviral Medication Pause) study, which combined more than 700 PWH who discontinued ART, reported posttreatment controller rates of up to 13% in early ART-treated individuals (Namazi et al., 2018); of note, less than 5% of posttreatment controllers were identified in those who initiated ART during chronic stages of infection.

Along these lines, the "Mississippi baby," a child born to a woman with HIV, was started on ART 30 hours after delivery and quickly achieved virologic suppression (Persaud et al., 2013). The child was lost to follow-up, however, and ART was discontinued by the caregiver. Despite stopping ART, the virus remained undetectable for 27 months, but the child ultimately suffered virologic rebound (Luzuriaga et al., 2015). These examples demonstrate that it is possible, under extraordinary circumstances, to eradicate HIV-1 (in the case of the Berlin and London patients) or control HIV-1 without ART (in the case of the VISCONTI and CHAMP cohorts and, temporarily, the Mississippi child). Now, the challenge is to extend the insights from these remarkable cases and cohorts to the development of practical interventions that will lead to ART-free remission in the large PWH population.

EARLY ESTABLISHMENT AND PERSISTENCE OF THE LATENT HIV-1 RESERVOIR

In 1995, Chun et al. identified integrated provirus as a persistent reservoir of infection in the resting CD4$^+$ T cells of PWH (Chun et al., 1995). While most activated memory CD4$^+$ T cells are destroyed during viral replication, a small fraction of infected cells survives to return to a resting and memory state. In the resting memory state, HIV-1 gene expression is shut down, resulting in latent infection of CD4$^+$ T cells (Nabel & Baltimore, 1987). As these cells do not express viral proteins, they remain hidden from the host immune response; moreover, without active replication, ARVs cannot act against the virus. While infected resting cells leave the quiescent memory pool at a steady rate, the pool of infected cells persists, perhaps in part because of homeostatic proliferation. It has also been suggested that specific CD4$^+$ T-cell memory subsets, including central memory, transitional memory, and memory stem cells, harbor the majority of integrated HIV-1 DNA and that eradication therapies may require targeting of specific CD4$^+$ T-cell populations (Buzon et al., 2014).

Reactivation of latently infected cells leads to viral gene expression and active viral replication. In patients on long-term ART, the percentage of latently infected cells is extremely low: less than 1 per million resting memory CD4$^+$ T cells harbor replication-competent HIV-1 (Finzi et al., 1997; Wong et al., 1997). Nevertheless, after a more rapid decline in the first year after infection, this latent pool decays very slowly: the mean half-life of this reservoir is approximately 44 months, and, as a result, suppressive ART would need to be maintained for more than 60 years to achieve viral eradication even if an infected person had only 100,000 latently infected cells (Besson et al., 2014; Finzi et al., 1999). In addition, it is conceivable that latent infection may persist in cells other than CD4$^+$ T cells; however, this has yet to be proven.

It was initially believed that early suppression of viral replication during primary infection might prevent reservoir formation. However, Chun et al. (1998) demonstrated that ART initiated within 10 days of primary infection did not prevent the generation of latently infected CD4$^+$ T cells, pointing toward an early seeding of the reservoir. Newer data from the rhesus macaque model demonstrate that the latent reservoir is established within days of virus exposure, even before virus can be detected in peripheral blood (Whitney et al., 2014); the implication of this finding is that it may be practically impossible to treat or even diagnose HIV-1 infection early enough to avoid reservoir seeding. Several studies, however, have demonstrated that initiating ART during the acute/early phase of the infection results in a smaller HIV-1 reservoir (Ananworanich et al., 2012; Hocqueloux et al., 2013; Saez-Cirion et al., 2013), suggesting that early treatment could be beneficial by reducing the barrier to cure (Henrich & Gandhi, 2013; Strain et al., 2005).

Persistence of the HIV-1 latent reservoir represents the biggest obstacle for cure approaches. For this reason, a deeper understanding of how latency is maintained and how this state can be reversed is critical to inform HIV-1 eradication strategies (Richman et al., 2009).

"KICK AND KILL" AND "BLOCK AND LOCK"

To achieve viral eradication, or at least a state of HIV-1 suppression without requiring continuous ART, different strategies have been proposed, including modification of the host immune response to achieve enhanced control of viral replication, interventions to prevent reactivation of virus latency (Mousseau et al., 2015), and gene therapy to increase the resistance of target cells to HIV-1 infection (Tebas et al., 2014). Currently, the strategy that is receiving the most attention is the "shock and kill" or "kick and kill" approach (Deeks, 2012). In this strategy, the first step is to flush out HIV-1 from the latent reservoir by activating proviral DNA expression in resting cells, leading to de novo viral protein production (the "shock" or "kick"). If this "kick" is successful, the next step is to enhance immune recognition and elimination of infected cells (the "kill"). This two-step approach, however, requires a latency-reversing strategy and an antiviral immune response in order to clear infected cells; both tasks are encumbered by substantial challenges.

A strategy that aims to achieve the opposite is named "block and lock." Here, HIV is locked into its latent form, eliminating or at least reducing the chance of viral reactivation and replication. This strategy does not require the help of the immune system as it does not seek viral eradication.

LATENCY-REVERSAL APPROACHES

Latently infected CD4$^+$ T cells evade immune surveillance as they do not express HIV-1 proteins (Hermankova et al., 2003). Reversal of HIV-1 latency and induction of virus expression may render infected cells susceptible to attack by cytolytic T lymphocytes or to destruction by viral cytopathic effects (Chun et al., 1997; Deeks, 2012). Several latency-reversing agents (LRAs) have been identified, perhaps the most promising being histone deacetylase inhibitors (HDACi) and Toll-like receptor (TLR) agonists (Kim et al., 2018). HDACi are currently approved as anti-cancer drugs, and several have been evaluated in ART-suppressed PWH for their latency-reversing potential (Archin et al., 2014; Elliott et al., 2014; Rasmussen et al., 2014). Vorinostat, the first HDACi to be studied in PWH on ART, was found to induce viral expression by an average of 4.8-fold in resting CD4$^+$ T cells after a single dose (Archin et al., 2014). Two other HDACi agents—panobinostat and romidepsin—have also been found to induce virus expression in PWH on suppressive ART (Rasmussen et al., 2014; Sogaard et al., 2015). Following administration of romidepsin, plasma HIV-1 RNA levels became detectable in some individuals, suggesting the LRA was inducing virus production (Sogaard et al., 2015). However, the size of the HIV-1 reservoir, based on measurements of HIV-1 DNA and virus outgrowth assay, remained unchanged following three weekly infusions of romidepsin.

In addition, in a recent trial, romidepsin alone failed to increase HIV-1 expression in persons on ART (McMahon et al., 2019), so clinical studies of romidepsin in combination with other agents or strategies are being explored (Mothe et al., 2020) and are discussed later in this chapter.

TLR agonists are another group of drugs being investigated. The TLR7 agonist vesatolimod was shown to induce transient increases in plasma viral load and decreases in cellular viral DNA levels in simian immunodeficiency virus (SIV)-infected rhesus macaques (Whitney et al., 2015). In a separate study in monkeys treated with ART during acute simian-human immunodeficiency virus (SHIV) infection, a combination of a TLR7 agonist with a broadly neutralizing antibody (PGT121) led to virologic control in 5 of 11 animals even after the interventions and ART were stopped (Borducchi et al., 2018). Trials using vesatolimod in ART-treated HIV-1–infected humans are being conducted (NCT02858401 and NCT03060447); one study in ART-suppressed PWH with low pre-ART viral loads demonstrated a modest increase in time to viral rebound after analytical treatment interruption (ATI) in the vesatolimod group (SenGupta et al., 2020). Furthermore, the TLR9 agonist lefitolimod increased HIV-1 transcription and enhanced cytotoxic natural killer (NK) cell activation in a small group of ART-suppressed individuals (Vibholm et al., 2017). Overall, it remains uncertain whether a single agent will be sufficient to effectively and completely purge the pool of replication-competent, integrated, latent HIV-1; rather, a combination of LRAs targeting distinct pathways, and potentially different cell types, might be required (Laird et al., 2015).

LATENCY SILENCING

In contrast to activating latency, it has been proposed that reinforcing a deep state of latency by permanently silencing HIV transcription could be an alternative approach for a functional cure (Mori & Valente, 2020). This concept, also known as the "block and lock" or "soothe and snooze" strategy, would apply latency-promoting agents (LPAs) to block the reactivation of latently infected HIV-1 proviruses. A potential agent that has been studied is the Tat inhibitor didehydro-cortistatin A, which, when added to ART, reduced viral mRNA in tissues of HIV-1–infected humanized mice and significantly delayed viral rebound following ART interruption (Kessing et al., 2017). More in vivo studies are needed to further determine the role of these interventions in HIV cure.

IMMUNE-ENHANCING AND/OR -MODULATING STRATEGIES

While latency reversal will be crucial for eradication strategies, inducing viral replication alone will most likely not be sufficient to eliminate HIV infection. Indeed, in an in vitro model, reversal of latency alone did not result in clearance of infected cells (Shan et al., 2012). For this reason, it is anticipated that, following reactivation, cells harboring the reservoir will need to be actively cleared, perhaps through a second line of attack by the host immune system. Strategies to enhance immune responses via active or passive immunization or via immunomodulation have been proposed. For example, it has been hypothesized that boosting T-cell responses will lead to enhanced viral control—similar to what is seen in so-called HIV-1 elite controllers, individuals who maintain undetectable viral loads in the absence of ART, where antiviral T cells have been associated with viral suppression (Deeks & Walker, 2007; McMichael et al., 2010). Vaccination strategies will be discussed later in this chapter; what follows next are other immunomodulatory approaches.

IMMUNE MODULATION: CHECKPOINT INHIBITORS

Given the challenge that the cellular dysfunction in PWH known as T-cell exhaustion poses for therapeutic vaccination strategies, novel immune-modulating concepts have been developed to reverse this state of exhaustion by inhibiting immune checkpoints. During progressive HIV-1 infection with persistent antigen exposure, increased expression of inhibitory receptors like PD-1 on HIV-1–specific T cells is associated with greater immune dysfunction (Day et al., 2006; Khaitan & Unutmaz, 2011), and it is thought that anti–PD-1 antibodies may be able to restore the function of exhausted $CD4^+$ and $CD8^+$ T cells by restoring host cell pathways needed for T-cell activation (Porichis & Kaufmann, 2012). Inhibiting the PD-1 pathway has shown efficacy in reversing T-cell exhaustion in the cancer field (Topalian et al., 2012), and recent data suggest that PD-1 blockade restores the ability of antiviral T cells to inhibit HIV-1 replication in animal models (Palmer et al., 2013; Velu et al., 2009). Moreover, PD-1 is believed to play an important role in the establishment and maintenance of latently infected cells (Evans et al., 2018), and PD-1 blockade might therefore lead to increased HIV transcription, a key step in latency reversal. A dose-escalation trial of an anti–PD-L1 antibody (BMS-936559) was shown in a trial of rhesus macaques to delay viral load rebound after ARV cessation and to significantly lower the viral load setpoint (Mason et al., 2014). In a phase 1 randomized clinical trial in eight HIV-1 patients on ART with $CD4^+$ T-cell counts of greater than 350 cells/mL and detectable viral load who received a single infusion of BMS-936559, two patients demonstrated an increase in HIV-specific T-cell responses. However, the trial was stopped prior to full enrollment as there was concern about antibody-associated retinal toxicity in animal studies (Gay et al., 2017). Another checkpoint inhibitor trial (ACTG 5370) was stopped early because of concern for two possible immune-related adverse event complications (Hardy, 2020). However, while these drugs are no longer in clinical development, these studies did demonstrate, as a proof of concept, the potential utility of immune checkpoint inhibitors in targeting the HIV reservoir. Intriguingly, repeated doses of the anti–PD-1 antibody pembrolizumab in a single HIV-positive individual with lung cancer were associated with an increase in functional HIV-specific $CD8^+$ T cells and a decline in cell-associated HIV DNA (Guihot et al., 2018).

Other immune checkpoint inhibitors have been approved as cancer therapies, including nivolumab, an anti–PD-1 antibody, which, as described in a case report, appeared to decrease the HIV reservoir (as suggested by a decrease in cell-associated HIV-DNA, increase in HIV-RT and Nef-specific CD8 cells, and increase in T-cell activation) in a 51-year-old man with non–small cell carcinoma and well-controlled HIV infection (Guihot et al., 2018). Data from several studies evaluating PD-1 blockade in HIV-infected participants on suppressive ART regimens and their effect on the virus reservoir in PWH on ART with concomitant malignant diseases are in progress (ClinicalTrials.gov identifiers: NCT02408861, NCT02595866, NCT03354936, NCT03367754, NCT04223804).

T-CELL TRAFFICKING

Early HIV infection of lymphocytes within gut-associated lymphoid tissue (GALT) and subsequent depletion of gut $CD4^+$ T cells appears to significantly contribute to the immune dysfunction observed in chronic HIV infection. Durable suppression of HIV replication with ART does not significantly reverse the damage caused to GALT during early infection. Accordingly, therapies aimed at attenuating HIV-mediated destruction of GALT may serve as an effective strategy to treat and/or prevent HIV-related immune dysfunction and have been suggested as a potential cure strategy. One such approach involves disruption of the interaction between $\alpha_4\beta_7$ gut homing receptors on $CD4^+$ T cells and the gut endothelial cell adhesion molecules to which these receptors bind via interaction with mucosal addressing cell adhesion molecules (MAdCAM). HIV interacts with $\alpha_4\beta_7$ via the V2 domain of the gp120 subunit, and $CD4^+$ T cells with high expression of $\alpha_4\beta_7$ appear to be preferentially infected during acute HIV or SIV infection. Treatment of SIV-infected ART-suppressed macaques with an anti-$\alpha_4\beta_7$ integrin monoclonal antibody resulted in persistent viral control following ART cessation (Byrareddy et al., 2016). However, other studies in macaques were unable to show this effect (Abbink et al., 2019; Iwamoto et al., 2019).

A commercially available humanized anti-$\alpha_4\beta_7$ mAb, vedolizumab (Act-1), is currently approved by the US Food and Drug Administration (FDA) for use in inflammatory bowel disease. This antibody blocks binding to MAdCAM at the b7 chain of $\alpha_4\beta_7$, thereby inhibiting the migration of lymphocytes into the gastrointestinal tract and reducing local inflammatory responses. Blocking of $CD4^+$ $\alpha_4\beta_7$ by this antibody may attenuate HIV-mediated damage to GALT by reducing the number of target cells in GALT that can be infected by HIV. Studies in nonhuman primates also suggested that vedolizumab may have a role in SIV prevention. Although in a phase 1 study evaluating vedolizumab in 20 participants with HIV infection undergoing analytical treatment interruption, the median duration of plasma viremia of less than 400 copies/mL was only 5.4 weeks, failing to show sustained viral suppression (Sneller et al., 2019), other studies are ongoing (ClinicalTrials.gov identifier: NCT03147859).

In contrast to preventing trafficking of HIV target cells into anatomic sites of high viral replication, an alternative approach is promoting cytotoxic CD8$^+$ T-cell migration into lymph node follicles to clear infected cells. In the non-human primate model, administration of an interleukin-15 super-agonist resulted in an increase of CXCR5 expression on CD8$^+$ T cells and increased frequency of such cells in the lymphoid tissues (Webb et al., 2018). This concept is now being examined in humans (ClinicalTrials.gov identifier: NCT02191098).

CYTOKINES

Interleukin (IL)-2, an autocrine T-cell growth factor, is produced by CD4$^+$ T cells and is therefore deficient and dysfunctional in PWH. Based on promising phase 2 trials showing increased CD4$^+$ T-cell counts in patients receiving recombinant IL-2 (rIL-2) (Pett et al., 2010), two phase 3 trials were performed. In the ESPRIT study, 4,111 PWH with CD4$^+$ T-cell counts of 300 cells/mL or more were randomized to receive SQ IL-2 (three 5-day cycles 8 weeks apart) with ART or ART alone (Abrams et al., 2009). Although the rIL-2 group had significantly higher CD4$^+$ T-cell counts, this difference declined with time, and clinical outcomes, including opportunistic infection/death and all-cause mortality, did not significantly differ between the two groups. In addition, there were more grade 4 adverse events in the group receiving IL-2, most notably deep venous thrombosis. Subsequent analysis also raised concern for an increased incidence of pneumonia in patients receiving rIL-2 less than 180 days previously (Pett et al., 2011). The second IL-2 phase 3 trial, SILCAAT, randomized 1,695 patients with CD4$^+$ T-cell counts of 50 to 299 cells/mm^3 to similar treatment arms, except the IL-2 group received six cycles at a lower dose (Abrams et al., 2009). CD4$^+$ T-cell counts were again higher in the IL-2 group, but statistically significant differences in opportunistic infection/death, all-cause mortality, and grade 4 clinical events were not seen.

IL-2 has also been studied as a means to eradicate HIV from latently infected CD4$^+$ T cells and reduce the viral reservoir. One randomized trial did not show an impact of rIL-2 with ART on proviral DNA in blood, lymph nodes, and cerebrospinal fluid compared to ART alone (Stellbrink et al., 2002), but the ongoing STARR study (ClinicalTrials.gov identifier: NCT03308786) will evaluate the effect of rIL-2 on levels of replication-competent CD4$^+$ T cells and on the size of the latent reservoir. Other potential uses of rIL-2, such as a means to delay ART initiation or facilitate ART treatment interruption or as a vaccine adjunct, have also been studied. However, in the STALWART study, a phase 2 trial in patients not on ART with CD4$^+$ T-cell counts greater than 300 cells/mL, rIL-2 use was associated with more opportunistic disease and death and a statistically significant increase in grade 3 or grade 4 events (Tavel et al., 2010). In summary, IL-2 does not appear to confer clinical benefit to patients with HIV infection, regardless of whether they are on ART, although this continues to be an area of investigation.

Other cytokines currently being studied for use in HIV include IL-7, IL-15, and IL-21. IL-7 plays a key role in T-cell homeostasis, leading to expansion and survival of naive and memory T cells and preventing apoptosis of CD4$^+$ and CD8$^+$ T cells in PWH in vitro. In early clinical trials, human recombinant IL-7 therapy was well tolerated and induced a significant and dose-dependent increase in functional naive and memory CD4$^+$ and CD8$^+$ T cells in lymphopenic PWH on ART (Levy et al., 2009; Sereti et al., 2009). In a randomized, placebo-controlled trial of recombinant IL-7 in ARV-treated PWH, there were brisk T-cell increases of naive and central memory T cells (averaging 323 cells/mL at 12 weeks) with a durable response seen up to 1 year (Levy et al., 2012). IL-7, however, appears to have a minimal impact on the HIV latent reservoir. A follow-up study of peripheral blood monocytes collected from 10 participants who participated in an IL-7 treatment trial failed to demonstrate activation of latently infected resting memory CD4$^+$ T cells (Vandergeeten et al., 2013).

In macaque models, IL-21 has demonstrated beneficial immune responses, such as improved NK and T-cell cytotoxicity and reduced levels of intestinal T-cell proliferation and microbial translocation. With this novel mechanism of action, it may become a useful treatment for augmenting immune response while ameliorating intestinal immune activation (Pallikkuth et al., 2011, 2013). To that end, preliminary work in SIV-uninfected rhesus macaques demonstrated that a combination of IL-21 and monoclonal $\alpha_4\beta_7$ was well tolerated and reduced intestinal immune activation (Pino et al., 2020).

IL-15, like IL-2, has lymphocyte stimulatory activity and is significantly increased in PWH with a virologic and immunologic response to ART compared to ARV-naive patients (Forcina et al., 2004), which has prompted interest in its role in immune therapy. Phase 1 studies are under way in PWH on ART evaluating N-803, a long-acting IL-15 super-agonist, in combination with broadly neutralizing antibodies.

CHIMERIC ANTIGEN RECEPTOR T CELLS

An alternative approach, which circumvents the problem of eliciting immune responses in PWH who have immune dysregulation, is the adoptive transfer of T cells with molecularly cloned high-affinity T-cell receptors (TCRs) and superior antiviral activity, targeting conserved and vulnerable regions of the virus (Varela-Rohena et al., 2008). The results of a phase 1 study testing the in vivo efficacy of these high-affinity gag-specific T cells in ART-treated patients are pending (ClinicalTrials.gov identifier: NCT00991224). Furthermore, chimeric antigen receptor (CAR) transduced T cells, which combine the specificity of an antibody with the signaling of a TCR, have shown promise in the cancer field (Hombach et al., 2013) and are now being studied in HIV (Lam & Bollard, 2013; Leibman et al., 2017). Specifically, two clinical trials are testing CAR T-cell therapy in ART-suppressed individuals including a broadly neutralizing anti–HIV-1 antibody, or bNAb (VRC01)-based CAR (ClinicalTrials.gov identifier: NCT03240328) and a CD4-CAR T cell modified by zinc-finger nuclease CCR5 disruption to induce HIV resistance (ClinicalTrials.gov identifier: NCT03617198).

MONOCLONAL ANTIBODY THERAPY

During the past decade, multiple monoclonal antibodies (mAbs) have been developed against various viral targets, including viral membrane targets (e.g., gp120 and gp41), the $CD4^+$ receptor, and the CCR5 coreceptor (Chen & Dmitrov, 2012). Very few of these mAbs showed clinical benefit despite efficacy in nonhuman primate models, largely due to the virus's ability to rapidly develop resistant variants. Nonetheless, several promising compounds and treatment approaches have evolved recently and are discussed here.

Leronlimab (PRO 140), a humanized CCR5 mAb, had potent activity in early clinical trials. Currently in a phase 2 study, participants who are suppressed on a stable ART regimen are switched to weekly subcutaneous injections of leronlimab as a single-agent maintenance therapy in patients with exclusively CCR5-tropic HIV-1. Preliminary results showed a failure rate of 65% in the 350-mg dose arm (Dhody et al., 2018; Dhody & Kazempour, 2019). However, in phase 2b/3, PRO 140 subcutaneous injections were added to a failing ART regimen. Of 52 participants, 64% versus 23% ($p = 0.0032$) had at least 0.5 log viral load drop after 1 week (Mascolini, 2018), with no treatment-related resistance.

UB-421 is a humanized IgG1 mAb that inhibits attachment of HIV-1 virus and entry into the cells by competitively binding to the $CD4^+$ receptor. In a phase 2 nonrandomized trial, 29 participants who had undetectable viral loads were enrolled and received either 10 mg/kg every week or 25 mg/kg biweekly after stopping their ART for 8 weeks, with 94% of the patients maintaining virologic suppression (Wang et al., 2019).

BROADLY NEUTRALIZING ANTIBODIES

HIV-1 immunotherapy with first-generation mAbs in the preclinical and clinical settings was largely ineffective. However, the recent identification of novel broadly neutralizing anti–HIV-1 antibodies (bNAbs), which are able to neutralize the majority of viral strains at very low concentrations, may provide another approach to target the HIV-1 reservoir. In preclinical studies, administration of bNAbs was shown to reduce plasma viremia in chimeric SHIV-infected macaques (Barouch et al., 2013b; Julg et al., 2017; Shingai et al., 2013); in fact, one particular bNAb, PGT121, also resulted in substantial reductions of proviral DNA in peripheral blood, lymph nodes, and gastrointestinal mucosa (Barouch et al., 2013b). Multiple different bNAbs have been tested in PWH and have shown promising reductions in plasma viremia (Caskey et al., 2015, 2017; Lynch et al., 2015). As a potential mechanism, it has been suggested that clearance of infected cells expressing viral antigen on their surfaces (Lu et al., 2016) is mediated through interactions between the Fc component of the antibody and its receptor on innate immune effectors cells like NK cells and macrophages (Bruel et al., 2016).

VRC01 is a bNAb that targets the CD4-binding site of the HIV envelope glycoprotein. In a phase 1 randomized placebo-controlled trial, VRC01 was safe and well tolerated but did not have any significant effects on plasma or cellular HIV-1 viremia (Riddler et al., 2018); nevertheless, VCR01 is undergoing phase 2b studies. A phase 1 study evaluating a long-acting form of VRC01 (VRC01LS) demonstrated that VRC01LS was safe and well tolerated, had a fourfold greater half-life, and elicited HIV-1 neutralizing activity (Gaudinski et al., 2018).

Administration of the antibodies 3BNC117 and VRC01 resulted in delayed viral rebound after ART cessation compared with historical controls, but the effects were modest and generally transient (Bar et al., 2016; Scheid et al., 2016). Not surprisingly, rapid selection of archived resistant viral strains reduced the therapeutic efficacy of single bNAbs; for this reason, bNAb combinations were proposed and a phase 1 clinical trial that combined the bNAbs 3BNC117 and 10-1074 demonstrated effective suppression of viral rebound for a median of 21 weeks (Mendoza et al., 2018). In addition, next-generation antibodies that incorporate the antigen specificity of different bNAbs by binding to multiple non-overlapping sites on the virus or attaching to both virus and $CD4^+$ receptors have been engineered (Huang et al., 2016; Xu et al., 2017). Triple combinations of bNAbs or a trispecific antibody (Xu et al., 2017) are currently being evaluated in early phase clinical trials (ClinicalTrials.gov identifiers: NCT03721510, NCT03705169).

These results will need to be studied further, especially with regard to impact on the latent reservoir and immune dysregulation, as chronic antigen stimulation should be reduced by these antibodies. Furthermore, the lack of accessibility of antibodies to certain anatomic reservoir sites, such as the central nervous system, will need to be overcome.

DUAL-AFFINITY RETARGETING

A novel method to combine antibody and T-cell activity against HIV-1–infected cells is through bispecific protein constructs (dual-affinity retargeting [DARTs]), which are designed to latch onto HIV-1 envelope proteins on the surface of infected cells while also binding to CD3 on T cells. This approach directs cytotoxic T cells to eliminate infected cells while obviating the need for the T cells to specifically bind to HIV-1 surface antigens (Pegu et al., 2015; Sung et al., 2015). Early in vitro studies of this approach are promising, and this concept is now being explored in a phase 1 study (ClinicalTrials.gov identifier: NCT03570918).

COMBINATION STRATEGIES

The first randomized human trial using the "shock and kill" cure strategy was the RIVER study that combined a therapeutic vaccine, ChAdV63.HIVconsv prime, with MVA. HIVconsv boost followed by administration of the LRA vorinostat. Disappointingly, no significant change in the viral reservoir was observed (Fidler et al., 2020). Another trial tested the combination of the HDACi romidepsin and the MVA. HIVconsv vaccine in early treated PWH, and a sustained suppression of viremia up to 32 weeks was reported (Mothe et al., 2020). In a randomized phase 1b/2a trial, the impact of latency reservoir romidepsin followed by 3BNC117 on reservoir size and time to viral rebound was compared to romidepsin alone. Twenty patients were enrolled; the combination did not reduce the reservoir size or delay viral rebound (Gruell et al., 2020). Another phase 2a trial is evaluating the efficacy of the TLR9 agonist lefitolimid with the bNAbs 3BNC117 and 10-1074 (ClinicalTrials.gov identifier: NCT03837756). There are also exciting results from a study combining a TLR-7 agonist with the broadly neutralizing antibody PGT121 in a nonhuman primate study, resulting in a subset of animals that did not have viral rebound upon ART interruption (Borducchi et al., 2018).

OTHER IMMUNOMODULATORY TREATMENTS

Because T-cell activation is controlled by several signaling pathways, inhibitors of these pathways may also play a role in reducing the size of the latent viral reservoir. Early preclinical research has shown that mTOR inhibitors (e.g., sirolimus, temsirolimus, and everolimus) may play a role in reducing T-cell activation and inflammation (Heredia et al., 2015; Martin & Siliciano, 2015; Palmer et al., 2015), although clinical trial data are lacking. A phase 4 study evaluated the impact of everolimus on HIV persistence after kidney or liver transplantation in patients who are stable on ART. The study failed to demonstrate significant change in low-level viremia or CD4+ T-cell associated HIV-DNA or RNA at 6 months after initiation of everolimus. However, the authors noted that participants who achieved a higher everolimus trough level of 5 during the first 2 months had significant sustained reduction in cellular RNA levels at 12 months. The study supported the hypothesis that there is a mechanistic interaction between mTOR inhibitor use and HIV persistence (Henrich et al., 2020).

GENE MODIFICATION

Gene therapy, also referred to as "intracellular immunization," involves the insertion of protective genes either mechanically or by viral vectors. Gene therapy research has focused on two areas: the disruption of cellular genes involved in HIV entry, such as the CCR5 coreceptor, and the introduction of genes to disrupt HIV replication. The goal of gene therapy in HIV is to have the target cells produce gene products that protect them and their progeny from HIV infection. The use of various technologies, including ribozymes, aptamers, RNA-based interference strategies, and zinc finger nucleases (ZFNs), is currently being investigated.

RENDERING THE HOST'S CD4+ T CELLS RESISTANT TO INFECTION

The Berlin patient and the London patient appear to be cured from HIV-1 after receiving stem cell transplants from CCR5Δ32 homozygous donors, which inspired attempts to generate HIV-1–resistant cells through gene therapy. ZFNs are bioengineered restriction enzymes with two functional domains—one that recognizes DNA and another that cleaves it. ZFNs can bind specific DNA sequences, produce a double-stranded break, and then lead to permanent gene disruption when cellular repair pathways lead to the addition or deletion of nucleotides at the break site. ZFNs have been shown to disrupt CCR5 expression in human stem cells administered in a mouse model of HIV and to be associated with lower HIV viral loads after HIV challenge (Holt et al., 2010; Perez et al., 2008).

SB-728T, an infusion of ZFN-modified autologous CD4+ T cells with the ability to knock out CCR5 expression, increased CD4+ T-cell counts, decreased proviral DNA, and restored the CD4+-depleted population of the gut mucosa in chronically infected patients with CD4+ T-cell counts of more than 200 cells/mL (June et al., 2012; Lalezari et al., 2012). One subject with the highest level of CCR5 modification had an undetectable viral load when ART treatment interruption occurred. Using the ZFN strategy, Tebas et al. (2014) modified the CCR5 gene ex vivo in autologous CD4+ T cells in 12 PWH and infused the cells back into the autologous donors. The study found that genetically modified CD4+ T cells were significantly increased and persisted in vivo with a half-life of nearly a year. While no dramatic difference was seen in viral load set points following interruption of ART in six study participants, the modified cells appeared to be protected from HIV-1 infection as unmodified cells showed a faster depletion. Six of these patients underwent 12-week ART interruption, but in only 1 patient (heterozygous for the CCR5Δ32 mutation) did the viral load decline to an undetectable level prior to ART reinitiation.

Additional studies of SB-728T are under way, with one examining CCR5Δ32 heterozygotes and another examining the use of cyclophosphamide prior to CD4+ T-cell infusion to decrease the number of existing CD4+ T cells. Early data from the latter trial have demonstrated that Cytoxan treatment is well tolerated with a dose-related increase in total CD4+ T-cell count and engraftment of CCR5-modified cells (Blick et al., 2014). While this approach did not lead to durable suppression of HIV after cessation of ART, it did appear to delay viral load rebound in study participants (Tebas et al., 2019). Additional research investigating HIV-1 coreceptor modulation is ongoing.

Recent data in SHIV-infected and ART-suppressed pigtail macaques demonstrated that CCR5 gene-edited hematopoietic stem/progenitor cells (HSPCs) persisted following transplantation and expansion through virus-dependent positive selection, resulting in a significant reduction of tissue-associated SHIV DNA and RNA levels in the transplanted animals compared to controls (Peterson et al., 2018). Gene-editing techniques carry a risk for off-target effects causing mutations at unintended sites in the genome, a currently relevant hurdle to their use in clinical trials (Cradick et al., 2013). The safety and feasibility of administration of clustered regularly interspaced short palindromic repeat (CRISPR)/Cas9 CCR5 gene-modified CD34+ HSPC and ZFN CCR5 modified autologous CD4+ T cells in ART-suppressed PWH is currently being evaluated (ClinicalTrials.gov identifiers: NCT02500849, NCT03164135, respectively). Of note, a 2019 report describes the case of an individual with HIV and acute lymphoblastic leukemia who was treated with an allogeneic bone marrow transplant in which the CCR5Δ32 mutation was introduced using CRISPR/Cas9. Cells with the deletion were found in only a small percentage of bone marrow engrafted cells. While the leukemia was subsequently in remission, the patient experienced viral rebound shortly after interrupting ART (Xu et al., 2019), perhaps because too few cells carried the protective mutation.

EXCISING THE HIV-1 PROVIRUS FROM THE HOST CELL GENOME

The CRISPR/Cas9 system permits targeted and precise genome editing in diverse cell types and organisms, including human cells (Cong et al., 2013). Recently, several research groups have successfully applied gene-editing technology to excise HIV-1 provirus from the host cell genome in vitro (Ebina et al., 2013; Hu et al., 2014; Liao et al., 2015). Importantly, the disruption of provirus expression not only restricted transcriptionally active provirus but also blocked the expression of latently integrated provirus (Ebina et al., 2013). Moreover, inserting the stably expressed CRISPR/Cas9 system into a T-cell line conferred long-term protection against HIV-1 infection (Liao et al., 2015). These results from in vitro cell culture models are promising, and this technology may open new avenues to developing antiviral therapies in the future.

RIBOZYMES, RNA-BASED INTERFERENCE, AND APTAMERS

Ribozymes are small, catalytically active RNA molecules that can be engineered to target specific RNA sequences. In HIV, they can target viral RNA during uncoating and after transcription, leading to RNA degradation. Although in vitro studies of ribozyme gene therapy have been promising, retroviral vectors delivering ribozymes targeting viral targets (e.g., tat and rev) have been plagued by problems with low transduction efficiency.

The first phase 2 randomized controlled trial of an anti-HIV ribozyme was conducted in 74 PWH on HAART receiving either autologous stem cells transduced with a ribozyme targeting the overlapping tat and vpr reading frames of HIV-1 (OZ1) or placebo (Mitsuyasu et al., 2009). No significant adverse events were reported with the infusion, but the subjects also had low engraftment levels and short persistence of the ribozyme. There was a trend, but no statistically significant difference, in HIV-1 viral load at the primary endpoint; however, after treatment interruption at 40 weeks, patients continuing to express OZ1 RNA had a statistically significant decrease in HIV-1 viral load.

RNA interference utilizes short RNAs that mediate the degradation of mRNAs in a sequence-specific manner. Theoretically, multiple short hairpin RNAs (shRNA) in a single vector are thought to prevent HIV-1 escape. With this strategy, antisense oligonucleotides bind mRNA and trigger degradation through an RNase H-dependent pathway or block ribosome binding, thus preventing gene expression. Clinical research in this field is evolving, but it has been limited by difficulty delivering the RNAs to the correct target cells, poor cellular uptake and stability, and viral escape (Zhou & Rossi, 2011). VRX496 (Lexgenleucel-T), antisense env in a lentiviral vector, has progressed to phase 2 trials, in which it has been delivered via autologous CD4+ T-cell infusion to both patients on failing regimens and patients on a fully suppressive ART regimen. In one trial, 17 patients received Lexgenleucel-T over 16 weeks, with ART interruption 1 month later in 13 of these patients (Tebas et al., 2013). Six of eight patients analyzed were noted to have a decrease in viral load set point. The use of a short-interfering RNA targeting a unique triple repeat of NF-κB was also shown to achieve long-term suppression of HIV-1 subtype C (Singh et al., 2014).

Aptamers are single-stranded RNA or DNA molecules that bind viral proteins, preventing them from carrying out their function in the viral life cycle (Figure 19.1). In clinical trials, when used alone, they have not been shown to be effective. However, strategies combining aptamers, ribozymes, and RNA interference, based on in vitro efficacy, require further investigation because they have been shown to exhibit potent inhibition of HIV-1 in vitro (Brake et al., 2008; Centlivre et al., 2013).

OTHER GENE STRATEGIES

One novel gene therapy approach currently in phase 1 trials is the use of MazF-T, autologous CD4+ T cells modified with the MAZF endoribonuclease gene, which can render T cells resistant to HIV replication (Saito et al., 2014). Additional trials using modified stem cells are also in early clinical stages for PWH with hematologic malignancies. Although promising, it will be difficult to develop these and other gene strategies for widespread use. Cost of the agents and technology, the development of an infrastructure for delivery, lack of availability of this technology in areas most affected by HIV-1, and patient insurance limitations all pose significant barriers to implementation.

Theoretically, gene therapy can also be used to inhibit viral fusion. C46, a structurally similar peptide to enfuvirtide, has been engineered to be expressed on autologous T cells and seems to be well tolerated in clinical trials, although clinical efficacy has not yet been demonstrated (van Lundzen et al., 2007). A dual-cassette, lentiviral vector expressing CCR5 shRNA (knockdown) and C46 (CAL-1) has been shown in preclinical studies to be nontoxic and to protect gene-modified cells from both CXCR4- and CCR5-tropic HIV-1 strains (Wolstein et al., 2014). The results of a phase 1/2a clinical trial using autologous, CAL-1–modified CD4+ T cells and hematopoietic progenitor/stem cells with and without bone marrow precondition (busulfan) in PWH demonstrated

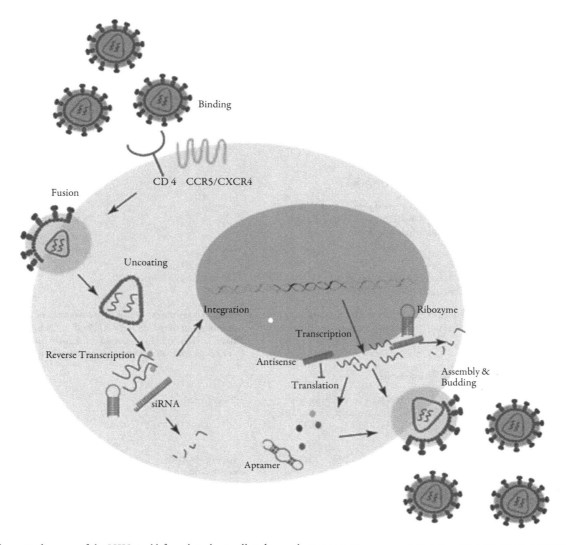

Figure 19.1 Schematic diagram of the HIV viral life cycle in host cell and gene therapy targets.   SOURCE: Zeller S, Kumar P. *Yale J Biol Med*. 2011;84(3):301–309.

safety but only transient evidence of bone marrow engraftment (Mitsuyasu et al., 2020).

NOVEL NONCURATIVE ARVS

ART remains the mainstay of treatment for patients chronically infected with HIV. Novel drugs, within both existing and new classes, are in various stages of development and testing (Table 19.1). Fostemsavir, an oral attachment inhibitor that was approved by the FDA in July 2020, binds to HIV-1 gp120, blocking viral attachment to host CD4⁺ T cells. The phase 3 BRIGHTE study evaluated fostemsavir in two cohorts of heavily treatment-experienced participants. In the randomized cohort, 272 participants were randomized 3:1 to receive 7 days of blinded therapy with either fostemsavir or placebo in addition to their failing background regimen. All participants then went on to receive open-label fostemsavir and an optimized background regimen for 96 weeks. A second nonrandomized cohort in this study evaluated open-label fostemsavir and optimized background therapy in 99 participants with limited treatment options (i.e., no fully

active approved agents) for 96 weeks. At 48 weeks, 54% and 38% patients in the randomized and nonrandomized cohorts, respectively, had virologic response with viral loads less than 400 copies/mL (Kozal et al., 2020).

Islatravir is a nucleoside reverse transcriptase translocation inhibitor in clinical development. MK-8591 triphosphate (MK-8591 TP) is the active phosphorylated form, which has a half-life of 78 to 128 hours in human peripheral blood mononuclear cells. In an open-label study, a single dose of MK-8591 in HIV-1 treatment-naive subjects showed a greater than 1 $\log_{10}$ viral load decline after 7 to10 days (Schürmann et al., 2020). A phase 2 randomized trial to evaluate the safety, tolerability, and ARV activity of MK-8591 in combination with doravirine and lamivudine is ongoing. Primate studies have demonstrated clinically relevant drug exposures for more than 6 months after a single dose of parenterally administered MK-8591, supporting evaluation of extended dosing formulations that may have utility as preexposure prophylaxis (PrEP) or maintenance treatment (Barrett et al., 2018).

Cenicriviroc is a novel oral CCR5 and CCR2 antagonist that showed potent antiviral activity in treatment-experienced

Table 19.1 ARVS IN CLINICAL TRIALS

AGENT	DESCRIPTION	STAGE OF DEVELOPMENT
Nucleoside Reverse Transcriptase Inhibitors (NRTIs)		
Elvucitabine	Cytosine nucleoside analog that can be used in case of resistance to emtricitabine (FTC) or lamivudine (3TC)	Phase 2 trials completed. Drug out-licensed for further development in China, Taiwan, and Hong Kong.
Islatravir (MK 8591)	Nucleoside reverse transcriptase translocation inhibitor	Phase 2
Nonnucleoside Reverse Transcriptase Inhibitors (NNRTIs)		
Elsulfavirine (VM 1500)	Elsulfavirine is the oral prodrug of VM 1500, which is available in a long-acting intramuscular formulation.	Phase 1
Entry and Fusion Inhibitors		
Fostemsavir	Attaches to HIV gp120 to prevent HIV attachment to the host CD4$^+$ T cell	FDA approved in July 2020
Cenicriviroc	Once-daily CCR5 antagonist that also has CCR2 activity (anti-inflammatory effect)	Phase 2 trial demonstrated improvement in neurocognition among participants with AIDS dementia complex. Phase 3 trials in HIV planned, currently undergoing phase 3 clinical trials in non-alcoholic steatohepatitis (NASH).
Inhibitors of Rev-Mediated Viral RNA Biogenesis		
ABX464	Enhances viral mRNA by interfering with these Rev-mediated functions (Campo, 2015)	Phase 2 trials
Capsid Inhibitors		
GS6207	Long-acting agent administered subcutaneously	Moving into phase 2 studies after phase 1 study demonstrated significant reduction in HIV-1 RNA

HIV-1 patients. In a phase 2 randomized controlled trial, 143 treatment-naive patients were randomized to receive cenicriviroc 100 mg or 200 mg or efavirenz. At 24 weeks, virologic suppression was achieved in 76%, 73%, and 71% of patients; these numbers declined to 68%, 64%, and 50% at 48 weeks (Thompson et al., 2016).

VM1500A (elsulfavirine) is a new oral prodrug nonnucleoside reverse transcriptase inhibitor (NNRTI) approved in Russia in 2017 for treatment of HIV-1 in combination with standard ART. A phase 1 study to assess the safety of a long-acting intramuscular formulation of VM1500A was recently presented at the Conference on Retroviruses and Opportunistic Infections (Yakubova et al., 2020).

Other interesting ARV agents in early stage development include a Rev inhibitor (ABX 464; Moron-Lopez et al., 2020); capsid inhibitor (GS-6207; Zheng et al., 2018); maturation inhibitor (GSK3640254; Krystal et al., 2016); entry inhibitor (combinectin-GSK3732394); and a new nucleoside reverse transcriptase inhibitor (NRTI) active against resistant virus (GS-9131; White et al., 2017). Phase 1 data of the capsid inhibitor GS-6207 demonstrated a significant reduction of 1.4 to 2.3 log viral load at day 10 after a single subcutaneous injection in patients who were experienced off ARV for 12 months. The most common side effect reported was a moderate reaction at the injection site. GS-6207 is now being investigated at a 6-month dosing interval in patients who are treatment naive and in those who are treatment experienced (Daar et al., 2020).

CONCLUSION

Although ARVs effectively treat HIV-1 infection, there are many compelling reasons to attempt to cure HIV-1, not the least of which is the stigma and isolation experienced by many PWH. The major barrier to HIV-1 cure is the persistence of a long-lived population of latently infected cells in people on suppressive treatment; because the latent reservoir is established soon after HIV-1 acquisition, even early initiation of ART cannot cure the infection. Current efforts to cure HIV-1 infection are centered on flushing HIV-1 out of the latent reservoir along with enhancing immune mechanisms to clear infected cells. We are still in the early days of this massively difficult undertaking, and it is too soon to tell whether the approaches being pursued will be effective. That being said, just as the development of combination ART was based on a series of advances that culminated in our ability to successfully treat HIV-1, the stepwise progress being made today will hopefully lead us to an even greater breakthrough: the capability to eradicate or control HIV-1 without the need for lifelong therapy.

RECOMMENDED READING

Ahlensteil CL, Suzuki K, Marks K, et al. Controlling HIV-1: non-coding RNA gene therapy approaches a functional cure. *Front Immunol.* 2015;6:474.

Arthos JA, Cicala C, Nawaz F, et al. The role of integrin $\alpha_4\beta_7$ in HIV pathogenesis and treatment. *Curr Opin HIV AIDS.* 2018;15:127–135.

Barouch DH, Deeks SG. Immunologic strategies for HIV-1 remission and eradication. *Science.* 2014;45(6193):169–174.

Chomont N, El-Far M, Ancuta P, et al. HIV reservoir size and persistence are driven by T cell survival and homeostatic proliferation. *Nat Med.* 2009;15(8):893–900.

Frater J. New approaches in HIV eradication research. *Curr Opin Infect Dis.* 2011;24(6):593–598.

Kitchen SG, Shimizu S, An DS. Stem cell-based anti-HIV gene therapy. *Virology.* 2011;411:260–272.

Levy J. Not an HIV cure but encouraging new directions. *N Engl J Med.* 2009;360:724–725.

Lewin S, Rouzioux C. HIV cure and eradication: how will we get from the laboratory to effective clinical trials? *AIDS.* 2011;25:885–897.

Olender SA, Taylor BS, Wong M, et al. CROI 2015: advances in antiretroviral therapy. *Top Antivir Med.* 2015;23(1):28–45.

Pace P, Markowitz M. Monoclonal antibodies to host cellular receptors for the treatment and prevention of HIV-1 infection. *Curr Opin HIV AIDS.* 2015;10(3):144–150.

Richman DD, Margolis DM, Delaney M., et al. The challenge of finding a cure for HIV infection. *Science.* 2009;323(5919):1304–1307.

THERAPEUTIC AND PREVENTIVE VACCINES

LEARNING OBJECTIVE

- Discuss the progression and status of research in HIV vaccines

WHAT'S NEW?

HIV vaccine research has seen a resurgence in recent years with different classes of vaccines showing promise in clinical trials.

KEY POINTS

- Therapeutic immunization is a strategy for boosting anti–HIV-1 immunity in chronically infected PWH.

- Recent therapeutic vaccines under study have provided more durable and diverse immune responses and lowering of viral load set points.

- Many different types of vaccines have progressed to phase 2 trials, including DNA, subunit, and dendritic cell vaccines.

OVERVIEW OF VACCINE TRIALS 1990–2015

Therapeutic immunization aims to induce a cellular immune response through vaccination with components of HIV-1 that will help contain viral replication through reconstitution of anti–HIV-1 immune responses. Data support the observation that the cellular immune response is critical in controlling HIV-1 replication, as reported in persons with primary HIV-1 infection and in HIV long-term nonprogressors (Borrow et al., 1994; Cao et al., 1995; Kroup et al., 1994; Rosenberg et al., 1997). Therapeutic vaccines can potentially be of benefit to ART-naive PWH by delaying progression to AIDS and time to initiation of ART. Among PWH on ART, development of a durable vaccine may intensify the effects of ART (accelerate response time to therapy, decrease risk of transmission, potentiate the immune effects of ART, reduce proviral DNA), simplify ART regimens, and support regimens with treatment interruption (Ensoli et al., 2014).

Clinical therapeutic vaccine research for HIV started prior to the introduction of ART, first with a gp120-depleted inactivated HIV-1 preparation and then with vectors expressing viral proteins (e.g., gag p17 and p24). Clinical trials of these agents largely failed to show efficacy and a sustained HIV-1–specific response (Hardy et al., 2007). Subsequent vaccines with recombinant HIV-1 glycoproteins (e.g., gp120 and gp160) also fared poorly, not altering the decline in CD4$^+$ T-cell count or halting disease progression in PWH in phase 2 trials (Eron et al., 1996; Pontesilli et al., 1998; Sandstrom et al., 1999; Tsoukas et al., 1998). In one of the largest of these trials, 608 PWH with CD4$^+$ T-cell counts of greater than 400 cells/mL were repeatedly immunized with a recombinant gp160 vaccine (VaxSyn HIV-1) or placebo and followed for 3 to 5 years. Although the vaccine had excellent immunogenicity (~70%), it failed to show a difference in reaching the primary clinical endpoints: a 50% decline in CD4$^+$ T-cell count or disease progression to Walter Reed stages 4, 5, and 6 (Birx et al., 2000).

ANRS 093, a study of 70 PWH, compared ART to immunization with recombinant canarypox vector expressing several HIV genes (env, gag, pol, and nef) and lipo-6T (HIV-1 lipopeptides) followed by subcutaneous IL-2. The vaccine elicited a statistically significant interferon (IFN)-γ–producing CD8$^+$ T-cell response that correlated with virologic control (Levy et al., 2005). The vaccine group had a lower viral set point and therefore a significantly greater number of days off ART (Levy et al., 2006), but the results of this study await validation in larger trials.

In ACTG 5197, administration of a replication-defective adenovirus type 5 HIV-1 gag vaccine to PWH with CD4$^+$ T-cell counts of more than 500 cells/mL failed to be sufficiently immunogenic and lacked statistically significant efficacy (Schooley et al., 2010). The finding that the plasma viral load was 0.5 $\log_{10}$ lower in the vaccine arm at 16 weeks after ART interruption prompted further analysis of the HLA class I alleles in all 110 participants because HLA classes have previously been shown to influence viral evolution and disease progression. Vaccinated PWH with neutral HLA alleles in this cohort had a lower plasma viral load than those of both PWH vaccinated with protective alleles and placebo participants with neutral alleles (Li et al., 2011).

A novel therapeutic vaccine strategy with promising results targeted Tat, a transactivator of HIV gene expression essential for viral replication that is relatively conserved among HIV-1 subtypes. This vaccine is aimed at PWH on ART with the hope of decreasing viral reservoirs and restoring immune homeostasis. In phase 2 trials, 168 PWH controlled on ART and anti-Tat antibody negative at baseline who were administered the vaccine three or five times monthly showed specific and durable immune responses when followed for up to 144 weeks (Ensoli et al., 2015). Most persons (79%) developed anti-Tat antibodies; this was associated with significant reduction of proviral DNA seen after week 72. The vaccine was also associated with a restoration of T, B, and NK cells and CD4[+] and CD8[+] T-cell central memory subsets.

A multinational phase 2 trial examined the safety and immunogenicity of Vacc-4x, a peptide-based HIV-1 therapeutic vaccine targeting the conserved domains of p24Gag (Pollard et al., 2014). In chronically infected PWH who were virologically suppressed on ART, the Vacc-4x vaccine did not alter time to ART resumption or lead to significant changes in CD4[+] T-cell count at week 28 during treatment interruption. However, there was a statistically significant difference in HIV viral load at both week 48 (23,000 vs. 71,800 copies/mL) and week 52 (19,500 vs. 51,000 copies/mL).

T-CELL VACCINES

The ability to enhance the host's immune responses by therapeutic vaccination faces several key challenges. The majority of PWH have dysfunctional virus-specific effector cells (Sauce et al., 2013) as a result of continuous antigenic stimulation prior to treatment; indeed, ART only incompletely restores T-cell functionality (Youngblood et al., 2013). Furthermore, in PWH who initiate ART during chronic infection, almost all of the proviral sequences in the latent reservoir contain escape mutations that prevent killing of infected cells by cytotoxic T lymphocytes (Deng et al., 2015; Papuchon et al., 2013). The implication is that an effective vaccination strategy, instead of just expanding preexisting responses that already had failed to control the infection, would need to improve the quality and functionality of HIV-1–specific immune response and elicit CD8[+] T-cell responses against previously untargeted epitopes or unmutated regions of the virus to avoid escape (reviewed in Chen & Julg, 2020). To achieve this goal, multiple approaches are currently being tested in preclinical and clinical studies, including:

- Viral-vector–based vaccines, such as adenovirus, poxvirus modified vaccinia Ankara (MVA), vesicular stomatitis virus (VSV), and modified cytomegalovirus (CMV). Some of these approaches to deliver HIV-1 antigens have demonstrated robust immunogenicity, inducing broad and durable cellular immune responses that were able to protect monkeys against SIV infection in preclinical challenge studies (Barouch et al., 2012, 2013a; Hansen et al., 2011, 2013) but, more importantly, significantly reduced the viral load set points in SIV-infected macaques following ART cessation when combined with a TLR7 agonist (Borducchi et al., 2016). A phase 1/2a clinical trial of an Ad26 prime/MVA boost combination with mosaic HIV inserts in a cohort that initiated ART during the acute infection, however, did not lead to viremic control after treatment interruption (Colby et al., 2020). Studies in individuals who started ART during chronic infection are ongoing (ClinicalTrials.gov identifier: NCT03307915). Another MVA-vectored vaccine trial expressing tHIV-consv3 and tHIVconsv4 immunogens was initiated last year to evaluate its safety and efficacy in adults with HIV (ClinicalTrials.gov identifier: NCT03844386).

- Plasmid DNA expressing HIV-1 genes (Hallengard et al., 2011; Ramirez et al., 2013; Rodriguez et al., 2013; Sneller et al., 2017). A phase w trial is currently evaluating whether the PENNVAX-B vaccine, a synthetic plasmid expressing HIV Gag, Pol, and Env, leads to a significant reduction of HIV reservoir size (ClinicalTrials.gov identifier: NCT03606213). Another vaccine with HIV-derived conserved element (CE) p24 Gag DNA showed promising immunogenicity in macaques (Hu et al., 2016), and a human study just completed enrollment (ClinicalTrials.gov identifier: NCT03560258). The DNA plasmid vaccine GTU-multiHIV B, aimed at inducing immune responses to HIV-1 regulatory genes, has shown efficacy in HIV-1 subtype C PWH not on ART. In a population of 63 persons, the vaccine was deemed safe and was associated with a statistically significant decline in log pHIV-RNA with an increase in CD4[+] T-cell counts nearing significance compared to placebo, especially after intramuscular injections (Vardas et al., 2012). The efficacy of GTU-multi-HIV B DNA vaccine and LIPO-5 vaccine in a prime-boost strategy for lowering viral set point after treatment interruption for PWH virologically suppressed on ART is currently being studied in phase 2 trials.

- Dendritic cell–based vaccines to deliver HIV-1 antigens. Significant attention has also focused on dendritic cells as cellular adjuvants for therapeutic HIV-1 vaccines because they have been shown to elicit strong CD4[+] and CD8[+] T-cell responses in vivo. One uncontrolled study of immunization of 18 treatment-naive PWH with dendritic cells pulsed with inactivated autologous virus reported a 90% decrease in viral load during the course of a year (Lu et al., 2004). A subsequent randomized controlled trial of 24 treatment-naive subjects with a similar vaccine, however, showed a weak HIV-1–specific response and a modest decrease in viral load compared to placebo (Garcia et al., 2011). In a trial of chronically infected PWH on ART with CD4[+] T-cell counts of more than 450 cells/mm[3], the use of a monocyte-derived dendritic cell pulse with heat-inactivated whole HIV helped lower plasma viral load set point after treatment interruption, with an associated increase in HIV-1–specific T-cell responses compared to placebo (Garcia et al., 2013). Recent trials have continued to demonstrate better vaccine responses and control of viral replication (Levy et al., 2014). Dendritic cells expressing the HIV proteins Gag, Tat, Rev, and Nef administered as a vaccine have been shown to elicit potent antiviral T-cell responses in PWH on ART, including a Gag-specific IFN-γ response that correlated with HIV-1 inhibitory activity (van Gulck et al., 2012). An ongoing trial aims to test if autologous dendritic cells loaded with a conserved HIV Gag and Pol peptide pool or inactivated autologous HIV will yield broader T-cell responses (ClinicalTrials.gov identifier: NCT03758625).

Although no therapeutic vaccine is currently FDA approved, the future of therapeutic vaccine research for both naive and ART-treated PWH remains promising. Recent data have been encouraging, but the results of therapeutic vaccine trials have yet to yield a therapeutic vaccine strategy that can be implemented. In addition to further clinical trials of the vaccines discussed previously, additional studies investigating the heterogeneity of response to vaccines (e.g., genetic determinants) and the immunologic correlates of vaccine efficacy are needed for the field to advance. Some of the key vaccines in development are highlighted in Table 19.2.

PREVENTIVE VACCINES

Although a preventive HIV-1 vaccine would help control the worldwide AIDS pandemic, there have been many obstacles to its development. HIV-1 has significant genetic and antigenic diversity, making it difficult to target with a vaccine. The failure to induce broadly neutralizing antibodies against the virus and the lack of clear immune correlates of protection have also been challenges. Additionally, the SIV/SHIV nonhuman primate models on which preclinical testing of the vaccines is typically done have often showed promising results not reproduced in human clinical trials.

Multiple phase 1 and 2 vaccine trials were conducted dating back to 1987, but very few reached phase 2b/3. Initial trials used recombinant proteins to induce neutralizing antibodies. In two large randomized controlled trials, VAX003 and VAX004, involving vaccination with recombinant gp120 subunits, there were no statistically significant reductions in HIV infection in the vaccinated groups (Flynn et al., 2005; Pitisuttithum et al., 2006). In subsequent analysis, these vaccines seemed to fail due to a lack of a broad neutralizing antibody response.

Table 19.2 SELECT THERAPEUTIC VACCINE TRIALS

VACCINE	DESCRIPTION	STAGE OF DEVELOPMENT	RESULTS
DNA Vaccines			
Dermavir	Topically applied DNA vaccine	Phase 2	Safe and immunogenic in ART-treated PWH with GAG-specific T-cell responses (Rodriguez et al., 2013)
GTU-multiHIV B	DNA plasmid vaccine, contains complete sequences of HIV-1 Rev, Nef, Tat, and Gag (p17/p24) and a number of T-cell epitopes from Pol and Env	Phase 2	Statistically significant decrease in log pHIV RNA in ART-naive PWH compared to placebo; currently being studied with LIPO-5 as a prime boost strategy for PWH on ART
Subunit Vaccines			
Tat protein vaccine	Recombinant biologically active HIV-1 B clade Tat protein	Phase 2	Induction of anti-Tat antibodies in most PWH on ART restoring T, B, and NK cells and CD4$^+$ and CD8^{VA} central memory subsets (Ensoli et al., 2015); significant reduction in proviral DNA seen at week 72
Vac-35	Peptide-based vaccine aimed at eliciting a humoral response against the highly conserved region of gp41	Phase 2	An increase in T-cell count was observed in PWH with higher antibody levels.
Vacc-4x	Peptide-based vaccine with four synthetic peptides based on the HIV-1 p24	Phase 2	Statistically significant lower HIV viral set point at week 48 compared to placebo in PWH on ART; no change in time to treatment interruption
HIV-v	T cell epitope HIV vaccine with synthetic peptides from conserved reions of Vpr, Vif, Rev, and Nef	Phase 1b/2	Safe, IgG responses in up to 75% of volunteers with 1 log reduction in viral load in ART-naive males with this response compared to placebo and nonresponders (Boffito et al., 2013)
Dendritic Cell Vaccines			
AGs-004	Patient-derived dendritic cells and loaded ex vivo with RNA encoding four (Gag, Nef, Rev, and Vpr) antigens plus CD40L	Phase 2	Delay in continuous ART resumption in 24 treated subjects, but no improvement in CD4$^+$ T-cell counts (DeBenedette et al., 2014). Greater effect on HIV-specific effector/memory CD8 T-cell responses but no effect on viral load after treatment interruption (Jacobson et al., 2016).
TJV-01 (THV01-1 and THV01-2)	Live lentiviral vector vaccines, carry transgene that induces cellular response and eliminates HIV infected cells	Phase 2	Able to elicit vaccine-specific CD4$^+$ and CD8$^+$ responses in patients on suppressive ART. Trials ongoing.

Vaccine development subsequently shifted toward the use of live viral or bacterial vectors engineered to carry genes encoding the HIV antigens. These antigens are expressed in the cytoplasm of the target cell, broken down, and then presented on the surface of the cell, priming a CD8$^+$ response. In the STEP trial, HIV-negative subjects received immunization with three injections of a replication-incompetent recombinant adenovirus vector expressing HIV-1 Gag, Pol, and Nef (Buchbinder et al., 2008). The vaccine did not show any benefit in preventing transmission or reducing early viral load after infection.

Surprisingly, however, vaccinated persons who were seropositive for AD-5 or uncircumcised had higher rates of HIV-1 infection than placebo, a finding prompting discontinuation of a contemporaneous clinical trial with the same vaccine. Subsequent genetic sequencing of the HIV-1 strains from the vaccine and placebo groups revealed that the virus infecting the vaccine group had different epitopes from those in the placebo group (Rolland et al., 2011). The divergence was confined to the vaccine components of the virus, supporting the notion of selective pressure from vaccine-induced T-cell responses.

More recent vaccine strategies have used a heterologous prime-boost strategy to activate both cellular and humoral immune arms by priming with a certain vaccine (e.g., DNA vaccine) and then boosting the immune response with another type of vaccine (e.g., live vector vaccine) (Girard et al., 2011). The RV144 trial, a phase 3 randomized controlled trial, primed subjects with two successive doses of a canarypox vector (ALVAC) encoding Gag/Pro and Env antigens followed by two additional immunizations with this vector and AIDSVAX B/E, a bivalent HIV gp120 envelope glycoprotein derived from a subtype B and subtype E envelope (Rerks-Ngarm et al., 2009). Seventy-four of 7,325 participants in the placebo group and 51 of 7,347 in the vaccine group developed HIV-1 infection at 96 weeks, offering a mildly statistically significant 31% efficacy. These results were encouraging, but there was not a significant broadly neutralizing antibody response, and the vaccine efficacy peaked in the first 6 to 12 months (50–60%) only to decrease thereafter. Analysis of the RV144 trial, however, showed two immune correlates of infection risk after vaccination (Haynes et al., 2012). Binding of IgG antibodies to the variable regions of Env inversely correlated with infection rates, while plasma IgA binding to Env was directly correlated.

Building on the RV144 data, the HIV Vaccine Trials Network implemented HVTN 100, a phase 1/2, randomized, controlled, double-blind trial in South Africa that compared a canarypox vector, ALVAC-HIV[vCP2438], in combination with an envelope glycoprotein (gp120), both adapted to circulating strains in South Africa and paired with a more potent adjuvant to placebo. This combination induced strong humoral and cellular responses (Bekker et al., 2018). These encouraging results led to the development of HVTN 702, a phase 2b/3 efficacy trial currently being implemented in South Africa.

Another strategy was evaluated in the APPROACH trial, a multicenter, randomized, double-blind, placebo-controlled phase 1/2a trial in Africa, South Africa, Thailand, and the US (Barouch et al., 2018). The participants received Ad26.Mos. HIV expressing mosaic HIV-1 envelope (Env)/Gag/Pol antigens and aluminum-adjuvanted clade C Env gp140 protein or placebo. Researchers evaluated the vaccine's safety, tolerability, and antibody responses at weeks 28 and 52. A parallel study was also conducted in rhesus monkeys. It elicited Env-specific binding antibody responses (100%) and antibody-dependent cellular phagocytosis responses (80%) at week 52 and T-cell responses at week 50 (83%) in humans. The most common adverse event was injection site reaction (69–88%). The encouraging results of these studies led to the development of HVTN 702 (Uhambo study), a phase 2b/3 efficacy trial undertaken in South Africa. This study evaluated the safety and efficacy of a subtype clade C vaccine regimen in 5,407 HIV-negative study participants in South Africa, but it was discontinued after an interim analysis (NIH press release, 2020) demonstrated that 129 infections occurred among 2,694 participants who received the experimental vaccine compared to 123 of 2,689 participants who received placebo.

Despite this setback, other vaccine work is ongoing evaluating Ad26 viral vectors–based vaccines. Currently, after promising phase 1/2a data demonstrated correlates of immunity comparable to protection against SHIV in primate models, two large global trials are under way evaluating Ad 26 viral vaccines that express mosaic Env/Gag and Pol antigens. In sub-Saharan Africa, HVTN 705 (Imbokodo trial) will investigate a trivalent Ad26 construct boosted with a clade C gp140 glycoprotein. In the Americas and Europe, HVTN 706 (Mosaico trial) will evaluate a tetravalent Ad26 vector boosted with a bivalent mosaic clade C gp140 glycoprotein with alum adjuvant (Stephenson et al., 2020).

In summary, recent progress has been made toward the development of a preventive HIV vaccine. Key issues in development remain the identification of the correlates of immunity, the induction of broadly neutralizing antibody responses, and the durability of these responses. Trials building on the results of RV144 are under way, and it is hoped that they will provide insight into the correlates of immunity and eventually lead to an effective preventive vaccine strategy.

RECOMMENDED READING

Ensoli B, Cafaro A, Monini P, et al. Challenges in HIV vaccine research for treatment and prevention. *Front Immunol*. 2014;5:417.

Gilliam BL, Redfield RR. Therapeutic HIV vaccines. *Curr Top Med Chem*. 2003;3(13):2536–1553.

Gotch FM, Imami N, Hardy G. Candidate vaccines for immunotherapy in HIV. *HIV Med*. 2001;2:260–265.

Levy Y. Therapeutic HIV vaccines: an update. *Curr HIV/AIDS Rep*. 2005;2(1):5–9.

Van Gulck E, Van Tendeloo VF, Berneman ZN, et al. Role of dendritic cells in HIV immunotherapy. *Curr HIV Res*. 2010;8(4):310–322.

ACKNOWLEDGMENTS

This chapter is based on previous versions with contributions from Drs. David Margolis, Adrian Majid, and Bruce Gilliam.

REFERENCES

Abbink P, Mercado NB, Nkolola JP, et al. Lack of therapeutic efficacy of an antibody to α4β7 in SIVmac251-infected rhesus macaques. *Science*. 2019;365(6457):1029–1033. doi:10.1126/science.aaw8562

Abrams D, Levy Y, Losso MH, et al.; INSIGHT-ESPRIT Study Group; SILCAAT Scientific Committee. Interleukin 2 therapy in patients with HIV infection. *N Engl J Med*. 2009;361(16):1548–1559.

Ananworanich J, Schuetz A, Vandergeeten C, et al. Impact of multi-targeted antiretroviral treatment on gut T cell depletion and HIV reservoir seeding during acute HIV infection. *PloS One*. 2012;7(3):e33948.

Archin NM, Bateson R, Tripathy MK, et al. HIV-1 expression within resting CD4⁺ T cells after multiple doses of vorinostat. *J Infect Dis*. 2014;210(5):728–735.

ART Collaboration Cohort. Life expectancy of individuals on combination antiretroviral therapy in high-income countries: a collaborative analysis of 14 cohort studies. *Lancet*. 2008;372:293–299.

Bar KJ, Sneller MC, Harrison LJ, et al. Effect of HIV antibody VRC01 on viral rebound after treatment interruption. *N Engl J Med*. 2016;375:2037–2050.

Barouch DH, Liu J, Li H, et al. Vaccine protection against acquisition of neutralization-resistant SIV challenges in rhesus monkeys. *Nature*. 2012;482(7383):89–93.

Barouch DH, Stephenson KE, Borducchi EN, et al. Protective efficacy of a global HIV-1 mosaic vaccine against heterologous SHIV challenges in rhesus monkeys. *Cell*. 2013a;155(3):531–539.

Barouch DH, Tomaka FL, Wegmann F, et al. Evaluation of a mosaic HIV-1 vaccine in a multicentre, randomised, double-blind, placebo-controlled, phase 1/2a clinical trial (APPROACH) and in rhesus monkeys (NHP 13–19). *Lancet*. 2018;392(10143):232–243.

Barouch DH, Whitney JB, Moldt B, et al. Therapeutic efficacy of potent neutralizing HIV-1-specific monoclonal antibodies in SHIV-infected rhesus monkeys. *Nature*. 2013b;503(7475):224–228.

Barrett SE, Teller RS, Forster SP, et al. Extended-duration MK-8591-eluting implant as a candidate for HIV treatment and prevention. *Antimicrob Agents Chemother*. 2018;62(10):e01058–18. doi:10.1128/AAC.01058-18

Bekker L-G, Moodie Z, Grunenberg N, et al. Subtype C ALVAC-HIV and bivalent subtype C gp120/MF59 HIV-1 vaccine in low-risk, HIV-uninfected, South African adults: a phase 1/2 trial. *Lancet HIV*. 2018;5(7):E366–E378.

Besson GJ, Lalama CM, Bosch RJ, et al. HIV-1 DNA decay dynamics in blood during more than a decade of suppressive antiretroviral therapy. *Clin Infect Dis*. 2014;59(9):1312–1321.

Birx D, Loomis-Price LD, Aronson N, et al. Efficacy of recombinant human immunodeficiency virus (HIV) gp160 as a therapeutic vaccine in early-stage HIV-1-infected volunteers. *J Infect Dis*. 2000;181:881–889.

Blick G, Lalezari J, Hsu R, et al. Cyclophosphamide enhances SB-728T engraftment to levels associated with HIV-RNA control [Abstract 141]. Paper presented at the 21st Conference on Retroviruses and Opportunistic Infections, Boston, MA, March 2014.

Boffito M, Folx J, Bowman C, et al. Safety, immunogenicity and efficacy assessment of HIV immunotherapy in a multi-centre, double-blind randomized placebo-controlled phase Ib human trial. *Vaccine*. 2013;31(48):5680–5686.

Borducchi E, Abbink P, Nkolola J, et al. PGT121 combined with GS-9620 delays viral rebound in SHIV-infected rhesus monkeys [Abstract 73LB]. Conference on Retroviruses and Opportunistic Infections, Boston, MA, March 4–7, 2018.

Borducchi EN, Cabral C, Stephenson KE, et al. Ad26/MVA therapeutic vaccination with TLR7 stimulation in SIV-infected rhesus monkeys. *Nature*. 2016;540(7632):284–287.

Borrow P, Lewicki H, Hahn BH, et al. Virus specific CD8 cytotoxic T-lymphocyte activity associated with control of viremia in primary human immunodeficiency virus type 1 infection. *J Virol*. 1994;68:6103–6110.

Brake OT, Hooft K, Liu YP, et al. Lentiviral vector design for multiple shRNA expression and durable HIV-1 inhibition. *Mol Ther*. 2008;16:557–564.

Bruel T, Guivel-Benhassine F, Amraoui S, et al. Elimination of HIV-1 infected cells by broadly neutralizing antibodies. *Nat Commun*. 2016;7:10844.

Buchbinder SP, Mehrotra DV, Duerr A, et al. Efficacy assessment of a cell-mediated immunity HIV-1 vaccine (the Step Study): a double-blind, randomised, placebo-controlled, test-of-concept trial. *Lancet*. 2008;372(9653):1881–1893.

Buzon MJ, Sun H, Li C, et al. HIV-1 persistence in CD4⁺ T cells with stem cell-like properties. *Nat Med*. 2014;20(2):139–142.

Byrareddy SN, Arthros J, Cicala C, et al. Sustained virologic control in SIV⁺ macaques after antiretroviral and α4β7 antibody therapy. *Science*. 2016;354:197–202.

Campo N, Myburgh R, Garcel A, et al. Long lasting control of viral rebound with a new drug ABX464 gettinging Rev-mediated viral RNA biogenesis. *Retrovirology*. 2015;12:30.

Cao Y, Qin L, Zhang L, et al. Virologic and immunologic characterization of long-term survivors of human immunodeficiency virus type 1 infection. *N Engl J Med*. 1995;332:201–208.

Caskey M, Klein F, Lorenzi JC, et al. Viraemia suppressed in HIV-1–infected humans by broadly neutralizing antibody 3BNC117. *Nature*. 2015;522(7557):487–491.

Caskey M, Schoofs T, Gruell H, et al. Antibody 10-1074 suppresses viremia in HIV-1-infected individuals. *Nat Med*. 2017;23(2):185–191.

Centlivre M, Legrand N, Klamer S, et al. Preclinical in vivo evaluation of the safety of a multi-shRNA-based gene therapy against HIV-1. *Mol Ther Nucleic Acids*. 2013; 2:e120.

Chen W, Dmitrov D. Monoclonal antibody-based candidate therapeutics against HIV type 1. *AIDS Res Hum Retroviruses*. 2012;28(5):425–434.

Chen Z, Julg B. Therapeutic vaccines for the treatment of HIV. *Transl Res*. 2020;223:61–75.

Chun TW, Engel D, Berrey MM, et al. Early establishment of a pool of latently infected, resting CD4⁺(⁺) T cells during primary HIV-1 infection. *Proc Natl Acad Sci USA*. 1998;95(15):8869–8873.

Chun TW, Finzi D, Margolick J, et al. In vivo fate of HIV-1–infected T cells: quantitative analysis of the transition to stable latency. *Nat Med*. 1995;1(12):1284–1290.

Chun TW, Stuyver L, Mizell SB, et al. Presence of an inducible HIV-1 latent reservoir during highly active antiretroviral therapy. *Proc Natl Acad Sci USA*. 1997;94(24):13193–13197.

ClinicalTrials.gov NCT00991224; NCT02191098; NCT02408861; NCT02500849; NCT02595866; NCT03147859; NCT03164135; NCT03240328; NCT03307915; NCT03308786; NCT003354936; NCT03367754; NCT03560258; NCT03570918; NCT03617198; NCT03705169; NCT03721510; NCT03758625; NCT03837756; NCT03844386; NCT04223804.

Colby DJ, Sarnecki M, Barouch DH, et al. Safety and immunogenicity of Ad26 and MVA vaccines in acutely treated HIV and effect on viral rebound after antiretroviral therapy interruption. *Nat Med*. 2020;26(4):498–501.

Cong L, Ran FA, Cox D, et al. Multiplex genome engineering using CRISPR/Cas systems. *Science*. 2013;339(6121):819–823.

Cradick TJ, Fine EJ, Antico CJ, et al. CRISPR/Cas9 systems targeting β-globin and CCR5 genes have substantial off-target activity. *Nucleic Acids Res*. 2013;41(20):9584–9592.

Daar E, McDonald C, Crofoot G, et al. Dose-response relationship of subcutaneous long-acting HIV capsid inhibitor GS-6207. Presented at the 27th Conference on Retroviruses and Opportunistic Infections, Boston, MA, March 2020.

Day CL, Kaufmann DE, Kiepiela P, et al. PD-1 expression on HIV-specific T cells is associated with T cell exhaustion and disease progression. *Nature*. 2006;443(7109):350–354.

DeBenedette M, Tcherepanova I, Gamble A, et al. Immune function and viral load post AGS-004 administration to chronic HIV subjects undergoing STI [Abstract 343]. Paper presented at the 21st

Conferences on Retroviruses and Opportunistic Infections, Boston, MA, March 2014.

Deeks SG. HIV: shock and kill. *Nature.* 2012;487(7408):439–440.

Deeks SG, Walker BD. Human immunodeficiency virus controllers: mechanisms of durable virus control in the absence of antiretroviral therapy. *Immunity.* 2007;27(3):406–416.

Deng K, Pertea M, Rongvaux A, et al. Broad CTL response is required to clear latent HIV-1 due to dominance of escape mutations. *Nature.* 2015;517(7534):381–385.

Dhody K, Kazempour K. PRO 140 SC: long-acting, single-agent, maintenance therapy for HIV-1 infection [Abstract 486]. Paper presented at Conferences on Retroviruses and Opportunistic Infections, Seattle, WA, March 2019.

Dhody K, Pourhassan N, Kazempour K, et al. PRO 140, a monoclonal antibody targeting CCR5, as a long-acting, single-agent maintenance therapy for HIV-1 infection. *HIV Clin Trials.* 2018;19(3):85–93.

Ebina H, Misawa N, Kanemura Y, et al. Harnessing the CRISPR/Cas9 system to disrupt latent HIV-1 provirus. *Sci Rep.* 2013;3:2510.

Elliott JH, Wightman F, Solomon A, et al. Activation of HIV transcription with short-course vorinostat in HIV-positive patients on suppressive antiretroviral therapy. *PLoS Pathog.* 2014;10(10):e1004473.

Engsig FN, Zangerle R, Katsarou O, et al. Long-term mortality in HIV-positive individuals virally suppressed for >3 years with incomplete CD4 recovery. *Clin Infect Dis.* 2014;58(9):1312–1321.

Ensoli B, Cafaro A, Monini P, et al. Challenges in HIV vaccine research for treatment and prevention. *Front Immunol.* 2014;5:417.

Ensoli F, Cafaro A, Casabianco A, et al. HIV-1 Tat immunization restores immune homeostasis and attacks the HAART-resistant blood HIV DNA: results of a randomized phase II clinical exploratory clinical trial. *Retrovirology.* 2015;12:33.

Eron JJ Jr, Ashby MA, Giordano MF, et al. Randomized trial of MNrgp120 HIV-1 vaccine in symptomless HIV-1 infection. *Lancet.* 1996;348:1547–1551.

Evans VA, van der Sluis RM, Solomon A, et al. Programmed cell death-1 contributes to the establishment and maintenance of HIV-1 latency. *AIDS.* 2018;32(11):1491–1497.

Fidler S, Stöhr W, Pace M, et al.; RIVER Trial Study Group. Antiretroviral therapy alone versus antiretroviral therapy with a kick and kill approach, on measures of the HIV reservoir in participants with recent HIV infection (the RIVER trial): a phase 2, randomised trial. *Lancet.* 2020;395(10227):888–898.

Finzi D, Blankson J, Siliciano JD, et al. Latent infection of CD4+ T cells provides a mechanism for lifelong persistence of HIV-1, even in patients on effective combination therapy. *Nat Med.* 1999;5(5):512–517.

Finzi D, Hermankova M, Pierson T, et al. Identification of a reservoir for HIV-1 in patients on highly active antiretroviral therapy. *Science.* 1997;278(5341):1295–1300.

Flynn NM, Forthal DN, Harro CD, et al. Placebo-controlled phase 3 trial of a recombinant glycoprotein 120 vaccine to prevent HIV-1 infection. *J Infect Dis.* 2005;191:654–665.

Forcina G, d'Ettorre G, Mastroianni C, et al. Interleukin-15 modulated interferon-γ and β-chemokine production in patients with HIV infection: implications for immune-based therapy. *Cytokine.* 2004;25:283–290.

Garcia F, Climent N, Assoumou L, et al. A therapeutic dendritic cell-based vaccine for HIV-1 infection. *J Infect Dis.* 2011;203:473–478.

Garcia F, Climent N, Guardo AC, et al. A dendritic cell–based vaccine elicits T cell responses associated with control of HIV-1 replication. *Sci Transl Med.* 2013;5:166ra62.

Gaudinski MR, Coates EE, Houser K, et al. Safety and pharmacokinetics of the Fc-modified HIV-1 human monoclonal antibody VRC01LS: a phase 1 open-label clinical trial in healthy adults. *PLoS Med.* 2018;15(1):e1002493. doi:10.1371/journal.pmed.1002493

Gay CL, Bosch RJ, Ritz J, et al. Clinical trial of the anti-PDL-L1 antibody BMS-936559 in HIV-1 infected participants on suppressive antiretroviral therapy. *J Infect Dis.* 2017;215(11):1725–1733.

Girard MP, Osmanov S, Assossou OM, et al. Human immunodeficiency virus (HIV) immunopathogenesis and vaccine development: a review. *Vaccine.* 2011;29:6191–6218.

Gruell H, Cohen Y, Gunst JD, et al. A randomized trial of the impact of 3BNC117 and romidepsin on the HIV-1 reservoir. [Abstract 38]. Paper presented at Conferences on Retroviruses and Opportunistic Infections, Boston, MA, 2020.

Guihot A, Marcelin AG, Massiani MA, et al. Drastic decrease of the HIV reservoir in a patient treated with nivolumab for lung cancer. *Ann Oncol.* 2018;29:517–518.

Gupta RK, Peppa D, Hill AL, et al. Evidence for HIV-1 cure after CCR5Δ32/Δ32 allogeneic haemopoietic stem-cell transplantation 30 months post analytical treatment interruption: a case report. *Lancet HIV.* 2020;7(5):e340–e347.

Hallengard D, Haller BK, Maltais AK, et al. Comparison of plasmid vaccine immunization schedules using intradermal in vivo electroporation. *Clin Vaccine Immunol.* 2011;18(9):1577–1581.

Hansen SG, Ford JC, Lewis MS, et al. Profound early control of highly pathogenic SIV by an effector memory T cell vaccine. *Nature.* 2011;473(7348):523–527.

Hansen SG, Piatak M, Jr., Ventura AB, et al. Immune clearance of highly pathogenic SIV infection. *Nature.* 2013;502(7469):100–104.

Hardy GA, Imami N, Nelson MR, et al. A phase I, randomized study of combined IL-2 and therapeutic immunization with antiretroviral therapy. *J Immune Based Ther Vaccines.* 2007;5:6.

Hardy WD. 2020. https://www.treatmentactiongroup.org/wp-content/uploads/2020/03/final_A5370_CROI_Presentations_030720.pdf

Haynes BF, Gilbert PB, McElrath MJ, et al. Immune-correlates analysis of and HIV-1 vaccine efficacy trial. *N Engl J Med.* 2012;366:1275–1286.

Henrich TJ, Gandhi RT. Early treatment and HIV-1 reservoirs: a stitch in time? *J Infect Dis.* 2013;208(8):1189–1193.

Henrich TJ, Schreiner C, Cameron C, et al. Everolimus, an mTORC1/2 inhibitor, in ART-suppressed individuals who received solid organ transplantation: a prospective study. *Am J Transplant.* 2020. doi:10.1111/ajt.16244

Heredia A, Le N, Gartenhaus RB, et al. Targeting of mTOR catalytic site inhibits multiple steps of the HIV-1 lifecycle and suppresses HIV-1 viremia in humanized mice. *Proc Natl Acad Sci USA.* 2015;112(30):9412–9417.

Hermankova M, Siliciano JD, Zhou Y, et al. Analysis of human immunodeficiency virus type 1 gene expression in latently infected resting CD4+ T lymphocytes in vivo. *J Virol.* 2003;77(13):7383–7392.

Hocqueloux L, Avettand-Fenoel V, Jacquot S, et al. Long-term antiretroviral therapy initiated during primary HIV-1 infection is key to achieving both low HIV reservoirs and normal T cell counts. *J Antimicrobial Chemother.* 2013;68(5):1169–1178.

Holt N, Wang J, Kim K, et al. Human hematopoietic stem/ progenitor cells modified by zinc-finger nucleases targeted to CCR5 control HIV-1 in vivo. *Nat Biotechnol.* 2010;28(8);839–847.

Hombach AA, Holzinger A, Abken H. The weal and woe of costimulation in the adoptive therapy of cancer with chimeric antigen receptor (CAR)-redirected T cells. *Curr Mol Med.* 2013;13(7):1079–1088.

Hu W, Kaminski R, Yang F, et al. RNA-directed gene editing specifically eradicates latent and prevents new HIV-1 infection. *Proc Natl Acad Sci USA.* 2014;111(31):11461–11466.

Hu X, Valentin A, Dayton F, et al. DNA prime-boost vaccine regimen to increase breadth, magnitude, and cytotoxicity of the cellular immune responses to subdominant Gag epitopes of simian immunodeficiency virus and HIV. *J Immunol.* 2016;197(10):3999–4013.

Huang Y, Yu J, Lanzi A, et al. Engineered bispecific antibodies with exquisite HIV-1-neutralizing activity. *Cell.* 2016;165:1621–1631.

Hutter G, Nowak D, Mossner M, et al. Long-term control of HIV by CCR5 Delta32/Delta32 stem-cell transplantation. *N Engl J Med.* 2009;360(7):692–698.

Iwamoto N, Mason RD, Song K, et al. Blocking α4β7 integrin binding to SIV does not improve virologic control. *Science.* 2019;365(6457):1033–1036.

Jacobson JM, Routy J-P, Welles S, et al. Dendritic cell immunotherapy for HIV-1 infection using autologous HIV-1 RNA: a randomized, double-blind, placebo-controlled clinical trial. *J AIDS.* 2016;72(1):31–38.

Julg J, Pequ A, Abbink P, et al. Virologic control by the CD4-binding site antibody N6 in simian-human immunodeficiency virus-infected rhesus monkeys. *J Virol.* 2017;91(16):e00498–17.

June C, Tebas P, Stein D, et al. Induction of acquired CCR5 deficiency with zinc finger nuclease-modified autologous CD4 T cells (SB-728-T) correlates with increases in CD4 count and effects on viral load in HIV-infected subjects [Abstract 155]. Paper presented at the 19th Conference on Retroviruses and Opportunistic Infection, Seattle, WA, February 2012.

Kessing CF, Nixon CC, Li C, et al. In vivo suppression of HIV rebound by didehydro-cortistatin A, a "block-and-lock" strategy for HIV-1 treatment. *Cell Rep.* 2017;21(3):600–611.

Khaitan A, Unutmaz D. Revisiting immune exhaustion during HIV infection. *Curr HIV/AIDS Rep.* 2011;8(1):4–11.

Kim Y, Anderson JL, Lewin SR. Getting the "kill" into "shock and kill": strategies to eliminate latent HIV. *Cell Host Microbe.* 2018;23(1):14–26.

Kozal M, Aberg J, Pialoux G, et al. Fostemsavir in adults with multidrug-resistant HIV-1 infection. *N Engl J Med.* 2020;382(13):1232–1243.

Kroup RA, Safrit JT, Cao Y, et al. Temporal association of cellular immune responses with the initial control of viremia in primary human immunodeficiency virus type 1 syndrome. *J Virol.* 1994;68:4650–4655.

Krystal M, Wensel D, Sun Y, et al. HIV-1 combinectin BMS-986197: a long-acting inhibitor with multiple modes of action [Abstract 97]. Presented at the 23rd Conference on Retroviruses and Opportunistic Infection, Boston, MA, February 22–25, 2016.

Laird GM, Bullen CK, Rosenbloom DI, et al. Ex vivo analysis identifies effective HIV-1 latency-reversing drug combinations. *J Clin Invest.* 2015;125(5):1901–1912.

Lalezari J, Mitsuyasu R, Wang S, et al. A single infusion of zinc finger nuclease CCR5 modified autologous CD4 T cells (SB-728T) increased CD4 counts and leads to decrease in HIV proviral load in an aviremic HIV-infect subject [Abstract 433]. Paper presented at the 19th Conference on Retroviruses and Opportunistic Infection, Seattle, WA, February 2012.

Lam S, Bollard C. T cell therapies for HIV. *Immunotherapy.* 2013;5(4):407–414.

Leibman RS, Richardson MW, Ellebrecht CT, et al. Supraphysiologic control over HIV-1 replication mediated by CD8 T cells expressing a re-engineered CD4-based chimeric antigen receptor. *PLoS Pathog.* 2017;13(10):e1006613.

Levy Y, Durier C, Lascaux AS, et al. Sustained control of viremia following therapeutic immunization in chronically HIV-1 infected individuals. *AIDS.* 2006;20:405–413.

Levy Y, Gahery-Segard H, Durier C, et al. Immunologic and virologic efficacy of therapeutic immunization combined with interleukin-2 in chronically HIV-1 infected patients. *AIDS.* 2005;19:279–286.

Levy Y, Lacabaratz C, Weiss L, et al. Enhanced T cell recovery in HIV-1 infected adults through IL-7 treatment. *J Clin Invest.* 2009;119(4)997–1007.

Levy Y, Sereti I, Tambussi G, et al. Effects of recombinant human interleukin 7 on T-cell recovery and thymic output in HIV-infected patients receiving antiretroviral therapy: results of a phase I/ IIa randomized, placebo-controlled multicenter study. *Clin Infect Dis.* 2012;55(2):291–300.

Levy Y, Thiebaut R, Montes M, et al. Dendritic cell-based therapeutic vaccine elicits polyfunctional HIV-specific T-cell immunity associated with control of viral load. *Eur J Immunol.* 2014;44:2802–2810.

Lewden C, Chene G, Morlat P, et al. HIV-infected adults with a CD4 cell count greater than 500 cells/μl on long-term combination antiretroviral therapy reach same mortality rates as the general population. *J AIDS.* 2007;46(1):72–77.

Li J, Brumme Z, Brumme C, et al. Factors associated with viral rebound in HIV-1 infected individuals enrolled in a therapeutic HIV-1 gag vaccine trial. *J Infect Dis.* 2011;203:976–983.

Liao HK, Gu Y, Diaz A, et al. Use of the CRISPR/Cas9 system as an intracellular defense against HIV-1 infection in human cells. *Nat Commun.* 2015;6:6413.

Lu CL, Murakowski DK, Bournazos S, et al. Enhanced clearance of HIV-1–infected cells by broadly neutralizing antibodies against HIV-1 in vivo. *Science.* 2016;352:1001–1004.

Lu W, Arraes C, Ferreira WT, et al. Therapeutic dendritic cell vaccination for chronic HIV-1 infection. *Nat Med.* 2004;10:1359–1365.

Luzuriaga K, Gay H, Ziemniak C, et al. Viremic relapse after HIV-1 remission in a perinatally infected child. *N Engl J Med.* 2015;372(8):786–788.

Lynch RM, Boritz E, Coates EE, et al. Virologic effects of broadly neutralizing antibody VRC01 administration during chronic HIV-1 infection. *Sci Transl Med.* 2015;7(319):319ra206.

Martin AR, Siliciano RF. Immune modulation with rapamycin as a potential strategy for HIV-1 eradication [Abstract 415]. Paper presented at the 22nd Conference on Retroviruses and Opportunistic Infections, Seattle, WA, February 2015.

Mascolini M. Primary efficacy results of PRO 140 SC in a pivotal phase 2b/3 study in heavily treatment-experienced HIV-1 patients. Paper presented at ASM Microbe, Atlanta, GA, June 2018.

Mason SW, Sanisetty S, Osuna Gutierrez C, et al. Viral suppression was induced by anti-PD-L1 following ARV-interruption in SIV-infected monkeys [Abstract 318LB]. Paper presented at the 21st Conference on Retroviruses and Opportunistic Infections, Boston, MA, March 2014.

McMahon DK, Zheng L, Cyktor JC, et al. Multidose IV romidepsin: no increased HIV-1 expression in persons on ART, ACTG A5315 [CROI Abstract 26]. *Top Antivir Med.* 2019;27(suppl 1):11s–12s.

McMichael AJ, Borrow P, Tomaras GD. The immune response during acute HIV-1 infection: clues for vaccine development. *Nat Rev Immunol.* 2010;10(1):11–23.

Mendoza P, Gruell H, Nogueira L, et al. Combination therapy with anti-HIV-1 antibodies maintains viral suppression. *Nature.* 2018;561(7724):479–484.

Mitsuyasu RT, Lalezari J, Burke B, et al. Phase I study of gene-modified CD4+ T cells and CD34+ cells with or without busulfan in HIV+ adults [CROI Abstract 338]. *Top Antivir Med.* 2020;28(1):116.

Mitsuyasu RT, Merigan TC, Carr A, et al. Phase 2 gene therapy trial of anti-HIV ribozyme in autologous CD34+ cells. *Nat Med.* 2009;15(3):285–292.

Mori L, Valente ST. Key players in HIV-1 transcriptional regulation: targets for a functional cure. *Viruses.* 2020;12(5):529.

Moron-Lopez S, Bernal S, Steens JM, et al. ABX464 decreases the total HIV reservoir and HIV transcription initiation in vivo [Poster Abstract 335]. Conference on Retroviruses and Opportunistic Infections, Boston, MA, 2020.

Mothe B, Rosás-Umbert M, Coll P, et al. HIVconsv vaccines and romidepsin in early-treated HIV-1-infected individuals: safety, immunogenicity and effect on the viral reservoir (Study BCN02). *Front Immunol.* 2020;11:823.

Mousseau G, Kessing CF, Fromentin R, et al. The tat inhibitor didehydro-cortistatin A prevents HIV-1 reactivation from latency. *MBio.* 2015;6(4).

Nabel G, Baltimore D. An inducible transcription factor activates expression of human immunodeficiency virus in T cells. *Nature.* 1987;326(6114):711–713.

Namazi G, Fajnzylber JM, Aga E, et al. The Control of HIV After Antiretroviral Medication Pause (CHAMP) study: posttreatment controllers identified from 14 clinical studies. *J Infect Dis.* 2018;218(12):1954–1963.

NIH Press Release. February 2, 2020. https://www.nih.gov/news-events/news-releases/experimental-hiv-vaccine-regimen-ineffective-preventing-hiv

Pallikkuth S, Micci L, Ende ZS, et al. Maintenance of intestinal Th17 cells and reduced microbial translocation in SIV-infected rhesus macaques treated with interleukin (IL)-21. *PLoS Pathog.* 2013;9:e1003471.

Pallikkuth S, Rogers K, Villinger F, et al. Interleukin-21 administration to rhesus macaques chronically infected with simian immunodeficiency viruses increases cytotoxic effector molecules in T cells and NK cells and enhances B cell function without increasing immune activation or viral replication. *Vaccine.* 2011;29:9929–9938.

Palmer BE, Neff CP, Lecureux J, et al. In vivo blockade of the PD-1 receptor suppresses HIV-1 viral loads and improves CD4+ T cell levels in humanized mice. *J Immunol.* 2013;190(1):211–219.

Palmer CS, Ostrowski M, Zhou J, et al. The mTORC1 inhibitors, temsirolimus and everolimus, suppress HIV-patient-derived CD4+ T-cell death and activation in vitro [Abstract 320]. Paper presented at the 22nd Conference on Retroviruses and Opportunistic Infections, Seattle, WA, February 2015.

Papuchon J, Pinson P, Lazaro E, et al. Resistance mutations and CTL epitopes in archived HIV-1 DNA of patients on antiviral treatment: toward a new concept of vaccine. PloS One. 2013;8(7):e69029.

Pegu A, Asokan M, Wu L, et al. Activation and lysis of human CD4 cells latently infected with HIV-1. Nature Commun. 2015;6:8447.

Perez EE, Wang J, Miller JC, et al. Establishment of HIV-1 resistance in CD4+ T cells by genome editing using zinc-finger nucleases. Nat Biotechnol. 2008;26(7):808–816.

Persaud D, Gay H, Ziemniak C, et al. Absence of detectable HIV-1 viremia after treatment cessation in an infant. N Engl J Med. 2013;369(19):1828–1835.

Peterson CW, Wang J, Deleage C, et al. Differential impact of transplantation on peripheral and tissue-associated viral reservoirs: implications for HIV gene therapy. PLoS Pathog. 2018;14(4):e1006956.

Pett SL, Carey C, Lin E, et al. Predictors of bacterial pneumonia in Evaluation of Subcutaneous Interleukin-2 in Randomized International TRIAL (ESPRIT). HIV Med. 2011;12(4):219–227.

Pett SL, Kelleher AD, Emery S. Role of interleukin-2 in patients with HIV infection. Drugs. 2010;70(9):1115–1130.

Pino M, Uppada SB, Pandey K, et al. Safety and immunological evaluation of interleukin-21 plus anti α4β7 mAb combination therapy in rhesus macaques. Front Immunol. 2020;11:1275.

Pitisuttithum P, Gilbert P, Gurwith M, et al. Randomized, double-blind, placebo-controlled efficacy trial of a bivalent recombinant glycoprotein 120 HIV-1 vaccine among injection drug users in Bangkok, Thailand. J Infect Dis. 2006;194:1661–1671.

Pollard RB, Rockstroh JK, Pantaleo G, et al. Safety and efficacy of the peptide-based therapeutic vaccine for HIV-1, Vacc-4x: a phase 2 randomised double-blind, placebo-controlled trial. Lancet Infect Dis. 2014;14(4):291–300.

Pontesilli I, Guerra ES, Ammassari A, et al. Phase II controlled trial of post-exposure immunization with recombinant gp160 versus antiretroviral therapy in asymptomatic HIV-1 infected adults. AIDS. 1998;12:473–480.

Porichis F, Kaufmann DE. Role of PD-1 in HIV pathogenesis and as a target for therapy. Curr HIV/AID Rep. 2012;9(1):81–90.

Ramirez LA, Arango T, Boyer J. Therapeutic and prophylactic DNA vaccines for HIV-1. Expert Opin Biol Ther. 2013;13(4):563–573.

Rasmussen TA, Tolstrup M, Brinkmann CR, et al. Panobinostat, a histone deacetylase inhibitor, for latent-virus reactivation in HIV-infected patients on suppressive antiretroviral therapy: a phase 1/2, single group, clinical trial. Lancet HIV. 2014;1(1):e14–e21.

Rerks-Ngarm S, Pitisuttithum P, Nitayaphan S, et al. Vaccination with ALVAC and AIDSVAX to prevent HIV-1 infection in Thailand. N Engl J Med. 2009;361(23):2209–2220.

Richman DD, Margolis DM, Delaney M, et al. The challenge of finding a cure for HIV infection. Science. 2009;323(5919):1304–1307.

Riddler SA, Zheng L, Durand CM, et al. Randomized clinical trial to assess the impact of the broadly neutralizing HIV-1 monoclonal antibody VRC01 on HIV-1 persistence in individuals on effective ART. Open Forum Infect Dis. 2018;5(10):ofy242.

Rodriguez B, Asmuth DM, Matining RM, et al. Safety, tolerability, and immunogenicity of repeated doses of dermavir, a candidate therapeutic HIV vaccine, in HIV-infected patients receiving combination antiretroviral therapy: results of the ACTG 5176 trial. J AIDS. 2013;64(4):351–359.

Rolland M, Tovanbutra S, Decamp AC, et al. Genetic impact of vaccination on breakthrough HIV-1 sequences from the STEP trial. Nat Med. 2011;17(3):366–371.

Rosenberg ES, Billingsley JM, Caliendo AM, et al. Vigorous HIV-1-specific CD4R T cell responses associated with control of viremia. Science. 1997;278:1447–1450.

Saez-Cirion A, Bacchus C, Hocqueloux L, et al. Post-treatment HIV-1 controllers with a long-term virological remission after the interruption of early initiated antiretroviral therapy ANRS VISCONTI Study. PLoS Pathog. 2013;9(3):e1003211.

Saito N, Chono H, Shibata H, et al. CD4+ T cells modified by endoribonuclease MazF are safe and can persist in SHIV-infected rhesus macaques. Mol Ther Nucleic Acids. 2014;3(6):e168.

Sandstrom E, Wahren B; Nordic Vac-04 Study Group. Therapeutic immunization with recombinant gp160 in HIV-1 infection: a randomized double-blind placebo-controlled trial. Lancet. 1999;353:1735–1742.

Sauce D, Elbim C, Appay V. Monitoring cellular immune markers in HIV infection: from activation to exhaustion. Curr Opin HIV AIDS. 2013;8(2):125–131.

Scheid JF, Horwitz JA, Bar-On Y, et al. HIV-1 antibody 3BNC117 suppresses viral rebound in humans during treatment interruption. Nature. 2016;535(7613):556–560.

Schooley RT, Spritzler J, Wang H, et al.; AIDS Clinical Trials Group 5197. A placebo-controlled trial of immunization of HIV-1-infected persons with a replication-deficient adenovirus type 5 vaccine expressing the HIV-1 core protein. J Infect Dis. 2010;202(5):705–716.

Schürmann D, Rudd DJ, Zhang S, et al. Safety, pharmacokinetics, and antiretroviral activity of islatravir (ISL, MK-8591), a novel nucleoside reverse transcriptase translocation inhibitor, following single-dose administration to treatment-naive adults infected with HIV-1: an open-label, phase 1b, consecutive-panel trial. Lancet HIV. 2020;7(3):e164–e172.

SenGupta D, Ramgopal M, Brinson C, et al. Safety and analytical treatment interruption outcomes of vesatolimod in HIV controllers [CROI Abstract 40]. Top Antivir Med. 2020;28(1):13–14.

Sereti I, Dunham RM, Spritzler J, et al. IL-7 administration drives T cell entry and expansion in HIV-1 infection. Blood. 2009;113(25):6304–6314.

Shan L, Deng K, Shroff NS, et al. Stimulation of HIV-1-specific cytolytic T lymphocytes facilitates elimination of latent viral reservoir after virus reactivation. Immunity. 2012;36(3):491–501.

Shingai M, Nishimura Y, Klein F, et al. Antibody-mediated immunotherapy of macaques chronically infected with SHIV suppresses viraemia. Nature. 2013;503(7475):277–280.

Singh A, Palanichamy JK, Ramalingam P, et al. Long-term suppression of HIV-1 C virus production in human peripheral blood mononuclear cells by LTR heterochromatization with a short double-stranded RNA. J Antimicrob Chemother. 2014;69:405–415.

Sneller MC, Clarridge KE, Seamon C, et al. An open-label phase 1 clinical trial of the anti-α4β7 monoclonal antibody vedolizumab in HIV-infected individuals. Sci Transl Med. 2019;11(509):eaax3447.

Sneller MC, Justement JS, Gittens KR, et al. A randomized controlled safety/efficacy trial of therapeutic vaccination in HIV-infected individuals who initiated antiretroviral therapy early in infection. Sci Transl Med. 2017;9(419):eaan8848.

Sogaard OS, Graversen ME, Leth S, et al. The depsipeptide romidepsin reverses HIV-1 latency in vivo. PLoS Pathog. 2015;11(9): e1005142.

Stellbrink HJ, van Lundzen J, Westby M, et al. Effects of interleukin-2 plus highly active antiretroviral therapy on HIV-1 replication and proviral DNA (COSMIC trial). AIDS. 2002;16:1479–1487.

Stephenson KE, Wagh K, Korber B, et al. Vaccines and broadly neutralizing antibodies for HIV-1 prevention. Ann Rev Immunol. 2020 38:673–703.

Strain MC, Little SJ, Daar ES, et al. Effect of treatment, during primary infection, on establishment and clearance of cellular reservoirs of HIV-1. J Infect Dis. 2005;191(9):1410–1418.

Sung JA, Pickeral J, Liu L, et al. Dual-affinity re-targeting proteins direct T cell-mediated cytolysis of latently HIV-infected cells. J Clin Invest. 2015;125(11):4077–4090.

Tavel JA; INSIGHT STALWART Study Group. Effect of intermittent IL-2 alone or with peri-cycle antiretroviral therapy in early HIV-1 infection: the STALWART study. PLoS One. 2010;5(2):e9334.

Tebas P, Jadlowski J, Shaw P, et al. Delayed viral rebound during ATI after infusion of CCR5 ZFN-treated CD4 T cells [Abstract 25]. Conference on Retroviruses and Opportunistic Infections, Seattle, WA, 2019.

Tebas P, Stein D, Binder-Scholl G, et al. Antiviral effects of autologous CD4 T cells genetically modified with a conditionally replicating lentiviral vector expressing long antisense to HIV. *Blood*. 2013;121(9):1524–1533.

Tebas P, Stein D, Tang WW, et al. Gene editing of CCR5 in autologous CD4 T cells of persons infected with HIV. *N Engl J Med*. 2014;370(10):901–910.

Thompson M, Saag M, DeJesus E, et al. A 48-week randomized phase 2b study evaluating cenicriviroc versus efavirenz in treatment-naive HIV-infected adults with C-C chemokine receptor type 5-tropic virus. *AIDS*. 2016;30(6):869–878.

Topalian SL, Hodi FS, Brahmer JR, et al. Safety, activity, and immune correlates of anti-PD-1 antibody in cancer. *N Engl J Med*. 2012;366(26):2443–2454.

Tsoukas CM, Raboud J, Bernard NF, et al. Active immunization of patients with HIV infection: a study of VaxSyn, a recombinant HIV envelope subunit vaccine, on progression of immunodeficiency. *AIDS Res Hum Retroviruses*. 1998;14:483–490.

Vandergeeten C, Fromentin R, DaFronseca S, et al. Interleukin-7 promotes HIV persistence during antiretroviral therapy. *Blood*. 2013;121(21):4321–4329.

Van Gulck E, Vlieghe E, Vekemans M, et al. mRNA-based dendritic cell vaccination induced potent antiviral responses in HIV-1 infected patients. *AIDS*. 2012;26:F1–F12.

Van Lundzen J, Glausinger T, Stahmer I, et al. Transfer of autologous gene-modified T cells in HIV-infected patients with advanced immunodeficiency and drug-resistant virus. *Mol Ther*. 2007;15:1024–1033.

Vardas E, Stanescu I, Leinonen M, et al. Indicators of a therapeutic effect in FIT-06, a phase II trial of a DNA vaccine, GTU-Multi-HIVB, in untreated HIV-1 infected subjects. *Vaccine*. 2012;30(27):4046–4054.

Varela-Rohena A, Molloy PE, Dunn SM, et al. Control of HIV-1 immune escape by CD8 T cells expressing enhanced T cell receptor. *Nat Med*. 2008;14(12):1390–1395.

Velu V, Titanji K, Zhu B, et al. Enhancing SIV-specific immunity in vivo by PD-1 blockade. *Nature*. 2009;458(7235):206–210.

Vibholm L, Schleimann MH, Hojen JF, et al. Short-course toll-like receptor 9 agonist treatment impacts innate immunity and plasma viremia in individuals with human immunodeficiency virus infection. *Clin Infect Dis*. 2017;64(12):1686–1695.

Wang CY, Wong WW, Tsai HC, et al. Effect of anti-CD4 antibody UB-421 on HIV-1 rebound after treatment interruption. *N Engl J Med*. 2019;380(16):1535–1545.

Webb GM, Li S, Mwakalundwa G, et al. The human IL-15 superagonist ALT-803 directs SIV-specific CD8+ T cells into B-cell follicles. *Blood Adv*. 2018;2:76–84.

White KL, Margot N, Stray K, et al. GS-9131 is a novel NRTI with activity against NRTI-resistant HIV-1 [Abstract 436]. Presented at the 24th Conference on Retroviruses and Opportunistic Infection, Seattle, WA, February 13–16, 2017.

Whitney JB, Hill AL, Sanisetty S, et al. Rapid seeding of the viral reservoir prior to SIV viraemia in rhesus monkeys. *Nature*. 2014;512(7512):74–77.

Whitney JB, Osuna CE, Sanisetty S, et al. Treatment with a TLR7 agonist induces transient viremia in SIV-infected ART-suppressed monkeys. Conference on Retroviruses and Opportunistic Infections, Seattle, WA, 2015.

Wolstein O, Boyd M, Millington M, et al. Preclinical safety and efficacy of an anti-HIV-1 lentiviral vector containing a short hairpin RNA to CCR5 and the C46 fusion inhibitor. *Mol Ther Methods Clin Dev*. 2014;1:11.

Wong JK, Hezareh M, Gunthard HF, et al. Recovery of replication-competent HIV despite prolonged suppression of plasma viremia. *Science*. 1997;278(5341):1291–1295.

Yakubova E, Mazus A, Kravchenko AV, et al. Safety and PK study of VM-1500A-LAI, a novel long-acting injectable therapy for HIV [Late-Breaking Poster Abstract 473LB]. Conference on Retroviruses and Opportunistic Infections, Boston, MA, 2020.

Youngblood B, Noto A, Porichis F, et al. Cutting edge: prolonged exposure to HIV reinforces a poised epigenetic program for PD-1 expression in virus-specific CD8 T cells. *J Immunol*. 2013;191(2):540–544.

Xu L, Pequ A, Rao E, et al. Trispecific broadly neutralizing HIV antibodies mediate potent SHIV protection in macaques. *Science*. 2017;358:85–90.

Xu L, Wang J, Liu Y, et al. CRISPR-edited stem cells in a patient with HIV and acute lymphocytic leukemia. *N Engl J Med*. 2019;381(13):1240–1247.

Yukl SA, Boritz E, Busch MB, et al. Challenges in detecting HIV persistence during potentially curative interventions: a study of the Berlin patient. *PLoS Pathog*. 2013;9(5):e1003347.

Zeller S, Kumar P. RNA-based gene therapy for the treatment and prevention of HIV: from bench to bedside. *Yale J Biol Med*. 2011;84(3):301–309.

Zheng J, Yant SR, Ahmadyar S, et al. GS-CA2: a novel, potent and selective first-in-class inhibitor of HIV-1 capsid function displays nonclinical pharmacokinetics supporting long-acting potential in humans [Abstract 539]. Presented at ID Week 2018, San Francisco, October 3–7, 2018.

Zhou J, Rossi JJ. Current progress in the development of RNAi based therapeutics for HIV-1. *Gene Ther*. 2011;18:1134–1138.

20.

ANTIRETROVIRAL RESISTANCE
EVALUATION AND CLINICAL MANAGEMENT

Carolyn Chu, Lealah Pollock, and Robert Shafer

CHAPTER GOALS

Upon completion of this chapter, the reader should be able to:

- Outline various types of HIV drug resistance (HIVDR) testing assays and clinical considerations for their use and interpretation

- Define transmitted HIVDR (TDR) and acquired HIVDR (ADR) and general principles/approaches to their management

- Describe unique considerations regarding HIVDR evaluation and management for select clinical scenarios, including antiretroviral treatment (ART) switches/simplification, pregnancy, recent use of pre-exposure prophylaxis (PrEP), "rapid ART," and care of persons with HIV (PWH) in low- and middle-income countries

---

WHAT'S NEW?

Approximately 37% of persons with diagnosed HIV infection in the US do not have a suppressed viral load (Harris et al., 2019), underscoring ongoing gaps in effective HIV treatment and prevention. In high-income countries, rates of TDR are relatively stable and rates of ADR appear to be falling; however, HIVDR remains a key contributor to treatment failure, and providers should be proficient in evaluating and managing resistance to help ensure appropriate antiretroviral drug (ARV) prescribing and monitoring. Proviral DNA sequencing is increasingly employed to guide decision-making for regimen switching/simplification; ongoing research will help fully elucidate its potential role in clinical practice. Next-generation sequencing, which allows for detection of low-abundance HIVDR mutations that would not be identified using traditional Sanger sequencing methods, has theoretical potential benefit, although its use in routine clinical practice remains limited at this time. Updated US guidelines incorporate specific ARV recommendations after first- and second-line treatment failures, accounting for commonly observed resistance patterns that emerge across varying treatment scenarios. Careful investigation and interpretation of HIVDR

findings are warranted for persons who acquire HIV in the setting of PrEP use to better understand the role that HIVDR might play in such cases of "PrEP failure."

KEY POINTS

- US treatment guidelines continue to recommend HIVDR testing at initial diagnosis and for persons who develop virologic failure on therapy.

- HIVDR testing is typically conducted with genotypic testing; supplemental phenotypic testing may be considered for PWH who have complicated drug resistance mutation (DRM) patterns.

- ADR remains an important issue even with increasing use of second-generation integrase strand transfer inhibitors (INSTIs); thus, clinicians should continue to emphasize treatment adherence and timely virologic monitoring.

INTRODUCTION

Before the availability of highly active combination treatment, HIVDR was the main obstacle to successful therapy. As newer ARVs became available, spanning different therapeutic classes, it became possible to overcome this obstacle. However, clinicians providing HIV care were required to become knowledgeable about HIVDR because ART failure and HIVDR were a part of everyday practice. As ART has continued to improve, many clinicians may now confront HIVDR less frequently. However, because HIV is a chronic, lifelong infection, cumulative development of resistance has the potential to limit treatment options over time and lead to poor health outcomes. HIVDR therefore remains an important problem that can complicate treatment if clinicians are not aware of basic HIVDR prevention and management approaches. Emerging trends in TDR and ADR, the continued introduction of new drugs, and increasing use of PrEP, dual therapy strategies, and rapid ART initiation all raise new considerations for how clinicians should incorporate knowledge about HIVDR into their clinical decision-making.

Table 20.1 HIVDR-ASSOCIATED TERMS AND DEFINITIONS

Drug resistance mutations (DRMs)	Amino acid changes selected by ARV therapy, reducing ARV susceptibility in vitro, and/or reducing virologic response to therapy
Polymorphism	Amino acid changes in the targets of ARV therapy that are often present in ART-naive persons. Although most polymorphisms do not influence ARV susceptibility, some are selected by therapy and contribute to reduced ARV susceptibility nearly always in combination with nonpolymorphic DRMs.
Transmitted drug resistance (TDR)	Presence of one or more nonpolymorphic DRMs in an ART-naive person
Pretreatment drug resistance	Presence of one or more nonpolymorphic DRMs in a PWH initiating or reinitiating ART in settings where pretherapy genotypic resistance testing is not routinely performed. Persons with pretreatment drug resistance may include ART-naive persons as well as pregnant persons who received ART for perinatal transmission prevention, persons receiving preexposure or postexposure prophylaxis, and persons who discontinued first-line ART without a documented history of virologic failure.
Acquired drug resistance (ADR)	DRMs that are selected during ARV therapy, which can happen when viral replication is not fully suppressed in the presence of drug
Genetic barrier to resistance	A function of the number of mutations required to reduce virus susceptibility to an ARV, the likelihood that these mutations will develop upon ARV drug exposure, and the impact of reduced ARV susceptibility on virologic outcome. Some mutations rarely occur because they are associated with markedly reduced virus replication. The impact of reduced ARV susceptibility on virologic outcome is highly heterogeneous
Genotyping	Analysis for HIVDR through examination of viral genetic structure, specifically involving the sequencing of molecular targets of therapy to determine the presence of mutations known to confer decreased ARV drug susceptibility
Phenotyping	Analysis for HIVDR that employs the measurement of drug susceptibility of virus by determining the concentration of drug that inhibits viral replication in tissue culture
Sanger sequencing	Sequencing method of choice for commercially available genotypic resistance testing for over 20 years: DNA sequencing method used following reverse transcription of the viral ribonucleic acid genome (based on selective incorporation of chain-terminating dideoxynucleotides by DNA polymerase during in vitro DNA replication)
Next-generation HIVDR testing	High-throughput DNA sequencing technologies, where millions of DNA strands can be sequenced in parallel, yielding substantially more throughput and minimizing need for the fragment-cloning methods often used in Sanger sequencing
Proviral DNA sequencing	Sequencing approach that samples the "archived" HIV viral reservoir found in PBMCs
Wild-type virus	Naturally occurring, nonmutated strain of a virus
Thymidine analogue mutations (TAM)	Nonpolymorphic mutations selected by the thymidine analogs AZT and d4T: the accumulation of TAMs leads to progressive decrease in drug susceptibility for all approved NRTIs

Adapted from Günthar°d HF, et al. *Clin Infect Dis.* 2019 Jan 15; 68(2): 177–187.

Table 20.1 includes a list of terms and definitions used in this chapter.

MECHANISMS OF HIVDR

HIV mutates at a high rate during virus replication, resulting in nearly one nucleotide change during each replication cycle (Abram et al., 2010). Among PWH receiving incompletely suppressive ART, some of these mutations result in amino acid changes that reduce susceptibility to one or more ARVs an individual is receiving (Coffin, 1995). In PWH on ART who do not maintain sufficiently high levels of medication adherence, viral variants possessing mutations that reduce ARV susceptibility will have a selective replication or "fitness" advantage. When strains harboring such mutations first emerge, they are part of a diverse swarm of viral variants often referred to as a *quasispecies*. The complexity of the HIV-1 quasispecies is also increased by the high recombination rate that occurs whenever more than one viral variant infects the same cell (Eberle & Gurtler, 2012b; Levy et al., 2004). With sufficient selective ARV pressure, these variants become the dominant quasispecies (Figure 20.1). By contrast, if a person maintains virus suppression through consistent ART use, HIV is unable to replicate to a level high enough to support ongoing evolution and the development of HIVDR (Siliciano & Siliciano, 2013; van Zyl et al., 2018).

HIVDR is mediated almost entirely by mutations in the molecular targets of ART, including the reverse transcriptase (RT) gene in persons receiving nucleoside RT inhibitors (NRTIs) or nonnucleoside RT inhibitors (NNRTIs), the protease gene in persons receiving protease inhibitors (PIs), the

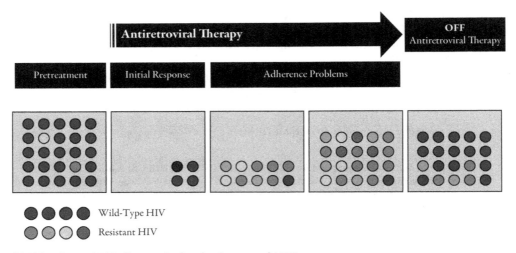

●●●● Wild-Type HIV

◐○◑◐ Resistant HIV

Figure 20.1 Suboptimal ART and poor ART adherence lead to development of ARV-resistant strains. SOURCE: National HIV Curriculum, available at https://www.hiv.uw.edu/go/antiretroviral-therapy/evaluation-management-virologic-failure/core-concept/all

integrase gene in persons receiving INSTIs; and the envelope genes (gp120 and gp41) in persons receiving entry inhibitors. The "genetic barrier to resistance" to an ARV is a useful yet loosely defined concept to indicate that ARVs differ in their vulnerability to HIVDR by virtue of the number of mutations required for clinically significant reductions in susceptibility and the likelihood that these mutations will develop upon drug exposure (Figure 20.2). Indeed, some HIVDR-associated mutations occur rarely because they are associated with markedly reduced virus replication.

During its replication cycle, HIV-1 integrates into host chromosomal DNA and is then usually expressed, leading to productive infection and cell killing. In resting memory CD4+ T cells, however, integrated proviral DNA may persist for many years, forming a stable reservoir. As a result, proviral DNA levels in peripheral blood mononuclear cells (PBMCs) remain detectable even in PWH on ART who have

undetectable plasma HIV-1 RNA levels. Therefore, in persons with stable virologic suppression, the DRMs present in proviral DNA will reflect resistance that emerged prior to the most recent regimen.

HIVDR is often caused by "major" DRMs that reduce drug susceptibility by themselves and accessory mutations that generally compensate for the reduced fitness associated with many of the major DRMs. With a few notable exceptions, major DRMs do not occur in previously untreated patients, whereas accessory mutations are often polymorphic. HIVDR emerges in viruses from PWH exposed to suboptimal inhibitory concentrations. As a result, most cases of virologic failure and drug resistance arise from incomplete adherence, which exposes a patient's virus to the incompletely suppressive ARV levels capable of exerting drug selective pressure. Accordingly, HIVDR appears to be less common in patients receiving fixed-dose combinations (FDCs) containing ARVs

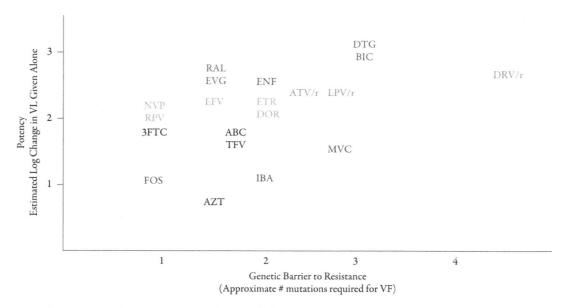

Figure 20.2 Schematic indicating genetic barrier to resistance (estimated) for select, approved ARV agents. VL = viral load; VF = viral failure

that have similar half-lives because incomplete adherence to these combinations is less likely to expose a virus to selective drug pressure (Llibre et al., 2011). Lower rates of HIVDR have also been associated with routine viral load monitoring programs/practices in which early detection of virologic rebound provides the opportunity for adherence assessment and counseling or regimen modification as necessary, prior to the evolution of multiple DRMs (Bachmann et al., 2019).

During its spread among humans, group M HIV-1 strains have evolved into many subtypes and circulating recombinant forms (Rambaut et al., 2004). However, none of the subtypes are intrinsically resistant to the main classes of ARVs (Gunthard et al., 2019). Although viruses belonging to different subtypes occasionally differ in the frequency with which they develop different DRMs, the phenotypic effect of these mutations appear to be subtype independent, and it is therefore not necessary to know the subtype of a patient's virus to select therapy or to interpret the results of HIVDR testing (Gunthard et al., 2019).

HIVDR TESTING

INDICATIONS FOR TESTING

Drug resistance testing is recommended at the time of initial diagnosis, regardless of whether the person starts ART soon thereafter, and in PWH who develop virologic failure on therapy (Department of Health and Human Services [DHHS], 2020; Gunthard et al., 2019). For ART-naive PWH, the role of baseline resistance evaluation is to guide initial regimen selection. For persons who do not immediately start ART, clinicians may consider repeat testing closer to the time of treatment initiation in PWH who are considered to be at high risk of having experienced superinfection (DHHS, 2020). For ART-experienced persons with virologic failure, the role of resistance testing is to help ascertain the cause of virologic failure as well as to determine which ARVs may have been compromised and which agents still retain activity, in order to design a new regimen.

The clinician who has performed HIV screening/testing is often the same care provider who notifies a PWH of their results. However, because many newly diagnosed PWH are referred to a specialist for care, the timeliness of baseline resistance testing may depend on access to local HIV service providers and insurance status. Therefore, early resistance testing should be prioritized particularly in certain populations such as persons with advanced disease at high risk of opportunistic infections, pregnant persons at risk of perinatal HIV transmission, and persons with acute HIV infection who are often at high risk of transmitting to others and in whom transmitted resistant variants are likely to recede.

With increasing use of first-line INSTI-containing regimens for most newly diagnosed PWH, the cost-effectiveness of baseline resistance testing may be less than it once was (Hyle et al., 2019). Nonetheless, baseline testing remains the standard of care and is valuable not only for persons starting a standard, contemporary dual NRTI- and INSTI-containing regimen but also for those who may require a subsequent regimen change, are considering a two-drug regimen, and who acquire HIV while on PrEP.

TIMING OF RESISTANCE TESTING

Timely resistance testing is recommended because resistant variants are less fit in the absence of ARV selection pressure compared to wild-type susceptible virus variants. Indeed, retrospective studies of stored samples from newly diagnosed PWH have shown that transmitted drug-resistant variants are frequently outcompeted by wild-type revertants (Castro et al., 2013; Jain et al., 2011; Pingen et al., 2014; Yanik et al., 2012). The speed with which transmitted mutations are replaced (i.e., no longer detectable within plasma) depends on the extent to which a mutation reduces virus fitness. Some mutations can be outcompeted by wild-type variants within several months, whereas others can persist as the dominant variant for years. In patients with virologic failure, resistance testing should be performed while the patient is still on ART because in this scenario DRMs may no longer be detected within weeks of treatment discontinuation—specifically, the mutations that emerged while on therapy will rapidly be replaced by archived wild-type variants that were present before therapy was initiated (Deeks et al., 2001; Devereux et al., 1999).

GENOTYPIC AND PHENOTYPIC RESISTANCE TESTING

HIVDR testing can be performed genotypically (by sequencing the molecular targets of therapy) or phenotypically (by determining drug susceptibility in cell culture). Both tests are performed using polymerase chain reaction (PCR) products directly amplified from cDNA that has been reverse-transcribed from plasma RNA. Genotypic resistance testing is recommended for ART-naive persons and involves direct sequencing of the viral genome using conventional Sanger sequencing methodologies to identify mutations in the reverse transcriptase (RT), protease (PR), and integrase strand transfer inhibitor (INSTI) genes of circulating plasma RNA. Although genotypic tests are more complex than typical antimicrobial susceptibility tests, their ability to detect mutations present as mixtures (i.e., co-circulating with wild-type variants), even if the mutation is present at a level too low to affect drug susceptibility in a phenotypic assay, provides insight into the potential for resistance to emerge. Sequencing tests can also detect transitional mutations that do not cause drug resistance by themselves but indicate the presence of selective drug pressure. Compared to phenotypic testing, additional advantages of genotypic testing include lower cost and shorter turnaround time.

Phenotypic susceptibility testing involves the identification of ARV concentration that inhibits HIV replication by 50% (EC_{50}). The EC_{50} of a clinically sampled virus is then compared to that of a drug-susceptible laboratory reference strain and expressed as a ratio, referred to as *fold change*, of the EC_{50} of the sampled virus relative to the reference control (Figure 20.3). Most phenotypic tests, including the main test

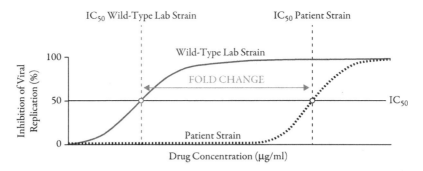

Figure 20.3 Calculating level of phenotypic resistance. This graph shows the method for calculating the level of phenotypic resistance of a single ARV. The ARV is tested on a patient's HIV isolate and a laboratory reference (wild-type strain). The IC_{50} represents the concentration of the ARV required to cause 50% inhibition of HIV replication. The fold change is calculated by dividing the IC_{50} of the patient's isolate by the IC_{50} of the wild-type laboratory strain. As shown, as the curve shifts to the right, a higher concentration of ARV would be required to inhibit HIV replication and thus the strain of HIV would be more resistant. The further the curve shifts to the right (for the patient's HIV strain tested), the greater the level of resistance. SOURCE: National HIV Curriculum, available at https://www.hiv.uw.edu/go/antiretroviral-therapy/evaluation-management-virologic-failure/core-concept/all

used in the US, use recombinant viruses created by inserting PCR-amplified clinical virus gene segments (protease/RT, integrase, envelope) into the backbone of a wild-type laboratory clone (Petropoulos et al., 2000). In general, phenotypic testing is not necessary as part of the baseline evaluation for newly diagnosed PWH. However, it may be a valuable complement to genotypic testing in persons who have developed virologic failure on multiple treatment regimens or who have complicated patterns of DRMs (DHHS, 2020; Gunthard et al., 2019). It may also be useful for PWH who have been primarily infected with a multiclass-resistant virus. When phenotypic testing is indicated, it should be performed in addition to genotypic testing (rather than on its own) because of the ability of genotypic testing to detect emerging resistance, as indicated earlier. Figure 20.4 depicts a sample genotype and phenotype testing report.

HIV THERAPEUTIC TARGETS FOR RESISTANCE TESTING

Sequencing of protease and the 5′ part of RT usually constitutes one assay, whereas sequencing of integrase usually constitutes a second, distinct assay. Whereas RT/PR genotypic testing is routinely recommended for all newly diagnosed PWH and in patients with virologic failure, integrase genotypic testing is recommended primarily in persons with virologic failure on an INSTI-containing regimen or persons with an incomplete or delayed virologic response on an INSTI-based regimen. Baseline INSTI resistance testing should be considered in select persons with TDR, such as those with reduced NRTI susceptibility or multiclass resistance and in persons who have been exposed to a PWH failing an INSTI-containing regimen (Gunthard et al., 2019).

Resistance testing for the four entry inhibitors is less widely available. Genotypic testing for HIV-1 tropism (to evaluate activity of the CCR5 antagonist maraviroc) and for enfuvirtide susceptibility is available in several reference laboratories, including Quest, Monogram Biosciences/LabCorp, and ARUP. Phenotypic testing for these two entry inhibitors is also available at Monogram Biosciences. Neither genotypic

nor phenotypic resistance tests are commercially available for the attachment inhibitor fostemsavir or the postattachment inhibitor ibalizumab.

HIV-1 RNA (VIRAL LOAD) THRESHOLDS FOR GENOTYPIC TESTING

Current DHHS guidelines recommend genotypic resistance testing for PWH with repeated viral loads greater than 500 to 1,000 copies/mL (DHHS, 2020). However, it is not uncommon for PWH to have repeated detectable viral load results between 50 and 500 copies/mL. Many studies have now demonstrated that repeated viral loads between 200 and 500 copies/mL are associated with an increased risk of HIVDR and/or subsequent further increases in viral load to higher levels (Elvstam et al., 2017; Fleming et al., 2019; Hermans et al., 2018; Joya et al., 2019; Li et al., 2012; Mackie et al., 2010; Ryscavage et al., 2014; Swenson et al., 2014; Vandenhende et al., 2015). Moreover, most genotypic assays that employ nested PCR are able to yield interpretable genotypic results for a large proportion of PWH with viral loads between 200 and 500 copies/mL (Gonzalez-Serna et al., 2014; Li et al., 2012; Mackie et al., 2010; Swenson et al., 2014).

PROVIRAL DNA SEQUENCING

Proviral DNA sequencing is being increasingly employed in PWH who are planning to modify their therapy while their virus levels are suppressed (Armenia et al., 2018; Ellis et al., 2019; van Wyk et al., 2020). There is a strong but imperfect correlation between the DRMs in PBMC proviral DNA and plasma HIV-1 RNA from the same blood samples (Derache et al., 2015; Devereaux et al., 2000; Verhofstede et al., 2004). In patients with suppressed plasma HIV-1 RNA levels, the proviral DNA genotyping will detect many but not all DRMs detected by previous plasma genotypic resistance testing (Allavena et al., 2018; Boukli et al., 2018; Delaugerre et al., 2012; Margot et al., 2020; Wirden et al., 2011; Zaccarelli et al., 2016). Proviral DNA testing has also been used in PWH with detectable viremia, but its clinical usefulness in this setting

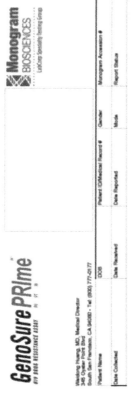

Figure 20.4 Sample HIV drug resistance testing (genotype and phenotype) reports. SOURCE: Monogram Biosciences. Available at: https://www.monogrambio.com/resources/

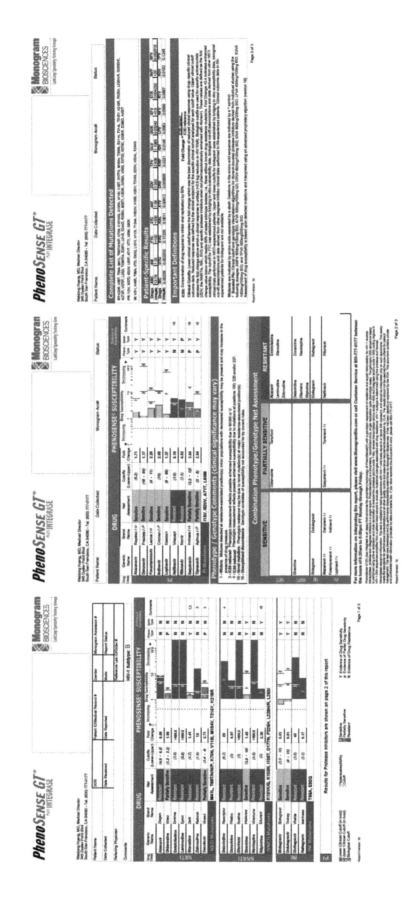

Figure 20.4 Continued.

has been less well studied (Boukli et al., 2018; Curanovic et al., 2020; Lubke et al., 2015; Zaccarelli et al., 2016).

NEXT-GENERATION SEQUENCING

Newer sequencing technologies—collectively referred to as next-generation sequencing (NGS)—are replacing Sanger sequencing for many applications in diagnostic microbiology laboratories. The cost of NGS can be considerably lower than that of Sanger sequencing should a sufficient number of samples be tested in the same sequencing run (Lapointe et al., 2015; Noguera-Julian et al., 2017). Additionally, the ability of NGS to detect low-abundance DRMs not detected by Sanger sequencing (i.e., present at a prevalence below 15–20%) has potential advantages for improving patient outcomes, particularly for the NNRTI class and for the detection of low-levels of CXCR4 tropic viruses (Avila-Rios et al., 2016; Boltz et al., 2011; Cozzi-Lepri et al., 2015; Li et al., 2011; Pou et al., 2014; Westby et al., 2006). Nonetheless, Sanger sequencing has been used for two decades to diagnose HIVDR and has been shown to be highly reproducible and interpretable in clinical settings, whereas the laboratory NGS procedures and approaches to sequence analysis continue to evolve (Avila-Rios et al., 2020; Mbunkah et al., 2020). Moreover, it has been difficult to translate the theoretical benefits of increased sensitivity for low-abundance variants into a practical clinical benefit, especially as ARV agents have become more potent and as most NGS assays have displayed reduced reproducibility at mutation detection thresholds below 5% (Avila-Rios et al., 2016; Huber et al., 2017; Inzaule et al., 2018). Although approaches to improve specificity are often used in research settings, these approaches are currently not used in clinical laboratories (Jabara et al., 2011).

INTERPRETATION OF RESISTANCE TESTING RESULTS

Genotypic resistance testing produces a list of DRMs, which is accompanied by a prediction of which ARVs are likely to have reduced activity. As the many known HIV-associated DRMs occur in complex patterns and cause varying levels of reduced drug susceptibility, interpretation systems are required to predict which ARVs are likely to retain activity. The four most commonly used publicly available interpretation systems are the Stanford HIVDB interpretation system (Paredes et al., 2017), the ANRS system (Eberle & Gurtler, 2012a), the Rega system (Eberle & Gurtler, 2012a), and HIV-GRADE (Obermeier et al., 2012). The International AIDS Study–USA (IAS-ISA) Antiviral group also maintains a list of DRMs considered to be the most clinically relevant (Wensing et al., 2019). This list has been used to track the development of resistance in clinical trials and cohorts and may also be helpful in the identification of key mutations associated with resistance to ARV drugs in order to guide ART decision-making for clinicians (Tables 20.2 and 20.3).

Genotypic resistance interpretation system rules are usually developed by considering several types of published data,

Table 20.2 SELECT RESOURCES ON HIVDR CLINICAL EVALUATION AND MANAGEMENT

U.S. DHHS Guidelines	https://clinicalinfo.hiv.gov/en/guidelines/adult-and-adolescent-arv/whats-new-guidelines
IAS-USA: Drug resistance mutations in HIV-1	https://www.iasusa.org/resources/hiv-drug-resistance-mutations/
Stanford HIV Database	https://hivdb.stanford.edu/
National HIV Curriculum (ART overview)	https://www.hiv.uw.edu/go/antiretroviral-therapy
National Clinician Consultation Center	https://nccc.ucsf.edu/
HIV-ASSIST	https://hivassist.com
Clinical Care Options (HIV portfolio)	https://clinicaloptions.com/hiv

including whether a DRM has been selected by a drug either in vitro or in PWH, whether a DRM reduces drug susceptibility in vitro, and whether there are data showing that a DRM interferes with virologic response to an ART regimen containing the relevant drug. Although one might expect that DRMs present at low levels would have a lesser clinical impact than those present at higher levels, there are no interpretation systems that treat low-abundance DRMs differently from those present at higher levels. Furthermore, interpretation systems often differ in the numbers of levels of resistance assigned. For example, most systems assign three levels: susceptible, low-level/possible resistance, and resistance. In contrast, the Stanford HIVDB system assigns five levels: susceptible, potential low-level resistance, low-level resistance, intermediate resistance, and high-level resistance. Overall, the systems are rarely completely discordant (i.e., a virus is rarely scored as being fully susceptible to a drug by one system but fully resistant by another system). Nonetheless, formal comparison of the various interpretation systems has found subtle differences (Rhee et al., 2009).

Phenotypic test results also require interpretation because the clinical significance of fold-reductions in susceptibility differ among ARVs (de Meyer et al., 2008; Eron et al., 2013; Vingerhoets et al., 2010; Winters et al., 2009). Whenever possible, phenotypic tests provides three thresholds for fold-reductions in drug susceptibility: (1) the reduction in susceptibility that exceeds the uppermost value for wild-type viruses, often referred to as the biological threshold (Parkin et al., 2004); (2) the lowest fold-reduction in susceptibility that indicates a PWH will have a reduced likelihood of responding to therapy (lower clinical threshold); and (3) the lowest fold-reduction in susceptibility that indicates a drug will likely be completely inactive (upper clinical threshold). Upper and lower clinical thresholds have been developed for ARVs that have been used in salvage therapy situations for the treatment of PWH with viruses containing DRMs affecting the same ARV class, including abacavir (Lanier et al., 2004), tenofovir (Miller et al., 2004),

Table 20.3 COMMON HIVDR MUTATIONS AND IMPACT ON ARV SUSCEPTIBILITY, BY CLASS AND MEDICATION

ARV DRUGS	DRUG RESISTANCE MUTATIONS (DRMS)
Nucleoside/nucleotide RT inhibitors	
Abacavir (ABC)	K65R, L74V/I, Y115F, M184V/I: 1 mutation confers low-level and 2 confer high-level resistance T215Y/F + 2 additional TAMS: intermediate- to high-level resistance MDR mutations: high-level resistance K70E/Q/N/T: low-level resistance
Lamivudine (3TC); emtricitabine (FTC)	M184V/I confer high-level resistance K65R, MDR mutations, and 4 or 5 TAMS confer intermediate levels of resistance
Tenofovir disoproxil fumarate (TDF); tenofovir alafenamide (TAF)	K65R: confers low-level phenotypic resistance but potentially high-level clinical resistance T215Y/F + 2 additional TAMS: intermediate- to high-level resistance MDR mutations: intermediate- to high-level resistance depending on the specific mutations K70E/Q/N/T: low-level phenotypic resistance
Zidovudine (AZT)	TAMs: confer intermediate- to high-level resistance MDR mutations: confer high-level resistance
	TAMs (thymidine analog mutations) are defined as M41L, D67N, K70R, L210W, T215F/Y, K219Q/E. T215F/Y is the most important of these, and the combination of M41L + L210W + T215Y has the greatest phenotypic and virologic impact. MDR mutations are defined as (i) Q151M usually in combination with ≥2 of the following: A62V, V75I, F77L, and F116Y; (ii) an amino acid insertion at position 69, which nearly always occurs with ≥1 TAM. M184V/I increase susceptibility to AZT, TDF, and TAF; K65R increases susceptibility to AZT. TAF and TDF have similar resistance profiles. However, TAF achieves >4-fold higher intracellular levels of the active inhibitor tenofovir (TFV) diphosphate, suggesting that it is likely to be more active than TDF at inhibiting both drug-susceptible and drug-resistant viruses. However, most genotypic resistance interpretation systems do not distinguish between the two TFV prodrugs. T215S/C/D/E/I/V are commonly transmitted mutations consistent with previous TAM selection pressure. These mutations have much less clinical significance than T215Y/F.
Nonnucleoside RT inhibitors	
Efavirenz (EFV)	L100I, K101E/P, K103N/S, V106A/M, Y188L/C/H, G190A/S/E/Q, P225H, F227C, M230L
Etravirine (ETR)	L100I, K101E/P, Y181C/I/V, G190E/Q, F227C, M230L
Rilpivirine (RPV)	ETR + E138A/G/K/Q/R, H221Y, Y188L
Doravirine (DOR)	V106A/M, Y188L, G190S/E, F227C/L, M230L, L234I, F318Y
General comments	Common accessory relatively nonpolymorphic DRMs: A98G, V106I, V108I, V179D/E/F, H221Y High-level DOR resistance usually requires V106A, Y188L, G190E, F227L/C, M230L, L234I, or a combination of ≥2 other NNRTI-resistance mutations, including some that do not cause resistance alone, including L100I, K101E, Y181C/I/V, and G190A/S. ETR usually requires ≥2 mutations for intermediate- or high-level resistance. The effect of E138 mutations on RPV is not well understood. Although E138K causes low-level RPV resistance, it is one of the most commonly emerging DRMs in persons developing virologic failure while receiving RPV. E138A, which is polymorphic in certain subtypes, minimally reduces RPV susceptibility but is of uncertain clinical significance. EFV has a higher genetic barrier to resistance than previously believed, with 2 mutations often required for high-level resistance.
Protease inhibitors	
Atazanavir (ATV/r)	V32I, M46I/L, I47V, G48V/M, I50L, I54V/T/A/S/L/M, V82A/C/F/M/S/T, I84V/A/C, N88S, L90M
Darunavir (DRV/r)	V32I, I47V/A, I50V, I54L/M, L76V, V82F, I84V/A/C
Lopinavir (LPV/r)	L24I, V32I, M46I/L, I47V/A, G48V/M, I50V, I54V/T/A/S/L/M, L76V, V82A/C/F/M/S/T, I84A/C/V, L90M
General comments	Common accessory nonpolymorphic DRMs: L10F, V11I/L, K20T, L33F, G73/S/T/C/A, T74P, L89V DRV/r has the highest genetic barrier to resistance, usually requiring 2 to 3 of the listed mutations and 2 or 3 of the accessory mutations to develop high-level resistance. LPV/r has a lower genetic barrier to resistance compared with DRV/r but likely a higher genetic barrier to resistance than ATV/r.

Table 20.3 CONTINUED

ARV DRUGS	DRUG RESISTANCE MUTATIONS (DRMS)

Integrase strand transfer inhibitors

Raltegravir (RAL)	T66K, E92Q, G118R, F121Y, E138A/K/T, G140A/S/C, Y143CRH, Q148H/R/K, N155H, S230R
Elvitegravir (EVG)	T66A/I/K, E92Q, G118R, F121Y, E138A/K/T, G140A/S/C, P145S, Q146P, S147G, Q148H/R/K, N155H, S230R, R263K
Dolutegravir (DTG)	G118R, E138A/K/T, G140A/S/C, Q148H/R/K, N155H, R263K
Bictegravir (BIC)	G118R, E138A/K/T, G140A/S/C, Q148H/R/K, N155H, R263K
Cabotegravir (CAB)	G118R, E138A/K/T, G140A/S/C/R, Q148H/R/K, N155H, R263K
Notes	Accessory slightly polymorphic DRMs: L74M, T97A, E157Q, G163K/E, D232N Many of the EVG and RAL-associated DRMs appear to be DTG and BIC-accessory DRMs. There are 3 somewhat overlapping RAL-resistance mutational pathways: Y143C/R/H vs. Q148H/R/K vs. N155H, often in combination with an additional mutation such as E92Q, E138K/A/T, G140S/A/C, and/or an accessory mutation. Persons receiving EVG are less likely to develop Y143 mutations and more likely to develop T66A/I/K, E92Q, and S147G, but there is a high-level of cross-resistance between RAL and EVG. There are somewhat overlapping DTG-resistance mutation pathways: Q148H/K/R + 1 or 2 additional mutations; N155H + ≥2 additional mutation; R263K; and G118R. Although R263K is the most commonly occurring DRM in persons developing DTG-associated virologic failure, it is associated with just a 2-fold reduction in susceptibility. BIC has a nearly identical resistance profile compared with DTG. High-level resistance to RAL and EVG usually requires just 1 or 2 DRMs, while high-level resistance to DTG and BIC appears to require 2 or 3 DRMs. Additionally, DRMs emerge less frequently in persons receiving DTG or BIC compared with those receiving RAL or EVG. DRMs associated with reduced DTG or BID susceptibility generally cause a greater reduction in CAB susceptibility.

Entry inhibitors

Enfuvirtide (fusion inhibitor)	Mutations in gp41 codons 36–45, the region to which enfuvirtide binds. The key mutations are G36D/E/V, V38E/A, Q40H, N42T, and N43D. A single mutation usually reduces susceptibility about 10-fold, whereas two mutations usually reduce susceptibility about 100-fold.
Maraviroc (CCR5 inhibitor)	CXCR4-tropic gp120 variants: positively charged residues at positions 11 and 25 of the V3 loop of gp120 and several other combinations of mutations primarily but not exclusively within the V3 loop are associated with CXCR4 tropism. The most common mechanism of resistance is the expansion of preexisting CXCR4-tropic variants that were not detected before therapy. Resistance can also emerge as a result of gp120 mutations that allow HIV-1 to bind to an altered CCR5 receptor. There is no consistent pattern of these mutations.
Ibalizumab (postattachment inhibitor)	Loss of potential N-linked glycosylation sites (PNGS) in the V5 loop of gp120 allows HIV-1 to bind CD4 and enter cells despite the presence of ibalizumab (Blair, 2010).
Fostemsavir	Several gp120 mutations, including M426L and S375M, are considered major fostemsavir-resistance mutations, while M434I and M475I are considered to have a lesser effect on susceptibility. The amino acids that explain why CRF01_AE viruses are usually resistant to fostemsavir map to 375H and 475I (Zhou et al., 2014).

etravirine (Vingerhoets et al., 2010), lopinavir (Kempf et al., 2002), darunavir (de Meyer et al., 2008), and dolutegravir (Eron et al., 2013).

Importantly, genotypic and phenotypic test interpretations alone do not contain sufficient information to construct a clinically appropriate ART regimen for an individual. In addition to the results of recent resistance testing, it is necessary to consider the results of previous resistance tests as well as previous ART a PWH was receiving at a time of virologic failure. PWH with high viral loads and low CD4 counts are also at increased risk of virologic failure and may require a more aggressive ART regimen than another PWH with similar results on resistance testing. Genotypic and phenotypic resistance interpretation systems also vary in how they take into account differences in ARV potency, and thus do not incorporate fundamental principles of how treatment regimens should be constructed. Therefore, clinicians must place the results of drug resistance assays within the context of current treatment guidelines.

REGULATORY STATUS

Currently there are two test kits approved by the US Food and Drug Administration (FDA) for HIVDR genotyping. The ViroSeq HIV-1 Genotyping System, v.2.0 (Abbott Molecular, Des Plaines, IL) for RT/protease and the ViroSeq

HIV-1 Integrase Genotyping Kit, Research Use Only (Abbott Molecular) for integrase use Sanger sequencing technology. The Sentosa SQ HIV-1 Genotyping Assay (Vela Diagnostics; Fairfield, NJ) uses Ion Torrent NGS technology to sequence RT, protease, and integrase in a single test. Most genotypic resistance tests, however, are likely being performed using laboratory-developed assays that comply with Clinical Laboratory Improvement Amendment (CLIA) guidelines, either in large reference laboratories or in laboratories affiliated with academic medical centers. Currently, nearly all phenotypic resistance testing is being performed using a CLIA-approved assay developed by Monogram BioSciences (LabCorp, South San Francisco).

TRANSMITTED HIVDR

EPIDEMIOLOGY

TDR is defined as the presence in an ART-naive person of one or more DRMs that are non-polymorphic in that they do not occur naturally in the absence of selective drug pressure. For practical purposes, non-polymorphic mutations have been defined as mutations that occur at a prevalence below 0.5% in all major HIV subtypes in ART-naive persons at times and in regions where TDR has been uncommon. The most common list of mutations used for surveillance of TDR was published in 2009 and is often referred to as the World Health Organization (WHO) list, as it was used in many WHO-sponsored studies (Bennett et al., 2009). It includes 34 NRTI mutations at 15 RT positions, 19 NNRTI mutations at 10 RT positions, and 40 PI mutations at 18 protease positions. The US Centers for Disease Control and Prevention uses a more expansive list of 108 DRMs that includes mutations that may be polymorphic in non-B subtypes (Wheeler et al., 2010). The subset of major IAS-USA mutations has also been used in several surveillance studies (Wensing et al., 2019).

Over the past 10 years, TDR prevalence has been approximately 15% in the US, 10% in Europe and the Latin American and Caribbean regions, and 5% in sub-Saharan Africa and Asia (Avila-Rios et al., 2016; Gupta et al., 2018; McClung et al., 2020; Rhee et al., 2015, 2020b). TDR prevalence has been stable in most geographic regions except for sub-Saharan Africa, where rates of transmitted NRTI and NNRTI resistance have been increasing, particularly among persons with pretreatment drug resistance, which includes ARV-naive persons as well as PWH who have received prior ARVs to prevent perinatal HIV transmission or who are reinitiating therapy without a documented history of virologic failure; see the section on resource-limited settings later in the chapter (Gupta et al., 2018; Rhee et al., 2020b).

Transmitted INSTI resistance has been below 1.0% in most regions, although recent increases may now be occurring in the US, where two nationwide studies have reported INSTI-associated TDR rates of 0.8% and one study in Florida reported rates of 1.4% in 2015 and 2.2% in 2016 (McClung et al., 2019, 2020; Poschman & Spencer, 2020).

Samples obtained from PWH in upper-income countries with identified NRTI, NNRTI, and PI-associated TDR generally contain DRMs associated with ARVs that are now used infrequently, such as thymidine analog mutations (TAMs), NNRTI-resistance mutations, and mutations associated with older PIs (Drescher et al., 2014; Machnowska et al., 2019; Margot et al., 2017; Pingen et al., 2014; Rhee et al., 2019a). Many of these circulating TDR strains are considered most likely to be established among ART-naive persons rather than reflecting direct transmission from persons experiencing virologic failure.

MANAGEMENT OF TDR

In the US and other high-income countries, the risk posed by TDR to the success of first-line therapy is low because, as noted earlier, most of the currently transmitted DRMs do not compromise currently recommended first-line ART regimens. Moreover, the routine performance of genotypic resistance testing makes it possible to identify those transmitted DRMs that would compromise currently recommended first-line ART regimens. For persons in whom baseline resistance evaluation suggests that a first-line regimen may not be effective, expert consultation may be useful. For example, the use of more than one anchor ARV may be considered, depending on which DRMs were identified.

No clinical trials have assessed approaches for treating persons in whom baseline genotypic resistance testing reveals the presence of TDR. However, several retrospective studies provide useful insight. First, because there is no cross-resistance between drug classes, persons with transmitted NNRTI resistance are expected to have an undiminished response to treatment using an INSTI- or PI-containing first-line ART regimen. Second, the presence of the most commonly transmitted NRTI-associated DRMs—TAMs other than T215Y/F—do not appear to influence the virologic response to first-line regimens containing tenofovir disoproxil fumarate (TDF) or tenofovir alafenamide (TAF) (Margot et al., 2017; Sörstedt et al., 2018). Third, although the presence of baseline TDR-associated DRMs suggests the possible presence of additional undetected transmitted DRMs (i.e., those that have faded to low levels following competition with wild-type revertants; Castro et al., 2013; Jain et al., 2011; Mbunkah et al., 2020; Pingen et al., 2014), such additional DRMs have not been detected frequently by sensitive NGS methods (Clutter et al., 2017; Dauwe et al., 2016; Toni et al., 2009; Varghese et al., 2009). Moreover, in retrospective studies, PWH with TDR detected by baseline genotypic resistance testing do not appear to have higher rates of virologic failure when the results of such testing are used to guide therapy (Borghetti et al., 2021; Geretti et al., 2019; Knyphausen et al., 2014; Margot et al., 2017; Metzner et al., 2010; Peuchant et al., 2008; Rhee et al., 2020a).

ACQUIRED HIVDR

EPIDEMIOLOGY

The increased use of ARVs with a high genetic barrier to resistance, particularly the second-generation INSTIs, and the use of FDCs often administered in a single-tablet regimen collectively make it less likely that medication nonadherence will result in a person's virus becoming exposed to an incompletely suppressive regimen. Many clinical trials and several longitudinal cohort studies in upper-income countries have reported that since 2000 fewer persons beginning ART have developed virologic failure or acquired HIVDR (Antiretroviral Therapy Cohort Collaboration, 2017; Carr et al., 2019; Davy-Mendez et al., 2018; Li et al., 2019; Lodi et al., 2018; Nance et al., 2018; Rhee et al., 2020a; Scherrer et al., 2016). Several laboratory-based studies have observed a decline in the proportion of submitted viruses with HIVDR and multiclass resistance (Kagan et al., 2019; Paquet et al., 2014), although much of this decrease reflects the likelihood that an increasing proportion of resistance test samples are from persons with newly diagnosed HIV rather than those with virologic failure. This is also supported by the decreasing proportion of PWH with extensive treatment histories (Bajema et al., 2019).

Nonetheless, adherence to a daily treatment regimen is a continuing challenge, particularly in populations that face logistical, social, and financial barriers to obtaining HIV care and accessing lifelong ARVs (Rich et al., 2020; Siefried et al., 2017, 2018). Moreover, despite the increased use of FDCs and ARVs with a high genetic barrier to resistance, such regimens are not available to many PWH, particularly those who have experienced previous virologic failure or who have coexisting medical conditions such as advanced liver/kidney disease that might preclude use of certain agents. A nationwide US surveillance study performed in 2017 reported that fewer than two-thirds of PWH had a suppressed viral load (Harris et al., 2019). The increasing practice of early ART administration and the anticipated use of long-acting ARVs—strategies designed to engage more PWH into care and to increase the proportion attaining long-term virologic suppression—may nonetheless pose an increased risk of ADR for some. As a result, ADR will remain a challenge for a significant proportion of PWH.

MANAGEMENT OF ADR

In PWH developing virologic failure on an initial ART regimen, those who develop HIVDR often have predictable patterns of DRMs. For example, persons receiving an NNRTI-containing regimen will usually have both NRTI- and NNRTI-associated DRMs, while those receiving a first-generation INSTI-containing regimen will often have both NRTI- and INSTI-associated DRMs (DHHS, 2020; Gregson et al., 2016; Rhee et al., 2020a). In these two scenarios, the most common NRTI-associated DRMs are the lamivudine (3TC)/emtricitabine (FTC) mutations M184V/I; additionally, approximately 30% of PWH will also develop a tenofovir-associated DRM (usually K65R or K70E/Q). In low- and middle-income countries, the proportion of persons developing a tenofovir-associated DRM on a first-line NRTI/NNRTI-containing regimen is higher and approaches 60% (Gregson et al., 2016). In contrast, among PWH receiving an initial boosted PI or second-generation INSTI-containing regimen, those who develop HIVDR will usually just acquire M184V/I (DHHS, 2020; Dolling et al., 2013; El Bouzidi et al., 2014; Lathouwers et al., 2020; Rhee et al., 2019b, 2020b; Scarsi et al., 2020). As a result of these predictable patterns, the DHHS has developed recommendations for first-line treatment failure scenarios: specific recommendations most commonly involve modifying therapy to include at least one active NRTI and either a second-generation INSTI or boosted darunavir (Table 20.4). McCluskey et al. (2019) have recently summarized published studies of second-line therapy; however, those often involved boosted lopinavir in combination with two NRTIs or raltegravir-based regimens that are no longer recommended in high-income countries; only one study involved dolutegravir plus two NRTIs (of which at least one had to be predicted to be active based on genotypic resistance testing) (Aboud et al., 2019).

In PWH who have experienced virologic failure on multiple ART regimens, the patterns of observed HIV-associated DRMs are often less predictable. In this scenario, the DHHS and IAS-USA guidelines recommend expert consultation and modification of therapy to include at least two fully active drugs from different ARV drug classes (DHHS, 2020; Saag et al., 2020). The vast majority of clinical trials performed in heavily treated PWH have been registration trials designed to study the impact of "salvage therapy" with ART regimens containing either boosted darunavir, boosted tipranavir, etravirine, dolutegravir, enfuvirtide, maraviroc, ibalizumab, or fostemsavir (McCluskey et al., 2019). Several additional trials have evaluated ART strategies that relied heavily on the use of the combination of boosted darunavir, raltegravir, and etravirine (Grinsztejn et al., 2019; Tashima et al., 2015; Yazdanpanah et al., 2009).

With the demonstration that both dolutegravir and boosted darunavir plus a single active NRTI are fully suppressive ART regimens, and with recent approval of several additional ARVs (i.e., doravirine, ibalizumab, fostemsavir), the prospects for constructing a fully suppressive regimen in nearly all PWH requiring salvage therapy are high. Among INSTI-naive PWH or among INSTI-experienced persons with viruses retaining complete susceptibility to dolutegravir, the combination of dolutegravir plus one fully active NRTI and/or fully active NNRTI (e.g., rilpivirine or doravirine) may be sufficient. Etravirine should not be combined with dolutegravir because it reduces dolutegravir levels, and guidelines recommend adding a boosted PI if etravirine and dolutegravir are used concurrently (DHHS, 2020). Bictegravir is also not used in this situation because, in contrast to dolutegravir, it has not been studied for salvage therapy and its dose cannot be doubled/adjusted to compensate for INSTI-related DRMs. Likewise, for PWH whose viruses retain complete or nearly complete susceptibility to boosted darunavir, the

CLINICAL SCENARIO	TYPE OF FAILING REGIMEN	HIVDR CONSIDERATIONS	NEW REGIMEN OPTIONS
First regimen failure	NNRTI + 2 NRTIs	Likely resistance to NNRTI ± XTC (i.e., NNRTI mutations ± M184V/I). Additional NRTI mutations may be present.	Boosted PI + 2 NRTIs (at least 1 active); *or* DTG + 2 NRTIs (at least one active); *or* Boosted PI + INSTI
	Boosted PI + 2 NRTIs	Most likely no resistance, or resistance limited to XTC (i.e., M184V/I without resistance to other NRTIs)	Continue same regimen; *or* Another boosted PI + 2 NRTIs (at least 1 active); *or* INSTI + 2 NRTIs (at least one active—if only one of the NRTIs is fully active or if adherence is a concern, DTG is preferred INSTI); *or* Another boosted PI + INSTI
	INSTI + 2 NRTIs	No INSTI resistance (can have XTC resistance, i.e., only M184V/I, usually without resistance to other NRTIs).	Boosted PI + 2 NRTIs (at least one active); *or* DTG + 2 NRTIs (at least one active); *or* Boosted PI + INSTI
		RAL or EVG ± XTC resistance. Resistance to first-line BIC or DTG is rare.	Boosted PI + 2 NRTIs (at least one active); *or* DTG twice daily (if virus is sensitive to DTG) + 2 active NRTIs; *or* DTG twice daily (if virus is sensitive to DTG) + boosted PI BIC has not been studied in this setting and therefore cannot be recommended.

XTC = 3TC/FTC; DTG = dolutegravir; RAL = raltegravir; EVG = elvitegravir; BIC = bictegravir; DRV = darunavir.

SOURCE: Panel on Antiretroviral Guidelines for Adults and Adolescents. Guidelines for the Use of Antiretroviral Agents in Adults and Adolescents with HIV. Department of Health and Human Services. Adapted from Table 11. Available at https://clinicalinfo.hiv.gov/sites/default/files/inline-files/AdultandAdolescentGL.pdf Accessed August 15, 2020.

combination of boosted darunavir plus one fully active NRTI and/or fully active NNRTI (e.g., etravirine or doravirine) may be sufficient.

In the presence of preexisting resistance to dolutegravir *and* boosted darunavir, current options for salvage therapy are more complicated. However, even in this scenario, there are several potentially useful treatment approaches, including the use of two or more drugs from the four main ARV classes and possibly the use of one or more entry inhibitors (Raymond et al., 2020).

Within the four main ARV classes, it should be possible to identify drugs with high genetic barriers to resistance that retain antiviral activity:

1. Boosted darunavir will likely retain significant activity because the prevalence of high-level boosted darunavir resistance has become increasingly rare (Brown et al., 2018). Although some boosted darunavir–resistant isolates will retain susceptibility to tipranavir, the overall lower inhibitory activity associated with tipranavir and its greater risk of toxicity (i.e., intracranial hemorrhage, severe hepatotoxicity) rarely make it a useful option.

2. INSTI-resistant viruses also often retain susceptibility to dolutegravir when dosed twice a day, although probably less often than they retain darunavir susceptibility (Akil et al., 2015; Castagna et al., 2014; Eron et al., 2013).

3. Few NRTI-resistant viruses will be highly resistant to tenofovir and resistant to AZT unless the sample contains the three TAMs M41L, L210W, and T215Y or one of the multiresistant DRM patterns (Parikh et al., 2006) (see Table 20.3). In the absence of these DRM patterns, tenofovir and/or zidovudine in combination with 3TC or FTC will likely retain residual activity. Although TAF yields approximately fourfold higher intracellular tenofovir triphosphate concentrations compared with TDF (Margot et al., 2020), these two prodrugs have not been compared for their use in salvage therapy.

4. Some NNRTI-resistant viruses may retain complete or partial susceptibility to etravirine or doravirine.

Among the entry inhibitors, enfuvirtide is a highly active treatment option for late salvage therapy, although it is now rarely used because of its requirement for twice-daily parenteral intramuscular administration. Although maraviroc is well tolerated, it is often not an option because highly treatment-experienced PWH tend to have advanced immunosuppression and an increased likelihood of harboring X4-tropic viruses. The postattachment inhibitor ibalizumab is almost certain to contribute to a salvage therapy regimen, although it is expensive and must be administered intravenously biweekly (Emu et al., 2018). In most PWH, fostemsavir may have a similar degree of antiviral activity as ibalizumab; however, a small subset of persons will harbor intrinsically resistant viruses (Kozal et al., 2020).

ARV RESISTANCE CONSIDERATIONS FOR SPECIAL CIRCUMSTANCES

There are a number of circumstances in which HIV treatment guidelines offer limited information on specific recommendations for evaluation and management of HIVDR. We will describe a few of these briefly.

ART SWITCH/SIMPLIFICATION (MODIFYING ART IN THE SETTING OF VIROLOGIC SUPPRESSION)

At times, providers and/or PWH may wish to consider changing a fully suppressive ARV regimen. This may be due to concerns regarding safety profile, side effects, new drug–drug interactions, pill burden, pregnancy status/intentions, or cost/access (including formulary changes). In these situations, providers should consider the person's complete treatment history and comprehensive resistance testing history to construct a cumulative resistance profile (DHHS, 2020; McCluskey et al., 2019; Saag et al., 2020). The fundamental clinical principle with regimen optimization/simplification is to maintain virologic suppression and not compromise future treatment options. If comprehensive resistance data are not available, clinicians may be able to extrapolate information from the treatment history—for example, a person with a history of virologic failure while taking ARVs with a relatively low barrier to resistance (most NNRTIs, first-generation INSTIs, lamivudine/emtricitabine) can be assumed to have accumulated resistance to these drugs (DHHS, 2020). Proviral DNA sequencing may be considered, but results should be interpreted with caution.

US guidelines list several specific optimization strategies that can be considered, based on available data, taking into account an individual's specific circumstance (e.g., reasons for considering a change in therapy, viral resistance profile, other concomitant disorders) (DHHS, 2020; Saag et al., 2020). Individuals with no suspected or documented history of HIVDR generally have multiple options for switching ARV drugs in their regimen, either between classes or within classes. However, clinicians should still exercise caution and generally avoid switching to an agent with a lower genetic barrier to resistance, given the risk of virologic failure if the patient actually has underlying TDR or ADR (DHHS, 2020; Eron et al., 2010). Of note, a number of two-drug regimens are currently identified as potential "switch" options; it would be especially prudent to have a high degree of confidence in a patient's full HIVDR profile when considering switching to a dual therapy regimen, to ensure that both ARV agents are active. For patients with a history of limited drug resistance, clinicians can consider a switch from one drug to another within the same class or in a different class, as long as the new drug has a high genetic barrier to resistance and there is no known or suspected resistance to the new agent. Based on data extrapolated from other studies, dolutegravir plus two NRTIs (one of which is fully active) should be effective as a switch strategy in virologically suppressed individuals without underlying dolutegravir resistance (DHHS, 2020).

Expert consultation may be especially helpful when considering regimen switching/simplification for PWH who are heavily ART-experienced, as individuals who have undergone multiple regimen modifications have often done so because of virologic failure and ADR (and often multiclass HIVDR development) (DHHS, 2020; Gudipati et al., 2020; Saag et al., 2020) (Table 20.5).

PREGNANCY AND YOUTH

The fundamental principles of HIVDR testing/evaluation and management for pregnant individuals and youth are the same as those in nonpregnant adults (i.e., perform drug resistance testing at diagnosis, at initiation or reinitiation of ART, and in the event of virologic failure) (DHHS, 2020).

With pregnancy, the main difference is the urgency of time: it is important to achieve virologic suppression early in pregnancy to minimize the risk of perinatal HIV transmission. Because resistance testing results can take multiple weeks, US guidelines recommend immediate ART initiation if HIV is diagnosed in pregnancy or in PWH who are not on ART when they become pregnant, even if resistance testing results are not yet available (DHHS, 2020). Initial therapy decisions should be guided by what is known about the person's previous ART regimens and responses, as well as previous resistance testing results, and should be modified (if indicated) once current resistance testing results are available—taking into account ARV safety and dosing in pregnancy. Pregnant persons who have documented zidovudine (ZDV) resistance should still receive intravenous ZDV during labor when indicated (i.e., HIV RNA >1,000 copies/mL near delivery).

Unique pregnancy-associated factors may increase the risk of incomplete viral suppression and HIVDR development, such as nausea and vomiting affecting adherence and pharmacokinetic changes such as increased plasma volume and renal clearance. Some ARVs require dose adjustment during pregnancy; US guidelines provide detailed information on use of specific ARVs in pregnancy. If perinatal HIV transmission does occur in the setting of incomplete maternal viral suppression, maternal HIVDR can be transmitted to the infant, limiting treatment options for the infant (Delaugerre et al., 2009). Decisions about ARV prophylaxis and/or treatment for infants exposed to drug-resistant virus should therefore be made in consultation with a pediatric HIV specialist.

For youth, one key consideration is that many acquired HIV perinatally and thus have been exposed to multiple ARVs. Because of limited infant and pediatric ARV treatment options and suboptimal adherence (often related to challenges of administering medications multiple times per day to younger individuals), many youth with HIV have experienced virologic failure on multiple regimens with development of ADR. For youth with known or suspected complex DRM patterns who are experiencing virologic failure, concurrent genotypic and phenotypic resistance testing should be considered. If maraviroc is being considered, coreceptor tropism testing should be obtained. In general, consultation with a pediatric HIV specialist is advisable when considering ART

Table 20.5 TREATMENT OPTIONS FOR OPTIMIZING ART IN THE SETTING OF VIROLOGIC SUPPRESSION

CLINICAL SCENARIO	TYPE OF SWITCH	STRATEGIES THAT HAVE EVIDENCE FOR SUCCESS
No suspected or documented HIVDR	Within-class switch	• TDF or ABC to TAF • RAL to DTG • DTG, EVG/c, or RAL to BIC • EFV to RPV or to DOR • Boosted ATV to unboosted ATV (when used with ABC/3TC)
	Between-class switch	• Replace a boosted PI with an INSTI (other than RAL) • Replace a boosted PI with RPV or DOR • Replace an NNRTI with an INSTI • Replace a boosted PI with MVC. When switching to MVC, coreceptor usage in patients with virologic suppression can be determined from proviral DNA.
	Switch from 3-drug to 2-drug regimen (both drugs should be fully active)	• DTG + RPV • DTG + 3TC • Boosted PI + 3TC • Boosted DRV + DTG
History of limited drug resistance	Within-class switch	• Switch from one drug with a high genetic barrier to resistance to another (i.e., from DTG to BIC) • Switch to a drug with a higher genetic barrier to resistance (i.e., from RAL to DTG or BIC)
	Between-class switch	• Switch from one drug with a high genetic barrier to resistance to another (i.e., from boosted PI to BIC or DTG) • Switch to a drug with a higher genetic barrier to resistance (i.e., from EFV to DTG or BIC or boosted PI)
History of complex underlying resistance	Proceed with caution; follow the same principles outlined under "Management of ADR" and consider expert consultation.	

TDF = tenofovir disoproxil fumarate; ABC = abacavir; TAF = tenofovir alafenamide; RAL = raltegravir; DTG = dolutegravir; EVG/c = elvitegravir/cobicistat; BIC = bictegravir; EFV = efavirenz; RPV = rilpivirine; DOR = doravarine; ATV = atazanavir; 3TC = lamivudine; MVC = maraviroc; DRV = darunavir

SOURCE: Panel on Antiretroviral Guidelines for Adults and Adolescents. Guidelines for the Use of Antiretroviral Agents in Adults and Adolescents with HIV. Department of Health and Human Services. Adapted from text. Available at http://www.aidsinfo.nih.gov/ContentFiles/AdultandAdolescentGL.pdf. Accessed August 15, 2020.

modification (including regimen switching/simplification) in infants and youth.

RAPID ART INITIATION AND RAPID ART REINITIATION

Rapid ART initiation immediately or very soon after HIV diagnosis is an approach that has gained increasing and widespread interest (Boyd et al., 2019). Individual clinical and public health benefits of rapid ART initiation include improved linkage to HIV medical care and ART uptake, decreased time to viral suppression, and decreased risk of HIV transmission to others (Ford et al., 2018; Mateo-Urdiales et al., 2019). Findings from several programs in the US as well as resource-limited settings have demonstrated its feasibility and acceptability (Coffey et al., 2019; Colasanti et al., 2018; Martin et al., 2020; Rodriguez et al., 2019). US guidelines currently recommend initiating ART at the time of diagnosis (when possible) or soon afterwards "to increase the uptake of ART, decrease the time required to achieve linkage to care and virologic suppression, and improve the rate of virologic suppression among individuals who have recently received HIV diagnoses" (DHHS, 2020).

Since regimen selection for rapid ART initiation occurs prior to the availability of baseline resistance testing results,

rapid ART options should have a suitably high likelihood of effectiveness and favorable safety and side-effect profiles; local TDR patterns may also need to be considered. To date, the most commonly used rapid ART combination options in the US include tenofovir (TDF or TAF, depending on clinical history and medication availability) plus emtricitabine (or lamivudine), paired with either a second-generation integrase inhibitor (i.e., bictegravir or dolutegravir) or (less frequently) once-daily boosted darunavir. If baseline resistance testing subsequently indicates potentially compromised ARV activity of any components of the selected regimen, providers are generally advised to consider treatment modification or, at minimum, frequent viral load monitoring until stable virologic suppression has been established. Most rapid ART studies have not provided detailed information on the frequency of, or reasons for, ART adjustments after initiation (Mateo-Urdiales et al., 2019), and very little has been published regarding the impact of baseline mutations on the efficacy of preselected rapid ART regimens. One study indicated ART was modified in less than 3% of participants after baseline genotype testing demonstrated transmitted resistance mutations (Coffey et al., 2019).

As of August 2020, the only specific medication recommendations provided in US guidelines on rapid ART selection were to avoid NNRTI-based regimens, abacavir, and the dual therapy combination of dolutegravir plus lamivudine. Preliminary findings of a single-arm study evaluating rapid ART initiation with dolutegravir plus lamivudine were released in fall 2020 (Rolle et al., 2020). Although some participants were able to achieve a viral load of less than 50 copies/mL at 6 months, further investigation and "real world" clinical experience (i.e., outside the context of a clinical trial) are warranted before this dual combination should be considered as an option for rapid ART initiation, especially given the potential impact of TDR on two-drug initial therapy approaches (Kessler et al., 2020).

For patients with chronic HIV infection who have been out of care and/or off ART, "rapid ART reinitiation" decisions may not be straightforward, especially if limited history is available. Depending on the individual's prior HIV treatment, some providers would consider obtaining resistance testing at the first clinical reengagement visit; however, as indicated earlier, testing performed in the absence of recent ART use may be of limited utility. Although it may provide useful information to guide therapy modification *after* rapid ART reinitiation (in the event that DRMs are identified), historically selected mutations may not be reflected accurately without the presence of selective drug pressure. In other words, the absence of detectable resistance must be viewed cautiously when interpreting results. Therefore, for treatment-experienced patients (especially heavily ART-experienced individuals), providers should obtain as much historical information as possible. Specific suggested practices include verifying pharmacy dispensing records, utilizing ART medication charts to see which agents are recognized, and obtaining prior medical records, including all resistance testing results.

For PWH who report achieving and maintaining an undetectable viral load on their last combination and who did not take ART intermittently before stopping (i.e., the provider has no concern for prior virologic failure), the same combination may potentially be considered for "rapid ART reinitiation" if no current contraindications are identified. Alternatively, providers/patients may wish to modify the patient's anchor agent by utilizing a newer drug within the same class if desired and clinically appropriate, or could consider one of the "rapid ART initiation" options described earlier if no resistance is suspected. In general, expert input is recommended for "rapid ART reinitiation" decisions since multiple factors should be taken into account (e.g., prior ART exposure and responses, previous resistance testing results, concern for potential untreated central nervous system opportunistic infections). After reinitiating therapy, and if the viral load does not decrease as anticipated, providers should have a low threshold to repeat resistance testing to guide further management.

HIV ACQUISITION IN THE SETTING OF PREP USE

There have been two main concerns regarding PrEP and HIVDR: (1) whether PrEP will remain effective in areas with high TDR prevalence and (2) whether PrEP will lead to an increased number of cases of HIVDR. Regarding the first issue, many studies have shown that the transmission of viruses resistant to tenofovir and/or 3TC/FTC is uncommon, with M184V/I occurring in 0.8% and K65R occurring in 0.1% of newly diagnosed PWH in the US (McClung et al., 2020). Likewise, approximately 0.5% of newly diagnosed PWH in the US are predicted to have cabotegravir resistance (McClung et al., 2020). However, among PWH experiencing virologic failure, approximately 15% have genotypic resistance to 3TC/FTC and/or tenofovir, while approximately 5% have genotypic resistance to cabotegravir. Therefore, the risk of PrEP failure will likely be higher if a PrEP user is directly infected with a virus transmitted from a PWH who is experiencing virologic failure.

Regarding the second concern of whether widespread PrEP use will increase HIVDR, data from PrEP clinical trials have indicated that there are two scenarios in which HIVDR can emerge: (1) persons who are undergoing acute infection at the time of PrEP initiation and (2) persons who acquire infection at a later time point (usually as a result of PrEP nonadherence). However, when HIVDR does occur, it is nearly always associated with M184V/I and 3TC/FTC resistance and very rarely with K65R and tenofovir resistance. A review of PrEP clinical trials reported that among persons who acquired HIV while receiving PrEP, about 5% had M184V/I and about 0.5% had K65R (Parikh & Mellors, 2016). "Real world" experience from New York City has suggested that the frequency of M184V/I is likely to be higher in clinical practice, with 29% of 71 persons with a new HIV diagnosis and a history of PrEP having M184V/I (compared with 2% in non-PrEP users) (Cox et al., 2020; Misra et al., 2019).

Importantly, baseline confirmation of negative HIV status via clinical assessment for acute HIV and standard HIV testing using reliable screening assays/algorithms and routine retesting remain the cornerstone for appropriate PrEP initiation and continuation. Nucleic acid testing may also be warranted in certain scenarios. Further, as newer agents (e.g., long-acting injectable cabotegravir) are investigated and utilized, the implications of HIVDR with PrEP may need to be further considered, especially in cases of HIV acquisition among persons who have been exposed to these novel ARV medications.

RESOURCE-LIMITED SETTINGS (LOW- AND MIDDLE-INCOME COUNTRIES)

The primary differences regarding evaluation and management of HIVDR between high-income countries and low-/middle-income countries include (1) the absence of universal access to routine genotypic resistance testing; (2) less frequent viral load monitoring; (3) high prevalence of infants and children with perinatally acquired HIV infection whose treatment options are limited due to transmitted or acquired DRMs; and (4) the large proportion of PWH who have failed first-line therapy (i.e., with resultant development of dual NRTI–NNRTI resistance) or who have failed first-*and* second-line therapy, with subsequent three-class drug resistance.

Pretreatment drug resistance refers to DRMs that are detected in PWH before they start ART. This may arise with either transmission of a drug-resistant strain (i.e., TDR) or DRMs due to previous ART exposure, such as with perinatal/postpartum ART use, preexposure or postexposure prophylaxis, or interrupted first-line ART. For low- and middle-income countries, global surveillance data have indicated a notable rise in pretreatment resistance to NNRTIs after ART scale-up, primarily due to use of first-generation NNRTIs with a low genetic barrier to resistance. Although the recent introduction of dolutegravir in many of these countries carries potential for improved individual and public health outcomes, concurrent scale-up of viral load and resistance testing may also be necessary to avoid inadvertently placing ART-experienced PWH on functional dolutegravir monotherapy. In addition, other prevalent, serious health conditions (i.e., tuberculosis coinfection) raise important and unique clinical challenges in resource-limited settings. The 2017–2021 WHO Global Action Plan for HIV drug resistance provides a framework to prevent HIVDR from undermining efforts to achieve desired public health outcomes in heavily impacted countries (Hamers et al., 2018).

HIV-2

HIV-2 infection (and HIV-1/-2 coinfection) remains rare in the US. However, HIV-2 is endemic in many regions experiencing high overall HIV prevalence, such as West Africa; providers should thus have some basic clinical knowledge of HIV-2. HIV-2 has demonstrated intrinsic, high-level resistance to NNRTIs and enfuvirtide. PIs exhibit variable activity against HIV-2: boosted lopinavir and darunavir are believed to have the most clinically useful potency. HIV-2 is susceptible to INSTIs as well as all NRTIs currently in clinical use; however, data suggest differences in INSTI and NRTI mutation selection and HIVDR mechanisms/pathways between HIV-2 and HIV-1 (Boyer et al., 2012; Gottlieb et al., 2009; Requena et al., 2017; Tzou et al., 2020). Outcomes of recent trials involving first- and second-generation INSTIs and PI-based regimens will help provide more evidence to shape first-line HIV-2 treatment recommendations (Gottlieb et al., 2018). Although the natural history of HIV-2 suggests lower virulence and less severe disease progression compared to HIV-1, RT, PR, and IN mutations all have been observed in ARV-naive as well as treatment-experienced persons. This highlights the need for ongoing surveillance efforts and clinical vigilance for HIV-2–related DRMs (Tzou et al., 2020). HIV-2 drug resistance testing is not commercially available in the US, but some research laboratories (e.g., University of Washington) have limited capacity to perform genotype testing under research protocols.

CONCLUSION

ADR and, to a lesser extent, TDR continue to pose challenges to the successful treatment of PWH. In the absence of selective drug pressure, DRMs can quickly be replaced by wild-type variants, so resistance testing should be performed as close to HIV diagnosis as possible and, ideally, while patients are still on ART when virologic failure is identified. Any DRMs identified should be documented and taken into account when considering ART reinitiation or modification. In most situations, genotypic testing is preferred over phenotypic testing. However, phenotypic testing can be helpful as an addition to genotypic testing in persons who have developed virologic failure on multiple treatment regimens or who have complicated DRM patterns. PBMC DNA sequencing, often known as "archive" genotyping, can be useful for ART switch/simplification in patients who are virologically suppressed on their current regimen, but results should be interpreted with caution. Management of ADR and TDR should take into account HIV-specific factors as well as non-HIV-specific factors to construct a clinically appropriate regimen that includes at least two fully active drugs from different ARV drug classes. With modern ARV options, almost all patients with ADR and TDR should still be able to access fully suppressive ART, although medication adherence may continue to pose challenges and should be an ongoing focus for HIV care teams. Rapid ART, HIV acquisition in the setting of recent PrEP use, virologic failure in highly treatment-experienced patients, and ART switch/simplification can all pose unique challenges for clinicians, and various resources are available to help guide treatment decisions.

REFERENCES

Aboud M, Kaplan R, Lombaard J, et al. Dolutegravir versus ritonavir-boosted lopinavir both with dual nucleoside reverse transcriptase inhibitor therapy in adults with HIV-1 infection in whom first-line therapy has failed (DAWNING): an open-label, non-inferiority, phase 3b trial. *Lancet Infect Dis.* 2019;19:253–264.

Abram ME, Ferris AL, Shao W, et al. Nature, position, and frequency of mutations made in a single cycle of HIV-1 replication. *J Virol.* 2010;84(19):9864–9878.

Akil B, Blick G, Hagins DP, et al. Dolutegravir versus placebo in subjects harbouring HIV-1 with integrase inhibitor resistance associated substitutions: 48-week results from VIKING-4, a randomized study. *Antivir Ther.* 2015;20:343–348.

Allavena C, Rodallec A, Leplat A, et al. Interest of proviral HIV-1 DNA genotypic resistance testing in virologically suppressed patients candidate for maintenance therapy. *J Virol Methods.* 2018;251:106–110.

Antiretroviral Therapy Cohort Collaboration. Survival of HIV-positive patients starting antiretroviral therapy between 1996 and 2013: a collaborative analysis of cohort studies. *Lancet HIV.* 2017;4:e349–e356.

Armenia D, Zaccarelli M, Borghi V, et al. Resistance detected in PBMCs predicts virological rebound in HIV-1 suppressed patients switching treatment. *J Clin Virol.* 2018;104:61–64.

Avila-Rios S, Garcia-Moralis C, Matias-Florentino M, et al.; HIVDR MexNet Group. Pretreatment HIV-drug resistance in Mexico and its impact on the effectiveness of first-line antiretroviral therapy: a nationally representative 2015 WHO survey. *Lancet HIV.* 2016;3:e57–591.

Avila-Rios S, Parkin N, Swanstrom R, et al. Next-generation sequencing for HIV drug resistance testing: laboratory, clinical, and implementation considerations. *Viruses.* 2020;12(6):617.

Avila-Rios S, Sued O, Rhee SY, et al. Surveillance of HIV transmitted drug resistance in Latin America and the Caribbean: a systematic review and meta-Analysis. *PLoS One.* 2016;11:e0158560.

Bachmann N, von Braun A, Labhardt ND, et al. Importance of routine viral load monitoring: higher levels of resistance at ART failure in Uganda and Lesotho compared with Switzerland. *J Antimicrob Chemother*. 2019;74(2):468–472.

Bajema KL, Nance RM, Delaney JAC, et al. Changing rates of heavily treatment experienced persons with HIV in the United States, 2000–2017 [Abstract MOPEB246]. Presented at the 10th International AIDS Society Conference on HIV Science, Mexico City, 2019. http://programme.ias2019.org/Abstract

Bennett DE, Camacho RJ, Otelea D, et al. Drug resistance mutations for surveillance of transmitted HIV-1 drug resistance: 2009 update. *PLoS One*. 2009;4(3):e4724,

Blair HA. Ibalizumab: a review in multidrug-resistant HIV-1 infection. *Drugs*. 2010;80:189–196.

Boltz VF, Zheng Y, Lockman S, et al. Role of low-frequency HIV-1 variants in failure of nevirapine-containing antiviral therapy in women previously exposed to single-dose nevirapine. *Proc Natl Acad Sci USA*. 2011;108:9202–9207.

Borghetti A, Cicculo A, Lombardi F, et al. Transmitted drug resistance to NRTIs and risk of virological failure in naïve patients treated with integrase inhibitors. *HIV Med*. 2021;22(1):22–27.

Boukli N, Boyd A, Collot M, et al. Utility of HIV-1 DNA genotype in determining antiretroviral resistance in patients with low or undetectable HIV RNA viral loads. *J Antimicrob Chemother*. 2018;73(11):3129–3136.

Boyd MA, Boffito M, Castagna A, et al. Rapid initiation of antiretroviral therapy at HIV diagnosis: definition, process, knowledge gaps. *HIV Med*. 2019;20(supp 1):3–11.

Boyer PL, Clark PJ, Hughes SH. HIV-1 and HIV-2 reverse transcriptases: different mechanisms of resistance to nucleoside reverse transcriptase inhibitors. *J Virol*. 2012;86(10):5885–5894.

Brown K, Steward L, Whitcomb JM, et al. Prevalence of darunavir resistance in the United States from 2010 to 2017. *AIDS Res Human Retroviruses*. 2018;34:1036–1043.

Carr A, Richardson R, Liu Z. Success and failure of initial antiretroviral therapy in adult: an updated systematic review. *AIDS*. 2019;33(3):443–453.

Castagna A, Maggiolo F, Penco G, et al. Dolutegravir in antiretroviral-experienced patients with raltegravir-and/or elvitegravir-resistant HIV-1: 24-week results of the Phase III VIKING-3 Study. *J Infect Dis*. 2014;210:354–362.

Castro H, Pillay D, Cane P et al.; UK Collaborative Group on HIV Drug Resistance. Persistence of HIV-1 transmitted drug resistance mutations. *J Infect Dis*. 2013;208:1459–1463.

Clutter DS, Zhou S, Varghese V, et al. Prevalence of drug resistant minority variants in untreated HIV-1-infected individuals with and those without transmitted drug resistance detected by Sanger sequencing. *J Infect Dis*. 2017;216(3):387–391.

Coffey S, Baccheti P, Sachdev D, et al. RAPID antiretroviral therapy: high virologic suppression rates with immediate antiretroviral therapy initiation in a vulnerable urban clinic population. *AIDS*. 2019;33(5):825–832.

Coffin JM. HIV population dynamics in vivo: implications for genetic variation, pathogenesis, and therapy. *Science*. 1995;267(5197):483–489.

Colasanti J, Sumitani J, Mehta CC, et al. Implementation of a rapid entry program decreases time to viral suppression among vulnerable persons living with HIV in the Southern United States. *Open Forum Infect Dis*. 2018;5(6):ofy104.

Cox S, Parukh U, Heaps A, et al. Deep sequencing with unique molecular identifiers for evaluation of HIV-1 drug resistance in the DISOCVER pre-exposure prophylaxis trial [Abstract PBD404]. Presented at the 23rd International AIDS Conference (Virtual), 2020.

Cozzi-Lepri A, Noguera-Julian M, Di Giallonardo F; CHAIN Minority HIV-1 Variants Working Group. Low-frequency drug-resistant HIV-1 and risk of virological failure to first-line NNRTI-based ART: a multicohort European case-control study using centralized ultrasensitive 454 pyrosequencing. *J Antimicrob Chemother*. 2015;70:930–940.

Curanovic D, Martens S, Rodriguez M, et al. HIV-1 DNA testing in viremic patients demonstrates a greater ability to detect drug resistance compared to plasma virus testing [Abstract PDB0402]. Presented at the 23rd International AIDS Conference (Virtual), 2020. https://www.aids2020.org/

Dauwe K, Staelens D, Vancoillie L, et al. Deep sequencing of HIV-1 RNA and DNA in newly diagnosed patients with baseline drug resistance showed no indications for hidden resistance and is biased by strong interference of hypermutation. *J Clin Microbiol*. 2016;54:1605–1615.

Davy-Mendez T, Eron JJ, Brunet L, et al. New antiretroviral agent use affects prevalence of HIV drug resistance in clinical care populations. *AIDS*. 2018;32(17):2593–2603.

Deeks SF, Wrin T, Liegler T, et al. Virologic and immunologic consequences of discontinuing combination antiretroviral-drug therapy in HIV-infected patients with detectable viremia. *N Engl J Med*. 2001;344:472–480.

Delaugerre C, Bruan J, Charreau I, et al.; ANRS 138-EASIER Study Group. Comparison of resistance mutation patterns in historical plasma HIV RNA genotypes with those in current proviral HIV DNA genotypes among extensively treated patients with suppressed replication. *HIV Med*. 2012:13:517–525.

Delaugerre C, Chaix ML, Blanche S, et al.; ANRS French Perinatal Cohort. Perinatal acquisition of drug-resistant HIV-1 infection mechanisms and long-term outcome. *Retrovirology*. 2009;6:85.

De Meyer S, Vangeneugden T, Van Baelen B, et al. Resistance profile of darunavir: combined 24-week results from the POWER trials. *AIDS Res Human Retroviruses*. 2008;24(3):379–388.

Department of Health and Human Services (DHHS). Panel on Antiretroviral Guidelines for Adults and Adolescents. Guidelines for the Use of Antiretroviral Agents in Adults and Adolescents with HIV. 2020. https://clinicalinfo.hiv.gov/sites/default/files/inline-files/AdultandAdolescentGL.pdf

Derache A, Shin HS, Balamane M, et al. HIV drug resistance mutations in proviral DNA from a community treatment program. *PLoS One*. 2015;10(1):30117430.

Devereux HL, Loveday C, Youle M, et al. Substantial correlation between HIV type 1 drug-associated resistance mutations in plasma and peripheral blood mononuclear cells in treatment-experienced patients. *AIDS Res Human Retroviruses*. 2000;16(11):1025–1030.

Devereux HL, Youle M, Johnson MA, et al. Rapid decline in detectability of HIV-1 drug resistance mutations after stopping therapy. *AIDS*. 1999;13:123–127.

Dolling DI, Dunn DT, Sutherland KA, et al.; UHDRD (UKHDRD) and the UCHCS (UK). Low frequency of genotypic resistance in HIV-1-infected patients failing an atazanavir-containing regimen: a clinical cohort study. *J Antimicrob Chemother*. 2013;68:2339–2343.

Drescher SM, von Wyl V, Yang WL, et al. Treatment-naïve individuals are the major source of transmitted HIV-1 drug resistance in men who have sex with men in the Swiss HIV Cohort Study. *Clin Infect Dis*. 2014;58(2):285–294.

Eberle J, Gurtler L. The evolution of drug resistance interpretation algorithms: ANRS, REGA and extension of resistance analysis to HIV-1 group O and HIV-2. *Intervirology*. 2012a;55(2):128–133.

Eberle J, Gurtler L. HIV types, groups, subtypes and recombinant forms: errors in replication, selection pressure and quasispecies. *Intervirology*. 2012b;55:79–83.

El Bouzidi K, White E, Mbisa JL, et al. Protease mutations emerging on darunavir in protease inhibitor-naïve and experienced patients in the UK. *J Int AIDS Soc*. 2014;17:19739. doi:10.7448/IAS.17.4.19739

Ellis KE, Nawas GT, Chan C, et al. Clinical outcomes following the use of archived proviral HIV-1 DNA genotype to guide antiretroviral therapy adjustment. *Open Forum Infect Dis*. 2019;7(1):ofz533.

Elvstam O, Medstrand P, Yilmaz A, et al. Virological failure and all-cause mortality in HIV-positive adults with low-level viremia during antiretroviral treatment. *PLoS One*. 2017;12(7): e0180761.

Emu B, Fessel K, Schrader S, et al. Phase 3 study of ibalizumab for multidrug-resistant HIV-1. *N Engl J Med*. 2018;379:645–654.

Eron JJ, Clotet B, Durant J, et al.; VIKING Study Group. Safety and efficacy of dolutegravir in treatment-experienced subjects with raltegravir-resistant HIV type 1 infection: 24-week results of the VIKING study. *J Infect Dis*. 2013;207:740–748.

Eron JJ, Young B, Cooper DA, et al. Switch to a raltegravir-based regimen versus continuation of a lopinavir-ritonavir-based regimen in stable HIV-infected patients with suppressed viraemic (SWITCHMRK 1 and 2): two multicenter-double-blind, randomized controlled trials. *Lancet*. 2010;375(9712):396–407.

Fleming J, Mathews WC, Rutstein RM, et al.; HIV Research Network. Low-level viremia and virologic failure in persons with HIV infection treated with antiretroviral therapy. *AIDS*. 2019;33:2005–2012.

Ford N, Migone C, Calmy A, et al. Benefits and risks of rapid initiation of antiretroviral therapy. *AIDS*. 2018;32(1):17–23.

Geretti AM, White E, Orkin C, et al. Virological outcomes of boosted protease inhibitor-based first-line ART in subjects harbouring thymidine analogue-association mutations as the sole form of transmitted drug resistance. *J Antimicrob Chemother*. 2019;74:746–753.

Gonzalez-Serna A, Min JE, Woods C, et al. Performance of HIV-1 drug resistance testing at low-level viremia and its ability to predict future virologic outcomes and viral evolution in treatment-naïve individuals. *Clin Infect Dis*. 2014;58:1165–1173.

Gottlieb GS, Dia Badiane NM, Hawed SE, et al.; University of Washington-Dakar HIV-2 Study Group. Emergence of multiclass drug resistance in HIV-2 in antiretroviral-treated individuals in Senegal: implications for HIV-2 treatment in resource-limited West Africa. *Clin Infect Dis*. 2009;48(4):476–483.

Gottlieb GS, Raugi DN, Smith RA. 90-90-90 for HIV-2? Ending the HIV-2 epidemic by enhancing care and clinical management of patients infected with HIV-2. *Lancet HIV*. 2018;5(7):e390–e399.

Gregson J, Tang M, Ndembi N, et al.; TenoRes Study Group. Global epidemiology of drug resistance after failure of WHO recommended first-line regimens for adult HIV-1 infection: a multicentre retrospective cohort study. *Lancet Infect Dis*. 2016;16(5):565–575.

Grinsztejn B, Hughes MD, Ritz J, et al. Third-line antiretroviral therapy in low-income and middle-income countries (ACTG A5288): a prospective strategy study. *Lancet HIV*. 2019;6:e588–e600.

Gudipati S, Brar I, Hanna Z, et al. Significance of archived HIV resistant associated mutations in the era of two drug ART therapy [Abstract #PEB0118]. Presented at the International AIDS Conference (Virtual), 2020. https://programme.aids2020.org

Günthard HF, Calvez V, Paredes R, et al. Human immunodeficiency virus drug resistance: 2018 recommendations of the International Antiviral Society–USA Panel. *Clin Infect Dis*. 2019;68(2):177–187.

Gupta RK, Gregson J, Parkin N, et al. HIV-1 drug resistance before initiation or re-initiation of first-line antiretroviral therapy in low-income and middle-income countries: a systematic review and meta-regression analysis. *Lancet Infect Dis*. 2018;18:346–355.

Hamers R, Rinke de Wit TF, Holmes CB. HIV drug resistance in low-income and middle-income countries. *Lancet HIV*. 2018;5(10):e588–e596.

Harris NS, Johnson AS, Huang YA, et al. Vital signs: status of human immunodeficiency virus testing, viral suppression, and HIV preexposure prophylaxis—United States, 2013–2018. *MMWR Morb Mortal Wkly Rep*. 2019;68:1117–1123.

Hermans LE, Moorhouse M, Carmona S, et al. Effect of HIV-1 low-level viraemia during antiretroviral therapy on treatment outcomes in WHO-guided South African treatment programmes: a muticentre cohort study. *Lancet Infect Dis*. 2018;18(2):130–131.

Huber M, Metzner KJ, Geissberger FD, et al. A rapid and versatile tool for HIV-1 drug resistance genotyping by deep sequencing. *J Virol Methods*. 2017;240:7–13.

Hyle EP, Scott JA, Sax PE, et al. Clinical impact and cost-effectiveness of genotype testing at human immunodeficiency virus diagnosis in the US. *Clin Infect Dis*. 2020;70(7):1353–1363.

Inzaule SC, Hamers RL, Noguera-Julian M, et al. Clinically relevant thresholds for ultrasensitive HIV drug resistance testing: a multicountry nested case-control study. *Lancet HIV*. 2018;5:e638–e646.

Jabara CB, Jones CD, Roach J, et al. Accurate sampling and deep sequencing of the HIV-1 protease gene using a primer ID. *Proc Natl Acad Sci USA*. 2011;108(50):20166–20171.

Jain V, Sucupira MC, Bacchetti P, et al. Differential persistence of transmitted HIV-1- drug resistance mutation classes. *J Infect Dis*. 2011;203:1174–1181.

Joya C, Won SH, Schofield C, et al. Persistent low-level viremia while on antiretroviral therapy is an independent risk factor for virologic failure. *Clin Infect Dis*. 2019;69(12):2145–2152.

Kagan RM, Dunn KJ, Snell GP, et al. Trends in HIV-1 drug resistance mutations from a U.S. reference laboratory from 2006 to 2017. *AIDS Res Hum Retroviruses*. 2019;35(8):698–709.

Kempf DF, Isaacson JD. King MS, et al. Analysis of the virological response with respect to baseline viral phenotype and genotype in protease inhibitor-experienced HIV-1-infected patients receiving lopinavir/ritonavir therapy. *Antivir Ther*. 2002;7:165–174.

Kessler HH, Stelzl E, Blazic A, et al. Antiretroviral treatment simplification with 2-drug regimens: impact of transmitted drug resistance mutations. *Open Forum Infect Dis*. 2020;7(1):ofz535.

Knyphausen F, Scheufele R, Kücherer C, et al. First line treatment response in patients with transmitted HIV drug resistance and well defined time point of HIV infection: updated results from the German HIV-1 Seroconverter Study. *PLoS One*. 2014;9:e95956.

Kozal M, Aberg J, Pialoux G, et al. Fostemsavir in adults with multidrug-resistant HIV-1 infection. *N Engl J Med*. 2020;382:1232–1243.

Lanier ER, Ait-Khaled M, Scott J, et al. Antiviral efficacy of abacavir in antiretroviral therapy-experienced adults harbouring HIV-1 with specific patterns of resistance to nucleoside reverse transcriptase inhibitors. *Antivir Ther*. 2004;9:37–45.

Lapointe HR, Dong W, Lee GQ, et al. High drug resistance testing by high-multiplex "wide" sequencing on the MiSeq instrument. *Antimicrob Agents Chemother*. 2015;59:6824–6833.

Lathouwers E, Seyedkazemi S, Lou D, et al. Pooled resistance analyses of darunavir once-daily regimens and formulations across 10 clinical studies of treatment-naïve and treatment-experienced patients with human immunodeficiency virus-1 infection. *HIV Res Clin Prac*. 2020;21:83–89.

Levy DN, Aldrovandi GM, Kutsch O, et al. Dynamics of HIV-1 recombination in its natural target cells. *Proc Natl Acad Sci USA*. 2004;101:4204–4209.

Li JZ, Gallien S, Do TD, et al. Prevalence and significance of HIV-1 drug resistance mutations among patients on antiretroviral therapy with detectable low-level viremia. *Antimicrob Agents Chemother*. 2012;56(11):5998–6000.

Li JZ, Paredes R, Ribaudo H, et al. Minority HIV-1 drug resistance mutations and the risk of NNRTI-based antiretroviral treatment failure: a systematic review and pooled analysis. *JAMA*. 2011;305(13):1327–1335.

Li X, Brown TT, Ho KS, et al. Recent trends and effectiveness of antiretroviral regimens among men who have sex with men living with HIV in the United States: the Multicenter AIDS Cohort Study (MACS) 2008-2017. *Open Forum Infect Dis*. 2019;6:ofz333. doi:10.1093/ofid/ofz333

Llibre JM, Arribas JR, Domingo P, et al. Clinical implications of fixed-dose coformulations of antiretrovirals on the outcome of HIV-1 therapy. *AIDS*. 2011;25(14):1683–1690.

Lodi S, Gunthard HF, Dunn D, et al. Effect of immediate initiation of antiretroviral treatment on the risk of acquired HIV drug resistance. *AIDS*. 2018;32(3):327–335.

Lubke N, Di Cristanziano V, Sierra S, et al.; Resina Study Group. Proviral DNA as a target for HIV-1 resistance analysis. *Intervirology*. 2015;58:184–189.

Machnowska P, Meixenberger K, Schmidt D, et al.; German HIV-1 Seroconverted Study Group. Prevalence and persistence of transmitted drug resistance mutations in the German HIV-1 Seroconverter Study Cohort. *PLoS One*. 2019;14(1):e0209605.

Mackie NE, Phillips AN, Kaye S, et al.; UK Resistance Database and the UK Collaborative HIV Cohort Study. Antiretroviral drug resistance in HIV-1-infected patients with low-level viremia. *J Infect Dis*. 2010;210(9):1303–1307.

Margot N, Ram R, Abram M, et al. Antiviral activity of tenofovir alafenamide against HIV-1 with thymidine analog-associated mutations and M184V. *Antimicrob Agents Chemother.* 2020;64(4): e02557-19.

Margot N, Ram R, McNicholl I, et al. Differential detection of M184V/I between plasma historical HIV genotypes and HIV proviral DNA from PBMCs. *J Antimicrob Chemother.* 2020;75:2249–2252.

Margot NA, Wong P, Kulkarni R, et al. Commonly transmitted HIV-1 drug resistance mutations in reverse-transcriptase and protease in antiretroviral treatment-naïve patients and response to regimens containing tenofovir disoproxil fumarate or tenofovir alafenamide. *J Infect Dis.* 2017;215(6):920–927.

Martin TCS, Abrams M, Anderson C, et al. Rapid antiretroviral therapy among individuals with acute and early HIV. *Clin Infect Dis.* 2020;ciaa1174. doi:10.1093/cid/ciaa1174

Mateo-Urdiales A, Johnson S, Smith R, et al. Rapid initiation of antiretroviral therapy for people living with HIV. *Cochrane Database Syst Rev.* 2019;6(6):CD012962.

Mbunkah HA, Bertagnolio S, Hamers RL; WHO HIVResNet Working Group. Low-abundance drug-resistant HIV-1 variants in antiretroviral drug-native individuals: a systematic review of detection methods, prevalence, and clinical impact. *J Infect Dis.* 2020;221:1584–1597.

McClung RP, Ocfemia CB, Saduvala N, et al. Integrase and other transmitted HIV drug resistance: 23 US jurisdictions, 2013–2016 [Abstract 3337]. Presented at the Conference on Retroviruses and Opportunistic Infections, Seattle, WA, 2019. https://www.croiconference.org/search-abstracts/

McClung RP, Ocfemia CB, Saduvala N, et al. U.S. HIV drug resistance: implications for current and future PrEP regimens [Abstract 512]. Presented at the Conference on Retroviruses and Opportunistic Infections, Boston, MA, 2020. https://www.croiconference.org/search-abstracts/

McCluskey SM, Siedner MJ, Marconi VC. Management of virologic failure and HIV drug resistance. *Infect Dis Clin North Am.* 2019;33(3):707–742.

Metzner KJ, Rauch P, von Wyl, et al. Efficient suppression of minority drug-resistant HIV type 1 (HIV-1) variants present at primary HIV-1 infection by ritonavir-boosted protease inhibitor-containing antiretroviral therapy. *J Infect Dis.* 2010;201:1063–1071.

Miller MD, Margot N, Lu B, et al. Genotypic and phenotypic predictors of the magnitude of response to tenofovir disoproxil fumarate treatment in antiretroviral-experienced patients. *J Infect Dis.* 2004;189:837–846.

Misra K, Huang J, Daskalakis DC, et al. Impact of PrEP on drug resistance and acute HIV infection, New York City, 2015–2017 [Abstract 107]. Presented at the Conference on Retroviruses and Opportunistic Infections, Seattle, WA, 2019. https://www.croiconference.org/search-abstracts/

Nance RM, Delaney JAC, Simoni JM, et al. HIV viral suppression trends over time among HIV-infected patients receiving care in the United States, 1997 to 2015. *Ann Intern Med.* 2018;169:376–384.

Noguera-Julian M, Edgil D, Harrigan PR, et al. Next-generation human immunodeficiency virus sequencing for patient management and drug resistance surveillance. *J Infect Dis.* 2017;216(suppl 9):S829–S833.

Obermeier M, Pironti A, Berg T, et al. HIV-GRADE: a publicly available, rules-based drug resistance interpretation algorithm integrating bioinformatics knowledge. *Intervirology.* 2012;55:102–107.

Paquet AC, Solberg OD, Napolitano LA, et al. A decade of HIV-1 drug resistance in the United States: trends and characteristics in a large protease/reverse transcriptase and co-receptor tropism database from 2003 to 2012. *Antivir Ther.* 2014;19:435–441.

Paredes R, Tzou PL, van Zyl G, et al. Collaborative update of a rule-based expert system for HIV-1genotypic resistance test interpretation. *PLoS One.* 2017;12(7):e0181357.

Parikh UM, Bacheler L, Koontz D, et al. The K65R mutation in human immunodeficiency virus type 1 reverse transcriptase exhibits bidirectional phenotypic antagonism with thymidine analog mutations. *J Virol.* 2006;80:4971–4977.

Parikh UM, Mellors JW. Should we fear resistance from tenofovir/emtricitabine preexposure prophylaxis? *Curr Opin HIV AIDS.* 2016;11:49–55.

Parkin NT, Hellmann NS, Whitcomb JM, et al. Natural variation of drug susceptibility in wild-type human immunodeficiency virus type 1. *Antimicrob Agents Chemother.* 2004;48:437–443.

Petropoulos CJ, Parkin NT, Limoli KL, et al. A novel phenotypic drug susceptibility assay for human immunodeficiency virus type 1. *Antimicrob Agents Chemother.* 2000;44(4):920–928.

Peuchant O, Thiebaut R, Capdepont S, et al. Transmission of HIV-1 minority-resistance variants and response to first-line antiretroviral therapy: transmission of minority resistant HIV-1. *AIDS.* 2008;22(12):1417–1423.

Pingen M, Wensing A, Fransen K, et al. Persistence of frequently transmitted drug-resistant HIV-1 variants can be explained by high viral replication capacity. *Retrovirology.* 2014;11:105.

Poschman K, Spencer EC. Prevalence of HIV-1 antiretroviral drug resistance in Florida, 2015–2016 [Abstract 526]. Presented at the Conference on Retroviruses and Opportunistic Infections, Boston, MA, 2020. https://www.croiconference.org/search-abstracts/

Pou C, Noguera-Julian M, Perez-Alvarez S, et al. Improved prediction of salvage antiretroviral therapy outcomes using ultrasensitive HIV-1 drug resistance testing. *Clin Infect Dis.* 2014;59(4):578–588.

Rambaut A, Posada D, Crandall KA, et al. The causes and consequences of HIV evolution. *Nature Rev Gen.* 2004;5:52–61.

Raymond S, Piffaut M, Bigot J, et al. Sexual transmission of an extensively drug-resistance HIV-1 strain. *Lancet HIV.* 2020;7(8):e529–e530.

Requena S, Trevino A, Cabeza T; Spanish HIV-2 Study Group. Drug resistance mutations in HIV-2 patients failing raltegravir and influence on dolutegravir response. *J Antimicrob Chemother.* 2017;72(7):2083–2088.

Rhee SY, Blanco JL, Jordan MR, et al. Geographic and temporal trends in the molecular epidemiology and genetic mechanisms of transmitted HIV-1 drug resistance: an individual-patient-and sequence-level meta-analysis. *PLoS Med.* 2015;12(4):e1001810. doi:10.1371/journal.pmed.1001810

Rhee S, Clutter D, Feddel WJ, et al. Trends in the molecular epidemiology and genetic mechanisms of transmitted human immunodeficiency virus type 1 drug resistance in a large US clinic population. *Clin Infect Dis.* 2019a;68(2):213–221.

Rhee SY, Clutter D, Hare CB, et al. Virological failure and acquired genotypic resistance associated with contemporary antiretroviral treatment regimens. *Open Forum Infect Dis.* 2020a;7(9):ofaa316.

Rhee SY, Fessel WJ, Liu TF, et al. Predictive value of HIV-1 genotypic resistance test interpretation algorithms. *J Infect Dis.* 2009;200(3):453–463.

Rhee SY, Grant PM, Tzou PL, et al. A systematic review of the genetic mechanisms of dolutegravir resistance. *J Antimicrob Chemother.* 2019b;74:3135–3149.

Rhee SY, Kassaye SH, Barrow G, et al. HIV-1 transmitted drug resistance surveillance: shifting trends in study design and prevalence estimates. *J Int AIDS Soc.* 2020b;23(9):e25611.

Rich SN, Poschman K, Hu H, et al. Sociodemographic, ecological, and spatiotemporal factors associated with HIV drug resistance in Florida: a retrospective analysis. *J Infect Dis.* 2020;jiaa413.

Rodriguez AE, Wawrzyniak AJ, Tookes HE, et al. Implementation of an immediate HIV treatment initiation program in a public/academic medical center in the US South: the Miami Test and Treat Rapid Response Program. *AIDS Behav.* 2019;23(suppl 3):287–295.

Rolle CP, Berge M, Singh T, et al. Feasibility, efficacy, and safety of using dolutegravir/lamivudine (DTG/3TC) as a first-line regimen in a test-and-treat setting for newly diagnosed people living with HIV (PLWH): the STAT Study [Abstract P020]. Presented at HIV Glasgow, 2020. https://onlinelibrary.wiley.com/toc/17582652/2020/23/S7

Ryscavage P, Kelly S, Li JZ, et al. Significance and clinical management of persistent low-level viremia and very-low-level viremia in HIV-1-infected patients. *Antimicrob Agents Chemother.* 2014;58(7):3585–3598.

Saag MS, Gandhi RT, Hoy JF, et al. Antiretroviral drugs for treatment and prevention of HIV infection in adults: 2020 recommendations of the International Antiviral Society-USA Panel. *JAMA.* 2020;324(16):1651–1669.

Scarsi KK, Havens JP, Podany AT, et al. HIV-1 integrase inhibitors: a comparative review of efficacy and safety. *Drugs.* 2020;80:1649–1676.

Scherrer AU, von Wyl V, Yang WL, et al. Emergence of acquired HIV-1 drug resistance almost stopped in Switzerland: a 15-year prospective cohort analysis. *Clin Infect Dis.* 2016;62:1310–1317.

Scherrer U, Yang WL, Kouyos RD, et al. Successful prevention of transmission of integrase resistance in the Swiss HIV Cohort Study. *J Infect Dis.* 2016;214(3):399–402.

Siefried KJ, Mao L, Cysique LA, et al. Concomitant medication polypharmacy, interactions and imperfect adherence are common in Australian adults on suppressive antiretroviral therapy. *AIDS.* 2018;32:35–48.

Siefried KJ, Mao L, Kerr S, et al.; PAART Study Investigators. Socioeconomic factors explain suboptimal adherence to antiretroviral therapy among HIV-infected Australian adults with viral suppression. *PLoS One.* 2017;12:e0174613.

Siliciano JD, Siliciano RF. Recent trends in HIV-1 drug resistance. *Curr Opin Virol.* 2013;3:487–494.

Sörstedt E, Carlander C, Flamholc L, et al. Effect of dolutegravir in combination with nucleoside reverse transcriptase inhibitors (NRTIs) on people living with HIV who have pre-existing NRTI mutations. *Int J Antimicrob Agents.* 2018;51:733–738.

Swenson LC, Min JE, Woods CK, et al. HIV drug resistance detected during low-level viremia is associated with subsequent virologic failure. *AIDS.* 2014;28(8):1125–1134.

Tashima KT, Mollan KR Na L, et al. Regimen selection in the OPTIONS trial of HIV salvage therapy: drug resistance, prior therapy, and race–ethnicity determine the degree of regimen complexity. *HIV Clin Trials.* 2015;16:147–156.

Toni TA, Asahchop EL, Moisi D, et al. Detection of human immunodeficiency virus (HIV) type 1 M184V and K103N minority variants in patients with primary HIV infection. *Antimicrob Agents Chemother.* 2009;53:1670–1672.

Tzou PH, Rhee SY, Descamps, et al.; WHO HIVResNet Working Groups. Integrase strand transfer inhibitor (INSTI)-resistance mutations for the surveillance of transmitted HIV-1 drug resistance. *J Antimicrob Chemother.* 2020;75:170–182.

Vandenhende MA, Perrier A, Bonnet F, et al. Risk of virological failure in HIV-1-infected patients experiencing low-level viraemia under active antiretroviral therapy (ANRS CO3 Cohort Study). *Antivir Ther.* 2015;20(6):655–660.

Van Wyk J, Orkin C, Rubio R, et al. Durable suppression and low rate of virologic failure 3 years after switch to dolutegravir + rilpivirine 2-drug regimen: 148-week results from the SWORD-1 and SWORD-2 randomized clinical trials. *J AIDS.* 2020;85(3):325–330.

Van Zyl G, Bale MJ, Kearney MF. HIV evolution and diversity in ART-treated patients. *Retrovirology.* 2018;15(1):14

Varghese V, Shahriar R, Rhee SY, et al. Minority variants associated with transmitted and acquired HIV-1 non-nucleoside RT (NNRTI) resistance: implications for the use of second generation NNRTIs. *J AIDS.* 2009;52(3):309–315.

Verhofstede C, Noe A, Demecheleer E, et al. Drug-resistance variants that evolve during nonsuppressive therapy persist in HIV-1-infected peripheral blood mononuclear cells after long-term highly active antiretroviral therapy. *J AIDS.* 2004;35:473–483.

Vingerhoets J, Tambuyzer L, Azijn H, et al. Resistance profile of etravirine: combined analysis of baseline genotypic and phenotypic data from the randomized, controlled Phase III clinical studies. *AIDS.* 2010;24(4):503–514.

Wensing AM, Calvez V, Ceccherini-Silberstein F, et al. 2019 update of the drug resistance mutations in HIV-1. *Top Antivir Med.* 2019;27(3):111–121.

Westby J, Lewis M, Whitcomb J, et al. Emergence of CXCR4-using human immunodeficiency virus type 1 (HIV-1) variants in a minority of HIV-1-infected patients following treatment with the CCR5 antagonist maraviroc is from a pretreatment CXCR4-using virus reservoir. *J Virol.* 2006;80(10):4909–4920.

Wheeler WH, Ziebell RA, Zabina H, et al. Prevalence of transmitted drug resistance associated mutations and HIV-1 subtypes in new HIV-1 diagnoses, U.S., 2006. *AIDS.* 2010;24:1203–1212.

Winters B, van Craenenbroeck E, van der Borght K, et al. Clinical cut-offs for HIV-1 phenotypic resistance estimates: update based on recent pivotal clinical trial data and a revised approach to viral mixtures. *J Virol Methods.* 2009;162:101–108.

Wirden M, Soulie C, Valantin MA, et al. Historical HIV-RNA resistance test results are more informative than proviral DNA genotyping in cases of suppressed or residual viraemia. *Antimicrob Chemother.* 2011;66:709–712.

Yanik EL, Napravnik S, Hurt CB, et al. Prevalence of transmitted antiretroviral drug resistance differs between acutely and chronically HIV-infected patients. *J AIDS.* 2012;61:258–262.

Yazdanpanah Y, Fagard C, Descamps D, et al. High rate of virologic suppression with ralteravir plus etravirine and darunavir/ritonavir among treatment-experienced patients infected with multidrug-resistant HIV: results of the ANRS. *Clin Infect Dis.* 2009;49:1441–1449.

Zaccarelli M, Santoro MM, Armenia D, et al. Genotypic resistance test in proviral DNA can identify resistance mutations never detected in historical genotypic test in patients with low level or undetectable HIV-RNA. *J Clin Virol.* 2016;82:94–100.

Zhou N, Nowicka-Sans B, McAuliffe B, et al. Genotypic correlates of susceptibility to HIV-1 attachment inhibitor BMS-626529, the active agent of the prodrug BMS-663068. *J Antimicrob Chemother.* 2014;69:573–581.

21.

ANTIRETROVIRALS DURING AND AFTER HOSPITALIZATION, INCLUDING BARIATRIC SURGERY

David E. Koren

CHAPTER GOALS

Upon completion of this chapter, the reader should be able to:

- Discuss issues in determining the relative priority of initiating and/or maintaining antiretroviral therapy (ART) in the context of hospitalized persons with HIV (PWH) with significant comorbid conditions, as well as issues of continuity of care after discharge from the inpatient setting

- Define antiretroviral stewardship and understand its potential benefit in implementation

- Describe important considerations in the perioperative care of a PWH

- Describe pharmacologic complications that may result from bariatric surgery

---

GENERAL HOSPITALIZATION CONCERNS IN PWH, INCLUDING ANTIRETROVIRAL STEWARDSHIP

LEARNING OBJECTIVE

- Discuss issues in determining the relative priority of initiating and/or maintaining ART in the context of the hospitalized PWH with significant comorbid conditions, the new concept of antiretroviral stewardship, and issues of continuity of care after discharge from the inpatient setting

WHAT'S NEW?

- An updated link to a reference table of available ART formulations is provided.

- New antiretroviral agents (ARVs) since last publication are incorporated.

- The American Academy of HIV Medicine partnered with the HIV Medicine Association and Infectious Diseases Society of America to establish a call to action for antiretroviral stewardship in the inpatient setting.

- Recent literature has suggested that initiation of ARVs in the inpatient setting may be associated with a more rapid linkage to care among people living with both HIV and substance use disorder.

The introduction of highly active antiretroviral therapy (HAART) has changed many root causes for hospitalization among PWH. In the pre-ART era, progressive opportunistic infections (OIs) and end-stage AIDS were the main causes of recurrent hospitalizations; however, these causes (as well as hospitalization rates) have dramatically declined in the ART era. Recent drivers for hospitalization have diversified and are now associated with an increased incidence of chronic, noncommunicable health conditions such as diabetes, cardiovascular disease, chronic kidney diseases, and malignancies (Paul et al., 2002). There are many considerations in the use of ART during hospitalization, and this issue can be divided into two main categories described here.

The first category consists of PWH not on ART at the time of admission, which may be due to nonadherence or not having been diagnosed with HIV until the hospitalization itself (possibly due to presentation with an OI). The general question in this case is whether to start ART during hospitalization. Concerns regarding additional pill burden, increased potential for side effects/drug interactions, and possible immune reconstitution inflammatory syndrome (IRIS) must be weighed against faster OI improvement and ultimate morbidity/mortality benefits. A 2009 randomized controlled trial helped inform the issue, concluding that early ART initiation resulted in less AIDS progression/death with no increase in adverse events or loss of virologic response compared to deferred ART (Zolopa et al., 2009). Additionally, current US Department of Health and Human Service (DHHS) guidelines, supported by clinical literature, including the START and TEMPRANO trials, recommend "initiating ART immediately (or as soon as possible) after HIV diagnosis in order to increase the uptake of ART and linkage to care, decrease the time to viral suppression for individual patients, and improve the rate of virologic suppression among persons with HIV." This may occur in a rapid start scenario, in which ARVs are initiated prior to return of all associated laboratory values (DHHS, 2020). Additionally, in a multisite cohort of 801 persons living with both HIV and substance use disorder, initiation of ART while hospitalized was associated with a shorter time to first HIV care visit (29 days among those who initiated ART while hospitalized compared to 54 days among those who did not, $p = 0.0145$) (Jacobs et al., 2020). These data, however, did not find an association between inpatient ART initiation and either retention or viral suppression over 12 months, demonstrating that further interventions may be required in this population.

A critical additional factor in deciding whether to initiate ART during hospitalization is the importance of ensuring that the PWH will be able to access and continue ART upon discharge to prevent lapses in adherence and potential resistance. This issue involves both the immediate availability of ART on discharge (i.e., if the PWH has access to outpatient medications via insurance coverage or the AIDS Drug Assistance Program) and whether the PWH is in a position to continue with successful adherence (i.e., housing stability, substance abuse treatment needs, mental healthcare optimization, and willingness to take ART). In all cases, it is essential to ensure that PWH will have streamlined access to ongoing outpatient HIV specialty care and that they are linked before discharge to prevent adherence lapses.

The second category consists of PWH with a known HIV diagnosis who are on ART at the time of admission. PWH who are on stable ART and admitted to the hospital should continue taking their regimen with few exceptions. Issues that impact ART continuation include the reason for admission and if it impacts the ability to take oral medications—that is, severe gastrointestinal (GI) disturbances such as intractable vomiting, diarrhea, or GI obstruction. In such cases, ART use may need to be temporarily suspended until the PWH's GI symptoms resolve sufficiently to tolerate oral medications again to avoid intermittent absorption and subtherapeutic drug levels predisposing to resistance. In addition, temporary ART discontinuation may need to be considered in presentations of severe lactic acidosis, pancreatitis, severe hepatic enzyme elevations, obtundation, or emergent surgical issues. ART dosing should be resumed as soon as safely possible when the PWH clinically improves from these initial severe presentations.

If possible, PWH who are *nihil per os* (NPO) should continue ART with water unless there is an acute GI problem that is rendering them NPO. PWH with nasogastric tubes should be given all ART in liquid form, when available, or crushed and reconstituted if no liquid form is available. An updated reference table based on a literature review for ARVs that can be crushed or sprinkled and also information on liquid formulation availability can be found at https://liverpool-hiv-hep.s3.amazonaws.com/prescribing_resources/pdfs/000/000/011/original/ARV_Swallowing_2018_Dec.pdf?1543916096.

Drug interaction issues need to be considered routinely during hospitalization. Any new medications given need to be checked for interactions with the PWH's current ART regimen, and dose adjustments or medication changes should be made as needed, ideally in concert with an HIV specialty pharmacist. Particular attention should be paid to proton pump inhibitor (PPI) interactions because PPIs are often started for ulcer prophylaxis or other reasons during hospitalization. Atazanavir and rilpivirine are particularly susceptible to subtherapeutic drug levels due to PPI interaction; therefore, extra care should be taken to mitigate problematic interactions. Additionally, integrase strand inhibitor agents (bictegravir, dolutegravir, elvitegravir, and raltegravir) may have decreased activity in the context of simultaneous administration with medications containing divalent cations. These examples are only some of many potential pharmacokinetic/dynamic interactions. An updated reference for drug–drug interactions concerning ARVs can be found at http://www.hiv-druginteractions.org.

Some other ART considerations during hospitalization include formulary availability, especially at smaller hospitals with less HIV experience, and adequate stock of all agents because the number and classes of ARVs have dramatically increased. It is important to work with the pharmacy to ensure that correct ART is available without delay in the correct dosing form and that, if there are any supply problems, appropriate class substitutions are given in consultation with an HIV expert. If a PWH is on an investigational medication via a research study, it is imperative that the treating physician and the research team administering the investigational drug are notified of the person's hospital admission because they must make arrangements to bring the drug to the hospital and arrange for its administration by the staff there.

To address all of these issues of inpatient HIV management, a joint call to action was published in 2020 by the American Academy of HIV Medicine, HIV Medicine Association, and Infectious Disease Society of America defining antiretroviral stewardship as "coordinated interventions designed to improve continuity of care of patients receiving ARVs through the utilization of evidence-based ARV practices including medication reconciliation, dosing, mitigation of drug interactions, and prevention of viral resistance." These activities, tailored to the needs of the individual institution, are generally conducted by stakeholders with experience in ART and may consist of clinical checklists to ensure safe prescribing practices, computerized physician order entry sets, and/or prospective review strategies by physician–pharmacist collaborations (Koren et al., 2020).

Currently, multiple long-acting injectable ARVs are being investigated; when these come into clinical use, they may play a significant role in the management of the hospitalized PWH in terms of expanding treatment options while decreasing pill burden.

PERIOPERATIVE CARE, SURGICAL ISSUES, AND THE BARIATRIC PWH

KEY POINTS

- The balance of data show no overall worse operation-associated morbidity and mortality in PWH undergoing surgical procedures.

- Perioperative complications may be more frequent or severe in very immunosuppressed PWH.

- There are some specific anesthesia considerations in PWH.

- Bariatric procedures may affect ARV absorption. Considerations should be made with regard to the person's specific ARV regimen and type of procedure during the evaluative workup.

Overall, data suggest that operation-associated morbidity and mortality in PWH are not different from those in uninfected people. Due to improvements in outcomes and overall OI reduction in the early ART era, the number of operations for AIDS-related surgical illnesses has decreased considerably (Saltzman et al., 2005). Additionally, given available data from the ART era, general data support that HIV infection does not increase the postoperative risk for complications or death (Cacala et al., 2006; Evron et al., 2004). Despite these positive attributes, given the vastly improved survival and longevity of people with HIV alongside ongoing comorbidities that increase with an aging HIV population, the need for non-HIV-related surgical operations and anesthesia has become far more common.

POSTOPERATIVE COMPLICATIONS AND HIV INFECTION

Uncontrolled or advanced HIV infection may influence postoperative wound healing and complication rates (Rose et al., 1998). Additionally, advanced HIV infection accompanied by OIs or malignancies may complicate the perioperative course and management. This may be due to debility and wasting as much as immunosuppression. A CD4$^+$ T-cell count and viral load measurement are useful when calculating surgical risks and developing a prognosis in PWH (Evron et al., 2004; Saltzman et al., 2005). Postoperative CD4$^+$ T-cell counts of 200 cells/mm^3 or less are associated with higher mortality rates (Saltzman et al., 2005). Irrespective of the surgical procedure, there is a 13.3% mortality rate in PWH with a CD4$^+$ T-cell count less than 50 cells/mm^3 and a 0.8% mortality rate with a CD4$^+$ T-cell count greater than 200 cells/mm^3 6 months postoperatively (Evron et al., 2004). Postoperative viral loads greater than 75,000 copies/mL are associated with higher complication and mortality rates (Saltzman et al., 2005). A 2006 Kaiser retrospective study showed that viral load suppression to less than 30,000 copies/mL reduced surgical complications (Horberg et al., 2006).

In a comprehensive literature review consisting mainly of literature from the pre-ART era, wound infection rates varied widely, especially for abdominal, anorectal, and general surgeries and central venous catheter insertions, whereas documented ophthalmologic surgery and splenectomies had consistently low morbidity rates (Rose et al., 1998). In 33% of the reports, complication rates were significantly higher in PWH with late-stage HIV compared to early-stage PWH. One study of dental extractions found that complication rates did not significantly differ by Centers for Disease Control and Prevention (CDC) stage of disease. A study of cesarean sections found that complication rates were not significantly different between CDC stages of disease but were significantly associated with CD4$^+$ T-cell counts (Rose et al., 1998).

To mitigate operative complications, PWH with a history or signs of cardiac or pulmonary dysfunction should undergo a more thorough evaluation prior to surgery (e.g., blood gases, pulmonary function tests, echocardiography, further cardiac testing, or even cardiac catheterization as appropriate). Relevant history of past treatment with potentially cardiotoxic therapies, such as chemotherapy for Kaposi's sarcoma or lymphoma, should be considered in assessing operative risk. PWH may be in a relatively hypercoagulable state, with accelerated coronary atherosclerosis and possibly decreased left ventricular contractility (Evron et al., 2004).

ANESTHESIA CONSIDERATIONS AND DRUG INTERACTIONS

Information about the relative general hazards of anesthesia and surgery for PWH is scarce (Evron et al., 2004). Many ARVs may interact directly with anesthetic drugs and can cause side effects that influence which anesthetics are used and the manner in which they are administered (Evron et al., 2004; Hughes, 2004). This issue is continually evolving given interaction profiles of each ARV.

Specific considerations when administering general anesthesia to PWH include the possible effects of anesthesia and opioids on the immune system, the cardiopulmonary and neurologic status of the person, and possible interactions with ARVs.

- *Opioids*: Although there is laboratory evidence that opioids may detrimentally affect immune function, the clinical significance of short-term opioid administration during general anesthesia is unclear, and not enough clinical data are available to justify its avoidance.

- *Neurologic considerations*: Neurologic manifestations, such as overt dementia, may impair the ability of PWH to provide preoperative consent and may increase brain sensitivity to sedative or psychoactive drugs such as opioids, benzodiazepines, and neuroleptics.

- *General central nervous system (CNS)*: Increased intracranial pressure (ICP) and CNS infections (i.e., meningitis, encephalopathy, or myelopathy) are contraindications to neuraxial anesthesia.

- *Cerebrospinal fluid analysis and nerve or muscle biopsy* may be required, and radiologic studies of the spinal cord should be performed as part of the neurologic evaluation to exclude compressive lesions in symptomatic PWH. OIs may be associated with increased ICP, especially in the case of toxoplasmosis or cryptococcal meningitis. Because these infections respond to medical therapy, surgery should be postponed whenever possible if they are present.

- *Pulmonary considerations*: Pulmonary complications can occur as a consequence of many OIs, leading to respiratory distress and hypoxemia.

Regional anesthesia has been shown to be associated with reduced morbidity and mortality in a wide range of patients, including PWH having cesarean delivery under spinal anesthesia. However, a high motor block with intercostal muscle paralysis may not be tolerated (Evron et al., 2004). Regional anesthesia is less likely to interfere with immune function or interact with ARVs. Sepsis and platelet abnormalities are contraindications to regional anesthesia, and neuropathy may also interfere. Post–dural puncture headache may occur after regional anesthesia and may necessitate an epidural blood patch. No increase in neurologic abnormalities in six PWH receiving an epidural blood patch during a follow-up period of 2 years was observed, and there is no evidence to contraindicate the use of a blood patch in PWH (Evron et al., 2004; Tom et al., 1992).

Some nonnucleoside reverse transcriptase inhibitors such as efavirenz or etravirine induce the cytochrome P450 enzyme system (CYP3A3/4) and may decrease serum levels of some anesthetic or sedative drugs that use this metabolic pathway, such as midazolam and fentanyl (Evron et al., 2004). Etomidate, atracurium, remifentanil, and desflurane are not dependent on CYP450 hepatic metabolism and may be preferable in persons receiving ART (Evron et al., 2004).

Protease inhibitors (PIs) primarily use the cytochrome P450 system as well (CYP3A4). Because PIs often inhibit, and may also induce, this enzyme, they may increase or decrease the effects of other drugs using the same metabolic pathway; any anesthetics used concomitantly should be carefully titrated. Ritonavir is the most potent inhibitor of CYP3A4 and CYP2D6. Another CYP3A inhibitor, cobicistat, is commonly used as an ART-boosting agent and has similar interactions to ritonavir, with a similar need for dosing considerations. Fentanyl is metabolized mainly by CYP3A4 (Evron et al., 2004); ritonavir can reduce fentanyl clearance by up to 67%. This strong interaction suggests that fentanyl (as well as other anesthetics) should be carefully titrated and monitored in a PWH on a concomitant boosting agent. These effects may be deleterious; respiratory monitoring should be maintained in the setting of this interaction as the risk of respiratory depression for an increased duration will likely be higher (Hughes, 2004).

BARIATRIC SURGERY IN PWH TAKING ART

Although bariatric surgeries have proven effective in reducing both obesity-related mortality and obesity-related comorbidities, they may bring about pharmacologic considerations/complications depending on the type of surgery performed on the PWH (e.g., Roux-en-Y gastric bypass or sleeve gastrectomy) (Cimino et al., 2018). Generally, these considerations consist of absorptive and dietary concerns. If the person's ART is known to be absorbed in the small intestine, and the small intestine is permanently bypassed due to surgical procedure,

the medication will not be absorbed. Additionally, if an ARV requires a caloric and/or fat requirement, and the stomach volume is reduced significantly due to the procedure, this will inevitably result in subtherapeutic absorption. Minimal data exist on this issue, generally consisting of collections of case reports given the broad array of potential bariatric procedures and ARV combinations. During the evaluative workup prior to a procedure, considerations should be made as to available formulations of the PWH's ART regimen (including whether the medication can be crushed), potential for drug–drug interactions (including acid suppression and di/polyvalent cations), and the type of bariatric procedure. While the exact site of absorption is known for only a few ARVs, among those that are, many are absorbed in the small intestine; thus, Roux-en-Y procedures may compromise absorption (Cimino et al., 2018).

RECOMMENDED READING

Cimino C, Binkley A, Swisher R, et al. Antiretroviral considerations in HIV-infected patients undergoing bariatric surgery. J Clin Pharm Ther. 2018;43:757–767.

Huesgen E, DeSear KE, Egelund EF, et al. A HAART-breaking review of alternative antiretroviral administration: practical considerations with crushing and enteral tube scenarios. Pharmacotherapy. 2016;36(11):1145–1165.

Koren DE, Scarsi KK, Farmer EK, et al. A call to action: the role of antiretroviral stewardship in inpatient practice: a joint policy paper of the Infectious Diseases Society of America, HIV Medicine Association, and American Academy of HIV Medicine. Clin Infect Dis. 2020;70(11):2241–2246.

REFERENCES

Cacala SR, Mafana E, Thompson SR, et al. Prevalence of HIV status and CD4 counts in a surgical cohort: their relationship to clinical outcome. Ann R Coll Surg Engl. 2006;88(1):46–51.

Cimino C, Binkley A, Swisher R, et al. Antiretroviral considerations in HIV-infected patients undergoing bariatric surgery. J Clin Pharm Ther. 2018;43:757–767.

Department of Health and Human Services. Panel on Antiretroviral Guidelines for Adults and Adolescents. Guidelines for the use of antiretroviral agents in adults and adolescents living with HIV. https://aidsinfo.nih.gov/guidelines/html/1/adult-and-adolescent-arv/0

Evron S, Glezerman M, Harow E, et al. Human immunodeficiency virus: anesthetic and obstetric considerations. Anesth Analg. 2004;98(2):503–511.

Horberg MA, Hurley LB, Klein DB, et al. Surgical outcomes in human immunodeficiency virus-infected patients in the era of highly active antiretroviral therapy. Arch Surg. 2006;141(12):1238–1245.

Hughes SC. HIV and anesthesia. Anesthesiol Clin North Am. 2004;22(3):379–404.

Jacobs P, Feaster DJ, Pan Y, et al. Initiation of antiretroviral therapy in the hospital is associated with linkage to human immunodeficiency virus (HIV) care for persons living with HIV and substance use disorder. Clin Infect Dis. 2020 [E-pub ahead of print]. doi:10.1093/cid/ciaa838

Koren DE, Scarsi KK, Farmer EK, et al. A call to action: the role of antiretroviral stewardship in inpatient practice: a joint policy paper of the Infectious Diseases Society of America, HIV Medicine Association, and American Academy of HIV Medicine. Clin Infect Dis. 2020;70(11):2241–2246.

Paul S, Gilbert HM, Lande L, et al. Impact of antiretroviral therapy on decreasing hospitalization rates of HIV-infected patients in 2001. AIDS Res Hum Retroviruses. 2002;18:501–506.

Rose D, Collins M, Kelban R. Complications of surgery in HIV-infected patients. AIDS. 1998;12:2243–2251.

Saltzman DJ, Williams RA, Gelfand DV, et al. The surgeon and AIDS: twenty years later. Arch Surg. 2005;140(10):961–967.

Tom DJ, Gulevich SJ, Shapiro HM, et al. Epidural blood patch in the HIV-positive patient. Review of clinical experience. San Diego HIV Neurobehavioral Research Center. Anesthesiology. 1992;76(6):943–947.

Zolopa AR, Anderson J, Powderly W, et al. Early antiretroviral therapy reduces AIDS progression/death in individuals with acute opportunistic infections: a multicenter randomized strategy trial. PLoS One. 2009;4(5)e5575. doi:10.1371/journal.pone.0005575

22.

SOLID ORGAN TRANSPLANTATION IN PERSONS WITH HIV

Christine M. Durand

INTRODUCTION

The advent of effective combination antiretroviral therapy (ART) has resulted in increased life expectancy for people with HIV (PWH). With declining opportunistic infections (OIs), end-organ disease—both directly and indirectly associated with HIV—has become a major cause of morbidity and mortality in this population. Solid organ transplantation, once considered contraindicated for individuals with HIV, has demonstrated success and is now considered the standard of care for end-stage organ disease in this population.

This chapter focuses on kidney and liver transplantation in persons with HIV, which have the most evidence and experience to date. Relatively few studies have described cardiothoracic transplant and HIV-associated outcomes. One study of 75 heart transplant recipients with HIV demonstrated equivalent survival between matched recipients with and without HIV; similarly, a multicenter international study including 21 heart, 7 lung, and 1 heart/lung transplant recipients with HIV showed similar survival between recipients with and without HIV (Doberne et al., 2020; Koval et al., 2019).

Chronic kidney disease can develop as a direct consequence of the HIV virus itself (i.e., HIV-associated nephropathy [HIVAN]), long-term ART toxicities, and/or other comorbidities such as hypertension and diabetes, which are common in PWH (Abraham et al., 2015; Althoff et al., 2019; Mocroft et al., 2016). Liver disease can occur due to common coinfections such as hepatitis C virus (HCV) and hepatitis B virus (HBV; Platt et al., 2016; Sun et al., 2014), alcoholic liver disease, or non-alcoholic fatty liver disease. Once end-stage kidney or liver disease has developed, the best treatment is organ transplantation; accordingly, there has been a growing need for kidney and liver transplantation among PWH (Locke et al., 2017; Shaffer & Durand, 2018).

LEARNING OBJECTIVES

- Discuss the evaluation and management of the kidney and liver transplant candidate with HIV and clinical outcomes for kidney and liver transplant recipients with HIV
- Explain key drug–drug interactions between immunosuppressive agents and ART in transplant recipients with HIV

WHAT'S NEW?

- Studies have found that patient and graft survival rates in kidney transplant recipients with HIV are equivalent to kidney recipients without HIV.

- Studies have found that patient and graft survival rates in liver transplant recipients with HIV are lower than those without HIV, although outcomes are improving over time and with the advent of highly effective HCV treatment.

- With the increase in number and availability of integrase strand transfer inhibitors (INSTIs), clinicians and patients can often select an ART regimen that minimizes risk of drug interactions while limiting side effects, maintaining ease of administration, and preserving a high barrier to ART resistance.

- The HIV Organ Policy Equity (HOPE) Act, which was signed into US law in 2013, allows organs from PWH to be used for transplant for recipients with HIV under research protocols.

KEY POINTS

- End-organ disease has become a major cause of morbidity and mortality in people with HIV due to increased life expectancy, thus increasing the demand for organ transplantation in this population.

- The care of transplant recipients with HIV warrants a multidisciplinary team approach, including the specific organ transplant team, pharmacists, infectious disease/HIV specialists, nurses, patients, and families.

- Transplant-related immunosuppression for recipients with HIV has not been associated with loss of virologic control or increased OIs.

- Protease inhibitors (PIs) and pharmacoenhancing ("boosting") agents are strong inhibitors of cytochrome P450 3A4 (CYP3A4); their use results in clinically significant drug interactions with some transplant medications. Patients who receive these ART medications should be monitored carefully; for some, ART modification may be preferable to avoid problematic interactions. Use of older nonnucleoside reverse transcriptase inhibitors (NNRTIs;

i.e., efavirenz, nevirapine, etravirine) also leads to significant drug interactions with some transplant medications.

- Kidney transplant recipients with HIV face an increased risk of allograft rejection after transplant.

- HCV treatment is essential to improve outcomes among liver and kidney transplant recipients with HIV and HCV coinfection.

PRETRANSPLANT EVALUATION

CRITERIA FOR TRANSPLANTATION

Many of the following recommendations are based on the National Institutes of Health (NIH)–funded Solid Organ Transplantation in HIV: Multi-site Study (HIVTR Study), which was a prospective observational study of kidney and liver transplantation in PWH conducted across 26 transplant centers in the US between 2002 and 2013 (Roland et al., 2016; Stock et al., 2010; Terrault et al., 2012).

- Any OIs or malignancies should be completely treated prior to transplant. There are limited data on outcomes of transplant recipients who have a history of progressive multifocal leukoencephalopathy, visceral Kaposi's sarcoma, chronic cryptosporidiosis, or primary central nervous system lymphoma, as these individuals were excluded from clinical trials of kidney and liver transplantation for PWH.

- Transplant candidates with HIV should meet standard criteria for transplantation.

- Transplant candidates with HIV should be on a stable ART regimen.

Kidney Transplant Candidate Criteria

- CD4$^+$ T-cell count should generally be at least 200 cells/mL prior to transplant.

- HIV RNA should be suppressed to below the assay's limit of detection (excluding viral "blips" of 20–200 copies/mL, which are common and unlikely to be clinically significant) (Nettles et al., 2005).

Liver Transplant Candidate Criteria

- CD4$^+$ T-cell count should generally be at least 100 cells/mL. A lower CD4$^+$ T-cell count has been allowed for liver transplant candidates due to the impact of portal hypertension and splenomegaly on lowering overall lymphocyte counts.

- HIV RNA should be suppressed to below the limit of detection of the assay (excluding viral "blips" of 20–200 copies/mL, which are common and unlikely to be clinically significant) (Nettles et al., 2005).

PRETRANSPLANT INFECTION SCREENING AND VACCINATIONS

Latent Tuberculosis

All candidates should be screened for latent tuberculosis (TB) prior to transplantation, with either a tuberculin skin test or interferon-gamma release assay (Blumberg & Roger, 2019; Centers for Disease Control and Prevention et al., 2020). Patients should be treated if they have evidence of latent TB. The preferred regimen is isoniazid (INH) ±vitamin B6 for 9 months, completing at least 6 of the 9 months prior to transplantation. For liver transplantation, when prophylactic treatment cannot be completed prior to transplant, or if the risk of toxicity is too high, treatment should be completed as soon as possible after transplant.

Syphilis

Patients should be tested and treated for syphilis prior to transplant.

Other infectious conditions

All candidates should be tested for cytomegalovirus (CMV), Epstein–Barr virus, herpes simplex virus, varicella zoster virus (VZV), and viral hepatitis serologies. In addition, *Coccidioides* and *Strongyloides* serologies should be tested if the recipient has exposure to endemic areas.

Vaccinations

- Whenever possible, vaccinations should be given pretransplant. Live vaccines such as varicella and mumps/measles/rubella (MMR) vaccines should not be given pretransplant if the CD4$^+$ T-cell count is less than 300 cells/mL (Miro et al., 2014). No live vaccines should be given post-transplant.

- All candidates should be vaccinated against hepatitis A and B if not already immune.

- Inactivated influenza vaccine should be given yearly. The high-dose vaccine has demonstrated better immunogenicity and is safe in solid organ transplant recipients (Mombelli et al., 2018).

- Both the pneumococcal conjugate vaccine (PCV13) and the polysaccharide vaccine (PPV23) should be given. PCV13 should be given for first vaccination and PPV23 can be given at least 8 weeks later. These vaccines should be administered every 3 to 5 years (Blumberg & Roger, 2019).

- Tdap vaccine should be given if not received in the past 10 years.

- Human papillomavirus (HPV) vaccine should be given for patients ages 9 to 45 years.

- Meningococcal conjugate vaccine (MenACWY) should be given to all candidates, and the serogroup B meningococcal vaccine should be given to candidates between 16 and 23 years of age.

- Varicella vaccine should be given to those who are VZV seronegative (and have a CD4$^+$ T-cell count of ≥300 cells/mL) prior to transplant.

- Recombinant zoster vaccine (RSV, Shingrix) has shown safety and immunogenicity in immunocompromised populations (Berkowitz et al., 2015; Stadtmauer et al., 2014) and should be considered to prevent zoster reactivation, which is common among PWH and transplant recipients.

WHEN TO REFER

All individuals with HIV who have a glomerular filtration rate of 25 mL/min or less should be referred to a kidney transplant center.

All individuals with HIV who have decompensated or symptomatic cirrhosis or hepatocellular carcinoma should be referred for liver transplant evaluation. Patients with an albumin of less than 3 g/dL, a prolonged prothrombin time, or a modified Child–Turcotte–Pugh score of 7 or higher should also be considered.

POSTTRANSPLANT MANAGEMENT AND CARE

All pretransplant, peritransplant, and posttransplant care should be coordinated among a multidisciplinary team consisting of the transplant surgeon, an infectious disease or HIV specialist, a nephrologist or hepatologist, a primary care provider, a transplant coordinator, a transplant pharmacist, a social worker, and nursing staff.

IMMUNOSUPPRESSION THERAPY

Induction Immunosuppression for Kidney Transplantation

For kidney transplantation, induction immunosuppression at the time of transplant typically includes lymphocyte depletion with antithymocyte globulin (ATG) or an interleukin-2 receptor antagonist (anti–IL-2R), a less potent monoclonal antibody that blocks early T-cell activation (Gabardi et al., 2011). There remains debate about which agent is optimal for transplant recipients with HIV. The multicenter HIVTR study suggested that ATG use was associated with a higher risk of graft loss and hospitalizations due to infections (Stock et al., 2010). However, subsequent studies found a 2.6-fold lower risk of acute rejection and equivalent graft survival in transplant recipients with HIV who received ATG induction (Locke et al., 2014). A subsequent study of 830 renal transplant recipients with HIV found a 40% lower rate of rejection among those who received ATG for induction compared to either no induction or anti–IL-2R induction, without

evidence of increased infections (Kucirka et al., 2016). The choice of induction therapy should be made on a case-by-case basis, accounting for the individual's risk of rejection, although recent evidence suggests ATG is generally safe in PWH undergoing kidney transplantation.

Maintenance Immunosuppression

Maintenance immunosuppression generally consists of triple therapy including calcineurin inhibitors (CNIs) (e.g., cyclosporine and tacrolimus) with an antimetabolite (e.g., mycophenolate mofetil) and corticosteroids. A mammalian target of rapamycin (mTOR) inhibitor (e.g., sirolimus and everolimus) may be substituted if a patient cannot tolerate CNIs or antimetabolites. The HIVTR study found an increased risk of rejection with the use of cyclosporine compared to tacrolimus (Stock et al., 2010), and sirolimus was found to be associated with a higher rate of rejection (Locke et al., 2014). Early steroid withdrawal has also been associated with a 60% higher risk of allograft rejection in kidney transplant recipients with HIV (Werbel et al., 2020).

ART MANAGEMENT AMONG TRANSPLANT RECIPIENTS

Managing interactions between immunosuppressive agents and ART can be challenging. In ambulatory settings, clinicians will most frequently encounter maintenance immunosuppressive regimens consisting of a combination of a CNI, antimetabolite, and corticosteroids as described previously. In some individuals, an mTOR inhibitor will be used in place of one of these agents or as adjunctive therapy. Understanding the pharmacokinetics of each of these drug classes is crucial to safely manage transplant recipients with HIV. CNIs are substrates as well as weak inhibitors of CYP3A4 and therefore have potential for significant interaction with antiretroviral agents (ARVs) that are CYP3A4 inhibitors or inducers. mTOR inhibitors are substrates of CYP3A4, and dosing must be adjusted in the presence of CYP3A4 inhibitors or inducers. The antimetabolites mycophenolate mofetil and azathioprine are not substrates for CYP3A4 and therefore have no expected or documented interactions with ART.

ART should not be interrupted in the posttransplant period. The optimal regimen for individual patients varies based on their ART resistance pattern and prior ART exposures as well as overall clinical profile. As indicated earlier, drug–drug interactions between CNIs, mTOR inhibitors, and some ARVs (i.e., PIs and some NNRTIs) may affect the metabolism of immunosuppressant medications and potentially contribute to drug toxicity or rejection (Frasetto et al., 2007; Trullas et al., 2011; van Maarseveen et al., 2012). General guidelines by class are provided later in the chapter. There are no absolute contraindications, as dosing modifications based on therapeutic drug monitoring of the immunosuppressants can compensate for the altered metabolism of these drugs.

Nucleoside Reverse Transcriptase Inhibitors (NRTIs)

When possible, older nucleoside reverse transcriptase inhibitors (NRTIs) with significant mitochondrial toxicity such as zidovudine and stavudine should be avoided, due to antagonism when used with mycophenolate, and zidovudine may exacerbate bone marrow suppression. Tenofovir disoproxil fumarate should be avoided when possible due to nephrotoxicity, though its newer formulation (tenofovir alafenamide) may be a safer alternative.

NNRTIS

Older NNRTIs such as efavirenz, nevirapine, and etravirine are strong CYP3A4 inducers, thus increasing the metabolism of CNIs and decreasing their serum levels (mTOR levels may be similarly affected). The dose of these immunosuppressive agents frequently needs to be increased with close monitoring of drug levels. Newer NNRTIs such as rilpivirine and doravirine are not potent inducers and are not expected to impact CNI levels significantly (Spagnuolo et al., 2019). For transplant recipients taking proton pump inhibitors, rilpivirine should not be used.

PIs AND PHARMACOENHANCERS

PIs given in combination with low-dose ritonavir or cobicistat, known as "boosted PIs," act as strong CYP3A4 inhibitors (and sometimes also weak inducers) and decrease the metabolism of CNIs and mTOR inhibitors, resulting in higher levels of these agents. Thus, if boosted PIs or cobicistat must be used, the dosages of both CNIs and mTOR inhibitors commonly must be decreased and the dosing interval increased with close monitoring of drug levels, both to avoid toxicity and to maintain therapeutic immunosuppressive drug levels. Additionally, use of boosted PIs in kidney transplant recipients has been linked to an increased risk of graft loss and death in one recent study, while in another study it was found to actually be associated with reduced graft failure rates (Sawinski et al., 2017; Sparkes et al., 2018). This suggests that PIs should be used sparingly and with careful monitoring.

Boosted PIs also decrease the clearance of glucocorticoids, which may cause a Cushing-like syndrome. In addition, they may exacerbate hyperlipidemia posttransplant and potentiate CNI-induced impaired glucose tolerance.

INSTIs

INSTIs have no or only minimal effects on CYP3A metabolism; thus, there are few potential drug interactions with immunosuppressants, making this class of ARVs well suited for use in PWH during solid organ transplantation. Although experience is greatest with raltegravir (Barau et al., 2014; Bickel et al., 2010; Di Biagio et al., 2009; Miro et al., 2010), the absence of interaction and stability of immunosuppressant dosing are likely to be similar for other INSTIs, including dolutegravir and bictegravir. Because dolutegravir and bictegravir interfere with tubular secretion of creatinine, mild elevations of creatinine may be observed after dolutegravir (or bictegravir) initiation, but these do not represent a decline in glomerular filtration rate (Lee et al., 2016). However, when INSTIs such as elvitegravir are given in combination with the pharmacoenhancer cobicistat, this will cause potent CYP3A4 inhibition (see the earlier section on PIs and pharmacoenhancers). Thus, cobicistat should be avoided if possible, for the reasons discussed earlier.

CCR5 ANTAGONISTS

The CCR5 antagonist maraviroc does not have significant drug interactions with immunosuppressants and represents a good option for individuals with R5 tropic virus. Notably, blockade of CCR5 expression leads to a reduction in lymphocyte chemotaxis and has been hypothesized to reduce inflammation and potentially allograft rejection. It has been shown to reduce severe graft-versus-host disease after bone marrow transplantation (Reshef et al., 2012) and is currently under study to reduce rejection among kidney transplant recipients with HIV.

NEWER ART AGENTS

Ibalizumab is a monoclonal antibody for the CD4 T-cell receptor that does not have drug–drug interactions with immunosuppressants. Fostemsavir is an HIV attachment inhibitor that blocks the interaction between the CD4 T-cell receptor and the HIV envelope protein gp120. Neither of these ARVs is expected to have problematic drug interactions with immunosuppressants, although there is limited experience with their use in transplant recipients at this time.

POSTTRANSPLANT INFECTION PROPHYLAXIS

In addition to standard posttransplant CMV prophylaxis, kidney and liver transplant recipients with HIV should receive the following prophylaxis:

- *Pneumocystis jirovecii*
  - Prophylaxis with trimethoprim/sulfamethoxazole (TMP/SMX) or dapsone (if sulfa allergy or bone marrow suppression is an issue, provided glucose-6-phosphate dehydrogenase [G-6PD] levels are normal). Atovaquone can also be used as a secondary alternative to TMP/SMX.
  - Prophylaxis is recommended for at least 1 year (Blumberg & Roger, 2019).
- *Mycobacterium avium* complex (MAC): Some experts recommend primary prophylaxis against MAC with azithromycin for persons with a CD4$^+$ T-cell count less than 50 cells/mL (Blumberg & Roger, 2019). However, recent OI guidelines have eliminated CD4-directed prophylaxis for MAC generally for PWH, due to low incidence

(i.e., primary prophylaxis is no longer recommended for persons who immediately initiate ART, and it may be discontinued in persons who are continuing on a fully suppressive ART regimen) (Centers for Disease Control and Prevention et al., 2020; Saag et al., 2018). This may also extend to transplant recipient populations.

- Toxoplasmosis: TMP/SMX should be used if the CD4[+] T-cell count is less than 100 cells/mL and if either the recipient or the donor carries IgG antibodies against *Toxoplasma gondii*. Atovaquone can be used if a patient cannot tolerate TMP/SMX or dapsone (Blumberg & Roger, 2019).

- Prior OIs: Continue secondary prophylaxis for OIs such as cryptococcus or coccidioidomycosis until CD4[+] T-cell counts are above the discontinuation threshold (i.e., CD4[+] >200 cells/mL) for approximately 3 to 6 months, although many may prefer lifelong secondary prophylaxis (Blumberg & Roger, 2019).

OUTCOMES

PATIENT AND GRAFT SURVIVAL AND REJECTION

Kidney Transplantation

A review of over 1,400 PWH listed for kidney transplant showed a 79% reduction in the risk of death at 5 years for those who received a transplant compared with those who remained on dialysis (Locke et al., 2017). Several studies have shown patient and graft survival rates for kidney transplant recipients with HIV that are largely comparable to the transplant population as a whole. The HIVTR study, a prospective, nonrandomized investigation funded by the NIH, included 150 kidney transplant recipients with well-controlled HIV and demonstrated excellent 1- and 3-year patient and graft survival rates that were above the rates for recipients over the age of 65 (Stock et al., 2010). The overall patient and graft survival rates of kidney transplant recipients with HIV in the HIVTR study were between the rates observed in HIV-uninfected, older recipients and all recipients, with rates of 94.6% ± 2% and 90.4% at 1 year and 88.2% ± 3.8% and 73.7% at 3 years, respectively. Kidneys from living donors were associated with improved survival, and the use of ATG, HCV coinfection, and older age were associated with decreased survival (Stock et al., 2010). Subsequently, the use of ATG induction was found to be associated with patient and graft survival rates equivalent to a cohort without HIV (Locke et al., 2014).

The HIVTR study also found the rate of acute rejection to be twofold to threefold higher, and acute rejection was more aggressive, with a rate of 31% at 1 year and 41% at 3 years in kidney transplant recipients with HIV compared to rates in recipients without HIV (Stock et al., 2010). ATG induction was associated with a 2.6-fold decrease in the rate of acute rejection compared to that of patients who did not receive any

induction (Locke et al., 2014) and a 40% lower rate of rejection compared to those who received either no induction or anti–IL-2R induction (Kucirka et al., 2016).

A study utilizing national data from the US Scientific Registry of Transplant Recipients (SRTR) that included 510 kidney transplant recipients with HIV showed that, in the absence of HCV coinfection, 5- and 10-year patient and graft survival rates for recipients with and without HIV were similar (Locke et al., 2015).

Liver Transplantation

Data also support liver transplantation in individuals with HIV. The HIVTR study included 125 liver transplant recipients with HIV and demonstrated a survival benefit of liver transplantation for individuals with end-stage liver disease and a Model for End-Stage Liver Disease (MELD) score greater than 15 (Roland et al., 2016). In this study, overall survival was acceptable, but it was lower for liver transplant recipients with HIV and HCV coinfection, with a 3-year survival of 60% versus 79% for those with HIV and HCV C coinfection versus HCV alone, respectively (Terrault et al., 2012). The findings of lower survival in those with HCV coinfection was confirmed in a multicenter Spanish study (Miro et al., 2012) and a larger US national registry study (Locke et al., 2016). Studies have also shown that simultaneous liver and kidney transplantation, a lower pretransplant body mass index, older age, and HCV coinfection were associated with decreased patient survival, although there was a survival benefit for liver recipients with a pretransplant MELD score of 15 or higher (Roland et al., 2016). A recent study using combined data from the US and European registries between 2008 and 2015 showed that outcomes have significantly improved among liver transplant recipients with HIV and HCV coinfection in the recent era (Campos-Varela et al., 2020). This is likely due to the advent of highly effective direct-acting antivirals (DAAs) for HCV, which have demonstrated efficacy including in liver transplant recipients with HIV and HCV coinfection (Manzardo et al., 2018).

HIV/HCV COINFECTION

KIDNEY TRANSPLANTATION

Kidney transplant recipients with HIV and HCV have lower 3-year patient survival and graft survival rates (73% and 60%, respectively) compared to recipients without infection (90% and 86%, respectively), with HIV infection only (89% and 81%, respectively), and with HCV infection only (84% and 78%, respectively) (Sawinski et al., 2015). Coinfected recipients are also at a higher risk of acute rejection at 1 year, and the use of induction in this population confers a survival benefit (Vivanco et al., 2013). These findings are consistent with those of other studies, suggesting that HCV coinfection has a negative impact on kidney transplantation outcomes. DAAs effectively cure HCV in kidney transplant recipients with HIV and HCV (Camargo et al., 2019), and with widespread use these disparities in outcomes are expected to improve.

LIVER TRANSPLANTATION

As discussed previously, liver transplant recipients with both HIV and HCV have worse outcomes compared to recipients with either virus alone. Initial studies of liver transplantation in recipients with HIV showed that the 3-year patient and graft survival rates for HIV/HCV coinfected patients were lower (53% and 74%, respectively) than those with HCV infection alone (60% and 79%, respectively) (Terrault et al., 2012). One explanation is that many of these patients will have recurrent HCV infection that can be very aggressive, leading to graft loss and death. Previously reported 5-year survival rates of approximately 50% to 55% may increase to 80% in coinfected liver recipients in whom HCV infection has been cleared (Miro et al., 2015). With the increasing use of DAAs, the negative patient and graft survival effects of HCV coinfection are predicted to decline, and more recent studies on temporal trends in liver transplant recipients with HIV have demonstrated this improvement (Campos-Varela et al., 2020).

HIV/HBV COINFECTION

KIDNEY TRANSPLANTATION

Kidney recipients with HBV infection have overall lower survival rates compared to noninfected recipients. The 10-year patient survival rate was 51.4% in recipients with HBV compared to 82.8% in recipients without HBV, and graft survival rates were 44% for recipients with HBV compared to 74.2% for recipients without HBV (Lee et al., 2001).

LIVER TRANSPLANTATION

The overall outcomes for liver transplant recipients with HIV/HBV coinfection recipients appear to be equivalent to recipients with HBV only. One small study found that no patients developed clinical evidence of HBV recurrence despite low-grade viremia in 54% of coinfected recipients when treated with HBV immunoglobulin (HBIg) with or without anti-HBV antiviral therapy (Coffin et al., 2010). The recommended management for liver recipients with HBV includes a nucleos(t)ide analog (e.g., lamivudine, tenofovir, entecavir) posttransplant with or without hepatitis B immunoglobulin at the time of transplantation, with HBV DNA monitoring every 6 months (Te & Doucette, 2019). This should be incorporated into or added to the ART regimen of HIV/HBV coinfected recipients.

PROGRESSION OF HIV DISEASE

The HIVTR study reported five cases of new OIs, including two cases of cutaneous Kaposi's sarcoma, one case of cryptosporidiosis, one presumed case of *P. jirovecii*, and one case of candidal esophagitis. Despite an initial decline in the CD4+ T-cell count posttransplant, which was more pronounced with ATG induction, there was no increase in complications associated with HIV disease or progression of HIV (Stock et al., 2010).

RISK OF INFECTION, IMMUNE RECOVERY, AND MALIGNANCY

Overall, 38% of kidney recipients had infections posttransplant in the HIVTR study. These infections consisted of predominantly genitourinary infections (26%), respiratory tract infections (20%), and bacteremia (19%). This study also found that HCV coinfected recipients had a higher rate of serious infections compared to recipients without HCV (Stock et al., 2010).

Another study found that individuals with pretransplant CD4+ T-cell counts of less than 350 cells/mL had a lower CD4+ T-cell nadir 4 weeks posttransplant, which was associated with prolonged CD4+ T-cell lymphopenia and increased risk for serious infections (Suarez et al., 2016). Induction with ATG is associated with a more significant CD4+ T-cell nadir posttransplant; however, larger observational studies have not identified an independent increased risk in infections with ATG use (Kucirka et al., 2016).

Based on available data, the incidence of new or recurrent cancer after transplantation in recipients with HIV is low and not significantly different from recipients without HIV. In the HIVTR study, 9% of patients (11.2% of liver recipients and 8.7% of kidney recipients) developed posttransplant malignancies (including skin cancer, cutaneous Kaposi's sarcoma, penile squamous cell cancer, head and neck cancer, renal cell cancer, lymphoma, recurrence of pretransplant hepatocellular carcinoma, and cholangiocarcinoma), and 3% of patients died from a cancer-related cause (Stock et al., 2010). The same study showed an increased risk of developing high-grade squamous intraepithelial lesions after transplantation in 89 patients followed for anal cytology; this requires further study (Nissen et al., 2012).

DONORS WITH HIV: THE HOPE ACT

With recognition of major advances in HIV and transplantation medicine, the HOPE Act of 2013 lifted the federal ban on the use of organs from donors with HIV. This legislation was also based on promising data from a cohort of transplant recipients in South Africa who had received organs from donors with HIV and who had good outcomes, with overall survival rates of 84% at 1 year, 84% at 3 years, and 74% at 5 years, with graft survival rates of 93% at 1 year and 84% at both 3 and 5 years and rejection rates of 8% at 1 year and 22% at 3 years (Muller et al., 2015). The HOPE Act allows transplantation from donors with HIV to recipients with HIV (D+/R+) within research protocols and was implemented in 2015.

The HOPE Act has received widespread support among the PWH community, with high rates of willingness both to donate (Nguyen et al., 2018) and to receive organ from donors with HIV (Seaman et al., 2020). The first HIV D+/R+ deceased donor kidney and liver transplants were performed in 2016 (Malani, 2016), and results of a multicenter pilot study were published in 2020 (Durand et al., 2020). This study of 75 kidney recipients with HIV directly compared outcomes between recipients of donors with and without HIV, finding excellent survival (100% in both arms) and no increased risk of graft failure, HIV viremia, OIs, or serious adverse events between groups (Durand et al., 2020). There have been a handful of successful international case reports of HIV D$^+$/R$^+$ liver transplantation (Calmy et al., 2016; Hathorn et al., 2016; Lauterio et al., 2019).

CONCLUSION

People living with HIV and end-stage organ disease can experience a survival benefit from transplantation, especially kidney transplantation and, in select cases, liver transplantation. Posttransplant immunosuppression does not appear to advance HIV disease or increase the risk of OIs. Recipients with HCV appear to have worse clinical outcomes, partially due to a more aggressive posttransplant HCV recurrence, which emphasizes the importance of HCV cure with DAAs prior to or immediately after the transplant now that newer, less toxic therapies are available. Anticipation and careful management of drug–drug interactions is crucial. Care of transplant recipients with HIV should include an integrated and coordinated group of providers, including the transplant team, pharmacists, infectious disease/HIV specialists, and nurses, in addition to patients and caregivers.

ACKNOWLEDGMENTS

This chapter is an extension of previous work and contributions made by authors involved with prior editions of this content: Jennifer Husson, Eurides Lopes, Carolyn Kramer, and Emily Blumberg.

REFERENCES

Abraham AG, Althoff KN, Jing Y, et al. End-stage renal disease among HIV-infected adults in North America. *Clin Infect Dis.* 2015;60(6):941–949.

Althoff KN, Gebo KA, Moore RD, et al. Contributions of traditional and HIV-related risk factors on non-AIDS-defining cancer, myocardial infarction, and end-stage liver and renal diseases in adults with HIV in the USA and Canada: a collaboration of cohort studies. *Lancet HIV.* 2019; 6(2):e93–e104.

Barau C, Braun J, Vincent C, et al. Pharmacokinetic study of raltegravir in HIV-infected patients with end-stage liver disease: the LIVERAL-ANRS 148 study. *Clin Infect Dis.* 2014;59(8): 1177–1184.

Berkowitz EM, Moyle G, Stellbrink H-J, et al. Safety and immunogenicity of an adjuvanted herpes zoster subunit candidate vaccine in HIV-positive adults: a phase 1/2a randomized, placebo-controlled study. *J Infect Dis.* 2015;211(8):1279–1287.

Bickel M, Anadol E, Vogel M, et al. Daily dosing of tacrolimus in patients treated with HIV-1 therapy containing a ritonavir-boosted protease inhibitor or raltegravir. *J Antimicrob Chemother.* 2010;65(5):999–1004.

Blumberg EA, Roger CC. Solid organ transplantation in the HIV-infected patient: guidelines from the American Society of Transplantation Infectious Diseases Community of Practice. *Clin Transplant.* 2019; 33:e13499.

Calmy A, van Delden C, Giostra E, et al.; Swiss HIV and Swiss Transplant Cohort Studies. HIV-positive-to-HIV-positive liver transplantation. *Am J Transplant.* 2016;16(8):2473–2478.

Camargo JF, Anjan S, Chin-Beckford N, et al. Clinical outcomes in HIV+/HCV+ coinfected kidney transplant recipients in the pre- and post-direct-acting antiviral therapy eras: 10-year single center experience. *Clin Transplant.* 2019;33(5)e13532.

Campos-Varela I, Dodge JL, Berenguer M, et al. Temporal trends and outcomes in liver transplantation for recipients with human immunodeficiency virus infection in Europe and United States. *Transplantation.* 2020;104(10):2078–2086.

Centers for Disease Control and Prevention, National Institutes of Health, and HIV Medicine Association of the Infectious Diseases Society of America. Panel on Opportunistic Infections in Adults and Adolescents with HIV. Guidelines for the prevention and treatment of opportunistic infections in adults and adolescents with HIV. 2020. https://clinicalinfo.hiv.gov/en/guidelines/adult-and-adolescent-opportunistic-infection/whats-new-guidelines

Coffin CS, Stock PG, Dove LM, et al. Virologic and clinical outcomes of hepatitis B virus infection in HIV–HBV co-infected transplant recipients. *Am J Transplant.* 2010;10:1268–1275.

Di Biagio A, Rosso R, Siccardi M, et al. Lack of interaction between raltegravir and cyclosporine in an HIV-infected liver transplant recipient. *J Antimicrob Chemother.* 2009;64(4):874–875.

Doberne JW, Jawitz OK, Raman V, et al. Heart transplantation survival outcomes of HIV positive and negative recipients. *Ann Thorac Surg.* 2020;S0003-4975(20):31484–31488.

Durand CM, Zhang W, Brown DM, et al. A prospective multicenter pilot study of HIV-positive deceased donor to HIV-positive recipient kidney transplantation: HOPE in action. *Am J Transplant.* 2020 [online ahead of print].

Frasetto LA, Browne M, Cheng A, et al. Immunosuppressant pharmacokinetics and dosing modifications in HIV-1 infected liver and kidney transplant recipients. *Am J Transplant.* 2007;7(12):2816–2820. https://www.ncbi.nlm.nih.gov/pubmed/17949460

Gabardi S, Martin ST, Roberts KL, et al. Induction immunosuppressive therapies in renal transplantation. *Am J Health Syst Pharm.* 2011;68:211–218.

Hathorn E, Smit E, Elsharkawy AM, et al. HIV-positive-to-HIV-positive liver transplantation. *N Engl J Med.* 2016;375(18):1807–1809.

Koval CE, Farr J, Krisl J, et al. Heart or lung transplant outcomes in HIV-infected recipients. *J Heart Lung Transplant.* 2019;38(12):1296–1305.

Kucirka LM, Durand CM, Bae S, et al. Induction immunosuppression and clinical outcomes in kidney transplant recipients infected with human immunodeficiency virus. *Am J Transplant.* 2016;16(8):2368–2376.

Lauterio A, Moioli MC, Di Sandro S, et al. HIV-positive to HIV-positive liver transplantation: to be continued. *J Hepatol.* 2019;70(4):788–789.

Lee DH, Malat GE, Bias TE, et al. Serum creatinine elevation after switch to dolutegravir in a human immunodeficiency virus-positive kidney transplant recipient. *Transpl Infect Dis.* 2016;18(4):625–627.

Lee WC, Shu KH, Cheng CH, et al. Long-term impact of hepatitis B, C virus infection on renal transplantation. *Am J Nephrol.* 2001;21:300–306.

Locke JE, Durand C, Reed RD, et al. Long-term outcomes after liver transplantation among human immunodeficiency virus-infected recipients. *Transplantation.* 2016;100(1):141–146.

Locke JE, Gustafson MD, Mehta S, et al. Survival benefit of kidney transplantation in HIV-infected patients. *Ann Surg.* 2017;265(3):604–608.

Locke JE, James NT, Mannon RB, et al. Immunosuppression regimen and the risk of acute rejection in HIV-positive kidney transplant recipients. *Transplantation.* 2014;97(4):446–450.

Locke JE, Mehta S, Reed RD, et al. A national study of outcomes among HIV-infected kidney transplant recipients. *J Am Soc Nephrol.* 2015;265:2222–2229.

Locke JE, Mehta S, Sawinski D, et al. Access to kidney transplantation among HIV-infected waitlist candidates. *Clin J Am Soc Nephrol*. 2017;12(3):467–475.

Malani P. HIV and transplantation: new reasons for HOPE. *JAMA*. 2016;316(2):136–138.

Manzardo C, Londoño MC, Castells L, et al. Direct-acting antivirals are effective and safe in HCV/HIV-coinfected liver transplant recipients who experience recurrence of hepatitis C: a prospective nationwide cohort study. *Am J Transplant*. 2018;18(10):2513–2522.

Miro JM, Agüero F, Duclos-Vallée JC, et al. Infections in solid organ transplant HIV-positive patients. *Clin Microbiol Infect*. 2014;20:119–130.

Miro JM, Montejo M. Castells L, et al. Outcomes of HCV/HIV-coinfected liver transplant recipients: a prospective and multicenter cohort study. *Am J Transplant*. 2012;12:1866–1876.

Miro JM, Ricart MJ, Trullas JC, et al. Simultaneous pancreas–kidney transplantation in HIV-infected patients: a case report and literature review. *Transplant Proc*. 2010;42(9):3887–3891.

Miro JM, Stock P, Teicher E, et al. Outcome and management of HCV/HIV coinfection pre- and post-liver transplantation: a 2015 update. *J Hepatol*. 2015;62:701–711.

Mocroft A, Lundgren JD, Ross M, et al. Cumulative and current exposure to potentially nephrotoxic antiretrovirals and development of chronic kidney disease in HIV-positive individuals with a normal baseline estimated glomerular filtration rate: a prospective international cohort study. *Lancet HIV*. 2016;3(1):e23–e32.

Mombelli M, Rettby N, Perreau M, et al. Immunogenicity and safety of double versus standard dose of the seasonal influenza vaccine in solid-organ transplant recipients: a randomized controlled trial. *Vaccine*. 2018;36(41):6163–6169.

Muller E, Barday Z, Kahn D. HIV-positive-to-HIV-positive kidney transplantation: results at 3 and 5 years. *N Engl J Med*. 2015;372:613–620.

Nettles RE, Kieffer TL, Kwon P, et al. Intermittent HIV-1 viremia (blips) and drug resistance in patients receiving HAART. *JAMA*. 2005;293(7):817–829.

Nguyen AQ, Anjum SK, Halpern SE, et al. Willingness to donate organs among people living with HIV. *J AIDS*. 2018;79(1):e30–e36.

Nissen NN, Barin B, Stock PG. Malignancy in the HIV-positive patients undergoing liver and kidney transplantation. *Curr Opin Oncol*. 2012;24:517–521.

Platt L, Easterbrook P, Gower E, et al. Prevalence and burden of HCV co-infection in people living with HIV: a global systematic review and meta-analysis. *Lancet Infect Dis*. 2016;16:797–808.

Reshef R, Luger SM, Hexner E, et al. Blockade of lymphocyte chemotaxis in visceral graft-versus-host disease. *N Engl J Med*. 2012;367(2):135–145.

Roland ME, Barin B, Huprikar S, et al.; HIVTR Study Team. Survival in HIV-positive transplant recipients compared with transplant candidates and with HIV-negative controls. *AIDS*. 2016;30(3):435–444.

Saag MS, Benson CA, Gandhi RT, et al. Antiretroviral drugs for treatment and prevention of HIV infection in adults. 2018 recommendations of the International Antiviral Society–USA Panel. *JAMA*. 2018;320(4):379–396.

Sawinski D, Forde KA, Eddinger K, et al. Superior outcomes in HIV-positive kidney transplant patients compared with HCV-infected or HIV/HCV co-infected recipients. *Kidney Int*. 2015;88:341–349.

Sawinski D, Goldberg DS, Blumberg E, et al. Beyond the NIH multicenter HIV transplant trial experience: outcomes of HIV⁺ liver transplant recipients compared to HCV⁺ or HIV⁺/HCV⁺ co-infected recipients in the United States. *Clin Infect Dis*. 2015;61(7):1054–1062.

Sawinski D, Shelton BA, Mehta S, et al. Impact of protease inhibitor-based anti-retroviral therapy on outcomes for HIV⁺ kidney transplant recipients. *Am J Transplant*. 2017;17(12):3114–3122.

Seaman SM, Van Pilsum Rasmussen SE, Nguyen AQ, et al. Brief report: willingness to accept HIV-infected and increased infectious risk donor organs among transplant candidates living with HIV. *J AIDS*. 2020;85(1):88–92.

Shaffer AA, Durand CM. Solid organ transplantation for HIV-infected individuals. *Curr Treat Options Infect Dis*. 2018;10(1):107–120.

Spagnuolo V, Uberti-Foppa C, Castagna A. Pharmacotherapeutic management of HIV in transplant patients. *Expert Opin Pharmacother*. 2019;20(10):1235–1250.

Sparkes T, Manitpisitkul W, Masters B, et al. Impact of antiretroviral regimen on renal transplant outcomes in HIV-positive recipients. *Transpl Infect Dis*. 2018;20(6):e12992.

Stadtmauer EA, Sullivan KM, Marty FM, et al. A phase 1/2 study of an adjuvanted varicella-zoster virus subunit vaccine in autologous hematopoietic cell transplant recipients. *Blood*. 2014;124(19):2921–2929.

Stock P, Barin B, Murphy B, et al. Outcomes of kidney transplantation in HIV-positive recipients. *N Engl J Med*. 2010;363:2001–2014.

Suarez JF, Rosa R, Lorio MA, et al. Pretransplant CD4 count influences immune reconstitution and risk of infectious complications in human immunodeficiency virus-infected kidney allograft recipients. *Am J Transplant*. 2016;16(8):2463–2472.

Sun H-Y, Sheng W-H, Tsai M-S, et al. Hepatitis B virus coinfection in human immunodeficiency virus-infected patients: a review. *World J Gastroenterol*. 2014;20:14598–614.

Te H, Doucette K. Viral hepatitis: guidelines by the American Society of Transplantation Infectious Disease Community of Practice. *Clin Transpl*. 2019;33:e13499.

Terrault N, Roland ME, Schiano T, et al. Outcomes of liver transplant recipients with hepatitis C and human immunodeficiency virus coinfection. *Liver Transpl*. 2012;18(6):716–726.

Trullas JC, Cofan F, Tuset M, et al. Renal transplantation in HIV-positive patients: 2010 update. *Kidney Int*. 2011;79(8):825–842. https://www.ncbi.nlm.nih.gov/pubmed/21248716

van Maarseveen EM, Rogers CC, Trofe-Clark J, et al. Drug–drug interactions between antiretroviral and immunosuppressive agents in HIV-positive patients after solid organ transplantation: a review. *AIDS Patient Care STDs*. 2012;26(10):568–581.

Vivanco M, Friedmann P, Zia Y, et al. Campath induction in HCV and HCV/HIV-seropositive kidney transplant recipients. *Transpl Int*. 2013;26(10):1016–1026.

Werbel WA, Bae S, Yu S, et al. Early steroid withdrawal in HIV-infected kidney transplant recipients: utilization and outcomes. *Am J Transplant*. 2020 [online ahead of print].

23.

SELECT TOPICS IN THE CARE OF WOMEN WITH HIV

Theresa Christensen, Jason J. Schafer, and William R. Short

CHAPTER GOALS

Upon completion of this chapter, the reader should be able to:

- Discuss family planning and preconception care considerations in serodifferent couples living with HIV

- Discuss the recommended frequency and specimen collection technique for cervical Pap smears in women with HIV, the role of human papillomavirus (HPV) testing, and indications for specialist referral for colposcopy

- Describe the appropriate management of antiretroviral therapy (ART) for pregnant women with HIV

CONTRACEPTION AND PRECONCEPTION CARE

WHAT'S NEW?

- Recommendations on the use of dolutegravir in women who are currently pregnant and those of childbearing potential who are trying to conceive have been updated.

- Prior to attempts at conception, maximal viral load suppression should be achieved to decrease the risk of sexual transmission to a partner without HIV and potentially to the infant if conception is achieved.

- In serodifferent couples who wish to conceive naturally, condomless intercourse on the day of ovulation and 2 to 3 days preceding ovulation may be considered if the person with HIV (PWH) is on ART and has maintained sustained viral suppression. This option for conception carries extremely low risk of transmission to the partner without HIV.

- For serodifferent couples who attempt to conceive naturally through condomless intercourse when the PWH has not maintained sustained viral suppression or their status is unknown, daily use of preexposure prophylaxis (PrEP) is recommended to reduce the risk of HIV transmission to the partner without HIV. Condomless sex should be limited to days of peak fertility.

- In serodifferent couples who wish to conceive naturally through condomless intercourse during peak fertility, it is unclear whether the use of PrEP for the partner without HIV further reduces the risk of sexual transmission when the PWH has achieved viral suppression.

KEY POINTS

- Healthcare providers need to be proactive in addressing issues related to preconception care and contraception in women living with HIV who are of childbearing age.

- PWH should strive to achieve long-term, maximal suppression of viral load prior to attempts at conception. New recommendations have been made to address situations in which maximal suppression has been achieved, has not been achieved, or is unknown in serodifferent couples.

- HIV infection does not preclude the use of any methods of hormonal contraception; however, providers must make themselves aware of any potential drug–drug interactions between hormonal contraceptive methods and ART.

- Emergency contraception, including emergency contraceptive pills or copper intrauterine devices (IUDs), may be offered to women with HIV when clinically appropriate. Drug–drug interactions must be considered when using hormonal emergency contraception in combination with ART.

Women now account for approximately 23% of PWH in the US, and in 2018 19% of new HIV diagnoses in the US were in females (Centers for Disease Control and Prevention [CDC] et al., 2019). Because of this, there is continued emphasis placed on family planning and preconception care. The goals of family planning and preconception care are to promote pregnancy planning, reduce unintended pregnancy, and support safer conception and pregnancy for mother, fetus/infant, and partner without HIV. All women of childbearing age who are living with HIV should be offered comprehensive family planning and preconception care as part of routine primary medical care (American College of Obstetricians and Gynecologists [ACOG] et al., 2016).

IMPORTANCE OF FAMILY PLANNING AND PRECONCEPTION CARE

It is increasingly important for healthcare providers to be proactive in addressing issues related to preconception care and contraception in PWH who are of childbearing age. In areas where antiretroviral drugs (ARVs) are widely available and accessible, HIV has become a chronic disease with life expectancy comparable to that of persons without HIV (van Sighem et al., 2010), and perinatal transmission rates have been reduced to less than 1% (ACOG, 2016). Fertility desires in women with HIV in many studies show little difference from those in women without HIV (Craft et al., 2007; Finocchario-Kessler et al., 2012; Loutfy et al., 2009; Nattabi et al., 2009; Squires et al., 2011). In the Women's Interagency HIV Study cohort there was a 150% increase in live birth rates among women with HIV in the ART era when compared to the pre-ART era (Sharma et al., 2007). Current estimates are that 500 women with HIV give birth annually.

Studies among women with HIV suggest that unintended pregnancies are approximately 50% or higher (Craft et al., 2007; Loutfy et al., 2009; Massad et al., 2004). Many pregnancies among women with HIV occur despite the use of contraception (Massad et al., 2004), implying that the pregnancies were unintended and highlighting the importance of adequate and accurate counseling about use of effective birth control. Patients with unintended pregnancies are more likely than those without to not have received obstetrical/gynecologic care or HIV monitoring in the past year (Sutton et al., 2018). Women living with HIV express the desire to talk about reproductive plans with their healthcare providers; however, data suggest that such counseling does not often occur until after conception (Finocchario-Kessler et al., 2010; Loutfy et al., 2013; Panozzo et al., 2003; Squires et al., 2011).

COUNSELING AND ASSESSMENT ABOUT CHILDBEARING AND CONTRACEPTION

Because they may change over time, childbearing desires and intentions, including timing of pregnancy, should be assessed during the initial evaluation and at intervals throughout the course of care. A comprehensive HIV, medical, and obstetrical/gynecologic history and understanding of patient goals are important areas on which to focus counseling and assist in decision-making. Women who wish to prevent or delay pregnancy should receive information about contraceptive options and their efficacy, adverse effects, and other advantages or disadvantages, including noncontraceptive benefits. Individuals who wish to conceive should be given information about risk, rates, and prevention of perinatal transmission and the potential effects of HIV or its treatment on pregnancy course and outcomes. For couples in serodifferent relationships, the PWH should be counseled about the benefits of ART in reducing HIV transmission (Cohen et al., 2011). Disclosure and/or knowledge of HIV status for both partners is particularly important when conception is planned and should be encouraged and supported. It is also important to reinforce with patients that there may be legal ramifications for nondisclosure in certain jurisdictions. Knowledge of the disclosure laws in your area is suggested for review with patients during counseling sessions.

CARE FOR WOMEN WITH HIV WISHING TO CONCEIVE

Interventions for women who wish to conceive include the following:

- Overall health should be optimized with attention to standard primary care and management of chronic diseases, as well as treatment of drug and alcohol abuse.

- Benefits of smoking cession and the elimination of other drugs and alcohol for mother and developing fetus should be reviewed and referrals to cessation services should be offered.

- All current medications, including prescription, over-the-counter, and complementary/alternative medications, should be reviewed, and potential adverse effects associated with use of these drugs in pregnancy should be assessed.

- The need to initiate or modify an ART regimen should be evaluated for all women living with HIV prior to conception. For women on ART, a stable, maximally suppressed maternal viral load should be achieved prior to conception. The choice of ART regimen should take into account current adult treatment guidelines, what is known about the use of specific drugs in pregnancy, and the risk of teratogenicity or other adverse effects. The current guidelines for ART management during conception and the prenatal period can be found at https://clinicalinfo.hiv.gov/guidelines/perinatal.

- Both partners should be screened for genital tract infections, and these should be treated if present. Genital tract inflammation is associated with genital tract shedding of HIV, even in the setting of fully suppressed HIV viral load, and may additionally increase plasma viremia (Johnson & Lewis, 2008).

- Immunizations should be reviewed and updated as indicated, and folic acid supplementation should be started.

- Education on the risks of breastfeeding and potential transmission of the HIV virus to the infant should be discussed. It is currently recommended that women living with HIV in the US not breastfeed their infants due to the availability of sustainable and safe formula alternatives.

DOLUTEGRAVIR (DTG)

In 2018, preliminary data from a National Institutes of Health (NIH) observational study in Botswana identified an increased signal of neural tube defects (NTDs) in infants whose mothers initiated DTG prior to or when becoming pregnant and were receiving it at the time of conception (Zash et al., 2019). The same study provided data that women who initiated a DTG-based regimen in the first trimester had no increased signal of NTDs. Similar findings were noted in 396 women who began an efavirenz (EFV)-based regimen during their first trimester of pregnancy (Zash et al., 2017).

Of note, the analysis has been sequentially updated with additional pregnancies and the signal for increased incidence of NTDs associated with pregnancies in women receiving DTG at the time of conception has decreased to be statistically not different than women receiving non-DTG regimens (Zash et al., 2020).

The US Department of Health and Human Services (DHHS) now recommends DTG as a "preferred" ARV throughout pregnancy, regardless of trimester, and as an "alternative" ARV for women who are trying to conceive. A summary of the recommendations can be found here: https://clinicalinfo.hiv.gov/en/guidelines/perinatal/appendix-d-dolutegravir-counseling-guide-health-care-providers.

For more details on these recommendations, a table summary of the recommendations, and detailed treatment alternatives, please refer to the original article or most recent DHHS guidelines (2020) at https://clinicalinfo.hiv.gov/en/guidelines/perinatal/appendix-d-dolutegravir-counseling-guide-health-care-providers.

EFV

Animal models have suggested an increased risk of NTDs with the use of EFV. Prospective follow-up trials have not detected an increased risk when EFV is used in the first trimester of pregnancy (ACOG, 2016). In prior updates to the DHHS guidelines, the use of EFV prior to 8 weeks of pregnancy was not recommended due to the perceived risk of NTDs. Newer data from the Antiretroviral Pregnancy Registry (2018) include defects in 29 of 990 first-trimester exposures to the drug (2.4%; 95% confidence interval [CI], 1.4, 3.3). The same data revealed defects in 3 of 190 with late exposure (1.6%; 95% CI, 0.3, 4.6). Current data on first-trimester exposures have been enough to rule out a twofold increase in NTDs with use of the drug (NIH et al., 2020b). Data from a multicohort analysis showed birth defects 19 of 2,000 live births to women exposed to EFV at conception (1.6%; 95% CI, 0.96, 2.5), with none of these birth defects being NTDs (Begoña et al., 2019). This has led to the DHHS lifting its restriction on the use of EFV prior to 8 weeks of gestation. This decision is in line with recommendations from both the World Health Organization (WHO) and the British HIV Association. It is also recommended that women who are tolerating EFV well and have suppressed viral loads continue its use throughout their pregnancy. It is of note that the caution remains in the product's package insert.

HIV-SEROPOSITIVE COUPLES

In couples where both partners are HIV positive, a crucial aspect of the reproductive effort is ensuring that both partners have optimized their individual health. This should be accomplished from both the general and HIV perspective. This includes regular visits to their primary care provider, gynecologist, and HIV specialist for the female partner and evaluation by a primary care provider and HIV specialist for the male partner. In both cases, sustained optimal viral suppression through ART is critical. Each partner should be evaluated and treated for sexually transmitted infections because their presence can cause inflammation in the genital tract, which can lead to shedding of the virus even when the plasma viral load is undetectable (DHHS, 2020b). Unprotected intercourse should be timed to coincide with ovulation.

A semen analysis should be strongly considered for any male partner with HIV prior to attempting conception. Semen abnormalities have been noted in male patients living with HIV. These include motility abnormalities, low sperm count, low volume of ejaculate, and abnormal morphology (Cardona-Maya et al., 2009). These abnormalities are thought to arise from ART use and/or because of viral exposure itself. Early detection of semen abnormalities can identify potential infertility issues and thus limit the risk of viral mutation from unprotected intercourse.

Along with discussions aimed at identifying potential fetal risks and benefits during pregnancy, it is also important to counsel patients on psychosocial issues. While there have been advances to allow couples to conceive with significantly lower risk of superinfection or viral mutation, other issues remain. Specifically, although ART has significantly extended life expectancy of PWH, it is unclear how well that correlates to life expectancy in uninfected control populations. Medication adherence, genetics, and other factors may still cause the loss of one or both parents with HIV prior to the child becoming an adult (American Society for Reproductive Medicine, 2015). This in and of itself is not enough to counsel against conception but should be a part of conversations on the risks and benefits of conception in HIV-positive parents.

HIV-SERODIFFFERENT COUPLES

In cases where the female partner is living with HIV and is not virologically suppressed, it is advised that artificial insemination is the safest route of conception. This may be achieved through consultation with a physician, or the patient may choose to inseminate herself during her ovulatory window.

In cases where the male partner is living with HIV, consultation with a reproductive health specialist may be beneficial in identifying the options available to the couple. As previously mentioned, a semen analysis is recommended for males with HIV prior to attempts at conception to evaluate for abnormalities. The safest option for conception is insemination with a sperm donor. If this method is unacceptable or undesirable, techniques such as intrauterine insemination or in vitro fertilization with intracytoplasmic sperm injection utilizing sperm that have gone through preparatory techniques may be a suitable alternative (American Society for Reproductive Medicine, 2015; DHHS 2020b). Each of these options provides an excellent chance for fertility, with low risk of seroconversion of the mother and fetus.

Although ART-related options greatly reduce or eliminate HIV transmission risk between serodifferent partners, many couples desire more natural options to conceive. In couples where one partner is HIV negative and natural conception is desired, the goal is to achieve pregnancy while minimizing the risk of HIV transmission to the HIV-negative partner and, if this partner is female, to the baby as well. It is estimated that the risk of transmission to an HIV-negative partner is approximately 1 in 500 to 1,000 episodes of unprotected intercourse. The risk depends on the viral load of the partner with HIV (Mandelbrot et al., 1997). In light of this, the partner with HIV should receive ART to achieve sustained, maximal viral suppression prior to attempting conception (DHHS, 2020b).

The PARTNERS 1 trial was conducted to investigate HIV transmission rates in serodifferent couples (both heterosexual and men who have sex with men [MSM]) when maximal viral suppression with ART was achieved in the partner living with HIV. A total of 1,166 couples in the trial practiced condomless sex. At the end of 1.3 years, no cases of HIV transmission to the HIV-negative partner were demonstrated (DHHS, 2020b; Rodger et al., 2016). Similar results were found in a study of 161 serodifferent couples attempting to conceive via natural means: 144 were successful, 107 babies were born, and no cases of vertical transmission or transmission of HIV to the uninfected partner were noted (Del Romero et al., 2016; DHHS, 2020b).

Based on the results of these trials, several new recommendations have been made regarding natural conception between serodifferent partners:

1. In serodifferent couples who wish to conceive naturally, unprotected (condomless) intercourse in the peri-ovulatory period (2–3 days preceding ovulation) and the day of ovulation may be considered if the PWH is on ART and has maintained sustained viral suppression. This option for conception carries extremely low risk of transmission to the HIV-negative partner.

2. In serodifferent couples who wish to conceive naturally through unprotected (condomless) intercourse when the PWH has not maintained sustained viral suppression or their status is unknown, daily use of PrEP is recommended to reduce the risk of HIV transmission to the partner without HIV. Unprotected (condomless) sex should be limited to days of peak fertility.

3. In serodifferent couples who wish to conceive naturally through unprotected (condomless) intercourse during peak fertility, it is unclear whether the use of PrEP for the uninfected partner further reduces the risk of sexual transmission when the PWH has achieved viral suppression.

Providers may present the optional use of ovulation kits to couples to better predict peak fertility and assist in timing of unprotected intercourse.

In serodifferent couples who elect to use PrEP during the conception period, the CDC recommends that the partner without HIV begin treatment with daily combination tenofovir/emtricitabine 1 month prior to attempting conception and continue for 1 month beyond attempted conception (DHHS, 2020b). As in patients who are using PrEP for routine HIV prophylaxis, baseline HIV and pregnancy testing should be performed and repeated at 3-month intervals and renal function assessed at baseline and 6-month intervals (DHHS, 2020b).

CARE FOR WOMEN WISHING TO PREVENT OR DELAY PREGNANCY

In 2014, an expert panel from the WHO reviewed the evidence on currently available methods of hormonal contraception and reaffirmed their 2009 statement that women living with HIV can potentially use all existing hormonal contraceptive methods without restriction (WHO, 2014). However, special care must still be taken to address any potential drug–drug interactions and alterations in pharmacokinetics that may occur when ART and contraceptives are used together.

The WHO and the CDC state that with use of methods involving spermicides containing nonoxynol-9, the risks generally outweigh the advantages of the method because of potential disruption of cervical mucosa, which may increase viral shedding and HIV transmission to HIV-negative partners. Both the copper IUD and the levonorgestrel-containing IUD can be initiated or continued in women living with HIV who are clinically doing well on ART therapy. Pharmacokinetic interactions between hormonal contraceptives (primarily studied with combined estrogen–progestin oral contraceptives) and some protease inhibitors (PIs) and nonnucleoside reverse transcriptase inhibitors (NNRTIs) may modify steroid levels and potentially decrease contraceptive effectiveness or increase risk of adverse effects, although the true clinical effect is not clear; an additional or alternative contraceptive method is generally advised if hormonal contraception is considered (Cohn et al., 2007; El-Ibiary & Cocohoba, 2008; DHHS, 2020b; Vogler et al., 2010). Specifically, women on ritonavir-boosted PI regimens should be placed on an additional or alternative method of contraception if using ART with combination hormonal contraceptives. These methods include patches, pills, rings, or progestin-only pills. Similarly, in patients taking EFV, an additional barrier contraceptive or alternative regimen can be considered in women using etonogestrel or levonorgestrel contraceptive implants or combined oral contraceptives (Landolt et al., 2013; DHHS, 2020b; Patel et al., 2015). For a detailed list of contraceptive drugs and their potential interactions with ARVs, please see the table labeled "Drug Interactions Between Antiretroviral Agents and Hormonal Contraceptives" in the most current DHHS "Recommendations for Use of Antiretroviral Drug in Pregnant HIV-1 Infected Women for Maternal Health and Interventions to Reduce Perinatal HIV Transmission in the United States" (DHHS, 2020b).

Emergency contraception, including emergency oral contraceptives or the copper IUD, may be offered to women with HIV if clinically appropriate. When oral contraceptives (either combination or levonorgestrel only) are used with ARVs, the potential for drug interactions seems to be similar to when they are used for routine contraception (DHHS, 2020b).

Currently, there are no data on interactions between ART and ulipristal acetate, but interactions should be anticipated due to the metabolism of ulipristal acetate through the CYP3A4 pathways (DHHS, 2020b).

Most studies have found no association between the use of hormonal contraception and HIV disease progression (Morrison et al., 2011; Polis et al., 2010; Stringer et al., 2009). Early observational studies indicated that certain types of hormonal contraception, particularly depot medroxyprogesterone acetate (DMPA), might increase risk of HIV infection among at-risk seronegative women. However, the ECHO trial recently showed no significant difference in HIV acquisition among 7,800 women using intramuscular DMPA, copper IUDs, or levonorgestrel implants (ECHO Trial Consortium, 2019). Based on this study, the WHO recently updated its recommendations to indicate that women at higher risk for HIV infection should have the option of using any reversible contraception method, including all hormonal options (WHO, 2019). Regardless of what hormonal contraception choice is made, family planning conversations should emphasize the importance of PrEP and condoms to prevent transmission of HIV and other sexually transmitted infections,

RECOMMENDED READING

Carten ML, Kiser JJ, Kwara A, et al. Pharmacokinetic interactions between the hormonal emergency contraception, levonorgestrel (Plan B), and Efavirenz. *Infect Dis Obstet Gynecol.* 2012;2012:137192.

Department of Health and Human Services, Panel on Treatment of Pregnant Women with HIV Infection and Prevention of Perinatal Transmission. Recommendations for Use of Antiretroviral Drugs in Pregnant Women with HIV Infection and Interventions to Reduce Perinatal HIV Transmission in the United States. 2020. https://clinicalinfo.hiv.gov/en/guidelines/perinatal

CERVICAL HPV INFECTION IN WOMEN WITH HIV

WHAT'S NEW?

The cervical cancer screening guidelines for women living with HIV have been updated by the DHHS to include new recommendations for follow-up of an atypical squamous cells of undetermined significance (ASCUS) Pap smear with negative reflex HPV and a new recommendation for screening in women living with HIV who are 65 and older.

KEY POINTS

- In women with HIV younger than 21 years of age, cervical cancer screening (with liquid-based Pap alone) should begin within 1 year of the onset of sexual activity and no later than age 21 years. If normal, the test is repeated every 12 months. If the patient has three consecutive normal screenings, the testing interval should be increased to every 3 years.
- In women with HIV older than 30 years of age, cervical cancer screening with either Pap alone or combined with HPV co-testing may be offered. The appropriate interval of follow-up screening is determined by the type of screening performed and the results returned.
- Unlike the general population, women living with HIV who are 65 and older should continue screening with Pap alone or Pap and HPV co-testing.

In general, infection with HPV, the cause of cervical cancer, is quite common in the United States, with an estimated 24.9 million women between the ages of 14 to 59 having the infection (Dunne et al., 2007). Compared with HIV-negative women, women with HIV have a higher prevalence and incidence of HPV (Ahdieh et al., 2001; Branca et al., 2003), longer persistence of HPV (Ahdieh et al., 2001; Sun et al., 1997), higher HPV levels (Jamieson et al., 2002), higher prevalence of multiple HPV subtypes (Firnhaber et al., 2009; Jamieson et al., 2002; Sahasrabuddhe et al., 2007), and higher prevalence of oncogenic subtypes (Firnhaber et al., 2009; Minkoff et al., 1998; Volkow et al., 2001). In addition, there is increased HPV prevalence and persistence of high-risk HPV with decreasing CD4+ T-cell counts (Denny et al., 2008; Palefsky et al., 1999) and increasing HIV RNA levels (Palefsky et al., 1999). Also, compared to HIV-negative women, women with HIV are more likely to have abnormal cervical cytology (Denny et al., 2008; Ellerbrock et al., 2000), and both frequency and severity of cervical dysplasia increase with declining CD4+ T-cell counts (Davis et al., 2001; Massad et al., 2001, 2008). Recurrent cervical dysplasia after treatment is more common among women with HIV (Boardman et al., 1999; Fruchter et al., 1996; Holcomb et al., 1999; Massad et al., 2001; Six et al., 1998). Rates of cervical cancer are also significantly higher among women with HIV compared to women in the general population (Chaturvedi et al., 2009; Clifford et al., 2005; Dal Maso et al., 2009; Grulich et al., 2007). Several HPV subtypes have been associated with the development of squamous intraepithelial lesions and cervical cancer, including most commonly HPV-16 (found in almost half of all cervical cancers) and HPV-18 (found in 10–12% of cervical cancers) and less commonly HPV-31, -33, -35, -39, -45, -51, -52, -56, -58, -59, and -68 (each accounting for <5% of cervical cancers) (Castle et al., 2009; Schiffman & Solomon, 2009).

CERVICAL PAP SMEARS

Due to the high level of HPV infection and higher prevalence of oncogenic subtypes, it is critical for women with HIV to be regularly screened for cervical dysplasia. Although a single Pap smear has historically been associated with high false-negative rates (10–25%), regular screening can significantly improve accuracy (Anderson et al., 2012), and Pap smear screening programs have been associated with marked reductions in cervical cancer incidence (Eddy, 1990; Nygard et al., 2002).

Since the 2017 edition of *Fundamentals of HIV Medicine*, new recommendations for the follow-up of ASCUS with negative high-risk HPV and screening for women older than 65 have been added. The cervical cancer screening recommendations reflect the paradigm shift in testing noted with HIV-negative women in the 2012 recommendations. Table 23.1 presents a summary of the cervical cancer screening recommendations from the NIH et al. The recommendations are categorized into three groups: those for women with HIV younger than 21 years, those between 21 and 30 years, and those older than 30 years.

Table 23.1 CERVICAL CANCER SCREENING RECOMMENDATIONS FOR WOMEN WITH HIV

AGE	SCHEDULE	FOLLOW-UP RECOMMENDATIONS FOR ABNORMAL RESULTS

<21 years	• Start liquid-based Pap screening within 1 year of onset of sexual activity or at age 21, whichever comes first.
	  • Regardless of method of exposure to HIV
	  • Co-testing not recommended due to high prevalence of HPV in this age group
	• Repeat screen 12 months after HIV diagnosis if screen is normal.
	  • Note: Some experts recommend screen after 6 months.
	• Increase screening interval to 3 years after 3 consecutive normal tests.
		• Reflex HPV test if cytology shows ASCUS or greater
		  • Colposcopy if HPV positive
		• Colposcopy if cytology shows low-grade squamous intraepithelial lesion (LGSIL) or greater regardless of HPV status

21–30 years	• Baseline liquid-based Pap at initial HIV diagnosis
	  • Co-testing not recommended due to high prevalence of HPV in this age group
	• Repeat screen 12 months after HIV diagnosis if screen is normal.
	  • Note: Some experts recommend screen after 6 months.
	• Increase screening interval to 3 years after 3 consecutive normal tests.
		• Reflex HPV test if ASCUS or greater
		  • Colposcopy if HPV positive
		• Colposcopy if cytology shows LGSIL or greater regardless of HPV status

>30 years	• Option 1: Pap without HPV test at initial HIV diagnosis
	  • Repeat screen 12 months after HIV diagnosis if screen is normal.
	  • Note: Some experts recommend repeat screen after 6 months.
	  • Increase screening interval to 3 years after 3 consecutive normal tests.
	• Option 2: Pap with HPV co-test at HIV diagnosis
	  • Repeat in 3 years if both negative.
	• *Do not discontinue screening for either option at 65 years—continue screening throughout lifetime in HIV-positive population.*
		• Repeat Pap in 6–12 months if Pap shows ASCUS and HPV is negative or unavailable. Colposcopy if ASCUS or greater on repeat cytology.
		• If normal Pap but positive HPV on co-test:
		  • Colposcopy if HPV subtype is HPV16 or HPV16/18 positive
		  • Otherwise, repeat co-test in 1 year. Colposcopy if repeat test abnormal (either Pap or HPV).
		• Colposcopy if cytology shows LGSIL or greater regardless of HPV status

SOURCE: Department of Health and Human Services (DHHS). Panel on Guidelines for the Prevention and Treatment of Opportunistic Infections in Adults and Adolescents with HIV. Guidelines for the Prevention and Treatment of Opportunistic Infections in HIV-infected Adults and Adolescents: Recommendations from the Centers for Disease Control and Prevention, the National Institutes of Health, and the HIV Medicine Association of the Infectious Diseases Society of America. 2020a. https://clinicalinfo.hiv.gov/sites/default/files/inline-files/adult_oi.pdf. Accessed October 15, 2020.

CONSIDERATIONS FOR GENDER-DIVERSE PATIENTS

Transgender and gender-diverse individuals who have cervixes are at risk of HPV infection but are less likely than cisgender women to receive regular Pap tests (Hsiao, 2016). Transgender persons are also disproportionately affected by HIV (Clark et al., 2017). Transgender men and gender-diverse persons living with HIV should receive cervical cancer screenings on the same schedule as cisgender women, as outlined previously. Screening procedures should be performed in a supportive and culturally sensitive manner, and providers should be aware that exogenous testosterone use may increase the likelihood of unsatisfactory testing results (Hsiao, 2016). More specific recommendations for Pap smears in transgender patients can be found at https://transcare.ucsf.edu/guidelines/cervical-cancer.

RECOMMENDED READING

erican College of Obstetricians and Gynecologists. Gynecologic care for women with human immunodeficiency virus. *ACOG Practice Bull.* 2016;167 (reaffirmed 2019).
Department of Health and Human Services, Panel on Opportunistic Infections in HIV-Infected Adults and Adolescents. Guidelines for the prevention and treatment of opportunistic infections in HIV-infected adults and adolescents: Recommendations from the Centers for Disease Control and Prevention, the National Institutes of Health, and the HIV Medicine Association of the Infectious Diseases Society of America. https://clinicalinfo.hiv.gov/en/guidelines/adult-and-adolescent-opportunistic-infection

ART IN PREGNANT WOMEN

LEARNING OBJECTIVE

• Review the clinical management of pregnant women with HIV, including recommendations for use of ARVs and drug disposition

WHAT'S NEW?

• Initial results from an ongoing study in Botswana that noted an increased risk of NTDs in infants whose mother became pregnant while receiving a DTG-based regimen as compared to an EFV-based regimen have been updated.

- When a pregnant woman presents on an elvitegravir/cobicistat regimen, providers should consider switching to a more effective regimen. If an elvitegravir/cobicistat regimen is continued, the viral load should be monitored more frequently, and therapeutic drug monitoring may be helpful.

- There are inadequate data to determine whether administration of zidovudine (ZDV) intravenously to women with HIV and a viral load between 50 and 999 copies/mL provides any additional protection against perinatal transmission, but some experts would still administer intravenous ZDV to women with HIV-1 RNA in this range, as the transmission risk is slightly higher when HIV RNA is in the range of 50 to 999 copies/mL compared to less than 50 copies/mL.

KEY POINTS

- ART should be initiated in all pregnant women with HIV regardless of CD4+ T-cell count or HIV-1 RNA level. ARVs should be given as combination therapy, similar to that prescribed for nonpregnant women with HIV, with the goal of complete virologic suppression.

- ART changes during pregnancy have been associated with the loss of virologic control and are independently associated with mother-to-child transmission (MTCT) of HIV.

- All cases of prenatal antiretroviral exposure should be reported to the APR (www.apregistry.com).

INTRODUCTION

Over time, research has demonstrated that proper prevention strategies and interventions during pregnancy, labor, and delivery can significantly reduce the rate of MTCT of HIV. In 1994, a pivotal study in the field of HIV medicine, the Pediatric AIDS Clinical Trials Group (PACTG) 076, demonstrated that the use of ZDV monotherapy during pregnancy substantially reduced the risk of HIV transmission to infants by 67% (Connor et al., 1994). The protocol is summarized in Table 23.2. It consisted of oral administration of ZDV initiated between 14 and 34 weeks of gestation and continued throughout pregnancy, followed by intrapartum administration of intravenous ZDV and oral administration of ZDV to the newborn for 6 weeks after delivery. Additional studies have demonstrated the effectiveness of the use of combination ART, further decreasing the risk of HIV transmission to 1% to 2% (Cooper et al., 2002). Based on recent data, there have been modifications to the original protocol, including a more selective use of intravenous ZDV based on maternal viral load and changes to postpartum administration of ART to the newborn.

PHYSIOLOGIC CHANGES DURING PREGNANCY

Physiologic changes that occur during pregnancy may alter drug disposition and lead to decreased drug exposure. These

Table 23.2 THREE-PART ZDV CHEMOPROPHYLAXIS REGIMEN BASED ON PACTG 076

TIME OF ZDV ADMINISTRATION	REGIMEN
Antepartum	Oral administration of 100 mg ZDV 5 times daily,[a] initiated at 14–34 weeks of gestation and continued throughout pregnancy
Intrapartum	During labor, intravenous administration of ZDV in a 1-hour initial dose of 2 mg/kg body weight, followed by a continuous infusion of 1 mg/kg body weight/hour until delivery
Postpartum	Oral administration of ZDV to the newborn (ZDV syrup at 2 mg/kg body weight/dose every 6 hours) for the first 6 weeks of life, beginning at 8–12 hours after birth[b]

[a] Oral ZDV administered as 200 mg three times daily or 300 mg twice daily is currently used in general clinical practice and is an acceptable alternative regimen to 100 mg five times daily.

[b] Intravenous dosage for full-term infants who cannot tolerate oral intake is 1.5 mg/kg body weight intravenously every 6 hours. ZDV dosing for infants of less than 35 weeks gestation at birth is 1.5 mg/kg/dose intravenously, or 2.0 mg/kg/dose orally, every 12 hours, advancing to every 8 hours at 2 weeks of age if greater than 30 weeks gestation at birth or at 4 weeks of age if less than 30 weeks gestation at birth.

SOURCE: Department of Health and Human Services, Panel on Treatment of Pregnant Women with HIV Infection and Prevention of Perinatal Transmission. Recommendations for Use of Antiretroviral Drugs in Pregnant Women with HIV Infection and Interventions to Reduce Perinatal HIV Transmission in the United States. 2020b. https://clinicalinfo.hiv.gov/en/guidelines/perinatal/whats-new-guidelines. Accessed October 15, 2020.

changes may be associated with incomplete virologic suppression, virologic failure, and/or the development of drug resistance (Mirochnick & Capparelli, 2004). An understanding of the pharmacokinetic changes that can occur with ARVs during pregnancy is essential for making proper dose modifications to maintain efficacy and minimize toxicity. Summarized in Box 23.1 are some of the physiologic changes that occur during pregnancy that could affect drug disposition.

TRANSPLACENTAL TRANSFER OF ARVS

The placenta functions to transfer nutrients and oxygen to the fetus and assist in the removal of waste products (Syme et al., 2004). In general, nucleoside reverse transcriptase inhibitors (NRTIs), NNRTIs, and integrase strand transfer inhibitors (INSTIs) readily cross the placenta. Protease inhibitors (PIs), such as darunavir/ritonavir (DRV/r), are highly protein bound and therefore only the small percentage of drug that is unbound is free to transfer (DHHS, 2020b).

BASIC PRINCIPLES OF ARV USE IN PREGNANCY

- ARVs should be initiated in all pregnant women with HIV regardless of CD4+ T-cell count or HIV-1 RNA level (viral load).

- The regimen should have optimal efficacy and safety and should be well tolerated.

- The regimen should contain at least one NRTI with good placental passage.

- The provider should consider multiple factors when selecting a regimen, including baseline ARV resistance (determined by HIV genotype and treatment history), comorbidities, convenience, adverse effects, drug interactions, pharmacokinetics, and experience in pregnancy.

- Women entering pregnancy on ARVs should continue their regimen if it is effective and well tolerated and does not contain agents that are teratogenic.

RECOMMENDATIONS

ARV-Naive Patients

All women with HIV should receive a potent ARV regimen to reduce the risk of perinatal transmission. For an updated list, please refer to the current DHHS *preferred* and *alternate* regimens for women who have never received ART and are pregnant. There is also a section about drug regimens that are no longer recommended and the rationale for the discontinuation of their use. See https://clinicalinfo.hiv.gov/sites/default/files/inline-files/AdultandAdolescentGL.pdf

Pregnant Women with HIV on ART

HIV-positive pregnant women who present for care in the first trimester should be counseled about the risks and benefits of ART. If possible, they should be maintained on their current ART regimen, as discontinuation may lead to loss of virologic control. This could adversely affect the health of the fetus, including HIV transmission. In a prospective cohort of 937 mother–infant pairs, interruption of ART during the first and third trimesters was independently associated with MTCT of HIV. The overall rate of MTCT of HIV was 1.3%, compared to the rates associated with first- and third-trimester interruptions of ART, which were 4.9% and 18.2%, respectively (Galli et al., 2009).

In the past, there has been concern over the teratogenic effects of EFV use in the first trimester. Preclinical primate data and retrospective reports raised concern about an increased risk of NTDs with EFV use in pregnancy. It is important to note that the neural tube closes at 36 to 39 days after the last menstrual period. Thus, the risk of NTDs is restricted to the first 5 to 6 weeks of pregnancy. Finally, a meta-analysis that included data on 1,437 first-trimester EFV exposures showed *no* overall increased risk of birth defects compared to women on other ARVs. There was one NTD, giving an incidence of 0.07% (Ford et al., 2011). The panel on treatment of pregnant women with HIV has recently updated its recommendation, noting that EFV is an alternative NNRTI regimen due to extensive experience in pregnancy. Coformulated efavirenz//tenofovir disoproxil fumarate/emtricitabine (EFV/TDF/FTC) is the preferred regimen in women who require coadministration of drugs with significant interactions with preferred agents or those who need the convenience of a single tablet and are not eligible for rilpivirine (RPV). It is important to screen for antenatal and postpartum depression (DHHS, 2020).

DTG Use in Pregnancy

The Tsepamo birth outcome study is an ongoing observational study funded by the NIH in Botswana comparing birth outcomes among pregnant women taking EFV- versus DTG-based regimens. In 2018, an interim analysis was reported on women who were taking a DTG-containing regimen before or during conception and revealed 4 out of 429 newborns (0.94%) had NTDs. In comparison, NTDs occurred in 14 out of 11,300 infants (0.0012%) born to women receiving non–DTG-based regimens at the time of conception and 3 out of 5,787 infants (0.05%) born to women on EFV-containing regimens (Zash et al., 2018a). In an updated analysis, there was a marked decrease in the prevalence of NTDs.

The Panel on Antiretroviral Guidelines for Adults and Adolescents, the Panel on Antiretroviral Therapy and Medical Management of Children Living with HIV, and the Panel on Treatment of Pregnant Women Living with HIV and Prevention of Perinatal Transmission have reviewed all updated data and have made recommendations regarding the use of DTG in adults and adolescents with HIV who are pregnant or of childbearing potential; see https://clinicalinfo.hiv.gov/en/guidelines

Pregnant Women with HIV Lacking Viral Suppression

In late pregnancy, lack of virologic suppression could be due to either inadequate time on ART, poor adherence, or virologic failure. Providers must consider several things when evaluating a pregnant woman with lack of viral suppression, including adherence, tolerability, correct dosing, drug interactions, and resistance. If there is a concern for resistance, ARV resistance studies should be sent and consultation with an expert is advised.

There have been case reports on the use of raltegravir-containing regimens in late pregnancy due to the rapid viral decay that has been demonstrated with INSTIs. There are data demonstrating superior viral-load suppression at the time of delivery in pregnant women with HIV receiving DTG-containing regimens versus those receiving EFV-based regimens (DHHS, 2020).

Intrapartum Zdv During Labor

Women with HIV-1 RNA counts of greater than 1,000 copies/mL or an unknown viral load near delivery should receive intravenous ZDV (Briand et al., 2013). In the past, all HIV-positive women were given intravenous ZDV during pregnancy regardless of viral load, as this was part of the PACTG 076 protocol noted earlier in the chapter (see Table 23.2).

The French Perinatal Cohort evaluated perinatal transmission in more than 11,000 pregnant women with HIV receiving ART. The overall rate of perinatal transmission was 0.9% in those who received intravenous ZDV and 1.8% without intravenous ZDV. Among women with HIV-1 RNA levels of more than 1,000 copies/mL, the risk of transmission without ZDV was 10.2% compared to 2.5% with intravenous ZDV if neonates received only ZDV for prophylaxis, but the risk was no different without or with intrapartum ZDV if the neonate received intensified prophylaxis with two or more ARVs. Among women with HIV-1 RNA levels of less than 1,000 copies/mL at delivery, zero transmissions occurred among 369 women who did not receive intravenous ZDV, compared to 0.6% of those receiving intravenous ZDV (Briand et al., 2013). A few additional studies were reported; based on these studies, intravenous ZDV should continue to be administered to women with HIV RNA counts of greater than 1,000 copies/mL near delivery regardless of intrapartum regimen. The panel recommends intrapartum ZDV administration to women with HIV-1 RNA levels in the range of 50 to 999 copies/mL as the risk of transmission is slightly higher (1–2% vs. 1% or less).

ANTIVIRAL PREGNANCY REGISTRY

Established in 1989, the APR collects data on pregnant women with HIV taking ARVs with the goal of detecting any major teratogenic effects. Registration is voluntary and confidential; however, providers are strongly encouraged to enroll pregnant patients in the registry at the time of the initial evaluation of the pregnant woman. This is an observational, exposure registration and follow-up study. The APR is an international registry that has received reports from 67 countries, mostly from the US. More information can be obtained at www.APRegistry.com.

REFERENCES

Ahdieh L, Klein RS, Burk R, et al. Prevalence, incidence, and type-specific persistence of human papillomavirus in human immunodeficiency virus (HIV)-positive and HIV-negative women. *J Infect Dis.* 2001;184:1682–1690.

American College of Obstetricians and Gynecologists. Gynecologic care for women with human immunodeficiency virus. *ACOG Practice Bull.* 2016;167 (reaffirmed 2019).

American Society for Reproductive Medicine. Human immunodeficiency virus (HIV) and infertility treatment: a committee opinion. 2015. https://www.asrm.org/globalassets/asrm/asrm-content/news-and-publications/ethics-committee-opinions/human_immunodeficiency_virus_and_infertility_treatment-pdfmembers.pdf

Anderson J, Lu E, Sanghvi H, et al. Cervical cancer screening and prevention for HIV-infected women in the developing world. In *Cancer Prevention: From Mechanisms to Translational Benefits.* IntechOpen, 2012.

Antiretroviral Pregnancy Registry Steering Committee. Antiretroviral Pregnancy Registry International interim report for 1 January 1989–31 July 2017. 2018. www.APRegistry.com

Begoña MT; European Pregnancy and Paediatric HIV Cohort Collaboration Study Group. Birth defects after exposure to efavirenz-based antiretroviral therapy at conception/first trimester of pregnancy: a multicohort analysis. *J AIDS.* 2019;80(3):316–324.

Boardman LA, Peipert JF, Hogan JW, et al. Positive cone biopsy specimen margins in women infected with the human immunodeficiency virus. *Am J Obstet Gynecol.* 1999;181(6):1395–1399.

Branca M, Garbuglia AR, Benedetto A, et al.; DIANAIDS Collaborative Study Group. Factors predicting the persistence of genital human papillomavirus infections and Pap smear abnormality in HIV-positive and HIV-negative women during prospective follow-up. *Int J STD AIDS.* 2003;14(6):417–425.

Briand N, Warszawski J, Mandelbrot L, et al. Is intrapartum intravenous zidovudine for prevention of mother-to-child HIV-1 transmission still useful in the combination antiretroviral therapy era? *Clin Infect Dis.* 2013;57(6):903–914.

Cardona-Maya W, Velilla P, Montoya CJ, et al. Presence of HIV-1 DNA in spermatozoa from HIV-positive patients: changes in the semen parameters. *Curr HIV Res.* 2009;7(4):418–424.

Castle PE, Rodriquez AC, Burk RD, et al. Short term persistence of human papillomavirus and risk of cervical precancer and cancer: population based cohort study. *BMJ.* 2009;339:b2569. doi:10.1136/bmj.b2569

Centers for Disease Control and Prevention. HIV Surveillance Report, 2018 (Preliminary). Published November 2019. http://www.cdc.gov/hiv/library/reports/hiv-surveillance.html

Chaturvedi AK, Madeleine MM, Biggar RJ, et al. Risk of human papillomavirus-associated cancers among persons with AIDS. *J Natl Cancer Inst.* 2009;101(16):1120–1230.

Clark H, Babu AS, Wiewel EW, et al. Diagnosed HIV infection in transgender adults and adolescents: results from the national HIV surveillance system, 2009–2014. *AIDS Behav.* 2017;21(9):2774–2783.

Clifford GM, Polesel J, Rickenbach M, et al. Cancer risk in the Swiss HIV Cohort Study: associations with immunodeficiency, smoking and highly active antiretroviral therapy. *J Natl Cancer Inst.* 2005;97(6):425–432.

Cohen MS, Chen YQ, McCauley M, et al. Prevention of HIV-1 infection with early antiretroviral therapy. *N Engl J Med.* 2011;365:493–505.

Cohn SE, Park JG, Watts DH, et al. Depo-medroxyprogesterone in women on antiretroviral therapy: Effective contraception and lack of clinically significant interactions. *Clin Pharmacol Ther.* 2007;81(2):222–227.

Connor EM, Sperling RS, Gelber R, et al. Reduction of maternal-infant transmission of human immunodeficiency virus type 1 with zidovudine treatment. *N Engl J Med.* 1994;331:1173–1180.

Cooper ER, Charurat M, Mofenson L, et al. Combination antiretroviral strategies for the treatment of pregnant women HIV-1 infected women and prevention of perinatal HIV-1 transmission. Women and Infants' Transmission Study Group. *J AIDS*. 2002;29(5):489–494.

Craft SM, Delaney RO, Bautista DT, et al. Pregnancy decisions among women with HIV. *AIDS Behav*. 2007;11(6):927–935.

Dal Maso L, Polesel J, Serraino D, et al. Pattern of cancer risk in persons with AIDS in Italy in the HAART era. *Br J Cancer*. 2009;100(5):840–847.

Davis AT, Chakraborty H, Flowers L, et al. Cervical dysplasia in women infected with the human immunodeficiency virus (HIV): a correlation with HIV viral load and CD4+ count. *Gynecol Oncol*. 2001;80(3):350–354.

Del Romero J, Baza MB, Rio I, et al. Natural conception in HIV-serodiscordant couples with the infected partner in suppressive antiretroviral therapy: a prospective cohort study. *Medicine*. 2016;95(30):e4398.

Denny L, Boa R, Williamson AL, et al. Human papillomavirus infection and cervical disease in human immunodeficiency virus-1-infected women. *Obstet Gynecol*. 2008;111(6):1380–1387. doi:10.1097/AOG.0b013e181743327

Department of Health and Human Services (DHHS). Panel on Guidelines for the Prevention and Treatment of Opportunistic Infections in Adults and Adolescents with HIV. Guidelines for the Prevention and Treatment of Opportunistic Infections in HIV-infected Adults and Adolescents: Recommendations from the Centers for Disease Control and Prevention, the National Institutes of Health, and the HIV Medicine Association of the Infectious Diseases Society of America. 2020a. https://clinicalinfo.hiv.gov/sites/default/files/inline-files/adult_oi.pdf

Department of Health and Human Services, Panel on Treatment of Pregnant Women with HIV Infection and Prevention of Perinatal Transmission. Recommendations for Use of Antiretroviral Drugs in Pregnant Women with HIV Infection and Interventions to Reduce Perinatal HIV Transmission in the United States. 2020b. https://clinicalinfo.hiv.gov/en/guidelines/perinatal/whats-new-guidelines.

Dunne EF, Unger ER, Sternberg M, et al. Prevalence of HPV infection among females in the United States. *JAMA*. 2007;297(8):813–819.

ECHO Trial Consortium. HIV incidence among women using intramuscular depot medroxyprogesterone acetate, a copper intrauterine device, or a levonorgestrel implant for contraception: a randomised, multicentre, open-label trial. *Lancet*. 2019;394(10195):303–313.

Eddy DM. Screening for cervical cancer. *Ann Intern Med*. 1990;113(3):214–226.

El-Ibiary SY, Cocohoba JM. Effects of HIV antiretrovirals on the pharmacokinetics of hormonal contraceptives. *Eur J Contracept Reprod Health Care*. 2008;13(2):123–132.

Ellerbrock TV, Chiasson MA, Bush TJ, et al. Incidence of cervical squamous intraepithelial lesions in HIV-infected women. *JAMA*. 2000;283(8):1031–1037.

Finocchario-Kessler S, Dariotis JK, Sweat MD, et al. Do HIV-infected women want to discuss reproductive plans with providers, and are those conversations occurring? *AIDS Patient Care STDs*. 2010;24(5):317–323.

Finocchario-Kessler S, Mabachi N, Dariotis JK, et al. "We weren't using condoms because we were trying to conceive": the need for reproductive counseling for HIV-positive women in clinical care. *AIDS Patient Care STDs*. 2012;26(11):700–707.

Firnhaber C, Zungu K, Levin S, et al. Diverse and high prevalence of human papillomavirus associated with a significant high rate of cervical dysplasia in human immunodeficiency virus-infected women in Johannesburg, South Africa. *Acta Cytol*. 2009;53(1):10–17.

Ford N, Calmy A, Mofenson L. Safety of efavirenz in the first trimester of pregnancy: an updated systematic review and meta-analysis. *AIDS*. 2011;25(18):2301–2304.

Fruchter RG, Maiman M, Sedlis A, et al. Multiple recurrences of cervical intraepithelial neoplasia in women with the human immunodeficiency virus. *Obstet Gynecol*. 1996;87:338–344.

Galli L, Puliti D, Chiappini E, et al. Is the interruption of antiretroviral treatment during pregnancy an additional major risk factor for mother-to-child transmission of HIV type 1? *Clin Infect Dis*. 2009;48:1310–1317.

Grulich AE, van Leeuwen MT, Falster MO, et al. Incidence of cancers in people with HIV/AIDS compared with immunosuppressed transplant recipients: a meta-analysis. *Lancet*. 2007;370(9581):59–67.

Holcomb K, Matthews RP, Chapman JE, et al. The efficacy of cervical conization in the treatment of cervical intraepithelial neoplasia in HIV-positive women. *Gynecol Oncol*. 1999;74(3):428–431.

Hsiao KT. Screening for cervical cancer in transgender men. UCSF Transgender Care. 2016. https://transcare.ucsf.edu/guidelines/cervical-cancer

Jamieson DJ, Duerr A, Burk R, et al. Characterization of genital human papillomavirus infection in women who have or are at risk for having HIV infection. *Am J Obstet Gynecol*. 2002;186(1): 21–27.

Johnson LF, Lewis DA. The effect of genital tract infections on HIV-1 shedding in the genital tract: a systematic review and meta-analysis. *Sex Transm Dis*. 2008;35(11):946–959.

Landolt NK, Phanuphak N, Ubolyam S, et al. Efavirenz, in contrast to nevirapine, is associated with unfavorable progesterone and antiretroviral levels when coadministered with combined oral contraceptives. *J AIDS*. 2013;62(5):534–539.

Loutfy MR, Blitz S, Zhang Y, et al. Self-reported preconception care of HIV-positive women of reproductive potential: a retrospective study. *J Intl Assoc Prov AIDS Care*. 2013;5:424–433.

Loutfy MR, Hart TA, Mohammed SS, et al. Fertility desires and intentions of HIV-positive women of reproductive age in Ontario, Canada: a cross-sectional study. *PLoS One*. 2009;4(12): e7925.

Mandelbrot L, Heard I, Henrion-Geeant E, et al. Natural conception in HIV-negative women with HIV-infected partners. *Lancet*. 1997;349:850–851.

Massad LS, Ahdieh L, Benning L, et al. Evolution of cervical abnormalities among women with HIV-1: evidence from surveillance cytology in the Women's Interagency HIV study. *J AIDS*. 2001;27:432–442.

Massad LS, Seaberg EC, Wright RL, et al. Squamous cervical lesions in women with human immunodeficiency virus: long-term follow-up. *Obstet Gynecol*. 2008;111(6):1388–1393.

Massad LS, Springer G, Jacobson L, et al. Pregnancy rates and predictors of conception, miscarriage and abortion in US women with HIV. *AIDS*. 2004;18(2):281–286.

Minkoff H, Feldman J, DeHovitz J, et al. A longitudinal study of human papillomavirus carriage in human immunodeficiency virus-infected and human immunodeficiency virus-uninfected women. *Am J Obstet Gynecol*. 1998;178:982–986.

Mirochnick M, Capparelli E. Pharmacokinetic of antiretrovirals in pregnant women. *Clin Pharmacokinetics*. 2004;43(15):1071–1087.

Morrison CS, Chen PL, Nankya I, et al. Hormonal contraceptive use and HIV disease progression among women in Uganda and Zimbabwe. *J AIDS*. 2011;57(2):157–164.

Nattabi B, Li J, Thompson SC, et al. A systematic review of factors influencing fertility desires and intentions among people living with HIV/AIDS: implications for policy and service delivery. *AIDS Behav*. 2009;13(5):949–968.

Nygard JF, Skare GB, Thoresen SO. The cervical cancer screening programme in Norway, 1992–2000: changes in Pap smear coverage and incidence of cervical cancer. *J Med Screen*. 2002;9(2):86–91.

Palefsky JM, Minkoff H, Kalish LA, et al, Cervicovaginal human papillomavirus infection in human immunodeficiency virus-1 (HIV)-positive and high-risk HIV-negative women. *J Natl Cancer Inst*. 1999;91(3):226–236.

Panozzo L, Friedl A, Vernazza PL. High risk behaviour and fertility desires among heterosexual HIV-positive patients with a serodiscordant partner-two challenging issues. *Swiss Med Wkly*. 2003;133(7–8):124–127.

Patel RC, Onono M, Gandhi M, et al. Pregnancy rates in HIV-positive women using contraceptives and efavirenz-based or nevirapine-based antiretroviral therapy in Kenya: a retrospective cohort study. *Lancet HIV*. 2015;2(11):e474–e482.

Polis CB, Wawer MJ, Kiwanuka N, et al. Effect of hormonal contraceptive use on HIV progression in female HIV seroconverters in Rakai, Uganda. *AIDS*. 2010;24(12):1937–1944.

Rodger AJ, Cambiano V, Bruun T, et al. Sexual activity without condoms and risk of HIV transmission in serodifferent couples when the HIV-positive partner is using suppressive antiretroviral therapy. *JAMA*. 2016;316(2):171–181.

Sahasrabuddhe VV, Mwanahamuntu MH, Vermund SH, et al. Prevalence and distribution of HPV genotypes among HIV-infected women in Zambia. *Br J Cancer*. 2007;96(9):1480–1483.

Schiffman M, Solomon D. Screening and prevention methods for cervical cancer. *JAMA*. 2009;302(16):1809–1810. doi:10.1001/jama.2009.1573

Sharma A, Feldman JG, Golub ET, et al. Live birth patterns among human immunodeficiency virus-infected women before and after the availability of highly active antiretroviral therapy. *Am J Obstet Gynecol*. 2007;196(6):541–e1.

Six C, Heard I, Bergeron C, et al. Comparative prevalence, incidence and short-term prognosis of cervical squamous intraepithelial lesions amongst HIV-positive and HIV-negative women. *AIDS*. 1998;12:1047–1056.

Squires KE, Hodder SL, Feinberg J, et al. Health needs of HIV-infected women in the United States: insights from the women living positive survey. *AIDS Patient Care STDs*. 2011;25(5):279–285.

Stringer EM, Giganti M, Carter RJ, et al. Hormonal contraception and HIV disease progression: a multicountry cohort analysis of the MTCT-Plus Initiative. *AIDS*. 2009;23(01):S69–S77.

Sun XW, Kuhn L, Ellerbrock TV, et al. Human papillomavirus infection in women infected with the human immunodeficiency virus. *N Engl J Med*. 1997;337(19):1343–1349.

Sutton MY, Zhou W, Frazier EL. Unplanned pregnancies and contraceptive use among HIV-positive women in care. *PLoS One*. 2018;13(5):e0197216.

Syme MR, Paxton JW, Keelan JA. Drug transfer and metabolism by the human placenta. *Clin Pharmacokinetics*. 2004;43(8):487–514.

van Sighem A, Gras L, Reiss P, et al. Life expectancy of recently diagnosed asymptomatic HIV-infected patients approaches that of uninfected individuals. *AIDS*. 2010;24(10):1527–1535.

Vogler MA, Patterson K, Kamemoto L, et al. Contraceptive efficacy of oral and transdermal hormones when co-administered with protease inhibitors in HIV-1–infected women: pharmacokinetic results of ACTG Trial A5188. *J AIDS*. 2010;55(4):473.

Volkow P, Rubí S, Lizano M, et al. High prevalence of oncogenic human papillomavirus in the genital tract of women with human immunodeficiency virus. *Gynecol Oncol*. 2001;82:27–31.

World Health Organization. Contraceptive eligibility for women at high risk of HIV: 2019 guidance statement. 2019.

World Health Organization. Hormonal contraceptive methods for women at high risk of HIV and living with HIV: 2014 guidance statement. 2014.

Zash R, Holmes L, Diseko M, et al. Neural-tube defects and antiretroviral treatment regimens in Botswana. *N Engl J Med*. 2019;381:827–840.

Zash R, Jacobson D, Maswabi K, et al. Dolutegravir/tenofovir/emtricitabine (DTG/TDF/FTC) started in pregnancy is as safe as efavirenz/tenofovir/emtricitabine (EFV/TDF/FTC) in nationwide birth outcomes surveillance in Botswana. Ninth IAS, Paris, France, 2017.

24.

ANTIRETROVIRAL THERAPY FOR CHILDREN AND NEWBORNS

Karin Nielsen-Saines

CHAPTER GOALS

Upon completion of this chapter, the reader should be able to:

- Understand the basics regarding pathogenesis of mother-to-child HIV transmission (MTCT) and be aware of landmark studies targeting prevention of MTCT

- Understand the concept of HIV exposure versus HIV infection

- Comprehend the specific challenges of early HIV diagnosis of infants and understand the importance of timing of transmission for diagnosis and pathogenesis

- Be aware of the concept of HIV remission in infants who are treated early

- Have a general idea of HIV disease course in children and surrogate markers of disease

- Be aware of specific caveats guiding the use of antiretroviral agents (ARVs) in children, particularly in newborns receiving presumptive HV therapy

INTRODUCTION

In the absence of interventions to curtail MTCT, HIV-1 infection in children parallels that of women of childbearing age. Perinatal transmission of HIV-1 accounts for nearly all worldwide cases of pediatric HIV-1 infection today, with the exception of adolescent acquisition of HIV-1 via adult risk behaviors. MTCT occurs in 25% to 30% of cases when there is no maternal ARV treatment (Newell, 1991; Scott et al., 1989); if breastfeeding until 12 months of age is included, transmission risk can be as high as 40%. Infection may be transmitted during pregnancy, at the time of labor and delivery, and via breastfeeding. Since 2019, the annual number of new HIV infections in children has decreased by over 50% due to provision of combination antiretroviral treatment (ART) to women living with HIV (AVERT, 2020). In 2019, approximately 82% of women living with HIV globally received combination ART to prevent MTCT (UNICEF, 2019). Considering there are approximately 1.3 million women living with HIV who become pregnant each year, roughly 234,000 women did not receive prevention of MTCT in 2019 (UNICEF, 2020). It is estimated that approximately 150,000 new HIV infections occurred in children in 2019, which equates to 410 children infected per day per year. Although combination ART can reduce the HIV MTCT rate to less than 1% (Dorenbaum et al., 2002; Flynn et al., 2018; Fowler et al., 2016), failure to recognize HIV-1 infection in women and/or unavailability of treatment still contributes to continuing MTCT worldwide. Management of HIV-1 infection in children has to take into consideration several factors. These include early diagnosis of infection, the natural history of HIV-1 infection in children and surrogate markers of disease, suitable pediatric drug formulations, drug metabolism and pharmacokinetics of ARVs in children, and the general paucity of pediatric treatment data as compared to adults.

LEARNING OBJECTIVES

- Discuss advances in ART for prevention of MTCT, particularly for postexposure infant prophylaxis

- Review pediatric-specific issues of early HIV diagnosis, timing and pathogenesis of HIV disease, and use of surrogate markers of HIV infection in this population

- Discuss current guidelines for management of ARVs in children within the context of what drugs to use, when to start, and when to change ART

WHAT'S NEW?

- ARV guidelines from the US Department of Health and Human Services (DHHS) now recommend presumptive HIV therapy for infants who are at higher risk of perinatal HIV acquisition. This is intended to be preliminary HIV treatment for a newborn who may later be documented to have HIV infection, but it may also serve as prophylaxis against HIV acquisition for infants who were exposed to HIV but did not acquire it perinatally. Presumptive HIV therapy differs from ARV prophylaxis, which is the administration of one or more ARVs to a newborn without documented HIV infection to reduce the risk of perinatal HIV acquisition. HIV therapy, on the other hand, is defined as administration of a three-drug ART regimen at treatment doses for treatment of infants with documented HIV infection.

- Infants at risk for HIV acquisition include neonates whose mothers did not receive antepartum or intrapartum ARVs or whose mothers only received intrapartum ARVs; infants whose mothers did not achieve virologic suppression near delivery; and infants of mothers with acute HIV infection during pregnancy or while breastfeeding.

- Infants of mothers with previously unknown HIV status who are found to be HIV positive by point-of-care testing during labor or delivery should start either presumptive HIV therapy or two-drug ARV prophylaxis based on clinical risk assessment. If supplemental testing excludes maternal HIV infection, the ARV regimen should be discontinued.

- ART should be initiated in all infants with confirmed HIV infection.

- A 4-week zidovudine (ZDV) ARV prophylaxis regimen is now recommended for HIV prophylaxis in newborns whose mothers received ART during pregnancy and had sustained viral suppression near delivery (defined as a confirmed HIV RNA level <50 copies/mL) and for whom there are no concerns related to maternal adherence. Originally a 6-week course of ZDV was recommended for the same purpose.

- Only ZDV, lamivudine, and nevirapine should be recommended in premature newborns of less than 37 weeks of gestational age because of lack of dosing and safety data.

- Preconception care should include testing of sexually active women for HIV. All pregnant women should be tested for HIV as early as possible during pregnancy. Partners of pregnant women should be encouraged to undergo HIV testing if their status is unknown.

- Repeat HIV testing in the third trimester of pregnancy is recommended for women with negative initial HIV antibody tests who are at increased risk of acquiring HIV. This includes women receiving care in facilities that have an HIV incidence of at least 1 case per 1,000 pregnant women per year, women who reside in jurisdictions with an elevated HIV incidence, or women who reside in states that require third-trimester testing.

- Women who were not tested for HIV before or during labor should undergo expedited HIV antibody testing during the immediate postpartum period (or their newborns should undergo expedited HIV antibody testing). If results for the mother or infant are positive, an appropriate infant ARV drug regimen should be initiated immediately, and the mother should not breastfeed unless supplemental HIV testing is negative. Expedited HIV testing should be available 24 hours a day during labor and delivery for any pregnant woman with undocumented HIV status, and results should be available within 1 hour.

- HIV testing is recommended for infants and children in foster care and adoptees for whom maternal HIV infection status is unknown.

- HIV antibody tests should not be used in children aged less than 18 months. For diagnosis of HIV in this younger population, virologic assays such as HIV RNA or HIV DNA nucleic acid tests are recommended. HIV RNA or HIV DNA nucleic acid tests are equally recommended.

- Assays that detect non-B subtype HIV or Group O HIV infections (HIV RNA NAT or a dual-target total DNA/RNA test) are recommended for use in infants born to mothers with known or suspected non-B subtype virus or Group O infections. If a mother of an infant acquired HIV outside the US and has had repeated undetectable HIV RNA by standard testing, consultation with a clinical virologist on more sensitive HIV nucleic acid testing is suggested.

- There are dosing guidelines for the use of raltegravir in infants with suspected or confirmed HIV infection. Nevertheless, DHHS guidelines continue to recommend that neonatal care providers who are considering a three-drug ART regimen for term infants younger than 2 weeks or premature infants contact a pediatric HIV expert for guidance and individual case assessment of the risk/benefit ratio of treatment and for the latest information on neonatal drug doses. The National Perinatal HIV Hotline (1-888-448-8765) provides free clinical consultation on perinatal HIV care.

- Studies have continued to demonstrate a significant benefit of early ART to infants less than 12 months of age in the prevention of HIV mortality and morbidity, and treatment is recommended to all HIV-infected infants in this age group in all geographic settings, regardless of clinical findings, CD4$^+$ T-cell counts, or viral load. The updated recommendation is that treatment of infants under 12 months of age who are diagnosed with HIV should be expedited; this characterizes an urgent situation. HIV diagnosis is an emergency, and infants identified as HIV exposed should be tested as soon as possible. Treatment should not be delayed and can be started as early as the first day of life if HIV diagnosis is confirmed. ARVs that can be used from birth for which there is pharmacokinetic data include ZDV, nevirapine, lamivudine, and raltegravir. Lopinavir/ritonavir can be used as early as 2 weeks of age, abacavir as early as 3 months.

- Initial combination therapy for ART-naive children includes the use of integrase strand transfer inhibitor (INSTI)-based regimens as agents to be used in combination with two nucleoside analog reverse transcriptase inhibitors (NRTIs). Bictegravir/emtricitabine/tenofovir alafenamide (BIC/FTC/TAF) is recommended as a preferred INSTI-based regimen for adolescents aged at least 12 years and weighing at least 25 kg and as an alternative

INSTI-based regimen for children aged at least 6 years and weighing at least 25 kg. elvitegravir/cobisistat/emtricitabine/tenofovir alafenamide (EVG/cobi/FTC/TAF) is recommended as a preferred INSTI-based regimen for children and adolescents weighing at least 25 kg who have creatinine clearance (CrCl) of at least 30 mL/min. Dolutegravir (DTG) plus a two-NRTI backbone is recommended as a preferred INSTI-based regimen for children and adolescents aged at least 3 years and weighing at least 25 kg. DTG plus a two-NRTI backbone is recommended as an alternative INSTI-based regimen for children aged at least 3 years and weighing between 20 and 25 kg. Raltegravir (RAL) plus a two-NRTI backbone is recommended as a preferred INSTI-based regimen for infants and children from birth to age 3 years who weigh at least 2 kg and for children aged at least 3 years and weighing less than 25 kg. It is an alternative INSTI-based regimen for children aged at least 3 years and weighing at least 25 kg. Once-daily dosing of RAL is not recommended for infants and children.

- Regarding the use of nonnucleoside analog reverse transcriptase inhibitors (NNRTIs) in children, efavirenz (EFV) plus a two-NRTI backbone is recommended as an alternative NNRTI-based regimen for initial treatment of HIV in children aged at least 3 years. Neverapine (NVP) plus a two-NRTI backbone is recommended as a preferred NNRTI-based regimen in infants aged less than 14 days and an alternative NNRTI-based regimen for children aged between 14 days and 3 years. Clinicians should consider switching from NVP to lopinavir/ritonavir (LPV/r) or RAL in children aged between 14 days and 3 years, as these drugs are the preferred ARVs for this age bracket. Rilpivirine (RPV) plus a two-NRTI backbone is recommended as an alternative NNRTI-based regimen for children and adolescents aged at least 12 years and weighing at least 35 kg who have HIV viral loads of 100,000 copies/mL or less.

- FTC/TAF is recommended as a preferred dual-NRTI combination in children and adolescents weighing at least 25 kg who have an estimated CrCl of at least 30 mL/min when this combination is used with an INSTI or NNRTI; this combination is considered a preferred dual-NRTI combination when used with a protease inhibitor (PI) in children and adolescents weighing at least 35 kg who have an estimated CrCl of at least 30 mL/min.

- The PI atazanavir boosted with ritonavir is an alternative PI in children aged between 3 months and 3 years and children at least 3 years old weighing at least 25 kg. Boosted atazanavir (ATV/r) plus a two-NRTI backbone is recommended as a preferred PI-based regimen for children aged at least 3 years and weighing less than 25 kg. Atazanavir/cobicistat plus a two-NRTI backbone is an alternative PI-based regimen for children weighing at least 35 kg. Boosted darunavir (DRV/r) plus a two-NRTI backbone is recommended as a preferred PI-based regimen for children aged at least 3 years and weighing between 10

and 25 kg, and as an alternative PI-based regimen for children aged at least 3 years and weighing at least 25 kg.

- DTG is recommended as a preferred ARV throughout pregnancy and as an alternative ARV in women who are trying to conceive. INSTI-based therapy has become the ART of choice during pregnancy.

KEY POINTS

- HIV-infected infants and children have a different, more progressive disease course as compared to adults given that early infection leads to sustained, high-magnitude viremia with significant seeding of reservoirs in the first months of life, prior to full maturation of the immune system.

- Early diagnosis of HIV infection is pivotal in the management of infants and in the prevention of HIV-associated morbidity and mortality.

- The availability of potent pediatric ARV formulations encompassing different classes of drugs for infected infants and young children is still limited and needs further development.

- Infant postexposure HIV prophylaxis varies according to the risk scenario; in some situations, presumptive therapy may be implemented.

- Early ART (i.e., at the time of diagnosis) is still the mainstay of pediatric HIV infection, particularly for infants less than 12 months of age, but is also highly recommended for older children.

- Early treatment of young infants diagnosed shortly after birth is the best approach to reduce the seeding of viral reservoirs and to potentially attain prolonged periods of HIV remission off ARVs, a strategy that has been evaluated in prospective clinical trials and is recommended by current guidelines.

ARVS TO THE HIV-EXPOSED INFANT

Advances in perinatal primary ART and antepartum, peripartum, and postpartum delivery of ZDV in non-breastfeeding, HIV-infected women without severe immunosuppression in the US led to a decrease in perinatal transmission rates. The US Centers for Disease Control and Prevention (CDC) estimates that the number of infants born annually with HIV in the US decreased from 1,650 in 1991 to 100 to 200 in 2004, with 91 cases of HIV in children younger than 13 years of age diagnosed in the US in 2018 (National Institutes of Health, 2020). The provision of ARVs to infants born to HIV-infected mothers as prophylaxis has been standard of care in the US since 1994, when results of Pediatric AIDS Clinical Trials Group study 076 (PACTG 076) were published (Connor et al., 1994). The study demonstrated that ZDV monotherapy given to the mother starting at 16 weeks' gestation, accompanied by an intravenous ZDV infusion during labor and delivery and followed by four-times-per-day dosing of ZDV to the infant from birth to 6 weeks of age was highly efficacious in preventing MTCT as compared to placebo (8% vs. 25% respectively, $p < 0.001$). In the developed-country setting, 4 to 6 weeks of ZDV to the infant initiated at birth, given at 2 mg/kg per dose four times a day or 4 mg/kg per dose twice a day, became standard of care (Ruane et al., 2013). The major toxicities of ZDV used as infant prophylaxis include anemia and neutropenia; however, these are dose-dependent and self-limiting, tend to occur toward the end of the course of treatment, and rarely require interruption of prophylaxis (Lahoz et al., 2010). In settings with limited resources, single-dose NVP to the infant (2 mg/kg) shortly after birth was used for many years as standard of care, following the publication of HIVNET 012 (Guay et al., 1999), which documented the efficacy of this approach in reducing MTCT when associated with single-dose nevirapine given to the mother at the time of labor. Nevertheless, this approach induced a large wave of ARV resistance in infants who ultimately became infected, rendering nevirapine use problematic for early infant treatment strategies in the developing world. Among HIV-infected infants whose mothers were not treated with ARVs throughout the course of pregnancy and are therefore at higher risk of HIV acquisition, double ARV prophylaxis initiated within 48 hours of birth with three doses of nevirapine in the first week of life concurrently with 6 weeks of ZDV has been shown to be more efficacious for the prevention of HIV intrapartum infection than ZDV alone (Nielsen-Saines et al., 2011). An alternative, equally efficacious regimen was the use of lamivudine (3TC) and nelfinavir in the first 2 weeks of life concurrent with 6 weeks of ZDV (Nielsen-Saines et al., 2011). LPV/r suspension is currently not recommended by the US Food and Drug Administration (FDA) for use in infants younger than 2 weeks of age; however, RAL has been used in this setting and has proven to be highly effective (Clarke et al., 2019). In resource-limited settings, the use of daily nevirapine prophylaxis to the HIV-exposed infant for prevention of MTCT has been evaluated up to 6 months of age and has been shown to be effective and safe in the prevention of postpartum HIV acquisition (Coovadia et al., 2012). At present, however, most settings in sub-Saharan Africa have transitioned to World Health Organization (WHO) Option B⁺, which recommends treatment with combination ART to all HIV-infected women during pregnancy, lactation, and onward with no further treatment interruption (WHO, 2014).

The selection of ART to reduce perinatal HIV transmission must include consideration of optimal treatment for the infected pregnant women and balance potential for fetal harm. Maternal factors that should be considered include the mother's viral load, degree of immunosuppression, medications for use in treatment of comorbid conditions (e.g., tuberculosis, hepatitis C virus), and the potential for inducing viral resistance. Transmission of resistant HIV to infants has been described in the literature, but it is an infrequent event (De Lourdes Teixeira et al., 2015; Yeganeh et al., 2018). Other considerations to prevent perinatal transmission of HIV include scheduled delivery to minimize prolonged rupture of membranes, including a recommendation from the American College of Obstetrics and Gynecology for scheduled cesarean section for women with viral loads exceeding HIV RNA levels of 1,000 copies/mL (Committee on Obstetric Practice, 2001). In a meta-analysis of 15 North American and European cohorts of HIV-infected pregnant women ($n = 100$), vertical transmission rates differed by 5% for those with scheduled delivery by cesarean section (transmission rate, 2%) as compared with those with other delivery modes (transmission rate, 7.3%; International Perinatal HIV Group, 1999). Evaluation of the morbidity and mortality related to such scheduled cesarean sections suggests that HIV-infected pregnant women may have a higher incidence of postpartum hemorrhage with resultant transfusion, sepsis, pneumonia, and death than do their noninfected pregnant peers undergoing the same scheduled procedure (odds ratio, 1.6) (Louis et al., 2007). HIV-infected pregnant women without detectable viral loads should be informed preoperatively of their risk for having morbidity related to cesarean section performed to prevent perinatal HIV transmission. Although intravenous ZDV was recommended in the past for use throughout labor and delivery, for women with an undetectable viral load during pregnancy, the current recommendation is to continue the current oral ARV regimen throughout labor and delivery without the need for intravenous ZDV.

Recently, INSTI-based ART has become the treatment of choice during pregnancy, and treatment recommendations emphasize that the same ART regimen should be used in both pregnant and nonpregnant women, with DTG and RAL being the preferred INSTI drugs of choice. The only exception is in women trying to conceive, where RAL is the preferred regimen and DTG is an alternative recommended drug. Bictegravir is not recommended during pregnancy because of paucity of data, and EVG/c is not recommended because of the cobi component (DHHS, 2020).

DIAGNOSIS

Early diagnosis of HIV-1 infection is crucial for identification of at-risk infants and consequent initiation of treatment. All HIV-1–exposed infants carry maternal HIV-1 antibodies until approximately 15 to 18 months of age. Thus, early pediatric diagnosis relies on identification of the virus, usually via HIV-1 DNA or RNA polymerase chain reaction (PCR) techniques. The former measures integrated virus in the host genome, and the latter measures circulating plasma virus. HIV-1 co-culture is not routinely performed because of cost and time, although it is also a reliable diagnostic method. Infants infected in utero usually have positive PCR results within the first 48 hours of birth, while infants infected at the time of labor and delivery may have a negative HIV DNA or RNA PCR result at birth, followed by a positive result 1 week to 2 months following birth (Bryson et al., 1992). Breastfed infants have continuing HIV exposure and thus can develop a positive HIV DNA or RNA PCR result at any time. The risk of transmission by breastfeeding from an HIV-positive mother is approximately 16% (Fowler & Newell, 2002). Therefore, repeat PCR testing in the first few months of life is critical for determining the timing of infection, with sensitivity of a PCR result reaching 96% by 4 weeks of life in the absence of breastfeeding (Dunn et al., 1992; Nielsen & Bryson, 2000). Infant HIV virologic diagnosis requires serial nucleic acid testing. Usually infants are tested within the first 48 hours of life to detect in utero infection. Current guidelines recommend that infants be tested between 14 and 21 days of life, between 1 and 2 months, and at 4 to 6 months of age (DHHS, 2020).

TIMING OF INFECTION

Acquisition of HIV infection may occur in utero, intrapartum, or through breastfeeding. Even before ART was recommended to pregnant women, two-thirds of HIV-exposed infants escaped HIV infection. Perinatal HIV infection rates have declined substantially in the developed world since 1994, following publication of the landmark PACTG 076 study, which demonstrated reduction of perinatal HIV transmission in women who used ZDV in pregnancy as compared to placebo (Connor et al., 1994). Approximately 30% to 50% of infants who contract HIV infection will acquire it in utero, and 50% to 70% will acquire it during the intrapartum period (Cao et al., 1997; Dickover et al., 1996; Mayaux et al., 1997). In order to characterize the timing of HIV infection, a working definition was created for acquisition of infection in utero and intrapartum (Bryson et al., 1992). An infant is considered to have in utero infection if virologic tests (HIV DNA or RNA PCR) are positive within 48 hours of life. Due to the risk of contamination with maternal blood, cord blood samples should not be used for diagnostic evaluations. Infants are considered to have intrapartum HIV infection if diagnostic tests within the first 48 hours of life are negative but further virologic testing after 1 week of life is positive. There is evidence that most cases of HIV transmission occur late in pregnancy or at delivery.

Postpartum transmission of HIV via breastfeeding has been a continuing problem for the prevention of MTCT efforts worldwide. HIV can be transmitted as cell-associated or cell-free virus in breast milk (Lyimo et al., 2012). Mastitis, which triggers migration of inflammatory cells, is also a known risk factor for HIV breast milk transmission (Semrau et al., 2013), as is nonexclusive breastfeeding (Coutsoudis et al., 1999) or the presence of oral thrush in the infant (Read et al., 2009). Longer duration of breastfeeding is also a well-known risk factor for transmission (Becquet et al., 2005), as is maternal primary infection during lactation (Morrison et al., 2015). In areas where safe alternatives to breastfeeding are not available, however, formula feeding is associated with higher morbidity and mortality. Provision of combination ART to lactating HIV-infected mothers has been demonstrated to significantly increase HIV-free survival in infants with improved infant outcomes in terms of growth and reduced infections (Inter-agency Task Team, 2015; Marazzi et al., 2007, 2009, 2010). Successful screening of pregnant women with availability of ART for HIV-positive pregnant and lactating women through the WHO B+ program (DHHS, 2020)

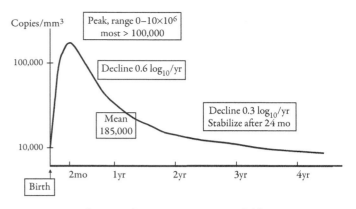

Figure 24.1 Natural course of HIV RNA viremia in children. SOURCE: Figure courtesy of Palumbo PE based on work from Palumbo PE, Raskino C, Riscus S, et al. Predictive value of quantitative plasma HIV RNA and CD4+ lymphocyte count in HIV-infected infants and children. *JAMA*. 1998. 279(10):756–761.

has decreased early and late postpartum HIV transmission via breastfeeding over time. In women with CD4+ T-cell counts higher than 350/mL in sub-Saharan Africa, the Promise Study observed a mother-to-child in utero transmission rate of HIV at 1 week of age of 0.5% when women received combination ART during pregnancy (Fowler et al., 2016). Follow-up of the same infants revealed very low breastfeeding transmission rates when mothers received combination ART during lactation (HIV transmission 0.57%) or infants received prophylactic infant nevirapine (HIV transmission 0.58%) during the first 18 months of life or following cessation of breastfeeding, whichever occurred first (Flynn et al., 2018).

The timing of HIV-1 infection (in utero vs. intrapartum) is somewhat predictive of the patient's subsequent clinical course (Dickover et al., 1994). Early onset of AIDS-defining conditions is more frequently observed in infants infected in utero who sustain early, prolonged elevated HIV RNA levels.

As in adults, prolonged periods of elevated HIV RNA levels are predictive of disease progression. HIV-infected infants undergo primary infection, either in utero or shortly after birth. Therefore, they tend to have very elevated virus loads in the first months of life (Figure 24.1).

MATERNAL RISK FACTORS FOR HIV TRANSMISSION

Maternal risk factors associated with enhanced perinatal HIV transmission identified include untreated HIV disease, seroconversion during pregnancy or breastfeeding, drug abuse, heterosexual infection by sexual partners with risk factors for acquiring HIV disease, presence of maternal syphilis (Yeganeh et al., 2015), other sexually transmitted infections (Adachi et al., 2015, 2016, 2018a, 2018b), risk of cytomegalovirus transmission (Adachi et al., 2017, 2018a, 2018b), and maternal transfusion before 1985. Prospective and retrospective evaluations of maternal predictors for perinatal HIV transmission have been the focus of multiple studies. Maternal transmission predictors identified to date include maternal viremia (measured as quantitative HIV RNA PCR or viral load; Gabiano et al., 1992; Magder et al., 2005), maternal immunosuppression, or an inadequate immune response (measured by the CD4+ T-cell count, neutralizing antibody production; Magder et al., 2005) and viral characteristics (chemokine receptor tropism, resistance patterns of maternal virus at delivery or infant virus at birth; Scarlatti, 2004). Pregnancy and placental variables (delivery mode, duration of rupture of membranes, chorioamnionitis) also may influence the risk for perinatal transmission of HIV (International Perinatal HIV Group, 1999; Mwanyumba et al., 2002; St. Louis et al., 1993). Infant variables evaluated as predictors of transmission of HIV include specific human leukocyte antigen (HLA) markers and the infant cellular immune response (cytokine production, activated T-cell function; European Collaborative Study, 1991; Luzuriaga et al., 1991; Magder et al., 2005; Polycarpou et al., 2002). In addition, immunogenetic factors (chemokine coreceptor expression) have been suggested to confer protection against progression of disease (Sei et al., 2001).

EARLY TREATMENT INITIATION AND HIV REMISSION IN HIV-EXPOSED INFANTS

ART to infants and children suppresses viremia, reduces the high infant mortality, and improves clinical outcome; however, children must continue lifelong ARV treatment. The major barrier to achieving HIV remission in children, as in adults, is the early establishment of long-lived latent cellular reservoirs in CD4+ T cells and other sites, with continued low-level replication and rebound viremia once taken off ARTs (Persaud et al., 2012). It is postulated that, through treatment of very early HIV infection, the establishment, quantity, or even elimination of latent reservoirs could be achieved by reducing viral spread into memory CD4+ T-cell reservoirs, which would potentially allow patients to thrive off of ARTs without viral rebound, as evidenced by the "Mississippi baby" who remained in ARV-free viral remission for 27 months after early combination ART (Luzuriaga et al., 2015; Persaud et al., 2013; Siliciano & Siliciano, 2014). Importantly, there are emerging data that very early therapy during acute HIV infection in both adult and children quantitatively modifies HIV persistence and may influence the rate of reservoir decay. This approach is being further evaluated in ongoing clinical trials.

DISEASE COURSE

The natural history of pediatric HIV-1 infection is bimodal (Scott, 1991). Studies conducted in developed countries prior to the availability of ARVs demonstrate that approximately 20% of children exhibit very rapid disease progression, with rapid loss of CD4+ T-cell counts and development of AIDS-defining conditions before 2 years of age (Nielsen et al., 1997). The majority of HIV-infected children, however (approximately 60–65%) will have intermediate disease progression,

with the presence of AIDS-defining events by 7 to 8 years of age. There is a small subset of children (as there is in adults), approximately 15% to 20% of patients, who have very slow to no disease progression by age 8 years, and an even smaller set of elite controllers (<5%) who enter adolescence with minimal to no symptoms of HIV disease. Studies conducted in Africa have demonstrated an even faster pace of disease progression, with the majority of pediatric patients having AIDS-defining conditions by age 5 years (Newell et al., 2004). This might be due to the higher overall burden of disease and presence of multiple coinfections. Combination ART makes it possible to alter the natural history of HIV disease and transform disease progressors into nonprogressors. This translates into improvements in the quality of life and reduction in HIV-associated morbidity and mortality.

Infants with in utero infection appear to have a more rapid disease course when compared to infants who acquire HIV infection intrapartum (Dickover et al., 1996). Infants infected in utero still have normal CD4+ T-cell values at birth and are usually born with a low virus load (as measured by DNA or RNA PCR) (Mayaux et al., 1996). In addition, even infants infected in utero are asymptomatic at birth. In utero HIV appears to result from transplacental passage of virus or ascending viral infection in patients with prolonged rupture of membranes (Minkoff et al., 1995). In the animal model, researchers have demonstrated that viral infection of the amniotic fluid with simian immunodeficiency virus (SIV) resulted in infection of all the offspring (Van Rompay et al., 1995). Intrapartum transmission of HIV infection is responsible for the majority of perinatal cases. In a prospective study of 271 HIV-infected infants using HIV DNA PCR, 38% of children were found to be positive within 48 hours of life, 93% were positive by 14 days of age, and 96% of the total number of infected children were positive by 4 weeks of age (Dunn et al., 1992). There are infants who might not have detectable virus as late as 3 months following delivery in selected cases. Untreated infants tend to maintain a very high virus burden throughout their first year of life, and immunologic patterns of primary viremia in infants have long been described (Luzuriaga et al., 1997). High-level viremia might persist for a longer period of time in infants than in adults undergoing primary infection; untreated early infection is associated with a high mortality risk (Violari et al., 2008). Many years prior to the advent of combination ART, discordant twin infections were reported, with the firstborn twin having a higher risk of infection (Duliege et al., 1995).

SURROGATE MARKERS OF DISEASE

The goal of ART is to reduce the HIV-1 viral load as much as possible while restoring or preserving immune function. Viral load is generally measured via plasma HIV-1 RNA reverse transcriptase (RT) PCR (Roche Molecular Systems), HIV RNA quantitation by branched (b) DNA (Chiron Corporation), or nucleic acid sequence-based amplification (NASBA) HIV-1 RNA quantitative (QT) assay (Organon Teknika). All three methods are reliable parameters for the measurement of free virus in plasma, with new-generation assays being able to identify virus isolates of different subtypes. Immune function in HIV disease is measured primarily by evaluating T-cell subsets, particularly CD4$^+$ T-cell absolute numbers and percentages. Three-color flow cytometry is generally the methodology employed for this purpose. Declining counts parallel disease progression, with declines in CD4$^+$ T cells usually following peak HIV RNA viremia. One important caveat in the management of HIV-infected children is that CD4$^+$ T-cell numbers, particularly in infants, differ significantly from adults and do not achieve similar levels until after 5 years. Therefore, an infant with a CD4$^+$ T-cell count of 750 cells/mm^3 or less is at significant risk for development of AIDS-defining conditions because normal values are generally greater than 2,000 cells/mm^3.

ARVS IN CHILDREN

One general principle in the use of ART is that continued viral replication in the presence of ARVs promotes development of drug resistance. Resistance to one specific ARV may in turn confer resistance to other drugs within the same class. Current standard of practice is that, once therapy is started, long-term or lifelong treatment is warranted. In children, the efficacy of ART often is extrapolated from data obtained from adult clinical trials because of lack of pediatric data. There are, however, significant age-related differences between children and adults. These encompass body composition, renal excretion, liver metabolism, and gastrointestinal function. This leads to differences in drug distribution and metabolism, drug clearance, drug dosing, and different toxicities between children and adults. In addition, protein binding and drug clearance of some specific ARVs may differ by race due to the presence of genetic polymorphisms. Nevertheless, often therapeutic doses for infants and children are not available. Liquid or palatable formulations for children do not exist for many ARVs, and adherence depends on adult caretakers. It is crucial when initiating ART to take into consideration the presence of comorbidities and concomitant medications in order to avoid overlapping drug toxicities. It is also important to consider cross-resistance and later therapeutic options.

GUIDELINES

Treatment guidelines have been developed over the years in order to address critical concerns about the use of ART in children. Major concerns have always included the optimal timing of initiation of ART, the preferred choice of ARVs, the best ways to monitor efficacy and toxicities, and when to change therapy. There are decreased variations in guidelines between developed and developing countries. In the US, traditionally, most children have been treated when identified as having HIV-1 infection, regardless of symptomatology. Given multiple therapeutic options and the general availability of viral load monitoring, guidelines in developed countries over the years have relied on virus load measures for predicting early switches in therapy (Panel on Antiretroviral Therapy, 2020). Randomized clinical trials, such as the CHER trial in South Africa, demonstrated that early ART to infants diagnosed before 12 months of age is clearly beneficial in reducing morbidity and mortality (Violari et al., 2008).

The current US pediatric ART guidelines panel has increased the strength of its recommendations for initiating ART in all children at the time of diagnosis and considers prompt initiation of treatment a medical emergency (Panel on Antiretroviral Therapy, 2020). Thus, the panel now recommends that all children receive ART, regardless of symptoms or CD4$^+$ T-cell count. WHO treatment guidelines for treatment of children with HIV infection also reflect the need for early treatment initiation (WHO, 2019).

TIMING OF INITIATION OF THERAPY

Early versus deferred initiation of ART in HIV-infected children was a controversial matter, but this is no longer a subject of debate. It is currently universally accepted in both the developed and developing world that ART should be started at the time of HIV diagnosis in all children, regardless of age. Starting therapy early in asymptomatic children controls viral replication before genetic mutations develop, leading to fewer circulating viral strains. It also prevents immune system destruction and avoids disease progression, including prevention of establishment of viral reservoirs in the brain. With this strategy, viral seeding of latent cells or CD4$^+$ T-cell reservoirs can often be circumvented. Given the significant repercussions to cognitive development when treatment is delayed, there is no justification at present to delay treatment to HIV-infected children.

CHANGE IN THERAPY

The decision to change ART varies slightly according to the pediatric guidelines employed. The variability is mostly due to the surrogate markers used. Nevertheless, most experts would agree that indicators of treatment failure include progression of HIV disease, growth failure, development of opportunistic infections while on established therapy, decline in CD4$^+$ percentiles, development of or worsening HIV encephalopathy, and significant increases in virus load. Tolerability, palatability, and drug toxicities are also reasons why ART regimens are switched in children, as in adults. Simplification of treatment regimens is recommended whenever possible, as the greatest predictor of achieving an undetectable plasma virus load is adherence.

SPECIFIC ARVS

ARVs currently available for use in the US are listed in Table 24.1. Optimal ARV combinations for children may differ slightly from those for adults. In infants, particularly those under 1 year of age, there is often a need to use very potent

ART regimens to reduce persistently elevated viral loads (Luzuriaga et al., 2004; Palumbo et al., 2010). Therefore, in this scenario, four-drug combinations including a PI, two NRTIs, and an NNRTI such as NVP may be indicated. The use of many ARVs is also limited in younger children (especially those aged <4 years) because of the lack of liquid formulations, as depicted in Table 24.1. Prevalent ART regimens in pediatrics include one PI such as ritonavir/lopinavir, or atazanavir or darunavir (in older children) in combination with a double-NRTI backbone. The PIs may be substituted with NNRTIs such as NVP or EFV (the latter in older children). Specific ARV regimens to be avoided include any type of monotherapy or dual therapy, or ATV without boosting. Treatment guidelines currently recommend use of integrase inhibitors in children as preferred regimens, contingent on availability of pediatric formulations. In resource-limited settings, treatment studies have demonstrated greater durability of viral load suppression in children treated with LPV/r-based

regimens as opposed to NVP-based regimens, although, interestingly, NVP has been shown to be associated with improved growth in this population (Chadwick et al., 2011). RAL and DTG have been increasingly recommended for use in the pediatric population in WHO guidelines. Pediatric guidelines for the US are extensively detailed in https://clinicalinfo.hiv.gov/en/guidelines/pediatric-arv.

TOXICITIES AND ADVERSE EFFECTS

The complications and side effects of specific ARVs are multiple. The most frequent toxicities of ZDV are hematologic, particularly anemia, and neutropenia. These may resolve with dose reduction. All NRTIs may cause some degree of mitochondrial toxicity. ZDV may cause myopathy, and peripheral neuropathy is seen with this drug and rarely with 3TC. Abacavir is famous for a fatal hypersensitivity reaction, which occurs in 1% of pediatric patients. It presents as flu-like symptoms with or without a rash, abdominal pain, sore throat, and myalgias. If the drug has been interrupted in this scenario, shock will ensue when it is restarted. The NNRTIs most commonly cause skin rashes (about 40%) and have rarely been associated with Steven-Johnson syndrome. There were concerns for the potential for EFV to be teratogenic, inducing neural tube defects (NTDs) when used in the first trimester of pregnancy, but they have not been demonstrated after large-scale use of the drug worldwide (Ford et al., 2014). EFV can induce central nervous system findings such as dizziness, insomnia, and nightmares, which have been reported shortly after initiation of treatment with this drug. There was concern about the use of NVP during pregnancy in women with CD4$^+$ T-cell counts greater than 250 cells/mm^3 due to an increased risk of hepatic failure (Hitti et al., 2004), but additional studies failed to demonstrate an association (De Lazzari et al., 2008).

PIs have multiple drug–drug interactions because of their cytochrome P450 metabolism in the liver. Their most common side effects are gastrointestinal symptoms. Hepatitis and hyperbilirubinemia are not uncommon. In adults, they have been shown to induce lipodystrophy, diabetes, and increased atherosclerosis because of lipid abnormalities. These findings are now being recognized in children, although complications are present to a lesser extent. There are also recent concerns about the potential for osteopenia and osteoporosis in children, either induced by ART (notably TDF) or HIV disease itself (Mora et al., 2004). With TAF increasingly replacing TDF use, it is likely that the concerns for osteopenia will decline over time.

INSTIs are generally well tolerated, with reduced toxicities. One major recent concern was the use of DTG during pregnancy and the potential for teratogenicity. Following the announcement of the launching of DTG to over 90 low- and middle-income countries at reduced pricing by UNAIDS and other partners in 2017, a report of NTDs following DTG treatment in pregnant women from the time of conception appeared in 2018 (Zash et al., 2018). This was data generated

Table 24.1 ARVS AVAILABLE FOR TREATMENT IN THE US

NRTIs	PIs
Zidovudine (ZDV/AZT) a	Saquinavir mesylate (SQV)
Lamivudine (3TC) a	Ritonavir a (RTV)
Abacavir (ABC) a	Lopinavir/ritonavir a (LPV/r)
Tenofovir disoproxil fumarate (TDF)	Atazanavir (ATV)
Tenofovir alafenamide (TAF)	Darunavir (DRV)
Emtricitabine (FTC)	Tipranavir (TPV)
NNRTIs	Fusion Inhibitors
Nevirapine a (NVP)	Enfuvirtide (ENF)
Efavirenz (EFV)	R-5 receptor inhibitors: maraviroc (MVC)
Etravirine (ETV)	Attachment inhibitors: fostemsavir (FTR)
Rilpivirine (RPV)	Post-attachment inhibitors: ibalizumab-uiyk (IBA)
Doravirine (DOV)	
Combination ARVs b	Integrase Inhibitors
ZDV/3TC	Raltegravir (RAL)
ZDV/3TC/ABC	Dolutegravir (DTG)
TDF/FTC or TAF/FTC	Elvitegravir (EVG)
3TC/TDF	Bictegravir (BIC)
ABC/3TC	
ABC/DTG/3TC	
EFV/TDF/FTC	
EFV/3TC/TDF	
FTC/RPV/TDF (or TAF)	
ATZ/cobi	
BIC/FTC/TAF	
DRV/cobi	
DRV/cobi/FTC/TAF	
DTG/3TC	
DTG/RPV	
DOR/3TC/TDF	
EVG/cobi/FTC/TDF (or TAF)	
LPV/r	

^{a} Pediatric formulation available

^{b} Additional formulations such as NVP/ZDV/3TC and NVP/D4T/3TC are available to children in pediatric formulations as generic drugs in resource-limited settings.

by the Tsepamo study in Botswana, which performed surveillance of birth outcomes at government maternity sites since 2014. The study was specifically designed to evaluate for potential NTDs following exposure to EFV at conception and for other adverse birth outcomes stratified by maternal HIV status and ART regimen. DTG was rolled out in Botswana in 2016. In May 2018, an NTD prevalence of 0.94% (4 cases in 426 participants) was noted in women who had been on DTG at conception. This contrasted with a prevalence of 0.12% for other women on non-DTG ART regimens at conception, 0.05% of women on EFV at conception, zero women who started DTG during pregnancy, and 0.09% of HIV-negative women (Zash et al., 2018). An update of study results in March 2019, when 1,683 participants had received DTG since the time of conception, demonstrated an NTD incidence of 0.30% (5 in 1,683 cases) (Zash et al., 2019). More recent data reported until April 2020 have shown a decline in the NTD incidence in women receiving DTG at conception, with an incidence of 0.19% (7 cases in 3,591 exposures). Subsequent studies have failed to demonstrate NTDs associated with DTG use during conception, including the IMPAACT 2010 and the VESTED trial, which compared regimens containing EFV and DTG during pregnancy (Chinula et al., 2020). Based on these findings, the WHO recommended DTG as the preferred HIV treatment option in all populations. DHHS guidelines also recommend the use of DTG during pregnancy but list the drug as an alternative drug regimen for women planning to conceive, with RAL being the preferred INSTI in this scenario (DHHS, 2020).

IMMUNE RECONSTITUTION INFLAMMATORY SYNDROME

One recognized potential complication of potent ARV therapy is the immune reconstitution inflammatory syndrome (IRIS). It is most frequently observed in patients who initiate ART with low CD4$^+$ T-cell counts. It is associated with a wide range of reactivation of previously latent pathogens, with tuberculosis being a common underlying condition. The underlying pathogenesis appears to start with unrecognized, low-level colonization of opportunistic pathogens in patients who have moderate to severe immunosuppression. With the initiation of ART and subsequent recovery of immunity to the organism, there is a paradoxical clinical deterioration due to a dysregulated, overly exuberant immune response. This syndrome usually presents in the first 6 weeks of ART and may resolve either with the use of steroids or temporary discontinuation of ART. It is infrequently seen in pediatric HIV practice in developed countries, particularly because children are generally treated earlier. However, it is prevalent in the developing world and may carry high morbidity and mortality. As more children are treated early and soon after diagnosis, it should become an increasingly rare complication of ART use in pediatric populations.

BENEFITS OF THERAPY

Despite the complications and controversies, the benefits of ART in children with HIV are overwhelming. In the US, the annual mortality in pediatric HIV patients decreased to less than 1% as of 1999 due to the availability of treatment (Gortmaker et al., 2001; Jeremy et al., 2005). ART decreases the virus load, preserves and restores the immune function, decreases the risk of comorbidities, decreases hospitalizations, improves survival, improves quality of life, and restores hope to children and their families. Many perinatally infected children who initiated treatment early in life are now adults who have families and children of their own. ART has also changed the AIDS paradigm. As one patient once said, HIV is no longer a disease you die from, but a disease you live with.

REFERENCES

Adachi K, Klausner JD, Bristow CC, et al.; NICHD HPTN 040 Study Team. Chlamydia and gonorrhea in HIV-infected pregnant women and infant HIV transmission. *Sex Transm Dis.* 2015;42(10):554–565.

Adachi K, Klausner JD, Xu J, et al.; NICHD HPTN 040 Study Team. *Chlamydia trachomatis* and *Neisseria gonorrhoeae* in HIV-infected pregnant women and adverse infant outcomes. *Pediatr Infect Dis J.* 2016;35(8):894–900.

Adachi K, Xu J, Ank B, et al. NICHD HPTN 040 Study Team. Congenital Cytomegalovirus and HIV Perinatal Transmission. *Pediatr Infect Dis J.* 2018a;37(10):1016–1021.

Adachi K, Xu J, Ank B, et al.; NICHD HPTN 040 Study Team. Cytomegalovirus urinary shedding in HIV-infected pregnant women and congenital cytomegalovirus infection. *Clin Infect Dis.* 2017;65(3):405–413.

Adachi K, Xu J, Yeganeh N, et al.; NICHD HPTN 040 Study Team. Combined evaluation of sexually transmitted infections in HIV-infected pregnant women and infant HIV transmission. *PLoS One.* 2018b;13(1):e0189851.

AVERT. Global information and education on HIV and AIDS. 2020. http://avert.org/professionals/hiv-social-issues/key-affected-populations/children

Becquet R, Ekouevi DK, Viho I, et al. Acceptability of exclusive breast-feeding with early cessation to prevent HIV transmission through breast milk, ANRS 1201/1202 Ditrame Plus, Abidjan, Cote d'Ivoire. *J AIDS.* 2005;40(5):600–608.

Bryson YJ, Luzuriaga K, Sullivan JL, et al. Proposed definitions for in utero versus intrapartum transmission of HIV-1. *N Engl J Med.* 1992;327:1246–1247.

Cao Y, Krogstad P, Korber BT, et al. Maternal HIV-1 viral load and vertical transmission of infection: the Ariel Project for the prevention of HIV transmission from mother to infant. *Nat Med.* 1997;3(5):549–552.

Chadwick EG, Yogev R, Alvero CG, et al.; International Pediatric Adolescent Clinical Trials Group (IMPAACT) P1030 Team. Long-term outcomes for HIV-infected infants less than 6 months of age at initiation of lopinavir/ritonavir combination antiretroviral therapy. *AIDS.* 2011;25:643–649.

Chinula L, Brummel SS, Zienba, L, et al. Abstract 130LB. Presented at Conference on Retroviruses and Opportunistic Infections, Boston, MA, 2020.

Clarke D, Acost EP, Cababasay M, et al.; International Pediatric Adolescent Clinical Trials Group (IMPAACT) P1110 Team. Raltegravir (RAL) in neonates: dosing, pharmacokinetics (PK), and safety in HIV-1–exposed neonates at risk of infection (IMPAACT P1110). *J AIDS.* 2020;84:70–77.

Committee on Obstetric Practice. ACOG committee opinion, scheduled cesarean delivery and the prevention of vertical transmission of HIV infection: number 234, May 2000 (replaces number 219, August 1999). *Int J Gynaecol Obstet*. 2001;73:279–281.

Connor EM, Sperling RS, Gelber R, et al.; Pediatric AIDS Clinical Trials Group Protocol 076 Study Group. Reduction of maternal-infant transmission of human immunodeficiency virus type 1 with zidovudine treatment. *N Engl J Med*. 1994;331(18):1173–1180.

Coovadia HM, Brown ER, Fowler MG, et al.; HPTN 046 Protocol Team. Efficacy and safety of an extended nevirapine regimen in infant children of breastfeeding mothers with HIV-1 infection for prevention of postnatal HIV-1 transmission (HPTN 046): a randomised, double-blind, placebo-controlled trial. *Lancet*. 2012;379(9812):221–228.

Coutsoudis A, Pillay K, Spooner E, et al.; South African Vitamin A Study Group. Influence of infant-feeding patterns on early mother-to-child transmission of HIV-1 in Durban, South Africa: a prospective cohort study. *Lancet*. 1999;354(9177):471–476.

De Lazzari E, León A, Arnaiz JA, et al. Hepatotoxicity of nevirapine in virologically suppressed patients according to gender and CD4 cell counts. *HIV Med*. 2008;9:221–226.

de Lourdes Teixeira M, Nafea S, Yeganeh N, et al. High rates of baseline antiretroviral resistance among HIV-infected pregnant women in an HIV referral centre in Rio de Janeiro, Brazil. *Int J STD AIDS*. 2015;26(13):922–928.

Department of Health and Human Services. Recommendations for the use of antiretroviral drugs in pregnant women with HIV infection and interventions to reduce perinatal HIV transmission in the United States. 2020. https://clinicalinfo.hiv.gov/en/guidelines/perinatal/whats-new-guidelines

Dickover RE, Dillon M, Gillette SG, et al. Rapid increases in load of human immunodeficiency virus correlate with early disease progression and loss of CD4 cells in vertically infected infants. *J Infect Dis*. 1994;170:1279–1284.

Dickover RE, Garratty EM, Herman SA, et al. Identification of levels of maternal HIV-1 RNA associated with risk of perinatal transmission: effect of maternal zidovudine treatment on viral load. *JAMA*. 1996;275(8):599–605.

Dorenbaum A, Cunningham CK, Gelber RD, et al. Two-dose intrapartum/newborn nevirapine and standard antiretroviral therapy to reduce perinatal HIV transmission: a randomized trial. *JAMA*. 2002;288:189–198.

Duliege AM, Amos CI, Felton S, et al.; International Registry of HIV-Exposed Twins. Birth order, delivery route, and concordance in the transmission of human immunodeficiency virus type 1 from mothers to twins. *J Pediatr*. 1995;126:625–632.

Dunn DT, Newell ML, Ades AE, et al. Risk of human immunodeficiency virus type 1 transmission through breastfeeding. *Lancet*. 1992;340:585–588.

European Collaborative Study. Children born to women with HIV-1 infection: natural history and risk of transmission. *Lancet*. 1991;337:253–260.

Ford N, Mofenson L, Shubber Z, et al. Safety of efavirenz in the first trimester of pregnancy: an updated systematic review and meta-analysis. *AIDS*. 2014;28:S123–S131.

Flynn PM, Taha TE, Cababasay M, et al. Prevention of HIV-1 transmission through breastfeeding: efficacy and safety of maternal antiretroviral therapy versus infant nevirapine prophylaxis for duration of breastfeeding in HIV-1-infected women with high CD4 cell count (IMPAACT PROMISE): a randomized, open-label, clinical trial. *J AIDS*. 2018;77(4):383–392.

Fowler MG, Newell ML. Breastfeeding and HIV-1 transmission in resource-limited settings. *J AIDS*. 2002;30:230–239.

Fowler MG, Qin M, Fiscus SA, et al. Benefits and risks of antiretroviral therapy for perinatal HIV prevention. *N Engl J Med*. 2016;375(18):1726–1737.

Gabiano C, Tovo PA, de Martino M, et al. Mother-to-child transmission of human immunodeficiency virus type 1: risk of infection and correlates of transmission. *Pediatrics*. 1992;90:369–374.

Gortmaker SL, Hughes M, Cervia J, et al.; Pediatric AIDS Clinical Trials Group Protocol 219 Team. Effect of combination therapy including protease inhibitors on mortality among children and adolescents infected with HIV-1. *N Engl J Med*. 2001;345(21):1522–1528.

Guay LA, Musoke P, Fleming T, et al. Intrapartum and neonatal single-dose nevirapine compared with zidovudine for prevention of mother-to-child transmission of HIV-1 in Kampala, Uganda: HIVNET 012 randomised trial. *Lancet*. 1999;354(9181):795–802.

Hitti J, Frenkel LM, Stek AM, et al.; PACTG 1022 Study Team. Maternal toxicity with continuous nevirapine in pregnancy: results from PACTG 1022. *J AIDS*. 2004;36:772–776.

Inter-agency Task Team on the Prevention and Treatment of HIV Infection in Pregnant Women Mothers and Children (IATT) CDC WHO and UNICEF. Monitoring & evaluation framework for antiretroviral treatment for pregnant and breastfeeding women living with HIV and their infants. 2015. http://www.who.int/hiv/mtct/iatt-me-framework/en/

International Perinatal HIV Group. The mode of delivery and the risk of vertical transmission of human immunodeficiency virus type 1—a meta-analysis of 15 prospective cohort studies. *N Engl J Med*. 1999;340(13):977–987.

Jeremy RJ, Kim S, Nozyce M, et al.; Pediatric AIDS Clinical Trials Group (PACTG) 338 & 377 Study Teams. Neuropsychological functioning and viral load in stable antiretroviral therapy-experienced HIV-infected children. *Pediatrics*. 2005;115:380–387.

Lahoz R, Noguera A, Rovira N, et al. Antiretroviral-related hematologic short-term toxicity in healthy infants: implications of the new neonatal 4-week zidovudine regimen. *Pediatr Infect Dis J*. 2010;29(4):376–379.

Louis J, Landon MB, Gersnoviez RJ, et al. Perioperative morbidity and mortality among human immunodeficiency virus infected women undergoing cesarean delivery. *Obstet Gynecol*. 2007;110(2 Pt 1):385–390.

Luzuriaga K, Bryson Y, Krogstad P, et al. Combination treatment with zidovudine, didanosine, and nevirapine in infants with human immunodeficiency virus type 1 infection. *N Engl J Med*. 1997;336:1343–1349.

Luzuriaga K, Gay H, Ziemniak C, et al. Viremic relapse after HIV-1 remission in a perinatally infected child. *N Engl J Med*. 2015;372:786–788.

Luzuriaga K, Koup RA, Pikora CA, et al. Deficient human immunodeficiency virus type 1-specific cytotoxic T cell responses in vertically infected children. *J Pediatr*. 1991;119:230–236.

Luzuriaga K, McManus M, Mofenson L, et al.; PACTG 356 Investigators. A trial of three antiretroviral regimens in HIV-1-infected children. *N Engl J Med*. 2004; 350(24):2471–2480.

Lyimo MA, Mosi MN, Housman ML, et al. Breast milk from Tanzanian women has divergent effects on cell-free and cell-associated HIV-1 infection in vitro. *PloS One*. 2012;7(8):e43815.

Magder LS, Mofenson L, Paul ME, et al. Risk factors for in utero and intrapartum transmission of HIV. *J AIDS*. 2005;38:87–95.

Marazzi MC, Germano P, Liotta G, et al. Implementing anti-retroviral triple therapy to prevent HIV mother-to-child transmission: a public health approach in resource-limited settings. *Eur J Pediatr*. 2007;166(12):1305–1307.

Marazzi MC, Liotta G, Nielsen-Saines K, et al. Extended antenatal antiretroviral use correlates with improved infant outcomes throughout the first year of life. *AIDS*. 2010;24(18):2819–2826.

Marazzi MC, Nielsen-Saines K, Buonomo E, et al. Increased infant human immunodeficiency virus-type one free survival at one year of age in sub-Saharan Africa with maternal use of highly active antiretroviral therapy during breast-feeding. *Pediatr Infect Dis J*. 2009;28(6):483–487.

Mayaux MJ, Burgard M, Teglas JP, et al.; The French Pediatric HIV Infection Study Group. Neonatal characteristics in rapidly progressive perinatally acquired HIV-1 disease. *JAMA*. 1996;275:606–610.

Mayaux MJ, Dussaix E, Isopet J, et al.; SEROGEST Cohort Group. Maternal virus load during pregnancy and mother-to-child transmission of human immunodeficiency virus type 1: the French perinatal cohort studies. *J Infect Dis*. 1997;175(1):172–175.

Minkoff H, Burns DN, Landesman S, et al. The relationship of the duration of ruptured membranes to vertical transmission of human immunodeficiency virus. *Am J Obstet Gynecol.* 1995;173:585–589.

Mora S, Zamproni I, Beccio S, et al. Longitudinal changes of bone mineral density and metabolism in antiretroviral-treated human immunodeficiency virus-infected children. *J Clin Endocrinol Metab.* 2004;89:24–28.

Morrison S, John-Stewart G, Egessa JJ, et al. Rapid antiretroviral therapy initiation for women in an HIV-1 prevention clinical trial experiencing primary HIV-1 infection during pregnancy or breastfeeding. *PloS One.* 2015;10(10):e0140773.

Mwanyumba F, Gaillard P, Inion I, et al. Placental inflammation and perinatal transmission of HIV-1. *J AIDS.* 2002;29:262–269.

Newell ML. The natural history of vertically acquired HIV infection. The European Collaborative Study. *J Perinat Med.* 1991;19(Suppl 1):257–262.

Newell ML, Coovadia H, Cortina-Borja M, et al.; Ghent International AIDS Society (IAS) Working Group on HIV Infection in Women and Children. Mortality of infected and uninfected infants born to HIV-infected mothers in Africa: a pooled analysis. *Lancet.* 2004;364:1236–1243.

Nielsen K, Bryson YJ. Diagnosis of HIV infection in children. *Pediatr Clin North Am.* 2000;47:39–63.

Nielsen K, McSherry G, Petru A, et al. A descriptive survey of pediatric human immunodeficiency virus-infected long-term survivors. *Pediatrics.* 1997;99:pe4.

Nielsen-Saines K, Watts DH, Veloso VG, et al.; NICHD HPTN 040/PACTG 1043 Protocol Team. Phase III randomized trial of the safety and efficacy of three neonatal antiretroviral regimens for prevention of intrapartum HIV-1 transmission (NICHD HPTN 040/PACTG 1043) [Late Breaker Abstract 124LB]. Presented at the 18th Conference on Retroviruses and Opportunistic Infections, Boston, MA, 2011.

National Institutes of Health. HIV and specific populations: HIV and children and adolescents. 2020. https://hivinfo.nih.gov/understanding-hiv/fact-sheets/hiv-and-children-and-adolescents

Palumbo P, Lindsey JC, Hughes MD, et al. Antiretroviral treatment for children with peripartum nevirapine exposure. *N Engl J Med.* 2010;363:1510–1520.

Palumbo PE, Raskino C, Fiscus S, et al. Predictive value of quantitative plasma HIV RNA and CD4+ lymphocyte count in HIV-infected infants and children. *JAMA.* 1998;279:756–761.

Panel on Antiretroviral Therapy and Medical Management of HIV-Infected Children. Guidelines for the use of antiretroviral agents in pediatric HIV infection. 2020. https://clinicalinfo.hiv.gov/en/guidelines/pediatric-arv/antiretroviral-management-newborns-perinatal-hiv-exposure-or-hiv-infection

Persaud D, Gay G, Ziemniak C, et al. Absence of detectable HIV-1 viremia after treatment cessation in an infant. *N Engl J Med.* 2013;369:1828–1835.

Persaud D, Palumbo PE, Ziemniak C, et al. Dynamics of the resting CD4+ T cell latent HIV reservoir in infants initiating highly active antiretroviral therapy less than six months of age. *AIDS.* 2012;26(12):1483–1490.

Polycarpou A, Ntais C, Korber BT, et al. Association between maternal and infant class I and II HLA alleles and of their concordance with the risk of perinatal HIV type 1 transmission. *AIDS Res Hum Retroviruses.* 2002;18:741–746.

Read JS, Mwatha A, Richardson B, et al. Primary HIV-1 infection among infants in sub-Saharan Africa: HPTN 024. *J AIDS.* 2009;51(3):317–322.

Ruane PJ, DeJesus E, Berger D, et al. Antiviral activity, safety, and pharmacokinetics/pharmacodynamics of tenofovir alafenamide as 10-day monotherapy in HIV-1-positive adults. *J AIDS.* 2013;63(4):449–455.

Scarlatti G. Mother-to-child transmission of HIV-1: advances and controversies of the twentieth century. *AIDS Rev.* 2004;6:67–78.

Scott GB. HIV infection in children: clinical features and management. *J AIDS.* 1991;4:109–115.

Scott GB, Hutto C, Makuch RW, et al. Survival in children with perinatally acquired human immunodeficiency virus type 1 infection. *N Engl J Med.* 1989;321:1791–1796.

Sei S, Boler AM, Nguyen GT, et al. Protective effect of CCR5 delta 32 heterozygosity is restricted by SDF-1 genotype in children with HIV-1 infection. *AIDS.* 2001;15:1343–1352.

Semrau K, Kuhn L, Brooks DR, et al. Dynamics of breast milk HIV-1 RNA with unilateral mastitis or abscess. *J AIDS.* 2013;62(3):348–355.

Siliciano JD, Siliciano RF. Recent developments in the search for a cure for HIV-1 infections: targeting the latent reservoir for HIV-1. *J Allergy Clin Immunol.* 2014;134:12–19.

St. Louis ME, Kamenga M, Brown C, et al. Risk for perinatal HIV-1 transmission according to maternal immunologic, virologic, and placental factors. *JAMA.* 1993;269:2853–2859.

UNICEF. Children, HIV and AIDS. Global snapshot. December 2019. Global AIDS Monitoring 2019, UNAIDS 2019 estimates and UNICEF Global Databases of nationally representative population-based surveys 2012–2018. https://data.unicef.org/topic/hivaids/global-regional-trends/

UNICEF. Elimination of mother-to-child transmission. 2020. https://data.unicef.org/topic/hivaids/emtct/

Van Rompay KK, Otsyula MG, Marthas ML, et al. Immediate zidovudine treatment protects simian immunodeficiency virus-infected newborn macaques against rapid onset of AIDS. *Antimicrob Agents Chemother.* 1995;39:125–131.

Violari A, Cotton MF, Gibb DM, et al.; CHER Study Team. Early antiretroviral therapy and mortality among HIV-infected infants. *N Engl J Med.* 2008;359:2233–2244.

World Health Organization. March 2014 Supplement to the 2013 Consolidated guidelines on the use of antiretroviral drugs for treating and preventing HIV infection recommendations for a public health approach. 2014. http://apps.who.int/iris/bitstream/10665/104264/1/9789241506830_eng.pdf?ua=1

World Health Organization. Update of recommendations on first- and second-line antiretroviral regimens. Geneva, Switzerland: World Health Organization; 2019. https://www.who.int/publications/i/item/WHO-CDS-HIV-19.15

Yeganeh N, Kerin T, Ank B, et al. HIV antiretroviral resistance and transmission in mother-infant pairs enrolled in a large perinatal study. *Clin Infect Dis.* 2018;66(11):1770–1777.

Yeganeh N, Watts HD, Camarca M, et al. Syphilis in HIV-infected mothers and infants: results from the NICHD/HPTN 040 study. *Pediatr Infect Dis J.* 2015;34(3):e52–e57.

Zash R, Holmes L, Diseko M, et al. Neural-tube defects and antiretroviral treatment regimens in Botswana. *N Engl J Med.* 2019;381(9):827–840.

Zash R, Makhema J, Shapiro RL. Neural-tube defects with dolutegravir treatment from the time of conception. *N Engl J Med.* 2018;379(10):979–981.

25.

UNDERSTANDING AND MANAGING ANTINEOPLASTIC AND ANTIRETROVIRAL THERAPY

Jason J. Schafer, Elizabeth M. Sherman, and Taylor K. Gill

LEARNING OBJECTIVE

- To review concepts regarding the safe and effective use of antineoplastic and antiretroviral therapy (ART) in people living with HIV and cancer

WHAT'S NEW?

To address the challenges of complicated interactions and toxicities associated with ARV and antineoplastic therapies, people with HIV and cancer should receive multidisciplinary care that includes primary care providers, infectious disease clinicians, hematologists/oncologists, and clinical pharmacists.

KEY POINTS

- The use of combination ART in people with HIV and malignancies is associated with improved HIV- and cancer-related outcomes.

- Combining ART and antineoplastic therapy is often complicated by significant drug–drug interactions, drug–disease state monitoring interactions, and overlapping toxicities.

- Definitive pharmacokinetic studies evaluating drug interactions between antineoplastics and antiretroviral agents (ARVs) are uncommon, and clinical judgment must often be used to determine the potential for significant interactions.

- Adjusting ART in response to significant drug interactions or overlapping toxicities is often more feasible than modifying antineoplastic protocols.

INTRODUCTION TO CANCER IN HIV

The incidence of cancer among persons with HIV (PWH) is nearly 50% greater than the general population (National Comprehensive Cancer Network [NCCN], 2020). The elevated risk of cancer in PWH is multifactorial and likely due to a combination of underlying immune deficiency, coinfection with oncogenic viruses, and a higher prevalence of other cancer-related risk factors such as the use of tobacco and alcohol products.

Before the widespread use of ART, AIDS-defining malignancies (ADMs) such as Kaposi's sarcoma, non-Hodgkin's lymphoma, and invasive cervical cancer accounted for the largest burden of cancer in PWH (Rubinstein et al., 2014). These malignancies occur most commonly in people with advanced HIV, and all are associated with oncogenic viruses. Following the widespread use of ART in the mid-1990s, there was a substantial decline in the number of new AIDS diagnoses and AIDS-related deaths (Rubinstein et al., 2014). The ability to reconstitute the immune system with ART also led to a decrease in ADMs. At the same time, the occurrence of non–AIDS-defining malignancies (NADMs) increased. These malignancies include Hodgkin's lymphoma, leukemia, and cancers of the head, neck, lung, kidney, liver, gastrointestinal tract, anus, and skin. Currently, NADMs cause more cancer-related morbidity and mortality than ADMs and will remain common among PWH, with lung and prostate cancer expected to emerge as the most prevalent cancer types in the next decade (Shiels et al., 2018).

Although ADMs most commonly occur in people with severe immune suppression, low $CD4^+$ T-cell counts (<500 cells/mm³) have been identified as a risk factor for both ADMs and NADMs (Torres & Mulanovich, 2014). This suggests that initiating ART to suppress HIV replication and reconstituting $CD4^+$ T-cell counts may reduce the overall risk of malignancies in PWH. Recently, viral suppression, particularly long-term suppression with ART, has been linked with ADM and NADM prevention. Despite this, cancer risk can remain elevated even in virally suppressed PWH in comparison to persons without HIV infection (Park et al., 2018).

In people with cancer, the use of ART alongside chemotherapy is now routinely recommended to improve overall survival. The administration of chemotherapy and ART concurrently can be complicated by a number of factors (Rudek et al., 2011), including limited data regarding safe and effective therapy combinations; significant drug–drug interactions among ART, antineoplastics, and supportive care medications; drug–disease state monitoring interactions; and overlapping drug toxicities. This chapter reviews contemporary information regarding the use of chemotherapy and ART in combination, including strategies for managing potential drug–drug interactions and considerations for preventing and/or monitoring for toxicity.

GENERAL CONSIDERATIONS FOR COMBINING ANTINEOPLASTIC THERAPY AND ART

DRUG INTERACTIONS: CYP450

Drug interactions between ART and antineoplastic agents may occur via several different mechanisms. The most common are the interactions that occur during metabolism of medications from active to inactive substances via the hepatic cytochrome P450 (CYP450) system. Medications may be substrates of the CYP450 system, meaning that they use this system for metabolism, and their concentrations may be altered by concurrent administration with other agents. In addition, medications may be inducers or inhibitors of individual CYP450 isoenzymes, such as 3A4. CYP450 inducers will increase the metabolism of CYP450 substrates, thus decreasing the concentration of medication, which may lead to subtherapeutic medication levels. Conversely, CYP450 inhibitors will decrease the metabolism of CYP450 substrates, thus increasing the medication concentration, which may lead to toxicity. The timing of the CYP450 interactions may also vary as enzyme inhibition occurs rapidly, with maximum effect occurring when a medication is at steady state and enzyme induction occurring more slowly due to the need for enzyme synthesis (Di Francia et al., 2014). Many ARV, antineoplastic, and supportive care medications utilize the CYP450 system for metabolism, and drug interactions are expected to be a challenge in this setting.

Several antineoplastic agents are substrates, inducers, or inhibitors of CYP3A4. The result is complex bidirectional interactions with ART (Rudek et al., 2011). Interacting agents include vinblastine, vincristine, paclitaxel, docetaxel, ifosfamide, cyclophosphamide, tyrosine kinase inhibitors, and corticosteroids that are metabolized by CYP3A4 (Rubinstein et al., 2014). HIV protease inhibitors (PIs), the integrase inhibitor elvitegravir, nonnucleoside reverse transcriptase inhibitors (NNRTIs), and the pharmacokinetic enhancers cobicistat and ritonavir have a higher likelihood of drug interactions because of their CYP450 metabolism. ART regimens containing integrase inhibitors without pharmacologic boosters are favored in the setting of malignancy due to a lower potential for drug interactions (NCCN, 2020).

DRUG INTERACTIONS: P-GLYCOPROTEIN

To add to the complexity of interactions that occur with medication metabolism, there may also be absorption interactions with the p-glycoprotein efflux pump in the gastrointestinal tract. Like the CYP450 interactions, medications may be p-glycoprotein substrates, inducers, or inhibitors. P-glycoprotein inducers stimulate the efflux of medications back into the gastrointestinal lumen, thus decreasing the absorption and plasma concentrations of these medications. Likewise, p-glycoprotein inhibitors will increase the absorption of medication and increase plasma concentrations of substrates, which could lead to toxicities. ARVs that affect, and are affected by, p-glycoprotein include maraviroc, NNRTIs, integrase inhibitors, and PIs. Literature has shown that p-glycoprotein is highly expressed in HIV-associated malignancies such as non-Hodgkin's lymphoma and plays a significant role in the effectiveness of both ART and antineoplastic therapy (Klibanov & Clark-Vetril, 2007). Clinicians should be aware of ARV, antineoplastic, and supportive care agents that affect p-glycoprotein and should realize the potential for drug interactions with medications that influence, or are influenced by, this mechanism.

MEDICATION TOXICITIES

Clinicians will also need to consider overlapping toxicities of medication classes. Some ART and antineoplastic agents are known for causing severe adverse effects that may become additive when used in combination. For example, the entry inhibitor maraviroc may cause hepatotoxicity; nucleoside reverse transcriptase inhibitors (NRTIs) may cause neutropenia, peripheral neuropathy, hepatotoxicity, or nephrotoxicity; various NNRTIs are associated with rash and hepatic transaminase elevations; and PIs may lead to greater gastrointestinal upset, including nausea, vomiting, and diarrhea (DHHS, 2020). PI may also potentiate the myelosuppressive effects of certain chemotherapy (Torres & Mulanovich, 2014). Integrase inhibitors, however, are well tolerated, and overlapping toxicities with antineoplastic agents are not projected to be a major concern. It is vitally important when devising medication regimens that serious adverse effects of all agents be identified and overlapping toxicities minimized when possible.

DRUG–DISEASE INTERACTIONS

The presence of drug–disease interactions will need to be recognized when combining ARVs and antineoplastic agents. Disease monitoring interactions are a concern because certain ARVs increase oncologic disease markers such as bilirubin. Bilirubin is often used as a means for determining dosage adjustments for a number of chemotherapeutic agents, such as docetaxel, paclitaxel, doxorubicin, etoposide, irinotecan, imatinib, and vincristine (Beumer et al., 2014). Atazanavir may cause unconjugated hyperbilirubinemia secondary to UGT1A1 inhibition, leading to possible inaccuracies in chemotherapy dosage calculations.

Conversely, there are also concerns that antineoplastic agents may affect the level of CD4+ T cells, rendering the monitoring parameters of both disease states inaccurate (Klibanov & Clark-Vetril, 2007). To supplement these monitoring parameter concerns, there may also be medication absorption concerns due to the presence of disease complications such as gastrointestinal tumors, mucositis, and graft-versus-host disease (Torres & Mulanovich, 2014). Clinicians may need to be creative in these situations, such as selecting medication regimens available in liquid formulations or alternative routes of administration.

The key concepts of drug interactions, overlapping toxicities, and drug–disease interactions are just a few examples of the complexity in utilizing combination ART and antineoplastic therapy. Specific literature and guideline recommendations to assist in the selection, dosing, and monitoring of these agents when used in combination are scarce. Thus, these concepts should be considered on a case-by-case basis and explored when crafting a medication regimen in the treatment of both HIV and oncologic diseases.

STRATEGIES FOR CLINICAL MANAGEMENT OF PEOPLE WITH CANCER AND HIV

Treatment of PWH and cancer is complex and a variety of management strategies should be considered. Examples of management strategies include alterations to the ART or chemotherapy regimens, changes in monitoring frequency, and optimization of opportunistic infection (OI) prophylaxis. To address the challenges, persons who have both HIV infection and cancer should be treated using a multidisciplinary approach that includes primary care providers, infectious disease clinicians, hematologists/oncologists, and clinical pharmacists. Communication among these professions is essential.

In combining ART and anticancer drug therapy, drug interactions and overlapping toxicities can be minimized or avoided by altering either the ART regimen or the chemotherapy regimen. In many instances, it is often simpler to substitute one or more components of a person's ART regimen in order to avoid the risk of drug interactions or additive toxicity. When determining interaction potential, drug interaction resources such as the following should be consulted: the Toronto General Hospital Immunodeficiency Clinic (https://hivclinic.ca/drug-information/antiretroviral-interactions-with-chemotherapy-regimens/) and the University of Liverpool HIV drug interaction website (http://www.hiv-druginteractions.org). ART regimen changes should always be carried out in conjunction with an HIV specialist utilizing the person's complete ART history, past adverse events, and resistance test results. Interruption of ART or a delay in ART initiation is not recommended because it has been associated with an increase in mortality. In addition, modifications to the medications in an antineoplastic regimen or their doses may also be considered based on the person's tolerance and response. Regardless, both ART and chemotherapy should be individualized according to the person's characteristics.

Increased monitoring for efficacy and toxicity is recommended when coadministering any ART regimen with chemotherapy. If an ARV regimen is modified, more intensive monitoring of tolerability, viral suppression, adherence, and laboratory changes is recommended during the first 3 months after a regimen switch. Identification and enhanced monitoring for toxicities is also recommended and should be assessed individually for each person.

Lastly, in persons with HIV infection and cancer, OI prophylaxis should be tailored and expanded with antimicrobials required for specific chemotherapy regimens or hematopoietic stem cell transplantation. The need for OI prophylaxis should be reevaluated on a regular basis and adjusted as needed via coordination among the infectious disease and the oncology providers. Prophylaxis may need to be modified as the person's CD4$^+$ T-cell count decreases with some chemotherapy regimens or increases after completion of therapy.

REFERENCES

Beumer JH, Venkataramanan R, Rudek MA. Pharmacotherapy in cancer patients with HIV/AIDS. *Clin Pharmcol Ther.* 2014;95(4):370–372.

Department of Health and Human Services (DHHS). Panel on Antiretroviral Guidelines for Adults and Adolescents. Guidelines for the use of antiretroviral agents in adults and adolescents with HIV. Department of Health and Human Services. 2020. https://clinicalinfo.hiv.gov/sites/default/files/inline-files/AdultandAdolescentGL.pdf

Di Francia R, Di Paolo M, Valente D, et al. Pharmacogenetic based drug–drug interactions between highly active antiretroviral therapy (HAART) and antiblastic chemotherapy. *World Cancer Res J.* 2014;1(2):e386.

Klibanov OM, Clark-Vetril R. Oncologic complications of human immunodeficiency virus infection: changing epidemiology, treatments, and special considerations in the era of highly active antiretroviral therapy. *Pharmacotherapy.* 2007;27(1):122–136.

National Comprehensive Cancer Network. Clinical practice guidelines in oncology: cancer in people living with HIV. Version 1. 2020. https://www.nccn.org/professionals/physician_gls

Park LS, Tate JP, Sigel K, et al. Association of viral suppression with lower AIDS-defining and non-AIDS-defining cancer incidence in HIV-infected veterans: a prospective cohort study. *Ann Intern Med.* 2018;169(2):87–96.

Rubinstein PG, Aboulafia DM, Zloza A. Malignancies in HIV/AIDS: from epidemiology to therapeutic challenges. *AIDS.* 2014;28(4):453–465.

Rudek MA, Flexner C, Ambinder RF. Use of antineoplastic agents in patients with cancer who have HIV/AIDS. *Lancet Oncol.* 2011;12(9):905–912.

Shiels MS, Islam JY, Rosenberg PS, et al. Projected cancer incidence rates and burden of incident cancer cases in HIV-infected adults in the United States through 2030. *Ann Intern Med.* 2018;168(12):866–873.

Torres HA, Mulanovich V. Management of HIV infection in patients with cancer receiving chemotherapy. *Clin Infect Dis.* 2014;59(1):106–114.

26.

SUBSTANCE USE IN HIV POPULATIONS

Elizabeth H. David and Thanh Thuy Truong

CHAPTER GOAL

Upon completion of this chapter, the reader should be able to:

- Discuss issues, implications, diagnosis, and treatment of substance use disorders in HIV-positive individuals.

INTRODUCTION

The relationship between substance use and HIV infection is complex and encompasses all stages, including transmission, diagnosis, progression, and treatment. Substance use can increase risk for exposure to HIV via needle sharing or by impairing judgment, which is linked to risky sexual behaviors. Among men who had sex with men (MSM), substance use was associated with an increased risk of HIV infection, particularly with binge drinking and use of crack/cocaine, methamphetamine, and inhalants. In a Centers for Disease Control and Prevention (CDC) report, MSM accounted for 66% of HIV diagnoses in the US. HIV diagnoses attributed to injection drug use increased from 2014 to 2018, which was likely due to the increase in prescription opioid use and heroin (CDC, 2020). Among persons with HIV (PWH), substance use can lead to a poor prognosis and progression to AIDS. Irregular follow-up with treatment, poor adherence to antiretroviral therapy (ART), and risk of acquiring other sexually transmitted infections and hepatitis C virus (HCV) through injection drug use increase morbidity and mortality (Cofrancesco et al., 2008; Stern et al., 2018).

Biological, psychological, and social factors influence the relationship between substance use disorders (SUDs) and HIV infection. Risk of substance use involves interactions between genes and the environment. Approximately 40% to 60% of vulnerability to addiction can be attributable to genetic variance. For example, while some genes have been associated with susceptibility to excess alcohol consumption, polymorphisms in alcohol-metabolizing enzymes like alcohol dehydrogenases ADH1B and ALDH2 are protective against alcohol use disorder (AUD) (Chen et al., 1999). Furthermore, certain periods of normal development have a higher risk of drug use. During adolescence, normal behaviors of novelty seeking, risk taking, and sensitivity to peer pressure may result in experimenting with legal and illegal substances. Adolescent brains have not completed development in areas involved in executive function, which is necessary for regulating impulses and emotions. Not surprisingly, high rates of use for most substances occur between age 18 and 24, prior to full development of frontal lobes and functional networks at age 25 (Miller et al., 2019). Adolescent neurological development is also more vulnerable to the long-term effects of chronic drug and alcohol exposure and can sustain dependence later in life. This interaction between biological and psychological development leads to risky behaviors such as multiple partners and inconsistent condom use that increase exposure to HIV (Hillfors et al., 2007). Socioeconomic disadvantage, low education, and unstable housing also contribute to unsafe sexual practices and limited access to preventive measures, thus increasing the prevalence of HIV in these populations (Millett et al., 2007).

Psychiatric illnesses and substance use are separate and additive risk factors for HIV infection. Psychiatric illnesses are more prevalent in PWH. For example, personality disorders are highly represented among PWH, likely due to traits such as impulsivity and maladaptive coping strategies to stress that perpetuate risky behaviors. Similarly, PWH are more likely to have a mental illness like anxiety or depression, whether resulting from HIV infection of neural tissue or a distinct comorbidity (Stern et al., 2018). One study of PWH revealed that those who have a dual diagnosis of mental illness and substance use have an HIV prevalence of 4.7% as opposed to 2.4% for those with a SUD diagnosis alone—almost double the rate. This highlights the importance of a comprehensive approach in the treatment of those with dual diagnoses. Problems with adherence to medical treatment seem to be more pronounced in this group (Moore et al., 2008; Sullivan et al., 2011). Finally, unhealthy substance use is associated with a host of medical sequelae (liver disease, infection, diabetes, cardiovascular disease, and neurocognitive changes) that add to the many potential medical complications associated with HIV and AIDS. Despite advancement in diagnosis and treatment among PWH since the 1990s (Bhaskaran et al., 2008), stigma, shame, and complacency continue to be significant barriers to care in PWH and SUDs. Routine voluntary testing in all individuals aged 13 to 64 is recommended by the CDC to facilitate early detection and treatment of HIV (Branson et al., 2006). Testing may be postponed in acute exacerbations of mental illness and substance use but should be offered once the person has the capacity to consent to testing and treatment. A comprehensive and harm-reduction approach involving patient education and collaboration in therapeutic decisions is critical for this complex patient population. Persistent risky substance use should prompt referral to drug treatment services and relapse prevention should be discussed at each patient encounter (CDC, 2003). Education about reducing risk of opportunistic infections should be provided. Resources may be limited in some areas for an interdisciplinary team approach, but if possible, care is best managed concurrently with an HIV treatment expert.

LEARNING OBJECTIVES

- Describe the bidirectional interactions between HIV and unhealthy substance use

- Recognize unhealthy substance use in PWH

- Provide an initial outline of potential approaches to the treatment of SUDs in this population.

WHAT'S NEW?

The chapter has been updated to reflect the terminology of the fifth edition of the *Diagnostic and Statistical Manual of Mental Disorders* (American Psychiatric Association, 2013). More thorough and specific treatment modalities and recommendations are included.

SCREENING AND DIAGNOSIS OF SUDS

Prior to conducting screening, assessment, or treatment planning, providers should evaluate their personal beliefs and attitudes toward PWH with SUDs. Working with this population often elicits difficult feelings that can be emotionally and physically demanding for staff. Examining countertransference reactions and biases such as homophobia and fear of infection can help decrease burnout and facilitate a stronger therapeutic alliance with the PWH. Providers must be comfortable discussing taboo topics such as sex, drug use, shame, and trauma. Cultural competency is also important because people from different ethnic groups, socioeconomic class, gender, and cultures have varying levels of comfort in discussing these topics. For example, asking personal questions about substance use and sexual risk factors may feel intrusive and disrespectful to some Asian and Pacific Islander individuals. Approaching screening by asking the least intrusive question first may ease the person into more detailed questions later. While HIV/AIDS disproportionately affects African Americans, many have mistrust of the healthcare system stemming from a long history of exploitation of their community by medical institutions. Providers should be aware of social, economic, and political issues such as institutional racism that continue to affect the African American community. Working with lesbian, gay, bisexual, and transgender (LGBTQ) populations requires understanding and sensitivity, as members of this population often face stigma, trauma, low self-esteem, and lack of family and social supports. Another group that needs special consideration is women.

Women present differently and often at later stages in the HIV/AIDS disease process compared to men. Factors such as identity (e.g., as a caregiver), stigma (e.g., "unfit mother"), and shame and guilt over being HIV positive may play a major role in a woman's care decisions. Lastly, while it is helpful to consider the common experiences of a group, providers should seek to understand the unique experience of each individual.

Although there are specific criteria for the diagnosis of SUD and physiologic dependence (American Psychiatric Association, 2013), assessing the impact of a substance is difficult and a comprehensive evaluation is needed to understand the individual's unique experience. Historically, addiction was viewed as a voluntary moral failing by the individual, which led to stigmatization that has been a significant barrier to appropriate care. However, research has advanced our understanding of the profound drug effects on neural networks involved in reward processing, motivation, and behavioral and emotional regulation that lead to compulsive behaviors. Definitions of SUD in the literature have reflected this progress, targeting biological, psychological, and social factors. After reviewing several definitions, one practical definition adopted by the European Monitoring Centre for Drugs and Drug Addiction is "a repeated powerful motivation to engage in a purposeful behavior that has no survival value, acquired as a result of engaging in that behavior, with significant potential for unintended harm" (West, 2013). The severity of substance use varies between individuals, encompassing low-risk, hazardous, harmful, and addiction levels. Generally, SUD is diagnosed when use of a substance results in an impairment of functioning in multiple areas (occupational, social, and recreational), loss of control over intake, and presence of a negative emotional state during abstinence.

Screening and brief intervention (SBI) for tobacco and alcohol use disorder in a variety of clinical settings have demonstrated significant benefit in reducing use of these substances. Routine screening of all adults and pregnant women for alcohol and tobacco use is recommended by the US Preventive Services Task Force (Campos-Outcalt, 2016). A variety of screening tools for unhealthy alcohol and illicit drug use are available through the National Institute on Alcohol Abuse and Alcoholism (NIAAA), the National Institute on Drug Abuse (NIDA), and other governmental agencies. The single question "How many times in the past year have you used an illegal drug or used a prescription medication for nonmedical reasons?" has been shown to accurately identify drug use. A response of at least one time is positive for unhealthy drug use. To prescreen for any alcohol use, asking "Do you sometimes drink beer, wine, or other alcoholic beverages?" can gently prepare the person for more detailed questions about unhealthy use. For heavy drinking, the question "How many times in the past year have you had five or more (for men) or four or more (for women) drinks in a day?" is sensitive and specific for identifying unhealthy alcohol use in primary care settings (NIAAA, 2017). A positive screen should prompt further assessment of the severity and impact on the individual's functioning to determine risk level. Differentiating between at-risk use or an SUD is relevant to guide clinical recommendations for treatment. Brief intervention such as advice and motivational interviewing may be appropriate for at-risk use, whereas more extensive follow-up and referral to an addiction specialist would be suitable for PWH meeting criteria for an SUD. Screening would be best accompanied by laboratory studies such as urine toxicology for drugs and serum carbohydrate and mean corpuscular volume for alcohol use.

TREATMENT

GENERAL PRINCIPLES

Successful treatment of PWH with SUD poses significant challenges and requires a multimodal approach. Chronic drug exposure leads to long-lasting neurological and behavioral changes that contribute to relapse, which can make PWH and providers feel frustrated and demoralized. Approaching SUD as a chronic disease such as diabetes or hypertension that necessitates long-term management represents a shift in ideology toward a harm-reduction model. Recognizing that the illness involves periods of recovery and relapse depending on compliance and efficacy of treatment helps PWH and the treatment team approach care rationally. Rather than failure, relapse can be reframed as a temporary setback as part of trial and error in achieving an effective care regimen. Some individuals may not be able to achieve abstinence despite appropriate treatment, so setting more achievable goals such as reducing the frequency and severity of use and relapse can improve overall functioning. Clarifying and communicating these expectations to the PWH and treatment team can lead to improved outcomes and retention in treatment (McLellan et al., 2000). A combination of psychosocial and pharmacological interventions is strongly recommended to target different facets of addiction. When possible, use of an interdisciplinary team including psychiatry, primary care, social work, substance use counseling, and case management is ideal for supporting individuals in their recovery and preventing relapse.

General principles of effective SUD treatment include easy access to care, collaborating with patients to create treatment plans to addresses their individual needs, monitoring for relapse, and treating psychiatric and medical comorbidities. Tests for HIV/AIDS, hepatitis B and C, tuberculosis, and other infectious diseases should be readily available. On-site availability of HIV testing can increase the likelihood of people being tested and receiving their results (NIDA, 1999). Individuals often present when seeking withdrawal management, which can be viewed as entry into treatment. Physicians should establish rapport with individuals and facilitate their motivation toward engaging in recommended addiction services. The appropriate treatment setting depends on the PWH's insight and physical and emotional ability to engage in care and the availability of necessary treatment (e.g., opioid-agonist therapy). Hospitalization is recommended for PWH who are a danger to themselves or others because of intoxication or acute psychiatric disorder, those who need intensive withdrawal management, or those who have life-threatening medical conditions. Residential treatment programs are best

for PWH who have fluctuating insight and need a highly structured and supportive environment. Partial hospitalization and intensive outpatient programs can be considered for persons who are transitioning out of a residential or hospital setting to a lower level of care but still need close monitoring to manage risk of relapse. PWH who have a history of relapse after treatment completion or have plans to return to high-risk environments would be best continued in a highly structured setting. Finally, for PWH who demonstrate insight into their disease, high compliance with treatment, and low severity of symptoms, outpatient programs are an appropriate and cost-effective option. Outpatient programs vary from low to high intensity; many of them have a multimodal approach, involving individual and group therapy as well as mental health and medical treatment (Miller et al., 2019).

THERAPY

Various psychotherapies have been shown to be effective for treatment of SUD through helping PWH modify the behaviors, feelings, thoughts, and social contexts that drive compulsive drug use. Therapeutic intervention can increase motivation, improve mood, and build a strong social support network, all of which improve the person's chances of recovery and prevent relapse. Motivational enhancement therapy is used to help PWH address their ambivalence about drug use and engaging in treatment. Motivational interviewing techniques enhance motivation and commitment for change or maintaining abstinence. Cognitive-behavioral therapy (CBT) has demonstrated efficacy in relapse prevention, helping individuals to identify and correct behaviors and thoughts that precede cravings and increase risk of relapse. Studies have demonstrated retention of CBT skills at least a year after discharge from treatment (Carroll et al., 1994). Individual counseling focuses on reducing or stopping substance use, addresses various areas of impaired functioning, and connects PWH to community resources such as 12-step programs (Alcoholics Anonymous, Narcotics Anonymous) or Self-Management and Recovery Training (SMART) recovery for patients who prefer a science-based and secular program. Among PWH with cocaine and opioid use disorders comorbid with psychiatric disorders, supportive expressive psychotherapy was shown to improve outcomes (Woody et al., 1995). Another strategy that has been shown to increase the duration of abstinence is voucher-based reinforcement therapy, where people are provided with a voucher that can be exchanged for retail goods and services that are consistent with a substance-free lifestyle each time they provide a drug-free urine sample. These voucher-based treatment approaches may provide individual, group, and family counseling; vocational counseling; and pharmacologic treatment.

ALCOHOL

Excessive use of alcohol, especially binge drinking, is an important risk factor for HIV infection. Alcohol intoxication is linked to risky sexual behaviors (e.g., not using a condom, multiple partners) that increase the risk of HIV infection. AUD also leads to poorer treatment outcomes due to nonadherence to ART and medical morbidities like liver and cardiovascular disease.

INTOXICATION/WITHDRAWAL

Alcohol intoxication is characterized by reversible psychological and behavioral changes that occur after alcohol consumption. A blood alcohol concentration of 0.08% is the limit for legal intoxication. However, significant impairment may occur at much lower levels in some PWH (younger or medically/mentally ill), while others may be functional at much higher levels due to tolerance. Intoxication is associated with physical symptoms of nausea and vomiting and neurological impairment (incoordination and ataxia). Overdose can result in respiratory depression, hypotension, hypothermia, profound central nervous system depression, coma, and death. Management of intoxication and overdose is supportive, with intravenous fluids and airway protection to prevent aspiration. The presence of other forms of alcohol, such as methanol, and other substances like opioids and benzodiazepines should prompt adjustments in clinical management. PWH with AUD may have a thiamine deficiency, which can precipitate Wernicke's encephalopathy and Korsakoff psychosis. Intravenous thiamine should thus be given, ideally before glucose to avoid central pontine myelinolysis. For behavioral dysregulation not responsive to verbal deescalation, antipsychotics such as haloperidol (e.g., 2–5 mg given intravenously, intramuscularly, or orally) and olanzapine should be considered. Benzodiazepines are commonly used to treat agitation but should be used with caution as they can further disinhibit the person and worsen agitation and respiratory depression.

Alcohol withdrawal begins 6 to 24 hours after the last drink or substantial reduction in drinking. Early symptoms include anxiety, irritability/restlessness, insomnia, nausea, headache, diaphoresis, and fine tremor. PWH may experience visual, auditory, and tactile hallucinations. Alcoholic hallucinosis may occur independently of other withdrawal symptoms that characterize delirium tremens (DTs). Alcohol withdrawal seizures may occur within 12 to 48 hours after the last drink, sometimes earlier. For most people, withdrawal does not progress beyond mild to moderate symptoms that remit after 48 hours. For a minority of individuals, withdrawal can progress to DTs, characterized by autonomic dysfunction (tachycardia, fever, hypertension) and delirium. Without proper management, DTs can be life-threatening. Pharmacologic treatment often involves benzodiazepines. Selection of the benzodiazepine should consider its pharmacokinetics, its abuse potential, and the presence of hepatic injury. Longer-acting agents (diazepam, chlordiazepoxide) may have a smoother withdrawal course but have higher risks of excessive sedation in some individuals (e.g., elderly). For PWH with significant hepatic dysfunction, a benzodiazepine that does not undergo first-pass metabolism (lorazepam, oxazepam) may be preferred. Phenobarbital can be used in PWH who are not responding to benzodiazepines. Other agents that have shown efficacy and are well tolerated include anticonvulsants such as gabapentin, carbamazepine, and valproate (Minozzi et al., 2010). However, there are limited data on their ability to prevent DTs and withdrawal seizures.

PHARMACOTHERAPY FOR AUD

Treatment for AUD involves medications that reduce the reinforcing effects of alcohol or deter use by causing adverse reactions with alcohol consumption. Commonly used agents are as follows:

- **Naltrexone** is a mu-opioid receptor antagonist that reduces the reinforcing effects of alcohol. This results in decreased craving as well as disruption of the euphoric feelings associated with alcohol intoxication. Naltrexone has been shown to reduce alcohol consumption and prevent relapse to heavy drinking (Miller et al., 2019). Naltrexone use is contraindicated in PWH with significant liver disease (hepatitis and liver failure), and all persons should have liver function tested prior to initiation of this drug. Monitoring for liver toxicity is recommended in PWH, who may have concurrent liver disease from substance use, concurrent hepatitis infection, or liver impairment from ART. Naltrexone is often well tolerated and does not have documented interactions with ART. Naltrexone should be avoided in individuals who require opioids for pain management or are in acute opioid withdrawal. PWH can be started on oral naltrexone at 50 to 100 mg/day. It is also available in an intramuscular formulation (Vivitrol) at doses of 380 mg every 4 weeks. Common early side effects (nausea and other gastrointestinal effects, headache, dizziness) are usually mild and transient. For the intramuscular formulation, swelling, pain, and other injection-site reactions may occur.

- **Acamprosate** works through modulating glutamate neurotransmission and increasing gamma-aminobutyric acid (GABA) activity. It has been shown to reduce alcohol consumption and increase the duration of abstinence (Stern et al., 2018). The medication is often well tolerated and safe in PWH with impaired liver function. However, because it is excreted renally, dose adjustments may be needed in persons with renal failure. Acamprosate is approved by the US Food and Drug Administration (FDA) at a dosage of 1,998 mg/day, or a 333-mg capsule three times daily. The frequent dosing is a barrier to using this medication in many people. Common side effects are often mild and transient and include gastrointestinal (e.g., nausea, diarrhea) and dermatologic (e.g., itching) symptoms. Acamprosate carries a warning for a possible increase in suicidal behavior; however, many of these events occurred in the context of alcohol relapse, and no consistent pattern of relationship between the clinical course of recovery from alcoholism and the emergence of suicidality was identified (Campral/acamprosate product information, Forest Pharmaceuticals, 2004).

- **Disulfiram** (Antabuse) discourages drinking by causing an adverse physical reaction with alcohol consumption. It acts by inhibiting acetaldehyde dehydrogenase, which prevents the metabolism of acetaldehyde (byproduct of alcohol breakdown). The increased acetaldehyde concentration causes temporary flushing, sweating, palpitations, hypotension, nausea, and vomiting. Severe reactions have resulted in cardiovascular compromise and death. Due to these effects, it is often used in selected PWH who are highly motivated or are closely supervised for compliance and abstinence. The daily dose is limited to 250 to 500 mg/day due to more adverse effects at higher doses. Disulfiram should not be administered to anyone who has not abstained from alcohol for at least 48 hours. It should also be avoided in PWH with a history of cardiovascular disease (e.g., myocardial infarction), pregnant women, and persons with end-stage liver disease. Caution should be used in PWH with a history of psychosis due to disulfiram's inhibition of dopamine dehydroxylase; the increase in dopamine concentrations may exacerbate psychotic symptoms. In PWH, disulfiram is often avoided due to a potential interaction with ART. However, a 2014 study indicated that there were no significant changes in adverse symptoms compared to baseline with coadministration of disulfiram and common antiretroviral medications (ARVs; i.e., ritonavir). Disulfiram should still be considered with close monitoring in some PWH to deter alcohol use (McCance-Katz et al., 2014).

- **Anticonvulsants** are becoming commonly used off-label in treatment of AUD. Among these are gabapentin, topiramate, carbamazepine, and divalproex; all have demonstrated efficacy in reducing drinking and/or relapse in placebo-controlled trials. These medications have different mechanisms of action, though it is likely that they work for AUD by antagonizing glutamate receptors and potentiating GABA receptors (Miller et al., 2019). Due to cognitive side effects, slow titration of topiramate is recommended. Gabapentin has demonstrated efficacy in reducing cravings, amount consumed, and alcohol withdrawal symptoms at 900 to 1,800 mg/day in divided doses (Anton et al., 2020).

OPIOIDS

Use of opioid-based drugs (e.g., heroin, morphine, oxycodone, fentanyl), particularly injection drug use, has long been associated with HIV infection and transmission. Opioids act on mu receptors and activate the reward system in the central nervous system, resulting in euphoria and dependence. The risk of developing an opioid use disorder (OUD) has been shown to be even higher in those who also have psychiatric illness. Depression in injection drug users has been linked to increased rates of sharing of needles and other paraphernalia, resulting in a greater risk for HIV infection. It is therefore crucial to treat both the psychiatric disorders and the behavioral risk factors in injection drug use (Ruiz & Strain, 2007).

THE US OPIOID EPIDEMIC AND HIV

In recent years, opioid addiction has emerged as one of America's most pressing public health concerns, prompting greater consideration of how this growing epidemic could be impacting the transmission and treatment of HIV and other bloodborne infections, such as HCV. In 2016, 2.1 million Americans were estimated to have an OUD, with nearly 12 million Americans estimated to have misused opioids during the preceding year (SAMHSA, 2016). Apart from the heightened morbidity and mortality associated with opioid overdose, this epidemic also places affected individuals at additional risk of contracting and transmitting infectious diseases during the course of their addiction. Research shows that people who misuse and abuse opioids commonly move from oral use to inhalation to injection use as they build tolerance to the drug's effects and require more potent concentrations to achieve their desired level of intoxication (Peters et al., 2016). Moreover, it is estimated that 10% to 20% of people who misuse prescription opioids move on to inject either opioids or heroin (Van Handel et al., 2016). Given the long-standing association between injection drug use and transmission of HIV and HCV via needle sharing, public health providers must remain vigilant in hopes of identifying co-occurring trends in these epidemics. One such instance was documented in 2015, in Scott County, Indiana, where opioid use was implicated in an HIV outbreak that resulted in 181 individuals being diagnosed with HIV, most of whom were coinfected with HCV (Van Handel et al., 2016). As individuals engaged in escalating drug use, they became more susceptible to transmission of HIV and HCV by way of high-risk sexual activity and injection drug use behaviors. This incident was integral in prompting the CDC to identify 220 jurisdictions that might be equally vulnerable to similar co-occurring outbreaks due to the preponderance of opioid addiction and high-risk needle sharing, as well as limited access to care in those geographic areas (Van Handel et al., 2016). Targeted interventions such as these must be undertaken not only in hopes of preventing and rapidly identifying subsequent epidemics, but also as a means of ensuring that individuals with comorbid opioid dependence and HIV have adequate access to both medication-assisted treatment (MAT) for OUD and ART. In 2016, a systematic review and meta-analysis of 4,685 articles and 32 studies revealed that MAT for OUD was associated with a 69% increase in recruitment into ART, a 54% increase in ART coverage, a twofold increase in ART adherence, a 23% decrease in the odds of attrition, and a 45% increase in odds of viral suppression (Low et al., 2016). Taken together, these striking statistics illustrate the importance of substance abuse recovery in both preventing the spread of HIV and improving the overall quality of life and treatment for PWH with OUD. It is imperative that individuals with opioid dependence are screened early for HIV/HCV and then promptly referred for MAT to reduce morbidity and mortality and mitigate the impact of these epidemics across the general population.

INTOXICATION/WITHDRAWAL

Acute intoxication with opioids is characterized by euphoria, slurred speech, sedation, and analgesia. Physical signs include miosis, constipation, respiratory depression, and sedation. Overdoses result in respiratory arrest, cardiovascular compromise, coma, and death. Naloxone, a short-acting opioid antagonist, at doses of 0.5 to 2 mg given intramuscularly or intravenously, is used in all cases of suspected opioid overdose. Multiple doses may be required in the presence of fentanyl. In severe cases, care in an intensive care unit is required.

Opioid withdrawal is extremely uncomfortable and a reason for continued use in many individuals. Symptoms usually begin 8 to 12 hours after the last dose. Early symptoms include yawning, sweating, rhinorrhea, lacrimation, and irritability. More severe symptoms such as gastrointestinal disturbance (abdominal cramps, diarrhea, vomiting), insomnia, tachycardia, and hypertension may occur 24 to 36 hours after the last dose. People on methadone (long half-life) may have a more protracted withdrawal lasting 2 to 4 weeks. This initial withdrawal phase is often followed by symptoms lasting for weeks or months. This "protracted abstinence syndrome" includes depressed mood, low energy, poor sleep, and anhedonia. Animal studies have implicated serotonin dysfunction in the development of this syndrome, which may respond to selective serotonin reuptake inhibitors (SSRIs; Goeldner et al., 2011).

Initial treatment of opioid dependence consists of a period of withdrawal management, which can be assisted by use of opioid agonists (e.g., methadone, buprenorphine) and/or supportive care for specific symptoms. Supportive care regimens may include acetaminophen for muscle aches, α2-adrenergic agonists (clonidine, guanfacine, lofexidine) for autonomic symptoms, ondansetron for nausea, dicyclomine for abdominal cramps, and lorazepam for anxiety/insomnia. Rapid and ultra-rapid withdrawal protocols use an opioid antagonist to precipitate withdrawal; then, symptoms are managed with supportive treatments (e.g., sedation procedures, anesthesia in ultra-rapid protocol, clonidine). Many PWH cannot tolerate withdrawal symptoms and opioid-replacement therapy with methadone or buprenorphine is initiated, then tapered.

PHARMACOTHERAPY FOR MAINTENANCE OF OUD

METHADONE

Developed in the 1960s, methadone is a mu-receptor agonist as well as a weak NMDA receptor antagonist, and it has proved to be a very effective treatment for opiate addiction. The use of methadone has been shown to decrease the use of intravenous opioid drugs and the spread of communicable diseases such as HIV, hepatitis B virus, and HCV by modifying behaviors such as intravenous drug use (Lollis et al., 2000). Methadone treatment for opioid dependence is provided in specialized opioid treatment programs that require federal licensing and certification. In addition to supplying methadone to its patients, these clinics also provide counseling, drug testing, and vocational training/assistance. It is illegal for noncertified healthcare entities to provide methadone maintenance treatment. Doses are carefully titrated to the needs of the individual (generally 60–100 mg/day). Studies have shown that methadone doses in the range of 20 to 40 mg/day are effective in suppressing symptoms of withdrawal, but they may not be effective in reducing or stopping symptoms of craving (Strain et al., 1993a, 1993b).

Unfortunately, there are many issues with the use of methadone in HIV-positive individuals because this medication has many side effects and drug–drug interactions. Methadone prolongs QT/QTc intervals; therefore, close monitoring is required in persons who are taking other QT interval-prolonging drugs. ARVs known to significantly interfere with methadone serum levels include lopinavir/ritonavir, efavirenz, and nevirapine. Other medications that have been shown to have drug–drug interactions with methadone include the anticonvulsants carbamazepine and phenytoin as well as some antibiotics, such as rifampin. In general, use of these medications should be avoided in persons who are being treated or plan to be treated with methadone. If such medication combinations are required, then methadone doses should be titrated upward to avoid withdrawal symptoms and continue maximized treatment. Methadone has been shown to be safe for use during pregnancy (especially relative to opioid use or withdrawal) and with breastfeeding. Some newborns may experience neonatal abstinence syndrome, which consists of blotchy skin coloring (mottling), diarrhea, high-pitched crying, excessive sucking, fever, hyperactive reflexes, increased muscle tone, irritability, poor feeding, and, in rare cases, seizures.

BUPRENORPHINE (SUBUTEX) AND BUPRENORPHINE PLUS NALOXONE (SUBOXONE)

Buprenorphine is a partial agonist to the mu-opioid receptor and an antagonist at the kappa-opioid receptor. When PWH are not taking opioids, buprenorphine acts as an agonist, whereas it acts as an antagonist when individuals attempt to take opioids. Naloxone is added to reduce the abuse potential of the drug. These medications require special certification for prescription, but they can be prescribed in an office setting. Initial doses are low (regardless of the person's wish to start at a higher dose) to avoid potential side effects—2 or 4 mg is standard, and ideally individuals should be in some form of opioid withdrawal. If well tolerated and there are still signs of withdrawal, this dosage can be repeated 1 or 2 hours later. Titration to the target dose (generally 8–16 mg/day, although up to 24 mg/day can be used) is done quickly to minimize patient dropout and withdrawal symptoms. If a person requires doses greater than 24 mg/day, issues of diversion or misuse must be considered. Suboxone has ceiling effects: unlike other opioid treatment drugs, it plateaus at a certain dose (32 mg/day), and a higher dose has no therapeutic benefit. Overdose can still occur, resulting in respiratory distress that may require airway management. Other potential side effects include central nervous system depression and hepatitis. Those with a history of traumatic brain injury should be monitored for increased intracranial pressure because all potent opioids may elevate cerebrospinal fluid pressure. Buprenorphine is metabolized by CYP450 3A4 enzyme, and there are several clinically significant drug–drug interactions. Those taking CYP450 3A4 inhibitors such as nefazodone, fluvoxamine, fluoxetine, ketoconazole, itraconazole, erythromycin, clarithromycin, grapefruit juice, and most protease inhibitors (PIs, especially ritonavir) should take reduced doses of buprenorphine.

NALTREXONE

As a mu-opioid receptor antagonist, naltrexone blocks the reinforcing effects of opioids. Oral and intramuscular formulations of naltrexone are effective for highly motivated individuals who have completed withdrawal and can maintain abstinence from opioids. Oral naltrexone should be initiated after 5 to 7 days of abstinence from short-acting opioids and 7 to 10 days for long-acting opioids to avoid precipitating withdrawal. It can be started at 25 mg and increased to 50 mg daily, or 350 mg weekly in three divided doses (100, 100, and 150 mg). While oral naltrexone is not effective for many people, the intramuscular formulation can improve abstinence and retention in treatment. It can be given at 380 mg every 4 weeks. See the earlier section on alcohol for more details on naltrexone.

COCAINE/CRACK

In addition to the increased incidence of risk behaviors in cocaine abusers, recent studies have shown that cocaine abuse may have broad-ranging effects on human immunity. Regarding HIV infection, in vitro studies have shown that cocaine enhances infection of stimulated lymphocytes. Moreover, cohort studies in the pre- and post-highly active ART (HAART) era have linked stimulant abuse with increased HIV pathogenesis (Baum et al., 2009). It is therefore crucial to treat PWH with cocaine dependence.

Cocaine blocks dopamine reuptake at the presynaptic site, thus increasing levels of dopamine at the nucleus accumbens, resulting in its addictive properties. Cocaine effects depend on the mode of use, with smoked (crack) and intravenous administration having the quickest effects (seconds to 30 minutes; peak, 15–30 minutes) and intranasal administration having slightly more delayed effects (5–90 minutes; peak, 30 minutes). Mild to moderate intoxication produces sympathomimetic symptoms—generally increased heart rate and blood pressure, decreased appetite, insomnia, euphoria, hyperalertness, and irritability. With severe intoxication, there is dilation of the pupils, and severe hypertension, hyperthermia, cardiac arrhythmias/myocardial infarction, stroke, seizures, coma, and death may occur. At any level of intoxication, there may also be psychiatric symptoms—auditory/visual/tactile hallucinations, delusions, paranoia, and aggression/violence. For individuals with severe cocaine intoxication (i.e., malignant hypertension, hyperthermia, and seizure), the goal is to stabilize vital signs and eliminate seizure activity. Phentolamine, cooling, and other supportive measures should be used for hypertensive crisis and hyperthermia; benzodiazepines should be given to prevent seizures and agitation. Antipsychotics may be useful for severe agitation/aggression/psychosis but should be avoided in persons with seizures because neuroleptics may further decrease the seizure threshold.

Research into medications for treating cocaine addiction has failed to show conclusive evidence of effectiveness, but efforts are ongoing. Recent research has focused on creating a cocaine vaccine that uses a modified cold virus attached to cocaine-like molecules to trigger the body to produce cocaine antibodies. Disulfiram has been studied as a potential treatment due to its inhibition of dopamine-β-hydroxylase, which prevents the conversion of dopamine to norepinephrine, thus increasing dopamine levels. However, data have been inconsistent regarding its efficacy. Doxazosin, an α1-adrenergic receptor antagonist, has shown some promise in decreasing cocaine use at doses of 8 mg/day in a small, clinically controlled trial (Shorter et al., 2013). Other promising agents include modafinil, topiramate, and desipramine, which may decrease cocaine craving.

METHAMPHETAMINE

Unlike many of the other drugs of abuse, which tend to predominate in urban areas, methamphetamine use has grown exponentially in both rural and urban areas during the past few decades. It is an extremely addictive drug that heightens sexual arousal with reduced inhibition and judgment, placing its users at risk of contracting sexually transmitted diseases such as HIV. It can be smoked, eaten, snorted, injected, or rectally inserted. It is a relatively inexpensive drug with rapid onset and a long-lasting high (half-life of 11–12 hours). Use increases the release of newly synthesized dopamine, norepinephrine, and serotonin. It is also an indirect catecholamine and serotonin (5-HT) agonist. Like cocaine, methamphetamine can deplete dopamine stores and lead to significant symptoms of depression and, in some cases, suicide. Other symptoms that may be experienced include psychosis (may last weeks to months), aggression, thought disorders, and gum disease with long-term use. Acute intoxication with methamphetamine is treated like cocaine intoxication with phentolamine, cooling, and other supportive measure for hypertensive crisis and hyperthermia; benzodiazepines are used to prevent seizures and agitation. Antipsychotics may also be required to control severe aggression/agitation. Addiction is more difficult to treat because there are no currently FDA-approved medications. Most controlled clinical trials have not demonstrated efficacy. A small controlled clinical trial for mirtazapine showed some promise in reducing methamphetamine use. Medications that have not shown efficacy include topiramate, SSRIs, serotonin and norepinephrine reuptake inhibitors (SNRIs), and ondansetron (Miller et al., 2019). Unlike other drugs of its kind, methamphetamine may induce sensitization, which results in an enhanced response to the drug because of prior exposure and thus a higher likelihood of overdosing.

ECSTASY OR "MOLLY" (MDMA)

Dubbed the "intimacy drug," Ecstasy use has been shown to produce profound feelings of closeness, which may lead to high-risk sexual behavior and HIV exposure. Some studies have shown that those using Ecstasy may perceive less danger of contracting HIV and other sexually transmitted diseases compared to nonusers (Theall et al., 2006). It is therefore critical that those with HIV and those at higher risk of contracting HIV be educated about the dangers of Ecstasy use in addition to the other known health issues that may result from its use. Currently, there is no FDA-approved medication for treatment of Ecstasy abuse, and acute management is geared toward treating life-threatening conditions such as serotonin syndrome and hyperthermia that are commonly seen in rave parties.

SPECIAL CONSIDERATIONS IN HIV POPULATIONS

Interactions between substances of abuse and ARVs have been reported. The toxicity of amphetamines, MDMA, meperidine, and GHB is dangerously increased by ritonavir. Barbiturates induce the cytochrome systems responsible for the metabolism of PIs, nonnucleoside reverse transcriptase inhibitors (NNRTIs), maraviroc, elvitegravir, and dolutegravir, significantly decreasing their effectiveness. Oral midazolam and triazolam are contraindicated with PIs, NNRTIs, and efavirenz. The toxicity of ketamine and phencyclidine (PCP) is dangerously increased by PIs and etravirine.

All the agents listed for use in withdrawal management and maintenance of sobriety have utility in the HIV population, but there are special considerations:

- Buprenorphine administration is office-based but requires special training and certification. Also, clinically significant interactions occur with ARVs, including atazanavir, darunavir, and ritonavir (increased buprenorphine activity and sedation, especially with atazanavir) and etravirine, nevirapine, and tipranavir (decreased buprenorphine activity, with tipranavir levels also significantly decreased). Fluconazole can increase the activity of buprenorphine, whereas phenobarbital, phenytoin, rifabutin, and rifampin decrease the effective amounts, sometimes causing withdrawal symptoms.

- Bupropion (used for nicotine use disorder) decreases the seizure threshold, particularly in individuals with weight loss or electrolyte instability.

- Disulfiram (Antabuse) has a high risk of hepatotoxicity and may interact with tipranavir/ritonavir capsules (they contain alcohol).

- Methadone maintenance cannot be done outside a registered clinic, and this agent has several clinically significant adverse interactions with ARVs. Blood levels of abacavir are decreased. Blood levels of zidovudine are increased. Abacavir increases blood levels of methadone and dose adjustment may be required to avoid sedation. Efavirenz, nevirapine, darunavir, lopinavir, ritonavir (even in boosting doses), and tipranavir all decrease methadone availability and may precipitate withdrawal symptoms. Drug interactions with other medications frequently used in the HIV population are also reported: carbamazepine, phenobarbital, phenytoin, and rifampin sharply decrease methadone levels, and fluconazole significantly increases methadone blood levels.

- Naltrexone cannot be used in individuals requiring narcotic pain control but does not seem to interact with ARVs.

SUBSTANCE USE AND HIV IN THE CORONAVIRUS (COVID-19) PANDEMIC

The COVID-19 pandemic has placed tremendous strain on the healthcare system, creating unique challenges for individuals with SUD. Currently there are limited data on the intersection between the COVID-19 pandemic, SUD, and HIV/AIDS. However, the pandemic involves social isolation, anxiety, stress, and boredom, all of which can increase risk for substance use. Many individuals with SUD are homeless, incarcerated, or actively seeking drugs, putting them at greater risk for contracting or transmitting COVID-19. As previously mentioned, substance use can increase exposure to HIV, which may be more likely with greater difficulty accessing community harm-reduction resources like syringe services programs that provide sterile injection equipment. In addition, persons with SUD and comorbid medical conditions may be more likely to develop severe illness with COVID-19 infection. The virus's attack on the lungs could be a serious threat for PWH who smoke and vape tobacco and marijuana. Individuals with OUD may be vulnerable to hypoxemia with concurrent opioid use and respiratory infections. Methamphetamine can cause lung damage from constriction of blood vessels and pulmonary hypertension. Preexisting respiratory conditions such as chronic obstructive pulmonary disease may increase mortality from the viral illness. Data from the Chinese Center for Disease Control and Prevention showed that the fatality rate for COVID-19 was 6.3% for those with chronic respiratory disease compared to a rate of 2.3% overall (Wu & McGoogan, 2020). PWH may also be at risk of developing severe disease based on their age, comorbid medical conditions, and immune status. Thus, compliance with ART and medical follow-up should be discussed at each visit. PWH should be provided education on these risks with practical recommendations to reduce or stop substance use. Those with ongoing substance use should be encouraged to practice harm-reduction behaviors such as using protective equipment (e.g., masks) when seeking drugs, practicing physical distancing when using, and using sterile needles when injecting. Although research is ongoing regarding the impact of COVID-19 on various populations, PWH with respiratory diseases may experience discomfort with breathing while wearing a mask. Another consideration is a history of trauma in this population, which means that mask wearing—depending on the trauma—may elicit traumatic memories and feelings of suffocation and helplessness. Providers attuned to these issues may guide the individual in finding solutions to practice safe behaviors.

Many residential/inpatient treatment centers have reduced the number of available beds to follow physical distancing guidelines. People who need residential treatment may have to be managed on an outpatient basis with close follow-up until space becomes available. Telehealth services have expanded in response to the pandemic, allowing continuation of care for those who need or want to maintain physical distancing. Collaboration between individuals and providers is key to determining if telehealth or in-person treatment is best. Careful balancing of risk of exposure to COVID-19 and benefits of in-person visits should be discussed with each person. PWH with ongoing substance use may require frequent in-person visits for comprehensive evaluation and physical exam, but stable PWH may be appropriate for telehealth management. For example, PWH with OUD on opioid-replacement therapy may need to continue in-person visits for urine toxicology screens and physical assessment. For those who have had a long period of stability, a combination of telehealth and in-person care may be appropriate (e.g., in-person visit with urine toxicology screen once every 3 months). Many clinics have adopted a hybrid telehealth/in-person model to provide care for different SUD populations. Whenever possible and appropriate, telehealth should be utilized to decrease exposure to COVID-19. Providers are encouraged to check the CDC, SAMHSA, NIDA, and other trusted organizations for updates on recommendations and research as the COVID-19 pandemic evolves.

SUMMARY

Substance use or misuse is common in the HIV population and requires early and aggressive diagnosis and treatment, both to minimize further spread of the disease through ungoverned risk behaviors and to maximize the ability of the individual to fully participate in HIV treatment. Successful management will decrease morbidity and mortality from both conditions. Adequate treatment of substance use can improve adherence to HIV regimens (clinic visits and ART) to levels comparable to those seen in nonaddicted HIV populations. These principles apply even more stringently in those with "triple diagnosis"—substance abuse, mental illness, and HIV. As with any treatment process, success involves establishing a collaborative alliance—a therapeutic relationship between treatment staff and the individual. This sets the stage for honest communication, mutual respect of boundaries, and continued participation in treatment (on both sides) despite temporary setbacks and failures. Integrated treatment of substance abuse and HIV (or substance abuse, HIV, and mental illness in the case of triple diagnosis) offers distinct advantages for these complex cases with multiple barriers to participation. Factors in a decision to start ART in individuals with active substance abuse are obviously complex, but substance use alone should not be an absolute contraindication to ART.

RECOMMENDED READING

Miller SC, Fiellin DA, Rosenthal RN, et al. *ASAM principles of addiction medicine*. Philadelphia: Wolters Kluwer; 2019.

Ruiz P, Strain EC. Alcohol abstinence pharmacotherapy treatment; Amphetamines and other stimulants; Buprenorphine treatment; Cocaine and crack; Methadone maintenance treatment; and Naltrexone and other pharmacotherapies for opioid dependence. In: *The substance abuse handbook*. Philadelphia: Lippincott Williams & Wilkins; 2014.

REFERENCES

American Psychiatric Association. *Diagnostic and statistical manual of mental disorders*. 5th ed. Washington, DC: APA Press; 2013.

Anton RF, Latham P, Voronin K, et al. Efficacy of gabapentin for the treatment of alcohol use disorder in patients with alcohol withdrawal symptoms: a randomized clinical trial. JAMA Intern Med. 2020;180(5):728–736.

Bhaskaran K, Hamouda O, Sannes M, et al. Changes in the risk of death after HIV seroconversion compared with mortality in the general population. JAMA. 2008;300(1):51–59.

Baum MK, Rafie C, Lai S, et al. Crack-cocaine use accelerates HIV disease progression in a cohort of HIV-positive drug users. J AIDS. 2009;50(1):93–99.

Branson BM, Handsfield HH, Lampe MA, et al. Revised recommendations for HIV testing of adults, adolescents, and pregnant women in health-care settings. MMWR Recomm Rep. 2006;55(RR-14):1–17.

Carroll K, Rounsaville B, Nich C, et al. One-year follow-up of psycho-therapy and pharmacotherapy for cocaine dependence: delayed emergence of psychotherapy effects. Arch Gen Psychiatry. 1994;51:989–997.

Campos-Outcalt D. 8 USPSTF recommendations FPs need to know about. J Fam Pract. 2016;65:338–342.

Campral (Acamprosate calcium) delayed release tablets [product information]. St. Louis, MO: Forest Pharmaceuticals; 2004.

Centers for Disease Control and Prevention. Incorporating HIV prevention into the medical care of persons living with HIV. Recommendations of CDC, the Health Resources and Services Administration, the National Institutes of Health, and the HIV Medicine Association of the Infectious Diseases Society of America. MMWR Recomm Rep. 2003;52(RR-12):1–24.

Centers for Disease Control and Prevention. *HIV Surveillance Report, 2018 (Updated)*; vol. 31. May 2020. http://www.cdc.gov/hiv/library/reports/hiv-surveillance.html

Chen CC, Lu R-B, Chen Y-C, et al. Interaction between the functional polymorphisms of the alcohol metabolism genes in protection against alcoholism. Am J Hum Genet. 1999;65:795–807.

Cofrancesco J Jr, Scherzer R, Tien PC, et al. Illicit drug use and HIV treatment outcomes in a US cohort. AIDS. 2008;22:237–245.

Goeldner C, Lutz PE, Darcq E, et al. Impaired emotional-like behavior and serotonergic function during protracted abstinence from chronic morphine. Biol Psychiatry. 2011;69(3):236–244.

Hillfors DD, Iritani BJ, Miller WC, et al. Sexual and drug behavior patterns and HIV and STD racial disparities: the need for new directions. Am J Public Health. 2007;97(1):125–132.

Lollis CM, Strothers HS, Chitwood DD, et al. Sex, drugs and HIV: does methadone maintenance reduce drug use and risky sexual behavior? J Behav Med. 2000;23(;6):545–557.

Low AJ, Mburu G, Welton NJ, et al. Impact of opioid substitution therapy on antiretroviral therapy outcomes: a systematic review and meta-analysis. Clin Infect Dis. 2016;63(8):1094–1104.

McCance-Katz EF, Gruber VA, Beatty G, et al. Interaction of disulfiram with antiretroviral medications: efavirenz increases while atazanavir decreases disulfiram effect on enzymes of alcohol metabolism. Am J Addict. 2014;23(2):137–144.

McLellan AT, Lewis DC, O'Brien CP, et al. Drug dependence, a chronic medical illness: implications for treatment, insurance, and outcomes evaluation. JAMA. 2000;284:1689–1695.

Miller SC, Fiellin DA, Rosenthal RN, et al. *The ASAM principles of addiction medicine*. Philadelphia: Wolters Kluwer; 2019.

Millett GA, Flores SA, Bakeman R. Explaining disparities in HIV infection among Black and White men who have sex with men: a meta-analysis of HIV risk behaviors. AIDS. 2007;21(15):2083–2091.

Minozzi S, Amato L, Vecchi S, et al. Anticonvulsants for alcohol withdrawal. Cochrane Database Syst Rev. 2010;(3):CD005064.

Moore RM, Gebo KA, Lucas GM, et al. Rate of co-morbidities not related to HIV infection or AIDS among HIV-positive patients by CD4 count and HAART use status. Clin Infect Dis. 2008;47(8):1102–1104.

National Institute on Alcohol Abuse and Alcoholism. *Helping patients who drink too much: a clinician's guide*. Washington, DC: Author, 2007. www.niaaa.nih.gov/guide

National Institute on Drug Abuse. *Principles of drug addiction treatment: a research-based guide*. 3rd ed. Rockville, MD: NIDA (NIH Publication No. 12–4180); 1999:2–5.

Peters P, Pontones P, Hoover KW, et al. HIV infection linked to injection use of oxymorphone in Indiana, 2014–2015. N Engl J Med. 2016;375:229–239.

Ruiz P, Strain EC. Psychiatric complications of HIV-1 infection and drug abuse. In: *The substance abuse handbook*. Philadelphia: Lippincott Williams & Wilkins; 2014.

Shorter D, Lindsay JA, Kosten TR. The alpha-1 adrenergic antagonist doxazosin for treatment of cocaine dependence: a pilot study. Drug Alcohol Depend. 2013;131(1-2):66–70.

Stern TA, Freudenreich O, Smith FA, et al. *Massachusetts General Hospital handbook of general hospital psychiatry*. Philadelphia: Elsevier; 2018.

Strain EC, Stitzer ML, Lisbon IA, et al. Dose–response effects of methadone in the treatment of opioid dependence. Ann Intern Med. 1993a;119:23–27.

Strain EC, Stitzer ML, Lisbon IA, et al. Methadone dose and treatment outcome. Drug Alcohol Depend. 1993b;33:105–117.

Sullivan LE, Goulet JL, Justice AC, et al. Alcohol consumption and depressive symptoms over time: a longitudinal study of patients with and without HIV infection. Drug Alcohol Depend. 2011;117:158–163.

Theall KP, Elifson KW, Sterk CE. Sex, touch, and HIV risk among Ecstasy users. AIDS Behav. 2006;10(2):169–178.

Van Handel M, Rose CE, Hallisey EJ, et al. County-level vulnerability assessment for rapid dissemination of HIV or HCV infections among persons who inject drugs, United States. J AIDS. 2016;73(3):323–331.

West R. Models of addiction. European Moderating Centre for Drugs and Drug Addiction. 2013. Models of addiction | www.emcdda.europa.eu

Woody GE, McLellan AT, Luborsky L, et al. Psychotherapy in community methadone programs: a validation study. Am J Psychiatry. 1995;152(9):1302–1308.

Wu Z, McGoogan JM. Characteristics of and important lessons from the coronavirus disease 2019 (COVID-19) outbreak in China: summary of a report of 72 314 cases from the Chinese Center for Disease Control and Prevention. JAMA. 2020;323(13):1239–1242.

27.

CARING FOR OLDER PEOPLE WITH HIV

Aroonsiri Sangarlangkarn Howell, John D. Zeuli, and Anchalee Avihingsanon

LEARNING OBJECTIVE

- Describe the differences in HIV care and management for persons with HIV (PWH) who are 50 years or older compared to their younger counterparts

WHAT'S NEW?

- Although the relationship between COVID-19 and HIV remains to be fully investigated, it is likely that social distancing efforts will result in increased psychosocial burden and limited access to care among older PWH.

- A practical guide on how to perform comprehensive geriatric assessment (CGA) is included.

KEY POINTS

- Each older PWH is a unique and complex individual, and disease-centric guidelines should not be applied the same way in every patient.

- Management of diseases in older PWH should be individualized based on aging phenotypes, interactions with multimorbidity, and patient preferences.

- The Veterans Aging Cohort Study (VACS) index may be used to identify aging phenotypes and can provide prognostic information to help prioritize interventions and guide shared decision-making with PWH and caregivers.

INTRODUCTION

There are increasing proportions of older PWH. It is estimated that at year-end 2018, persons aged 50 to 54 years made up the largest percentage of PWH (15%). From 2011 to 2015, the largest increase in rates of PWH was among persons aged 65 years and older (57%, from 94.2 in 2011 to 148.0 in 2015) (Centers for Disease Control and Prevention [CDC], 2020). Part of this group consisted of individuals who have aged with chronic HIV infection, but a large proportion also resulted from new HIV diagnosis, with 16.6% of all new HIV transmissions in 2016 diagnosed in PWH aged 50 years or older (CDC, 2020).

Although many of the recommendations on the management of HIV infection are not age-specific, PWH over 50 years old differ from their younger counterparts in many aspects, including diagnostic considerations, immune response to antiretroviral therapy (ART), and multimorbidity. In this chapter, we outline these differences, offer a strategy on how to care for this unique population, provide a practical guide on how to perform CGA, and describe special considerations for problem-based management of PWH over 50 years old.

DIFFERENCES IN OLDER PWH COMPARED TO YOUNGER PWH

The most common mode of HIV transmission among adults 50 years and older is through sexual contact. Among men, male-to-male sexual contact is the most common transmission risk, while heterosexual contact is the most common among women (CDC, 2018). This may be due to a false sense of security among older adults who view sexually transmitted illness as a condition of the young and may forgo safe sex practices based on this perception (Pilowsky & Wu, 2015). They may also forgo barrier contraceptives when unwanted pregnancy is no longer a concern. Even though sexual exposure is the most common mode of HIV transmission among PWH 50 years and older, prior research has found that healthcare professionals often underestimate the level of sexual activity among older adults and their risk of exposure to sexually transmitted diseases (Lindau et al., 2007; Pilowsky & Wu, 2015).

Moreover, many symptoms of early HIV transmission mimic those of old age and may be difficult for clinicians to tease apart. Symptoms of acute HIV transmission such as headache, loss of energy, loss of appetite, flu-like symptoms, or weight loss are common in older adults and can be caused by a myriad of conditions associated with old age, such as malignancy or frailty.

With inaccurate perception of HIV exposure risk and symptom mimicry, underdiagnoses and late diagnoses of HIV transmission are common among older adults (Dai et al., 2015; Pilowsky & Wu, 2015). Late diagnosis is associated with delayed treatment, impaired response to ART, increased morbidity and mortality, lost opportunity to prevent onward transmission, and increased cost of healthcare (British HIV Association, 2015). As a result, clinicians must maintain a high suspicion and routinely screen older adults for HIV, regardless of risk perception. Although CDC guidelines recommend routine screening up to the age of 64 years old (CDC, 2020), the rationale or research evidence for this age cutoff was not included, and we recommend routine screening for all older adults as risk perception may be inaccurate in this population.

Despite successful viral suppression with ART, older adults have less robust immunologic recovery compared to their younger counterparts, with an associated increase in mortality (Mpondo et al., 2016; Semeere et al., 2014; Vinikoor et al., 2014). Consequently, early HIV diagnosis and treatment is of great importance.

MULTIMORBIDITY

Older PWH are at increased risk of multimorbidity (Guaraldi et al., 2014), defined as the development of multiple chronic conditions that do not simply coexist but interact to worsen health outcomes. Compared to their uninfected peers, older PWH have higher burdens of cardiovascular, metabolic, pulmonary, renal, bone, and malignant diseases (Schouten et al., 2014). Multimorbidity is likely contributed to by both lifestyle risk factors and chronic HIV infection, with a longer duration of severe immunodeficiency (CD4 counts <200 cells/mL), correlating with a higher comorbidity burden (Schouten et al., 2014).

Multimorbidity has important ramifications on health outcomes. It is associated with self-reported poor health, declines in self-rated health status, and increased mortality (adjusted odds ratio 11.87; 95% confidence interval, 5.72–24.62) (Koroukian et al., 2015). With increasing disease burden, PWH with multimorbidity are also at risk of fragmentation in care due to involvement of multiple clinicians in multiple settings. Guidelines for one disease may clash with another, as most are disease-centric recommendations based on the ideal patient without multimorbidity (Tinetti et al., 2012). Treatments for one disease may inadvertently worsen other conditions, and increased treatment burden stemming from efforts to adhere to all relevant disease-centric guidelines without prioritization may not bring improvement in mortality or quality of life.

MANAGEMENT STRATEGY FOR THE CARE OF OLDER PWH

Each HIV-positive older adult is a unique and complex individual. Older PWH cannot be described fully by one-dimensional classifications such as chronological age or single disease entities. Aging occurs at different rates in different individuals, and within the same individual in different organs (Emory University, 2015), resulting in different aging phenotypes that cannot be predicted by chronological age alone. Additionally, viewing PWH by a single disease entity ignores the importance of multimorbidity and the often-multifactorial nature of their diseases. Most importantly, different PWH have different goals and preferences. Consequently, applying disease-centric guidelines uniformly to every patient without considering aging phenotypes, multimorbidity, or individual preference ignores the unique care needs of each patient and likely will not lead to desirable patient-centered outcomes.

Understanding that not all PWH aged 50 years and older should be approached the same way, clinicians may utilize the VACS index (Justice et al., 2013) to distinguish between those who are aging well and those who may appear phenotypically older than their chronological age. The VACS index has been shown to correlate with functional status (John et al., 2014), provide insight to clinician assessment of severity of illness (Justice et al., 2013), and predict cause-specific (Justice et al., 2012) as well as all-cause (Justice et al., 2013) mortality. Based on prognosis predicted by the VACS index, clinicians can elicit patient preferences, identify diseases and risk factors that affect these goals, calculate the likely effects and lag time to benefit (Lee et al., 2013) of various disease-centric guidelines on these goals, and use this information to prioritize interventions and guide shared decision-making with patients and caregivers.

COMPREHENSIVE GERIATRIC ASSESSMENT

CGA is defined as a multidisciplinary diagnostic and treatment process that evaluates medical, psychosocial, and functional deficits in order to develop a coordinated intervention/plan to maximize overall health with aging (Stuck et al., 1993). CGA is based on the idea that a systematic evaluation of an older patient may lead to early detection of geriatric problems, help prevent complications, and aid the formation of comprehensive treatment plans (Bellera et al., 2012).

There is no peer-reviewed literature to demonstrate the efficacy of CGA in older PWH, although due to increased risks of geriatric syndromes in older PWH, many studies advocate for CGA in this population. In the uninfected, CGA in the home may improve functional status, prevent institutionalization, and reduce mortality (Huss et al., 2012). CGA in the hospital, especially in dedicated units, may improve survival (Ellis et al., 2017). However, CGA in outpatient settings has not been found to consistently show benefits (Stuck et al., 1993), possibly due to variability in adherence to CGA recommendations. CGA as part of inpatient geriatric consultation (except for specific conditions such as hip fracture) has shown little benefit (Ellis et al., 2017; Stuck et al., 1993). Studies have shown that more complex CGA programs that address adherence or target patients at higher risk of admission may improve outcomes such as physical functioning, social functioning, pain, mental/physical/emotional health, and overall well-being (Reuben et al., 1999).

PERFORMING CGA

Consider avoiding assessing all domains of CGA in a single visit—this could be overwhelming and tiring for elderly patients and their family members. It may make sense to prioritize domains that are most likely to be abnormal or most urgent (i.e., likely to cause complications or catastrophic outcomes). Once the most urgent domains have been managed, patients can be brought back to complete the remaining non-urgent domains at subsequent visits. Various team members may be delegated certain domains of the CGA based on their expertise or availability. For example, it may make sense for a pharmacist to assess patients for polypharmacy instead of a physician.

There is no consensus on selection criteria for patients who may benefit from CGA However, prior programs have used criteria such as age, medical comorbidities/complexity, specific geriatric syndromes such as falls/dementia, previous or predicted high utilization rates, or at times of transition, such as from hospital to home or from home to nursing home.

There is no consensus on what domains should be included in CGA and what tools are appropriate for each domain. However, most programs include some or all of the following domains. Except when noted, corresponding interventions are described in more details in the European AIDS Clinical Society guideline, accessible through website or mobile app at https://www.eacsociety.org/guidelines/eacs-guidelines/eacs-guidelines.html (EACS, 2020).

FUNCTION

Asking older PWH about activities of daily living (ADLs) and instrumental activities of daily living (IADLs) can readily identify essential deficits that may guide interventions. To assess function, providers may ask about ADLs/IADLs and determine who does them (the patient or others). ADLs consist of bathing, dressing, grooming, toileting, transferring, and eating. IADLs consist of cooking, shopping, managing medications, using the phone, doing housework, doing laundry, driving or using public transportation, and managing finances (Katz et al., 1963).

MOBILITY/FALLS

For subjective measures, PWH may be asked if they had a fall in the past 12 months, defined as unexpectedly dropping to the floor or ground from a standing, walking, or bending position (Erlandson et al., 2012, 2016; Ruiz et al., 2013, 2016). For objective measures, providers may use the Timed Get-Up-and-Go (TUG) test (Podsiadlo & Richardson, 1991), in which the patient is timed while he/she rises from a chair, walks 3 meters, turns, walks back, and sits down again. The TUG has been used in prior HIV studies (Grinspoon et al., 1996, 1998) and explores multiple components of mobility, including gait speed, balance, and proximal muscle strength. The TUG has also been shown to correlate with functional capacity and more formal tests on balance and gait speed (Podsiadlo & Richardson, 1991). Although various cutoffs have been used in prior studies, the CDC (2017) recommends that an older adult who takes 12 seconds or more to complete the TUG should be considered at risk of falling.

FRAILTY

There is no consensus on the best tools to assess for frailty in older PWH (Brothers & Rockwood, 2019; Conroy, 2009). The Fried frailty phenotype (Fried et al., 2001) is commonly used in HIV research and has been operationalized for clinical practice (Rockwood et al., 2007) to consist of five components (no items = robust, 1 or 2 items = pre-frail, 3 to 5 items = frail):

1. Weight loss: defined as loss of either 10 pounds or more or 5% or more of body weight in the past year

2. Exhaustion (poor endurance and energy): defined as self-reporting of feeling "tired all the time"

3. Low physical activity levels and energy expenditure: defined as needing assistance with walking to being unable to walk

4. Slowness: defined as a time of 19 seconds or more on the TUG

5. Weakness: defined as abnormal strength on physical examination

The VACS index is another frailty tool specifically validated in PWH, with more details described later in this chapter. An online calculator is accessible at https://vacs-apps2.med.yale.edu/calculator. Prior HIV studies have also used the frailty index. However, because it follows the cumulative deficit approach and assesses for at least 30 and up to 75 health variables (Searle et al., 2008), this may prove cumbersome in clinical practice.

COGNITION/SAFETY CONCERNS

Age is a risk factor for cognitive impairment associated with HIV as well as other causes (Chan & Brew, 2014). Many studies of cognitive impairment screening in PWH focus on the entity of HIV-associated neurocognitive disorder (HAND), although in clinical practice providers would likely need to screen for cognitive impairment from all causes as older PWH are not immune from Alzheimer's disease or vascular dementia. Providers may consider using the Montreal Cognitive Assessment (MoCA), since it has been studied extensively in PWH (Rosca et al., 2019; Sangarlangkarn et al., 2019) and is commonly used to screen for other causes of cognitive impairment. The HIV Dementia Scale (Power et al., 1995) and the International HIV Dementia Scale (Sacktor et al., 2005) were developed to screen for HAND, but their effectiveness in screening for other causes of dementia is unclear. Even though the Mini-Mental Status Exam (MMSE) is regularly used in HIV-negative individuals, it does not assess for executive function, which may be impaired in patients with HAND (Valcour et al., 2011). Neuropsychological testing may be inaccessible or cumbersome for older PWH to complete.

MOOD

Depression and posttraumatic stress disorder (PTSD) are common in older PWH, especially women and men who have sex with men (Gallagher et al., 2008). Screening for depression and assessment of its severity are important, since depression affects quality of life and medical compliance. Multiple tools have been used in PWH to screen for depression, including a screening Patient Health Questionnaire (PHQ-2) with subsequent diagnostic PHQ-9 (Chibanda et al., 2016; EACS, 2020), the Beck Depression Inventory II (BDI-II) (Rodkjaer et al., 2016), or the Center for Epidemiological Studies Depression Scale (CES-D) (Mueses-Marín et al., 2019). Although as many as 14 tools have been used to screen for PTSD in PWH (Gallagher et al., 2008), the PTSD Checklist (PCL-5) was validated for use in HIV primary care (Verhey et al., 2018). Because the understanding and perception of depression or other mental illnesses can be affected by culture, it is important to use tools that have been validated locally if available (Sangarlangkarn et al., 2019).

POLYPHARMACY

Older PWH face a unique challenge of managing the burden of HIV disease in the context of chronic multidrug ART, increased risk of polypharmacy due to multimorbidity, decreasing end-organ function, and physiologic pharmacodynamic changes resulting in a narrower therapeutic index for many drug therapies. HIV providers need to be aware of polypharmacy in older PWH and take steps to optimize medication safety and effective medication use.

The term "polypharmacy" has been variably defined in the literature, but it usually means that a patient's medication profile has reached a threshold number of medications (often six or more), with the degree of polypharmacy correlated to a larger number of absolute medications, though it has also been associated with duration of time on multiple medications, and characterized as to whether multiple medications were appropriate for a given condition (i.e., appropriate vs. inappropriate polypharmacy) (Masnoon et al., 2017). The nature of chronic combined ART for PWH in an aging population already at risk of higher medication burden predisposes to potential drug therapy issues (e.g., drug interaction, additive adverse effects/toxicities, pharmacodynamic sensitivity, pill burden, medication errors). Consequently, it has been shown that the burden of polypharmacy is greater in older PWH than older patients in the general population (Kong et al., 2019) and also greater than in younger PWH (Holtzman et al., 2013; Marzolini et al., 2011).

ART-SPECIFIC CLINICAL CONSIDERATIONS

Multiple factors (e.g., ART history, viral resistance, history of adverse effects, drug interactions, comorbid conditions) will dictate the selection of appropriate ART and are covered in detail elsewhere, but considerations can be employed to mitigate age-related concerns in older PWH. Table 27.1 lists relevant class- and drug-specific considerations for older PWH.

ADVERSE EFFECT CONSIDERATIONS

We often have limited data on the prevalence of specific adverse effect rates of ART in older PWH, since these patients are often excluded from clinical trials on the basis of confounding illness/multimorbidity, decreased drug clearance, drug–drug interactions that may affect primary outcomes, discontinuation rates, or adverse effect assessment. Although more data evaluating ART in older PWH is being published (Ramgopal et al., 2020), clinicians still need a heightened awareness of adverse effects of ART, taking into account the extended duration of therapy, potential additive adverse effects from other drug therapy, historical toxicities from older ART regimens, and increased risk of complications due to certain disease states (i.e., cardiovascular disease, diabetes, osteopenia/osteoporosis).

MEDICATION CLEARANCE CONSIDERATIONS

Aging is associated with loss of function in both the kidney and liver, which can lead to reduced drug metabolism and excretion, increased drug exposure, and predisposition for potentially more drug toxicity (Knobel et al., 2001; Lindeman et al., 1985; Schmucker, 2001, Wellons et al., 2002). Declining drug clearance with age highlights the need to monitor glomerular filtration rate and adjust ART dosages as well as other drug therapy accordingly. The CKD-EPI equation has been postulated in a small subset of HIV patients on stable ART to best predict glomerular filtration rate (Vrouenraets et al., 2012), but the Cockcroft-Gault estimated creatinine clearance remains the standard in clinical trial evaluation and should be used for medication dosing where renal adjustments are required (Abrass et al., 2012). The Child–Pugh score should be calculated for those with chronic liver disease. The Department of Health and Human Services (DHHS) guidelines (Panel on Antiretroviral Guidelines for Adults and Adolescents, 2019) provide a summary table for dosing adjustments of ART based on estimated creatinine clearance and liver compromise.

COMPREHENSIVE MEDICATION ASSESSMENT

A defined systematic approach to routine medication review will enable identification of medication concerns, guide intervention to address medication issues, optimize prescribing practices, and mitigate or prevent complications arising from polypharmacy in older PWH. Routine and regular medication review should be performed at every care visit, and detailed medication reconciliation should occur at least annually.

Table 27.1 CLASS- AND DRUG-SPECIFIC CONSIDERATIONS FOR THE SELECTION OF ART IN OLDER PWH

Integrase strand transfer inhibitors (INSTIs)	Often INSTIs are preferred agents given limited drug interactions (except for EVG/c) and favorable adverse effect profile. Potential association with weight gain. Possible neuropsychiatric adverse effects (dizziness, depression, insomnia), though rare. Polyvalent mineral supplements (calcium, iron, etc.) should be spaced accordingly to avoid chelation. BIC and DTG inhibit tubular secretion of creatinine and may cause a stable increase in serum creatinine levels of 0.1–0.2 mg/dL without effect on GFR. BIC and DTG have been associated with weight gain.
Non-nucleoside reverse transcriptase inhibitors (NNRTIs)	EFZ may be a concern in older PWH due to the high incidence of neuropsychiatric adverse effects (dizziness, altered sensorium, worsening depression, vivid dreams/nightmares), notable drug interactions (CYP2B6/3A4 inducer), and association with metabolic abnormalities (dysglycemia, lipid abnormalities). RPV has activity against the common EFZ-associated K103N mutation. However, acid suppression will decrease RPV absorption (proton pump inhibitors are contraindicated with use), and the food requirement for RPV administration may be inconvenient for older patients. RPV has been associated with QT prolongation, which may be more relevant in older PWH. DOR has fewer clinical data but may be a favorable option given minimal adverse events and activity in the setting of other NNRTI mutations (K103N/Y181C).
Protease inhibitors (PIs)	Notable drug interactions must be accounted for with the PI and boosting agent combinations. PIs as a class have both inhibition and induction effects on cytochrome P450 enzymes. The PI class is also associated with lipid abnormalities, metabolic abnormalities, and cardiovascular events. Both DRV and ATV require food for administration. ATV has been shown to have a lower association with cardiovascular events than DRV, but ATV absorption is reduced with acid suppression therapy. ATV inhibits UGT and leads to increased indirect serum bilirubin. Skin yellowing, scleral icterus, and bile salt deposition of the skin/consequent pruritus can occur in some patients. Risk is higher based on UGT1A1 genotype.
Boosting agents	Both ritonavir (RTV) and cobisistat (cobi) pose noteworthy drug interactions as potent CYP3A4 and 2D6 inhibitors. Cobi lacks any relevant CYP induction (RTV induces several CYP enzymes) and may produce fewer gastrointestinal adverse effects. Cobi may also have a lower risk of lipid effect given the independent association of RTV with hypertriglyceridemia. Cobi also inhibits tubular secretion of creatinine and may cause a stable increase in serum creatinine levels of 0.1–0.2 mg/dL without effect on GFR.
Nucleoside reverse transcriptase inhibitors (NRTIs)	Older NRTIs (ddI, D4T) should not be used given the high risk of mitochondrial toxicity (lactic acidosis, hepatotoxicity, lipodystrophy) and availability of alternatives. AZT can contribute to macrocytic anemia and peripheral neuropathy and should generally be avoided in older PWH. Tenofovir is associated with nephrotoxicity, Fanconi syndrome, and bone mineral density decreases. TAF affords a lower systemic exposure of tenofovir versus TDF, and TAF has demonstrated less effect on serum creatinine levels and fewer bone mineral density changes during treatment, but may increase lipids. TAF has been associated with weight gain. ABC has been associated with cardiovascular disease and cardiovascular-associated mortality in some studies, though its role as a risk factor is unclear.

EVG/c, elvitegravir/cobicistat; BIC, bictegravir; DTG, dolutegravir; GFR, glomerular filtration rate; EFZ, efavirenz; RPV, rilpivirine; PI, protease inhibitor; DRV, darunavir; ATV, atazanavir; RTV, ritonavir; ddI, didanosine; d4T, stavudine; AZT, zidovudine; TAF, tenofovir alafenamide; TDF, tenofovir disoproxil fumarate; ABC, abacavir.

We recommend the following systematic approach to medication review in older PWH:

1. Obtain a comprehensive, accurate medication list to perform medication reconciliation.

2. Discontinue unnecessary medication therapy or supplements and optimize nonpharmacologic approaches to aid disease management.

3. Consider new medication therapy for needed indications.

4. Screen for drug interactions.

5. Confirm dosing appropriateness based on renal/liver function and relevant drug interactions.

6. Optimize and simplify the dosing regimen.

The "brown bag review" (Weiss et al., 2016) is a helpful approach to medication reconciliation where patients are encouraged to bring all medications, herbal medications/supplements, creams/ointments, inhalers, and eye drops—essentially any item that they use regularly to optimize their health—in a brown bag to their appointment for discussion and review. An advantage to the brown bag approach is that patients can physically point out specific medications and describe how they physically take them, which is particularly helpful when actual administration differs from the instructions printed on the prescription label. Other helpful ways to garner the medication list can be to (1) obtain a medication profile and dispensing history from their pharmacy for the last 3 to 6 months and (2) screen health information networks (i.e., Surescripts) to garner medication dispensing histories, which can be viewed/pulled in by certain electronic health record systems.

After confirming an up-to-date medication list, providers need to align each medication with an indication for therapy, enabling assessment of appropriateness for the indication. Furthermore, each indication for drug therapy can be assessed for nonpharmacologic measures to reduce medication need. The Beers Criteria (American Geriatrics Society, 2019), the Medication Appropriateness Index (Hanlon et al., 1992; Hanlon & Schmader, 2013), and STOPP/START (Gallagher et al., 2008) can be utilized to effectively determine inappropriate medications in older PWH that can be discontinued or changed to safer alternatives. The Beers Criteria provide guidance on inappropriate medication selection in older patients, while the Medication Appropriateness Index utilizes a 10-item assessment to determine degree of medication appropriateness. STOPP (Screening Tool of Older Persons' Prescriptions) helps identify inappropriate medications in the setting of specific diseases, and START (Screening Tool to Alert to Right Treatment) advocates for utilizing appropriate, effective therapy for a given condition. While inappropriate or harmful medications should be removed, appropriate and indicated medications (e.g., aspirin for prophylaxis of cardiovascular stent thrombosis) should most certainly be added where appropriate.

Interaction screening will assess for additive toxicity of multiple therapies, determine if increased/decreased exposure of drugs is expected, or identify if efficacy concerns may arise from the medication profile. Electronic drug database platforms (e.g., Micromedex, Lexi-Comp, Efacts) often have drug interaction screening tools to assist clinicians, though reviewing the metabolic pathways and the enzyme inhibitor/inducer status of profile medications will also help identify potential problems (see Table 20 of the DHHS guidelines; Panel on Antiretroviral Guidelines for Adults and Adolescents, 2019). Tables 21a–22b in the DHHS guidelines and the University of Liverpool website (www.hiv-druginteractions.org/) offer in-depth interaction details and recommendations for ART.

Finally, medications need to be dosed appropriately for medication clearance (using estimated creatinine clearance and Child–Pugh scores where appropriate), with medication regimens simplified to reduce complexity. Simplification may mean combining administration times to reduce the number of times a day the patient takes medication and/or offering coformulated tablets to reduce pill burden.

The drug therapy evaluation will need to continually screen for adverse effects, toxicity, and barriers to adherence to maximize safe medication use, ensure efficacy of therapy, and reduce complications related to polypharmacy. This requires providers to:

1. Screen any new clinical sign/symptom as a potential adverse drug effect

2. Monitor for changes in renal/liver function and adjust the medication dosage appropriately

3. Monitor for socioeconomic barriers (i.e., loss of job/insurance/income) to appropriate medication therapy, engaging social services as able

4. Continue to discuss goals of care and perceived treatment burden, adjusting or stopping medication therapy that may no longer be congruent with the patient's wishes

Clinically trained HIV pharmacists are key care team members that can aid in providing optimal care to older PWH (Schafer et al., 2016). Poised to assist in the provision of medication therapy management services, pharmacists are optimal providers to comprehensively reconcile patient medication profiles, screen for drug interactions, and assist with screening of toxicities related to ART and other drugs. When HIV clinical pharmacy services are available, we recommend integrating pharmacists into the care team to aid with the comprehensive and systemic medication review in older PWH.

SOCIAL/FINANCIAL ISSUES

A complete social history should be taken. Providers should also ask with whom the patient lives and what types of help/services (nursing, physical therapy, home health aides) he/she has in the home at baseline to determine the types of support that are currently available and what additional services may be needed. Caregivers should be screened periodically for caregiver burnout (Adelman et al., 2014). Elder mistreatment/abuse should be evaluated when there are worrisome signs such as bruises, burn/bite marks, pressure ulcers, or malnutrition without clinical explanation (National Center on Elder Abuse, 2018). A financial history should include determination of health insurance and identification of financial power of attorney in case patients become too ill to manage their finances.

NUTRITION/WEIGHT CHANGES

There is no consensus on an appropriate nutritional screening tool in older PWH, since there are few studies in this area (Ruiz & Kamerman, 2010). The Rapid Nutrition Screening for HIV disease (RNS-H) is the only validated tool in PWH (Wright & Epps, 2020). It has seven questions, takes 10 minutes to administer, and includes important outcomes such as food security, anthropometric measures, and nutritional complications such as dysphagia or diarrhea.

SYMPTOM BURDEN/PAIN

The HIV Symptom Index (Justice et al., 2001) assesses bothersome HIV symptoms (Kilbourne et al., 2002; Ruiz et al., 2010; Whalen et al., 1994) and demonstrates strong associations with disease severity and physical and mental health (Justice et al., 2001). These scales can help providers determine the symptoms present, evaluate the overall symptom burden, and track the severity of the symptoms over time.

The first step in pain management involves assessing the characteristics of the pain and conducting biopsychosocial diagnostic evaluation of the pain, including assessing for associated conditions such as depression/anxiety or substance abuse. The Infectious Disease Society of America recommends using the Brief Pain Inventory-Short Form (BPI-SF) (Goodin et al., 2018) or the PEG (average pain intensity, interference with enjoyment of life, and interference with general activity) (Merlin et al., 2018) to understand the functional impact of pain. Using this information, providers can develop treatment plans that improve not only pain but also physical as well as emotional functions.

ADVANCE CARE PLANNING

Advance care planning is defined as a process of communication between individuals and their healthcare agents to understand, reflect on, discuss, and plan for future healthcare decisions for a time when individuals are not able to make their own healthcare decisions in order to help maximize patient autonomy (International Society of Advance Care Planning & End of Life Care, 2020). With increased risk of neurocognitive impairment and debility from multimorbidity, advance care planning is essential among older PWH. Without clear documentation of a surrogate decision maker for healthcare and finances, decisions regarding emergent or end-of-life care may be legally deferred to estranged family members who are unaware of the patient's preferences or HIV status (Sangarlangkarn et al., 2015). Although there are no specific guidelines for PWH, DHHS recommends advance care planning in all patients with chronic life-limiting illness or anyone over 55 years old regardless of health status (Agency for Health Research and Quality: National Guideline Clearinghouse, 2015).

There is no formal guideline on the optimal time to initiate advance care planning in PWH. However, it is important to keep in mind that a conversation that is too early may result in changing patient preferences over time or the discussion becoming too abstract/far off in the future, while a conversation that is too late may result in patients being too sick or cognitively impaired to communicate preferences, leading to care that does not match patient preferences. With the lack of validated tools in PWH, providers may use the well-established "Respecting Choices" (Pecanac et al., 2014) paradigm detailing three stages of planning based on the patient's state of health. In cases of late diagnosis with advanced disease at the time of ART initiation, short-term prognosis depends on the severity of the acute illness (such as opportunistic infections), while long-term prognosis depends on the patient's adherence to ART and their retention in HIV primary care. As a result, advance care planning in this setting needs to balance the optimism surrounding the effectiveness of ART against the severity of the acute illness and the long-term challenges of retention in HIV primary care.

If a patient appears to have cognitive impairment, either from baseline dementia or delirium related to other comorbid disease, capacity should be assessed. Patients with cognitive impairment/delirium/dementia should not be dismissed as lacking capacity. Any provider can determine capacity, not just psychiatrists or geriatricians. Capacity is specific to the treatment or scenario and is defined as the ability to use information regarding a proposed intervention to make a choice that is congruent with the patient's values and preferences. Despite cognitive impairment, a patient who can demonstrate understanding, expressing a choice, appreciation, and reasoning, is deemed to have capacity to make medical decisions.

SPECIAL CONSIDERATIONS FOR PROBLEM-BASED MANAGEMENT OF OLDER PWH

DIABETES

Although primary care guidelines for the management of PWH by the Infectious Disease Society of America (IDSA) did not include age-specific glycemic goals for PWH, the American Academy of HIV Medicine (2014) recommends a target hemoglobin A1C of 8% for older PWH with frailty, less than a 5-year life expectancy, high risk for hypoglycemia, or high risk for polypharmacy. This recommendation mirrors the guideline on standards of medical care in diabetes from the American Diabetes Association (2015).

HYPERTENSION

Goal blood pressure for hypertensive patients in the general population remains controversial and presents a challenge for clinicians, with even less evidence to guide management among the HIV-positive population. The Systolic Blood Pressure Intervention Trial (SPRINT) was halted early in September 2015 due to benefits of lowering systolic blood pressure to below 120 mmHg (Ambrosius et al., 2014), and the results of SPRINT have effected a change in guidelines in the US and other countries. The American College of Cardiology and the American Heart Association guidelines currently recommend a blood pressure cutoff of 130/80 mmHg (Whelton et al., 2017). The 2018 Canadian Hypertension Education Program Guidelines recommend a target systolic blood pressure of 140 mmHg or less (Grade A) (Narenberg et al., 2018), while the 2016 Australian guideline (National Heart Foundation, 2016) also recommends a target systolic blood pressure of 120 mmHg or less (strong recommendation, Class II) for patients with high cardiovascular risk without diabetes, including patients with chronic kidney disease and those older than 75 years. However, the Eighth Joint National Committee (JNC 8) recommendation has not been updated since SPRINT, and the goal remains less than 150/90 mmHg in hypertensive adults aged 60 years and older, and a blood pressure goal of less than 140/90 mmHg for all hypertensive adults with diabetes or nondiabetic chronic kidney disease (James et al., 2014). Current gaps include lack of specific recommendations for the HIV-positive population and lack of consensus among varying guidelines. A sensible approach may include a careful uptitration of blood pressure medications to achieve the goal blood pressure of 125/90 mmHg as long as the patient does not experience medication side effects such as dizziness or falls.

BONE

Certain lifestyle and HIV-related factors put PWH at higher risk of osteoporosis, including smoking, alcohol abuse, glucocorticoid therapy, low consumption of calcium and vitamin D, low physical activity, immune dysfunction and persistent inflammation, and side effects of ART (Castronuovo et al., 2015). Modifiable risk factors should be addressed, and viral suppression should be achieved with ART. The IDSA recommends baseline bone densitometry (DXA) screening for osteoporosis in HIV-positive postmenopausal women and men aged 50 years and up (Aberg et al., 2014). If osteoporosis is detected, bisphosphonates may be considered, with a follow-up DXA screening 1 year afterward to monitor response to therapy. Providers should also ensure patients ingest adequate amounts of calcium (1,200 mg/day total diet plus supplement) and vitamin D (800 IU/day) (UpToDate, 2020).

PERIPHERAL NEUROPATHY

Age is a risk factor for peripheral neuropathy (Kaku & Simpson, 2014). As a result, pain should be considered the fifth vital sign and should be assessed at every visit. Currently, trials on symptomatic and disease-modifying treatments for HIV-associated distal symmetric polyneuropathy have had limited success, and at present there are no treatments approved by the US Food and Drug Administration.

AGE-RELATED SEXUAL CHANGES

Age-related sexual changes in PWH include menopause in women and hypogonadism in men.

The IDSA guideline advises that although hormone replacement therapy may be considered in patients with severe menopausal symptoms, it should be used only for a limited period of time at the lowest effective dose. This is because hormone replacement therapy has been associated with a small increased risk of breast cancer, cardiovascular disease, and thromboembolic morbidity (Aberg et al., 2014).

Morning serum testosterone level may be assessed in older HIV-positive men with decreased libido, erectile dysfunction, reduced bone mass or low-trauma fractures, hot flashes, or sweats. Low levels should be confirmed with repeat testing. Full recommendations are included in the IDSA guidelines (Aberg et al., 2014).

MALIGNANCY

As with the uninfected population, age is a risk factor for multiple types of malignancies among PWH. According to the IDSA, mammography should be performed annually in HIV-positive women aged 50 years and up, and colorectal cancer screening should be performed at age 50 years in asymptomatic PWH with average risk (Aberg et al., 2014). The US Preventive Services Task Force recommends annual screening for lung cancer with low-dose computed tomography (CT) in adults aged 55 to 80 years who have a 30 pack-year smoking history and currently smoke or have quit within the past 15 years. The screening should be discontinued once the patient has not smoked for 15 years or develops a health problem that limits life expectancy or the ability/willingness to have curative lung surgery (Agency for Health Research and Quality, 2018). Although there was concern that PWH would have a higher false-positive rate from chronic lung changes related to immunosuppression-related pulmonary infections, a prior study has shown that this may not be true (Sigel et al., 2014). There was a similar likelihood of pulmonary nodules meeting National Lung Screening Trial (NLST) criteria for a positive computed tomography (CT) scan among PWH and the uninfected population. There were also similar patterns of clinical evaluation triggered by the CT scan, suggesting that follow-up may not be more aggressive among PWH (Sigel et al., 2014).

IMMUNIZATIONS

Live attenuated varicella vaccination can be given to adult PWH without evidence of immunity with CD4⁺ T-cell counts of 200 cells/mL or more (Grohskopf et al., 2019), as no transmission of vaccine strain varicella-zoster virus (VZV) has been documented in PWH with CD4⁺ T-cell counts above this threshold (Shafran, 2016).

Regarding zoster prevention, recombinant zoster vaccine (RZV) has higher and more long-lasting efficacy against herpes zoster and postherpetic neuralgia than herpes zoster live-attenuated vaccine (ZVL), and the CDC preferentially recommends RZV in all persons aged at least 50 years. However, the efficacy studies did not include immunocompromised persons, and the CDC does not make recommendations regarding use of RZV in this population, although it may be reasonable to vaccinate PWH aged 50 years or older with CD4⁺ T-cell counts 200 cells/mL or more (Aberg et al., 2014). We recommend RZV over ZVL in older PWH due to its superior immunogenicity.

A recent study showed superior immunogenicity in adults 65 years and older who received high-dose inactivated influenza vaccine (Fluzone High-Dose HD-IIV3) compared to standard dosing (Fluzone SD-IIV3). Similar results were shown in a small clinical trial among PWH aged 18 years and older (McKittrick et al., 2013). Currently, the CDC recommends any IIV formulation (standard dose or high dose, trivalent or quadrivalent, unadjuvanted or adjuvanted) for patients aged 65 years and older regardless of HIV status (Grohskopf et al., 2019). We recommend high-dose IIV in older PWH due to its superior immunogenicity.

COVID-19

The severe acute respiratory syndrome coronavirus 2 (SARS-CoV-2) emerged in December 2019, causing the coronavirus disease 2019 (COVID-19). Preliminary studies found that although higher mortality from COVID-19 is reported among persons with immunosuppression, HIV infection was not identified as an important comorbid condition in hospitalized COVID-19 patients (del Amo et al., 2020). Moreover, despite risk factors for severe COVID-19 being common among older PWH—older age, male sex, hypertension, diabetes mellitus, kidney disease, chronic obstructive pulmonary disease—PWH do not seem to experience increased risk for serious COVID-19. It is speculated that PWH may not develop the intense immunologic response that leads to complications in COVID-19 (Borobia et al., 2020), despite preserved CD4⁺ T-cell counts (Guo et al., 2020). ART may also provide a protective factor. Studies have shown that certain nucleos(t)ide reverse transcriptase inhibitors (NRTIs), such as tenofovir disoproxil fumarate (TDF), tenofovir alafenamide (TAF), abacavir (ABC), and lamivudine (3TC), may be effective against SARS-CoV-2 (del Amo et al., 2020). The relation between HIV and SARS-CoV-2 remains to be further investigated.

The psychosocial burden and limited healthcare access among older PWH are expected amidst social distancing and physical isolation recommended by the CDC to reduce the spread of COVID-19 (Shiau et al., 2020). HIV infection and COVID-19 share many psychosocial drivers common among marginalized populations, including mental illness, illicit drug use, lower socioeconomic status, medical mistrust, food insecurity, and homelessness. These factors may worsen in older PWH with COVID-19, while limited access to care brought on by social distancing can also threaten ART adherence, successful viral suppression, and long-term health outcomes. The loneliness and social isolation experienced by older PWH will also likely be worsened by social distancing efforts.

CONCLUSION

There are an increasing proportion of older PWH, and they differ from their younger counterparts in many ways, including the risk for late diagnosis or underdiagnosis, decreased immunologic recovery, and increased multimorbidity. However, each older PWH is a unique and complex individual, and disease-centric guidelines should not be applied the same way in every patient. Management of diseases in older PWH should be individualized based on aging phenotypes, interactions with multimorbidity, and patient preferences. The VACS index may be used to identify aging phenotypes and can provide useful prognostic information to help prioritize interventions and guide shared decision-making with patients and caregivers.

RECOMMENDED READING

American Academy of HIV Medicine. Recommended treatment strategies for clinicians managing older patients with HIV. 2014. https://aahivm-education.org/sites/default/files/projects/aging/HIVandAgingConsensusProject051815.pdf

Boyd CM, Lucas GM. Patient-centered care for people living with multimorbidity. Curr Opinion HIV AIDS. 2014;9(4):419–427.

Calcagno A, Nozza S, Muss C, et al. Aging with HIV: a multidisciplinary review. Infection. 2015;43(5):509–522.

REFERENCES

Aberg JA, Gallant JE, Ghanem KG, et al. Primary care guidelines for the management of persons infected with HIV: 2013 update by the HIV Medicine Association of the Infectious Diseases Society of America. Clin Infect Dis. 2014;58(1):e1–e34. doi:10.1093/cid/cit665

Abrass C, Appelbaum J, Boyd C, et al. Summary report from the Human Immunodeficiency Virus and Aging Consensus Project: treatment strategies for clinicians managing older individuals with the human immunodeficiency virus. J Am Geriatr Soc. 2012;60(5):974–979.

Adelman RD, Tmanova LL, Delgado D, et al. Caregiver burden: a clinical review. JAMA. 2014;311(10):1052–1060. doi:10.1001/jama.2014.304

Agency for Health Research and Quality. Recommendations: screening for lung cancer. 2018. https://epss.ahrq.gov/ePSS/RecomDetail.do?method=search&sid=256&age=65&sex=Male&sexuallyActive=yes&tobacco=yes

Agency for Health Research and Quality: National Guideline Clearinghouse. Advanced care planning guideline. 2015. http://www.guideline.gov/content.aspx?id=47803

Ambrosius WT, Sink KM, Foy CG, et al. The design and rationale of a multicenter clinical trial comparing two strategies for control of systolic blood pressure: the Systolic Blood Pressure Intervention Trial (SPRINT). Clin Trials. 2014;11(5):532–546.

American Academy of HIV Medicine. Recommended treatment strategies for clinicians managing older patients with HIV. 2014. https://aahivm-education.org/sites/default/files/projects/aging/HIVandAgingConsensusProject051815.pdf

American Diabetes Association. Standards of medical care in diabetes—2015 abridged for primary care providers. Clin Diabet. 2015;33(2):97–111.

American Geriatrics Society. Updated AGS Beers Criteria for potentially inappropriate medication use in older adults. J Am Geriatr Soc. 2019;67(4):674–694.

Bellera CA, Rainfray M, Mathoulin-Pelissier S, et al. Screening older cancer patients: first evaluation of the G-8 geriatric screening tool. Ann Oncol. 2012;23:2166–2172.

Borobia A, Carcas A, Arnalich F, et al. A cohort of patients with COVID-19 in a major teaching hospital in Europe. J Clin Med. 2020;9:1733. doi:10.3390/jcm9061733

Brothers TD, Rockwood K. Frailty: a new vulnerability indicator in people aging with HIV. Eur Geriatr Med. 2019;10(2):219–226. doi:10.1007/s41999-018-0143-2

Castronuovo D, Pinzone MR, Moreno S, et al. HIV infection and bone disease: a review of the literature. Infect Dis Trop Med. 2015;1(2):e116

Centers for Disease Control and Prevention. Assessment Timed Up & Go (TUG). 2017. https://www.cdc.gov/steadi/pdf/TUG_Test-print.pdf

Centers for Disease Control and Prevention. Diagnoses of HIV infection among adults aged 50 years and older in the United States and dependent areas, 2011–2016. HIV Surveillance Supplemental Report. 2018;18(No. 3). https://www.cdc.gov/hiv/pdf/library/reports/surveillance/cdc-hiv-surveillance-supplemental-report-vol-23-5.pdf

Centers for Disease Control and Prevention. HIV Surveillance Report, 2018 (Updated); vol. 31. May 2020. http://www.cdc.gov/hiv/library/reports/hiv-surveillance.html

Chan P, Brew BJ. HIV associated neurocognitive disorders in the modern antiviral treatment era: prevalence, characteristics, biomarkers, and effects of treatment. Curr HIV/AIDS Rep. 2014;11(3):317–324. doi:10.1007/s11904-014-0221-0

Chibanda D, Verhey R, Gibson LJ, et al. Validation of screening tools for depression and anxiety disorders in a primary care population with high HIV prevalence in Zimbabwe. J Affect Disord. 2016;198:50–55. doi:10.1016/j.jad.2016.03.006

Conroy S. Defining frailty—the holy grail of geriatric medicine. J Nutr Heal Aging. 2009;13(4):389. doi:10.1007/s12603-009-0050-9

Dai SY, Liu JJ, Fan YG, et al. Prevalence and factors associated with late HIV diagnosis. J Med Virol. 2015;87(6):970–977. doi:10.1002/jmv.24066

del Amo J, Polo R, Moreno S, et al. Incidence and severity of COVID-19 in HIV-positive persons receiving antiretroviral therapy. Ann Intern Med. 2020;173(7):536–541. doi:10.7326/m20-3689

Ellis G, Gardner M, Tsiachristas A, et al. Comprehensive geriatric assessment for older adults admitted to hospital. Cochrane Database Syst Rev. 2017;9(9):CD006211. doi:10.1002/14651858.CD006211.pub3

Erlandson KM, Allshouse AA, Jankowski CM, et al. Risk factors for falls in HIV-infected persons. J AIDS. 2012;61:484–489.

Emory University, Division of Geriatric Medicine and Gerontology. The Emory "Big 10" basics in geriatrics. 2015. http://medicine.emory.edu/documents/geriatrics-big10.pdf#Emory

Erlandson KM, Plankey MW, Springer G, et al. Fall frequency and associated factors among men and women with or at risk for HIV infection. HIV Med. 2016;17:740–748.

European AIDS Clinical Society. Guidelines Version 10.0. 2020. https://www.eacsociety.org/guidelines/eacs-guidelines/eacs-guidelines.html

Fried LP, Tangen CM, Walston J, et al. Frailty in older adults: evidence for a phenotype. J Gerontol A Biol Sci Med Sci. 2001;56(3):M146–M157. doi:10.1093/gerona/56.3.M146

Gallagher P, Ryan C, Byrne S, et al. STOPP (Screening Tool of Older Person's Prescriptions) and START (Screening Tool to Alert Doctors to Right Treatment). Consensus validation. Int J Clin Pharmacol Ther. 2008;46(2):72–83.

Goodin BR, Owens MA, White DM, et al. Intersectional health-related stigma in persons living with HIV and chronic pain: implications for depressive symptoms. AIDS Care. 2018;30(supp 2):66–73. doi:10.1080/09540121.2018.1468012

Grinspoon S, Corcoran C, Askari H, et al. Effects of androgen administration in men with the AIDS wasting syndrome: a randomized, double-blind, placebo-controlled trial. Ann Intern Med. 1998;129:18–26.

Grinspoon S, Corcoran C, Lee K, et al. Loss of lean body and muscle mass correlates with androgen levels in hypogonadal men with acquired immunodeficiency syndrome and wasting. J Clin Endocrinol Metab. 1996;81:4051–4058.

Grohskopf LA, Alyanak E, Broder KR, et al. Prevention and control of seasonal influenza with vaccines: recommendations of the Advisory Committee on Immunization Practices—United States, 2019–20 influenza season. MMWR Recomm Rep. 2019;68(RR-3):1–21. http://dx.doi.org/10.15585/mmwr.rr6803a

Guaraldi G, Silva AR, Stentarelli C. Multimorbidity and functional status assessment. Curr Opin HIV AIDS. 2014;9(4):386–397. doi:10.1097/COH.0000000000000079

Guo W, Ming F, Dong Y, et al. A survey for COVID-19 among HIV/AIDS patients in two districts of Wuhan, China. Lancet. March 13, 2020. [E-pub before print]. doi:10.2139/ssrn.3550029

Hanlon JT, Schmader KE. The medication appropriateness index at 20: where it started, where it has been, and where it may be going. Drugs Aging. 2013;30(11):893–900.

Hanlon JT, Schmader KE, Samsa GP, et al. A method for assessing drug therapy appropriateness. J Clin Epidemiol. 1992;45(10):1045–1051.

Holtzman C, Armon C, Tedaldi E, et al. Polypharmacy and risk of antiretroviral drug interactions among the aging HIV-infected population. J Gen Intern Med. 2013;28(10):1302–1310.

Huss A, Stuck AE, Rubenstein LZ, et al. Multidimensional preventive home visit programs for community-dwelling older adults: a systematic review and meta-analysis of randomized controlled trials. J Gerontol A Biol Sci Med Sci. 2008;63(3):298.

International Society of Advance Care Planning & End of Life Care. The definition of advance care planning. 2020. https://www.acp-i.org/mission/

James PA, Oparil S, Carter BL, et al. 2014 evidence-based guideline for the management of high blood pressure in adults: report from the Panel Members Appointed to the Eighth Joint National Committee (JNC 8). JAMA. 2014;311(5):507–520. doi:10.1001/jama.2013.284427

John M, Hessol N, Hare CB, et al. Veterans Aging Cohort Study (VACS) index, functional status, and other patient reported outcomes in older HIV-positive (HIV+) adults. Open Forum Infect Dis. 2014;1(supp 1):S428–S429. doi:10.1093/ofid/ofu052.1153

Justice AC, Holmes H, Gifford AL, et al. Development and validation of a self-completed HIV symptom index. J Clin Epidemiol. 2001;54(12):S77–S90.

Justice AC, Modur SP, Tate JP, et al. Predictive accuracy of the Veterans Aging Cohort Study index for mortality with HIV infection: a North American cross cohort analysis. J AIDS. 2013;62(2):149–163. doi:10.1097/QAI.0b013e31827df36c

Justice A, Tate J, Brown S, et al. Can the Veterans Aging Cohort Study Index improve clinical judgment for both HIV infected and uninfected veterans? J Gen Intern Med. 2013;28:S39.

Justice AC, Tate J, Freiberg M, et al. Reply to Chow et al. Clin Infect Dis. 2012;55(5):751–752.

Kaku M, Simpson DM. HIV neuropathy. Curr Opin HIV AIDS. 2014;9(6):521–526. doi:10.1097/COH.0000000000000103

Katz S, Ford AB, Moskowitz RW, et al. Studies of illness in the aged. The Index of ADL: a standardized measure of biological and psychosocial function. JAMA. 1963;185:914–919.

Kilbourne AM, Justice AC, Rollman BL, et al. Clinical importance of HIV and depressive symptoms among veterans with HIV infection. J Gen Intern Med. 2002;17(7):512–520.

Knobel H, Guelar A, Valldecillo G, et al. Response to highly active antiretroviral therapy in HIV-infected patients aged 60 years or older after 24 months follow-up. AIDS 2001;15(12):1591–1593.

Kong AM, Pozen A, Anastos K, et al. Non-HIV comorbid conditions and polypharmacy among people living with HIV age 65 or older compared with HIV-negative individuals age 65 or older in the United States: a retrospective claims-based analysis. AIDS Patient Care STDs. 2019;33(3):93–103.

Koroukian SM, Warner DF, Owusu C, et al. Multimorbidity redefined: prospective health outcomes and the cumulative effect of co-occurring conditions. Prev Chronic Dis. 2015;12:E55. doi:10.5888/pcd12.140478

Lee SJ, Leipzig RM, Walter LC. Incorporating lag time to benefit into prevention decisions for older adults. JAMA. 2013;310(24):2609–2610.

Lindau ST, Schumm LP, Laumann EO, et al. A study of sexuality and health among older adults in the United States. N Engl J Med. 2007;357(8):762–774. doi:10.1056/NEJMoa067423

Lindeman RD, Tobin J, Shock NW. Longitudinal studies on the rate of decline in renal function with age. J Am Geriatr Soc. 1985;33(4):278–285.

Marzolini C, Back D, Weber R, et al. Ageing with HIV: medication use and risk for potential drug-drug interactions. J Antimicrob Chemother. 2011;66(9):2107–2111.

Masnoon N, Shakib S, Kalisch-Ellett L, et al. What is polypharmacy? A systematic review of definitions. BMC Geriatr. 2017;17(1):230.

McKittrick N, Frank I, Jacobson JM, et al. Improved immunogenicity with high-dose seasonal influenza vaccine in HIV-infected persons: a single-center, parallel, randomized trial. Ann Intern Med. 2013;158(1):19–26. doi:10.7326/0003-4819-158-1-201301010-00005

Merlin JS, Westfall AO, Long D, et al. A randomized pilot trial of a novel behavioral intervention for chronic pain tailored to individuals with HIV. AIDS Behav. 2018;22(8):2733–2742. doi:10.1007/s10461-018-2028-2

Mpondo BC, Gunda DW, Kilonzo SB, et al. Immunological and clinical responses following the use of antiretroviral therapy among elderly HIV-positive individuals attending care and treatment clinic in Northwestern Tanzania: a retrospective cohort study. J Sex Transm Dis. 2016;2016:5235269.

Mueses-Marín H, Montaño D, Galindo J, et al. Psychometric properties and validity of the Center for Epidemiological Studies Depression Scale (CES-D) in a population attending an HIV clinic in Cali, Colombia. Biomedica. 2019;39(1):33–45. doi:10.7705/biomedica.v39i1.3843

Narenberg KA, Zarnke KB, Leung AA, et al. Hypertension Canada's 2018 Canadian Hypertension Education Program guidelines for blood pressure measurement, diagnosis, assessment of risk, prevention, and treatment of hypertension. Can J Cardiol. 2018;34:506–525.

National Center on Elder Abuse. 2018. https://ncea.acl.gov/

National Heart Foundation. Guideline for the diagnosis and management of hypertension in adults—2016. https://www.heart-foundation.org.au/images/uploads/publications/PRO-167_Hypertension-guideline-2016_WEB.pdf

Panel on Antiretroviral Guidelines for Adults and Adolescents. Guidelines for the use of antiretroviral agents in adults and adolescents living with HIV. Department of Health and Human Services. 2019. AdultandAdolescentGL.pdf (hiv.gov)

Pecanac KE, Repenshek MF, Tennenbaum D, et al. Respecting Choices® and advance directives in a diverse community. J Palliat Med. 2014;17(3):282–287. doi:10.1089/jpm.2013.0047

Pilowsky D, Wu L-T. Sexual risk behaviors and HIV risk among Americans aged 50 years or older: a review. Subst Abuse Rehabil. 2015;6:51. doi:10.2147/sar.s78808

Podsiadlo D, Richardson S. The Timed Up & Go: a test of basic functional mobility for frail elderly persons. J Am Geriatr Soc. 1991;39:142–148.

Power C, Selnes OA, Grim JA, et al. HIV Dementia Scale: a rapid screening test. J AIDS Retrovirol. 1995;8(3):273–278. doi:10.1097/00042560-199503010-00008

Ramgopal M, Maggiolo F, Ward D, et al. Pooled analysis of 4 international trials of bictegravir/emtricitabine/tenofovir alafenamide (B/F/TAF) in adults aged 65 or older demonstrating safety and efficacy: week 48 results. J Int AIDS Soc. 2020;23(supp 4):e25547.

Reuben DB, Frank JC, Hirsch SH, et al. A randomized clinical trial of outpatient comprehensive geriatric assessment coupled with an intervention to increase adherence to recommendations. J Am Geriatr Soc. 1999;47(3):269.

Rockwood K, Andrew M, Mitnitski A. A comparison of two approaches to measuring frailty in elderly people. J Gerontol A Biol Sci Med Sci. 2007;62(7):738–743. doi:10.1093/gerona/62.7.738

Rodkjaer L, Gabel C, Laursen T, et al. Simple and practical screening approach to identify HIV-infected individuals with depression or at risk of developing depression. HIV Med. 2016;17(10):749–757. doi:10.1111/hiv.12381

Rosca EC, Albarqouni L, Simu M. Montreal Cognitive Assessment (MoCA) for HIV-associated neurocognitive disorders. Neuropsychol Rev. 2019;29(3):313–327. doi:10.1007/s11065-019-09412-9

Ruiz M, Kamerman LA. Nutritional screening tools for HIV-infected patients: implications for elderly patients. J Int Assoc Physicians AIDS Care. 2010;9:362–367.

Ruiz MA, Reske T, Cefalu C, et al. Falls in HIV-infected patients: a geriatric syndrome in a susceptible population. J Int Assoc Provid AIDS Care. 2013;12:266–269.

Sacktor NC, Wong M, Nakasujja N, et al. The International HIV Dementia Scale: a new rapid screening test for HIV dementia. AIDS. 2005;19(13):1367–1374.

Sangarlangkarn A, Apornpong T, Justice AC, et al. Screening tools for targeted comprehensive geriatric assessment in HIV-infected patients 50 years and older. Int J STD AIDS. 2019;30(10):1009–1017. doi:10.1177/0956462419841478

Sangarlangkarn A, Merlin JS, Tucker RO, et al. Advance care planning and HIV infection in the era of antiretroviral therapy: a review. Top Antivir Med. 2016;23(5):174–180.

Schafer JJ, Gill TK, Sherman EM, et al. ASHP guidelines on pharmacist involvement in HIV care. Am J Health Syst Pharm. 2016;73(7):468–494.

Schmucker DL. Liver function and phase I drug metabolism in the elderly: a paradox. Drugs Aging. 2001;18(11):837–851.

Schouten J, Wit FW, Stolte IG, et al. Cross-sectional comparison of the prevalence of age-associated comorbidities and their risk factors between HIV-infected and uninfected individuals: the AGEhIV cohort study. Clin Infect Dis. 2014;59(12):1787–1797. doi:10.1093/cid/ciu701

Searle SD, Mitnitski A, Gahbauer EA, et al. A standard procedure for creating a frailty index. BMC Geriatr. 2008;8:24. doi:10.1186/1471-2318-8-24

Semeere AS, Lwanga I, Sempa J, et al. Mortality and immunological recovery among older adults on antiretroviral therapy at a large urban HIV clinic in Kampala, Uganda. J AIDS. 2014;67(4):382–389. doi:10.1097/QAI.0000000000000330

Shafran SD. Live attenuated herpes zoster vaccine for HIV-infected adults. HIV Med. 2016;17(4):305–310.

Shiau S, Krause KD, Valera P, et al. The burden of COVID-19 in people living with HIV: a syndemic perspective. AIDS Behav. 2020;24(8):2244–2249. doi:10.1007/s10461-020-02871-9

Sigel K, Wisnivesky J, Shahrir S, et al. Findings in asymptomatic HIV infected patients undergoing chest computed tomography testing: implications for lung cancer screening. AIDS. 2014;28(7):1007–1014.

Stuck AE, Siu AL, Wieland GD, et al. Comprehensive geriatric assessment: a meta-analysis of controlled trials. Lancet. 1993;342(8878):1032–1036. doi:10.1016/0140-6736(93)92884-V

Tinetti ME, Fried TR, Boyd CM. Designing health care for the most common chronic condition: multimorbidity [published correction appears in JAMA. 2012 Jul 18;308(3):238]. JAMA. 2012;307(23):2493–2494. doi:10.1001/jama.2012.5265

UpToDate. Calcium and vitamin D supplementation in osteoporosis. 2020. https://www.uptodate.com/contents/calcium-and-vitamin-d-supplementation-in-osteoporosis?search=calcium%20vit%20d%20osteoporosis&source=search_result&selectedTitle=3~150&usage_type=default&display_rank=3

Valcour V, Paul R, Chiao S, et al. Screening for cognitive impairment in human immunodeficiency virus. Clin Infect Dis. 2011;53(8):836–842. doi:10.1093/cid/cir524

Verhey R, Chibanda D, Gibson L, et al. Validation of the Posttraumatic Stress Disorder Checklist—5 (PCL-5) in a primary care population with high HIV prevalence in Zimbabwe. BMC Psychiatry. 2018;18(1):109. doi:10.1186/s12888-018-1688-9

Vinikoor MJ, Joseph J, Mwale J, et al. Age at antiretroviral therapy initiation predicts immune recovery, death, and loss to follow-up among HIV-infected adults in urban Zambia. AIDS Res Hum Retroviruses. 2014;30(10):949–955. doi:10.1089/AID.2014.0046

Vrouenraets SM, Fux CA, Wit FW, et al. A comparison of measured and estimated glomerular filtration rate in successfully treated HIV-patients with preserved renal function. Clin Nephrol, 2012;77(4):311–320.

Weiss BD, Brega AG, LeBlanc WG et al. Improving the effectiveness of medication review: guidance from the Health Literacy Universal Precautions Toolkit. J Am Board Fam Med. 2016;29(1):18–23.

Wellons MF, Sanders L, Edwards LJ, et al. HIV infection: treatment outcomes in older and younger adults. J Am Geriatr Soc. 2002;50(4):603–607.

Whalen CC, Antani M, Carey J, et al. An index of symptoms for infection with human immunodeficiency virus: reliability and validity. J Clin Epidemiol. 1994;47(5):537–546.

Whelton PK, Carey RM, Aronow WS, et al. 2017 ACC/AHA/AAPA/ABC/ACPM/AGS/APhA/ASH/ASPC/NMA/PCNA guideline for the prevention, detection, evaluation, and management of high blood pressure in adults: a report of the American College of Cardiology/American Heart Association Task Force on Clinical Practice Guidelines. J Am Coll Cardiol. 2018;71(19):e127–e248. doi:10.1016/j.jacc.2017.11.006

Wright L, Epps JB. Development and validation of a HIV disease–specific nutrition screening tool. Top Clin Nutr. 2020;35(3):264–269.

28.

OPPORTUNISTIC INFECTIONS

Lisa Y. Armitage, Karen J. Vigil, and Manali Pednekar

CHAPTER GOAL

Upon completion of this chapter, the reader should be able to:

- Recognize and manage the most common opportunistic infections (OIs) found in persons with HIV (PWH).

TIMING OF ANTIRETROVIRAL THERAPY INITIATION AND IMPACT ON OIS

LEARNING OBJECTIVES

- Describe the issues concerning starting antiretroviral therapy (ART) in the setting of an OI

- Summarize the recommendations for starting ART in the setting of an OI

WHAT'S NEW?

Data and guidelines on starting ART in patients with cryptococcal meningitis have been updated.

KEY POINTS

- Early initiation of ART was associated with a decrease in AIDS progression and death in AIDS Clinical Trials Group (ACTG) A5164.

- Early initiation of ART near the time of starting treatment for an OI should be considered for most patients, with the possible exception of patients with cryptococcal or tuberculous meningitis.

The question of when to initiate ART in the setting of an acute or ongoing OI has been controversial. On the one hand, the immediate initiation of ART in the presence of an OI may provide better clinical outcomes as the immune system improves. On the other hand, rapidly decreasing viral load has been associated with the immune reconstitution inflammatory syndrome (IRIS), which may lead to further complications in the setting of an OI. There are also questions of increasing pill burden, potential drug–drug interactions,

additive toxicity and adverse events, and the more practical problem of continuity of care if ART is started in a hospital setting for a newly diagnosed patient with HIV, without established outpatient care already in place. This problem could be particularly troublesome for patients who do not have health insurance or otherwise do not have affordable access to ART in the outpatient setting.

Some OIs associated with severe immunosuppression, such as cryptosporidiosis, microsporidiosis, and progressive multifocal leukoencephalopathy (PML), do not have adequate specific treatment other than ART. For these patients, the only way to improve the condition is by starting ART, so it makes sense to start ART immediately. Similarly, in patients with mild to moderate Kaposi's sarcoma, this condition may improve after the initiation of ART even without chemotherapy. However, for OIs such as *Pneumocystis jirovecii* pneumonia (PCP), *Cryptococcus neoformans* meningitis, or *Mycobacterium tuberculosis* meningitis, targeted antimicrobial treatment is available to stabilize the condition, and the patient can improve in the absence of ART. It is for these patients that controversy has existed about the optimal time to start ART.

CLINICAL TRIAL RESULTS

ACTG A5164 was designed to address the question of the optimal timing of ART initiation for individuals presenting with AIDS-defining OIs or serious bacterial infections (BIs), other than tuberculosis, for which effective antimicrobial therapies were available. This was a randomized, open-label strategy trial to evaluate early (defined as within 14 days of starting acute OI treatment) versus deferred (given after OI treatment is completed) initiation of ART in patients starting treatment of acute OIs or BIs, using clinical and virologic endpoints at 48 weeks (Zolopa et al., 2009). A total of 282 patients were evaluable, with 141 in each arm. Most study participants were from racial/ethnic minority groups (73%) and male (85%), with a median age of 38 years, a median CD4$^+$ T-cell count of 29 cells/mm^3, and a median HIV RNA of 5.07 log$_{10}$ copies/mL. The most common entry OIs included PCP (63%), cryptococcal meningitis (12%), and BIs (12%). ART was initiated a mean of 12 days after starting OI treatment in the "early" arm and a mean of 45 days after OI treatment in the "deferred" arm.

The study found a statistically significant decrease in the proportion of participants experiencing a second

AIDS-defining disease and/or death (composite endpoint) in the early treatment arm (14.2%) compared to the deferred arm (24.1%) (odds ratio [OR], 0.51; 95% confidence interval [CI], 0.27–0.94). The time to AIDS progression and death was also longer in the early treatment arm compared to the deferred group (hazard ratio, 0.53; 95% CI, 0.30–0.92). The impact of these differences was seen most prominently in the first 6 months after diagnosis of the OI. The number of adverse events was not different in the two arms, and IRIS was reported in 8 participants in the early arm and 12 participants in the deferred arm. Based on these data, it is clear that early initiation of ART during treatment for an acute OI or serious BI is life-saving or at least serious morbidity–reducing if there are no major contraindications to starting ART. A cost-effectiveness analysis, supportive of this early treatment strategy, has also been published (Sax et al., 2010).

The overall rates of IRIS in A5164 were lower than rates observed in previous retrospective trials. This was possibly because of the types of the OIs in this study (largely PCP) and because patients with *M. tuberculosis* infection were excluded from entry due to the fact that it was the subject of separate trials. Factors that were found to be associated with IRIS in A5164 were the presence of fungal infections (*Cryptococcus* or *Histoplasma*), lower baseline CD4$^+$ T-cell counts, and higher baseline HIV RNA levels. IRIS was also associated with higher CD4$^+$ T-cell counts and lower HIV RNA levels while on ART. Early initiation of ART did not increase the incidence of IRIS in this study.

However, recommendations regarding the timing of starting ART specifically in the setting of meningitis due to *C. neoformans* or *M. tuberculosis* have been more complex. A study of IRIS-related meningitis associated with *C. neoformans* was published in 2009 (Sungkanuparph et al., 2009). Although this study of 101 participants employed a different methodology than A5164, it also found no association between the timing of ART initiation and the diagnosis of IRIS. Rather, it found that an increased baseline serum cryptococcal antigen titer was a risk factor for IRIS. In contrast, a study of 54 participants in Zimbabwe showed that early initiation of ART (within 72 hours of diagnosis) in persons with cryptococcal meningitis versus delayed initiation (after 10 weeks of treatment with fluconazole alone) was associated with increased mortality; in the study's setting, optimal management of increased intracranial pressure (i.e., decreasing cerebrospinal fluid [CSF] volume by lumbar puncture or other sterile procedure) may not be available (Makadzange et al., 2010). Furthermore, the 2014 Cryptococcal Optimal ART Timing (COAT) trial of 177 participants with HIV from Uganda and South Africa with cryptococcal meningitis reported increased mortality (hazard ratio, 1.73) at 26 weeks for participants who started ART within 1 or 2 weeks compared to those who had deferral of ART for 5 weeks (Boulware et al., 2014). Participants in the early group started ART a median of 8 days after antifungal therapy, and patients in the deferred group started ART at a median of 36 days. Most of the increase in mortality was observed within the first 8 to 30 days of the study. The differences in mortality were especially pronounced in patients who had white blood cell (WBC) counts

of less than 5 cells/mL in their CSF, although it was unclear if the increase in mortality in this study was due to progression of cryptococcal disease or IRIS. Current US Department of Health and Human Services (2019) guidelines recommend a short delay in initiating ART in the presence of cryptococcal meningitis (discussed later).

Implementation of the findings of A5164 and similar studies may prove difficult in practice, particularly in settings in which patients may not have existing linkage to primary care and may have limited access to ongoing treatment with ART after the resolution of the acute OI. However, effective implementation of early ART was accomplished and published by an academic medical center, and this may be a model for bringing early ART to a "real-world" population (Geng et al., 2011).

RECOMMENDATIONS OF GUIDELINES

The guidelines for prevention and treatment of OIs in adults and adolescents with HIV were updated in May 2018, revised in June 2019, February 2020, and May 2020, and are available in the latest form online (https://clinicalinfo.hiv.gov/en/guidelines/adult-and-adolescent-opportunistic-infection/whats-new-guidelines). These guidelines provide recommendations regarding the timing of initiation of ART in the setting of specific opportunistic conditions, and they should be referenced for guidance in the treatment of patients with those conditions. These guidelines generally reiterate the findings of A5164, suggesting that, unless contraindications are present, early initiation of ART near the time of treatment of an OI should be considered for most patients with an acute OI. Other elements that should be considered are degree of immunosuppression, availability of treatment for the OI, drug–drug interactions and overlapping toxicities, and the risk and potential consequences of IRIS.

In many instances, it is recommended that ART should be started as soon as possible. These conditions include PML, which is caused by the John Cunningham (JC) virus; cryptosporidiosis; microsporidiosis; and fungal infections other than meningitis caused by *C. neoformans*. For PCP and invasive BIs, the guidelines recommend starting ART within 2 weeks of diagnosis, although the panel notes that no patients with respiratory failure requiring mechanical ventilation were enrolled in A5164. For *Toxoplasma gondii* encephalitis, the panel cites expert opinion to start ART within 2 or 3 weeks after diagnosis and initiation of specific treatment for toxoplasmosis based on the data from A5164, in which only 5% of participants were diagnosed with toxoplasmosis. For disseminated *Mycobacterium avium* complex (MAC), the panel cites expert opinion to consider starting ART after the first 2 weeks of antimycobacterial therapy in order to decrease the overall initial pill burden and also to decrease the possibility for IRIS. For cytomegalovirus (CMV) retinitis, the panel notes that many experts would not delay ART for more than 2 weeks after the start of CMV-specific treatment.

Regarding cryptococcal meningitis, the panel notes that it would be prudent to defer ART at least until the initial 2-week antifungal induction is complete and possibly until the completion of the consolidation phase at 10 weeks, especially if the patient has increased intracranial pressure or a low CSF WBC count. The panel also notes that if ART is started prior to 10 weeks of antifungal treatment, then the clinician should be prepared to promptly investigate and treat manifestations of IRIS, including increased intracranial pressure. Last, there is very limited evidence from randomized clinical trials to guide the optimal time for initiation of ART in the setting of concomitant tuberculous meningitis. Expert opinion remains relevant in managing these patients.

SUMMARY

Although substantial barriers to early initiation of ART in the setting of an acute OI exist, the weight of the available evidence falls on the side of starting ART as soon as possible for most patients with acute OIs and invasive BIs, with the notable exception of meningitis due to *C. neoformans* or *M. tuberculosis*.

RECOMMENDED READING

Abdool Karim SS, Naidoo K, Grobler A, et al. Timing of initiation of antiretroviral drugs during tuberculosis therapy. *N Engl J Med.* 2010;362(8):697–706. http://www.ncbi.nlm.nih.gov/pubmed/20181971

Blanc FX, Sok T, Laureillard D, et al. Earlier versus later start of antiretroviral therapy in HIV-positive adults with tuberculosis. *N Engl J Med.* 2011;365(16):1471–1481. http://www.ncbi.nlm.nih.gov/pubmed/22010913

Boulware DR, Meya DB, Muzoora C, et al. Timing of antiretroviral therapy after diagnosis of cryptococcal meningitis. *N Engl J Med.* 2014;370(26):2487–2498.

Havlir DV, Kendall MA, Ive P, et al. Timing of antiretroviral therapy for HIV-1 infection and tuberculosis. *N Engl J Med.* 2011;365(16):1482–1491. http://www.ncbi.nlm.nih.gov/pubmed/22010914

Mfinanga SG, Kirenga BJ, Chanda DM, et al. Early versus delayed initiation of highly active antiretroviral therapy for HIV-positive adults with newly diagnosed pulmonary tuberculosis (TB-HAART): a prospective, international, randomised, placebo-controlled trial. *Lancet Infect Dis.* 2014;14(7):563–571. http://www.ncbi.nlm.nih.gov/pubmed/24810491

Temprano ANRS Study Group. A trial of early antiretrovirals and isoniazid preventive therapy in Africa. *N Engl J Med.* 2015;373(9):808–822. http://www.ncbi.nlm.nih.gov/pubmed/26193126

Zolopa A, Andersen J, Powderly W, et al. Early antiretroviral therapy reduces AIDS progression/death in individuals with acute opportunistic infections: a multicenter randomized strategy trial. *PLoS One.* 2009;4(5):e5575.

MYCOBACTERIAL INFECTIONS

LEARNING OBJECTIVE

• Discuss the available tests and treatment modalities to appropriately manage PWH with *M. tuberculosis*, MAC, and *M. kansasii*, the most common mycobacterial diseases associated with HIV infection

WHAT'S NEW?

• Shorter latent tuberculosis infection (LTBI) regimens such as 3 months of weekly isoniazid (INH)–rifapentine show higher completion rates when given with compatible antiretroviral (ARV) regimens.

• Primary prophylaxis to prevent disseminated MAC disease is no longer recommended for PWH who immediately initiate ART.

KEY POINTS

• HIV infection markedly increases the likelihood of a person progressing from LTBI to active TB disease.

• Rifamycins are a critical component of effective TB therapy in PWH but have many drug–drug interactions.

• MAC should be treated with multidrug therapy, including clarithromycin and ethambutol optimally.

• Optimal treatment of MAC disease should include medications for both MAC and HIV (to reconstitute the immune system).

• *M. kansasii* infection closely resembles TB, with more frequent pulmonary presentation than MAC.

• Diagnosis and treatment of *M. kansasii* as outlined in the American Thoracic Society guidelines are the same for people with and without HIV.

M. TUBERCULOSIS

Epidemiology

There were 10.0 million new cases of TB worldwide in 2019; 8.6% of these cases were in PWH (World Health Organization, 2019). Recognition of the vulnerability of the HIV population to TB and increased awareness of the need to rapidly diagnose and treat persons coinfected with TB and HIV have led to a steady decrease in HIV-associated TB deaths since the numbers peaked globally in 2004. Deaths from TB in PWH have declined from 540,000 in 2004 to 251,000 in 2018. Despite these gains, TB still kills an estimated one in three persons with AIDS annually worldwide (World Health Organization, 2019).

The total number of TB cases in the US peaked in 1992 and has been steadily declining since. The Centers for Disease Control and Prevention (CDC) recommends testing for HIV in all active cases of TB (CDC, 2012). HIV testing was completed for 88% of reported TB cases in the US, with 5.1% of total cases reported as HIV positive in 2018 (CDC, 2019). This is down significantly from the peak in 1992, when nearly two-thirds of TB cases in 25- to 44-year-olds were HIV positive. Attention to screening and treatment of TB as well as increasing focus on HIV treatment in the US has resulted in a decrease in HIV-associated TB cases and a faster decline than in the general population (CDC, 2019). The percent of TB patients with HIV in the US has remained stable for the past 4 years.

Unlike other HIV-related OIs, the CD4⁺ T-cell count does not predict risk of TB infection. Rates of TB in PWH are higher than those in HIV-negative individuals at all CD4⁺ T-cell counts.

Clinical Presentation

Infection with *M. tuberculosis* generally occurs after inhalation of infectious particles coughed into the air by a person with active pulmonary TB disease. A less common route of infection involves ingestion of unpasteurized dairy products produced from the milk of *Mycobacterium bovis*-infected cows (bovine TB). Once infected, individuals will either progress to active disease (progressive primary disease) or their immune system will contain growth of the organism but not kill it (LTBI). Host immune factors play a major role in which route initial infection will take. Host factors also play a role in whether individuals with LTBI will progress to active TB disease (postprimary or reactivation disease).

TB in HIV-negative persons typically presents as pulmonary disease. Often, the upper lobes of the lung are involved, and cavitary lesions are characteristic. Pulmonary disease is frequently accompanied by constitutional symptoms such as fever, night sweats, and weight loss. These findings are more typical of reactivation disease rather than progressive primary infection found when there is poor containment of the infecting organism by the immune system.

The CD4⁺ T-cell count plays a pivotal role in the containment of *M. tuberculosis*. As HIV infection progresses and there is a decline in the number of these cells, there is less containment of infecting organisms. The clinical presentation of TB in PWH differs based on the CD4⁺ T-cell count. PWH with CD4⁺ T-cell counts of more than 350 cells/mm³ often present with the classic pulmonary presentation described. As the CD4⁺ T-cell count decreases, the clinical presentation can look more like progressive primary disease. In PWH with CD4⁺ T-cell counts below 200 cells/mm³, pulmonary lesions may involve any lobe of the lungs and range from infiltrates to pneumonia. Cavitary lesions become less common with advanced HIV disease, and a number of persons with HIV and TB will have no abnormalities on chest radiograph at all.

Another feature of HIV-associated TB is extrapulmonary disease. Extrapulmonary disease is found in up to 50% of individuals in some series. Lymph node disease is the most common extrapulmonary site. Disseminated (miliary) disease and mycobacteremia are far more common in PWH with low CD4⁺ T-cell counts.

Diagnosis

Diagnosis of TB infection in PWH requires a high index of suspicion. Recent advances in diagnostic tests for TB, such as interferon-gamma release assays (IGRAs), have not translated into a major improvement in the diagnosis of TB infection in PWH. Diagnosis of TB disease requires the HIV physician to remain vigilant.

Traditionally, screening for TB infection has been via the tuberculin skin test (TST). The assay involves injection of 0.1 mL (comprising 5 tuberculin units) of purified protein derivative subcutaneously into the volar surface of the forearm. Individuals who have been previously infected with *M. tuberculosis* develop a delayed-type hypersensitivity reaction to the injected proteins. Induration caused by this reaction is measured after 48 to 72 hours. A TST measurement of 5 mm of induration or greater is considered positive in PWH. The sensitivity of this test has always been poor in PWH, and it can be as low as 30% in TB patients with CD4⁺ T-cell counts of less than 200 cells/mm³. It is also important to note that the TST will not distinguish between persons with LTBI and those with active TB, and it may be falsely positive in persons vaccinated with Bacillus Calmette–Guérin (BCG) due to cross-reaction with the antigens found in the BCG vaccine.

IGRAs are diagnostic blood tests for detection of *M. tuberculosis* infection. These tests are based on immune responses to antigens unique to *M. tuberculosis*. IGRAs have the benefits of negating the false positives seen with BCG vaccination and offering a blood draw that requires a single visit. There are two commercially available IGRAs that have been approved by the US Food and Drug Administration (FDA)—the QuantiFERON-TB Plus (QFT-Plus) and the T.SPOT.*TB* (T-spot). The QFT-Plus assay replaced the QFT Gold In Tube (QFT-GIT) and tests CD4 and CD4/CD8 responses to *M. tuberculosis*-specific antigens. All indications are that the QFT-Plus and QFT-GIT assays perform similarly. Meta-analyses (Cattamanchi et al., 2011; Santin et al., 2012) show the sensitivity to be approximately 60% for the QFT-GIT and 70% for the T-spot in detecting *M. tuberculosis* infection. Although this appears to be an improvement over the TST, there was not a significant difference in head-to-head sensitivity with either test compared to the TST. The studies highlight the fact that there are still a large number of cases of LTBI or active TB disease that may be missed by these tests, so a high index of suspicion is still warranted. As highlighted in the recommendations on IGRAs issued by the American Thoracic Society, CDC, and Infectious Diseases Society of America (Nahid et al., 2016), these tests are most useful in BCG-vaccinated populations (adding greater specificity) and in populations with poor rates of return (negating the need for a return visit for reading). These same guidelines state clearly that routine testing with both a TST and an IGRA is not generally recommended.

People with HIV should be screened for TB infection by a TST or an IGRA at the time of HIV diagnosis and, if at high risk for exposure, regularly thereafter. Individuals who travel to countries with a high TB burden or who reside in areas with high rates of TB should be tested annually. All others should be tested when there is suspicion of exposure to an active case after their initial testing. Individuals with CD4⁺ T-cell counts below 200 cells/mm³ at HIV diagnosis should be tested at baseline and, if they test negative, should have a repeat diagnostic test after CD4⁺ T-cell count recovery to above 200 cells/mm³ to confirm they are truly negative.

An individual with a positive TB diagnostic test (TST or IGRA) without evidence of active TB disease should be given a diagnosis of LTBI. People with HIV and LTBI are at very high risk for advancing to active TB. Individuals with LTBI without HIV have a 5% to 10% lifetime risk of developing active TB, whereas PWH and LTBI are 19 (15–22) times more likely to progress to active disease than persons without HIV (World Health Organization, 2018). LTBI treatment in this population is paramount and has formed the cornerstone of progress in reducing global HIV-associated TB cases.

Diagnosis of active TB disease requires utilization of many pieces of data. A thorough history is useful in most cases. Important information to note includes exposure to an active TB case, residence in high-risk settings such as jail or homeless shelters, and prior diagnosis of untreated LTBI. Signs and symptoms of active disease may include cough lasting longer than 3 weeks, unexplained weight loss, fevers, and/or night sweats. There are no physical exam findings specific for TB, but a thorough physical exam may reveal suspicious lymphadenopathy, draining fistulas, abnormal respiratory sounds, or signs of meningitis.

Diagnostic tests such as the TST and IGRA can add to available data but cannot be relied on entirely. One may also consider performing more than one of these tests to increase sensitivity, especially when the individual has a low $CD4^+$ T-cell count. In general, a positive TST or IGRA result should be taken as evidence of infection.

All PWH suspected of having active TB should receive a chest radiograph because the lungs are the most common entry point and a frequent site of infection. Though the chest radiograph can be normal in patients with culture-positive pulmonary TB, a high-resolution computed tomography (CT) scan may show early miliary-type lesions. Any person with respiratory symptoms, regardless of chest radiograph findings, should have sputum collected (at least three specimens) 8 to 24 hours apart, with at least one specimen being an early morning specimen and, preferably, at least one observed.

Individuals with lower $CD4^+$ T-cell counts are more likely to have extrapulmonary TB with infection in tissues that are more difficult to access and that have fewer organisms. It may be necessary to obtain biopsy specimens from lymph nodes, bone marrow, or lung tissue to make the diagnosis. CSF or ascitic or abscess fluid may provide important diagnostic information. All tissue from suspected sites of infection should be submitted for smear and culture analysis for acid-fast bacilli and, if indicated, histopathologic analysis searching for characteristic granulomas on pathology.

TREATMENT

Treatment of LTBI in PWH is essentially the same as that in people without HIV. The mainstay of treatment for LTBI in PWH has been 9 months of INH dosed daily self-administered or intermittently (twice weekly) by directly observed therapy (DOT). In PWH, 9 months of treatment is considered optimal as there have been no studies comparing 6 versus 9 months of INH therapy. While treatment with INH has the benefit of compatibility with nearly all HIV treatment regimens, completion rates tend to be lower with longer courses of treatment for LTBI. Newer, shorter treatment regimens using rifamycins have been shown to be equally effective with increased rates of completion.

Rifampin taken for 4 months is an acceptable and effective LTBI treatment, especially in patients who are intolerant of INH or who are exposed to an INH-resistant case. Rifampin interacts with almost all of the ARVs. This interaction excludes all of the nucleoside analogs except tenofovir alafenamide (TAF). *TAF use is contraindicated with all rifamycins.* In many cases, rifabutin can be substituted for rifampin. When a rifamycin is used in the treatment of a patient on ART, drug–drug interactions must be carefully considered. Guidance is available in a regularly updated document at https://aidsinfo.nih.gov.

The most recently approved treatment regimen for LTBI is INH–rifapentine dosed weekly for 12 weeks (3HP). This regimen can be given by DOT or can be self-administered. This regimen is highly desirable as it can provide cure for LTBI with only 12 weekly doses. Initially, this regimen could not be given to any patients taking ARVs, but newer pharmacokinetic data show 3HP use to be compatible with raltegravir- and efavirenz-based regimens (Borisov et al., 2018).

The BRIEF-TB study evaluated 1 month of daily INH–rifapentine for the treatment of LTBI in PWH. Endpoints of the study included progression to active TB disease, death from TB, and death from other causes. Though the outcomes of treatment with 1 month of daily INH–rifapentine were similar to treatment with 9 months of INH, only 21% of enrollees had a positive screening TST at baseline, indicating a low risk of progression in the study group as a whole (Swindells et al., 2019).

Treatment of active TB disease in PWH is also essentially the same as that for HIV-negative patients. All patients diagnosed in the US with active TB should be started on a four-drug regimen consisting of INH, rifampin, ethambutol, and pyrazinamide unless there is known resistance or baseline severe impairment of hepatic or renal function. After 2 months of this four-drug therapy (initial phase) and if the patient's organism is not resistant, the regimen can be reduced to INH and rifampin for the duration of treatment (continuation phase). Length of treatment will depend on the site and extent of disease. Most cases can be treated with 6 to 9 months of total therapy, whereas infections involving the bones or meninges should be treated for a total of 9 to 12 months. Infections of the central nervous system should be treated with steroids in addition to anti-TB medications. Prior recommendations were to treat infections of the pericardium with steroids, though new data suggest the addition of steroids in these cases does not impact outcomes (Nahid et al., 2016).

The most significant differences between treatment of PWH and that of HIV-negative patients involve use of the rifamycins and frequency of dosing. As previously noted, there is significant interaction between rifampin and most ARVs, so care must be taken in introducing this class of medications into the regimen. Treatment regimens for active TB that do not contain a rifamycin require up to 18 to 24 months of therapy and have very high rates of relapse. Every effort should be made to include a rifamycin in the treatment of

PWH and TB. Regularly updated guidance on how to manage drug interactions can be found at https://aidsinfo.nih.gov.

DOT is highly recommended for all cases of active TB treated in the US to support the individual's efforts at cure. Patients can receive intermittent dosing but only if receiving DOT. Highly intermittent dosing of TB therapy (once- or twice-weekly dosing) is associated with an increased risk of relapse with rifampin-resistant disease and should be avoided in PWH (Nahid et al., 2016). This is especially noted in patients with CD4+ T-cell counts below 100 cells/mm³. New cases of active TB disease in persons with HIV should receive daily dosing for the first 2 months of therapy, then daily or thrice-weekly dosing to complete therapy (Nahid et al., 2016).

The question of when to initiate ART in a person with HIV and TB is not a trivial one. Treatment for both diseases simultaneously can result in a large pill burden, potential for multiple drug interactions, and potential for multiple drug toxicities. Although it is clear that patients who are diagnosed with TB should be started immediately on anti-TB medications, until recently the timing of adding ART was less clear. Several studies (Blanc et al., 2011; Karim et al., 2011; Havlir et al., 2011, Martinson et al., 2011) conducted at multiple sites have shown a survival benefit (reduced mortality) when starting ART within 2 weeks of starting TB medications in patients with CD4+ T-cell counts below 50 cells/mm³. Of note, a single study (Mfinanga et al., 2014) showed ART could be delayed until completion of 6 months of TB therapy in patients with CD4+ T-cell counts above 220 cells/mm³. At CD4+ T-cell counts below 50 cells/mm³, the incidence of IRIS events increased. Though these same studies did not show a survival benefit to starting ART earlier in patients with CD4 counts of 50 cells/mm³ or more, there was no demonstration of harm and there were many other documented benefits to starting ART. Expert opinion is that ART should be started by 8 weeks of starting treatment for TB in patients with CD4+ T-cell counts of 50 cells/mm³ or more.

If IRIS does occur in the course of treatment, it is important that both ART and TB treatment be continued. Mild cases of IRIS can be observed or treated with nonsteroidal anti-inflammatory agents; if more severe, a short course of steroids may be necessary. A randomized trial showed a lower incidence of TB-associated IRIS in PWH, TB, and median CD4+ T-cell counts of approximately 50 cells/mm³ started empirically on steroids (Meintjes et al., 2018). In patients where TB-associated IRIS is likely, empiric steroids may be considered.

Special consideration should be given to PWH and TB meningitis. IRIS involving central nervous system disease leads to worse outcomes. People with HIV and TB meningitis must be monitored carefully and treated with steroid therapy and a slow wean to reduce the inflammatory effects associated with disease. ART should be added with careful monitoring of the patient with TB meningitis for any evidence of IRIS.

Drug-resistant disease in PWH requires individualized therapy and should be approached with an expert in drug-resistant TB. Patients with multidrug-resistant or extensively drug-resistant TB should have ART initiated within 2 to 4 weeks after initiation of second-line TB drug therapy.

PREVENTION

People with HIV should be screened for TB by a TST or an IGRA at the time of diagnosis and as needed thereafter. People with HIV who are found to have a positive TST or IGRA without evidence of active disease should be treated for LTBI to prevent progression to active disease.

People with HIV who are contacts to an infectious pulmonary case of TB and have no evidence of active disease should be treated with a full course of therapy for LTBI, even with a negative diagnostic test. As outlined previously, available diagnostic tests are not sensitive enough to rule out TB infection, and patients exposed to an infectious case are highly susceptible. Active disease should be ruled out in all patients prior to initiation of treatment for LTBI.

Patients who have a history of untreated or inadequately treated TB who do not have evidence of currently active disease should receive treatment for LTBI. This may be manifest as old fibrotic lesions on chest x-ray noted during routine screening.

MAC
EPIDEMIOLOGY

MAC, also known as MAI, consists of *M. avium* and *M. intracellulare*, two organisms so similar that they can only be differentiated using DNA probes. MAC infections are the most common nontuberculous mycobacteria (NTM) infections in both people with and without HIV infection (Griffith et al., 2007).

These organisms are ubiquitous and are found environmentally in water, soil, and animal sources. Despite the many places from which the organisms can be isolated, the actual route of infection in PWH is unclear. There is no evidence for human-to-human or animal-to-human transmission.

Disseminated disease is the most common presentation of MAC infection associated with HIV and occurs almost exclusively in individuals with profound immunosuppression who are not yet receiving ART. Disseminated disease is most commonly found in PWH with CD4+ T-cell counts of less than 50 cells/mm³. Having a high HIV RNA level (>100,000 copies/mm³) has also been identified as a risk factor. The incidence of disseminated MAC has declined steadily since the introduction of effective ART, with most cases occurring in individuals who have not accessed care.

CLINICAL PRESENTATION

As stated previously, the most common presentation of MAC infection in PWH is disseminated disease. Symptoms tend to be nonspecific and typically include fever, night sweats, anorexia, weight loss, and gastrointestinal symptoms such as nausea, vomiting, diarrhea, and abdominal pain. It is important to remember that these same symptoms can be associated with other OIs, such as TB and fungal disease.

Disseminated MAC infection tends to involve the reticuloendothelial system; subsequently, physical exam findings may include hepatomegaly, splenomegaly, and lymphadenopathy.

Pulmonary disease is rare, even with disseminated disease, but occasionally can manifest as nodules, infiltrates, cavities, or mediastinal/hilar adenopathy. Pulmonary findings are more likely to be associated with infection due to *M. tuberculosis* or *M. kansasii*.

Immune reconstitution in patients newly started on ART may "unmask" preexisting, previously undetected disease. The presentation in this case may manifest as disseminated disease or perhaps localized disease.

DIAGNOSIS

Isolation of MAC from a normally sterile site, such as the blood or tissue, should be considered diagnostic for disseminated disease. In the absence of a positive blood culture, other more invasive approaches, such as lymph node, liver, or bone marrow biopsy, may be necessary to obtain an adequate specimen for diagnosis.

Isolation of MAC from nonsterile sites such as the respiratory or gastrointestinal tracts may represent true pathology but can also represent colonization. In these cases, it is important to make an effort to determine if other pathogens may be at play.

TREATMENT

Optimally, the approach to treatment of disseminated MAC disease should include treatment of both MAC and HIV. Like treatment of TB and other NTM infections, treatment of MAC infection should include multidrug therapy and ART should be started and optimized as soon as possible. Drug susceptibility testing should be performed as macrolide susceptibility is associated with greater treatment success when using this class of drug. Only macrolide and amikacin susceptibilities are associated with treatment outcomes.

Clarithromycin should be the first drug added to a MAC treatment regimen. Studies have shown treatment with clarithromycin to be associated with faster clearance of bacteremia than treatment with azithromycin. In the event of clarithromycin intolerance or unacceptable drug interaction with other medications, azithromycin may be substituted.

The second drug added should be ethambutol. Addition of ethambutol to a macrolide is associated with decreased relapse in the treatment of MAC. Rifabutin can also be added to the MAC treatment regimen, especially in situations where the risk of mortality is high and/or emergence of resistance is likely. Addition of rifabutin also adds the potential for significant interaction with many ARVs and can lower serum drug levels of clarithromycin when used in combination. Prior to addition of rifabutin to the treatment of a mycobacterial infection, TB must be ruled out to prevent the emergence of rifampin-resistant TB disease.

Based on data from HIV-negative persons, fluoroquinolones such as moxifloxacin or levofloxacin and injectable antibiotics such as amikacin and streptomycin can be utilized if there is a need for additional medication options due to resistance or toxicity. While there are in vitro data showing susceptibility to these drugs, there are no randomized controlled trials evaluating efficacy in the setting of macrolide susceptibility or effective ART.

IRIS has been documented with treatment of MAC disease, as it has with TB. The presentation generally manifests as a return of fever and worsening lymphadenitis with negative blood cultures. Mild cases can be simply monitored or treated with a nonsteroidal anti-inflammatory agent or, in severe cases, a short course of steroids. Treatment for both MAC and HIV should be continued during management of IRIS reactions.

Treatment of disseminated disease should continue until there is a response to ART. Repeat blood cultures should be reserved for those without a clinical response after 4 to 8 weeks of treatment. PWH who complete a 12-month course of therapy, who remain free of signs or symptoms of disease, and who show a sustained increase in CD4+ T-cell count to above 100 cells/mm³ for at least 6 months have a low risk of relapse. A previously treated person who experiences a decrease in CD4+ T-cell count to less than 100 cells/mm³ or is not on a fully suppressive ART regimen should be placed back on preventive (secondary) prophylactic treatment.

PREVENTION/PROPHYLAXIS

No direct route for infection with MAC has been identified and, thus, there is no specific action known to prevent exposure to MAC. Primary prophylaxis to prevent disseminated MAC disease is no longer recommended for patients who immediately initiate ART. If primary prophylaxis is initiated, it should be discontinued once the patient is on a fully suppressive ART regimen. Primary prophylaxis for disseminated MAC is reserved for patients with a CD4+ T-cell count of less than 50 cells/mm³ who are not receiving ART, who remain viremic, or for whom a fully suppressive ART regimen is not an option. Before starting primary prophylaxis, disseminated MAC should be ruled out.

Azithromycin dosed at 1,200 mg weekly is the preferred regimen for both primary and secondary prophylaxis. Clarithromycin dosed at 500 mg twice daily is effective but, due to the increased pill burden and higher number of drug interactions, is considered an alternative to azithromycin.

Rifabutin is an alternative when there is evidence of macrolide-resistant disease and secondary prophylaxis is needed or when there is macrolide intolerance, but rifabutin is less effective in this capacity and adds the increased risk of drug interactions with many of the ARVs. Before using rifabutin, every effort should be made to rule out active TB.

M. KANSASII

EPIDEMIOLOGY

M. kansasii infection is the second most common NTM infection in PWH (after MAC infection). Tap water appears to be the most likely environmental reservoir for strains causing human disease (Griffith, 2002). Lung disease caused by

M. kansasii closely resembles disease caused by *M. tuberculosis* in both people with and without HIV. Despite its similarities to TB, there is no evidence of human-to-human transmission of *M. kansasii*. Similar to MAC, infection with *M. kansasii* is most commonly found in individuals with CD4$^+$ T-cell counts below 50 cells/mm^3.

CLINICAL PRESENTATION

Unlike MAC disease, which is most commonly disseminated and rarely pulmonary, *M. kansasii* can be disseminated but is more commonly pulmonary. Radiographically, *M. kansasii* infection closely resembles infection with *M. tuberculosis*, with symptoms that include cough, fever, night sweats, weight loss, and hemoptysis.

DIAGNOSIS

Diagnosis requires isolation of the organism from a sterile site or meeting the criterion outlined in the guidelines set forth by the American Thoracic Society (Griffith et al., 2007). Briefly, the American Thoracic Society criteria for both people with and without HIV require that the individual in question have pulmonary symptoms with suggestive radiography, exclusion of other diagnoses, positive culture results from two separate expectorated sputum samples, or at least one bronchoalveolar lavage specimen or bronchial biopsy with suggestive histopathology.

M. kansasii, like other mycobacteria, will stain positive by acid fast staining, which, when isolated from the sputum of a person with pulmonary lesions, can trigger an unnecessary public health investigation for TB. Testing with a nucleic acid amplification test can rule out TB in these cases.

TREATMENT

Most studies guiding treatment of *M. kansasii* infection are conducted in individuals without HIV. *M. kansasii* responds well to anti-TB medications, although the organism is widely resistant to pyrazinamide. Treatment with a rifamycin, ethambutol, and either isoniazid or a macrolide is recommended for at least 12 months. Prior studies suggested treatment for 12 months after culture conversion, but there is no evidence that treatment for longer than 12 total months prevents relapse (Daley et al., 2020). Two studies demonstrated good outcomes with clarithromycin substituted for isoniazid (Daley et al., 2020). Rifamycins in the treatment regimen of *M. kansasii* patients (unlike those with MAC disease) provide clear benefit and prevent relapse. The choice and dose of rifamycin should be guided by the patient's ART, with special attention to potential drug interactions.

As with infections caused by other mycobacteria, IRIS has been documented with treatment of *M. kansasii*. Mild cases can be simply monitored or treated with a nonsteroidal anti-inflammatory agent or, in severe cases, a short course of steroids. It is important that treatment for both *M. kansasii* and HIV be continued during management of IRIS reactions.

RECOMMENDED READING

Department of Health and Human Services. Guidelines for prevention and treatment of opportunistic infections in HIV-infected adults and adolescents. 2020. https://aidsinfo.nih.gov/guidelines/html/4/adult-and-adolescent-opportunistic-infection/325/tb

Department of Health and Human Services, Panel on Antiretroviral Guidelines for Adults and Adolescents. Guidelines for the use of antiretroviral agents in HIV-1-infected adults and adolescents. 2020. https://clinicalinfo.hiv.gov/sites/default/files/inline-files/AdultandAdolescentGL.pdf

Griffith DE, Aksamit T, Brown-Elliott BA, et al. An official ATS/IDSA statement: diagnosis, treatment, and prevention of nontuberculous mycobacterial diseases. *Am J Respir Crit Care Med*. 2007;175:367–416.

OIS: VIRAL INFECTIONS

LEARNING OBJECTIVE

• Discuss the established and evolving science regarding diagnosis, treatment, and prophylaxis of opportunistic viral infections associated with HIV infection to improve quality of life and length of survival

WHAT'S NEW?

A new recombinant zoster vaccine was approved in October 2017. The Advisory Committee for Immunization Practices is still evaluating recommendations for PWH.

KEY POINTS
HERPES SIMPLEX VIRUS

• Herpes simplex virus (HSV) is a very common disease in PWH, typically presenting with orolabial, genital, and/or anorectal ulcers that may be very severe in the setting of advanced immunosuppression. HSV could also manifest as proctitis (particularly in men who have sex with men [MSM]), esophagitis, keratitis, meningitis, encephalitis, radiculitis, and retinitis (presenting as acute retinal necrosis).

• Treatment is generally with acyclovir or one of its derivatives. Acyclovir resistance is more common among PWH. HSV suppression should be considered for individuals with frequent or severe recurrent episodes.

VARICELLA ZOSTER VIRUS

• Varicella zoster reactivation disease in PWH is often more severe, multidermatomal, or disseminated. Severe complications such as progressive outer retinal necrosis must be treated quickly to prevent permanent sequelae. For mild disease, oral therapy with acyclovir or one of its derivatives is appropriate; in severe cases, however, intravenous therapy is required.

CMV

- CMV may cause a variety of clinical manifestations in PWH with CD4$^+$ T-cell counts of less than 50 cells/mm^3. Retinitis and colitis are the most common manifestations. Ganciclovir (or the oral prodrug valganciclovir), cidofovir, and foscarnet are the most common therapies, but they carry significant risk of toxicity. Primary prophylaxis is not recommended.

JC VIRUS

- JC virus causes progressive multifocal leukoencephalopathy, a progressive, demyelinating disease of the central nervous system that leads to relatively rapid accumulation of neurologic deficits with dementia, coma, and death. Diagnosis is generally made clinically with the support of typical magnetic resonance imaging (MRI) findings and polymerase chain reaction (PCR) testing for JC virus in the CSF. Definitive diagnosis is made by brain biopsy. No specific antiviral therapy exists for JC virus. ART often results in stabilization or regression of disease.

HERPES SIMPLEX VIRUS

In the US, the seroprevalence of HSV types 1 and 2 (HSV-1 and HSV-2) is 47.8% and 11.9%, respectively, in the age group 14 to 49 years (McQuillan et al., 2016). HSV-1 and HSV-2 are highly prevalent in PWH. Classically, HSV-1 caused oral ulcers whereas HSV-2 caused genital ulcers; currently, however, both are recognized as a cause of genital infection, especially in young women and MSM. The incidence of HSV-1 as the etiology of primary infection in genital herpes has been increasing, with lesions identical to HSV-2 (Ryder et al., 2009).

HSV-2 is one of the most common sexually transmitted infections worldwide and the primary cause of genital ulcer disease. The overall national HSV-2 prevalence was reported as 16.2% in 2010 (Xu et al., 2006); however, seroprevalence rates near 70% have been reported in PWH (Corey et al., 2004). The primary mode of transmission is through direct contact with oral secretions or genital secretions. Clinical HSV disease is common in the absence of HIV infection, but manifestations are more common, more severe, or atypical in the setting of HIV infection.

CLINICAL PRESENTATION

The classical presentation of herpes infection is large, painful, grouped vesicles with an erythematous base typically in the orolabial, genital, and anorectal regions; however, they may involve any areas of the body. Inguinal lymphadenopathy is commonly seen in primary infection (Corey et al., 1983). In patients with advanced HIV-associated immunosuppression, anogenital lesions may be severe, and they may be refractory to treatment or secondary to acyclovir-resistant virus (Safrin et al., 1994). Dissemination is possible, but it is rarely seen in PWH. Hypertrophic genital herpes, which is an atypical presentation, often resembles neoplasia, and a biopsy is needed to

confirm the diagnosis (Yudin et al., 2008). Proctitis (particularly in MSM), keratitis, meningitis, encephalitis, radiculitis, and retinitis (presenting as acute retinal necrosis) are possible complications. HSV esophagitis may occur in people with CD4$^+$ T-cell counts of less than 50 cells/mm^3 and typically presents with retrosternal chest pain and odynophagia.

Reactivation of HSV is more common in PWH. Recurrent lesions are often more frequent, more extensive, and of longer duration in this population. In addition, there is prolonged shedding of the virus even in the absence of lesions, especially in patients with lower CD4$^+$ T-cell counts and higher plasma HIV-1 RNA levels.

DIAGNOSIS

HSV DNA PCR and viral culture are the recommended modalities for diagnosis for all suspected HSV mucosal infections, with PCR having the highest sensitivity (Workowski & Berman, 2010). Type-specific serologic assays are available and recommended, but false-positive HSV-2 serologic tests have been reported with enzyme immunoassay antibody tests with low index values (1.1–3.5) and repeat testing is recommended in such cases for confirmation (Workowski & Bolan, 2015). Culture specimens can also be tested for antiviral drug susceptibility.

PREVENTION

Consistent use of latex condoms decreases acquisition of HSV-2 in HSV-2-discordant heterosexual couples according to the 2018 Panel on Opportunistic Infections in HIV-Positive Adults and Adolescents (Panel on Guidelines for the Prevention and Treatment of Opportunistic Infections in Adults and Adolescents with HIV, 2018 [OI Guidelines], AII). Suppressive acyclovir is not recommended in people with HIV/HSV-2 coinfection who are not on ART as it did not prevent transmission of HSV-2 to the susceptible partner in HSV-2-discordant couples (OI Guidelines, AI). There is no vaccine available for prevention of HSV infection.

TREATMENT

Table 28.1 shows the current treatment recommendations from the OI Guidelines. Oral acyclovir, valacyclovir, and famciclovir are comparable alternatives. In patients with extensive mucocutaneous lesions, it is recommended to use intravenous acyclovir. No sign of resolution of herpes lesions in 7 to 10 days after starting anti-HSV therapy raises suspicion for acyclovir resistance, and viral culture of the lesion with phenotypic testing and susceptibility testing should be performed (OI Guidelines, AII).

Resistance to acyclovir has been reported in up to 5% of PWH with HSV-2 infection and is more common in patients with prolonged acyclovir use. Acyclovir inhibits HSV-specific DNA polymerase after incorporation into the growing DNA, resulting in a chain termination due to the absence of the 3′ hydroxyl group. It requires phosphorylation by a virally encoded thymidine kinase in order to be active. Altered, reduced, or absent thymidine kinase or altered viral DNA polymerase

Table 28.1 HSV TREATMENT RECOMMENDATIONS

CONDITION	FIRST-CHOICE TREATMENT	ALTERNATIVE TREATMENT
Orolabial lesions	Valacyclovir 1 g PO b.i.d. *or* Famciclovir 500 mg PO b.i.d. *or* Acyclovir 400 mg PO t.i.d. for 5–10 days	
Initial or recurrent genital lesions	Valacyclovir 1 g PO b.i.d. *or* Famciclovir 500 mg PO b.i.d. *or* Acyclovir 400 mg PO t.i.d. for 5–10 days	
Severe mucocutaneous lesions	Acyclovir 5 mg/kg IV every 8 hours until lesions regress, then switch to acyclovir 400 mg PO t.i.d. until lesions are healed	
Esophagitis	Valacyclovir 1 g PO t.i.d. *or* Famciclovir 500 mg PO t.i.d. *or* Acyclovir 400 mg PO 5 times daily for 14–21 days	
Encephalitis and hepatitis	Acyclovir 10–15 mg/kg IV every 8 hours for 21 days	
Acyclovir-resistant herpes	Foscarnet 80–120 mg/kg/day IV 2 or 3 times daily until clinical response Cidofovir 5 mg/kg/week IV for 3 weeks, then 5 mg/kg every other week with saline hydration and probenecid 2 g PO 3 hours before the dose followed by 1 g 2 hours and 8 hours after the dose (total of 4 g) until clinical response (off label)	Topical trifluridine *or* Cidofovir 1% gel *or* Topical imiquimod 5% 3 times weekly for 21–28 days or longer based on clinical response

confers resistance to acyclovir and all the class, including ganciclovir. In these cases, foscarnet is the drug of choice. Cidofovir is a reasonable alternative for thymidine kinase–negative HSV. Pritelivir, a helicase-primase inhibitor, is a novel agent that is being studied in clinical trials for treatment of acyclovir-resistant herpes in immunocompromised patients. Prolonged application (21–28 days or longer) of topical agents like trifluridine, foscarnet, cidofovir, and imiquimod can effectively treat external lesions (OI Guidelines, CIII).

PROPHYLAXIS

Condoms are recommended to prevent transmission of HSV-2. The use of 1% tenofovir vaginal gel has been shown to be associated with a 50% risk reduction of HSV-2 acquisition in women at high risk of HIV infection. However, this has not been confirmed in other studies. In addition, in patients taking oral tenofovir, the rates of vaginal shedding of HSV-1 and HSV-2 are similar. Suppressive therapy with oral acyclovir, valacyclovir, or famciclovir is effective in preventing genital herpes recurrences, and it should be discussed with all HSV-2-infected patients (Table 28.2). Immune reconstitution improves the frequency and severity of clinical episodes of genital herpes, but it does not decrease shedding.

In individuals with a CD4+ T-cell count of less than 250 cells/mm^3 who will start ART, there is an increased risk of HSV-2 shedding and genital ulcer diseases in the first 6 months. It is recommended to give suppressive antiviral therapy because it decreases the risk of genital ulcer diseases by 60%.

VARICELLA ZOSTER VIRUS

Varicella zoster virus (VZV) causes initial infection in childhood (chickenpox) and later reactivates, causing herpes zoster. The prevalence of herpes zoster is 3% to 5% in the general population, but it is 15 to 25 times higher in PWH (Buchbinder et al., 1992). Lower CD4+ T-cell counts have been associated with more atypical presentations of the disease, but not with increased incidence.

CLINICAL PRESENTATION

The initial clinical presentation is similar to that in immunocompetent patients. It manifests as a prodrome of cutaneous burning or pain, followed by a cutaneous eruption of grouped vesicles on an erythematous base along a dermatome. However, PWH are at increased risk for multidermatomal or disseminated zoster, including neurologic and ophthalmologic complications. Approximately 20% to 30% of PWH will experience subsequent episodes of herpes zoster, either in the same or in different dermatomes. The probability of a recurrence of herpes zoster within 1 year of the index episode is 10% (Gebo et al., 2005). Postherpetic neuralgia is reported

Table 28.2 HSV SUPPRESSIVE THERAPY RECOMMENDATIONS

CONDITION	FIRST-CHOICE TREATMENT
Genital lesions	Valacyclovir 500 mg PO b.i.d. *or* Famciclovir 500 mg PO b.i.d. *or* Acyclovir 400–800 mg PO b.i.d. or t.i.d.

in 10% to 15% of PWH (Gebo et al., 2005; Harrison et al., 1999).

Atypical VZV presentations such as chronic hyperkeratotic lesions or chronic disseminated ecthyma have also been reported. Meningitis, multifocal leukoencephalitis, ventriculitis, myelitis, cranial nerve palsies, and focal brainstem lesions are possible neurologic complications.

Involvement of the ophthalmic division of the trigeminal nerve causes anterior uveitis, corneal scarring, and vision loss. Ocular involvement with acute retinal necrosis and progressive outer retinal necrosis is syndromes similar to CMV retinitis but of faster progression that typically occurs in those with CD4⁺ T-cell counts of less than 100 cells/mm³ and may result in retinal blindness (Engstrom et al., 1994).

DIAGNOSIS

The diagnosis is made clinically. Laboratory confirmation could be done by viral culture, direct immunofluorescence testing, and the PCR assay, which is the most sensitive test.

TREATMENT

VZV treatment is summarized in Table 28.3.

PREVENTION

Long-term prophylaxis or suppressive treatment is not recommended. VZV vaccine is recommended for PWH with CD4⁺ T-cell counts of 200 cells/mm³ or higher who have no documented history of vaccination or laboratory confirmation of disease. Primary varicella vaccination (Varivax) requires two doses administered 3 months apart. In the event that vaccination results in disease, acyclovir is recommended.

Postexposure prophylaxis is recommended for PWH who are susceptible to VZV and who have had close contact with a person who has active varicella or herpes zoster. The preferred regimen is a single intramuscular dose of VariZIG dosed on body weight (maximum of 625 IU) administered as soon as possible and within 10 days after exposure. Alternatively, acyclovir or valacyclovir could be given starting 7 to 10 days after exposure.

There are two vaccines available for the prevention of zoster: a live attenuated virus zoster vaccine (ZVL) and a non-live recombinant vaccine (RZV). ZVL was studied in a phase 2, randomized, double-blind, placebo-controlled clinical trial designed to evaluate its safety, tolerability, and immunogenicity in PWH on ART with CD4⁺ T-cell counts of 200 cells/mm³ or higher and virologic suppression (Benson et al., 2018). A total of 295 participants received the vaccine. ZVL was safe and immunogenic. Those with CD4⁺ T-cell counts of 350 cells/mm³ or higher developed the highest zoster antibody levels after vaccination. A small phase 1/2a, randomized, observer-masked, placebo-controlled study evaluated the safety and immunogenicity of RZV in 123 PWH. The vaccine was found to have a clinically acceptable safety profile and elicited strong gE-specific cell-mediated and anti-gE humoral immune responses that persisted at least 1 year after the last vaccination (Berkowitz et al., 2015). The Advisory Committee for Immunization Practices does not recommend

Table 28.3 VZV TREATMENT RECOMMENDATIONS

CONDITION	FIRST-CHOICE TREATMENT
VZV infection, immunocompromised patients	SEVERE: Acyclovir 10–15 mg/kg IV every 8 hours for 7–10 days. May switch to PO if no evidence of visceral involvement. UNCOMPLICATED: Valacyclovir (1 g PO 3 times daily) *or* famciclovir (500 mg PO 3 times daily) for 5 to 7 days.
Herpes zoster, acute localized dermatomal	Valacyclovir 1 g t.i.d. *or* Famciclovir 500 mg t.i.d. *or* Acyclovir 800 mg PO 5 times daily, each administered for 7–10 days Consider longer duration if lesions slow to resolve.
Herpes zoster, extensive cutaneous lesion or visceral involvement	Acyclovir 10–15 mg/kg IV every 8 hours After clinical improvement is evident, switch to oral therapy: Valacyclovir 1 g t.i.d. *or* Famciclovir 500 mg t.i.d. *or* Acyclovir 800 mg 5 times daily, each administered for 10–14 days
Acute retinal necrosis	Acyclovir 10 mg/kg IV every 8 hours for 10–14 days, followed by oral valacyclovir 1 g t.i.d. for 6 weeks *plus* Ganciclovir 2 mg/0.05 mL intravitreal twice weekly × 1 or 2 doses
Progressive outer retinal necrosis	Ganciclovir 5 mg/kg IV *and/or* Foscarnet 90 mg/kg IV every 12 hours *plus* Ganciclovir 2 mg/0.05 mL intravitreal twice weekly × 1 or 2 doses
Acyclovir-resistant VZV infection	Foscarnet 90 mg/kg IV every 12 hours

using RZV in PWH due to limited data. However, experts do recommend administering RZV to PWH who are older than 50 years, considering the increased risk of herpes zoster in PWH. RZV is preferred over ZLV due to higher efficacy data in immunocompetent patients (OI Guidelines, AIII). ZLV can be given as an alternative in PWH with CD4 counts above 200 cells/mm³ in case of unavailability of RZV or intolerance to it (OI Guidelines, BIII). ZVL is contraindicated in PWH with CD4 counts below 200 cells/mm³ as it can lead to disseminated ZVL vaccine strain infection (OI Guidelines, AIII).

CMV

CMV is a DNA herpesvirus and the largest virus that infects humans. It is typically acquired from close contact during youth or adolescence. In the general population, the percentage of people with evidence of previous CMV infection ranges from 40% to 100% and varies with ethnicity and country. Active disease associated with HIV typically results from reactivation of latent infection in the setting of advanced immunosuppression with CD4⁺ T-cell counts of less than 50 cells/mm³ (Dieterich et al., 1991). Other risk factors for CMV disease include plasma HIV RNA levels of more than 100,000 copies/mL and the presence of other OIs.

Before the use of ART, CMV retinitis was the most common intraocular infection in patients with AIDS, occurring in up to 40% of patients (Whitcup et al., 2000). Currently, the incidence of new cases of CMV end-organ disease has declined to fewer than 6 cases/100 person-years (Jabs et al., 2007).

CLINICAL PRESENTATION AND DIAGNOSIS

CMV can infect different organs of the body. Retinitis accounts for 85% of CMV manifestations and is the leading cause of vision loss among people with AIDS. Other CMV clinical syndromes include esophagitis, colitis, polyradiculopathy, ventriculoencephalitis, pneumonitis, adrenalitis, and pancreatitis.

Chorioretinitis
CMV chorioretinitis presents with painless progressive loss of vision, floaters, and/or visual field cut defects. Symptoms are unilateral at first, but without treatment they can become bilateral. The diagnosis is exclusively made by recognition of typical retinal changes during a funduscopic examination: creamy or yellow-white granular areas with perivascular exudates and hemorrhage. These lesions initially are found in the periphery of the fundus but can later involve the macula and the optic disc, resulting in blindness.

Colitis
CMV colitis is the second most common manifestation of CMV infection in people with AIDS. Patients present with severe diarrhea, abdominal pain and cramping, anorexia, weight loss, and fever. The diagnosis is made by detection of mucosal ulcerations on endoscopic examination combined with colonoscopic or rectal biopsy. Pathology will reveal intracytoplasmic or intranuclear inclusions. A positive culture itself does not confirm the diagnosis. Mucosal hemorrhage and perforation rarely occur, but they are life-threatening.

Esophagitis
CMV esophagitis causes odynophagia, nausea, fever, and retrosternal pain. Diagnosis is made by endoscopic examination that reveals diffuse inflammation of the esophagus and/or esophageal ulcers. Biopsy specimens also reveal intranuclear inclusions. A positive culture itself does not make the diagnosis.

CMV Polyradiculopathy
CMV polyradiculopathy presents with sacrolumbar radicular pain and lower limb paresthesia that may develop into progressive flaccid paralysis of the legs with decreasing and ultimately absent tendon reflexes. Urinary retention and stool incontinence may occur. If untreated, the condition rapidly advances up the spine, causing ascending sensory loss and growing flaccidity in the upper limbs, similar to Guillain–Barré paralysis. The CSF may have a pleocytosis with a predominance of polymorphonuclear cells, elevated protein, and moderately low glucose. Lumbar MRI reveals gadolinium enhancement of the cauda equina in 33% of patients. Diagnosis is made by viral culture, CMV antigen assays, and detection of CMV DNA via PCR in the CSF.

Ventriculoencephalitis
CMV ventriculoencephalitis is a late manifestation of CMV disease. It presents with fever, lethargy, confusion, and an acute course consisting of cranial nerve palsies, nystagmus, and other focal neurologic deficits that rapidly leads to death. CT and MRI scans show white matter enhancement. MRI with gadolinium may reveal a characteristic periventricular ring-like enhancement. Viral culture of the CSF is not always positive, although CMV DNA can often be detected in CSF using PCR.

Dementia
CMV dementia can present with fever, lethargy, and confusion, and it may be clinically similar to dementia caused directly by HIV. CSF reveals pleocytosis that may be polymorphonuclear, low to normal glucose, and normal to high protein. CT and MRI scans may show cerebral atrophy.

Pneumonia
CMV pneumonitis is uncommon in patients with AIDS. Symptoms include shortness of breath, dyspnea, dry nonproductive cough, and hypoxia. Imaging studies show diffuse interstitial infiltrates. A definitive diagnosis is made when multiple CMV inclusion bodies are seen in lung tissue. CMV may be isolated in bronchial washings and lavage fluid from approximately 50% of PWH undergoing bronchoscopy secondary to viral shedding.

CMV viremia is common in asymptomatic persons with low CD4⁺ T-cell counts (<100 cells/mm³). Viremia is typically present in active disease but may also be present in the absence of end-organ disease, so the tests are of limited value.

The absence of CMV antibody may be helpful in excluding CMV disease; however, active disease can rarely present during primary CMV infection with negative antibodies, and immunoglobin G antibody tests may revert to negative in individuals with advanced immunosuppression.

TREATMENT

Table 28.4 shows the current treatment recommendations from the Guidelines for the Prevention and Treatment of Opportunistic Infections (Department of Health and Human Services, 2020).

For CMV chorioretinitis, treatment consists of an induction phase of high-dose drug given for at least 2 weeks. Once retinitis is stable, patients are placed on chronic maintenance therapy until there is evidence of immune recovery (sustained CD4$^+$ T-cell counts >100 cells/mm^3 for at least 6 months). In the absence of antiretroviral-mediated immune reconstitution, most patients will have a reactivation of CMV infection despite suppressive therapy and will require reinduction therapy. Intraocular therapy may be useful in salvage therapy for patients who cannot tolerate systemic therapy. Any local therapy should be accompanied by systemic anti-CMV therapy. Systemic therapy has been shown to decrease CMV involvement of the contralateral eye, to reduce the risk of CMV disease in other organs, and to increase survival rates. Intraocular therapy alone has been associated with progression of CMV to the contralateral eye, as well as with systemic disease (Martin et al., 1994).

Ganciclovir and valganciclovir, foscarnet, and cidofovir carry significant risk for toxicity. Ganciclovir and valganciclovir can cause neutropenia, thrombocytopenia, nausea, diarrhea, renal dysfunction, and central venous catheter infection. Foscarnet more commonly causes nephrotoxicity, electrolyte abnormalities, seizures, genital ulcers, and central venous catheter infection. Cidofovir, when used, is associated with nephrotoxicity and intraocular hypotony.

PREVENTION/PROPHYLAXIS

In patients with CD4$^+$ T-cell counts of less than 100 cells/mm^3, early recognition of the manifestations of end-organ CMV disease is the primary method of prevention. Primary prophylaxis against CMV is not recommended. Patients with CD4$^+$ T-cell counts of less than 100 cells/mm^3 should have an annual ophthalmology exam. Secondary prophylaxis is done with valganciclovir until the CD4$^+$ T-cell count has been greater than 100 cells/mm^3 for 3 to 6 months and the lesions

Table 28.4 CMV TREATMENT RECOMMENDATIONS

CONDITION	FIRST-CHOICE TREATMENT	ALTERNATIVE TREATMENT
CMV retinitis	*For sight-threatening lesions:* Intravitreal injections Ganciclovir or foscarnet *plus* Valganciclovir 900 mg PO b.i.d. for 14–21 days, then once daily *For small peripheral lesions:* Valganciclovir 900 mg PO bid for 14–21 days, then 900 mg once daily *Or any of the alternative treatments*	Intravitreal injections Ganciclovir or foscarnet *plus* Ganciclovir 5 mg/kg IV every 12 hours for 14–21 days, then 5 mg/kg IV daily *or* Ganciclovir 5 mg/kg IV every 12 hours for 14–21 days, then valganciclovir 900 mg PO daily Foscarnet 60 mg/kg IV every 8 hours *or* Foscarnet 90 mg/kg IV every 12 hours for 14–21 days, then 90–120 mg/kg IV every 24 hours *or* Cidofovir 5 mg/kg/week IV for 2 weeks, then 5 mg/kg every other week with saline hydration and probenecid 2 g PO 3 hours before the dose followed by 1 g 2 hours and 8 hours after the dose (total of 4 g)
Secondary prophylaxis (previously called maintenance therapy) for CMV retinitis	Valganciclovir 900 mg PO daily *or* Ganciclovir implant (replaced every 6–8 months if CD4$^+$ count remains <100 cells/mm^3) *plus* Valganciclovir 900 mg PO daily until immune recovery	Ganciclovir 5 mg/kg IV 5–7 times weekly *or* Foscarnet 90–120 mg/kg body weight IV once daily *or* Cidofovir 5 mg/kg body weight IV every other week as above
CMV colitis or esophagitis	Ganciclovir IV *or* Foscarnet IV for 21–28 days	
CMV neurologic disease	Ganciclovir IV *plus* Foscarnet IV until symptomatic improvement	

IV, intravenous; PO, orally.

are not life-threatening. If the CD4$^+$ T-cell count decreases to less than 100 cells/mm^3, secondary prophylaxis should be reinstituted.

HUMAN HERPESVIRUS-8

The prevalence of human herpesvirus-8 (HHV-8) ranges between 1% and 5% in the general population but is between 20% and 77% in MSM (Pauk et al., 2000). HHV-8 is associated with all forms of Kaposi's sarcoma, primary effusion lymphoma, and lymphoproliferative disorders such as multicentric Castleman's disease (see Chapter 29).

JC VIRUS

JC virus causes PML, a disease characterized by focal demyelination. Approximately 85% of adults worldwide are seropositive for JC virus. Most individuals usually are exposed to JC virus in childhood, which causes asymptomatic infection and chronic asymptomatic carrier state (Antonsson et al., 2010; Knowles et al., 2006). The incidence of PML has decreased significantly since the widespread use of ART. However, PML has also been reported in PWH with CD4$^+$ T-cell counts of greater than 300 cells/mm^3 and as a complication of IRIS (Berger et al., 1998; Cinque et al., 2003).

CLINICAL PRESENTATION

The clinical presentation of PML depends on the location of brain lesions, and the specific deficits vary from patient to patient. Commonly involved areas are the occipital lobe, which presents with hemianopsia; the frontal and parietal lobes, which can present with aphasia, hemiparesis, and hemisensory deficits; and the cerebellar peduncles and deep white matter, which can present with dysmetria and ataxia (Richardson et al., 1983). The spinal cord is rarely involved. The optic nerves are spared (Bernal-Cano et al., 2007). Patients present with symptoms ranging from diffuse encephalopathy to focal deficits such as ataxia, hemiparesis, or speech difficulties. Symptoms tend to progress rapidly over several weeks to months. Seizures are seen in 20% of cases. Headache and fever are unusual in PML; if present, the possibility of another OI should be considered.

DIAGNOSIS

MRI of the brain demonstrates distinct white matter lesions in areas of the brain corresponding to the clinical deficits. The lesions are usually white on T2 images, and they are also characteristically dark on T1 images. PCR detection of the JC virus in CSF is recommended to confirm the diagnosis and has diagnostic sensitivity of 70% to 80% and specificity of 100% (Cinque et al., 1997). Brain biopsy, which is used to make a definitive diagnosis, will reveal the typical findings of focal myelin loss with characteristic astrocytes and lipid-laden macrophages. Due to high JC virus seroprevalence, serologic testing is not recommended.

PREVENTION

Early initiation of ART in order to prevent HIV-related immunosuppression is the only effective modality for prevention of PML (OI Guidelines, AII).

TREATMENT

Initiation of effective ART is the treatment of choice. It prolongs survival and improves neurologic deficits when immune reconstitution is achieved. The early use of a five-drug ARV regimen after PML diagnosis appears to improve survival (Gasnault et al., 2011). Other treatments have been attempted with no improvement in survival. Recrudescence after remission of PML with ART is extremely rare, but a couple of cases have been reported (Cinque et al., 2001; Crossley et al., 2016).

PML-IRIS

PML-IRIS may occur after ART initiation in people with advanced HIV infection with low CD4 counts and presents with different clinical and radiologic findings as compared to classical PML. Radiologic findings of lesions with contrast enhancement, edema, and mass effect have been reported (Post et al., 2013). Both onset and paradoxical worsening of PML can occur in ART-induced IRIS, and in many studies, empiric use of corticosteroids has been seen to be beneficial. The dose and duration of treatment with corticosteroids are yet to be established (Cinque et al., 2009; Fournier et al., 2017; Tan et al., 2009).

REFERENCES

Antonsson A, Green AC, Mallitt KA, et al. Prevalence and stability of antibodies to the BK and JC polyomaviruses: a long-term longitudinal study of Australians. *J Gen Virol.* 2010;91(Pt 7):1849–1853.

Benson CA, Andersen JW, Macatangay BJC, et al. Safety and immunogenicity of Zoster [JWOY1] vaccine live in HIV-positive adults with CD4+ cell counts above 200 cells/mL virologically suppressed on antiretroviral therapy. *Clin Infect Dis.* 2018;67(11):1712–1719.

Berger JR, Levy RM, Flomenhoft D. Predictive factors for prolonged survival in acquired immunodeficiency syndrome-associated progressive multifocal leukoencephalopathy. *Ann Neurol.* 1998;44:341–349.

Berkowitz EM, Moyle G, Stellbrink HJ, et al. Safety and immunogenicity of an adjuvanted herpes zoster subunit candidate vaccine in HIV-positive adults: a phase 1/2a randomized, placebo-controlled study. *J Infect Dis.* 2015;211(8):1279–1287.

Bernal-Cano F, Joseph JT, Koralnik IJ. Spinal cord lesions of progressive multifocal leukoencephalopathy in an acquired immunodeficiency syndrome patient. *J Neurovirol.* 2007;13(5):474–476. https://www.ncbi.nlm.nih.gov/pubmed/17994433

Blanc FX, Sok T, Laureillard, D, et al. Earlier versus later start of antiretroviral therapy in HIV-positive adults with tuberculosis. *N Engl J Med.* 2011;365(16):1471–1481.

Borisov AS, Bamrah Morris S, Njie GJ. Update of recommendations for use of once-weekly isoniazid-rifapentine regimen to treat latent *Mycobacterium tuberculosis* infection. *MMWR Morb Mortal Wkly Rep.* 2018;67(25):723–726.

Cattamanchi A, Smith R, Steingart KR, et al. Interferon-gamma release assays for the diagnosis of latent tuberculosis infection in HIV-infected individuals: a systematic review and meta-analysis. *J AIDS.* 2011;56(3):230–238.

Centers for Disease Control and Prevention. Recommendations for human immunodeficiency virus (HIV) screening in tuberculosis (TB) clinics. Factsheet. Atlanta, GA: US Department of Health and Human Services, CDC; 2012. https://www.cdc.gov/tb/publications/factsheets/testing/HIVscreening.pdf

Centers for Disease Control and Prevention. Reported tuberculosis in the United States, 2018. Atlanta, GA: US Department of Health and Human Services, CDC; 2019.

Daley CL, Iaccarino JM, Lang C, et al. Treatment of nontuberculous mycobacterial pulmonary disease: an official ATS/ERS/ESCMID/IDSA clinical practice guideline. *Clin Infect Dis*. 2020;71(4):e1–e36.

Department of Health and Human Services. Guidelines for prevention and treatment of opportunistic infections in HIV-infected adults and adolescents. 2020. https://aidsinfo.nih.gov/guidelines/html/4/adult-and-adolescent-opportunistic-infection/325/tb

Griffith DE. Management of disease due to *Mycobacterium kansasii*. *Clin Chest Med*. 2002;23:613–621.

Griffith DE, Aksamit T, Brown-Elliott BA, et al. An official ATS/IDSA statement: diagnosis, treatment, and prevention of nontuberculous mycobacterial diseases. *Am J Respir Crit Care Med*. 2007;175:367–416.

Karim SSA, Naidoo K, Grobler A, et al. Integration of antiretroviral therapy with tuberculosis treatment. *N Engl J Med*. 2011; 365(16):1492–1501.

Martinson NA, Hoffmann CJ, Chaisson RE. Epidemiology of tuberculosis and HIV. *Proc Am Thorac Soc*. 2011;8:288–293.

Meintjes G, Stek C, Blumenthal L, et al. Prednisone for the prevention of paradoxical tuberculosis-associated IRIS. *N Engl J Med*. 2018;379:1915–1925.

Mfinanga SG, Kirenga BJ, Chanda DM, et al. Early versus delayed initiation of highly active antiretroviral therapy for HIV-positive adults with newly diagnosed pulmonary tuberculosis (TB-HAART): a prospective, international, randomised, placebo-controlled trial. *Lancet Infect Dis*. 2014;14:563–571.

Nahid P, Dorman SE, Alipanah N, et al. Official American Thoracic Society/Centers for Disease Control and Prevention/Infectious Diseases Society of America clinical practice guidelines: treatment of drug-susceptible tuberculosis. *Clin Infect Dis*. 2016;63(7):e147–e195. doi:10.1093/cid/ciw376

Santin M, Munoz L, Rigau D. Interferon-γ release assays for the diagnosis of tuberculosis and tuberculosis infection in HIV-infected adults: a systematic review and meta-analysis. *PLoS One*. 2012;7(3):332482.

Swindells S, Ramchandani R, Gupta A, et al. One month of rifapentine plus isoniazid to prevent HIV-related tuberculosis. *N Engl J Med*. 2019;380:1001–1011. doi:10.1056/NEJMoa1806808

Workowski KA, Berman S. Sexually transmitted diseases treatment guidelines, 2010. *MMWR Recomm Rep*. 2010;59(RR-12):1–110.

Workowski KA, Bolan GA. Sexually transmitted diseases treatment guidelines, 2015. *MMWR Recomm Rep*. 2015;64(RR-03):1–137.

World Health Organization. Global tuberculosis report 2019. https://apps.who.int/iris/bitstream/handle/10665/329368/9789241565714-eng.pdf?ua=1

World Health Organization. HIV-associated tuberculosis factsheet 2018. https://www.who.int/tb/areas-of-work/tb-hiv/tbhiv_factsheet.pdf?ua=1

29.

MALIGNANCIES IN HIV

Eva H. Clark and Elizabeth Y. Chiao

CHAPTER GOALS

Upon completion of this chapter, the reader should be able to:

- Review the epidemiology and role of antiretroviral therapy (ART) on the impact of AIDS-defining malignancies, which remain common among people with HIV (PWH)

- Discuss the role of human herpes virus-8 (HHV-8) in the development of Kaposi's sarcoma (KS), which remains the most common tumor associated with HIV infection

- Discuss the role of Epstein–Barr virus (EBV) in primary central nervous system (CNS) lymphoma and other HIV-associated lymphomas

- Review the role of human papillomavirus (HPV) vaccination in virally mediated anogenital squamous cell cancers in both men and women

- Discuss non–AIDS-defining malignancies, including lung, prostate, oropharyngeal, liver, breast, and pancreatic cancer

- Emphasize that ART initiation is of utmost importance for all AIDS-defining malignancies and non–AIDS-defining malignancies and summarize National Cancer Center Network Guidelines for HIV malignancies

INTRODUCTION

LEARNING OBJECTIVE

- Discuss the role of virally mediated and non-virally mediated AIDS-associated and non–AIDS-associated malignancies

WHAT'S NEW?

Use of integrase inhibitors, the newest class of antiretrovirals (ARVs), makes concurrent chemotherapeutic options safer and more feasible for many patients.

KEY POINTS

- Malignancies in PWH remain a major health concern and are one of the leading causes of death among PWH.

- ART continues to influence the epidemiology of malignancies, with decreasing rates overall.

Malignancies were one of the earliest recognized manifestations that led to the eventual description of the AIDS epidemic. KS became one of the first entities described in association with AIDS (Ziegler et al., 1984). Subsequently, intermediate-grade and high-grade non-Hodgkin's lymphoma (NHL), invasive cervical cancer, and primary central nervous system lymphoma (PCNSL) were defined by the US Centers for Disease Control and Prevention (CDC, 2008) as "AIDS-defining conditions." Since the advent of combination ART, several other cancers that are not AIDS-defining have been found to have an increased incidence in PWH. These include, but are not limited to, Hodgkin's disease and anal, liver, lung, oropharyngeal, colorectal, and renal cancers (Patel et al., 2008). They are generally referred to as "non–AIDS-defining cancers" (NADCs). The increasing longevity of PWH as well as concurrent modifiable risk factors such as tobacco use may also influence the epidemiology of these malignancies.

The introduction of combination ART in the mid-1990s has significantly impacted the clinical history and outcomes of PWH. In addition to changing the natural history of HIV disease in terms of survival and incidence of opportunistic diseases, it has also dramatically decreased the incidence of viral-mediated HIV-associated malignancies, such as KS and PCNSL (Silverberg et al., 2015). Even so, cancer remains a significant concern for PWH. A large US registry linkage study during the post-ART era included 448,258 PWH from 1996 to 2012 (Hernández-Ramírez et al., 2017). It found an elevated risk for development of cancer overall (standardized incidence ratio [SIR], 1.69; 95% confidence interval [CI], 1.67–1.72), AIDS-defining cancers (KS [498.11, 477.82–519.03], NHL [11.51, 11.14–11.89], and cervical cancer [3.24, 2.94–3.56]), most other virus-related cancers (e.g., anal [19.06, 18.13–20.03], liver [3.21, 3.02–3.41], and Hodgkin's lymphoma [7.70, 7.20–8.23]), as well as several virus-unrelated cancers (e.g., lung [1.97, 1.89–2.05]) (Hernández-Ramírez et al., 2017). However, their SIRs significantly decreased over the study period for KS, two subtypes of NHL, and cancers of the anus, liver, and lung, although they remained elevated above that of the general population. SIRs did not increase over time for any cancer. In addition, cancer risk appears to be higher for older PWH. When this same dataset was stratified by age, PWH older than 50 years were more likely to develop KS (SIR, 103.34), NHL (3.05), Hodgkin's lymphoma (7.61), and cervical (2.02), anal (14.00), lung (1.71), liver (2.91), and oral cavity/pharyngeal (1.66) cancers but were less likely to develop breast (0.61), prostate (0.47), and colon (0.63) cancers (Mahale et al., 2018) compared to the general population. Furthermore, recent data indicate that PWH have an increased risk for not only these cancers initially, but also for developing a second primary cancer (Hessol et al., 2018; Mahale et al., 2020).

Although cancer mortality remains high in PWH, it has declined over time. A recent US population-based HIV and cancer registry study found that cancer-attributed mortality for PWH was 386.9 per 100,000 person-years (including 9.2% of deaths from NADCs and 5.0% of deaths from AIDS-defining cancers) (Horner et al., 2020). In this study, most cancer deaths were due to NHL (3.5%), lung cancer (2.4%), KS (1.3%), liver cancer (1.1%), and anal cancer (0.6%), and cancer mortality was highest among PWH 60 years or older.

Management of malignancies in PWH presents the clinician with many challenges, including the risk of further compromise to the immune system of PWH receiving chemotherapy, toxicities of treatment, pharmacologic interaction between ART and chemotherapy drugs, and the risk of intercurrent opportunistic infections (Reid et al., 2018). The safety profile and the feasibility of ART administration with concurrent chemotherapy have improved with the introduction and increased use of integrase inhibitors during the past several years. Guidelines for managing cancer in PWH were released in 2018 by the National Comprehensive Cancer Network (NCCN) (Reid et al., 2018). They advise that PWH who develop cancer should be cared for by both an oncologist and an HIV specialist and should receive cancer therapy according to standard guidelines developed for the general population. The patient's ART may need to be modified if there are potential interactions with the proposed cancer therapy, but generally ART should be continued during cancer therapy.

This chapter reviews the malignancies most commonly associated with HIV, along with other non-HIV-associated cancers that PWH often develop.

RECOMMENDED READING

Horner MJ, Shiels MS, Pfeiffer RM, et al. Deaths attributable to cancer in the United States HIV population during 2001–2015. *Clin Infect Dis*. 2020;ciaa1016 [E-pub before print]. doi:10.1093/cid/ciaa1016

Reid E, Suneja G, Ambinder RF, et al. Cancer in people living with HIV, Version 1.2018, NCCN clinical practice guidelines in oncology. *J Natl Compr Canc Netw*. 2018;16(8):986–1017.

Shiels MS, Islam JY, Rosenberg PS, et al. Projected cancer incidence rates and burden of incident cancer cases in HIV-infected adults in the United States through 2030. *Ann Intern Med*. 2018;168(12):866–873. doi:10.7326/M17-2499

Silverberg MJ, Lau B, Achenbach CJ, et al. Cumulative incidence of cancer among persons with HIV in North America. *Ann Intern Med*. 2015;163(7):507–518.

Silverberg MJ, Leyden W, Hernandez-Ramirez RU, et al. Timing of antiretroviral therapy initiation and risk of cancer among persons living with HIV. *Clin Infect Dis*. 2020;ciaa1046 [E-pub before print]. doi:10.1093/cid/ciaa1046

KAPOSI'S SARCOMA

LEARNING OBJECTIVES

- Discuss the epidemiology of KS
- Discuss the pathogenesis and clinical manifestations
- Review the treatments for KS, including local and systemic therapies

WHAT'S NEW?

The incidence of KS continues to decline with the use of ART, but it remains significantly elevated in areas with endemic disease, such as sub-Saharan Africa. Several novel therapies have been studied for HIV-related KS.

KEY POINTS

- The presence of HHV-8 and advanced immunosuppression are both associated with risk of KS development and other lymphoproliferative states, such as multicentric Castleman's disease and primary body cavity lymphoma.
- Treatment for KS includes ART, local therapy, and systemic therapy.
- The goals of treatment are suppressive and generally noncurative.

Chemotherapy and radiotherapy are palliative treatments for KS. In general, treatment decisions and referrals to oncology should be based on evidence of symptomatic or systemic disease. Radiotherapy should be avoided in the pelvis and lower extremities because of damage to the lymphatics and the potential for lymphedema and skin breakdown.

EPIDEMIOLOGY

KS was first described in 1872 by Moritz Kaposi, a Hungarian dermatologist. Four types of KS have been described: classic, endemic, transplant-associated, and AIDS-associated or epidemic KS. Classic KS is typically seen in elderly men of Mediterranean or Eastern European descent and is characterized by cutaneous lesions of the lower extremities (Iscovich et al., 2000). The endemic form, found primarily in sub-Saharan Africa, often is more aggressive and morbid, with visceral involvement (Friedman-Kien & Saltzman, 1990).

Transplant-associated KS was first described in the 1970s and is seen in immunosuppressed allograft recipients. Although cutaneous disease is often the most common presentation, visceral disease has been described in multiple organs (Penn, 1979).

AIDS-associated KS was first described in gay men in the early 1980s, at the advent of the HIV epidemic (Friedman-Kien, 1981). This malignancy disproportionately affected gay men with AIDS, who were estimated to have a 20-fold higher risk of developing KS compared to other HIV transmission risk groups (Beral et al., 1990; Hoover et al., 1993). KS is rarely reported in intravenous drug users or other HIV risk groups (Mitsuyasu et al., 1984; Safai et al., 1987).

The incidence of KS in resource-abundant countries has declined markedly since the early 1990s with the widespread use of ART. Of 85,922 cases of KS in the US evaluated by Shiels et al. between 1990 and 2007, the proportion of KS in persons with AIDS declined from 89% in 1990 to 1995 to 67% in 2001 to 2007 ($p < 0.001$) (Shiels et al., 2011). Cumulative incidence of KS by age 75 years was among the highest compared to other cancers (lung, anal, colorectal, Hodgkin's lymphoma, liver, and oropharyngeal) from 1995 to 2009 at 4.1%. However, there were significant decreases in incidence of KS by 4% per year from 2005 to 2009 compared to 1996–1999 rates ($p < 0.01$) (Silverberg et al., 2015). Similarly, the Swiss HIV Cohort Study showed that the KS incidence was 33.3 per 1,000 patient-years (py) in 1984–1986 and did not change significantly in the subsequent periods until 1996–1998, when it declined to 5.1 per 1,000 py (95% CI, 3.9–6.5) during that time period and then further decreased to 1.4 per 1,000 py in 1999–2001 and remained constant thereafter (Franceschi et al., 2008). A Brazilian retrospective cohort also described a decreased incidence of KS from 1998 to 2010, with an incidence rate ratio per year of 0.89 (95% CI, 0.83–0.97) (Castilho et al., 2015). In 2010, KS accounted for approximately 12% of cancers diagnosed in PWH (Robbins et al., 2015).

Despite the overall decline in KS, there remain concerning differences in improvement in traditionally underserved racial and geographic groups. Between 2001 and 2013, Royse et al. evaluated 4,455 KS cases in US men and determined that the annual percent change (APC) for KS incidence significantly decreased for White men between 2001 and 2013 (APC −4.52, $p = 0.02$); however, the APC for African American men was not significant (APC −1.84, $p = 0.09$), and the APC among Southern African American men significantly increased (+3.0, $p = 0.03$) (Royse et al., 2017).

In areas of southern Africa where KS is endemic, this cancer reached epidemic proportions during the initial AIDS epidemic due to lack of ART. For instance, in Zimbabwe, KS was reported to represent 40% of all cancers in men (Chokunonga et al., 2000). A prospective cohort from 2004 to 2010 found that the incidence in Zimbabwe, Botswana, South Africa, and Zambia reached 413 per 100,000 py (95% CI, 342–497), with higher rates among age groups older than 60 years (Rohner et al., 2014). Despite the increased availability of ART in these countries, estimates of KS have minimally decreased in the HIV population on ART, with the incidence of KS remaining high at 164 per 100,000 py (95% CI, 151–178) (Rohner et al., 2014). Individuals with KS in this geographic region have high tumor burdens and aggressive disease progression, and survival from time of diagnosis is often less than 6 months (Campbell et al., 2003).

PATHOGENESIS

In 1994, Chang and Moore (Chang, 1994) discovered a new herpesvirus, HHV-8 or KS herpes virus (KSHV), in more than 90% of AIDS-KS tissue samples. Although the KS types vary in epidemiology and clinical presentation, all are associated with HHV-8. In 2003, HHV-8 viremia was shown to be an early marker of KS, and the risk of developing disease was demonstrated to increase with HHV-8 antibody titers (Engels et al., 2003; Newton et al., 2003). HHV-8 also is associated with rare lymphoproliferative diseases most often seen in individuals with HIV, including multicentric Castleman's disease and a rare form of NHL called primary effusion or body cavity lymphoma. Although infection with KSHV is necessary for the development of KSHV-associated disease, it is not sufficient; in fact, HHV-8 viremia is prevalent only in a subset of cases. In an analysis of 335 patients with HIV-associated KS, only 130 (39%) were viremic, and the mean HHV-8 viral load was only moderate with 6,630 DNA copies/mL (Haq et al., 2016). Among individuals with HIV, immunosuppression confers the greatest risk and is most predictive of development of KS (Jacobson et al., 2000; Renwick et al., 1998).

The pathogenesis of KS is complex and involves viral processes and dysregulation of cytokine pathways. The HHV-8 genome encodes many homologs of human cellular gene products that are involved in inflammation, cell cycle regulation, and angiogenesis, such as viral cyclin-D1, vascular endothelial growth factor (VEGF), basic fibroblast growth factor, and interleukin-6 (IL-6) (Cannon et al., 2000). Much work has been done on the tumorigenesis of KS. KSHV infection leads to upregulation of Toll-like receptor 4 (TLR4), its adaptor MyD88, and coreceptors CD14 and MD2 (Gruffaz et al., 2018). The TLR4 pathway seems to be activated constitutively in KSHV-transformed cells, resulting in chronic induction of IL-6, IL-1β, and IL-18. IL-6 production in turn results in activation of the STAT3 pathway, an essential event for uncontrolled cellular proliferation and transformation. Gruffaz et al. have shown that TLR4 stimulation with lipopolysaccharides or live bacteria enhanced tumorigenesis, while TLR4 antagonist CLI095 inhibited it. A regulatory transactivating (tat) protein of HIV is released by infected cells and guards KS cells from apoptosis (Deregibus et al., 2002), stimulates growth and angiogenesis (Barillari & Ensoli, 2002; Ensoli et al., 1990), and also increases the production and release of matrix metalloproteinases (MMPs) from endothelial and inflammatory cells. MMPs contribute to the angiogenesis found in KS lesions (Impola et al., 2003; Lafrenie et al., 1996). Clinically, KSHV-mediated systemic inflammation that develops in patients without Kaposi Sarcoma Herpesvirus (KSHV)-Associated Multicentric Castleman Disease (-MCD) is recognized as KSHV-inflammatory cytokine syndrome (KICS) (Polizzotto et al., 2016a).

The mechanism of HHV-8 transmissibility remains unclear. HHV-8 has been detected in semen, prostate tissue (Monini et al., 1996), and breast milk (Dedicoat et al., 2004). The virus is often shed from the oropharynx of both immunocompetent and immunocompromised men and women in areas where KSHV is endemic (Casper et al., 2004, 2007). Behaviors associated with exposure to saliva are correlated with a higher risk of KSHV infection, implicating both sexual and horizontal transmission (Casper et al., 2006; Plancoulaine et al., 2000). A relatively high KSHV seroprevalence has been described among injection drug users, and an increased incidence of KSHV infection has been noted among transfusion recipients in areas where KSHV is endemic, suggesting that parenteral transmission may be possible (Cannon et al., 2001; Hladik et al., 2006). Finally, transmission of KSHV from donors of solid organs has been described (Barozzi et al., 2003; Luppi et al., 2000).

CLINICAL MANIFESTATIONS

KS is an angioproliferative disease varying from an indolent to fulminant disease with potential for significant morbidity and mortality. The disease can occur in patients with a wide range of CD4+ cell counts but becomes increasingly common as immune function declines. The progression of disease may be rapid or slow. Patients with limited disease and controlled HIV infection usually do reasonably well. However, in the setting of uncontrolled HIV viral replication and low CD4+ counts, KS progresses rapidly.

The skin is the most common site of presentation. Visceral involvement also occurs, and, as the disease progresses, KS frequently involves the gastrointestinal (GI) tract. At autopsy, almost every organ system can show involvement. Visceral disease is rare in the absence of extensive cutaneous disease.

The cutaneous presentation of KS occurs in 95% of cases. Lesions may occur anywhere on the skin. Common sites include the face (particularly the periorbital area and tip of the nose), external ear, mouth, torso, and lower extremities. They can evolve from macules or nodular tumors to large plaque-like tumor masses that involve extensive cutaneous surfaces and eventually evolve into ulcerating tumors. Their color may vary from violaceous in light-skinned individuals to brownish-black in dark-skinned individuals. These lesions are generally nonblanching, and nonpruritic. Lesions of KS may be associated with some pain, particularly in the setting of immune reconstitution inflammatory syndrome (IRIS).

Lymphedema associated with KS usually appears in patients with visible cutaneous lesions, and edema may be out of proportion to the extent of visible lesions. Lymphedema also may occur in patients with no visible skin lesions. Common sites include the face, neck, external genitals, and lower extremities. A contiguous area of skin usually is involved as well.

Oral cavity involvement is seen in approximately one-third of KS patients and is the initial site of diagnosis 15% of the time (Dezube et al., 2004). These lesions may be flat or nodular and are red or purplish. They usually appear on the hard palate, but they may develop on the soft palate, gingival areas, and tongue. Oral lesions, if extensive, may cause tooth loss, pain, and ulceration. Involvement of the oral cavity correlates with KS in the GI tract.

GI KS has been reported in 40% of cases at initial diagnosis (Dezube et al., 2004) with any segment of the GI tract involved. Visceral spread of KS that involves the GI tract is rarely symptomatic. However, with disease progression, patients may have symptoms of abdominal pain, nausea, vomiting, or GI bleeding (Danzig et al., 1991). Rare cases of obstruction, perforation, or protein-losing enteropathy have been reported (Friedman, 1988). In those with advanced immunosuppression (CD4+ T-cell count <100 cells/mm³), GI KS may be more severe with complications. Some believe that screening endoscopy to detect occult disease may be warranted in these patients (Nagata et al., 2012).

Pulmonary KS is also common; however, in contrast to KS at other visceral sites, lung involvement is generally symptomatic. Common symptoms include cough, bronchospasm, dyspnea, and hemoptysis. This complication tends to occur in the setting of advanced AIDS, with most individuals having CD4+ cell counts of less than 100 cells/mm³ (Gill et al., 1989), and in patients with more extensive cutaneous disease (e.g., with >50 lesions). Of note, it can occur in patients with minimal and absent cutaneous KS. The disease is often rapidly progressive when it involves the lungs, with a median survival time of only 2 to 6 months in the pre-ART era (Kaplan et al., 1988). Respiratory failure is often the cause of death. The radiographic appearance is variable, with the characteristic reticulonodular pattern seen in approximately one-third of patients (Kaplan et al., 1988). Otherwise, diffuse interstitial infiltrates, pleural effusions, and hilar adenopathy may be seen (Levine & Tulpule, 2001).

Once KS is clinically suspected, diagnosis is made by biopsy and histologic examination or by presumptive diagnosis based on the endoscopic appearance of a visceral lesion (Aboulafia, 2001). A histologic confirmation is essential to exclude other conditions that can mimic KS. Endoscopically, the classic appearance of small submucosal vascular nodules establishes the diagnosis of GI KS. It may be difficult to establish a diagnosis of GI KS by biopsy because many of the lesions are submucosal (Hengge et al., 2002). In patients with suspected pulmonary KS, violaceous endobronchial lesions typically are observed on bronchoscopic examination. A presumptive diagnosis of pulmonary KS can be made based on characteristic radiographic and endobronchial findings in patients who have had KS at other sites (Kaplan et al., 1988). Endobronchial biopsy is discouraged because of the risk of hemorrhage. Gallium scanning may be helpful in differentiating KS from pulmonary infection because KS is not gallium-avid (Kaplan et al., 1988).

In the pre-ART era, the AIDS Clinical Trials Group (ACTG) developed a staging system based on tumor extent (T), severity of immunosuppression (I), and the presence of systemic illness (S) (Krown et al., 1997). Two different risk categories were noted based on this staging system: a good risk, defined as T0I0S0, and a poor risk, defined as T1I1S1 (Table 29.1).

Table 29.1 AIDS CLINICAL TRIALS GROUP (ACTG) TUMOR STAGING SYSTEM

CHARACTERISTIC	GOOD RISK (0)	POOR RISK (1)
	All of the following:	*Any of the following:*
Tumor (T)	Tumor confined to skin and/or lymph nodes and/or minimal oral disease[a]	Tumor-associated edema or ulceration; extensive oral KS; GI KS; other visceral KS
Immune system (I)	CD4 count ≥150 cells/mm^3	CD4$^+$ T-cell count <150 cells/mm^3
Systemic illness (S)	No history of OI or thrush; no systemic symptoms; Karnofsky Performance Status ≥70	History of OI and/or thrush; systemic symptoms; Karnofsky Performance Status <70; other HIV-related illnesses

[a]Non-nodular KS confined to the palate.

GI, gastrointestinal; KS, Kaposi's sarcoma; OI, opportunistic infection.

Adapted from Krown (1989) and incorporating revision by Krown (1997), with permission from the American Society of Clinical Oncology.

Based on epidemiologic, clinical, staging, and survival data of patients in two Italian prospective cohort studies (*n* = 211), Nasti et al. (2003) concluded that, in the era of ART, a refinement of the ACTG staging system is needed. Patient CD4$^+$ T-cell counts in this study did not provide prognostic information, and only the combination of T1S1 identified patients with unfavorable prognosis. The 3-year survival rate for patients with T1S1 was 53%, which was significantly lower compared to the 3-year survival rates of patients with T0S0, T1S0, and T0S1, which were 88%, 80%, and 81%, respectively. Several studies have found other prognostic markers for KS. Stebbing et al. (2006) developed a prognostic index predicting poor survival, including not having KS as the AIDS-defining illness, decreasing CD4$^+$ T-cell count, age 50 years or older, and having another AIDS-associated illness at the same time. Other variables, including CD8$^+$ cell count (Stebbing et al., 2007) and detectable HHV-8 DNA in plasma at the time of diagnosis (El Amari et al., 2008), have also been associated with poor KS prognosis.

TREATMENT

IMPACT OF ART

ART is a key component in the treatment of KS and should be initiated or optimized to achieve complete HIV RNA suppression in all patients with AIDS-associated KS. The inhibition of HIV replication, decreased production of the tat protein, restored immunity to HHV-8, and the direct antiangiogenic activity of some protease inhibitors (PIs) are among the many benefits of ART (Dubrow et al., 2017; Noy, 2003). Some older data suggested that PIs have an anti-KS effect (Sgadari et al., 2003); however, non-PI-containing ART regimens also lead to KS regression.

Combination ART has been associated with a lengthening of time to treatment failure with either local or systemic therapy for KS. A retrospective study found a median time of 20.4 months from the initiation of ART plus chemotherapy versus 6 months with just chemotherapy to detect treatment failure among PWH with KS (Bower et al., 1999). PWH who were receiving ART at KS diagnosis have a less aggressive presentation versus individuals who were ART-naïve at the time of KS diagnosis (Nasti et al., 2003). Another retrospective analysis from 1990 to 1999 found an 81% reduction in the risk of death among PWH with KS after the initiation of ART (Tam et al., 2002).

KS-associated IRIS has been well described. Some patients may experience painful enlarged lesions or progression of KS lesions during the first months of ART. In a prospective study of 69 patients with HIV and KSHV coinfection, approximately 12% of patients experienced IRIS-KS after initiation of ART (Letang et al., 2010).

LOCAL TREATMENT

Local treatment should be reserved for patients with minimal or locally symptomatic disease. These patients should concurrently receive ART. Current options for local treatment include the following:

- Radiotherapy has been the mainstay of local therapy for KS. It is best suited for patients with a single or a few locally symptomatic areas or for symptomatic disease that requires rapid tumor reduction. Electron beam radiation applied to the entire face is highly effective in relief of facial edema. Radiotherapy also can be useful for treatment of dysphagia caused by pharyngeal lesions and tumor masses of the eye or the extremities (Hill, 1987). Radiotherapy, whether given as whole-body electron beam therapy, fractionated focal radiation therapy, or single treatments, has produced complete remissions in 50% to 80% of patients (Cooper et al., 1991; Pluda et al., 1992). Complications such as severe mucositis, radiotherapy fibrosis, loss of skin compliance, and chronic lymphedema may occur with these treatments and radiotherapy is not recommended for the lower extremities due to potential skin changes and the high risk for cellulitis.

- With intralesional chemotherapy, vinblastine has been most commonly used, with a reported response rate of 70% in older studies (Boudreaux et al., 1993). Small cutaneous lesions can be treated with intralesional chemotherapy for cosmetic purposes. Repeated treatments may be necessary. Intralesional chemotherapy can cause significant pain and areas of hyperpigmentation after treatment.

- Alitretinoin gel (Panretin) is a topical treatment that may be used for relatively asymptomatic patients with KS lesions that do not respond to ART alone and for whom the KS is predominantly an issue of cosmesis. A response rate of 49% ($n = 184$) in a phase 3 study was reported (Walmsley et al., 1999). Adverse effects include dry skin and light hypersensitivity.

- Cryotherapy with liquid nitrogen and laser therapy have been used successfully for the treatment of isolated small KS lesions. Given the significant mucosal toxicity associated with radiotherapy in the treatment of oral lesions, laser surgery may be substituted for radiation.

- There are several new therapies being explored for KS. One is a phase 1 trial of intralesional nivolumab therapy, which is an immune checkpoint inhibitor (NCT03316274; Bender-Ignacio et al., 2018).

SYSTEMIC TREATMENT

Treatment of KS is generally not considered curative and was not shown to have a significant impact on survival in the pre-ART era. An older retrospective review of 194 cases of KS (Volberding et al., 1989) showed no significant difference in survival time between patients treated with chemotherapy or interferon-α (IFN-α) and untreated patients. In a more recent randomized trial done in South Africa of ART alone versus ART plus chemotherapy for KS, there was a significant difference in KS response but no difference in survival between the two arms (Mosam et al., 2012). Although starting ART is strongly recommended for all PWH with KS, adjunct therapies for patients with mild to moderate disease have not been well studied. One recent multicenter trial evaluated the use of oral etoposide (given "as needed" vs. immediately [as eight cycles of therapy]) and found that only about 30% of patients in both groups responded to therapy overall (Hosseinipour et al., 2018). Immediate treatment with oral etoposide resulted in early clinical benefits that were no longer observed 48 weeks after therapy. The researchers subsequently conducted a post-hoc analysis of that study to evaluate the effects of oral etoposide on the development of KS-IRIS and early progressive disease (KS-PD) after starting ART and found that etoposide decreased the development of KS-IRIS and KS-PD after ART initiation.

Systemic intravenous chemotherapy is used for more severe disease, including symptomatic visceral disease, extensive skin involvement, significant edema, or rapidly progressive KS. As described previously, the goal of systemic chemotherapy is mainly palliation of symptoms. Large, randomized studies have established liposomal anthracyclines (doxorubicin and daunorubicin) as first-line single-agent chemotherapy agents with promising results compared to combination chemotherapy treatment (Gill et al., 1996; Northfelt et al., 1998; Stewart et al., 1998). These studies found that liposomal anthracyclines alone can achieve response rates

equal to or better than those of combination chemotherapy with a lower incidence of toxicity such as nausea, fatigue, alopecia, and neuropathy. Neutropenia, however, occurred as frequently with the liposomal agent as with the standard combination regimen. Prognosis is good; in one study of 140 patients with T1 disease who were treated with ART and liposomal anthracycline chemotherapy, the 5-year overall survival was 85% (Bower et al., 2014).

Paclitaxel is a highly active agent that is often used as second-line therapy. It has significant antitumor activity in patients with previously untreated (Gill et al., 1995) and refractory (Saville et al., 1995) KS.

Liposomal doxorubicin is currently not available in many low-middle-income countries (LMICs), so other regimens including bleomycin and vincristine have been utilized for KS treatment. However, a recent three-arm randomized clinical trial conducted by the ACTG/AIDS Malignancy Consortium in 11 sites in Brazil, Kenya, Malawi, South Africa, Uganda, and Zimbabwe compared oral etoposide plus ART and bleomycin plus vincristine plus ART to paclitaxel plus ART. The study was stopped early because the paclitaxel arm demonstrated superior progression-free survival at week 48 compared to the other two arms (Krown et al., 2020). The most significant side effects of paclitaxel are hypersensitivity, myelosuppression, peripheral neuropathy, alopecia, and drug interactions with ART. This agent is the treatment of choice for refractory KS or if there are contraindications to the use of anthracyclines. Regarding comparison of liposomal anthracyclines versus taxanes, Cianfrocca et al. (2010) conducted a small, randomized trial of paclitaxel compared to liposomal doxorubicin. They found that both therapies improved symptoms such as pain and swelling in PWH with advanced KS and found comparable response rates, progression-free survival, and median survival between the two arms. There was a slightly higher rate of grade 3 to 5 toxicity in the paclitaxel arm. A 2014 Cochrane review indicated no observed difference between liposomal doxorubicin, liposomal daunorubicin, and paclitaxel for patients on ART (Gbabe et al., 2014). In the US, because long-term cure of KS is difficult to measure given the fact that hyperpigmented inactive lesions can often remain, the primary goals of treatment for patients with KS are palliation of symptoms and improved cosmesis. Consultation with a KS-experienced oncologist or dermatologist should be considered for most patients diagnosed with this malignancy.

Several newer therapies are currently being studied for severe KS. Inhibition of the KS-activated mammalian target of rapamycin (mTOR) signaling pathway has been examined in an AIDS Malignancy Consortium study and has shown promising therapeutic results (Krown et al., 2012). Imatinib, a platelet-derived growth factor receptor/c-kit inhibitor, induced responses in 10 of 30 patients with KS when given up to 1 year in a multicenter phase 2 trial (Koon et al., 2014). The vascular endothelial growth factor-A inhibitor, bevacizumab, was shown in another phase 2 trial to produce complete and partial responses in 3 and 2 of 16 patients, respectively (Uldrik et al., 2012). Two immunomodulatory agents with antiangiogenic effects, pomalidomide (oral) and lenalidomide (intravenous), were recently evaluated in phase 1/2 trials. Pomalidomide was found to be well tolerated and active in KS regardless of HIV status (Polizzotto et al., 2016b; NCT02659930). Lenalidomide was well tolerated in ART-experienced patients with progressive KS previously treated with chemotherapy, but its phase 2 trial was halted due to lack of responses in this study population (Pourcher et al., 2017). Several other targeted therapies for KS are currently being evaluated in clinical trials (Bender-Ignacio et al., 2018).

RECOMMENDED READING

Cianfrocca M, Lee S, Von Roenn J, et al. Randomized trial of paclitaxel vs. pegylated liposomal doxorubicin for advanced human immunodeficiency virus-associated Kaposi sarcoma: evidence of symptom palliation from chemotherapy. *Cancer.* 2010;116(16):3969–3977.

Hosseinipour MC, Kang M, Krown SE, Bukuru A, et al. As-needed vs. immediate etoposide chemotherapy in combination with antiretroviral therapy for mild-to-moderate AIDS-associated Kaposi sarcoma in resource-limited settings: A5264/AMC-067 randomized clinical trial. *Clin Infect Dis.* 2018;67(2):251–260.

Krown SE, Moser CB, MacPhail P, et al. Treatment of advanced AIDS-associated Kaposi sarcoma in resource-limited settings: a three-arm, open-label, randomised, non-inferiority trial. *Lancet.* 2020;395(10231):1195–1207. doi:10.1016/S0140-6736(19)33222-2

Reid E, Suneja G, Ambinder RF, et al. Cancer in people living with HIV, Version 1.2018, NCCN clinical practice guidelines in oncology. *J Natl Compr Canc Netw.* 2018;16(8):986–1017.

Shiels MS, Pfeiffer RM, Hall HI, et al. Proportions of Kaposi sarcoma, selected non-Hodgkin lymphomas, and cervical cancer in the United States occurring in persons with AIDS, 1980–2007. *JAMA.* 2011;305(14):1450–1459.

HIV-RELATED PRIMARY CENTRAL NERVOUS SYSTEM LYMPHOMA

LEARNING OBJECTIVES

- Review the epidemiology of PCNSL in PWH
- Review the pathophysiology and clinical presentation
- Review chemotherapeutic strategies for treatment
- Discuss survival among these patients

WHAT'S NEW?

Fluorodeoxyglucose–positron emission tomography (FDG-PET) and magnetic resonance spectroscopy provide less invasive strategies to characterize invasiveness of disease and distinguish it from other pathologies.

KEY POINTS

- Epstein–Barr virus (EBV)-mediated oncogenesis in the setting of advanced immunosuppression is largely responsible for PCNSL.

- Treatment with ART should be initiated and maintained for all PWH with PCNSL.

- Despite improved survival in the ART era, overall survivability remains poor.

PCNSL is a rare type of NHL, accounting for 1% to 2% of all NHLs and less than 5% of all primary brain tumors (Lister et al., 2002). PCNSL has been diagnosed in 1.6% to 9.0% of patients with AIDS and represents the second most common intracranial mass lesion in this population (Rosenblum et al., 1988; Welch et al., 1984). The vast majority of PCNSL has been linked to EBV-infected B cells that reach the CNS during advanced immunodeficiency (Cingolani et al., 2005). MacMahon et al. (1991) noted that EBV genes important for oncogenesis are abundant in patients with PCNSL, suggesting a pathogenic role of EBV in this setting. This association suggests that the pathogenesis of PCNSL might differ from systemic NHL, which has a 40% to 50% association with EBV (Ballerini et al., 1993; Hamilton-Dutoit et al., 1989).

EPIDEMIOLOGY

In the era before effective ART, the relative risk of PCNSL was approximately 1,000-fold and as high as 3,600-fold in individuals with AIDS compared to the general population (Cote et al., 1996).

The age-adjusted incidence of PCNSL in the US had increased substantially since the 1970s, from 0.16 per 100,000 py in 1973–1984 to 0.48 per 100,000 py in 1985–1997 (Olson et al., 2002). However, with the introduction of ART in the mid- to late 1990s, the incidence of PCNSL in AIDS significantly decreased (Hoffman et al., 2001; Wolf et al., 2005). In the Multicenter AIDS Cohort Study, the incidence rate in 2,734 HIV-positive men declined from 4.3 to 0.4 per 100,000 py (Sacktor et al., 2001). In another study, PCNSL accounted for only 1% of lymphoma diagnoses in PWH in the period 2006–2015 (Gopal et al., 2013). Despite this dramatic decrease in incidence, survival rates have not significantly improved, especially compared to those of HIV-negative individuals (Bayraktar et al., 2011; Conti et al., 2000).

CLINICAL PRESENTATION

The clinical presentation of CNS lymphoma is similar irrespective of HIV status. Symptoms may include headaches, confusion, lethargy, memory loss, personality changes, and seizures. On examination, patients may present with hemiparesis, aphasia, and cranial nerve palsies. Lesions are most common in the cerebrum, basal ganglia, and brainstem. More diffuse and multifocal involvement is seen in HIV-related PCNSL (Gage et al., 2000). These lesions are contrast-enhancing on computed tomography (CT) and MRI. Before ART, the median CD4$^+$ cell count at presentation was less than 50 cells/mm^3 (Levine et al., 1991).

Polymerase chain reaction (PCR) to detect EBV DNA in the cerebrospinal fluid is useful for diagnosing AIDS-associated CNS lymphoma. Identification of EBV by PCR can detect most cases of AIDS-related PCNSL with a sensitivity of 80% to 100% and specificity for lymphoma of 93% to 100% (Bossolasco et al., 2002). Cerebrospinal fluid cytology alone has limited utility due to poor sensitivity and specificity (Ekstein et al., 2006).

Single-photon emission CT has been suggested as a less invasive technique for diagnosis. However, due to conflicting results in terms of sensitivity and specificity, its role in the diagnosis of PCNSL remains limited (Licho et al., 2002; Ruiz et al., 1994). FDG-PET and magnetic resonance spectroscopy are two other imaging modalities that can aid in the diagnosis of cerebral PCNSL lesions apart from other infectious CNS pathologies such as toxoplasmosis. Magnetic resonance spectroscopy typically shows decreased N-acetyl aspartate and increased choline, which reflects neoplastic cell proliferation (Westwood et al., 2013). FDG-PET can also help identify extracerebral systemic disease involvement (Lewitschnig et al., 2013). Currently, the gold standard for diagnosis of PCNSL is stereotactic brain biopsy. In patients in whom a brain biopsy is unobtainable, the combination of imaging, negative toxoplasma serology, previous toxoplasmosis prophylaxis, and positive EBV cerebrospinal fluid by PCR may be sufficient to make a presumptive diagnosis.

TREATMENT AND SURVIVAL

The relative rarity of PCNSL precludes large-scale randomized trials; therefore, the optimal treatment for PCNSL has not been determined. Norden et al. (2011) showed that HIV positivity significantly reduced median overall survival to 2 months versus 12 months in HIV-negative patients. Despite good initial response rates to treatment, median survival times with treatment remain only 2 to 5.5 months (Baumgartner et al., 1990). The previous standard treatment of patients with AIDS-related PCNSL was palliative corticosteroids and whole-brain radiation that achieved a complete response in 20% to 50% of patients (Cote et al., 1996). Radiation alone can improve symptoms and extend median survival, but this is likely affected by a patient's baseline functional status and not the dose of radiation received (Goldstein et al., 1991).

Regarding chemotherapy for AIDS-related PCNSL, an uncontrolled pilot study published in 1997 used high-dose intravenous methotrexate in 15 patients, including 10 with histologically confirmed PCNSL. The median time since clinical onset was 27 days (range 7–69 days), and the mean CD4+ T-cell count was 30 cells/mm³. Complete responses, defined as clinical improvement and disappearance of contrast-enhancing brain abnormalities on CT or MRI, were obtained in 7 of 15 patients (3 of 10 patients with histologic diagnosis and 4 of 5 patients without histologic confirmation). One patient relapsed at 6 months. Six patients failed to respond, and 2 patients died of severe sepsis. The median survival time was 290 days for the 10 patients with histologic diagnosis and 347 days for the 5 patients without histologic confirmation. In addition, steroids were also administered and individuals ultimately received ART including a PI (Jacomet et al., 1997). More recently, Gupta et al. (2017) retrospectively studied 20 PWH treated with methotrexate-based regimens. Some of these patients were treated with high-dose methotrexate alone, some with high-dose methotrexate and rituximab, and some with regimens that included a variety of other agents. The median survival in patients treated before ART and without high-dose methotrexate was 2 months, whereas with ART and high-dose methotrexate-based regimens, the median survival had not yet been reached with a median follow-up of 27 months. In HIV-negative individuals with PCNSL, high-dose intravenous methotrexate remains the standard of care for those who can tolerate the therapy, and available evidence supports this strategy, combined with ART, in PWH as well. In 2016, the IELSG32 trial provided a high level of evidence supporting the use of MATRix combination (methotrexate, cytarabine, and rituximab with or without thiotepa) as the new standard chemoimmunotherapy for patients aged up to 70 years with newly diagnosed PCNSL (Ferreri et al., 2016). A phase 2 trial is under way evaluating induction with rituximab, high-dose methotrexate, and leucovorin every 2 weeks for six cycles, followed by consolidation with high-dose methotrexate alone (NCT00267865). Whole-brain radiation is traditionally reserved for those with poor performance status (NCCN, 2015a); however, in the second randomization of the IELSG32 trial, both whole-brain radiotherapy and autologous stem-cell transplantation were found to be feasible and effective as consolidation therapies after high-dose methotrexate-based chemoimmunotherapy (Ferreri et al., 2017). Finally, a recent small prospective series conducted by Lurain et al. (2020) at the National Cancer Institute demonstrated that 8 of the 12 PWH and PCNSL who received ART, rituximab, and high-dose methotrexate had sustained complete response (67%), including 3 participants who received second-line therapy without relapse at 2 years. They demonstrated that for all 12 participants, the estimated 60-month overall survival was 67% (95% CI, 32–86%), and with median potential follow-up of 82 months, the median overall survival was not reached. They concluded that treatment with ART, rituximab, and high-dose methotrexate is associated with a high response rate, CD4+ lymphocyte reconstitution, and long-term survival with preservation or improvement of neurocognitive function. In addition, the treatment regimen was tolerable, even for those with advanced HIV, significant comorbidities, and CNS infections.

ROLE OF ART

Combination ART should be initiated in all individuals with AIDS-related PCNSL who are undertaking treatment because it is associated with significant improvement in survival. In the pre-ART era, radiotherapy prolonged survival for 2 to 5.5 months compared to palliative care (Donahue et al., 1995). McGowan and Shah (1998) were the first to describe a case of remission maintained for more than 2 years after treatment with ART alone in an individual who had PCNSL. Other case reports have also reported similar PCNSL response to ART (Aboulafia & Puswella, 2007; Corales et al., 2000; Travi et al., 2012). In a retrospective analysis, Hoffman et al. (2001) showed that survival times of patients receiving ART in addition to radiotherapy differed significantly from those of patients receiving radiotherapy or palliative care alone. Four of the six patients receiving ART survived for more than 1.5 years. In another retrospective analysis, Skiest and Crosby (2003) demonstrated a prolonged median survival of 667 days in individuals who received ART. These findings strongly suggest that immune recovery contributes to longer remission in HIV patients with PCNSL.

RECOMMENDED READING

Cingolani A, Fratino L, Scoppettuolo G, et al. Changing pattern of primary cerebral lymphoma in the highly active antiretroviral therapy era. *J Neurovirol.* 2005;11(Suppl 3):38–44.

Ferreri AJM, Cwynarski K, Pulczynski E, et al. Whole-brain radiotherapy or autologous stem-cell transplantation as consolidation strategies after high-dose methotrexate-based chemoimmunotherapy in patients with primary CNS lymphoma: results of the second randomisation of the International Extranodal Lymphoma Study Group-32 phase 2 trial. *Lancet Haematol.* 2017;4(11):e510–e523.

Gupta NK, Nolan A, Omuro A, et al. Long-term survival in AIDS-related primary central nervous system lymphoma. *Neuro Oncol.* 2017;19:99–108.

Westwood TD, Hogan C, Julyan PJ, et al. Utility of FDG-PETCT and magnetic resonance spectroscopy in differentiating between cerebral lymphoma and non-malignant CNS lesions in HIV-infected patients. *Eur J Radiol.* 2013;82(8):e374–e379.

SYSTEMIC NON-HODGKIN'S LYMPHOMA

LEARNING OBJECTIVES

- Review the epidemiology of NHL

- Review the pathophysiology and clinical manifestations of NHL

- Review the treatment of NHL and survival outcomes

WHAT'S NEW?

- Survival for NHL continues to improve in the ART era; however, incidence continues to be significantly higher compared to that for HIV-negative persons.

- Intensive chemotherapy and autologous hematopoietic cell transplantation (HCT) are safe in patients with HIV and are associated with improved outcomes.

KEY POINTS

- NHL development likely involves a multifactorial interplay among host immune factors as well as the presence of viral mediators including EBV and HHV-8. Disease can occur in a variety of nodal and extranodal sites, and some forms of NHL are more aggressive than others, such as primary effusion lymphoma (PEL).

- Prognostic factors include host immunity, the presence of injection drug use, performance status, and the degree of tumor burden.

- Treatment with ART and intensive chemotherapy with consideration of HCT are cornerstones of NHL treatment.

Box 29.1. AIDS-RELATED LYMPHOMAS: WORLD HEALTH ORGANIZATION CLASSIFICATION

Lymphomas also occurring in immunocompetent people with HIV
Burkitt's lymphoma
Diffuse large B-cell lymphoma: centroblastic, immunoblastic, and anaplastic variants

Lymphomas occurring specifically in PWH
Primary effusion lymphoma
Plasmablastic lymphoma

Lymphomas also occurring in other immunodeficiency states
Polymorphic or posttransplant lymphoproliferative disorder-like B-cell lymphoma

---

The first cases of AIDS-related NHL were described in 1982 (Ziegler et al., 1982). In 1985, NHL was added to the list of AIDS-defining malignancies. Before the ART era, it was estimated to occur in approximately 8% of all HIV cases (Kaplan et al., 1989), and it is currently the second most common neoplasm occurring among PWH (Knowles, 2001).

The World Health Organization (WHO) has divided AIDS-related lymphomas (ARLs) into three categories (Box 29.1):

1. Lymphomas also occurring in immunocompetent patients, such as Burkitt's lymphoma (BL) and diffuse large B-cell lymphoma (DLBCL)

2. Lymphomas occurring specifically in PWH, such as PEL and plasmablastic lymphoma

3. Lymphomas also occurring in other immunodeficiency states, such as polymorphic or posttransplant lymphoproliferative disorder–like B-cell lymphoma

DLBCL and BL are the most common ARLs, representing approximately 90% of these malignancies (Besson et al., 2001). Only intermediate-grade or high-grade lymphomas are considered AIDS-defining.

EPIDEMIOLOGY

There are more than 30 types of NHLs, including DLBCL and BL. Individuals with impaired cell-mediated immunity show a marked increase in the incidence of NHL. This has been best described in immunosuppressed allograft recipients. Similar trends were seen in PWH in the pre-ART era. The CDC examined data of 2,824 NHL cases occurring in 97,258 PWH between 1981 and 1989 in the US. The risk was 60 times greater in PWH (Beral et al., 1991). The risk also varies by histologic subtype, with up to 600-fold excess risk for immunoblastic lymphoma (IBL) (Cote, 1997). In a recent study evaluating the cumulative incidence of NHL in persons with HIV living in the US and Canada ($n = 86,620$), the incidence of NHL from 1996 to 2009 was 4.5% by age 75 years compared to only 0.7% in HIV-negative persons

(n = 196,987) (Silverberg et al., 2015). Gopal et al. (2013) evaluated data from the US Centers for AIDS Research network including 23,050 PWH diagnosed between 1996 and 2011 and found that lymphomas developed in 2.1% of these patients. Most of these were DLBCL (42.2%), followed by Hodgkin's lymphoma (16.6%), BL (11.8%), PCNSL (11.3%), and other NHLs (18.1%).

PATHOGENESIS

The pathogenesis of HIV NHL is most likely multifactorial, involving HIV, immune dysfunction, cytokine dysregulation, and other viral antigens, including EBV and HHV-8 (Gates et al., 2003). EBV is present in approximately 40% to 50% of cases of AIDS-related systemic NHL (Hamilton-Dutoit et al., 1989). This contrasts with a report by Ballerini et al. (1993), who reported 100% EBV coinfection in the IBL variant of DLBCL. The expression of the latent EBV transforming proteins EBNA-2 and LMP-1 is known to play a central role in the initiation and maintenance of EBV-induced B-cell growth and proliferation (Liebowitz et al., 1989). Both EBNA-2 and LMP-1 can serve as targets for cytotoxic T cells; thus, their expression induces T-cell immune surveillance and regulates lymphomagenesis in individuals who are immunocompetent. With immunodeficiency states such as late-stage HIV, EBNA-2 and LMP-1 expression may become unregulated and subsequently lead to uncontrolled proliferation of EBV-infected cells (Gaidano & Dalla-Favera, 1995). Genetic alterations involving oncogenes and tumor suppressor genes may also occur, and often *MYC* and *BCL6* translocations are implicated in neoplastic development (Chadburn et al., 2013).

Expression of HHV-8 also is associated with PEL, which often presents as malignant effusions in both the chest and the abdomen with a paucity of nodal masses. It is aggressive and often refractory to chemotherapy. HHV-8 has been universally found in malignant cells, often in conjunction with EBV (Komanduri et al., 1996). Neoplastic cells have an immunoblastic to plasmablastic appearance. Most PELs have lymphocyte activation markers (CD30 and CD38) without normal B-cell markers (CD19 and CD20).

CLINICAL CHARACTERISTICS

Approximately two-thirds of ARLs are classified as DLBCL (Navarro & Kaplan, 2006). AIDS-related systemic NHL usually presented as widespread disease involving extranodal sites in the pre-ART era (Knowles et al., 1988). The most common sites of extranodal disease are the GI tract, CNS, bone marrow, and liver. Ziegler et al. (1984) reported that 95% of patients from several institutions had evidence of extranodal disease, including 42% with CNS involvement and 33% with bone marrow involvement. In a multicenter retrospective review of pooled data from 886 HIV patients with DLBCL, CNS involvement was found in 13% of patients and was not associated with reduced overall survival (Barta et al., 2016). However, CNS relapse was associated with a median overall survival of only 1.6 months. GI NHL occurs in approximately 30% of PWH with NHL. Most of these cases involve the stomach, but virtually any site in the GI tract or hepatobiliary tree can be involved (Burkes et al., 1986). Interestingly, plasmablastic lymphomas are associated with characteristic development of oral cavity lesions in the majority of cases and predominate in mucosal sites (Chadburn et al., 2013). In the ART era, among patients with undetectable plasma HIV RNA levels, Gerard et al. (2009) found that NHL occurred at a median CD4+ T-cell count of 297 cells/mm³. In addition, they found that 65% of the cases occurred within 18 months of initiating HIV treatment with ART. Other studies have shown that PEL and immunoblastic NHL are seen in patients with lower CD4+ cell counts, of older age, and with a prior diagnosis of AIDS, whereas Burkitt NHL tends to occur in patients with more preserved immune function (Knowles, 1996). In a more recent study of 23,050 patients with HIV infection diagnosed between 1996 and 2011, Gopal et al. (2013) found that patients with Hodgkin's lymphoma and Burkitt NHL had the highest CD4+ T-cell counts, while patients with PCNSL had the lowest. In 2010, NHL accounted for approximately 21% of cancers diagnosed in PWH (Robbins et al., 2015).

PROGNOSTIC FEATURES

Historically, poor prognostic factors for patients with HIV-related NHL have included age older than 35 years, CD4+ T-cell count of less than 100 cells/mm³, history of injection drug use, history of AIDS-defining condition, poor performance status, elevated lactate dehydrogenase, tumor bulk or stage of disease, and International Prognostic Index (IPI) (Straus et al., 1998). The IPI includes clinical features that reflect the growth and invasive potential of the tumor (tumor stage, serum lactate dehydrogenase [LDH] level, and number of extranodal disease sites), the patient's response to the tumor (performance status), and the patient's ability to tolerate intensive therapy (age and performance status). The simplified model for younger patients (the age-adjusted IPI) uses a subgroup of these clinical features (tumor stage, LDH level, and performance status).

Lim et al. (2005) compared the prognostic factors for survival and the use of the IPI in pre- and post-ART PWH with DLBCL. In groups with low-, low-intermediate-, and high-intermediate-risk IPI disease, the 3-year overall survival rates were 20%, 22%, and 5% in the pre-ART era and improved to 64%, 64%, and 50% in the post-ART era, respectively.

Of note, PEL and extracavity PEL are known to be aggressive malignancies with a traditionally dismal prognosis. An early study found a median survival time of 6 months and few survivors beyond 12 months. Poor performance status and lack of ART portend poorer prognosis (Boulanger et al., 2005). However, PEL prognosis may be improving. A 2015 single-center retrospective study of 15 patients found that complete remission was achieved in 14 (93.3%) (Cattaneo et al., 2015). Subsequently 4 patients relapsed, and 2 patients died. The overall survival rate at 3 years was 66.7%.

More recently, Barta et al. (2014) have developed an AIDS-related lymphoma IPI that combines the age-adjusted IPI with an HIV severity score including CD4+ T-cell count, viral load, and prior history of AIDS to risk-stratify HIV-related lymphomas. Using this scoring system, this group evaluated patients enrolled in HIV-associated lymphoma trials between 2005 and 2010 and found that individual HIV-related factors such as low CD4$^+$ T-cell counts (<50 cells/mm^3) and prior history of AIDS were no longer associated with poorer outcomes (Barta et al., 2015).

TREATMENT

The treatment for AIDS-related lymphoma is similar to that of HIV-negative individuals, with some exceptions (Reid et al., 2018). Intrathecal chemotherapy prophylaxis is necessary because patients with HIV are at an increased risk for CNS involvement. Those cases include lymphomas with aggressive pathologic features, including BL, plasmablastic lymphoma, and presentations consistent with possible CNS involvement (Chari et al., 2005). The use of hematopoietic stimulants such as granulocyte colony-stimulating factor (G-CSF) may aid in reducing chemotherapy-induced cytopenic complications. *Pneumocystis jirovecii* pneumonia prophylaxis is administered with standard-dose chemotherapy, irrespective of CD4$^+$ T-cell count.

CHEMOTHERAPY IN THE PRE-ART ERA

In the pre-ART era, PWH with NHL had a poor prognosis, were managed on low-dose chemotherapy regimens because of concern for toxicity, and had a median survival of 5 to 8 months (Kaplan et al., 1997; Sandler et al., 1996). In addition to persistent neoplasia contributing to death, many patients in this era died due to the infectious complications of opportunistic diseases (Lowenthal et al., 1988).

CHEMOTHERAPY IN THE ART ERA

In the ART era, more recent standard chemotherapy regimens have been reported without excessive toxicity due to restored immunity. The AIDS Malignancy Consortium reported on 65 patients who were given reduced doses of cyclophosphamide and doxorubicin combined with vincristine and prednisone (modified CHOP) or full doses of CHOP combined with G-CSF with concomitant ART. Complete response rates were 30% and 48% in the reduced- and full-dose groups, respectively (Ratner et al., 2001). No long-term outcomes were reported in this study. Other studies of CHOP-based chemotherapy and concurrent ART have reported median survival of 2 years. In patients with BL, a particularly aggressive form of NHL, intensive chemotherapy with cyclophosphamide, doxorubicin, high-dose methotrexate/ifosfamide, etoposide, and high-dose cytarabine (CODOX-M/IVAC) resulted in rates of event-free survival and remission similar to those of their HIV-negative counterparts (Wang et al., 2003).

Risk-adaptive chemotherapy has also been studied comparing the post- to pre-ART era. A total of 485 PWH were assigned randomly to chemotherapy after risk stratification based on an HIV score (comprising performance status, prior AIDS, and CD4$^+$ T-cell counts <100 cells/mm^3). Of these

patients, there were 218 good-risk patients (HIV score 0) who received doxorubicin, cyclophosphamide, vindesine, bleomycin, and prednisone (ACVBP) or CHOP; 177 intermediate-risk patients (HIV score 1) who received CHOP or low-dose CHP; and 90 poor-risk patients (HIV score 2 or 3) who received low-dose CHOP or vincristine and steroids. Five-year overall survival in the good-risk group was 51% for ACVBP versus 47% for CHOP ($p = 0.85$), that in the intermediate-risk group was 28% for CHOP versus 24% for low-dose CHOP ($p = 0.19$), and that in the poor-risk group was 11% for low-dose CHOP versus 3% for vincristine and steroid ($p = 0.14$). The significant factors in this study for overall survival were ART (relative risk [RR], 1.6; $p = 0.0002$), HIV score (RR, 1.7; $p = 0.0001$), and IPI score (RR, 1.5; $p = 0.0012$) but not the intensity of chemotherapy (Mounier et al., 2006).

An infusional regimen of cyclophosphamide, doxorubicin, and etoposide with or without ART (only didanosine) resulted in a complete response rate of 45% and median overall survival of 12.8 months. At the time of the analysis, 30% in the pre-ART group were alive, compared with 47% in the ART group. Furthermore, patients in the ART group experienced less nonhematologic toxicity (22% vs. 42%), thrombocytopenia (31% vs. 52%), and anemia (9% vs. 27%) (Sparano et al., 2004). A similar regimen, etoposide, prednisone, vincristine, and doxorubicin (EPOCH), has been used more commonly and with perhaps even more success in the latter portion of the ART era. In two retrospective pooled analyses, Barta et al. (2012, 2013) concluded that EPOCH is superior to CHOP; however, these studies were limited by the potential confounder that experience with CHOP occurred in earlier time periods than that with EPOCH.

Regarding treatment of PEL, a 2012 multicenter retrospective study found no survival benefit from regimens that were more intensive than CHOP (Castillo et al., 2012). A 2015 retrospective single-institution study of 15 patients treated with CHOP or CHOP-like regimens found that complete remission was achieved in 14 patients (93.3%); 4 of these subsequently relapsed (Cattaneo et al., 2015).

REGIMENS THAT INCLUDE RITUXIMAB

In the early 2000s, uncertainty existed around the use of rituximab in PWH with low CD4$^+$ T-cell counts due to concern for increased infection risk (Avivi et al., 2003; Kaplan et al., 2003). However, with subsequent experience there is now a consensus that outcomes are improved when rituximab is added to the chemotherapy regimens discussed earlier. Thus, rituximab should be regarded as the standard of care for both DLBCL and BL. Two recent multicenter retrospective analyses of DLBCL patients with and without HIV infection treated with rituximab plus CHOP (R-CHOP) have been completed. Coutinho et al. (2014) evaluated patients treated between 2003 and 2011 and found that HIV positivity was associated with an improved 5-year overall survival rate (78% vs. 64% in patients without HIV infection). In contrast, Baptista et al. (2015) evaluated patients treated between 2001 and 2011 and found that HIV positivity was associated with a worse 5-year survival rate (56% vs. 74% in HIV-negative patients). However, in the latter study the PWH had a worse performance status and higher Ann Arbor stages than did HIV-negative patients, and, when complete response rates were compared among patients with high tumor burdens, there was no difference between the two groups. Although R-CHOP has become a commonly used regimen in the developed world, there is a paucity of data from low-resource settings. Currently, a phase 2 trial of R-CHOP in HIV-positive and -negative patients with DLBCL is under way in Malawi to establish the safety of this regimen in that population (NCT02660710).

Sparano et al. (2010) examined rituximab plus infusional etoposide, vincristine, doxorubicin, cyclophosphamide, and prednisone (R-EPOCH) given either concurrently or sequentially. In the concurrent arm, 35 of 48 evaluable patients (73%; 95% CI, 58–85%) had a complete response, whereas 29 of 53 evaluable patients in the sequential arm (55%; 95% CI, 41–68%) had a complete response. Toxicity was comparable in the two arms, although patients with a baseline CD4$^+$ T-cell count of less than 50 cells/mm^3 had a high infectious death rate in the concurrent arm. There is an ongoing phase 2 trial of short-course R-EPOCH in PWH with untreated NHL (NCT00006436). It is a dose-escalation study in which patients receive treatment every 3 weeks with R-EPOCH for one cycle beyond complete response of all detectable tumors for a minimum of three and a maximum of six cycles. Finally, there is a phase 2 trial of ibrutinib (a small molecule drug that binds permanently to Bruton's tyrosine kinase) in combination with R-EPOCH in stage II to IV DLBCL (NCT03220022). Evidence remains unclear whether R-CHOP or R-EPOCH is best for patients with AIDS-related lymphomas. A large multicenter trial recently addressed this question in the HIV-negative population and showed no difference between R-CHOP and dose-adjusted R-EPOCH in event-free survival or overall survival (Wilson et al., 2016). Despite a paucity of large studies in PWH, treatment with both R-CHOP and R-EPOCH is usually effective at achieving remission in HIV patients with DLBCL, and most patients who achieve remission remain lymphoma-free.

Regarding BL, a 2012 study examined CODOX-M, followed by IVAC with or without rituximab (Rodrigo et al., 2012). Most patients were on ART and had a median CD4$^+$ T-cell count of 375 cells/mm^3. Ten of the 14 patients who received ART, intensive chemotherapy, and rituximab survived to the follow-up period of nearly 12 months. Complications included late neutropenia, which responded well to G-CSF. Due to predilection of herpesvirus reactivation with rituximab, prophylaxis for herpes simplex and varicella zoster and preemptive monitoring of cytomegalovirus were given. More recently, a prospective multicenter trial showed that modified CODOX-M/IVAC with rituximab was safe and effective in PWH receiving ART, and the 2-year overall survival rate for 34 patients with HIV-related BL was 69.0% (Noy et al., 2015). A 2013 study of short-course low-intensity R-EPOCH in 13 patients with BL, including 11 PWH, found that the overall survival at a median follow-up of 73 months was even better, 90% (Dunleavy et al., 2013). No randomized data are available to determine which of the two regimens is better in PWH with BL; however, both appear to be effective, although the efficacy of R-EPOCH in patients with CNS involvement has not yet been established.

INTRATHECAL CHEMOTHERAPY FOR AIDS-RELATED NHL

CNS involvement by systemic DLBCL has long been recognized as a problem, especially in PWH. To date there have not been any formal studies to evaluate the role of intrathecal prophylaxis in HIV patients with DLBCL. In the absence of definitive data, clinicians routinely administer prophylaxis to patients with the following characteristics: extranodal involvement of two or more sites, elevated lactate dehydrogenase levels, or bone marrow or testicular involvement.

ALTERNATIVE THERAPIES FOR AIDS-RELATED NHL

Newer, targeted anticancer therapies are currently being explored for several types of uncommon but aggressive ARLs, but currently data are sparse. One systematic review published in 2017 evaluated the use of bortezomib (a 26S proteasome inhibitor that is traditionally used for multiple myeloma) in 21 patients with plasmablastic lymphoma, of whom 11 received bortezomib as initial treatment and 10 received bortezomib for relapsed disease. Eleven patients were HIV positive and 10 were HIV negative. The overall response rate to bortezomib-containing regimens was 100% as initial therapy and 90% in the relapsed setting, and the 2-year survival of patients treated with bortezomib initially was 55% (Guerrero-Garcia et al., 2017). Daratumumab, a CD38-directed human IgG1κ monoclonal antibody that is typically used for multiple myeloma, has been shown to be effective in controlling a case of refractory PEL (Shah et al., 2018). Pembrolizumab is a biologic agent currently in phase 1 trials for patients with advanced NHL (NCT02595866). Chimeric antigen receptor (CAR) T-cell therapy is also being evaluated as a treatment for PWH and hematologic malignancies (Rust et al., 2020).

HCT FOR AIDS-RELATED NHL

Autologous HCT has long been the optimal therapy for high-risk and refractory NHL in non-HIV patients, and now a sufficient number of PWH have undergone autologous HCT to determine that it is a safe and feasible approach for ARL patients who meet criteria for transplantation (Navarro & Kaplan, 2006). A multicenter study to evaluate the safety and efficacy of autologous HCT for PWH and lymphoma evaluated 40 patients with persistent or recurrent ARLs (DLBCL, plasmablastic lymphoma, Burkitt's or Burkitt's-like lymphoma, or classical Hodgkin's lymphoma) (Alvarnas et al., 2016). Overall survival and time to progression were not different for PWH when compared with matched HIV-negative controls. Uninterrupted ART should be continued in these patients during the peritransplant period, when feasible, to maintain virologic suppression and to avoid untoward effects of acute virologic rebound, including acute retroviral syndrome and opportunistic infections (Woolfrey et al., 2008). Administration of ART is generally considered safe, with minimal effect on the transplantation course, including adverse drug–drug interactions or other significant adverse events (Johnston et al., 2016).

One study showed that low CD4[+] T-cell count, marrow involvement, and poor performance status independently affected survival with HCT (Re et al., 2009). Overall survival has been reported to be 50% to 55% at 9 months (Gabarre et al., 2000; Re et al., 2003), 71% at 21 months (Diez-Martin et al., 2003), and 85% at 32 months (Krishnan et al., 2005). All studies except a French series (Diez-Martin et al., 2003) have required HIV disease to be under control for HCT, either by low to undetectable HIV RNA levels or by CD4[+] T-cell counts of more than 100 cells/mm^3. In another study, Diez-Martin et al. (2009) showed a similar incidence of relapse, overall survival, and progression-free survival in cohorts of HIV-positive and HIV-negative lymphoma patients who received HCT. Long-term survival of autologous HCT for relapsed/refractory lymphoma was examined in a 2015 retrospective review of HIV-positive survivors (Zanet et al., 2015). This study found a survival of 65% at 5 years for 37 patients. Among 26 patients who achieved complete remission, overall survival at 10 years was 91% and event-free survival was 36%. Nine patients developed opportunistic infections at a median of 0.4 years after HCT.

Regarding allogeneic bone marrow transplant (alloBMT), one famous case reported in 2009 demonstrated that allogeneic HCT with donor cells that are resistant to HIV infection (in this case, because of a homozygous deletion polymorphism in the donor's CCR5 gene) can cure HIV infection (Hutter et al., 2009). Although fascinating, this outcome is the exception rather than the rule with allogeneic HCT. Importantly, caution must be observed because, in typical alloBMTs, the HIV reservoir disappears along with the patient's T cells but can aggressively rebound if ART is discontinued (Henrich et al., 2014; Sugarman et al., 2016). More research is required to thoroughly explore the mechanism and frequency of this phenomenon. The first prospective multicenter trial of matched related or unrelated allogeneic HCT in PLWH was recently completed and included 17 patients with acute leukemias, myelodysplasia, Hodgkin's lymphomas, and NHLs (Ambinder et al., 2017). There were no deaths at 100 days posttransplant, and the overall survival rate at 1 year was 57%. Deaths were due to relapsed or progressive disease in five patients, acute graft-versus-host disease, adult respiratory distress syndrome, and liver failure. The overall conclusion from this trial was that allogeneic HCT should be considered the standard of care for PWH who meet usual transplant eligibility criteria. Other studies are currently being conducted to explore gene-modified autologous and alloBMT with HIV-resistant cells (Bender-Ignacio et al., 2018; DiGiusto et al., 2016; Lederman et al., 2016). Other recent studies have contributed important observations on the latent HIV reservoir dynamics after stem cell transplant. Eberhard et al. (2020) found strong CD4[+] and CD8[+] T-cell activation (as measured by coexpression of CD38 and HLA-DR) followed alloHSCT that peaked between months 2 and 3 after HSCT, demonstrating that there is a period of high immune activation and a potential window of vulnerability for HIV reservoir reseeding during that time. In another small study of allogeneic transplant patients where posttransplant cyclophosphamide was used for graft-versus-host disease prophylaxis to expand donor options, Durand et al. (2020) demonstrated that among six patients who had longitudinal measurements available, the HIV latent reservoir was not detected after alloBMT in four patients with more than 95% donor chimerism, consistent with a 2.06 to 2.54 log$_{10}$ reduction in the HIV latent reservoir. However, the HIV latent reservoir remained stable in the two patients with less than 95% donor chimerism. Although three of the six patients ultimately died after alloBMT, this study supports the use of alloBMT for PWH and reinforces the observation that alloBMT alone diminishes but does not eliminate the HIV latent reservoir.

CHEMOTHERAPY–ART INTERACTIONS

ART interruption during cancer treatment should generally be avoided because it increases the risk of severe consequences (including immunologic compromise, opportunistic infection, and death) (El-Sadr et al., 2006) and it improves tolerance and outcomes of cancer treatment. However, interactions between ART and proposed anticancer therapeutic options must always be checked as many medications used for chemotherapy (such as cyclophosphamide and vincristine) and immunotherapy are metabolized via the CYP3A4 isoenzyme. PIs (including ritonavir), non-nucleoside reverse transcriptase inhibitors, and pharmacokinetic boosters such as cobicistat inhibit and induce CYP3A4, with the potential for altered chemotherapeutic and cytotoxic effects. Thus, chemotherapy without ARVs has been studied due to concerns of drug interactions with chemotherapy and noncompliance with ART resulting in increased resistance (Powles et al., 2000). Furthermore, PIs (in ART regimens) have been associated with increased incidence of neutropenia with concomitant chemotherapy (Bower et al., 2004). In one study of 39 patients receiving dose-adjusted EPOCH, ARVs were not given until after the final cycle of chemotherapy; a complete remission rate of 74% was achieved (Little et al., 2003).

There are many types of ART regimens that are unlikely to lead to problematic drug–drug interactions with chemotherapeutic agents. Among those with the fewest potential interactions are the integrase inhibitors (raltegravir, elvitegravir, dolutegravir, and bictegravir). Raltegravir, an integrase inhibitor that is metabolized via glucuronidation, has been given simultaneously with CHOP and with other antimetabolites such as gemcitabine and methotrexate, as well as with monoclonal antibodies rituximab and trastuzumab, with good tolerability and durable viral suppression (Bañon et al., 2014). The class of integrase inhibitors, particularly raltegravir, improves virologic and immunologic responses in ART-naïve patients and is considered in the US Department of Health and Human Services (USDHHS) ART guidelines for HIV disease as an acceptable first-line therapy; thus, it could be a suitable alternative for preventing chemotherapy–ART interactions (Fulco et al., 2010).

IMPACT OF ART

Most studies have shown that the incidence of HIV NHL, like that for most other AIDS-defining cancers, has declined over time. In a meta-analysis by Appleby et al. (2000) that included 47,936 PWH with NHL (including PCNSL), the incidence declined from 6.2 cases per 1,000 py in the pre-ART era to 3.6 cases per 1,000 py in the post-ART era ($p < 0.0001$).

In a population-based, record-linkage study of cancer in 472,378 individuals with AIDS from 1980 to 2006, the cumulative incidence of NHL declined from 3.8% during 1990–1995 to 2.2% during 1996–2006. Of note, NHL was the most common AIDS-defining cancer during the ART era (53%) (Simard et al., 2011). In addition, the Swiss Cohort Study examined 429 NHL cases of 12,959 PWH from 1993 to 2006. NHL incidence reached 13.6 per 1,000 py in 1993–1995 and declined to 1.8 in 2002–2006. Combination ART use was associated with a decline in NHL incidence (hazard ratio [HR], 0.26; 95% CI, 0.20–0.33) (Polesel et al., 2008).

A retrospective study using US and Canadian data from 1996 to 2009 showed a significant decline in the annual hazard rate of NHL (−8%) in PWH compared to that of HIV-negative individuals, signifying a narrowing of the gap of NHL burden between PWH and HIV-negative groups (Silverberg et al., 2015). This reduction also represents the benefit of immunologic recovery and viral control.

RECOMMENDED READING

Alvarnas JC, Le Rademacher J, Wang Y, et al. Autologous hematopoietic cell transplantation for HIV-related lymphoma: results of the BMT CTN 0803/AMC 071 trial. *Blood.* 2016;128:1050–1058.

Bañon S, Machuca I, Araujo S, et al. Efficacy, safety, and lack of interactions with the use of raltegravir in HIV-infected patients undergoing antineoplastic chemotherapy. *J Intern AIDS Soc.* 2014;17(4 Suppl 3):19590.

Rust B, Kiem HP, Uldrick T. CAR T-cell therapy for cancer and HIV through novel approaches to HIV-associated haematological malignancies. *Lancet Haematol.* 2020;7(9):E690–696. doi:10.1016/S2352-3026(20)30142-3

Zanet E, Taborelli M, Rupolo M, et al. Postautologous stem cell transplantation long-term outcomes in 26 PLWH affected by relapsed/refractory lymphoma. *AIDS.* 2015;29(17):2303–2308.

NON–AIDS-DEFINING CANCERS

LEARNING OBJECTIVES

- Review the risk factors and epidemiology of NADCs

- Review the impact of anogenital neoplasias and squamous cell cancer of the anus (SCCA) in men and women

- Discuss treatment of anogenital neoplasias and SCCA, including the role of ART

WHAT'S NEW?

- Women are more recognized as a high-risk group for SCCA, and predisposing factors include positivity for high-risk human papillomavirus (HPV) serotypes.

- HPV vaccination in women with HIV (WWH) has demonstrated durable immunogenicity and safety.

- HPV vaccination for HIV-positive men beyond recommended ages may be beneficial and cost-effective in preventing invasive neoplasia.

KEY POINTS

- Due to the aging HIV population, NADCs are responsible for an increasing number of deaths. Immunologic control with ART, however, has decreased the incidence of some cancers, including anogenital cancers.

- Screening with either cervical Papanicolaou (Pap) smear or high-risk HPV in women is a key surveillance measure for detecting precancerous lesions. Screening with anal Pap smear in men and women with risk factors is also recommended, although uptake of this practice may be contingent on the availability of high-resolution anoscopy.

- HPV vaccination for HIV-positive men and women is safe and efficacious.

Since the advent of widely available ART in the US, PWH have had significantly improved survival and decreased mortality from AIDS-related infections and AIDS-defining cancers (ADCs). However, with longer survival, it has become evident that PWH are now at increased risk for NADCs. Multiple risk factors for NADCs include degree and duration of viremia, low $CD4^+$ T-cell nadir, coinfection with oncogenic viruses (e.g., HPV and HBV), and personal carcinogenic exposure, which also should be considered when implementing risk mitigation strategies (Kowalkowski et al., 2014; Vallet-Pichard & Pol, 2004).

Simard et al. (2011) confirmed the benefits of immunologic control in a population-based, record-linkage study examining cancers in 472,378 individuals with AIDS from 1980 to 2006. The cumulative incidence of AIDS-defining conditions declined sharply across three AIDS calendar periods (from 18% in 1980–1989 to 11% in 1990–1995 and 4.2% in 1996–2006). The cumulative incidence of NADC increased from 1.1% to 1.5%, with no change thereafter (1% in 1996–2006). However, the cumulative incidence increased steadily over time for specific NADCs (anal cancer, Hodgkin's lymphoma, and liver cancer) (Simard et al., 2011). Another study (Simard et al., 2010b) showed an elevated incidence for the following NADCs in patients 3 to 10 years after the onset of AIDS: Hodgkin's lymphoma and cancers of the oral cavity and/or pharynx, tongue, anus, liver, larynx, lung and/or bronchus, and penis. These data demonstrate that having previously diagnosed advanced immunosuppression appears to increase the risk for NADCs as well as ADCs.

The increased risk of NADCs among PWH has been reported by Patel et al. (2008). The incidences of the following cancers were significantly higher: anal (standardized rate ratio [SRR], 42.9; 95% CI, 34.1–53.3), vaginal (SRR, 21.0; CI, 11.2–35.9), Hodgkin's lymphoma (SRR, 14.7; CI, 11.6–18.2), liver (SRR, 7.7; CI, 5.7–10.1), lung (SRR, 3.3; CI, 2.8–3.9), melanoma (SRR, 2.6; CI, 1.9–3.6), oropharyngeal (SRR, 2.6; CI, 1.9–3.4), leukemia (SRR, 2.5; CI, 1.6–3.8), colorectal (SRR, 2.3; CI, 1.8–2.9), and renal (SRR, 1.8; CI, 1.1–2.7). The incidence of prostate cancer was significantly lower among PWH compared to the general population (SRR, 0.6; CI, 0.4–0.8). Only the relative incidence of anal cancer increased over time (Patel et al., 2008). Of particular note, none of the AIDS–cancer match studies found an increased risk of breast, colon, or prostate cancer. It is unclear if there is a definite link between the level of immunodeficiency and certain NADCs. Some studies have failed to show such a relationship (Burgi et al., 2005). Conversely, Reekie et al. (2010) utilized data from 4,453 patients in the prospective, multinational EuroSIDA cohort. The incidence of NADCs in this cohort from 1994 to 2007 was 4.3 per 1,000 py of follow-up. After adjustment, a higher current CD4+ T-cell count was independently associated with a decreased incidence of NADCs. In addition, an increased rate of virus-related cancers and non–virus-related epithelial cancers was found in immunodeficient patients. Hodgkin's lymphoma, anal cancer, and lung cancer were all found at a higher rate in patients with lower current CD4+ T-cell counts after adjustment for other demographic and traditional risk factors (Reekie et al., 2010). More recently, data from the US Veterans Aging Cohort Study also showed that increased risk of lung cancer is associated with lower CD4+ T-cell counts, lower CD4:CD8 ratios, and increased viral load (Sigel et al., 2017).

It has also been previously hypothesized that individuals with HIV are at higher risk for malignancies at younger ages. Shiels et al. (2010) used the national US AIDS Cancer Registry Match to demonstrate that individuals with HIV are not at increased risk for colon, prostate, or breast cancer at younger ages, but they were younger at the time of diagnosis for lung and anal cancers. They also found that the age of diagnosis of Hodgkin's lymphoma was significantly older than that of the general population. A study using data from the HIV/AIDS Cancer Match study found that PWH with cancer tended to be younger than age 50 years compared to their uninfected counterparts, whose cancer occurred more often after age 60 years. This study also found that those with HIV presented with more advanced-stage cancers with distant disease (32.2%) compared to uninfected patients (17.7%), and they experienced higher cancer-specific mortality (Coghill et al., 2015). By comparing data from both the North American AIDS Cohort Collaboration on Research and Design (NAACCRD) and the SEER program, Shiels et al. (2017) found that PWH were diagnosed with lung cancer, anal cancer, head and neck cancer, kidney cancer, and myeloma at earlier ages than their HIV-negative counterparts.

NADCs are responsible for an increasingly large proportion of deaths in patients with HIV disease in the ART era, which is likely due to longer survival among individuals with HIV. A study conducted by the Data Collection on Adverse Events of Anti-HIV Drugs (D:A:D) evaluated factors associated with mortality due to NADCs and ADCs (Monforte et al., 2008). The study included 23,437 patients followed from 1999 to 2001. It was found that the overall mortality rate due to NADCs was higher than that due to ADCs. The death rate from NADCs was 1.8 per 1,000 py of follow-up (95% CI, 1.5–2.1) compared to 1.1 per 1,000 py of follow-up (95% CI, 0.9–1.2) for ADCs. In addition, based on multivariable analysis, it was found that most recent CD4+ T-cell count and increasing age were associated with an increased risk of death from ADCs and NADCs. Other factors, such as ART utilization, increased the risk of death for NADCs only. It is unlikely that HIV treatment itself increases the risk for NADCs. Rather, this finding underscores the complex relationship between prolonged survival with HIV disease, immunosuppression, and the diagnosis of and survival from NADCs.

The Mortalité study in France captured the changing patterns of AIDS-related deaths in that country (Bonnet et al., 2005; Lewden et al., 2005). Lewden reported on cancer deaths among PWH in the original study and found that, in 2000, NADCs were the third leading cause of death. It was also found that as the patient population increased above age 45 years, deaths due to malignant disease eclipsed those due to infectious etiologies. The study was updated in 2005 and it found that the rate of death from non-AIDS/hepatitis-related cancers increased from 38% in 2000 to 50% in 2005. A follow-up study found that the combination of ADCs and NADCs has become the leading cause of death in France (Morlat et al., 2014). Similarly, a more recent Tanzanian study showed that NADCs increased by 33.8% from 2002 to 2014, while the proportion of NADCs relative to all cancers significantly decreased from 6.8% in 2002 to 5.6% in 2014 (APC = −2.74%) (Campbell et al., 2016). Most of these increases were due to lung and liver cancers, although the number of head and neck cancers also increased. More recently, a large US population registry-based study found that most cancer deaths among PWH were due to NADCs, including lung cancer (2.4%), liver cancer (1.1%), and anal cancer (0.6%) (Horner et al., 2020).

Regardless of etiology, as the HIV-positive population ages, the risk of NADCs will also undoubtedly increase. A US retrospective study found that cancer-related mortality among PWH compared to HIV-negative individuals (1996–2010) was significantly elevated for colorectal cancer (HR, 1.49; 95% CI, 1.2–1.8), pancreatic cancer (HR, 1.7; CI, 1.35–2.18), lung cancer (HR, 1.28; CI, 1.17–1.3), melanoma (HR, 1.72; CI, 1.09–2.7), breast cancer (HR, 2.61; CI, 2.06–3.3), and prostate cancer (HR, 1.57; CI, 1.02–2.41) (Coghill et al., 2015). Some evidence suggests that treatment of these individuals may be more difficult than that of the general population, that PWH may present with more advanced disease, and that PWH may not tolerate cancer therapies as well as HIV-negative patients (Bower et al., 2003). Screening for early signs of malignancy may be an important method for earlier diagnosis. However, no studies of screening approaches have been performed, and no specific recommendations for alternative screening practices different from what is recommended for the general population exist for PWH for most cancers.

Most studies of treatment outcomes for NADCs in the ART era demonstrate that PWH have outcomes similar to those of HIV-negative individuals. Simard and Engels (2010) evaluated cause of death in the pre-ART and ART eras and showed that death from NADCs (lung, Hodgkin's lymphoma, anal cancers, and other unspecified cancers) decreased steadily from 1980 to 2006. For all NADCs, the number of deaths per 1,000 py from 1980 to 1989 and then from 1996 to 2006 significantly declined from 2.21 to 0.84 (Simard & Engels, 2010). However, while more recent population-based studies such as that of Horner et al. also show overall cancer mortality for PWH declining (from 484.0 per 100,000 py during 2001–2005 to 313.6 per 100,000 py during 2011–2015), their population-attributable fractions for NADCs increased from 7.2% to 11.8% in 2011–2015. Due to the benefit of ART on cancer outcomes in PWH, it is recommended that most patients be treated similarly to those without HIV infection and that ART should be administered concurrently with chemotherapy or radiotherapy (Chiao et al., 2010; Reid et al., 2018).

ANOGENITAL NEOPLASIA

Anogenital neoplasia refers to anal and cervical carcinomas and their precursor lesions. One of the most important risk factors associated with anogenital neoplasia is HPV infection. HPV is a DNA virus and generally infects stratified squamous epithelium. More than 100 HPV serotypes have been identified to date, and at least 30 of these have a high predilection for the anogenital tract. HPV serotypes 6 and 11 have been associated with benign disease, whereas serotypes 16, 18, and 31 are associated with high-grade cervical or anal squamous intraepithelial lesions (SILs) or cervical and anal carcinomas.

For PWH, HPV infection has a well-established relationship with the increased risk of developing anogenital neoplasia (Bjorge et al., 2002; Palefsky et al., 1991). Invasive and in situ forms of not only cervical and anal cancer but also vulvar/vaginal and penile cancers are reported among PWH (Frisch et al., 2000a; Frisch & Bigger, 2000b; Smith et al., 2019).

PATHOGENESIS OF HPV IN HIV INFECTION

The increased prevalence of HPV disease associated with HIV infection may be mediated by impaired T-cell and antigen-presenting cell function. However, local effects of HIV infection may also upregulate HPV replication and oncogenesis. The HPV viral oncogenes E6 and E7 can immortalize primary keratinocytes and transform cells in culture (Barbosa & Schlegel, 1989; Munger et al., 1989). In an animal model of estrogen-stimulated HPV-induced cervical cancer, expression of E7 alone resulted in precancers and cancer, whereas the expression of E6 and E7 together resulted in larger cancers (Riley et al., 2003). Although the exact mechanisms of HIV-related immunosuppression and HPV coinfection have not been determined, several in vitro studies have shown that the HIV tat protein can drive the replication of HPV-16 and HPV-18 through the overexpression of E7 and other genes in the early region (Tornesello et al., 1993; Vernone et al., 1993).

EPIDEMIOLOGY OF HIV-ASSOCIATED CERVICAL INTRAEPITHELIAL NEOPLASIA

The relationship between HIV infection and increased prevalence of cervical intraepithelial neoplasia (CIN) has been shown in many studies. Mandelblatt et al. (1999) performed a meta-analysis of 15 cross-sectional studies published between 1986 and 1998 that evaluated prevalence of cervical neoplasia, HPV infection, and HIV infection among women. They found that among women infected with HPV, WWH were significantly more likely to develop cervical neoplasia, and this effect was related to the degree of immunodeficiency. Several other studies have also shown that WWH are at higher risk for CIN, including that by Ahdieh et al. (2000), who found that 13% of WWH versus 2% of HIV-negative women had abnormal cytologic findings. They also found that WWH had a much lower rate of HPV clearance on follow-up exams and that, in a multivariate model, the increased rate of CIN among WWH was fully accounted for by HPV persistence (Ahdieh et al., 2000). A 2016 study from the Kaiser group found that WWH had twofold higher odds of CIN grade 2$^+$ (CIN2$^+$) and CIN3$^+$, but this was only in women with a recent CD4$^+$ count of less than 500 cells/mm^3 (Silverberg et al., 2016).

EPIDEMIOLOGY OF HIV-ASSOCIATED CERVICAL CARCINOMA

Since 1993, invasive cervical cancer has been listed by the CDC (2008) as an "AIDS-defining" condition. In the US, where the incidence of cervical cancer in general is relatively low, the incidence in WWH is 66% higher than in women without HIV (Brickman et al., 2015). However, in some areas of Africa, the cervical cancer incidence is much higher, nearly 168 per 100,000 women (Lince-Deroche et al., 2015). Cervical cancer mortality remains higher in WWH than in HIV-negative women, especially in resource-limited settings (Ferlay et al., 2013). However, quantifying the contribution of HIV infection to the development of cervical cancer among WWH was challenging in the pre-ART era. A 1996 study that evaluated the relationship between HIV and cervical cancer found no conclusive evidence that HIV per se increased the risk of cervical cancer among WWH (International Agency for Research on Cancer, 1996). Subsequent studies continue to yield conflicting results. In developed countries with access to ART, several studies have shown an increased risk of cervical cancer. Using a national AIDS–cancer linked registry database of cases through 1998, Frisch et al. (2001) found a relative risk of 5.4 for invasive cervical cancer among WWH compared to the general population. However, no increased risk in cervical cancer has been noted in case–control studies from multiple sub-Saharan African countries, where endemic rates of cervical cancer are higher and women have shorter survival (Gichangi et al., 2002; La Ruche et al., 1998; Patil et al., 1995).

As noted previously, with the use of ART since the mid-1990s, there have been definite declines in the incidence of AIDS-related cancers. This has been attributed to the improved immune function and control of oncogenic viruses seen with ART. This declining trend has not been consistently seen in AIDS-related cervical cancer. Shiels et al. (2011) showed an increasing proportion of cervical cancers in persons with AIDS from 0.11% in 1980–1989 (95% CI, 0.08–0.13) to 0.69% in 2001–2007 (95% CI, 0.49–0.89).

EFFECT OF ART ON HIV-ASSOCIATED CERVICAL DYSPLASIA

Although ART has significantly improved the survival of PWH through immune reconstitution and has decreased the incidence of opportunistic infections, the effects of ART on HPV infection and CIN among WWH remain unclear. Whereas three older studies did not find a significant reduction in risk of cervical dysplasia among women on ART (Lillo et al., 2001; Moore et al., 2002; Orlando et al., 1999), a recent prospective study did find a reduction in cervical dysplasia risk related to ART (Minkoff et al., 2010).

The largest retrospective analysis, performed by the Women's Interagency HIV Study (WIHS) group, found that, among 741 WWH, those on ART were 40% (95% CI, 4–81%) more likely to exhibit a regression of cervical lesions and were also significantly less likely to have progression of CIN (odds ratio [OR], 0.68) (Minkoff et al., 2001). The same group subsequently prospectively evaluated 286 WWH who initiated ART (Minkoff et al., 2010). They were assessed semiannually for HPV infection (by PCR) and SILs. Combination ART initiation among adherent women was associated with a significant reduction in HPV prevalence, incident detection of oncogenic HPV infection, and decreased prevalence and more rapid clearance of oncogenic HPV-positive SILs. Effects were smaller among nonadherent women (Minkoff et al., 2010). More recently, a large systematic review evaluated WWH with high-grade cervical lesions (high-grade squamous intraepithelial lesions [HSIL]-CIN2$^+$) (Kelly et al., 2020). WWH on ART had lower prevalence of high-risk HPV than did those not on ART. Their review included 17 studies that reported the association of ART with longitudinal cervical lesion outcomes and determined that ART was associated with a decreased risk of HSIL-CIN2$^+$ incidence, SIL progression, and increased likelihood of SIL or CIN regression. Furthermore, three of their studies indicated that ART was associated with a reduction in invasive cervical cancer incidence. Collectively, the data suggest that treating HIV infection with ART has a beneficial effect on progression of HPV-related cervical disease.

SCREENING, TREATMENT, AND PREVENTION OF HIV-ASSOCIATED CERVICAL DYSPLASIA

SCREENING

Current US Public Health Service and Infectious Diseases Society of America guidelines recommend that WWH undergo a complete history and physical that includes a pelvic exam and Pap test at the time of initial evaluation. The Pap test is the primary mode for cervical cancer screening for WWH. Screening for these women should commence within 1 year of the onset of sexual activity regardless of mode of HIV transmission (e.g., sexual activity and perinatal exposure) but no later than age 21 years. Women aged 21 to 29 years should have a Pap test at the time of initial diagnosis with HIV. Co-testing (Pap test and HPV test) is not recommended for women with HIV younger than 30 years. If the initial Pap test for young (or newly diagnosed) WWH is normal, the next Pap test should be performed in 12 months (although some experts still recommend a repeat Pap test at 6 months after baseline testing). If the results of the three consecutive Pap tests are normal, follow-up Pap tests can be done every 3 years. For women age 30 years or older, either Pap testing alone or co-testing with both Pap and HPV are acceptable screening strategies. For women who undergo Pap testing alone, the protocol is identical to that just described for women younger than 30. For women who undergo co-testing, Pap and HPV testing should be done at the time of HIV diagnosis (or starting at age 30 years). If the Pap is normal and the HPV screening test is negative, repeat cervical cancer screening can be done in 3 years. Women who have a normal Pap test but are positive for HPV should have repeat co-testing in 1 year (unless genotype testing for 16 or 16/18 is positive, in which case the patient should be referred for colposcopy). If either of the co-tests at 1 year is abnormal (i.e., abnormal cytology or positive HPV), referral to colposcopy is recommended. Any WWH with an abnormal Pap smear that shows atypical squamous cells of undetermined significance (ASCUS) or higher-grade lesions should undergo colposcopy (DHHS, 2020). Cervical cancer screening in WWH should continue throughout their lifetime (and not end at age 65 years, as in the general population).

TREATMENT

Treatment options for CIN include cryotherapy, loop electrosurgical excision procedure (LEEP), and cold knife conization (Santesso et al., 2016). These options are generally safe and effective. Cryotherapy is an especially important option for women living in low-resource settings. A recent South African study evaluated 220 WWH who were randomized to cryotherapy ($n = 112$) or no treatment ($n = 108$) (Firnhaber et al., 2017). Ninety-four percent were receiving ART, their median CD4$^+$ T-cell counts were 499 cells/mm^3, and 59% were high-risk HPV positive. Cryotherapy reduced progression to HSIL (2 of 99 [2%] progressed in the cryotherapy group vs. 15 of 103 [15%] in the no treatment group; 86% reduction [95% CI, 41–97%; $p = 0.002$]). Participants in the cryotherapy arm experienced greater regression to normal histology and improved cytologic outcomes. Of note, endocervical extension is more frequent among WWH (Foulot et al., 2008). Therefore, LEEP is thought to be less effective and recurrence rates are higher in WWH than in HIV-negative women, although another recent South African study found that rates of cumulative CIN2$^+$ were lower after LEEP than cryotherapy treatment at 6 months (Smith et al., 2017). Importantly, in this study, both treatments appeared effective in reducing CIN2+ by more than 70% at 12 months.

Invasive cervical cancer diagnosed in WWH is treated using the same criteria and protocols as those for HIV-negative women as long as no other contraindications for treatment exist (Reid et al., 2018). Limited data exist on the treatment of cervical cancer in WWH (Ntekim et al., 2015). One prospective cohort study of 348 patients with cervical cancer in Botswana compared outcomes between WWH (66%) and HIV-negative women (Dryden-Peterson et al., 2016). The WWH group had a median CD4+ T-cell count of 397 cells/mm³ (interquartile range, 264–555). HIV infection was significantly associated with an increased risk of death among all women (HR, 1.95; 95% CI, 1.20–3.17) and among the subset of those who received guideline-concordant curative therapy (HR, 2.63; 95% CI, 1.05–6.55). These results suggest that HIV infection has an adverse effect on cervical cancer survival. That this effect was greater for women with a lower CD4+ T-cell count ($p = 0.036$) suggests that immune suppression plays a significant role. Of note, the study was conducted in a resource-limited environment, and survival of both WWH and HIV-negative women with cervical cancer was lower than would be expected in the US. Regarding newer therapies, there is an ongoing phase 3 trial evaluating standard chemoradiotherapy with or without modulated electrohyperthermia (a noninvasive intervention using 13.56-MHz radiofrequency treatment) for locally advanced cervical cancer in South Africa that includes WWH (NCT03332069).

PREVENTION

There are currently three HPV vaccines that have been approved by the US Food and Drug Administration (FDA): bivalent, quadrivalent, and 9-valent. All three prevent HPV-16 and HPV-18 infections and prevent precancers (and likely cancers) caused by HPV-16 and HPV-18. In addition, the quadrivalent and 9-valent HPV vaccines prevent HPV-6 and HPV-11 infections and genital warts due to these types. The 9-valent vaccine also prevents infection and precancers due to five additional types (31, 33, 45, 52, and 58). The CDC currently recommends the HPV vaccine for PWH 9 to 26 years old. For individuals 9 to 14 years old, the vaccine can be given as two doses 6 to 12 months apart (CDC, HPV Fact Sheet). Older individuals should receive the three-dose series (0, 2, and 6 months). Although the CDC has not yet released recommendations for older individuals, the FDA has approved the HPV vaccine for individuals up to 45 years old. Additionally, starting ART early likely reduces the risk of high-risk HPV infection and cervical cancer development.

EPIDEMIOLOGY OF HIV-ASSOCIATED ANAL INTRAEPITHELIAL NEOPLASIA

Unlike cervical HPV infection, which peaks in the third decade in women, anal HPV infection is highly prevalent throughout adult life among men who have sex with men (MSM) well into the sixth decade (Chin-Hong et al., 2004;

Schiffman et al., 2003). Several studies have reported the prevalence of anal intraepithelial neoplasia (AIN) among HIV-positive men and women. Palefsky et al. (2001) found that the relative risk of developing HSILs was 3.7 for HIV-positive compared to HIV-negative MSM. Sixteen studies demonstrated that between 41% and 97% of HIV-positive men are found to have anal dysplasia on anal Pap smear screening (Kiviat et al., 2002; Palefsky et al., 2001; Piketty et al., 2008). In a meta-analysis of 31 studies, Machalek et al. (2012) showed that the pooled prevalence of anal HPV detected by PCR was 89% in HIV-positive compared to 53.6% in HIV-negative men ($p = 0.047$). In addition, the prevalence of HPV-16 and HPV-18, associated with high-grade neoplasia and malignancy, was also significantly higher in HIV-positive compared to HIV-negative men.

EPIDEMIOLOGY OF HIV-ASSOCIATED SCCA

Even before the HIV epidemic, anal cancer incidence among MSM was estimated to be as high as approximately 35 cases per 100,000 py. This rate is comparable to the incidence of cervical cancer in the US before the advent of routine cervical cytology (Daling et al., 1987; Melbye et al., 1994). In the 1960s, the annual incidence of SCCA among men in the United States was relatively low and stable, with approximately 0.5 cases per 100,000 persons. Since then, studies have shown a steady increase. A US population-based analysis of the Surveillance, Epidemiology and End Results (SEER) program data found that the incidence of SCCA in the US among men increased from 1.06 per 100,000 persons from 1973 to 1979 to 2.04 per 100,000 persons from 1996 to 2004 (Johnson et al., 2004).

Many studies have shown that the incidence of SCCA is higher in PWH. In a meta-analysis, Machalek et al. (2012) examined nine studies published before November 2011 reporting anal cancer incidence in MSM. Six were linkage studies based on data obtained from HIV/AIDS and cancer registries, and three were observational cohort studies. The incidence of anal cancer was significantly higher in HIV-positive men than in HIV-negative men ($p = 0.011$). This result has been mirrored in several studies in the US and Europe, which show that the incidence of anal cancer among PWH ranges from 42 to 137 cases per 100,000 py, a rate 30 to 100 times higher than that of the general population (D'Souza et al., 2008; Patel et al., 2008; Piketty et al., 2008).

SCCA may be overlooked in the female population; however, the rate of HPV-related anal cancers among women appears to be higher than that in men (1.8 vs. 1.2 per 100,000 persons) (CDC, 2012a). Other publications have found incidence rates as high as 18 to 30 per 100,000 persons (Piketty et al., 2012; Silverberg et al., 2012). Incidence of anal cancer in WWH in higher-income countries is also high (3.9–30 per 100,000 persons) (Stier et al., 2015). Women with CD4+ T-cell counts of less than 200 cells/mm³ have a nearly 15-fold higher risk of developing invasive SCCA compared to the general population (SIR 14.5; 95% CI, 8.8–22.4) (Chaturvedi et al., 2009). Like the effects of HPV on cervical endothelium, the virus can lead to high-grade precancerous lesions and anal cancer. A recent systematic review of SCCA in women revealed higher prevalence of HPV in the anus versus cervix in most studies reviewed (16–85% vs. 17–70%, respectively) and that concordant HPV genotypes were found in 9% to 16% of women. Risk factors for anal HPV included cervical HPV, low CD4+ cell count, smoking, and perianal warts (Stier et al., 2015). Furthermore, Machalek et al. (2012) found that the incidence of anal cancer was actually higher in the ART era. For example, from 1996 onward, the annual incidence of SCCA was 78 per 100,000 persons compared to 22 per 100,000 persons prior to this time. The reason for this increase is unclear. Improved survival associated with ART may allow for sufficient time for men with chronic HPV infection to develop anal cancer. Increases in screening are unlikely to explain this trend because routine screening is not yet currently recommended or routinely implemented in most clinical practice settings (Machalek et al., 2012). However, risk factors associated with SCCA have been shown to be associated with greater immunosuppression, including nadir CD4+ T-cell count and median HIV RNA levels of greater than 500,000 copies/mL (Guiguet et al., 2009).

SCREENING, TREATMENT, AND PREVENTION OF HIV-ASSOCIATED ANAL DYSPLASIA

As discussed previously, PWH are at an increased risk for SCCA and AIN; however, there is no standard screening protocol for anal cancer. SCCA shares many biological similarities with cervical cancer, including detectable dysplastic precursor lesions and high-risk HPV infection. Consequently, many have recommended annual anal Pap screening for PWH (Bosch et al., 1995). Anal Pap smears are acquired by randomly obtaining squamous cells from the anal canal using a Dacron swab. They are then fixed in liquid cytology media. Like cervical cytology protocols, abnormal anal cytologic findings are confirmed by high-resolution anoscopy-directed

biopsy of visualized lesions (Figure 29.1). HPV DNA testing remains controversial due to the high prevalence of high-risk HPV infection in PWH (Benevolo et al., 2016; Berry et al., 2009). However, presence of high-risk HPV genotype 16 is associated with concurrent high-grade anal lesions in WWH (Heard et al., 2015, 2016). A recent study in which high-resolution anoscopy was performed on 156 PWH who tested negative for high-risk HPV by anal swab found that an approximately 8% risk of anal precancer remains for PWH who test high-risk HPV negative by anal swab (Wang et al., 2020). Anal cytology is categorized according to the Bethesda system for cervical cytology: ASCUS, low-grade squamous intraepithelial lesion (LSIL), and HSIL. Anal Pap smears have a similar sensitivity and specificity as cervical Pap smears. Note that there are no definitive clinical studies showing that anal Pap smears decrease SCCA-related morbidity and mortality among PWH. Furthermore, anal cytology should not be performed if evaluation with high-resolution anoscopy is not available for the patient. Women with a history of cervical or vulvar neoplasias are more likely to have anal HPV infection and abnormal anal cytology (Stier et al., 2015). The presence of anal warts or condyloma acuminata may also be an indicator for HPV infection of the anal canal and may warrant further screening. High-risk patients should be followed every 6 months for at least 5 years, ideally with periodic photographic documentation of the perianal region. There should be a low threshold to repeat biopsies of any changing lesion.

There is a lack of consensus and rigorous evidence regarding recommendations for performing annual digital rectal exam (DRE) in patients at risk for SCCA, such as MSM. The 2020 European AIDS Clinical Society (EACS) guidelines recommend DRE with or without an anal Pap smear every 1 to 3 years in MSM (EACS, 2020). The 2020 Guidelines for Prevention and Treatment of Opportunistic Infections in HIV-Positive Adults and Adolescents suggest that annual DRE is only a class B, grade III recommendation (USDHHS,

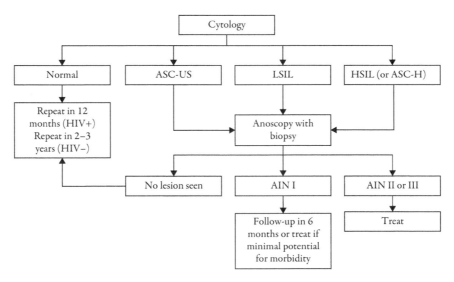

Figure 29.1 Screening protocol for anal intraepithelial neoplasia (AIN). ASC-H, atypical squamous cells, cannot rule out HSIL; ASC-US, atypical squamous cells of undetermined significance; HSIL, high-grade squamous intraepithelial lesion; LSIL, low-grade squamous intraepithelial lesion. SOURCE: From Park IU, et al. *Curr Infect Dis Rep*. 2010 March; 12(2): 126–133.

2020). Recently, a phase 2 clinical trial was conducted to assess the feasibility of teaching MSM to recognize palpable masses in the anal canal using self- or partner exams (Nyitray et al., 2018). Results indicated that tumors 3 mm or larger may be detectable by self- or partner exams, which is significant as there is a high cure rate for tumors 10 mm or smaller.

TREATMENT

The surveillance of patients with AIN II and III is predominantly aimed at the identification of early invasive carcinoma that can be treated by local excision or localized chemotherapy and radiation. Few data exist regarding the management of AIN, but it is thought that, like CIN, if AIN can be eradicated, then malignant transformation can be prevented. Targeted biopsies using high-resolution anoscopy and 3% acetic acid to the anal canal mucosa (like colposcopy) can help identify areas of AIN.

Treatment options for anal dysplasia are similar for PWH and HIV-negative individuals. These include topical trichloroacetic acid, liquid nitrogen, imiquimod, infrared coagulation, electrocautery, carbon dioxide (CO_2) laser, and surgical excision. One randomized trial of 156 HIV-positive MSM showed that electrocautery is better than imiquimod and fluorouracil in the treatment of AIN but recognized that recurrence rates were substantial (Richel et al., 2013). Of note, there are several new therapies being evaluated for PWH with anal dysplasia. These include two Australian studies: a phase 2 trial evaluating the immunomodulator pomalidomide in anal HSIL (NCT03113942) and a phase 1 study evaluating a new topical drug with direct anti-HPV activity, ABI-1968 (NCT03202992).

Currently, the recommended treatment for PWH with anal cancer is the same as that recommended for the general population (Reid et al., 2018). In the general population, concurrent chemoradiotherapy with 5-fluorouracil (5-FU) infusion and mitomycin (or cisplatin) has been established as the standard-of-care regimen for nonmetastatic anal cancer (Leiker et al., 2020). In the ART era, reports on clinical outcomes of PWH with anal cancer have been conflicting. Some studies have shown that PWH and HIV-negative people had comparable disease control and survival (Blazy et al., 2005; Chiao et al., 2008; Fraunholz et al., 2011), whereas others have suggested that PWH (particularly those with increased time between anal cancer diagnosis and treatment and those with lower posttreatment CD4+ T-cell counts) may do worse in terms of treatment-related toxicity and/or an increased risk for local relapse (Grew et al., 2015; Oehler-Janne et al., 2008; Susko et al., 2020). Existing evidence is limited by mostly retrospective data as well as small numbers of patients studied; thus, further investigation into this question would be beneficial.

PREVENTION

Routine vaccination with quadrivalent HPV or the 9-valent HPV vaccine is now available for all individuals aged 9 to 45 years to prevent genital warts and the development of precancerous and cancerous HPV-mediated lesions (FDA, 2018). Advisory Committee on Immunization Practices (2016) recommendations for individuals older than age 26 have not yet been updated. Starting ART early likely reduces the risk of high-risk HPV infection and anal cancer development (Kelly et al., 2020).

EFFECT OF ART ON ANAL DYSPLASIA

Like studies evaluating the effect of ART on cervical dysplasia, studies evaluating the effect of HIV therapy on anal dysplasia have found conflicting results. This may be related to the significant design and methodologic differences among these studies. There are two small case series ($n = 4$ and 26 patients, respectively) describing outcomes of HIV-associated SCCA, with 5-year survival rates of 47% to 60% (Jephcott et al., 2004; Myerson et al., 2001). In studies that specifically compared survival among patients with SCCA in the pre-ART versus ART eras, there was a nonsignificant trend toward improved survival, better tolerability of chemoradiotherapy, and improved local tumor control in the ART era (Bower et al., 2004; Cleator et al., 2000; Stadler et al., 2004).

A study linking the New York State cancer registry with the New York City HIV/AIDS registry found that in the early ART era (1990–1996), the 24-month survival was 76% for patients with AIDS compared to 78% for patients without AIDS, suggesting that, at least during this time period, PWH with SCCA had equivalent survival with HIV-negative patients.

Palefsky et al. (2001) compared the rates of progression and regression of anal dysplasia after 6 months of ART. They found that the likelihood of lesion progression or regression was not affected by ART initiation, but they noted that among the patients starting ART at higher CD4+ T-cell counts, ART demonstrated a nonsignificant benefit on anal dysplasia lesions. In contrast, Wilkin et al. (2004) conducted a cross-sectional study evaluating anal HPV infection and anal dysplasia in 98 HIV-positive men. In a multivariate analysis, they found that ART and higher nadir CD4+ T-cell count were significantly protective for anal dysplasia by histology but were not protective for anal HPV infection. A Canadian study retrospectively evaluated 1,691 HIV-positive MSM and found that immunosuppression with nadir CD4+ T-cell count of less than 100 cells/mm³ was a risk factor for anal cancer (OR, 3.08; $p = 0.01$). They also found that men treated during the pre-ART era had a higher incidence (370 vs. 93 per 100,000 py) and shorter lead time to development of anal cancer compared to those in the post-ART era (Duncan et al., 2015). Therefore, it remains unclear if ART initiation influences the natural history of AIN in PWH. However, ART is beneficial for men undergoing treatment for HPV-related disease.

RECOMMENDED READING

Kojic EM, Kang M, Cespedes MS, et al. Immunogenicity and safety of the quadrivalent human papillomavirus vaccine in HIV-1-infected women. *Clin Infect Dis*. 2014;59(1):127–135.

Leiker AJ, Wang CJ, Sanford NN, et al. Feasibility and outcome of routine use of concurrent chemoradiation in PLWH with squamous cell anal cancer. *Am J Clin Oncol.* 2020;43(10):701–708. doi:10.1097/COC.0000000000000736

Piketty C, Selinger-Leneman H, Grabar S, et al. Marked increase in the incidence of invasive anal cancer among HIV-infected patients despite treatment with combination antiretroviral therapy. *AIDS.* 2008;22(10):1203–1211.

Smith AJB, Varma S, Rositch AF, et al. Gynecologic cancer in HIV-positive women: a systematic review and meta-analysis. *Am J Obstet Gynecol.* 2019;221(3):194–207. doi:10.1016/j.ajog.2019.02.022

Stier EA, Sebring MC, Mendez AE, et al. Prevalence of anal human papillomavirus infection and anal HPV-related disorders in women: a systematic review. *Am J Obstet Gynecol.* 2015;213(3):278–309.

LUNG CANCER

LEARNING OBJECTIVES

- Review the epidemiology and risks of lung cancer in PWH

- Review the pathogenesis of lung cancer

- Discuss the treatment of lung cancer

- Discuss the treatment outcomes and mortality associated with lung cancer in PWH

WHAT'S NEW?

- PWH have an increasing incidence of lung cancer during the ART era.

- Surgery, chemotherapy, and radiation are mainstays of standard treatment for PWH.

- Treatment disparities between PWH and HIV-negative patients may contribute to poor survivability of those with lung cancer.

KEY POINTS

- Tobacco cessation is of utmost importance in preventing lung cancers in PWH.

- PWH have a higher incidence of lung cancer than the general population, although a predominant histology of non-small cell lung cancer (NSCLC) is common in both groups.

- PWH have worse survival, which may be due to frequent presentation with advanced disease.

- No specific guidelines for treating PWH and lung cancer exist, and more rigorous studies evaluating standards of care are needed.

Lung cancer is the leading cause of death due to cancer in the general US population, and it also represents the most common NADC (Frisch et al., 2001). Lung cancers in HIV are primarily NSCLC types, including adenocarcinoma and squamous cell carcinoma. This largely reflects the trend of histology types among the general population in Western settings (Cadranel et al., 2006). Mortality from lung cancer remains high in PWH compared to the general population, especially for patients presenting at advanced stages (Coghill et al., 2015; Shiels et al., 2010).

The incidence of lung cancer, like that of other NADCs, has increased for several reasons, including increased life expectancy in the era of ART and longer cumulative exposure to carcinogens known to be associated with lung cancer development, namely tobacco smoke. Notably, tobacco exposure in the HIV population remains a significant health problem, with disproportionate use compared to the general population (Altekruse et al., 2018; Clifford et al., 2012; Rahmanian et al., 2011). Due to this increased risk, smoking cessation is of utmost importance in this patient population (Shepherd et al., 2018). Immunosuppression may also be a contributing factor; however, this relationship is not clearly understood.

EPIDEMIOLOGY OF LUNG CANCER IN HIV

Engels et al. (2008) examined data from large HIV and cancer registries in the US to estimate the incidence of lung cancer. They found the incidence in the HIV population to be 59 per 100,000 py during the period from 1991 to 2002 (Engels et al., 2008). This same study found that the incidence of lung cancer increased from 51 per 100,000 py to 126 per 100,000 py in those with HIV compared to those with an AIDS diagnosis (Engels et al., 2008). In another study including Canadian data, researchers found that, from 1996 to 2009, the incidence of lung cancer in PWH was 129 per 100,000 py compared to 45.4 per 100,000 py in HIV-negative individuals. The incidence of lung cancer was higher for persons aged 75 years than for those aged 65 years (3.4% vs. 2.2%), which supports the increased risk of cancer development as the population ages (Silverberg et al., 2015). Marcus et al. (2017) evaluated a Californian cohort of 24,768 PWH compared to 257,600 HIV-negative individuals between 1996 and 2011 and found that the lung cancer rate was 66 per 100,000 py for PWH and 33 per 100,000 py for HIV-negative individuals (rate ratio 2.0, 95% CI: 1.7–2.2).

A Ugandan study evaluating overall cancer incidence (ADC and NADCs) in PWH from 1988 to 2002 found the incidence over time to be increased, with a SIR of 5 (Mbulaiteye et al., 2006). Another study using the Swiss HIV Cohort Study and Swiss cancer registries found that cancers of the trachea, lung, and bronchus were significantly elevated compared to those of the general population, with a SIR of 3.2 (Clifford et al., 2005).

The impact of ART on the incidence and risk of lung cancer remains unclear. Studies attempting to evaluate the incidence of lung cancer during the pre-ART and ART eras have found mixed results, with increased incidence in both eras. The previously cited study by Silverberg et al. (2015) showed that cumulative incidence of lung cancer in North America continues to increase in the ART era. They found a cumulative incidence of 3.7% from 2005 to 2009 compared to 1.8% from 1996 to 2009 (Silverberg et al., 2015). Another study that examined data from 34 states showed similar results, with a steady increase in the number of lung cancers (35 to 283 cases) from 1991 to 2005, which largely occurred in persons older than 50 years (Shiels et al., 2011). This phenomenon speaks to the increasing longevity of the HIV population and accumulation of malignant comorbidities.

RISK FACTORS ASSOCIATED WITH LUNG CANCER IN HIV

Risk factors for lung cancer are multiple and include tobacco exposure, injection drug use, and possibly HIV infection itself. Other comorbid pulmonary diseases, such as chronic obstructive pulmonary disease and bacterial pneumonia, are more common in PWH than in HIV-negative individuals and may place PWH at higher risk for cancer due to persistent states of inflammation (Crothers et al., 2011; Shebl et al., 2010). Inflammatory markers circulating in the blood have been associated with theoretical risk of lung cancer; these include C-reactive protein, serum amyloid, soluble tumor necrosis factor receptor-2, lymphoid differentiation cytokine interleukin-7, and various leukocyte-derived chemokines (Shiels et al., 2013). However, it remains to be determined exactly how these inflammatory states that are not confounded by smoking or other traditional risks factors like pneumonia impact the risk of lung cancer.

Cigarette smoking has repeatedly been implicated as a major risk factor for lung cancer in the general population as well as in the HIV population (Altekruse et al., 2018; Shepherd et al., 2018). Prevalence of cigarette smoking among PWH is estimated to be between 42% and 59%, and it greatly exceeds that of the general population by two- to threefold (Altekruse et al., 2018; Mdodo et al., 2015; Tesoriero et al., 2010). In a Swiss study, Clifford et al. (2005) reported that all persons with cancer of the respiratory tract were smokers, and there was a threefold higher excess risk of these cancers. A similar finding was demonstrated in a US study that showed patients with HIV and lung cancer were 1.3 times more likely to be current or former smokers and to have greater pack-year tobacco consumption history compared to those with HIV but without cancer (D'Jaen et al., 2010). Shiels et al. (2010) also examined the role of cigarette smoking in the development of lung cancer in HIV. They found that those with HIV who smoked more than 1.43 packs per day had twice the risk of lung cancer compared to those with HIV who smoked less. Compared to HIV-negative patients who smoked less than 1.43 packs per day, those with HIV and who smoked more than 1.43 packs per day had a 7.2 times higher risk of developing lung cancer (Shiels et al., 2010). A more recent study using the North American AIDS Cohort Collaboration on Research and Design consortium evaluated 52,441 PWH including 2,306 who were diagnosed with cancer between 2000 and 2015 (Altekruse et al., 2018). They found that PWH diagnosed with cancer were more likely to have been smokers (79%) compared to those without cancer (73%). Furthermore, in PWH smoking was associated with increased risk of cancer overall (HR =1.33 [95% CI, 1.18–1.49]), smoking-related cancers (HR= 2.31 [1.80–2.98]), and lung cancer (HR =17.80 [5.60–56.63]). Reddy et al. (2017) recently used an HIV microsimulation model to evaluate cumulative lung cancer mortality by smoking exposure and found that PWH who continue to smoke have a 16.6% to 29.8% estimated mortality depending on sex and smoking intensity, while estimated mortality decreased to 3.7% to 7.9% for those who quit smoking and to 1.2% to 1.6% for never smokers. Even PWH who were adherent to ART were 6 to 13 times more likely to die from lung cancer than from traditional AIDS-related causes. When the authors applied this model to the current US HIV-positive population, they found that 9.3% could die from lung cancer if their smoking habits do not change.

Other studies have not found the same association with smoking. Engels et al. (2006) studied 5,238 PWH and found that the overall smoking-adjusted SIR for lung cancer was 2.5 times higher than that of the general population (95% CI, 1.6–3.5). However, in an analysis that assumed that all participants smoked, the smoking-adjusted SIR was only 1.7. This suggests that smoking did not account for all excess risk of lung cancer in HIV (Engels et al., 2006). In the mortality analysis by Shiels et al. (2010), it was found that, after adjusting for smoking and other patient characteristics, the risk of death was 3.8 times higher for PWH versus HIV-negative patients. A large Veterans Administration study found that the incidence rate ratio (1.7) of lung cancer in HIV patients remained significantly elevated after multivariable adjustment for confounders including smoking compared to persons without HIV (Sigel et al., 2012). These studies suggest that, independent of smoking, HIV positivity portends a higher incidence and mortality risk for lung cancer.

Injection drug use among PWH has also been associated with an increased risk of lung cancer compared with that for nonusers in several studies. One study in particular demonstrated that those with injection drug use, with or without HIV, had an increased risk of lung cancer, with SIRs of 14.3 and 6.2, respectively (Serraino et al., 2000). Other studies have found little evidence to support this risk factor, however. In a study by Kirk et al. (2007) that included 2,086 participants (the AIDS Link to the Intravenous Experience Study), injection drug use was not associated with increased risk of lung cancer.

HIV itself may also be associated with the development of lung cancer due to directly acting oncogenic effects. HIV-1 replication depends on tat protein expression, which can upregulate expression of protooncogenes c-myc, c-fos, and c-jun to enhance cellular proliferation, including human adenocarcinoma cell lines (El-Solh et al., 1997). Allelic loss and changes in microsatellites, which are short tandem repeat DNA sequences, have also been described in other malignancies, such as KS, NHL, and SCCA, and have been found in lung cancers of PWH (Wistuba et al., 1998). These genetic alterations may lead to activation of oncogenes and loss of tumor suppressor genes. However, the lack of HIV viral integration into cellular DNA of somatic neoplastic cells challenges this hypothesis of oncogenesis because cancer cells can have background genetic alterations and immunosuppression can also be associated with microsatellite changes (Bedi et al., 1995). Poor control of HIV also could contribute to the development of lung cancer. A study of PWH included in the

US Veterans Aging Cohort Study found that increased risk of lung cancer was associated with low CD4+ T-cell count, low CD4/CD8 ratio, high HIV viral load, and more cumulative episodes of bacterial pneumonia (Sigel et al., 2017). Another recent study similarly noted that a CD4+ cell count of less than 200 cells/mm³ was associated with a younger age at lung cancer diagnosis (Shiels et al., 2017). In contrast, a large Californian cohort study by Marcus et al. (2017) did not find an association between increased development of lung cancer and CD4+ T-cell count of less than 200 cells/mm³.

Although men historically have been considered at higher risk for lung cancer, women also share a significant proportion of lung cancer diagnoses. This may be due to the increase in women tobacco smokers in the population or the increase in the number of WWH. The WIHS compared data from the National Health and Nutritional Examination (NHANES) II and SEER. Researchers found that WWH have higher lifetime cigarette consumption as well as an elevated SIR of 3 (95% CI, 1.7–5.1) compared to the general population, which has a SIR of 2.11 (95% CI, 0.25–7.61). Furthermore, these data did not vary by pre-ART versus ART era (Levine et al., 2010). A French study evaluating cancer in PWH in the pre-ART and ART eras found that the SIR of women was three times higher than that of men in the ART era (6.28 vs. 2.12) (Herida et al., 2003). Several additional studies have shown greater incidence in women with SIR ranging from 1.6 to 16.7 (Calabresi et al., 2013; Clifford et al., 2005; Ramirez-Marrero et al., 2010).

DIAGNOSIS AND CLINICAL PRESENTATION OF LUNG CANCER IN HIV

Despite the increased risk of cancer with aging, PWH and lung cancer tend to be younger. In several studies, age at presentation ranged from 38 to 57 years. This is far below the age of presentation among the general population, which is closer to the seventh decade of life (Winstone et al., 2013). Stage at presentation also tends to be advanced in PWH, with a majority presenting with stages III or IV. This likely contributes to the poor survivability of these patients (Sigel et al., 2012; Winstone et al., 2013).

The majority of histologic types mirror those of the general population, with greater than 50% consisting of NSCLC. Adenocarcinoma is the predominant NSCLC (36%), followed by squamous cell carcinoma (30%) (Sigel et al., 2012). Many patients present with advanced disease and have symptoms of persistent cough and chest pain (Karp et al., 1993). Early diagnosis of lung cancer improves prognosis; however, screening with plain chest radiography at any interval has not been shown to be effective and is not recommended. Use of low-dose chest CT (LDCT) may be beneficial in these patients. The recommendation of the US Preventive Services Task Force (USPTF) to screen high-risk patients for lung cancer with LDCT was based on the findings from the National Lung Screening Trial (2011). This large randomized trial found a 20% reduction in lung cancer mortality after implementing annual screening by LDCT in patients aged 55 to 74 years with at least a 30 pack-year smoking history. Because of improved mortality benefit, current USPTF guidelines recommend lung cancer screening with LDCT for people aged 55 to 80 in the general population with at least a 30 pack-year smoking history who currently smoke or who have quit within 15 years, regardless of gender (Moyer, 2014). Of note, a handful of studies that have evaluated LDCT in PWH have suggested that these patients, especially those with low CD4+ counts, are more likely to have false-positive LDCT findings due to prior lung infections (Ronit et al., 2017; Sigel et al., 2014). A recent modeling study evaluating HIV-infected patients with CD4+ T-cell counts of at least 500 cells/mm³ found that screening using the Centers for Medicare and Medicaid Services criteria (age 55–77, 30 pack-years of smoking, current smoker or quit within 15 years of screening) would reduce lung cancer mortality by 18.9% in this population, similar to the mortality reduction of uninfected individuals (Kong et al., 2018). Thus, the benefit and cost-effectiveness of LDCT in patients infected with HIV remain unknown, but following the USPTF and NCCN guidelines for the general population is reasonable after discussing risks (e.g., false positives and radiation exposure) and benefits (e.g., early detection and better prognosis) with patients (Reid et al., 2018). Currently, a French multicenter prospective pilot study (ANRS EP48 HIV-CHEST cohort) is evaluating the utility of LDCT in PWH (NCT01207986; Makinson et al., 2015).

Understanding the mechanisms underlying the development of lung cancer in PWH could lead to improved lung cancer screening methodologies. Zheng et al. (2018) recently studied the molecular mechanisms underlying the gene expression profiles of lung cancer in PWH and identified 758 differentially expressed genes in HIV-associated lung cancer. Specifically, they found that expression levels of SIX1 and TFAP2A mRNA are increased in HIV-associated lung cancer and expression levels of ADH1B, INMT, and SYNPO2 mRNA are decreased.

TREATMENT OF LUNG CANCER

There are no alternative or specific treatment guidelines for lung cancer in the HIV population. Most randomized trials for lung cancer have historically excluded PWH due to concerns regarding immune suppression, toxicity, and drug interactions with ART (Persad et al., 2008). Current treatment strategies are mainly with protocols for patients without HIV and depend on tumor histology, stage of disease, and underlying host factors such as comorbidities and pulmonary function. Patients with NSCLC are staged (I–IV) based on the tumor node metastasis (TNM) system, with stage I disease confined to localized tumor without invasion into the chest wall, diaphragm, mediastinum, or surrounding structures and stage IV indicating metastatic disease (Shepherd et al., 2007). MRI of the brain should also be pursued for stage II or higher to identify intracranial metastasis. For localized, nonmetastatic disease, surgical resection is the preferred strategy with intent to cure for those patients able to undergo surgery. Surgery (lobectomy, sublobular resection, and video-assisted thoracoscopy) may be followed by adjuvant chemotherapy or radiation for those with more advanced stages or invasion

(NCCN, 2015c). For nonsurgical candidates, ablation with radiotherapy can be considered. Studies evaluating surgery in PWH have been described in mainly small case–control series and case reports. Patients undergoing surgery for localized disease (stage I or stage II) tolerated surgery well with minimal complications (Cadranel et al., 2006).

For patients with advanced NSCLC or recurrence after initial definitive therapy, goals of therapy are largely palliative. For patients with solitary metastasis or recurrence, curative intention with additional surgery or radiotherapy may be indicated and beneficial to help prolong survival. However, risks and benefits must be weighed in advanced disease to avoid undue adverse events and toxicities. Systemic therapy with combination chemotherapy using a platinum-based regimen is the mainstay of treatment with or without additional agents, such as the vascular endothelial growth factor inhibitor bevacizumab (NCCN, 2015c).

While HIV infection is often an exclusion criterion in lung cancer clinical trials, use of chemotherapy for lung cancer treatment in PWH is feasible, and it has been used in patients to treat metastatic disease and as an adjuvant therapy in combination with radiation for locally advanced disease. One large retrospective study found similar rates of treatment modality between HIV and non-HIV patients (Sigel et al., 2013). Limited data from case series have provided heterogeneous results regarding use of chemotherapeutic agents, efficacy, and drug toxicities in HIV patients with lung cancer (Bower et al., 2003; Powles et al., 2003; Spano et al., 2004). Recently a French phase 2 trial of PWH with advanced non-squamous NSCLC showed that first-line four-cycle induction with carboplatin plus pemetrexed followed by pemetrexed maintenance was effective and reasonably well tolerated (Lavole et al., 2020). Additional studies to evaluate efficacy, tolerability, and safety of chemotherapy in HIV patients are needed.

Additional molecular and genetic mutation analysis for potential genetic-directed therapy targets has been explored. These should be performed when possible in patients with advanced-stage NSCLC, namely for the presence of epidermal growth factor receptor (EGFR) and anaplasmic lymphoma kinase (NCCN, 2015c). Other targets include RAS family oncogenes, the mTOR signaling pathway, and the MEK signaling pathway. Treatment with EGFR tyrosine kinase inhibitors such as erlotinib may also be considered for patients with this specific EGFR mutation in the tumor. However, long-term survival has yet to be established with use of these agents (Okuma et al., 2014). Several novel treatment regimens are being studied in PWH with advanced lung cancer. Immunotherapies such as nivolumab, ipilimumab, and durvalumab are being evaluated in patients with advanced solid tumors, including NSCLC (NCT03304093, NCT02408861) and solid tumors (NCT03094286); Bender-Ignacio et al., 2018).

SURVIVAL OF LUNG CANCER IN HIV

Survival among PWH and lung cancer is worse compared to that of their HIV-negative counterparts. Coghill et al. (2015) analyzed data from 1996 to 2010 and found that all-cause mortality and cancer-specific mortality risk were respectively 85% and 28% higher for PWH with lung cancer compared to HIV-negative patients. For patients with local-stage NSCLC receiving standard cancer therapy, PWH continued to have greater cancer-related deaths compared to HIV-negative patients (HR, 1.8; 95% CI, 1.21–2.7) (Coghill et al., 2015). Another large study utilizing SEER registry data compared 267 PWH to 1,428 HIV-negative patients with similar cancer stage and histology of NSCLC (Sigel et al., 2013). Both groups with stage I to IIIA disease received surgery, chemotherapy, and radiotherapy at similar rates. Among the PWH group, 82% died during follow-up compared to 66% of the HIV-negative group (p < 0.001). Median overall survival for PWH was only 6 months compared to 20 months for the HIV-negative cohort. Overall 5-year survival was also poor for PWH at 9% compared to 23% for the HIV-negative group. PWH and advanced disease (stage IIIB to IV) had the worst survival, with 9 to 20 times greater risk of death compared to PWH with only localized disease. Moreover, a major proportion of PWH also died from non–cancer-related causes (31% vs. 9%; p < 0.001).

Such disparity in outcomes in the previously discussed studies may be explained by several hypotheses, including the fact that PWH experience overall greater mortality than the general population. It may be that tumors behave more aggressively in PWH due to tumor effect or poor immunologic surveillance due to lack of fully intact cellular immunity. Evaluation of the North American AIDS Cohort Collaboration on Research and Design dataset found that PWH with a history of an AIDS-defining illness at lung cancer diagnosis had higher mortality and poorer survival after diagnosis compared to those without (Grover et al., 2018). Poor tolerability of surgery and chemotherapy may also contribute to worse outcomes. More studies are needed to clarify these issues.

Last, health disparities in treatment between PWH and HIV-negative populations may contribute to poor survivability. Data from the Texas Cancer Registry from 1995 to 2009 showed that PWH and NSCLC less frequently received any cancer treatments despite greater numbers presenting at younger ages and with distant-stage disease (Suneja et al., 2013). PWH and local-stage NSCLC were less likely to receive surgery (45.5% vs. 62.5%; p = 0.04) than HIV-negative patients. PWH with regional disease were less likely to receive systemic chemotherapy. For distant disease, PWH received less chemotherapy or radiation (31.1% vs. 45.5%; p = 0.0009) (Suneja et al., 2013).

RECOMMENDED READING

Coghill AE, Shiels MS, Suneja G, et al. Elevated cancer-specific mortality among HIV-infected patients in the United States. *J Clin Oncol.* 2015;33(21):2376–2383.

Grover S, Desir F, Jing Y, et al. Reduced cancer survival among adults with HIV and AIDS-defining illnesses despite no difference in cancer stage at diagnosis. *J AIDS.* 2018;79(4):421–429.

Lavole A, Greillier L, Mazieres J, et al. First-line carboplatin plus pemetrexed with pemetrexed maintenance in HIV+ patients with advanced non-squamous non-small cell lung cancer: the phase II IFCT-1001 CHIVA trial. *Eur Respir J*. 2020;56(2):1902066. doi:10.1183/13993003.02066-2019

Sigel K, Crothers K, Dubrow R, et al. Prognosis in HIV-infected patients with non-small cell lung cancer. *Br J Cancer*. 2013;109:1974–1980.

Suneja G, Shiels MS, Melville SK. Disparities in the treatment and outcomes of lung cancer among HIV-infected individuals. *AIDS*. 2013;27(3):459–468.

PROSTATE CANCER

LEARNING OBJECTIVES

- Review the epidemiology and risk factors for prostate cancer in men with HIV

- Review the current screening recommendations for prostate cancer

- Discuss the treatment options for prostate cancer in men with HIV

WHAT'S NEW?

- Since the advent of prostate-specific antigen (PSA) testing, the incidence of prostate cancer has increased in HIV-positive men. However, the true incidence may be lower than that of HIV-negative men.

- Routine prostate cancer screening with PSA testing is not recommended.

KEY POINTS

- Prostate cancer represents a significant burden of neoplastic disease and mortality in HIV-positive men and also men in the general population.

- Prostate cancer appears to be associated with states of immunologic control.

- Screening with serum PSA testing should not routinely be implemented, having a "D" recommendation by the USPSTF.

- Decision to treat early-stage cancer versus watchful waiting should be carefully considered because evidence of long-term mortality benefits remains unclear.

- First-line therapies include radical prostatectomy and radiation.

Prostate cancer remains the leading cancer diagnosis among men in the US and other industrialized countries. It is the second leading cause of cancer deaths after lung cancer. Increased screening efforts in the US led to increased incidence after the PSA test became widely available in 1992. However, screening and treatment among HIV-negative and PWH have been controversial due to the occult and often indolent nature of untreated prostate cancer, especially in older men with limited life expectancy. The mortality benefit of diagnosis and treatment of early-stage prostate cancer remains unproved; thus, emphasis on screening and early detection has waned in recent years. Compared to other NADCs, such as lung or anal cancer, some studies have demonstrated HIV infection to be associated with a reduced risk of prostate cancer (Sun et al., 2020). Regardless, diagnosis of prostate cancer carries a significant clinical impact on patients' sexual, genitourinary, and overall health.

EPIDEMIOLOGY OF PROSTATE CANCER IN HIV

HIV-positive men in the US experienced an increased incidence of prostate cancer after 1990 compared to the preceding decade, from 0.2% to 2.2% of all cancers in a retrospective study of population-based registry data (Engels et al., 2006). In the same study, the incidence increased during the pre-ART and post-ART eras, which may be explained by the introduction of the PSA screening test. Another study that was a large retrospective review also found that prostate cancer in HIV-positive men increased during the time from 1992 to 2003 (Patel et al., 2008). However, the HIV-positive group had statistically significantly lower rates of cancer compared to the general population in the pre-ART era (15 vs. 47 per 100,000 py) and the ART era (38 vs. 61 per 100,000 py) (Patel et al., 2008). Another study that examined the PSA testing era (1992–2007) found an incidence of 28 per 100,000 py in HIV-positive men. However, the incidence in HIV-positive men compared to the expected rate in the general population during this same time period was significantly reduced, with a SIR of only 0.5 (95% CI, 0.44–0.57) (Shiels et al., 2010). Of note, some disparity remains when prostate cancer diagnoses are compared among races. One study that evaluated men enrolled in the Multicenter AIDS Cohort Study (MACS) from 1996 to 2010 found an incidence of 169 per 100,000 py among all men 40 to 70 years old compared to 276 per 100,000 py among African American HIV-positive men (Dutta et al., 2017). In this study prostate cancer risk was similar by HIV-infection status (IRR 1.0; 95% CI, 0.55–1.82) but nearly threefold higher in African Americans compared to non-African Americans in adjusted models (IRRs 2.66 and 3.22; 95% CIs, 1.36–5.18 and 1.27–8.16 for all or HIV-positive men, respectively).

RISK FACTORS FOR PROSTATE CANCER

Postulated risk factors that promote development of prostate cancer in HIV-positive men include exposure to carcinogens and use of androgen supplementation to treat hypogonadism. Coinfection with oncogenic viruses may also promote neoplasia (Montgomery et al., 2006). Chronic inflammatory states promoted by HIV systemically and localized to the prostate, as well as chronic prostatitis, may contribute to cancer development (Leport et al., 1989; Smith et al., 2004).

Prostate cancer and risk of death have been associated with tobacco exposure in several studies. However, other studies have demonstrated conflicting data. Two large meta-analyses examined this issue and found similar results (Huncharek et al., 2010; Islami et al., 2014). Huncharek et al. found a dose-dependent relationship with incidence of prostate cancer in HIV-negative patients. The heaviest smokers had a 13% increased risk of cancer. These data were derived from seven prospective cohort studies. Based on 19 prospective studies, Islami et al. (2014) found smoking to be associated with an increased risk of death (RR, 1.24) from prostate cancer, which was dose-dependent. The incidence of prostate cancer, however, was not statistically significant overall. In fact, baseline cigarette smoking was inversely associated with incidence of prostate cancer (Islami et al., 2014).

Unlike other malignancies in HIV, immunologic control with increasing $CD4^+$ T-cell count has been associated with increased risk of prostate cancer, with a relative risk that is threefold greater in the ART era (Shiels et al., 2010). In several studies, HIV-positive men with prostate cancer had robust $CD4^+$ T-cell counts of greater than 300 cells/mm^3 (Hsiao et al., 2009; Marcus et al., 2014; Pantanowitz et al., 2008). Overall, data from numerous studies suggest that variations in prostate cancer deficits in HIV-positive men are due to differential PSA screening in this population and not to immunologic status.

PROSTATE CANCER SCREENING

The primary tools for diagnosis of prostate cancer include serum PSA measurement, DRE, and, ultimately, prostate biopsy for definitive histologic diagnosis. Both European and US guidelines have recommended against routine screening with PSA in both HIV-negative and HIV-positive men (Heidenreich et al., 2014; Moyer, 2012). Rather, whether to perform individual screening with PSA for early detection should be a well-informed, mutual decision between physician and patient based on possible benefits and harms of a positive PSA test. Optimal interval of PSA screening has also not been established. DRE alone has limited sensitivity (6–8%) of detecting prostate cancer (Gosselaar et al., 2009; Okotie et al., 2007). The combination of an abnormal DRE versus normal DRE with PSA level of higher than 3 ng/mL may enhance positive predictive value of cancer detection at 48% versus 22% (Gosselaar et al., 2008).

CLINICAL PRESENTATION

Prostate cancer diagnosis in HIV often occurs in the fifth and sixth decades of life, and patients often have a positive family history of prostate cancer (Hsiao et al., 2009; Ong et al., 2015; Shiels et al., 2010). Men with HIV may present more often with late-stage disease compared to the general population, although this is supported by limited data (Shiels et al., 2015). A large California cohort found more localized cancer compared to regional or distant disease among HIV-positive men (88% vs. 7%), which was similar to the pattern found in HIV-negative men (Marcus et al., 2014). Other studies have found no difference in presentation with early or advanced disease (Hsiao et al., 2009; Riedel et al., 2015). HIV-negative African Americans have a greater likelihood of presenting with advanced-stage prostate cancer in the general population (Siegel et al., 2012). Within the HIV population, African Americans may represent a higher-risk group for prostate cancer because they represent a large proportion of HIV prevalence and annual HIV diagnoses in the US.

TREATMENT AND TREATMENT OUTCOMES OF PROSTATE CANCER

Treatment of prostate cancer in HIV-positive men is similar to that of HIV-negative men and is based on stage and grade of disease with use of the Gleason score (ranging from 2 to 10). For localized disease (stage I and stage II) not spread to lymph nodes or distant sites, strategies include active surveillance (PSA monitoring and/or repeat biopsy), radical prostatectomy, or radiation therapy (external beam radiation therapy [EBRT] and/or brachytherapy) with or without androgen deprivation. For locally advanced disease (stage III) that has spread outside the prostate gland, surgery or radiation with androgen deprivation therapy are alternatives. A Gleason score greater than 8 represents high-risk neoplasia, even if disease is localized. The optimal choice between surgical intervention and radiation is unclear for these patients, and careful consideration of individual risks and benefits should be discussed on a case-by-case basis (Grimm et al., 2012).

Treatment of disseminated disease, which often involves osteoblastic lesions, typically involves androgen deprivation therapy, castration (medical or surgical), and systemic chemotherapy. Two phase 3 trials examining the use of abiraterone and enzalutamide for treatment of metastatic, castration-resistant prostate cancer have shown clinical benefit with these agents, which target the androgen-synthesis pathway (Loriot et al., 2015; Ryan et al., 2015). Chemotherapy with taxane-based regimens has also shown success in prolonging survival in men with castration-resistant prostate cancer. Docetaxel plus prednisone is currently the standard, initial cytotoxic chemotherapy used in metastatic, castration-resistant disease (Berthold et al., 2008).

Few studies have evaluated the safety, tolerability, and efficacy of treatments for prostate cancer in men with HIV. Most studies have been small and limited to evaluation of EBRT with heterogeneity of dosing. One Veterans Administration study reported 15 patients who received an EBRT dose-escalation approach (75.6–79.2 Gy) for localized disease. Of the 15 patients, 13 were treated with concomitant ART, and the 5-year event-free survival was 92.3% (Schreiber et al., 2014). Toxicities included urinary frequency and rectal bleeding. Eight patients on ART had a transient decline in $CD4^+$ cell count, which returned to near or above baseline in the follow-up period. Another study evaluating EBRT (72–81 Gy) for localized prostate cancer in HIV-positive compared to HIV-negative men found that 26% of men with HIV had biochemical failure compared to 12% of matched HIV-negative controls. At a mean of 36 months, there were no deaths in the HIV group. Genitourinary and anal adverse events were overall mild (Kahn et al., 2012).

The risk of death from prostate cancer is associated with advanced disease compared to local or regional prostate cancer (Shiels et al., 2010). In a large retrospective study of HIV and cancer registries from 1996 to 2010, mortality of prostate cancer was significantly higher for HIV-positive versus HIV-negative men (HR, 1.57; 95% CI, 1.02–2.41) even after adjusting for patient characteristics and cancer stage (Coghill et al., 2015). Cancer deaths were also greater in HIV-positive men after adjusting for treatment, but not significantly so (HR, 1.64; 95% CI, 0.93–2.89). One study that used data from 1996 to 2002 found a 2.1-fold increased risk of death from prostate cancer in HIV-positive compared to HIV-negative men. Interestingly, in this study, HIV-positive men had more localized disease (Marcus et al., 2014).

RECOMMENDED READING

Coghill AE, Shiels MS, Suneja G, et al. Elevated cancer-specific mortality among HIV-infected patients in the United States. *J Clin Oncol*. 2015;33(21):2376–2383.

Marcus JL, Chao CR, Leyden WA, et al. Prostate cancer incidence and prostate-specific antigen testing among HIV-positive and HIV-negative men. *J AIDS*. 2014;66:495–502.

Moyer VA. Screening for prostate cancer: US Preventive Services Task Force recommendation statement. *Ann Intern Med*. 2012; 157(2):120–135.

Shiels MS, Goedert JJ, Moore RD, et al. Risk of prostate cancer in U.S. men with AIDS. *Cancer Epidemiol Biomarkers Prev*. 2010;19(11): 2910–2915.

Sun D, Cao M, Li H, et al. Risk of prostate cancer in men with HIV/AIDS: a systematic review and meta-analysis. *Prostate Cancer Prostatic Dis*. 2020 [E-pub before print]. doi:10.1038/s41391-020-00268-2

COLORECTAL ADENOCARCINOMA

LEARNING OBJECTIVES

- Review the epidemiology of colorectal cancer (CRC) in the HIV population

- Discuss the screening methods for CRC

- Review treatment modalities and outcomes in HIV patients with CRC

WHAT'S NEW?

- CRC incidence has increased in the HIV population compared to the general population in the ART era, and mortality remains high compared to that of the HIV-negative population.

- Patients with HIV disproportionately receive less CRC screening than the general population.

- Standard chemoradiation and surgical approaches for treating CRC appear to be well tolerated in patients with HIV, although more research is needed in this area.

KEY POINTS

- CRC presents a major health and mortality burden in the HIV population.

- CRC presentation occurs often in younger patients and with more advanced disease compared to the general population.

- Significant disparities exist in screening HIV patients for CRC compared to HIV-negative patients.

- Standard CRC treatment includes surgery and neoadjuvant and/or adjuvant chemoradiation.

- Survival is significantly worse compared to that of HIV-negative patients with CRC.

In the US, CRC is the third leading cause of cancer death in the general population for both men and women. It has been the focus of large-scale primary prevention screening efforts to identify patients with early disease (Siegel et al., 2014). Non-AIDS cancers such as colorectal adenocarcinoma in the HIV population have become increasingly recognized as a significant health problem as patients are living longer and may accrue greater risk factors for cancer development. Vigilance for neoplastic processes such as CRC must be maintained in HIV patients because they are often diagnosed at advanced stages and can be overlooked due to presentation at a younger age and lack of traditional risk factors such as family history (Chapman et al., 2009; Yegüez et al., 2003). This phenomenon was characterized by early case reports of colorectal adenocarcinoma in HIV. Patients were often males, aged 20s to 40s, and with advanced immunosuppression (Cappell et al., 1988; Klugman & Schaffner, 1994; Ravalli et al., 1989).

HIV patients who are considered "average" risk are offered screening less frequently than the general population (Nayudu & Balar, 2012). Furthermore, disparities in cancer treatment between PWH and HIV-negative patients are also prevalent. PWH are less likely to receive treatment for CRC than their HIV-negative counterparts (Suneja et al., 2013). The lack of screening and treatment is likely to contribute to poorer outcomes and excess mortality in PWH.

EPIDEMIOLOGY OF COLON CANCER IN HIV

Patients with HIV have incurred a higher incidence of CRC than the general population. A large US study that examined cancer incidence in HIV patients compared to the general population from 1992 to 2003 found an increased SIR during the early time period of 1992 to 1995 (39.9 per 100,000 py) compared to the later time period of 2000 to 2003 (66.2 per 100,000 py). During both time periods, the rates were greater than those of the general population (20.4 and 21.1 per 100,000 py, respectively) (Patel et al., 2008). In a more recent study using US and Canadian data from 2006 to 2009, the incidence rate of CRC in PWH was 36.4 per 100,000 py compared to 27.7 per 100,000 py in HIV-negative patients. During this study period, the cumulative incidence declined by 6% per year for HIV-negative patients but increased in those with HIV by 5% per year. This may reflect the declining death rate among persons with HIV (Silverberg et al., 2015).

A large Taiwanese study that used the National Health Insurance Research Database from 1998 to 2009 found that, among 1,282 persons with HIV and cancer, the incidence of CRC, excluding anal cancer, was 51 per 100,000 py with a SIR of 5.9 (95% CI, 4.15–8.37). Interestingly, colon cancer was the most common NADC in females, with an incidence of 156 per 100,000 py (Chen et al., 2014). In the US surveillance study using the HIV/AIDS Cancer Match Study registry data from 1991 to 2002, the incidence of CRC, excluding anal cancer, was 15 per 100,000 py (Engels et al., 2008).

Immunosuppression likely plays a role in the epidemiology of CRC, as demonstrated in the previously discussed case reports from the pre-ART era. A study by Silverberg et al. (2011) stratified groups by $CD4^+$ T-cell count and found that those with HIV and less than 200 cells/mm^3 had an 80% higher relative risk compared to a protective effect of higher $CD4^+$ T-cell counts. Another study that used flexible sigmoidoscopy for CRC screening in HIV patients found that patients with duration of HIV of greater than 10 years and $CD4^+$ T-cell counts of less than 200 cells/mm^3 had greater odds of having distal colon neoplastic lesions compared to those with higher $CD4^+$ T-cell counts (Bini et al., 2006). On the contrary, many other studies have not shown significant differences in rates among AIDS patients or reduction of CRC in the ART era. Several studies support increases in CRC in the ART era. The lack of reporting of CRC in advanced immunosuppression coupled with the increase in CRC in the ART era may be explained by increased longevity of the HIV population as well as an increase in screening measures allowing for more diagnoses.

An Australian study that used national HIV and cancer registry data in the pre-ART era evaluated the incidence of cancer among those with HIV. It did not find significantly increased incidence rates among PWH before and after developing advanced immunosuppression (Gulrich et al., 2002). A US study examined cancer data from patients with an AIDS diagnosis from 1978 to 1996 (Frisch et al., 2001). It found the relative risk of colon cancer in patients with newly diagnosed AIDS to be no different in the period prior to AIDS or in the 5 years thereafter (RR, 0.9) (Frisch et al., 2001). A prospective study at the University of Alabama at Birmingham followed HIV patients from 1989 to 2002. It demonstrated an incidence during that period of 60 cases of NADC, with an increase in annual incidence of 0.65 cases per 1,000 py in the pre-ART era and 2.34 cases per 1,000 py in the ART era. Although the study found an increase in the incidence of the relative risk in the ART era of 3.6 (95% CI, 0.8–16.3), this difference was not statistically significant (Bedimo et al., 2004). These findings can likely be attributed to improved longevity and screening methods in the ART era. However, a lack of information on screening efforts reported in many of these studies is a major limitation in accurately measuring the true CRC incidence in the HIV population.

CRC SCREENING IN THE HIV POPULATION

Screening for CRC in HIV patients reflects that recommended for the general population with normal cancer risk. This is defined as no personal history of CRC, adenomatous polyps, or inflammatory bowel disease and no first-degree relative with a history of CRC. The USPSTF recommends that for adults with an average risk of CRC, screening with fecal occult blood testing, flexible sigmoidoscopy, or colonoscopy should begin at age 50 years and continue until age 75 years. The current screening interval for colonoscopy is 10 years. These recommendations have been effective for reducing the incidence and mortality of CRC. For those with increased risk, such as an immediate family member with a history of CRC, screening should begin at age 40 years or 10 years prior to the relative's age at onset of CRC, whichever occurs first (Whitlock et al., 2008). Interestingly, even in the general population, screening is underutilized. The CDC found that only 64.5% of screening-eligible people aged 50 to 75 years surveyed in the Behavioral Risk Factor Surveillance System reported having one of the recommended tests (Joseph et al., 2012).

Screening the HIV population based on standard guidelines has been more challenging, with significant disparity compared to the general population. A retrospective study in New York identified 565 screening-eligible HIV patients with average risk and found that only 25% underwent screening colonoscopy within 10 years of the review. The median age was 58 years, and most of these patients had well-controlled HIV compared to those who did not have colonoscopy. Among those who had colonoscopy and biopsy, 32% of biopsies were of tubular adenomas, which exceeds the detection rate of tubular adenomas in the general population for men (34%) and women (27%) (Nayudu & Balar, 2012). A prospective study performed among New York veterans from 1998 to 2003 sought to describe the prevalence of adenomas or CRC in the distal colon with flexible sigmoidoscopy (Bini et al., 2006). The study included 2,217 HIV-negative controls and 165 PWH (85.5% on ART and 45.5% with undetectable HIV viral load). Among the PWH eligible for CRC screening, 91.9% underwent flexible sigmoidoscopy, which was similar to the percentage who underwent it in the HIV-negative cohort. More polyps were identified in the HIV group compared to the control group (30.9% vs. 23%; $p = 0.2$), and polyps in the HIV group were more likely to have neoplastic features compared to those of the controls (25.5% vs. 13.1%; $p < 0.001$; OR, 2.27; 95% CI, 1.57–3.29). The study found that duration of HIV more than 10 years and lower $CD4^+$ cell count were significantly associated with having distal neoplasias. Those with positive sigmoidoscopy went on to have full colonoscopy, which showed a higher prevalence of proximal colon neoplastic lesions in the HIV group compared to the HIV-negative controls (61.2% vs. 47.8%; $p = 0.07$) (Bini et al., 2006). Although not statistically significant, it appears that PWH are at higher risk for malignant potential compared to their HIV-negative counterparts. Another study comparing CRC screening in HIV patients and controls demonstrated similar results as those obtained in the New York veterans' study. This study compared 302 PWH to 302 HIV-negative patients and found that PWH were significantly less likely to have any type of screening modality (55.6% vs. 77.8%; $p <$ 0.0001). Undetectable HIV RNA levels, older age, and a family history were variables associated with having at least one CRC screening (Reinhold et al., 2005).

Appropriate use of screening for eligible persons is of utmost importance for PWH because polyps may have more high-risk features than those of the general population. Barriers to colonoscopy referral and screening should be identified and managed. Increased provider and patient education may also be beneficial. One pilot study randomizing screening-eligible HIV patients to receive educational material and in-person decision-making support showed increased screening colonoscopy uptake (Ferron et al., 2015). Based on this evidence, efforts to increase on-time screening in eligible PWH should be undertaken.

CLINICAL PRESENTATION OF CRC

With regard to early presentations of CRC, one recent study compared the prevalence, type, and location of neoplastic lesions found on colonoscopy in 263 PWH matched with 657 HIV-negative patients and found that PWH were less likely to have any neoplastic lesions (21.3% vs. 27.7%, $p < 0.05$), adenoma (20.5% vs. 27.1%, $p = 0.04$), tubular adenomas greater than 10 mm (0.4% vs. 2.9%, $p = 0.02$), and serrated adenomas (0.0% vs. 2.6%, $p < 0.01$) (Fantry et al., 2016). They also found a nonsignificant increased prevalence of adenocarcinoma in PWH compared with HIV-negative individuals (1.5% vs. 0.8%, $p = 0.29$). However, at the time of diagnosis in HIV patients, CRC is often advanced and occurs in younger patients compared to the general population. Researchers from the Italian Cooperative Group AIDS and Tumors evaluated 27 PWH and 54 matched, HIV-negative patients who were diagnosed with CRC between 1985 and 2003 (Berretta et al., 2009). The majority were diagnosed in the ART era, with a median age of 48 years in both groups. However, most patients in the HIV cohort were younger than age 45 years. Median CD4+ T-cell count at the time of diagnosis was 325 cells/mm³. In PWH, the stage was predominantly Dukes stage D (distant metastasis) compared to those without HIV (74% vs. 35%; $p = 0.002$). Histopathology showed poorly differentiated adenocarcinoma in 66% of the HIV cohort compared to 26% in the HIV-negative matched controls (Berretta et al., 2009).

A case–control study from Southern California also found that CRC of PWH occurred mainly in those younger than age 50 years (72%) and with advanced disease (stages III and IV). HIV patients had a younger to older age ratio of 3:1 compared to the population controls, whose ratio was 1.33. In most patients, biopsy findings revealed poorly differentiated adenocarcinoma (64%). Of note, the mean CD4+ cell count at time of diagnosis was robust at 467 cells/mm³ (Wasserberg et al., 2007).

One multicenter retrospective study of 17 HIV patients with confirmed CRC from 1988 to 2003 reported that patients had a mean age of 43 years and a majority had a CD4+ cell count of less than 500 cells/mm³ (not specified further) (Chapman et al., 2009). Most tumors arose in the right side of the colon (57%) and with advanced stage IV disease (47%) and histopathology with grade 2 or 3 adenocarcinomas (79%). Most metastatic sites were to the liver but also included lung, peritoneum, and subcutaneous sites (Chapman et al., 2009). Sigel et al. (2016) more recently evaluated 184 patients with CRC (38 PWH and 146 HIV-negative patients) and found that PWH were more likely to have smoked ($p = 0.001$), have right-sided colorectal cancer (37% vs. 14%; $p = 0.003$), and tumor-infiltrating lymphocytes (TIL) above 50/10 high-power fields (21% vs. 7%). They also evaluated mismatch repair protein (MMR) expression levels between the two groups (as MMR is a marker for microsatellite instability) but found no difference between the two groups ($p = 0.6$) (Sigel et al., 2016). Given the presence of right-sided colonic tumors, colonoscopy in HIV patients may have a greater diagnostic yield compared to flexible sigmoidoscopy. Further prospective studies should be performed to evaluate the various screening techniques in the HIV-positive population.

CRC TREATMENT IN PWH

Treatment for CRC in PWH is the same as that for those without HIV and primarily depends on clinical staging of the malignancy, which is determined by physical exam and radiographic imaging. CT scanning is mandatory for determining regional extension, nodal involvement, or distant metastasis in the TNM staging system. Stages range from I to IV as the disease advances from confined disease to the colonic mucosa, regional lymph node involvement, and involvement of one or more distant organs including peritoneal seeding. For patients with stage II to IV disease, imaging with CT scan of the chest, abdomen, and pelvis is recommended (NCCN, 2015d). Further imaging with MRI may be useful for better characterization of the liver for metastatic disease, especially in the setting of background steatosis (Shahani et al., 2014). Testing with the tumor marker carcinoembryonic antigen (CEA) should be performed prior to treatment to help serve as a guide in the posttreatment follow-up. This test has not been validated for use specifically in the HIV population, nor has there been robust evidence supporting survival benefit in the general population, but CEA remains a standard pre- and posttreatment test for its prognostic utility (Locker et al., 2006).

SURGERY IN TREATMENT OF CRC

Treatment for localized disease can be curative with endoscopic resection of a carcinomatous polyp or surgical resection with simple colectomy and anastomosis. Surgery remains the cornerstone of therapy for localized disease, and margins should be free of cancer. Locally advanced disease or poorly differentiated polypoid lesions may warrant more invasive or radical surgery. If invasion involves surrounding structures, larger resection of contiguous, multivisceral structures is indicated to ensure negative margins in the affected noncolonic organs (NCCN, 2015b). This approach has yielded improved prognosis and outcomes in patients with locally advanced disease (Govindarajan et al., 2006; Lehnert et al., 2002). Tumor location is also an important aspect in consideration of surgical approach because management of CRC involving the rectum (especially the lower rectum) may compromise anal sphincter tone and genitourinary function. If the anus is involved, sphincter-sparing surgery may be considered with adjuvant or neoadjuvant chemotherapy and radiation (NCCN, 2015b; Sauer et al., 2012).

Colorectal adenocarcinoma typically metastasizes to the liver, lung, lymph nodes, and peritoneum. With limited metastatic disease, curative surgery remains an option to improve survival; however, recurrence of disease is a reality for some patients (Neef et al., 2009; Shah et al., 2006).

CHEMORADIOTHERAPY IN CRC

Neoadjuvant and adjuvant chemotherapies are generally considered for patients with advanced or metastatic disease when the expectation of noncurative surgery is present. Neoadjuvant chemoradiotherapy (CRT) is a standard approach to therapy in locally advanced rectal cancer (T3 or N1-2) prior to surgery or in rectal cancer that is unresectable or medically inoperable. This consists of fractionated radiation therapy usually with a 5-FU-based regimen in combination with other agents, such as capecitabine or oxaliplatin and leucovorin (NCCN, 2015b; Sauer et al., 2012). Adjuvant CRT following resection to eliminate microscopic foci of tumors and promote recurrence-free survival has been most beneficial in patients with nodal involvement (stage III), which has been shown in randomized controlled trials (Smith et al., 2004). Typical regimens include 5-FU/leucovorin- or capecitabine-based regimens (NCCN, 2015d). Other adjuvant therapies in metastatic disease include the vascular endothelial and epidermal growth factor inhibitor bevacizumab and cetuximab, respectively. Overall survival benefit of these agents remains controversial, and they may cause excess adverse events (da Gramont et al., 2012; Taieb et al., 2014).

TREATMENT OUTCOMES AND SURVIVAL OF PWH AND CRC

There is a paucity of data on the efficacy, tolerability, and treatment outcomes of CRC for PWH. Case series have provided most of the data on this population. As previously discussed, patients with HIV tend to present with more advanced disease, which may require both surgery and chemoradiation. In one case series, 10 PWH with stage III or IV disease underwent segmental colon or rectal resection; one of these patients underwent complete pelvic exenteration (Wasserberg et al., 2007). All patients also received first-line adjuvant chemotherapy with 5-FU/leucovorin. Four of the patients received additional CPT-11 or irinotecan for metastatic disease. Of the patients with rectal involvement, one patient received neoadjuvant 5-FU/leucovorin-based chemoradiation, and three patients received adjuvant radiation. Overall, chemotherapy was tolerated well, but some patients

did experience grade 3 adverse events with neutropenia and anemia (Wasserberg et al., 2007).

Another case series from Italy reported on 27 PWH, the majority with metastatic CRC (Berretta et al., 2009). Of those with metastatic disease, three received neoadjuvant oxaliplatin-based chemotherapy for liver metastasis, seven underwent palliative chemotherapy, and two were treated with 5-FU chemoradiation. The remaining patients with metastatic disease underwent palliation. One patient who received radiation incurred hemorrhagic proctitis, which prompted treatment cessation (Berretta et al., 2009). Overall, chemotherapy was tolerated well in the group, with few grade 3 neutropenic events.

Surgical resection provides the best curative treatment for localized colon cancer, and this has been demonstrated with SEER data (2005–2011) showing 5-year survival rates of 90% for localized disease. However, survival declines steeply with regional or nodal involvement (70%) and with distant metastasis (13%) (Howlader et al., 2015). Patients with HIV may not receive surgery when indicated, giving them a survival disadvantage. This disparity was highlighted in a follow-up study by the previously mentioned Italian group. In 2010, the group released a brief report on its experience treating HIV patients with liver metastasis (Berretta et al., 2010). They reported on 14 patients who had HIV and CRC-related liver metastasis. Only 3 patients initially had unresectable liver metastasis as determined by a multidisciplinary team; however, the other 11 patients underwent FOLFOX-4 treatment. Three patients in the group who were able to undergo surgery received neoadjuvant chemotherapy with FOLFOX-4 or FOLFIRI, followed by liver segmentectomy (2 patients) and liver segmentectomy plus radiofrequency ablation (1 patient). These 3 patients tolerated the treatments well and remained on ART without any grade 3 or 4 toxicities, and 2 of the 3 patients remained disease-free at 21-month follow-up. Although the number of patients was small, these researchers demonstrated that an aggressive surgical approach for metastatic CRC can be successfully performed in patients with HIV. Narrowing the treatment gap between the HIV population and the general population remains an important goal in the care of malignancies in HIV that may help improve survival outcomes for this group.

Mortality for HIV patients with CRC remains high compared to that for the general population. A large retrospective study estimated that those with HIV and CRC have a 50% higher risk of mortality compared to uninfected patients (Coghill et al., 2015). Smaller case–control studies have shown markedly poorer survival for HIV patients compared to negative controls, with 4-year survival of 15% and 49%, respectively (Berretta et al., 2009). A more recent study found that PWH and CRC had reduced overall survival ($p = 0.02$) when compared to their HIV-negative counterparts but no difference in progression-free survival (Sigel et al., 2016). It has been hypothesized that PWH are less likely to receive therapy and therefore, on a population level, will have poorer survival. HIV positivity should not preclude delivery of the standard of care, and further studies are needed to rigorously evaluate the standard of care delivered to these patients. Disparities in screening and treatment of HIV patients with CRC are likely to perpetuate their less-than-optimal survival outcomes relative to those of HIV-negative patients.

RECOMMENDED READING

Berretta M, Cappellani A, Di Benedetto F, et al. Clinical presentation and outcome of colorectal cancer in HIV-positive patients: a clinical case–control study. *Onkologie.* 2009;32:319–324.

Bini EJ, Park J, Francois F. Use of flexible sigmoidoscopy to screen for colorectal cancer in HIV-infected patients 50 years of age or older. *JAMA Intern Med.* 2006;166(15):1626–1631.

IMMUNE CHECKPOINT INHIBITOR THERAPY FOR NADC

LEARNING OBJECTIVE

- Review the mechanism and proposed use of immune check point inhibitor (ICPI) therapy for NADCs

WHAT'S NEW?

ICPI therapy is currently being evaluated in PWH and, in patients with well-controlled HIV infection, is thought to be just as efficacious for the treatment of various NADCs as for the general population.

KEY POINTS

- ICPIs target key immune regulatory pathways and thus can untether T-cell-mediated antitumor responses, which could help target certain cancers in PWH.

- ICPIs like programmed cell death-1 (PD-1) inhibitors may also be able to help eliminate the cells that carry HIV proviral DNA, thus contributing to elimination of the patient's HIV reservoir.

- PD-1/PD-L1 inhibitors have been approved for melanoma, NSCLC and other lung cancers, renal cell carcinoma, Hodgkin's lymphoma, head and neck squamous cell cancers, several types of breast cancers, gastric cancer, urothelial cancer, and CRC in the general population; studies evaluating their use in PWH are ongoing.

ICPIs are a relatively new class of immunotherapy medications that inhibit suppression of effector T-cell responses. In other words, they help to turn the cancer or infectious agent-suppressed cell-mediated immunity on again. Most of these are monoclonal antibodies directed against immune checkpoints that block the interaction between the immune checkpoint and their respective checkpoint ligands. One type of immune checkpoint is programmed cell death-1 (PD-1), which is predominantly expressed on T cells. The interaction of PD-1 with its ligands (PD-L1 and -L2) expressed on antigen-presenting cells and tumors sends a negative signal to T cells, which can lead to T-cell exhaustion or dysfunction.

T-cell exhaustion is now recognized as a key mechanism contributing to impaired T-cell responses against tumors and some pathogens.

ICPI therapies are an appealing treatment option for many cancers that express PD-1 because they have broad activity with good response rates, they frequently induce long-term disease control, and they are relatively nontoxic. So far, six monoclonal antibodies that target PD-1 or PD-L1 have been approved by the FDA. The first, a PD-1 inhibitor, pembrolizumab, was approved in September 2014 for the treatment of advanced or unresectable melanoma in patients failing other treatments and was so successful that it later became the first-line treatment (Robert et al., 2014). It is now approved for NSCLC (Garon et al., 2015), head and neck squamous cell cancers, refractory Hodgkin's lymphoma, primary mediastinal large B-cell lymphoma, advanced urothelial carcinoma, advanced gastric cancer, some types of CRCs, and advanced cervical cancer. A second PD-1 inhibitor, nivolumab, was approved in 2015 for the treatment of melanoma and is now also approved for NSCLC, renal cell carcinoma, Hodgkin's lymphoma, head and neck squamous cell cancers, advanced urothelial carcinomas, certain CRCs, and hepatocellular carcinoma. The third, fourth, and fifth approvals were for PD-L1 inhibitors (atezolizumab, durvalumab, and avelumab) for the treatment of advanced bladder cancer and NSCLC. The sixth and most recent (September 2018) approval was for cemiplimab, another PD-1 monoclonal antibody, for patients with metastatic or locally advanced cutaneous squamous cell carcinoma, with many more in the pipeline.

Therapies with ICPIs are an exciting prospect for PWH because they have the potential not only to treat the patient's cancer but also to eliminate or reduce the HIV reservoirs that persist despite ART (Day et al., 2006; Trautmann et al., 2006). The concept behind this latter theoretical use is that HIV persistence is thought to stem primarily from the presence of integrated copies of the proviral genome within long-lived cells. Because active viral gene expression causes cell death due to viral cytopathic effects and the immune response, long-lived cells likely harbor transcriptionally silent, latent provirus, which is the remaining major barrier to finding a cure for HIV. Several studies offer evidence as to why PD-1 may be an important part of this process. PD-1 has been found to be upregulated on HIV-specific CD8$^+$ T cells and has been correlated with disease progression (Day et al., 2006). Blockade of PD-L1 was shown to enhance IFN-γ secretion by HIV-specific CD8$^+$ T cells, suggesting that PD-1 signaling might play a role in limiting T-cell responses against HIV (Petrovas et al., 2006; Zhang et al., 2007). Checkpoints that are considered markers of T-cell exhaustion, such as PD-1, TIM-3, and LAG-3, have been used to predict time of viremia rebound after treatment interruption (Hurst et al., 2015). Another study suggested a role for the immune checkpoint TIGIT in limiting antiviral T-cell responses in HIV (Chew et al., 2016). This study also showed that TIGIT expression was coexpressed with PD-1 and upregulated on T cells from both PWH and simian immunodeficiency virus (SIV)-infected macaques. The AIDS Clinical Trials 5326 Study Team recently demonstrated that treatment with an anti-PD-L1 antibody enhanced HIV-specific CD8$^+$ T-cell response in two of eight HIV-infected patients on ART (Gay et al., 2017). Although these studies suggest that immune checkpoints may limit T-cell responses during HIV infection and that immune checkpoint blockade might be beneficial in PWH, larger studies are required to determine the therapeutic benefit of immune checkpoint blockade in PWH on ART.

With regard to cancer therapy, treatment with PD-1/PD-L1 inhibitors may be even more useful in PWH and cancer than in HIV-negative cancer patients because at least one study recently observed that while PD-L1 expression is high in tumor cells from both PWH and HIV-negative patients with NSCLC, it was associated with poor prognosis only in PWH (Okuma et al., 2018). However, to date, only a handful of case reports and small case series offer data about PWH treated with these new medications (Heppt et al., 2017; Guihot et al., 2018; Le Garff et al., 2017; Wightman et al., 2015). Many of the PD-1/PDL-1 inhibitor therapies currently in use or being tested in PWH have been mentioned throughout the text of this chapter. In addition, there are several larger clinical trials under way that will be emphasized here (Bender-Ignacio et al., 2018). The Cancer Immunotherapy Trials Network (CITN) conducted a trial of pembrolizumab in PWH with solid tumors and Hodgkin's lymphoma (NCT02595866). They accrued 30 patients with HIV and multiple different types of both AIDS-defining and non-AIDS defining cancers and found that pembrolizumab had acceptable safety in patients with cancer, treated with ART and a CD4$^+$ T-cell count of greater than 100 cells/mm^3. Despite the report of a treatment-emergent episode of B-cell clonal proliferation in a patient with KS, there was a clinical benefit participants with lung cancer, NHL, and KS (Uldrick et al., 2019). Other trials are still pending, including one that will evaluate pembrolizumab in patients with HIV and advanced cancers, although it requires patients to have a CD4$^+$ T-cell count of greater than 200 cells/mm^3 (NCT02595866). A French trial will evaluate therapy with nivolumab in PWH with NSCLC; they are accepting patients with any CD4$^+$ T-cell count but require a HIV viral load of less than 200 copies/mL (NCT03304093). Another French study is following PWH who receive ICPIs as part of routine cancer care to evaluate their safety and effects on the HIV reservoir (NCT03354936). Pending the results of these trials, HIV positivity is not thought to be a contraindication to treatment with PD-1 inhibitors, although PWH with low CD4$^+$ T-cell counts should be monitored closely both for treatment response and for IRIS.

REFERENCES

Aboulafia DM. Kaposi's sarcoma. *Clin Dermatol.* 2001;19(3):269–283.

Aboulafia DM, Puswella AL. Highly active antiretroviral therapy as the sole treatment for AIDS-related primary central nervous system lymphoma: a case report with implications for treatment. *AIDS Patient Care STDs.* 2007;21(12):900–907.

Advisory Committee on Immunization Practices. Recommended adult immunization schedule: United States, 2013. *Ann Intern Med.* 2013;158:191–199.

Ahdieh L, Munoz A, Vlahov D, et al. Cervical neoplasia and repeated positivity of human papillomavirus infection in human immunodeficiency virus-seropositive and -seronegative women. *Am J Epidemiol.* 2000;151(12):1148–1157.

Altekruse SF, Shiels MS, Modur SP, et al. Cancer burden attributable to cigarette smoking among HIV-infected people in North America. *AIDS.* 2018;32(4):513–521.

Alvarnas JC, Le Rademacher J, Wang Y, et al. Autologous hematopoietic cell transplantation for HIV-related lymphoma: results of the BMT CTN 0803/AMC 071 trial. *Blood.* 2016;128:1050–1058.

Ambinder RF, Wu J, Logan B, et al. Allogeneic hematopoietic cell transplant (alloHCT) for hematologic malignancies in human immunodeficiency virus infected (HIV) patients (pts): Blood and Marrow Transplant Clinical Trials Network (BMT CTN 0903)/AIDS Malignancy Consortium (AMC-080) trial. *J Clin Oncol.* 2017;35(15 Suppl):abstr 7006.

Appleby P, Beral V, Newton R, et al. Highly active antiretroviral therapy and incidence of cancer in human immunodeficiency virus-infected adults. *J Natl Cancer Inst.* 2000;92:1823–1830.

Avivi I, Robinson S, Goldstone A. Clinical use of rituximab in hematological malignancies. *Br J Cancer.* 2003;89(8):1389–1394.

Ballerini P, Gaidano G, Gong JZ, et al. Multiple genetic lesions in acquired immunodeficiency syndrome-related non-Hodgkin's lymphoma. *Blood.* 1993;81(1):166–176.

Bañon S, Machuca I, Araujo S, et al. Efficacy, safety, and lack of interactions with the use of raltegravir in HIV-infected patients undergoing antineoplastic chemotherapy. *J Intern AIDS Soc.* 2014;17(4 Suppl 3):19590.

Baptista MJ, Garcia O, Morgades M, et al. HIV-infection impact on clinical-biological features and outcome of diffuse large B-cell lymphoma treated with R-CHOP in the combination antiretroviral therapy era. *AIDS.* 2015;29:811–818.

Barbosa MS, Schlegel R. The E6 and E7 genes of HPV-18 are sufficient for inducing two-stage in vitro transformation of human keratinocytes. *Oncogene.* 1989;4(12):1529–1532.

Barillari G, Ensoli B. Angiogenic effects of extracellular human immunodeficiency virus type 1 Tat protein and its role in the pathogenesis of AIDS-associated Kaposi's sarcoma. *Clin Microbiol Rev.* 2002;15(2):310–326.

Barozzi P, Luppi M, Facchetti F, et al. Post-transplant Kaposi sarcoma originates from the seeding of donor-derived progenitors. *Nature Med.* 2003;9(5):554–561.

Barta SK, Joshi J, Mounier N, et al. Central nervous system involvement in AIDS-related lymphomas. *Br J Haematol.* 2016;173:857–866.

Barta SK, Lee JY, Kaplan LD, et al. Pooled analysis of AIDS malignancy consortium trials evaluating rituximab plus CHOP or infusional EPOCH chemotherapy in HIV-associated non-Hodgkin lymphoma. *Cancer.* 2012;118:3977–3983.

Barta SK, Samuel MS, Xue X, et al. Changes in the influence of lymphoma- and HIV-specific factors on outcomes in AIDS-related non-Hodgkin lymphoma. *Ann Oncol.* 2015;26:958–966.

Barta SK, Xue X, Wang D, et al. Treatment factors affecting outcomes in HIV-associated non-Hodgkin lymphomas: a pooled analysis of 1546 patients. *Blood.* 2013;122:3251–3262.

Barta SK, Xue X, Wang D, et al. A new prognostic score for AIDS-related lymphomas in the rituximab era. *Haematologica.* 2014;99:1731–1737.

Baumgartner JE, Rachlin JR, Beckstead JH, et al. Primary central nervous system lymphomas: natural history and response to radiation therapy in 55 patients with acquired immunodeficiency syndrome. *J Neurosurg.* 1990;73(2):206–211.

Bayraktar S, Bayraktar UD, Ramos JC, et al. Primary CNS lymphoma in HIV positive and negative patients: comparison of clinical characteristics, outcome and prognostic factors. *J Neurooncol.* 2011;101:257–265.

Bedi GC, Westra WH, Farzedegan H, et al. Microsatellite instability in primary neoplasms from HIV+ patients. *Nature Med.* 1995;1(1):65–68.

Bedimo R, Chen RY, Accortt NA, et al. Trends in AIDS-defining and non-AIDS defining malignancies among HIV-infected patients: 1989–2002. *Clin Infect Dis.* 2004;39(9):1380–1384.

Bender-Ignacio R, Lin LL, Rajdev L, et al. Evolving paradigms in HIV malignancies: review of ongoing clinical trials. *J Natl Compr Canc Netw.* 2018;16(8):1018–1026.

Benevolo M, Donà MG, Ravenda PS, et al. Anal human papillomavirus infection: prevalence, diagnosis and treatment of related lesions. *Expert Rev Anti Infect Ther.* 2016;14(5):465–477.

Beral V, Peterman TA, Berkelman RL, et al. Kaposi's sarcoma among persons with AIDS: a sexually transmitted infection? *Lancet.* 1990;335(8682):123–128.

Beral V, Peterman T, Berkelman R, et al. AIDS-associated non-Hodgkin lymphoma. *Lancet.* 1991;337(8745):805–809.

Berretta M, Cappellani A, Di Benedetto F, et al. Clinical presentation and outcome of colorectal cancer in PLWH: a clinical case–control study. *Onkologie.* 2009;32:319–324.

Berretta M, Zanet E, Basile F, et al. HIV positive patients with liver metastasis from colorectal cancer deserve the same therapeutic approach as the general population. *Onkkologie.* 2010;33:203–204.

Berry JM, Palefsky JM, Jay N, et al. Performance characteristics of anal cytology and human papillomavirus testing in patients with high-resolution anoscopy-guided biopsy of high-grade anal intraepithelial neoplasia. *Dis Colon Rectum.* 2009;52(2):239–247.

Berthold DR, Pond GR, Soban F, et al. Docetaxel plus prednisone or mitoxantrone plus prednisone for advanced prostate cancer: updated survival in the TAX 327 study. *J Clin Oncol.* 2008;26(2):242–245.

Besson C, Goubar A, Gabarre J, et al. Changes in AIDS-related lymphoma since the era of highly active antiretroviral therapy. *Blood.* 2001;98(8):2339–2344.

Bini EJ, Park J, Francois F. Use of flexible sigmoidoscopy to screen for colorectal cancer in HIV-infected patients 50 years of age or older. *JAMA Intern Med.* 2006;166(15):1626–1631.

Bjorge T, Engeland A, Luostarinen T, et al. Human papillomavirus infection as a risk factor for anal and perianal skin cancer in a prospective study. *Br J Cancer.* 2002;87(1):61–64.

Blazy A, Hennequin C, Gornet JM, et al. Anal carcinomas in PLWH: high-dose chemoradiotherapy is feasible in the era of highly active antiretroviral therapy. *Dis Colon Rectum.* 2005;48(6):1176–1181.

Bonnet F, Burty C, Lewden C, et al. Changes in cancer mortality among HIV-infected patients: the Mortalité 2005 Survey. *Clin Infect Dis.* 2009;48(5):633–639.

Bosch FX, Manos MM, Munoz N, et al. Prevalence of human papillomavirus in cervical cancer: a worldwide perspective. *J Natl Cancer Inst.* 1995;87(11):796–802.

Bossolasco S, Cinque P, Ponzoni M, et al. Epstein–Barr virus DNA load in cerebrospinal fluid and plasma of patients with AIDS-related lymphoma. *J Neurovirol.* 2002;8(5):432–438.

Boudreaux AA, Smith LL, Cosby CD, et al. Intralesional vinblastine for cutaneous Kaposi's sarcoma associated with acquired immunodeficiency syndrome: a clinical trial to evaluate efficacy and discomfort associated with infection. *J Am Acad Dermatol.* 1993;28(1):61–65.

Boulanger E, Gerard L, Gabarre J, et al. Prognostic factors and outcome of human herpesvirus 8-associated primary effusion lymphoma in patients with AIDS. *J Clin Oncol.* 2005;23(19):4372–4380.

Bower M, Dalla Pria A, Coyle C, et al. Prospective stage-stratified approach to AIDS-related Kaposi's sarcoma. *J Clin Oncol.* 2014;32:409–414.

Bower M, Fox P, Fife K, et al. Highly active anti-retroviral therapy (HAART) prolongs time to treatment failure in Kaposi's sarcoma. *AIDS.* 1999;13(15):2105–2111.

Bower M, McCall-Peat N, Ryan N, et al. Protease inhibitors potentiate chemotherapy-induced neutropenia. *Blood.* 2004;104(9):2943–2946.

Bower M, Powles T, Nelson M, et al. HIV-related lung cancer in the era of highly active antiretroviral therapy. *AIDS.* 2003;17(3):371–375.

Bower M, Powles T, Newsom-Davis T, et al. HIV-associated anal cancer: has highly active antiretroviral therapy reduced the incidence or improved the outcome? *J AIDS.* 2004;37(5):1563–1565.

Brickman C, Palefsky JM. Review: human papillomavirus in the HIV-infected host: epidemiology and pathogenesis in the antiretroviral era. *Curr HIV/AIDS Rep.* 2015;12(1):6–15.

Burgi A, Brodine S, Wegner S, et al. Incidence and risk factors for the occurrence of non-AIDS-defining cancers among human immunodeficiency virus-infected individuals. *Cancer.* 2005;104(7):1505–1511.

Burkes RL, Meyer PR, Gill PS, et al. Rectal lymphoma in homosexual men. *Arch Intern Med.* 1986;146(5):913–915.

Cadranel J, Garfield D, Lavole A, et al. Lung cancer in HIV infected patients: facts, questions, and challenges. *Thorax.* 2006;61:1000–1008.

Calabresi A, Ferraresi A, Festa A, et al. Incidence of AIDS-defining cancers and virus-related and non-virus-related non-AIDS-defining cancers among HIV-infected patients compared with the general population in a large health district of northern Italy, 1999–2000. *HIV Med.* 2013;14(8):481–490.

Campbell JA, Soliman AS, Kahesa C, et al. Changing patterns of lung, liver, and head and neck non-AIDS-defining cancers relative to HIV status in Tanzania between 2002–2014. *Infect Agent Cancer.* 2016;11:58.

Campbell TB, Borok M, White IE, et al. Relationship of Kaposi sarcoma (KS)-associated herpesvirus viremia and KS disease in Zimbabwe. *Clin Infect Dis.* 2003;36(9):1144–1151.

Cannon MJ. Kaposi's sarcoma-associated herpesvirus and acquired immunodeficiency syndrome-related malignancy. *Semin Oncol.* 2000;27:408–419.

Cannon MJ, Dollard SC, Smith DK, et al. Blood-borne and sexual transmission of human herpesvirus 8 in women with or at risk for human immunodeficiency virus infection. *N Engl J Med.* 2001;344(9):637–643.

Cappell MS, Yao F, Cho KC. Colonic adenocarcinoma associated with the acquired immune deficiency syndrome. *Cancer.* 1988;62:616–619.

Casper C, Carrell D, Miller KG, et al. HIV serodiscordant sex partners and the prevalence of human herpesvirus 8 infection among HIV negative men who have sex with men: baseline data from the EXPLORE Study. *Sex Transm Infect.* 2006;82(3):229–235.

Casper C, Krantz E, Selke S, et al. Frequent and asymptomatic oropharyngeal shedding of human herpesvirus 8 among immunocompetent men. *J Infect Dis.* 2007;195(1):30–36.

Casper C, Redman M, Huang ML, et al. HIV infection and human herpesvirus-8 oral shedding among men who have sex with men. *J AIDS.* 2004;35(3):233–238.

Castilho JL, Luz PM, Shepherd BE, et al. HIV and cancer: a comparative retrospective study of Brazilian and US clinical cohorts. *Infect Agent Cancer.* 2015;10(4):1–10.

Castillo JJ, Furman M, Beltrán BE, et al. Human immunodeficiency virus–associated plasmablastic lymphoma. *Cancer.* 2012;118:5270–5277.

Cattaneo C, Re A, Ungari M, et al. Plasmablastic lymphoma among human immunodeficiency virus-positive patients: results of a single center's experience. *Leuk Lymphoma.* 2015;56:267–269.

Centers for Disease Control and Prevention. AIDS-defining conditions. 2008. https://www.cdc.gov/mmwr/preview/mmwrhtml/rr5710a2.htm

Centers for Disease Control and Prevention. Human papillomavirus-associated cancers—United States, 2004–2008. *Morbid Mortal Wkly Rep.* 2012a;61(15):258–261.

Centers for Disease Control and Prevention. Human papilloma virus (HPV) fact sheet. 2021. w.cdc.gov/std/hpv

Chadburn A, Abdul-Nabi AM, Teruya BS, et al. Lymphoid proliferations associated with human immunodeficiency virus infection. *Arch Path Lab Med.* 2013;137(3):360–370.

Chang Y, Cesarman E, Pessin MS, et al. Identification of herpesvirus-like DNA sequences in AIDS-associated Kaposi's sarcoma. *Science.* 1994;266(5192):1865–1869.

Chapman C, Aboulafia DM, Dezube BJ, et al. Human immunodeficiency virus-associated adenocarcinoma of the colon: clinicopathologic findings and outcome. *Clin Colorectal Cancer.* 2009;8(4):215–219.

Chari A, Kaplan L, Volberding PA, et al. Diagnosis and management of non-Hodgkin's lymphoma and Hodgkin's lymphoma. 2005.

Chaturvedi AK, Madeleine MM, Biggar RJ, et al. Risk of human papillomavirus-associated cancers among persons with AIDS. *J Natl Cancer Inst.* 2009;101(16):1120–1130.

Chen YH, Lin MW, Bhatia K, et al. Cancer incidence in a nationwide HIV/AIDS patient cohort in Taiwan in 1998–2000. *J AIDS.* 2014;65(4):463–472.

Chew GM, Fujita T, Webb GM, et al. TIGIT marks exhausted T cells, correlates with disease progression, and serves as a target for immune restoration in HIV and SIV infection. *PLoS Pathog.* 2016;12:e1005349.

Chiao EY, Dezube BJ, Krown SE, et al. Time for oncologists to opt in for routine opt-out HIV testing? *JAMA.* 2010;304(3):334–339.

Chiao EY, Giordano TP, Richardson P, et al. Human immunodeficiency virus-associated squamous cell cancer of the anus: epidemiology and outcomes in the highly active antiretroviral therapy era. *J Clin Oncol.* 2008;26(3):474–479.

Chin-Hong PV, Vittinghoff E, Cranston RD, et al. Age-specific prevalence of anal human papillomavirus infection in HIV-negative sexually active men who have sex with men: the EXPLORE study. *J Infect Dis.* 2004;190(12):2070–2076.

Chokunonga E, Levy LM, Bassett MT, et al. Cancer incidence in the African population of Harare, Zimbabwe: second results from the cancer registry 1993–1995. *Int J Cancer.* 2000;85(1):54–59.

Cianfrocca M, Lee S, Von Roenn J, et al. Randomized trial of paclitaxel vs. pegylated liposomal doxorubicin for advanced human immunodeficiency virus-associated Kaposi sarcoma: evidence of symptom palliation from chemotherapy. *Cancer.* 2010;116(16):3969–3977.

Cingolani A, Fratino L, Scoppettuolo G, et al. Changing pattern of primary cerebral lymphoma in the highly active antiretroviral therapy era. *J Neurovirol.* 2005; 11(Suppl 3):38–44.

Cleator S, Fife K, Nelson M, et al. Treatment of HIV-associated invasive anal cancer with combined chemoradiation. *Eur J Cancer.* 2000;36(6):754–758.

Clifford GM, Lise M, Franceschi S, et al. Lung cancer in the Swiss HIV Cohort Study: role of smoking, immunodeficiency, and pulmonary infection. *Br J Cancer.* 2012;106:448–452.

Clifford GM, Polesel J, Richenbach M, et al. Cancer risk in the Swiss HIV Cohort Study: associations with immunodeficiency, smoking, and highly active antiretroviral therapy. *J Natl Cancer Inst.* 2005;97(6):425–432.

Coghill AE, Shiels MS, Suneja G, et al. Elevated cancer-specific mortality among HIV-infected patients in the United States. *J Clin Oncol.* 2015;33(21):2376–2383.

Conti S, Masocco M, Pezzotti P, et al. Differential impact of combined antiretroviral therapy on the survival of Italian patients with specific AIDS-defining illnesses. *J AIDS.* 2000;25(5):451–458.

Cooper JS, Steinfeld AD, Lerch I. Intentions and outcomes in the radiotherapeutic management of epidemic Kaposi's sarcoma. *Int J Radiat Oncol Biol Phys.* 1991;20(3):419–422.

Corales R, Taege A, Rehm S, et al. Regression of AIDS-related CNS lymphoma with HAART [Abstract MoPpB1086]. Proceedings of the XIII International AIDS Conference, Durban, South Africa, 2000.

Cote TR, Biggar RJ, Rosenberg PS, et al. Non-Hodgkin's lymphoma among people with AIDS: incidence, presentation and public health burden. *Int J Cancer.* 1997;73(5):645–650.

Cote TR, Manns A, Hardy CR, et al.; AIDS/Cancer Study Group. Epidemiology of brain lymphoma among people with or without acquired immunodeficiency syndrome. *J Natl Cancer Inst.* 1996;88(10):675–679.

Coutinho R, Pria AD, Gandhi S, et al. HIV status does not impair the outcome of patients diagnosed with diffuse large B-cell lymphoma treated with R-CHOP in the cART era. *AIDS.* 2014;28:689–697.

Crothers K, Huang, L, Goulet JL, et al. HIV infection and risk for incident pulmonary diseases in the combination antiretroviral therapy era. *Am J Respir Crit Care Med.* 2011;183(3):388–395.

Da Gramont A, Van Cutsem E, Schmoll HJ, et al. Bevacizumab plus oxaliplatin-based chemotherapy as adjuvant treatment for colon cancer (AVANT): a phase 3 randomised controlled trial. *Lancet Oncol.* 2012;13(12):1225–1233.

Daling JR, Weiss NS, Hislop TG, et al. Sexual practices, sexually transmitted diseases, and the incidence of anal cancer. *N Engl J Med.* 1987;317(16):973–977.

Danzig JB, Brandt LJ, Reinus JF, et al. Gastrointestinal malignancy in patients with AIDS. *Am J Gastroenterol.* 1991;86(6):715–718.

Day CL, Kaufmann DE, Kiepiela P, et al. PD-1 expression on HIV-specific T cells is associated with T-cell exhaustion and disease progression. *Nature.* 2006;443:350–354.

Dedicoat M, Newton R, Alkharsah KR, et al. Mother-to-child transmission of human herpesvirus-8 in South Africa. *J Infect Dis.* 2004;190(6):1068–1075.

Department of Health and Human Services, Panel on Guidelines for the Prevention and Treatment of Opportunistic Infections in Adults and Adolescents with HIV. Guidelines for the Prevention and Treatment of Opportunistic Infections in HIV-infected Adults and Adolescents: Recommendations from the Centers for Disease Control and Prevention, the National Institutes of Health, and the HIV Medicine Association of the Infectious Diseases Society of America. 2020. https://clinicalinfo.hiv.gov/sites/default/files/inline-files/adult_oi.pdf

Deregibus M, Cantalupp IV, Doublier S, et al. HIV-1-Tat protein activates phosphatidylinositol 3-kinase/AKT-dependent survival pathways in Kaposi's sarcoma cells. *J Biol Chem.* 2002;277(28):25195–25202.

Dezube BJ, Pantanowitz L, Aboulafia DM. Management of AIDS-related Kaposi sarcoma: advances in target discovery and treatment. *AIDS Reader.* 2004;14(5):236–238, 243.

Diez-Martin J, Balsalobre P, Carrion R. et al. Long term survival after autologous stem cell transplant (ASCT) in AIDS related lymphoma patients [Abstract 868]. *Blood.* 2003;247a:102.

Diez-Martin JL, Balsalobre P, Re A, et al. Comparable survival between HIV+ and HIV- non-Hodgkin and Hodgkin lymphoma patients undergoing autologous peripheral blood stem cell transplantation. *Blood.* 2009;113(23):6011–6014.

DiGiusto DL, Cannon PM, Holmes MC, et al. Preclinical development and qualification of ZFN-mediated CCR5 disruption in human hematopoietic stem/progenitor cells. *Mol Ther Methods Clin Dev.* 2016;3:16067.

D'Jaen GA, Pantanowitz L, Bower M, et al. Human immunodeficiency virus-associated primary lung cancer in the era of highly active antiretroviral therapy: a multi-institutional collaboration. *Clin Lung Cancer.* 2010;11(6):396–404.

Donahue BR, Sullivan JW, Cooper JS. Additional experience with empiric radiotherapy for presumed human immunodeficiency virus-associated primary central nervous system lymphoma. *Cancer.* 1995;76(2):328–332.

Dryden-Peterson S, Bvochora-Nsingo M, Suneja G, et al. HIV infection and survival among women with cervical cancer. *J Clin Oncol.* 2016;34:3749–3757.

D'Souza G, Wiley D, Li X, et al. Incidence and epidemiology of anal cancer in the multicenter AIDS cohort study. *J AIDS.* 2008;48:491–499.

Dubrow R, Qin L, Lin H, et al. Association of CD4+ T-cell count, HIV-1 RNA viral load, and antiretroviral therapy with Kaposi sarcoma risk among HIV-infected persons in the United States and Canada. *J AIDS.* 2017;75(4):382–390.

Duncan KC, Chan KJ, Chiu CG, et al. HAART slows progression to anal cancer in HIV-infected MSM. *AIDS.* 2015;29:305–311.

Dunleavy K, Pittaluga S, Shovlin M, et al. Low-intensity therapy in adults with Burkitt's lymphoma. *N Engl J Med.* 2013;369:1915–1925.

Durand CM, Capoferri AA, Redd AD, et al. Allogeneic bone marrow transplantation with post-transplant cyclophosphamide for patients with HIV and haematological malignancies: a feasibility study. *Lancet HIV.* 2020;7(9):e602–e610. doi:10.1016/S2352-3018(20)30073-4

Dutta A, Uno H, Holman A, et al. Racial differences in prostate cancer risk in young HIV-positive and HIV-negative men: a prospective cohort study. *Cancer Causes Control.* 2017;28(7):767–777.

Eberhard JM, Angin M, Passaes C, et al. Vulnerability to reservoir reseeding due to high immune activation after allogeneic hematopoietic stem cell transplantation in individuals with HIV-1. *Sci Transl Med.* 2020;12(542):eaay9355. doi:10.1126/scitranslmed.aay9355

Ekstein D, Ben-Yehuda D, Slyusarevsky E, et al. CSF analysis of IgH gene rearrangement in CNS lymphoma: relationship to the disease course. *J Neurol Sci.* 2006;247:39–46.

El Amari EB, Toutous-Trellu L, Gayet-Ageron A, et al. Predicting the evolution of Kaposi sarcoma in the highly active antiretroviral therapy era. *AIDS.* 2008;22(9):1019–1028.

El-Sadr WM, Lundgren J, Neaton JD, et al. CD4+ count-guided interruption of antiretroviral treatment. *N Engl J Med.* 2006;355:2283–2296.

El-Solh A, Kumar NM, Nair MP, et al. An RDG-containing peptide from HIV-1 TAT-(65–80) modulates protooncogene expression in human bronchoalveolar carcinoma cell line, A549. *Immunol Invest.* 1997;26(3):351–370.

Engels EA, Biggar RJ, Hall I, et al. Cancer risk in people infected with human immunodeficiency virus in the United States. *Intern J Cancer.* 2008;123:187–194.

Engels EA, Biggar RJ, Marshall VA, et al. Detection and quantification of Kaposi's sarcoma-associated herpesvirus to predict AIDS-associated Kaposi's sarcoma. *AIDS.* 2003;17(12):1847–1851.

Ensoli B, Barillari G, Salahuddin S, et al. Tat protein of HIV-1 stimulates growth of cells derived from Kaposi's sarcoma lesions of AIDS patients. *Nature.* 1990;345(6270):84–86.

European AIDS Clinical Society. Guidelines version 10.1. October 2020. https://www.eacsociety.org/files/guidelines-10.1_5.pdf

Fantry LE, Nowak RG, Fisher LH, et al. Colonoscopy findings in HIV-infected men and women from an urban US cohort compared with non-HIV-infected men and women. *AIDS Res Hum Retroviruses.* 2016;32(9):860–867

Ferlay J, Soerjomataram I, Ervik M, et al. GLOBOCAN 2012 v1.0, Cancer incidence and mortality worldwide: IARC CancerBase No. 11. Lyon, France: International Agency for Research on Cancer. 2013. http://globocan.iarc.fr

Ferreri AJM, Cwynarski K, Pulczynski E, et al. Chemoimmunotherapy with methotrexate, cytarabine, thiotepa, and rituximab (MATRix regimen) in patients with primary CNS lymphoma: results of the first randomisation of the International Extranodal Lymphoma Study Group-32 (IELSG32) phase 2 trial. *Lancet Haematol.* 2016;3(5):e217–e227.

Ferreri AJM, Cwynarski K, Pulczynski E, et al. Whole-brain radiotherapy or autologous stem-cell transplantation as consolidation strategies after high-dose methotrexate-based chemoimmunotherapy in patients with primary CNS lymphoma: results of the second randomisation of the International Extranodal Lymphoma Study Group-32 phase 2 trial. *Lancet Haematol.* 2017;4(11):e510–e523.

Ferron P, Asfour SS, Metsch LR, et al. Impact of a multifaceted intervention on promoting adherence to screening colonoscopy among persons in HIV primary care: a pilot study. *Clin Transl Sci.* 2015;8(4):290–297.

Firnhaber C, Swarts A, Goeieman B, et al. Cryotherapy reduces progression of cervical intraepithelial neoplasia grade 1 in South African HIV-infected women: a randomized, controlled trial. *J AIDS.* 2017;76(5):532–538.

Foulot H, Heard I, Potard V, et al. Surgical management of cervical intraepithelial neoplasia in HIV-infected women. *Eur J Obstet Gynecol Reprod Biol.* 2008;141:153–157.

Franceschi S, Dal Maso L, Rickenbach M, et al. Kaposi sarcoma incidence in the Swiss HIV Cohort Study before and after highly active antiretroviral therapy. *Br J Cancer.* 2008;99(5):800–804.

Fraunholz I, Rabeneck D, Gerstein J, et al. Concurrent chemoradiotherapy with 5-fluorouracil and mitomycin C for anal carcinoma: are there differences between HIV-positive and HIV-negative patients in the era of highly active antiretroviral therapy? *Radiother Oncol.* 2011;98(1):99–104.

Friedman SL. Gastrointestinal and hepatobiliary neoplasms in AIDS. *Gastroenterol Clin North Am.* 1988;17(3):465–486.

Friedman-Kien AE. Disseminated Kaposi's sarcoma syndrome in young homosexual men. *J Am Acad Dermatol.* 1981;5(4):468–471.

Friedman-Kien AE, Saltzman BR. Clinical manifestations of classical, endemic African, and epidemic AIDS-associated Kaposi's sarcoma. *J Am Acad Dermatol.* 1990; 22(6 Pt 2):1237–1250.

Frisch M, Biggar RJ, Engels EA, et al.; AIDS–Cancer Match Registry Study Group. Association of cancer with AIDS-related immunosuppression in adults. *JAMA.* 2001;285(13):1736–1745.

Frisch M, Biggar RJ, Goedert JJ. Human papillomavirus-associated cancers in patients with human immunodeficiency virus infection and acquired immunodeficiency syndrome. *J Nat Cancer Inst.* 2000a;92(18):1500–1510.

Frisch M, Goodman MT. Human papillomavirus-associated carcinomas in Hawaii and the mainland U.S. *Cancer.* 2000b;88(6):1464–1469.

Fulco PP, Hynicka L, Rackley D. Raltegravir-based HAART regimen in a patient with large B-cell lymphoma. *Ann Pharmacother.* 2010;44(2):377–382.

Gabarre J, Azar N, Autran B, et al. High-dose therapy and autologous haematopoietic stem-cell transplantation for HIV-1-associated lymphoma. *Lancet.* 2000;355(9209):1071–1072.

Gage JT, Vance EA, Hildenbrand PG, et al. Brain lesion and AIDS. *Proc Baylor Univ Medical Center.* 2000;13(4):424–429.

Gaidano G, Dalla-Favera R. Molecular pathogenesis of AIDS-related lymphomas. *Adv Cancer Res.* 1995;67:113–153.

Garon EB, Rizvi NA, Hui R, et al. Pembrolizumab for the treatment of non-small-cell lung cancer. *N Engl J Med.* 2015;372:2018–2028.

Gates AE, Kaplan LD. Biology and management of AIDS-associated non-Hodgkin's lymphoma. *Hematol Oncol Clin North Am.* 2003;17(3):821–841.

Gay CL, Bosch RJ, Ritz J, et al. Clinical trial of the anti-PD-L1 antibody BMS-936559 in HIV-1 infected participants on suppressive antiretroviral therapy. *J Infect Dis.* 2017;215(11):1725–1733.

Gbabe OF, Okwundu CI, Dedicoat M, et al. Treatment of severe or progressive Kaposi's sarcoma in HIV-infected adults. *Cochrane Database Syst Rev.* 2014;(9):CD003256.

Gerard L, Meignin V, Galicier L, et al. Characteristics of non-Hodgkin lymphoma arising in HIV-infected patients with suppressed HIV replication. *AIDS.* 2009;23(17):2301–2308.

Gichangi P, De Vuyst H, Estambale B, et al. HIV and cervical cancer in Kenya. *Intern J Gynaecol Obstet.* 2002;76(1):55–63.

Gill ON, Weinberg JR, Fisher IS, et al. Meta-surveillance—safer cyber-surveillance. *Lancet.* 1995;346(8977):776.

Gill PS, Akil B, Colletti P, et al. Pulmonary Kaposi's sarcoma: clinical findings and results of therapy. *Am J Med.* 1989;87(1):57–61.

Gill PS, Wernz J, Scadden DT, et al. Randomized phase III trial of liposomal daunorubicin vs. doxorubicin, bleomycin, and vincristine in AIDS-related Kaposi's sarcoma. *J Clin Oncol.* 1996;14(8):2353–2364.

Goldstein JD, Dickson DW, Moser FG, et al. Primary central nervous system lymphoma in acquired immune deficiency syndrome: a clinical and pathologic study with results of treatment with radiation. *Cancer.* 1991;67(11):2756–2765.

Gopal S, Patel MR, Yanik EL, et al. Temporal trends in presentation and survival for HIV-associated lymphoma in the antiretroviral therapy era. *J Natl Cancer Inst.* 2013;105:1221–1229.

Gosselaar C, Roobol MJ, Roemeling S, et al. The role of the digital rectal examination in subsequent screening visits in the European Randomized Study of Screening for Prostate Cancer (ERSPC), Rotterdam. *Eur Urol.* 2008;54:581–588.

Gosselaar C, Roobol MJ, van den Bergh RC, et al. Digital rectal examination and the diagnosis of prostate cancer—a study based on 8 years and three screenings within the European Randomized Study of Screening for Prostate Cancer (ERSPC), Rotterdam. *Eur Urol.* 2009;55(1):139–146.

Govindarajan A, Coburn NH, Kiss A, et al. Population-based assessment of the surgical management of locally advanced colorectal cancer. *J Natl Cancer Inst.* 2006; 98(20):1474–1481.

Grew D, Bitterman D, Leichman CG, et al. HIV infection is associated with poor outcomes for patients with anal cancer in the highly active antiretroviral therapy era. *Dis Colon Rectum.* 2015;58(12):1130–1136.

Grimm P, Billiet I, Bostwick D, et al. Comparative analysis of prostate specific antigen free survival outcomes for patients with low, intermediate, and high risk prostate cancer treatment by radical therapy: results from the Prostate Cancer Results Study Group. *Br J Urol Int.* 2012;109(Suppl 1):22–29.

Grover S, Desir F, Jing Y, et al. Reduced cancer survival among adults with HIV and AIDS-defining illnesses despite no difference in cancer stage at diagnosis. *J AIDS.* 2018;79(4):421–429.

Gruffaz M, Vasan K, Tan B, et al. TLR4-mediated inflammation promotes KSHV-induced cellular transformation and tumorigenesis by activating the STAT3 pathway. *Cancer Res.* 2017;77(24):7094–7108.

Guerrero-Garcia TA, Mogollon RJ, Castillo JJ. Bortezomib in plasmablastic lymphoma: a glimpse of hope for a hard-to-treat disease. *Leuk Res.* 2017;62:12–16.

Guiguet M, Boue F, Cadranel J, et al. Effect of immunodeficiency, HIV viral load, and antiretroviral therapy on the risk of individual malignancies (FHDH-ANRS CO4): a prospective cohort study. *Lancet Oncol.* 2009;10(12):1152–1159.

Guihot A, Marcelin, AG, Massiani MA, et al. Drastic decrease of the HIV reservoir in a patient treated with nivolumab for lung cancer. *Ann Oncol.* 2018;29(2):517–518.

Gulrich AE, Yueming L, McDonald A, et al. Rates of non-AIDS defining cancers in people with HIV infection before and after AIDS diagnoses. *AIDS.* 2002;16:1155–1161.

Gupta NK, Nolan A, Omuro A, et al. Long-term survival in AIDS-related primary central nervous system lymphoma. *Neuro Oncol.* 2017;19:99–108.

Hamilton-Dutoit SJ, Pallesen G, Karkov J, et al. Identification of EBV-DNA in tumour cells of AIDS-related lymphomas by in-situ hybridisation. *Lancet.* 1989;1(8637):554–555.

Haq IU, Dalla Pria A, Papanastasopoulos P, et al. The clinical application of plasma Kaposi sarcoma herpesvirus viral load as a tumour biomarker: results from 704 patients. *HIV Med.* 2016;17:56–61.

Heard I, Etienney I, Potard V, et al. High prevalence of anal human papillomavirus-associated cancer precursors in a contemporary cohort of asymptomatic HIV-infected women. *Clin Infect Dis.* 2015;60(10):1559–1568.

Heard I, Pizot-Martin I, Potard V, et al. Prevalence of and risk factors for anal oncogenic human papillomavirus infection among HIV-infected women in France in the combination antiretroviral therapy era. *J Infect Dis.* 2016;213(9):1455–1461.

Heidenreich A, Bastian PJ, Bellmunt J, et al. European Association of Urology (EAU) guidelines on prostate cancer: part 1. Screening, diagnosis, and local treatment with curative intent—update 2013. *Eur Urol.* 2014;65(1):124–137.

Hengge UR, Ruzicka T, Tyring SK, et al. Update on Kaposi's sarcoma and other HHV8 associated diseases: part 1. Epidemiology, environmental predispositions, clinical manifestations, and therapy. *Lancet Infect Dis.* 2002;2(5):281–292.

Henrich TJ, Hanhauser E, Marty FM, et al. Antiretroviral-free HIV-1 remission and viral rebound after allogeneic stem cell transplantation: report of 2 cases. *Ann Intern Med.* 2014;161:319–327.

Heppt MV, Schlaak M, Eigenler TK, et al. Checkpoint blockade for metastatic melanoma and Merkel cell carcinoma in PLWH. *Ann Oncol.* 2017;28(12):3104–3106.

Herida M, Mary-Krause M, Kaphan R, et al. Incidence of non-AIDS defining cancers before and during the highly active antiretroviral therapy era in a cohort of human immunodeficiency virus-infected patients. *J Clin Oncol.* 2003;21:3447–3453.

Hernández-Ramírez RU, Shiels MS, Dubrow R, et al. Cancer risk in HIV-infected people in the USA from 1996 to 2012: a population-based, registry-linkage study. *Lancet HIV.* 2017;4(11):e495–e504.

Hessol NA, Whittemore H, Vittinghoff E, et al. Incidence of first and second primary cancers diagnosed among people with HIV, 1985–2013: a population-based, registry linkage study. *Lancet HIV.* 2018;5(11):e647–e655.

Hill DR. The role of radiotherapy for epidemic Kaposi's sarcoma. *Semin Oncol.* 1987;14:1207.

Hladik W, Dollard SC, Mermin J, et al. Transmission of human herpesvirus 8 by blood transfusion. *N Engl J Med.* 2006;355(13):1331–1338.

Hoffmann C, Tabrizian S, Wolf E, et al. Survival of AIDS patients with primary central nervous system lymphoma is dramatically improved by HAART-induced immune recovery. *AIDS.* 2001;15(16):2119–2127.

Hoover DR, Black C, Jacobson LP, et al. Epidemiologic analysis of Kaposi's sarcoma as an early and later AIDS outcome in homosexual men. *Am J Epidemiol.* 1993;138(4):266–278.

Horner MJ, Shiels MS, Pfeiffer RM, et al. Deaths attributable to cancer in the United States HIV population during 2001–2015. *Clin Infect Dis.* 2020;ciaa1016 [E-pub before print]. doi:10.1093/cid/ciaa1016

Hosseinipour MC, Kang M, Krown SE, Bukuru A, et al. As-needed vs immediate etoposide chemotherapy in combination with antiretroviral therapy for mild-to-moderate AIDS-associated Kaposi sarcoma in resource-limited settings: A5264/AMC-067 randomized clinical trial. *Clin Infect Dis.* 2018;67(2):251–260.

Howlader N, Noone AM, Krapcho M, et al. *SEER statistics review, 1975–2012.* Bethesda, MD: National Cancer Institute. 2015. http://seer.cancer.gov/archive/csr/1975_2012

Hsiao W, Anastasia K, Hall J, et al. Association between HIV status and positive prostate biopsy in a study of US veterans. *Scientific World J.* 2009;9:102–108.

Huncharek M, Haddock KS, Reid R, et al. Smoking as a risk factor for prostate cancer: a meta-analysis of 24 prospective cohort studies. *Am J Pub Health.* 2010;100(4):693–701.

Hurst J, Hoffmann M, Pace M, et al. Immunological biomarkers predict HIV-1 viral rebound after treatment interruption. *Nat Commun.* 2015;6:8495.

Hutter G, Nowak D, Mossner M, et al. Long-term control of HIV by CCR5 Delta32/Delta32 stem-cell transplantation. *N Engl J Med.* 2009;360:692–698.

Impola U, Cuccuru MA, Masala MV, et al. Preliminary communication: matrix metalloproteinases in Kaposi's sarcoma. *Br J Dermatol.* 2003;149(4):905–907.

International Agency for Research on Cancer. *Human immunodeficiency viruses and human T-cell lymphotropic viruses.* Geneva: World Health Organization; 1996.

Iscovich J, Boffetta P, Franceschi S, et al. Classic Kaposi sarcoma: epidemiology and risk factors. *Cancer.* 2000;88(3):500–517.

Islami F, Moreira DM, Boffetta P, et al. A systematic review and meta-analysis of tobacco use and prostate cancer mortality and incidence in prospective cohort-studies. *Eur Urol.* 2014;66(6):1054–1064.

Jacobson LP, Jenkins FJ, Springer G, et al. Interaction of human immunodeficiency virus type 1 and human herpesvirus type 8 infections on the incidence of Kaposi's sarcoma. *J Infect Dis.* 2000;181(6):1940–1949.

Jacomet C, Girard PM, Lebrette MG, et al. Intravenous methotrexate for primary central nervous system non-Hodgkin's lymphoma in AIDS. *AIDS.* 1997;11(14):1725–1730.

Jephcott CR, Paltiel C, Hay J. Quality of life after non-surgical treatment of anal carcinoma: a case–control study of long-term survivors. *Clin Oncol.* 2004;16(8):530–535.

Johnson LG, Madeleine MM, Newcomer LM, et al. Anal cancer incidence and survival: the Surveillance, Epidemiology, and End Results experience, 1973–2000. *Cancer.* 2004;101(2):281–288.

Johnston C, Harrington R, Jain R, et al. Safety and efficacy of combination antiretroviral therapy in human immunodeficiency virus-infected adults undergoing autologous or allogeneic hematopoietic cell transplantation for hematologic malignancies. *Biol Blood Marrow Transplant.* 2016;22:149–156.

Joseph DA, King JB, Miller JW, et al. Prevalence of colorectal cancer screening among adults—behavioral risk factor surveillance system, United States, 2010. *MMWR.* 2012;61(2):51–56.

Kahn S, Jani A, Edelman S, et al. Matched cohort analysis of outcomes of definitive radiotherapy for prostate cancer in human immunodeficiency virus-positive patients. *Int Radiat Oncol Biol Physics.* 2012;83(1):16–21.

Kaplan LD, Abrams DI, Feigal E, et al. AIDS-associated non-Hodgkin's lymphoma in San Francisco. *JAMA.* 1989;261(5):719–724.

Kaplan LD, Hopewell PC, Jaffe H, et al. Kaposi's sarcoma involving the lung in patients with the acquired immunodeficiency syndrome. *J AIDS.* 1988;1(1):23–30.

Kaplan LD, Straus DJ, Testa MA, et al. Low-dose compared with standard-dose m-BACOD chemotherapy for non-Hodgkin's lymphoma associated with human immunodeficiency virus infection. National Institute of Allergy and Infectious Diseases AIDS Clinical Trials Group. *N Engl J Med*. 1997;336(23):1641–1648.

Karp J, Profeta G, Marantz PR, et al. Lung cancer in patients with immunodeficiency syndrome. *Chest*. 1993;103(2):410–413.

Kelly H, Chikandiwa A, Vilches LA, et al. Association of antiretroviral therapy with anal high-risk human papillomavirus, anal intraepithelial neoplasia, and anal cancer in people living with HIV: a systematic review and meta-analysis. *Lancet HIV*. 2020;7(4):e262–e278. doi: 10.1016/S2352-3018(19)30434-5

Kirk GD, Merlo C, O'Driscoll P, et al. HIV infection is associated with an increased risk for lung cancer, independent of smoking. *Clin Infect Dis*. 2007;45(1):103–110.

Kiviat NB, Hawes S, Lampinen T, et al. The effect of HAART on detection of anal HPV and squamous intraepithelial lesions among HIV infected homosexual men. Paper presented at the 6th International Conference on Malignancies in AIDS and Other Immunodeficiencies, Bethesda, MD, 2002.

Klugman AD, Schaffner J. Colon adenocarcinoma in HIV infection: a case report and review. *Am J Gastroenterol*. 1994;89(2):254–256.

Knowles DM. Etiology and pathogenesis of AIDS-related non-Hodgkin's lymphoma. *Hematol Oncol Clin North Am*. 1996;10(5):1081–1109.

Knowles DM. *Neoplastic hematopathology*. Philadelphia: Lippincott Williams & Wilkins; 2001.

Knowles DM, Chamulak GA, Subar M, et al. Lymphoid neoplasia associated with the acquired immunodeficiency syndrome (AIDS): the New York University Medical Center experience with 105 patients (1981–1986). *Ann Intern Med*. 1988; 108(5):744–753.

Komanduri KV, Luce JA, McGrath MS, et al. The natural history and molecular heterogeneity of HIV-associated primary malignant lymphomatous effusions. *J AIDS*. 1996;13(3):215–226.

Kong CY, Sigel K, Criss SD, et al. Benefits and harms of lung cancer screening in HIV-infected individuals with CD4+ cell count at least 500 cells/µl. *AIDS*. 2018;32(10):1333–1342.

Koon HB, Krown SE, Lee JY, et al. Phase II trial of imatinib in AIDS-associated Kaposi's sarcoma: AIDS Malignancy Consortium Protocol 042. *J Clin Oncol*. 2014;32(5):402–408.

Kowalkowski MA, Day RS, Chan W, et al. Cumulative HIV viremia and non-AIDs-defining malignancies among a sample of HIV-infected male veterans. *J AIDS*. 2014;62(2):204–211.

Krishnan A, Molina A, Zaia J, et al. Durable remissions with autologous stem cell transplantation for high-risk HIV-associated lymphomas. *Blood*. 2005;105(2):874–878.

Krown SE, Metroka C, Wernz JC. Kaposi's sarcoma in the acquired immune deficiency syndrome: a proposal for uniform evaluation, response, and staging criteria. AIDS Clinical Trials Group Oncology Committee. *J Clin Oncol*. 1989;7(9):1201–1207.

Krown SE, Moser CB, MacPhail P, et al. Treatment of advanced AIDS-associated Kaposi sarcoma in resource-limited settings: a three-arm, open-label, randomised, non-inferiority trial. *Lancet*. 2020;395(10231):1195–1207. doi:10.1016/S0140-6736(19)33222-2

Krown SE, Roy D, Lee JY, et al. Rapamycin with antiretroviral therapy in AIDS-associated Kaposi sarcoma: an AIDS Malignancy Consortium Study. *J AIDS*. 2012;59(5):447–454.

Krown SE, Testa MA, Huang J. AIDS-related Kaposi's sarcoma: prospective validation of the AIDS Clinical Trials Group staging classification. AIDS Clinical Trials Group Oncology Committee. *J Clin Oncol*. 1997;15(9):3085–3092.

Lafrenie RM, Wahl LM, Epstein JS, et al. HIV-1-Tat modulates the function of monocytes and alters their interactions with microvessel endothelial cells: a mechanism of HIV pathogenesis. *J Immunol*. 1996;156(4):1638–1645.

La Ruche G, You B, Mensah-Ado I, et al. Human papillomavirus and human immunodeficiency virus infections: relation with cervical dysplasia–neoplasia in African women. *Int J Cancer*. 1998;76(4):480–486.

Lavole A, Greillier L, Mazieres J, et al. First-line carboplatin plus pemetrexed with pemetrexed maintenance in HIV+ patients with advanced non-squamous non-small cell lung cancer: the Phase II IFCT-1001 CHIVA Trial. *Eur Respir J*. 2020;56(2):1902066. doi:10.1183/13993003.02066-2019

Lederman MM, Cannon PM, Currier JS, et al. A cure for HIV infection: "not in my lifetime" or "just around the corner"? *Pathog Immun*. 2016;1:154–164.

Le Garff G, Samri A, Lambert-Niclot S, et al. Transient HIV-specific T cells increase inflammation in an HIV-infected patient treated with nivolumab. *AIDS*. 2017;31(7):1048–1051.

Lehnert T, Methner M, Pollok A, et al. Multivisceral resection for locally advanced primary colon and rectal cancer: an analysis of prognostic factors in 201 patients. *Ann Surg*. 2002;235(2):217–225.

Leiker AJ, Wang CJ, Sanford NN, et al. Feasibility and outcome of routine use of concurrent chemoradiation in PLWH with squamous cell anal cancer. *Am J Clin Oncol*. 2020;43(10):701–708. doi:10.1097/COC.0000000000000736

Leport C, Rousseau F, Perronne C, et al. Bacterial prostatitis in patients infected with the human immunodeficiency virus. *J Urol*. 1989;141(2):334–336.

Letang E, Almeida J, Miró J, et al. Predictors of immune reconstitution inflammatory syndrome-associated with Kaposi sarcoma in Mozambique: a prospective study. *J AIDS*. 2010;53(5):589–597.

Levine AM, Seaberg EC, Hessol NA, et al. HIV as a risk factor for lung cancer in women: data from the Women's Interagency HIV Study. *J Clin Oncol*. 2010;28(9):1514–1519.

Levine AM, Sullivan-Halley J, Pike MC, et al. Human immunodeficiency virus-related lymphoma: prognostic factors predictive of survival. *Cancer*. 1991;68(11):2466–2472.

Levine AM, Tulpule A. Clinical aspects and management of AIDS-related Kaposi's sarcoma. *Eur J Cancer*. 2001;37(10):1288–1295.

Lewden C, Salmon D, Morlat P, et al. Causes of death among human immunodeficiency virus (HIV)-infected adults in the era of potent antiretroviral therapy: emerging role of hepatitis and cancers, persistent role of AIDS. *Int J Epidemiol*. 2005;34(1):121–130.

Lewitschnig S, Gedela K, Toby M, et al. 18F-FDG PET/CT in HIV-related central nervous system pathology. *Eur J Nucl Mol Imaging*. 2013;40(9):1420–1427.

Licho R, Litofsky NS, Senitko M, et al. Inaccuracy of Tl-201 brain SPECT in distinguishing cerebral infections from lymphoma in patients with AIDS. *Clin Nuclear Med*. 2002;27(2):81–86.

Liebowitz D, Kieff E. Epstein–Barr virus latent membrane protein: induction of B-cell activation antigens and membrane patch formation does not require vimentin. *J Virol*. 1989;63(9):4051–4054.

Lillo FB, Ferrari D, Veglia F, et al. Human papillomavirus infection and associated cervical disease in human immunodeficiency virus-infected women: effect of highly active antiretroviral therapy. *J Infect Dis*. 2001;184(5):547–551.

Lim S-T, Karim R, Tulpule A, et al. Prognostic factors in HIV-related diffuse large-cell lymphoma: before versus after highly active antiretroviral therapy. *J Clin Oncol*. 2005;23(33):8477–8482.

Lince-Deroche N, Phiri J, Michelow P, et al. Costs and cost effectiveness of three approaches for cervical cancer screening among HIV-positive women in Johannesburg, South Africa. *PloS One*. 2015;10(11):e0141969.

Lister A, Abrey LE, Sandlund JT. Central nervous system lymphoma. *Hematology Am Soc Hematol Educ Prog*. 2002;283–296.

Little RF, Pittaluga S, Grant N, et al. Highly effective treatment of acquired immunodeficiency syndrome-related lymphoma with dose-adjusted EPOCH: impact of antiretroviral therapy suspension and tumor biology. *Blood*. 2003;101(12):4653–4659.

Locker GY, Hamilton S, Harris J, et al. ASCO 2006 update of recommendations for the use of tumor markers in gastrointestinal cancer. *J Clin Oncol*. 2006:24(33):5313.

Loriot Y, Miler K, Sternberg CN, et al. Effect of enzalutamide on health-related quality of life, pain, and skeletal-related events in asymptomatic and minimally symptomatic, chemotherapy-naïve patients with metastatic castration-resistant prostate cancer (PREVAIL): results from a randomised, phase 3 trial. *Lancet Oncol.* 2015;16(5):509–521.

Lowenthal DA, Straus DJ, Wise Campbell S, et al. AIDS-related lymphoid neoplasia: the Memorial Hospital experience. *Cancer.* 1988;61(11):2325–2337.

Luppi M, Barozzi P, Santagostino G, et al. Molecular evidence of organ-related transmission of Kaposi sarcoma-associated herpesvirus or human herpesvirus-8 in transplant patients. *Blood.* 2000;96(9):3279–3281.

Lurain K, Uldrick TS, Ramaswami R, et al. Treatment of HIV-associated primary CNS lymphoma with antiretroviral therapy, rituximab, and high-dose methotrexate. *Blood.* 2020;136(19):2229–2232. doi:10.1182/blood.2020006048

Machalek DA, Poynten M, Jin F, et al. Anal human papillomavirus infection and associated neoplastic lesions in men who have sex with men: a systematic review and meta-analysis. *Lancet Oncol.* 2012;13(5):487–500.

MacMahon EM, Glass JD, Hayward SD, et al. Epstein–Barr virus in AIDS-related primary central nervous system lymphoma. *Lancet.* 1991;338(8773):969–973.

Mahale P, Engels EA, Coghill AE, et al. Cancer risk in older persons living with human immunodeficiency virus infection in the United States. *Clin Infect Dis.* 2018;67(1):50–57.

Mahale P, Ugoji C, Engles EA, et al. Cancer risk following lymphoid malignancies among HIV-infected people. *AIDS.* 2020;34(8):1237–1245. doi:10.1097/QAD.0000000000002528

Makinson A, Cheret A, Abgrall S, et al. *Early lung cancer diagnosis in HIV infected population with an important smoking history with low-dose Ct: a pilot study (EP48 HIV CHEST).* Bethesda, MD: National Library of Medicine; 2015. https://www.clinicaltrials.gov/ct2/show/NCT01207986?term=NCT01207986&rank=1. NLM Identifier: NCT 01207986.

Mandelblatt JS, Kanetsky P, Eggert L, et al. Is HIV infection a cofactor for cervical squamous cell neoplasia? *Cancer Epidemiol.* 1999;8(1):97–106.

Marcus JL, Chao CR, Leyden WA, et al. Prostate cancer incidence and prostate-specific antigen testing among HIV-positive and HIV-negative men. *J AIDS.* 2014;66:495–502.

Marcus JL, Leyden WA, Chao CR, et al. Immunodeficiency, AIDS-related pneumonia, and risk of lung cancer among HIV-infected individuals. *AIDS.* 2017;31(7):989–993.

Mbulaiteye SM, Katabira ET, Wabinga H, et al. Spectrum of cancers among HIV-infected persons in Africa: the Uganda AIDS-Center Registry Match Study. *Int J Cancer.* 2006;118(4):985–990.

McGowan JP, Shah S. Long-term remission of AIDS-related primary central nervous system lymphoma associated with highly active antiretroviral therapy. *AIDS.* 1998;12(8):952–954.

Mdodo R, Frazier EL, Dube SR, et al. Cigarette smoking prevalence among adults with HIV compared with the general adult population in the United States: cross-sectional surveys. *Ann Intern Med.* 2015;162(5):335–344.

Melbye M, Rabkin C, Frisch M, et al. Changing patterns of anal cancer incidence in the United States, 1940–1989. *Am J Epidemiol.* 1994;139(8):772–780.

Minkoff H, Ahdieh L, Massad LS, et al. The effect of highly active antiretroviral therapy on cervical cytologic changes associated with oncogenic HPV among HIV-infected women. *J AIDS.* 2001;15(16):2157–2164.

Minkoff H, Zhong Y, Burk RD, et al. Influence of adherent and effective antiretroviral therapy use on human papillomavirus infection and squamous intraepithelial lesions in human immunodeficiency virus-positive women. *J Infect Dis.* 2010;201(5):681–690.

Mitsuyasu RT, Groopman JE. Biology and therapy of Kaposi's sarcoma. *Semin Oncol.* 1984;11(1):53–59.

Monforte A, Abrams D, Pradier C, et al. HIV-induced immunodeficiency and mortality from AIDS-defining and non-AIDS-defining malignancies. *AIDS.* 2008;22(16):2143–2153.

Monini P, de Lellis L, Fabris M, et al. Kaposi's sarcoma-associated herpesvirus DNA sequences in prostate tissue and human semen. *N Engl J Med.* 1996;334(18):1168–1172.

Montgomery JD, Jacobson LP, Dhir R, et al. Detection of human herpesvirus 8 (HHV-8) in normal prostates. *Prostate.* 2006;66(12):1302–10.

Moore AL, Sabin CA, Madge S, et al. Highly active antiretroviral therapy and cervical intraepithelial neoplasia. *AIDS.* 2002;16(6):927–929.

Morlat P, Roussillon C, Henard S, et al. Causes of death among HIV-infected patients in France in 2010 (national survey): trends since 2000. *AIDS.* 2014;28(8):1181–1191.

Mosam A, Shaik F, Uldrick TS, et al. A randomized controlled trial of HAART versus HAART and chemotherapy in therapy-naive patients with HIV-associated Kaposi sarcoma in South Africa. *J AIDS.* 2012;60(2):150.

Mounier N, Spina M, Gabarre J, et al. AIDS-related non-Hodgkin lymphoma: final analysis of 485 patients treated with risk-adapted intensive chemotherapy. *Blood.* 2006;107(10):3832–3840.

Moyer VA. Screening for prostate cancer: US Preventive Services Task Force recommendation statement. *Ann Intern Med.* 2012;157(2):120–135.

Moyer VA. Screening for lung cancer. US Preventative Services Task Force recommendation statement. *Ann Intern Med.* 2014;160(5):330–338.

Munger K, Phelps WC, Bubb V, et al. The E6 and E7 genes of the human papillomavirus type 16 together are necessary and sufficient for transformation of primary human keratinocytes. *J Virol.* 1989;63(10):4417–4421.

Myerson RJ, Kong F, Birnbaum EH, et al. Radiation therapy for epidermoid carcinoma of the anal canal: clinical and treatment factors associated with outcome. *Radiother Oncol.* 2001;61(1):15–22.

Nagata N, Shimbo T, Yazaki H, et al. Predictive clinical factors in the diagnosis of gastrointestinal Kaposi's sarcoma and its endoscopic severity. *PLoS One.* 2012;7(11):1–7.

Nasti G, Martellotta F, Berretta M, et al. Impact of highly active antiretroviral therapy on the presenting features and outcome of patients with acquired immunodeficiency syndrome-related Kaposi sarcoma. *Cancer.* 2003;98(11):2440–2446.

Nasti G, Talamini R, Antinori A, et al. AIDS-related Kaposi's sarcoma: evaluation of potential new prognostic factors and assessment of the AIDS Clinical Trial Group Staging System in the HAART Era—the Italian Cooperative Group on AIDS and Tumors and the Italian Cohort of Patients Naive from Antiretrovirals. *J Clin Oncol.* 2003;21(15):2876–2882.

National Comprehensive Cancer Network. NCCN clinical practice guidelines in oncology. Primary CNS lymphoma version 1.2015. 2015a. https://www.nccn.org/professionals/physician_gls/pdf/cns.pdf

National Comprehensive Cancer Network. NCCN clinical practice guidelines in oncology. Rectal cancer version 1.2016. November 4, 2015b. https://www.nccn.org/professionals/physician_gls/pdf/rectal.pdf

National Comprehensive Cancer Network. NCCN clinical practice guidelines in oncology. Non-small cell lung cancer version 2.2016. November 23, 2015c. https://www.nccn.org/professionals/physician_gls/pdf/nscl.pdf

National Comprehensive Cancer Network. NCCN clinical practice guidelines in oncology. Colon cancer version 2.2016. November 23, 2015d. https://www.nccn.org/professionals/physician_gls/pdf/colon.pdf

National Lung Screening Trial Research Team. Reduced lung-cancer mortality with low-dose computed tomographic screening. *N Engl J Med.* 2011;365(5):395–409.

Navarro WH, Kaplan LD. AIDS-related lymphoproliferative disease. *Blood.* 2006;107(1):13–20.

Nayudu SK, Balar B. Colorectal cancer screening in human immunodeficiency virus populations: are they at average risk? *World J Gastrointestinal Oncol.* 2012;4(12):259–264.

Neef H, Horth W, Makowiec F, et al. Outcome after resection of hepatic and pulmonary metastasis of colorectal cancer. *J Gastrointest Surg.* 2009;13(10):1813–1820.

Newton R, Ziegler J, Bourboulia D, et al. Infection with Kaposi's sarcoma-associated herpesvirus (KSHV) and human immunodeficiency virus (HIV) in relation to the risk and clinical presentation of Kaposi's sarcoma in Uganda. *Br J Cancer.* 2003;89(3):502–504.

Norden AD, Drappatz J, Wen PY, et al. Survival among patients with primary central nervous system lymphoma, 1973–2004. *J Neurooncol.* 2011;101(3):487–493.

Northfelt DW, Dezube BJ, Thommes JA, et al. Pegylated-liposomal doxorubicin versus doxorubicin, bleomycin, and vincristine in the treatment of AIDS-related Kaposi's sarcoma: results of a randomized phase III clinical trial. *J Clin Oncol.* 1998;16(7):2445–2451.

Noy A. Update in Kaposi sarcoma. *Curr Opin Oncol.* 2003;15(5):379–381.

Noy A, Lee JY, Cesarman E, et al. AMC 048: modified CODOX-M/IVAC-rituximab is safe and effective for HIV-associated Burkitt lymphoma. *Blood.* 2015;126:160–166.

Ntekim A, Campbell O, Rothenbacher D. Optimal management of cervical cancer in PLWH: a systematic review. *Cancer Med.* 2015;4:1381–1393.

Nyitray AG, Hicks JT, Hwang LY, et al. A phase II clinical study to assess the feasibility of self and partner anal examinations to detect anal canal abnormalities including anal cancer. *Sex Transm Infect.* 2018;94(2):124–130.

Oehler-Janne C, Huguet F, Provencher S, et al. HIV-specific differences in outcome of squamous cell carcinoma of the anal canal: a multicentric cohort study of PLWH receiving highly active antiretroviral therapy. *J Clin Oncol.* 2008;26(15):2550–2557.

Okotie OT, Roehl KA, Han M, et al. Characteristics of prostate cancer detected by digital rectal examination only. *Urology.* 2007;70(6):1117–1120.

Okuma Y, Hishima T, Kashima J, et al. High PD-L1 expression indicates poor prognosis of HIV-infected patients with non-small cell lung cancer. *Cancer Immunol Immunother.* 2018;67(3):495–505.

Okuma Y, Hosomi Y, Imamura A. Lung cancer patients harboring epidermal growth factor receptor mutation among those infected by human immunodeficiency virus. *Onco Targets Ther.* 2014;31:111–115.

Olson JE, Janney CA, Rao RD, et al. The continuing increase in the incidence of primary central nervous system non-Hodgkin lymphoma: a surveillance, epidemiology, and end results analysis. *Cancer.* 2002;95(7):1504–1510.

Ong WL, Manohar P, Millar J, et al. Clinicopathological characteristics and management of prostate cancer in the human immunodeficiency virus (HIV)-positive population: experience in an Australian major HIV center. *Br J Urol Int.* 2015; 116(Suppl 3):5–10.

Orlando G, Fasolo MM, Schiavini M, et al. Role of highly active antiretroviral therapy in human papillomavirus-induced genital dysplasia in HIV-1-infected patients. *AIDS.* 1999;13(3):424–425.

Palefsky JM, Holly EA, Gonzales J, et al. Detection of human papillomavirus DNA in anal intraepithelial neoplasia and anal cancer. *Cancer Res.* 1991;51(3):1014–1019.

Palefsky JM, Holly EA, Ralston ML, et al. Effect of highly active antiretroviral therapy on the natural history of anal squamous intraepithelial lesions and anal human papillomavirus infection. *J AIDS.* 2001;28(5):422–428.

Pantanowitz L, Bohac G, Cooley T, et al. Human immunodeficiency virus-associated prostate cancer: clinicopathological findings and outcome in a multi-institutional study. *Br J Urol Int.* 2008;101:1519–1523.

Patel P, Hanson DL, Sullivan PS, et al. Incidence of types of cancer among HIV-infected persons compared with the general population in the United States, 1992–2003. *Ann Intern Med.* 2008;148(10):728–736.

Patil P, Elem B, Zumla A. Pattern of adult malignancies in Zambia (1980–1989) in light of the human immunodeficiency virus type 1 epidemic. *J Trop Med Hyg.* 1995;98(4):281–284.

Penn I. Kaposi's sarcoma in organ transplant recipients: report of 20 cases. *Transplantation.* 1979;27(1):8–11.

Persad GC, Little RF, Grady C. Including persons with HIV infection in cancer clinical trials. *J Clin Oncol.* 2008;26(7):1027–1032.

Petrovas C, Casazza JP, Brenchley JM, et al. PD-1 is a regulator of virus-specific CD8+ T cell survival in HIV infection. *J Exp Med.* 2006;203:2281–2292.

Piketty C, Seliger-Leneman H, Bouvier AM. Incidence of HIV-related anal cancer remains increased despite long-term combined antiretroviral treatment: results from the French Hospital Database on HIV. *J Clin Oncol.* 2012;30(35):4360–4366.

Piketty C, Selinger-Leneman H, Grabar S, et al. Marked increase in the incidence of invasive anal cancer among HIV-infected patients despite treatment with combination antiretroviral therapy. *AIDS.* 2008;22(10):1203–1211.

Plancoulaine S, Abel L, van Beveren M, et al. Human herpesvirus 8 transmission from mother to child and between siblings in an endemic population. *Lancet.* 2000;356(9235):1062–1065.

Pluda J, Broder S, Yarchoan R. Therapy of AIDS and AIDS-associated neoplasms. *Cancer Chemother Biol Response Modif.* 1992;13:404–439.

Polesel J, Clifford GM, Rickenbach M, et al. Non-Hodgkin lymphoma incidence in the Swiss HIV Cohort Study before and after highly active antiretroviral therapy. *AIDS.* 2008;22(2):301–306.

Polizzotto MN, Uldrick TS, Wyvill KM, et al. Clinical features and outcomes of patients with symptomatic Kaposi sarcoma herpesvirus (KSHV)-associated inflammation: prospective characterization of KSHV inflammatory cytokine syndrome (KICS). *Clin Infect Dis.* 2016a;62(6):730–738. doi:10.1093/cid/civ996

Polizzotto MN, Uldrick TS, Wyvill KM, et al. Pomalidomide for symptomatic Kaposi's sarcoma in people with and without HIV infection: a phase I/II study. *J Clin Oncol.* 2016b;34(34):4125–4131.

Pourcher V, Desnoyer A, Assoumou L, et al. Phase II trial of lenalidomide in HIV-infected patients with previously treated Kaposi's sarcoma: results of the ANRS 154 Lenakap Trial. *AIDS Res Hum Retroviruses.* 2017;33(1):1–10.

Powles T, Matthews G, Bower M. AIDS related systemic non-Hodgkin's lymphoma. *Sex Transm Infect.* 2000;76(5):335–341.

Powles T, Thirwell C, Newsom-Davis T, et al. Does HIV adversely influence the outcome in advanced non-small-cell lung cancer in the era of HAART? *Br J Cancer.* 2003;89:457–459.

Rahmanian S, Wewers ME, Koletar S, et al. Cigarette smoking in the HIV-infected population. *Proc Am Thorac Soc.* 2011;8(3):313–319.

Ramirez-Marrero FA, Smit E, de la Torre-Feliciano T, et al. Risk of cancer among Hispanics with AIDS compared with the general population in Puerto Rico: 1987–2003. *Puerto Rico Health Sci J.* 2010;29(3):256–264.

Ratner L, Lee J, Tang S, et al. Chemotherapy for human immunodeficiency virus-associated non-Hodgkin's lymphoma in combination with highly active antiretroviral therapy. *J Clin Oncol.* 2001;19(8):2171–2178.

Ravalli S, Chabon A, Khan A. Gastrointestinal neoplasia in young HIV antibody-positive patients. *Am J Clin Pathol.* 1989;91:458–461.

Re A, Cattaneo C, Michieli M, et al. High-dose therapy and autologous peripheral-blood stem-cell transplantation as salvage treatment for HIV-associated lymphoma in patients receiving highly active antiretroviral therapy. *J Clin Oncol.* 2003;21(23):4423–4427.

Re A, Michieli M, Casari S, et al. High-dose therapy and autologous peripheral blood stem cell transplantation as salvage treatment for AIDS-related lymphoma: long-term results of the Italian Cooperative Group on AIDS and Tumors (GICAT) study with analysis of prognostic factors. *Blood.* 2009;114(7):1306–1313.

Reddy KP, Kong CY, Hyle EP, et al. Lung cancer mortality associated with smoking and smoking cessation among people living with HIV in the United States. *JAMA Intern Med.* 2017;177(11):1613–1621.

Reekie J, Kosa C, Engsig F, et al. Relationship between current level of immunodeficiency and non-acquired immunodeficiency syndrome-defining malignancies. *Cancer.* 2010;116(22):5306–5315.

Reid E, Suneja G, Ambinder RF, et al. Cancer in people living with HIV, Version 1.2018, NCCN clinical practice guidelines in oncology. *J Natl Compr Canc Netw.* 2018;16(8):986–1017.

Reinhold JP, Moon M, Tenner CT, et al. Colorectal cancer screening in HIV-infected patients 50 years of age and older: missed opportunities for prevention. *Am J Gastroenterol.* 2005;100:1805–1812.

Renwick N, Halaby T, Weverling GJ, et al. Seroconversion for human herpesvirus 8 during HIV infection is highly predictive of Kaposi's sarcoma. *AIDS.* 1998;12(18):2481–2488.

Richel O, de Vries HJ, van Noesel CJ, et al. Comparison of imiquimod, topical fluorouracil, and electrocautery for the treatment of anal intraepithelial neoplasia in HIV-positive men who have sex with men: an open-label, randomised controlled trial. *Lancet Oncol.* 2013;14:346–353.

Riedel DJ, Cox ER, Stafford KA, et al. Clinical presentation and outcomes of prostate cancer in an urban cohort of predominantly African American, human immunodeficiency virus-infected patients. *Urology.* 2015;85(2):415–421.

Riedel DJ, Rositch AF, Redfield RR. Patterns of HIV viremia and viral suppression before diagnosis of non-AIDS-defining cancers in HIV-infected individuals. *Infect Agent Cancer.* 2015;38(10):1–7.

Riley RR, Duensing S, Brake T, et al. Dissection of human papillomavirus E6 and E7 function in transgenic mouse models of cervical carcinogenesis. *Cancer Res.* 2003;63(16):4862–4871.

Robbins HA, Pfeiffer RM, Shiels MS, et al. Excess cancers among HIV-infected people in the United States. *J Natl Cancer Inst.* 2015;107(4):dju503.

Robert C, Ribas A, Wolchok JD, et al. Anti-programmed-death-receptor-1 treatment with pembrolizumab in ipilimumab-refractory advanced melanoma: a randomised dose-comparison cohort of a phase 1 trial. *Lancet.* 2014;384:1109–1117.

Rodrigo JA, Hicks LK, Cheung MC, et al. HIV-associated Burkitt lymphoma: good efficacy and tolerance of intensive chemotherapy including CODOX-M/IVAC with or without rituximab in the HAART era. *Adv Hematol.* 2012;2012:1–9.

Rohner E, Valeri F, Maskew M, et al. Incidence rate of Kaposi sarcoma in HIV-infected patients on antiretroviral therapy in southern Africa: a prospective multicohort study. *J AIDS.* 2014;67(5):547–554.

Ronit A, Kristensen T, Klitbo DM, et al. Incidental lung cancers and positive computed tomography images in people living with HIV. *AIDS.* 2017;31:1973–1977

Rosenblum ML, Levy RM, Bredesen DE, et al. Primary central nervous system lymphomas in patients with AIDS. *Ann Neurol.* 1988;23(Suppl):S13–S16.

Royse K, El Chaer F, Amirian ES, et al. Disparities in Kaposi sarcoma incidence and survival in the United States: 2000–2013. *PLoS One.* 2017;12(8):e0182750.

Ruiz A, Ganz WI, Post MJ, et al. Use of thallium-201 brain SPECT to differentiate cerebral lymphoma from toxoplasma encephalitis in AIDS patients. *Am J Neuroradiol.* 1994;15(10):1885–1894.

Rust B, Kiem HP, Uldrick T. CAR T-cell therapy for cancer and HIV through novel approaches to HIV-associated haematological malignancies. *Lancet Haematol.* 2020;7(9):E690–696. doi:10.1016/S2352-3026(20)30142-3

Ryan CJ, Smith MR, Fizazi K, et al. Abiraterone acetate plus prednisone versus placebo plus prednisone in chemotherapy-naïve men with metastatic castration-resistant prostate cancer (COU-AA-302): final overall survival analysis of a randomised, double-blind, placebo-controlled phase 3 study. *Lancet Oncol.* 2015;16(2):152–160.

Sacktor N, Lyles RH, Skolasky R, et al. HIV-associated neurologic disease incidence changes: multicenter AIDS cohort study, 1990–1998. *Neurology.* 2001;56(2):257–260.

Safai B. Pathophysiology and epidemiology of epidemic Kaposi's sarcoma. *Semin Oncol.* 1987;2:7–12.

Sandler AS, Kaplan LD. Diagnosis and management of systemic non-Hodgkin's lymphoma in HIV disease. *Hematol Oncol Clin North Am.* 1996;10(5):1111–1124.

Santesso N, Mustafa RA, Schunemann HJ, et al. World Health Organization guidelines for treatment of cervical intraepithelial neoplasia 2-3 and screen-and-treat strategies to prevent cervical cancer. *Int J Gynaecol Obstet.* 2016;132:252–258

Sauer R, Liersch T, Merkel S, et al. Preoperative versus postoperative chemoradiotherapy for locally advanced rectal cancer: results of the German CAO/ARO/AIO-94 randomized phase III trial after a median follow-up of 11 years. *J Clin Oncol.* 2012;20(16):1926–1933.

Saville M, Lietzau J, Pluda J, et al. Activity of placlitaxel (Taxol) as therapy for HIV-associated Kaposi's sarcoma. *Lancet.* 1995;346:26–28.

Schiffman M, Kjaer SK. Natural history of anogenital human papillomavirus infection and neoplasia. *JNCI Monographs.* 2003;2003(31):14–19.

Schreiber D, Chhabra A, Rineer J, et al. Outcomes and tolerance of human immunodeficiency virus-positive veterans undergoing dose-escalated external beam radiotherapy for localized prostate cancer. *Clin Genitourin Cancer.* 2014;12(2):94–99.

Serraino D, Boschini A, Carrieri P, et al. Cancer risk among men with, or at risk of, HIV infection in southern Europe. *AIDS.* 2000;14(5):553–559.

Sgadari C, Monini P, Barillari G, et al. Use of HIV protease inhibitors to block Kaposi's sarcoma and tumour growth. *Lancet Oncol.* 2003;4(9):537–547.

Shah NN, Singavi AK, Harrington A. Daratumumab in primary effusion lymphoma. *N Engl J Med.* 2018;379(7):689–690.

Shah R, Al-Sukhni W, Kim RD, et al. Resection of hepatic and pulmonary metastasis from colorectal carcinoma. *J Am Coll Surg.* 2006;202(3):468–475.

Shebl FM, Engels EA, Goedert JJ, et al. Pulmonary infections and risk of lung cancer among persons with AIDS. *J AIDS.* 2010;55:375–379.

Shepherd FA, Crowley J, van Houtte P, et al.; the IASLC Lung Cancer Staging Project. Clinical staging of small cell lung cancer in the forthcoming (seventh) edition of the Tumor, Node, Metastasis Classification for Lung Cancer. *J Thoracic Oncol.* 2007;2(12):1067–1077.

Shepherd L, Ryom L, Law M, et al. Cessation of cigarette smoking and the impact on cancer incidence in HIV-positive persons: the D:A:D study. *Clin Infect Dis.* 2018;68(4):650–657. doi:10.1093/cid/ciy508

Shiels MS, Althoff KN, Pfeiffer RM, et al. HIV infection, immunosuppression, and age at diagnosis of non-AIDS-defining cancers. *Clin Infect Dis.* 2017;64(4):468–475.

Shiels MS, Cole SR, Mehta SH, et al. Lung cancer incidence and mortality among HIV-infected and HIV-uninfected injection drug users. *J AIDS.* 2010;55(4):510–515.

Shiels MS, Copeland G, Goodman M, et al. Cancer stage at diagnosis in patients infected with the human immunodeficiency virus and transplant recipients. *Cancer.* 2015;121(12):1063–2071.

Shiels MS, Goedert JJ, Moore RD, et al. Reduced risk of prostate cancer in US men with AIDS. *Cancer Epidemiol Biomarkers Prev.* 2010;19(11):2910–2915.

Shiels MS, Pfeiffer RM, Engels EA. Age at cancer diagnosis among persons with AIDS in the United States. *Ann Intern Med.* 2010;153(7):452–460.

Shiels MS, Pfeiffer RM, Gail MH, et al. Cancer burden in the HIV-infected population in the United States. *J Natl Cancer Inst.* 2011;103:753–762.

Shiels MS, Pfeiffer RM, Hall HI, et al. Proportions of Kaposi sarcoma, selected non-Hodgkin lymphomas, and cervical cancer in the United States occurring in persons with AIDS, 1980–2007. *JAMA.* 2011;305(14):1450–1459.

Shiels MS, Pfeiffer RM, Hildesheim A, et al. Circulating inflammation markers and prospective risk for lung cancer. *J Natl Cancer Inst.* 2013;105(24):1871–1880.

Siegel R, DeSantis C, Jemal A. Colorectal cancer statistics, 2014. *CA Cancer J Clin.* 2014;64(2):104–117.

Siegel R, Naishadham D, Jemal A. Cancer statistics, 2012. *CA Cancer J Clin.* 2012;62(1):10–29.

Sigel C, Cavalcanti MS, Daniel T, et al. Clinicopathologic features of colorectal carcinoma in PLWH. *Cancer Epidemiol Biomarkers Prev.* 2016;25:1098–1104.

Sigel K, Crothers K, Dubrow R, et al. Prognosis in HIV-infected patients with non-small cell lung cancer. *Br J Cancer.* 2013;109:1974–1980.

Sigel K, Wisnivesky J, Crothers K, et al. Immunological and infectious risk factors for lung cancer in US veterans with HIV: a longitudinal cohort study. *Lancet HIV.* 2017;4(2):e67–e73.

Sigel K, Wisnivesky J, Gordon K, et al. HIV as an independent risk factor for incident lung cancer. *AIDS.* 2012;26;1017–1025.

Sigel K, Wisnivesky J, Shahrir S, et al. Findings in asymptomatic HIV-infected patients undergoing chest computed tomography testing: implications for lung cancer screening. *AIDS.* 2014;28(7):1007–1014.

Silverberg MJ, Lau B, Achenbach CJ, et al. Cumulative incidence of cancer among persons with HIV in North America. *Ann Intern Med.* 2015;163(7):507–518.

Silverberg MJ, Lau B, Justic AC, et al. Risk of anal cancer in HIV-infected and HIV-uninfected individuals in North America. *Clin Infect Dis.* 2012;54(17):1026–1034.

Silverberg MJ, Leyden W, Gregorich S, et al. Is intensive cervical cancer screening justified in immunosuppressed women? [Abstract 162] Paper presented at the Conference on Retroviruses and Opportunistic Infections (CROI), Boston, February 22–25, 2016.

Silverberg MJ, Leyden W, Hernandez-Ramirez RU, et al. Timing of antiretroviral therapy initiation and risk of cancer among persons living with HIV. *Clin Infect Dis.* 2020;ciaa1046 [E-pub before print]. doi:10.1093/cid/ciaa1046

Simard EP, Engels EA. Cancer as a cause of death among people with AIDS in the United States. *Clin Infect Dis.* 2010a;51(8):957–962.

Simard EP, Pfeiffer RM, Engels EA. Spectrum of cancer risk late after AIDS onset in the United States. *Arch Intern Med.* 2010b;170(15):1337–1345.

Simard EP, Pfeiffer RM, Engels EA. Cumulative incidence of cancer among individuals with acquired immunodeficiency syndrome in the United States. *Cancer.* 2011;117(5):1089–1096.

Skiest DJ, Crosby C. Survival is prolonged by highly active antiretroviral therapy in AIDS patients with primary central nervous system lymphoma. *AIDS.* 2003;17(12):1787–1793.

Smith AJB, Varma S, Rositch AF et al. Gynecologic cancer in HIV-positive women: a systematic review and meta-analysis. *Am J Obstet Gynecol.* 2019;221(3):194–207. doi:10.1016/j.ajog.2019.02.022

Smith DM, Kingery JD, Wong JK, et al. The prostate as a reservoir for HIV-1. *AIDS.* 2004;18(11):1600–1602.

Smith JS, Sanusi B, Swarts A, et al. A randomized clinical trial comparing cervical dysplasia treatment with cryotherapy vs loop electrosurgical excision procedure in HIV-seropositive women from Johannesburg, South Africa. *Am J Obstet Gynecol.* 2017;217(2):183.e1–183.e11.

Smith RE, Colangelo L, Wieand HS, et al. Randomized trial of adjuvant therapy in colon carcinoma: 10-year results of NSABP Protocol C-01. *J Natl Cancer Inst.* 2004;96(15):1128–1132.

Spano JP, Massiani MA, Bentata M, et al. Lung cancer in patients with HIV infection and review of the literature. *Med Oncol.* 2004;21:109–115.

Sparano JA, Lee S, Chen MG, et al. Phase II trial of infusional cyclophosphamide, doxorubicin, and etoposide in patients with HIV-associated non-Hodgkin's lymphoma: an Eastern Cooperative Oncology Group Trial (E1494). *J Clin Oncol.* 2004;22(8):1491–1500.

Sparano JA, Lee JY, Kaplan LD, et al. Rituximab plus concurrent infusional EPOCH chemotherapy is highly effective in HIV-associated B-cell non-Hodgkin lymphoma. *Blood.* 2010;115(15):3008–3016.

Stadler RF, Gregorcyk SG, Euhus DM, et al. Outcome of HIV-infected patients with invasive squamous-cell carcinoma of the anal canal in the era of highly active antiretroviral therapy. *Dis Colon Rectum.* 2004;47(8):1305–1309.

Stebbing J, Sanitt A, Nelson M, et al. A prognostic index for AIDS-associated Kaposi's sarcoma in the era of highly active antiretroviral therapy. *Lancet.* 2006;367(9521):1495–1502.

Stebbing J, Sanitt A, Teague A, et al. Prognostic significance of immune subset measurement in individuals with AIDS-associated Kaposi's sarcoma. *J Clin Oncol.* 2007;25(16):2230–2235.

Stewart S, Jablonowski H, Goebel FD, et al. Randomized comparative trial of pegylated liposomal doxorubicin versus bleomycin and vincristine in the treatment of AIDS-related Kaposi's sarcoma: International Pegylated Liposomal Doxorubicin Study Group. *J Clin Oncol.* 1998;16(2):683–691.

Stier EA, Sebring MC, Mendez AE, et al. Prevalence of anal human papillomavirus infection and anal HPV-related disorders in women: a systematic review. *Am J Obstet Gynecol.* 2015;213(3):278–309.

Straus DJ, Huang J, Testa MA, et al. Prognostic factors in the treatment of human immunodeficiency virus-associated non-Hodgkin's lymphoma: analysis of AIDS Clinical Trials Group protocol 142—Low-dose versus standard-dose m-BACOD plus granulocyte-macrophage colony-stimulating factor; National Institute of Allergy and Infectious Diseases. *J Clin Oncol.* 1998;16(11):3601–3606.

Sugarman J, Lewin SR, Henrich TJ, et al. Ethics of ART interruption after stem-cell transplantation. *Lancet HIV.* 2016;3:e8–e10.

Sun D, Cao M, Li H, et al. Risk of prostate cancer in men with HIV/AIDS: a systematic review and meta-analysis. *Prostate Cancer Prostatic Dis.* 2020 [E-pub before print]. doi:10.1038/s41391-020-00268-2

Suneja G, Shiels MS, Melville SK. Disparities in the treatment and outcomes of lung cancer among HIV-infected individuals. *AIDS.* 2013;27(3):459–468.

Susko M, Wang, CJ, Lazar AA, et al. Factors impacting differential outcomes in the definitive radiation treatment of anal cancer between HIV-positive and HIV-negative patients. *Oncologist.* 2020;25(9):772–779. doi:10.1634/theoncologist.2019-0824

Taieb J, Tabernero J, Mini E, et al. Oxaliplatin, fluorouracil, and leucovorin with or without cetuximab in patients with resected stage III colon cancer (PETACC-8): an open-label, randomised phase III trial. *Lancet Oncol.* 2014;15(8):862–873.

Tam HK, Zhang Z-F, Jacobson LP, et al. Effect of highly active antiretroviral therapy on survival among HIV-infected men with Kaposi sarcoma or non-Hodgkin lymphoma. *Int J Cancer.* 2002;98(6):916–922.

Tesoriero JM, Gieryic SM, Carrascal A, et al. Smoking among HIV-positive New Yorkers: prevalence, frequency, and opportunities for cessation. *AIDS Behav.* 2010;14(4):824–835.

Tornesello ML, Buonaguro FM, Beth-Giraldo E, et al. Human immunodeficiency virus type 1 tat gene enhances human papillomavirus early gene expression. *Intervirology.* 1993;36(2):57–64.

Trautmann L, Janbazian L, Chomont N, et al. Upregulation of PD-1 expression on HIV-specific CD8+ T cells leads to reversible immune dysfunction. *Nat Med.* 2006;12:1198–1202.

Travi G, Ferreri A, Cinque P, et al. Long term remission of HIV-associated primary CNS lymphoma achieved with highly active antiretroviral therapy alone. *J Clin Oncol.* 2012;30(10):e119–e121.

Uldrick TS, Gonçalves PH, Abdul-Hay M, et al. Assessment of the safety of pembrolizumab in patients with HIV and advanced cancer: a phase 1 study. *JAMA Oncol.* 2019;5(9):1332–1339. doi:10.1001/jamaoncol.2019.2244

Vallet-Pichard A, Pol S. Hepatitis viruses and human immunodeficiency virus co-infection: pathogenesis and treatment. *J Hepatol.* 2004;41(1):156–166.

Vernone SD, Hart CE, Reeves WC, et al. The HIV-1 tat protein enhances E2-dependent human papillomavirus 16 transcription. *Virus Res.* 1993;27(2):133–145.

Volberding P, Kusick P, Feigal D. Effects of chemotherapy for HIV-associated Kaposi's sarcoma on long-term survival. *Proc Am Soc Clin Oncol.* 1989;3(9):abstract 11.

Walmsley S, Northfelt DW, Melosky B, et al. Treatment of AIDS-related cutaneous Kaposi's sarcoma with topical alitretinoin (9-cis-retinoic acid) gel: Panretin Gel North American Study Group. *J AIDS.* 1999;22(3):235–246.

Wang ES, Straus DJ, Teruya-Felstein J, et al. Intensive chemotherapy with cyclophosphamide, doxorubicine, high-dose methotrexade/ifosfamide, etoposide, and high-dose cytarabine (CODOX-M/IVAC) for human immunodeficiency virus-associated Burkett lymphoma. *Cancer.* 2003;98(3):1196–1205.

Wang Y, Wang Y, Gaisa MM, et al. Negative predictive value of human papillomavirus testing: implications for anal cancer screening in people living with HIV/AIDS. *J Oncol.* 2020;2020:6352315. doi:10.1155/2020/6352315

Wasserberg N, Nunoo-Mensah JW, Gonzalez Ruiz C, et al. Colorectal cancer in HIV-infected patients: a case control study. *Colorectal Dis.* 2007;22(10):1217–1221.

Welch K, Finkbeiner W, Alpers CE, et al. Autopsy findings in the acquired immune deficiency syndrome. *JAMA.* 1984;252(9):1152–1159.

Westwood TD, Hogan C, Julyan PJ, et al. Utility of FDG-PETCT and magnetic resonance spectroscopy in differentiating between cerebral lymphoma and non-malignant CNS lesions in HIV-infected patients. *Eur J Radiol.* 2013;82(8):e374–e379.

Whitlock EP, Lin JS, Liles E, et al. Screening for colorectal cancer: a targeted, updated systematic review for the US Preventive Services Task Force. *Ann Intern Med.* 2008;149(9):638–658.

Wightman F, Solomon A, Kumar SS, et al. Effect of ipilimumab on the HIV reservoir in an HIV-infected individual with metastatic melanoma. *AIDS.* 2015;29(4):504–506.

Wilkin TJ, Palmer S, Brudney KF, et al. Anal intraepithelial neoplasia in heterosexual and homosexual HIV-positive men with access to antiretroviral therapy. *J Infect Dis.* 2004;190(9):1685–1691.

Wilson WH, Sin-Ho J, Pitcher BN, et al. Phase III randomized study of R-CHOP versus DA-EPOCH-R and molecular analysis of untreated diffuse large B-cell lymphoma: CALGB/Alliance 50303. *Blood.* 2016;128:469.

Winstone TA, Man SF, Hull M, et al. Epidemic of lung cancer in patients with HIV infection. *Chest.* 2013;143(2):305–314.

Wistuba IL, Behrens C, Milchgrub S, et al. Comparison of molecular changes in lung cancers in HIV-positive and HIV-indeterminate subjects. *JAMA.* 1998;279(19):1554–1559.

Wolf T, Brodt H-R, Fichtlscherer S, et al. Changing incidence and prognostic factors of survival in AIDS-related non-Hodgkin's lymphoma in the era of highly active antiretroviral therapy (HAART). *Leuk Lymphoma.* 2005;46(2):207–215.

Woolfrey AE, Malhotra U, Harrington RD, et al. Generation of HIV-1-specific CD8+ cell responses following allogeneic hematopoietic cell transplantation. *Blood.* 2008;112(8):3484–3487.

Yegüez JF, Martinez SA, Sands DR, et al. Colorectal malignancies in PLWH. *Am Surg.* 2003;69(11):981–987.

Zanet E, Taborelli M, Rupolo M, et al. Postautologous stem cell transplantation long-term outcomes in 26 PLWH affected by relapsed/refractory lymphoma. *AIDS.* 2015;29(17): 2303–2308.

Zhang JY, Zhang Z, Wang X, et al. PD-1 up-regulation is correlated with HIV-specific memory CD8+ T-cell exhaustion in typical progressors but not in long-term nonprogressors. *Blood.* 2007;109: 4671–4678.

Zheng J, Wang L, Cheng Z, et al. Molecular changes of lung malignancy in HIV infection. *Sci Rep.* 2018;8(1):13128.

Ziegler JL, Drew WL, Miner RC, et al. Outbreak of Burkitt's-like lymphoma in homosexual men. *Lancet.* 1982;2(8299):631–633.

Ziegler JL, Templeton AC, Vogel CL. Kaposi's sarcoma: a comparison of classical, endemic, and epidemic forms. *Semin Oncol.* 1984;11(1):47–52.

30.

DERMATOLOGIC COMPLICATIONS OF HIV

Kudakwashe Mutyambizi and Philip Bolduc

OVERVIEW OF CUTANEOUS FINDINGS IN HIV INFECTION

LEARNING OBJECTIVE

- Review the approach to skin findings in the context of acute and chronic HIV infection

WHAT'S NEW?

Multiple biopsies increase diagnostic yield for identification of cutaneous complications of HIV.

KEY POINTS

- Dermatoses that are rare in the general population but common in HIV populations should prompt testing for HIV when there is no preexisting diagnosis.

- Correct diagnosis and management of skin complaints can improve the quality of life of persons with HIV (PWH) who have increased longevity with antiretroviral therapy (ART).

- The appearance of AIDS-defining cutaneous illnesses in previously immune-reconstituted patients on ART should prompt a reassessment of CD4+ T-cell count and HIV RNA levels.

- In patients who have been on ART for less than 24 weeks, the appearance or worsening of dermatoses may be due to immune reconstitution inflammatory syndrome (IRIS).

The hallmark of HIV infection is immune dysregulation and immunosuppression. As the immune system deteriorates, inflammatory dermatoses, metabolic dysregulation, adverse drug reactions, opportunistic infections (OIs), and cutaneous malignancies become more common, atypical in presentation, and recalcitrant to therapy. Both acute and chronic skin complaints contribute significantly to reduced quality of life for HIV patients (Mirmirani et al., 2002).

The US Centers for Disease Control and Prevention (CDC) recommends that individuals between ages 13 and 64 years be tested for HIV at least once in their lifetime, with increased screening of high-risk individuals and testing based on symptoms. The presence of dermatoses uncommon in the general population but concentrated in the HIV population, or dermatoses strikingly recalcitrant to therapy, should warrant suspicion and testing for HIV. In patients with known HIV/AIDS, there is a correlation between CD4+ T-cell count and the occurrence of characteristic dermatoses (Goldstein et al., 1997; Rigopoulos et al., 2004). Direct CD4+ T-cell testing is the gold standard assessment of immune function; however, the World Health Organization's (WHO) clinical staging provides guidelines regarding skin findings that should raise suspicion for immune deterioration, thus prompting CD4+ T-cell testing, and have significance in international settings in which CD4+ T-cell testing is of limited availability (Baveewo et al., 2011; Weinberg & Kovarik, 2010). The occurrence of AIDS-defining illnesses such as Kaposi's sarcoma (KS) or acute systemic illnesses and infections in patients previously immunocompetent by CD4+ T-cell count or previously well controlled on ART should prompt an assessment of CD4+ T-cell count and HIV RNA levels to evaluate for immune deterioration. In patients who have been on ART for less than 24 weeks, acute systemic illnesses may be due to IRIS or treatment toxicity and, during this period, do not closely parallel the WHO clinical staging guidelines (Ratnam et al., 2006). With these caveats, the dermatoses discussed in this chapter are presented along with the corresponding CD4+ T-cell count at which they typically occur (Zancanaro et al., 2006).

HIV practitioners can competently diagnose many of the dermatologic conditions discussed in this chapter as well as perform diagnostic biopsies and minor cosmetic procedures. Busy HIV practices sometimes maintain a supply of liquid nitrogen to treat warts and an electrocautery machine known as a hyfrecator to electrodesiccate lesions such as molluscum contagiosum. Referral to a dermatologist is recommended when presented with diagnostic or management uncertainty, particularly in the acutely ill PWH,

Box 30.1 INDICATIONS FOR REFERRAL TO A
DERMATOLOGIST

Diagnostic uncertainty
Management uncertainty
Life-threatening differential diagnoses
Rapid progression
Persistence or recurrence despite therapy
Requires specialized medications
Requires specialized procedures
Suspected skin cancer
Indications for skin cancer screening
Pigmented lesions
Improve compliance
Patient request

with common or chronic dermatoses recalcitrant to therapies familiar to the HIV practitioner, and for optimal tissue procurement when the clinician is uncertain of appropriate biopsy site or method.

It is important for HIV practitioners to be aware that several serious disseminated OIs, some of which may be fatal, may first manifest as an acute cutaneous eruption. Therefore, it is important for a skin biopsy to be performed in an acutely febrile PWH with a newly developed skin eruption. The biopsy should be accompanied with a request for urgent processing with special stains for bacteria, atypical mycobacteria, fungi, and viruses as appropriate. Tissue is placed in 10% formalin for routine processing, but a portion should be placed in normal saline so that cultures for microorganisms can be performed to aid in definitive diagnosis.

In general, when sampling a lesion, especially one that is papular or pustular, an early, new lesion that is not excoriated is most likely to yield tissue with changes that afford the dermatopathologist the best opportunity to make an accurate diagnosis (Altman et al., 2015). A pertinent exception in this population is biopsy of suspected KS because early lesions can present a confusing picture histologically. An older, more mature lesion, if present, will have greater diagnostic yield (Maurer, 2005). When in doubt, one should consider taking multiple biopsies from the lesion in different stages of evolution and from different cutaneous sites. If the practitioner is not comfortable performing a good skin biopsy, dermatologic referral for evaluation and biopsy determination should be made. Box 30.1 provides guidelines for referral.

RECOMMENDED READING

Altman K, Vanness E, Westergaard RP. Cutaneous manifestations of human immunodeficiency virus: a clinical update. *Curr Infect Dis Rep.* 2015;17(3):464.

Mirmirani P, Maurer TA, Berger TG, et al. Skin-related quality of life in HIV-infected patients on highly active antiretroviral therapy. *J Cutan Med Surg.* 2002;6(1):10–15.

INFLAMMATORY DERMATOSES AND HIV

LEARNING OBJECTIVE

- Discuss the incidence, presentation, and management of inflammatory dermatoses in HIV

WHAT'S NEW?

Traditional immunosuppressants and newer biological therapies have both been used safely in controlled settings and for short courses in PWH with refractory psoriasis and debilitating psoriatic arthritis who are on concurrent ART.

KEY POINTS

- ART, ultraviolet B (UVB), and oral retinoids are good initial therapies for PWH with psoriatic arthritis.

- Topical tacrolimus inhibitors and UV light have both been used safely in PWH.

- PWH receiving systemic biologics for debilitating psoriatic arthritis should be carefully selected and closely monitored.

- Papular pruritic eruption of AIDS and HIV-associated eosinophilic pustular folliculitis are HIV/AIDS-associated dermatologic illnesses and should prompt testing for HIV in a previously undiagnosed person.

SEBORRHEIC DERMATITIS

Seborrheic dermatitis is a common skin disorder, with a prevalence of approximately 5% in the general population. It was noted to be the most common dermatosis in PWH, with a prevalence of greater than 83% in HIV/AIDS populations in the pre-ART era (Sadick et al., 1990). Seborrheic dermatitis is seen at all clinical stages of disease. *Malassezia* species are the causative organisms. The typical presentation is of episodic variably pruritic, thin, erythematous plaques with branny or greasy yellow-white scale involving the scalp and central face, particularly the eyebrows and nasolabial folds. Scalp involvement ranges from light "dandruff" to crusted plaques. Involvement of the anterior chest and groin areas is common. HIV should be considered in rapid and exaggerated presentations with thick, extensive plaques and also in cases recalcitrant to advanced treatment regimens. The clinical differential for facial seborrheic dermatitis includes rosacea; an overlapping presentation with psoriasis called sebopsoriasis that is often more difficult to treat than standard seborrheic dermatitis; contact dermatitis; tinea faciei; and connective tissue disease. In tinea faciei, a potassium hydroxide (KOH) preparation can identify dermatophytes exhibiting characteristic hyphae. In contrast, seborrheic dermatitis is thought to be an inflammatory response to the commensal yeast *Malassezia* species (thus, KOH evaluation has no role), with the increased presentation in PWH thought to be due to a more vigorous inflammatory response as the yeast proliferate in the setting of CD4+ T-cell lymphopenia (Oble et al., 2005; Pedrosa et al., 2014). Seborrheic dermatitis is a clinical diagnosis; thus, biopsy is infrequently performed. Histology reveals psoriasiform hyperplasia, neutrophilic spongiosis, perifollicular mound parakeratosis with necrotic keratinocytes, and plasma cells, which occasionally present in HIV-associated seborrheic dermatitis (Soeprono et al., 1986). Treatment does not differ between PWH and HIV-negative persons; first-line therapy is with low- to mid-potency topical steroids for the face and trunk respectively, topical antifungals such as ketoconazole, or combinations thereof (Osborne et al., 2003). More refractory cases can be treated with oral itraconazole 200 mg QD, although attention must be paid to interactions with ART agents. ART therapy improves seborrheic dermatitis occurring in the setting of HIV/AIDS; however, PWH typically continue to experience episodic flares.

PSORIASIS

Psoriasis also presents at all clinical stages of HIV, but more frequently at CD4+ T-cell counts of less than 350 cells/mm³ (Bartlett et al., 2007). Psoriasis has a prevalence of approximately 2% or 3% in the general population, with various series suggesting a similar or higher incidence in HIV populations (Mallon & Bunker, 2000; Obuch et al., 1992). The prevalence of psoriatic arthritis in the general population has previously been underestimated and is now thought to be approximately 11% in the US psoriasis population, and it is more concentrated in PWH (Dover & Johnson, 1991; Gelfand et al., 2005). Psoriasis characteristically presents as variably pruritic, episodic, well-demarcated plaques with silvery white scale anywhere on the body but with a predilection for the scalp, elbows, lower back, gluteal folds, external genitalia, and acral sites. Preexisting psoriasis can worsen with HIV infection and immune deterioration, and psoriasis can develop de novo with HIV infection. De novo psoriasis in HIV often involves palmar-plantar locations with pustules, nail dystrophy, and psoriatic arthritis that can be debilitating. Inverse psoriasis (involving intertriginous areas), generalized pustular psoriasis, and erythrodermic psoriasis also occur more frequently in HIV (Obuch et al., 1992). Erythrodermic psoriasis can be difficult to distinguish from other causes of erythroderma, including atopic dermatitis, drug-induced erythroderma, pityriasis rubra pilaris, Sézary syndrome, and a paraneoplastic presentation or HIV presentation; thus, it typically warrants a biopsy. Histology reveals parakeratosis, collections of neutrophils in the stratum corneum and epidermis, and a diminished granular layer. Whereas increased defensins and canthelicidins in the skin of psoriatics in the general population have been associated with a relatively low frequency of bacterial superinfection compared to other chronic dermatoses that also result in a compromised skin barrier, such as atopic dermatitis, there is an increased frequency of bacterial superinfection in HIV psoriatics (Mallon & Bunker, 2000; Zheng et al., 2007). Theories regarding the increased incidence and severity of psoriasis in HIV include the fact that overexpression of tumor necrosis factor (TNF) occurs in both

psoriasis and HIV. Furthermore, CD4+ T-cell depletion in HIV skews the T-cell population to CD8 cells, the effector cells in psoriasis, and the HIV tat gene directly induces epidermal proliferation (Duvic, 1990; Kim et al., 1992).

In treating psoriasis, exacerbating medications should be discontinued. Of note, systemic steroids exacerbate psoriasis. Topical treatments including topical steroids, vitamin D analogs, and topical calcineurin inhibitors such as tacrolimus are first-line therapies for mild to moderate plaque psoriasis. A "black box" warning on tacrolimus and malignancy risk has not identified a causal relationship, and studies have shown that topical calcineurin inhibitors can be safely used in the immunosuppressed HIV population (de Moraes et al., 2007; Toutous-Trellu et al., 2005). Randomized controlled studies have not been conducted to evaluate the efficacy and safety of systemic treatments for psoriasis in the HIV setting; thus, many of the following data are derived from case reports and case series.

Systemic therapies can be used in combination with each other and with topical treatments to optimize efficacy. ART can effectively treat both moderate to severe psoriasis and psoriatic arthritis, and it is a first-line treatment, as is UV light, for this severity category (Duvic et al., 1994; Menon et al., 2010; Meola et al., 1993). UVB is preferentially used over psoralens plus UVA (PUVA) given its more favorable side-effect profile. Although in vitro studies have shown that UVB light can activate latent HIV in chronically infected monocytes, it has not been associated with short-term changes in immune function in vivo or changes in HIV RNA levels in PWH receiving concomitant suppressive ART therapy (Breuer-McHam et al., 1999; Meola et al., 1993; Stanley et al., 1989). Oral retinoids, particularly acitretin, are an attractive second-line therapy because they are non-immunosuppressants with efficacy for moderate to severe psoriasis and psoriatic arthritis. Acitretin use is limited by hypertriglyceridemia; liver function test elevation, particularly in combination with some antiretroviral medications (ARVs); and an extended 3-year teratogenicity period in women of childbearing age due to re-esterification to etretinate (Dogra & Yadav, 2014).

PWH with refractory or debilitating psoriatic arthritis are candidates for immunosuppressant therapies, including low-dose methotrexate and brief courses of cyclosporine and TNF-α inhibitors. In a case report, dramatic improvement of HIV-associated psoriatic arthritis was achieved, but frequent polymicrobial infections were experienced on etanercept (Aboulafia et al., 2000). In a 2018 Cochrane review of 25 reported cases of systemic immunosuppressives used to treat psoriatic disease in PWH, including methotrexate, cyclosporine, etanercept, adalimumab, infliximab, and ustekinumab, evidence suggests that these biological therapies may be effective for refractory psoriasis and may actually have a positive effect on CD4+ T-cell counts and HIV viral load when used in combination with ART (Nakamura et al., 2018). Rigorous patient selection, concomitant ART therapy, strict prophylaxis against OIs, monitoring of CD4+ T-cell counts and HIV RNA levels, and close clinical monitoring are advised when treating HIV-associated psoriasis with immunosuppressant therapy.

ATOPIC DERMATITIS AND XEROSIS

The prevalence of eczema in the US adult population is estimated at 10.7%, with approximately 17% of the population experiencing at least one of four eczematous symptoms (Hanifin et al., 2007). An atopic dermatitis-like condition occurs frequently in HIV populations, often despite never having had a history of atopic dermatitis in childhood. One series reported that 29% of PWH who attended an urban HIV clinic in the pre-ART era had this condition (Lin & Lazarus, 1995). This atopic dermatitis–like condition is characterized by pruritus and a spectrum of generalized scaling from xerosis to ichthyosis, with variable plaques and lichenification involving extremities and flexural areas (Singh et al., 2003). Often, this xerotic condition initially presents when the CD4+ T-cell count is still higher than 400 cells/mm³ and is thus an early clinical sign of HIV/AIDS, typically preceding the other HIV-related papulosquamous disorders. The generalized ichthyotic form typically occurs with CD4+ T-cell counts less than 50 cells/mm³ (Sadick et al., 1990). Decreased cellular immunity and a switch to the TH2-like cytokine profile resulting in polyclonal activation of B cells with increased IgE production are thought to contribute to the increase in atopic conditions in HIV (Nissen et al., 1999). In addition, nutritional deficits and autonomic nervous dysfunction causing alterations in sweating, sebaceous gland secretion, and reduction in natural moisturizing factor secretion are thought to contribute to xerosis and ichthyosis (Cockerell & Calame, 2013). Decreased lipids and increased water are found in the dermis of PWH compared to HIV-negative reference groups, as well as excessive levels of epidermal carotenoids, mainly lycopene, potentially leading to these adverse effects and premature skin aging (Mischo et al., 2014). Biopsy, which is not regularly performed for this diagnosis, shows variable hyperkeratosis and parakeratosis, spongiosis, and superficial perivascular lymphocytic infiltrate. The clinical differential diagnosis includes scabies, psoriasis, and contact dermatitis. For erythematous plaques, topical steroid preparations, preferably ointments, and topical calcineurin inhibitors are appropriate first-line therapies. Topical keratolytics such as urea and lactic acid formulations are useful for areas of lichenification. Widespread flares may require short courses of systemic steroids, bridging to phototherapy for more sustained flares. Oral antihistamines and a dry skin care regimen of short lukewarm showers, frequent use of nonallergic emollients, and avoidance of allergens should be used in conjunction. Bacterial superinfection is common and should be managed with antibiotics.

PAPULAR PRURITIC ERUPTION OF AIDS

Papular pruritic eruption (PPE) is a markedly pruritic papulosquamous eruption characterized by symmetric crops of nonfollicular, often urticarial erythematous papules involving the extensor extremities. Excoriations and prurigo nodularis are frequently associated secondary changes due to marked pruritus in this condition. PPE is uncommon in the general adult population but has a prevalence in the HIV population of 11% to 46%, thus the designation *PPE of AIDS* (Eisman, 2006). It has a greater prevalence in HIV/AIDS cohorts in sub-Saharan Africa than in the US. Among other theories, PPE is hypothesized to be due to an exaggerated response to arthropod antigens that occurs in the setting of immune dysregulation (Resneck et al., 2004). PPE can develop well before other symptoms and serologic diagnosis of HIV is made; however, its occurrence has historically been correlated with lower CD4+ T-cell counts, particularly less than 100 cells/mm³ (Boonchai et al., 1999; Cockerell & Calame, 2013). However, studies from India found otherwise: one-third of cases occurred in PWH with CD4+ T-cell counts above 350 (Farsani et al., 2013) and 86% above 200 (Mohammed et al., 2019). This difference is yet unexplained but highlights that PPE can be seen at any CD4+ count.

The clinical differential of PPE includes eosinophilic folliculitis, which, in contrast, affects the face and upper trunk, and prurigo nodularis, which also may also be pruritic. The diagnosis is typically made clinically based on the distribution of lesions. Early lesions without secondary changes carry the highest histologic diagnostic yield; they may show a dense perivascular and interstitial infiltrate of lymphocytes and some eosinophils and neutrophils, which may extend deeply around adnexa and vessels, although nonspecific findings occur (Calonje et al., 2012). The disease has a chronic waxing-and-waning course and is associated with decreased quality of life due to pruritus (Hevia et al., 1991; Liu et al., 2013). Given its association with low CD4+ T-cell counts, initiation of ART may improve the disease, although it can also flare with immune reconstitution. UVB has been shown to decrease both papules and pruritus, and it may have greater efficacy in regimens combining other modalities including oral antihistamines, pentoxifylline, topical steroids, topical tacrolimus, and topical anti-itch preparations (Bellavista et al., 2013). Reducing exposure to bites by wearing clothing that covers skin and application of insect repellant is also recommended.

HIV-ASSOCIATED EOSINOPHILIC PUSTULAR FOLLICULITIS

Eosinophilic pustular folliculitis (EPF, or Ofugi's disease) is rare in the general adult population but common in the HIV/AIDS population, particularly once the CD4+ T-cell count declines below 250 cells/mm³. HIV-associated eosinophilic folliculitis is characterized by persistent, markedly pruritic erythematous, mostly follicular papules and occasional pustules on the face, trunk, and upper extremities. Urticarial plaques and nonfollicular erythematous papules are also described. Peripheral eosinophilia can also be common along with elevated IgE levels (Rosenthal et al., 1991). It is thought to be an exaggerated cutaneous reaction to *Malassezia* yeast or other microorganisms colonizing the follicular infundibulum and reflects TH1/2 immune dysregulation. CD163+ macrophages have been implicated in the pathogenesis (Okada et al., 2013). Additional theories include autoimmune activation against antigens in sebocytes in HIV-positive individuals (Fearfield et al., 1999). The clinical differential includes PPE as well as acne, molluscum, and drug reactions. Biopsy may be useful, with erythematous nonexcoriated follicular lesions carrying the highest diagnostic yield. Spongiosis involving the follicular epithelium and intra- and perifollicular mixed infiltrate is typically seen, with eosinophilic abscess formation in longstanding lesions. Treatment is often difficult, with pruritus contributing to reduced quality of life. Phototherapy (UVB or UVA), oral antihistamines, itraconazole, isotretinoin, and metronidazole are all reported treatments; however, no controlled clinical trials have been performed. Whereas classic EPF is preferentially treated with oral indomethacin, topical steroids are preferred for HIV-related EPF (Nomura et al., 2016), and other potential treatments include UVB phototherapy and oral antihistamines.

RECOMMENDED READING

Cockerell CC, Calame A. *Cutaneous manifestations of HIV disease.* London: Manson; 2013.

Toutous-Trellu L, Abraham S, Pechere M, et al. Topical tacrolimus for effective treatment of eosinophilic folliculitis associated with human immunodeficiency virus infection. *Arch Dermatol.* 2005;141(10):1203–1208.

HIV DRUG REACTIONS AND INTERACTIONS

LEARNING OBJECTIVE

- Describe common and important cutaneous adverse drug reactions in PWH and pertinent factors in their management

WHAT'S NEW?

In recent years, several adverse drug reactions to ARVs have been identified that were not observed or were underrepresented in preapproval trials.

KEY POINTS

- Nonnucleoside reverse transcriptase inhibitors (NNRTIs) are the most common ARVs that cause morbilliform skin eruptions.

- Abacavir hypersensitivity reaction (AHR) can be fatal, and predisposed individuals can be identified by testing for the HLA-B5701 allele prior to commencing abacavir therapy.

- The injectable fillers poly-l-lactic acid and calcium hydroxyapatite are approved for facial fat loss treatment in HIV.

- Ritonavir, a CYP34A inhibitor often used to boost other ARVs, increases the levels of corticosteroids, which can result in hypothalamic–pituitary–adrenal (HPA) axis dysfunction and Cushing syndrome.

Historically, the incidence of medication-related skin rashes in the HIV-positive population was approximately 50% (Davis & Shearer, 2008), although literature is lacking on the incidence with newer ARVs. Drug hypersensitivity reactions are classified into two categories: those secondary to ART regimens and those secondary to other medications taken by PWH. Since its inception, ART has revolutionized the management of HIV/AIDS, with new drug classes and single-tablet combination formulations designed to decrease pill burden now available. However, ARVs have been complicated by adverse drug reactions, including reactions that may not have been recognized or underrepresented in preapproval clinical trials (Introcaso et al., 2010). Thus, recognition of known and identification of previously unreported drug reactions are extremely important in the management of ARV-related drug hypersensitivity reactions. It can be a particular challenge to differentiate between drug hypersensitivity reactions, IRIS, and worsening HIV infection when patients are commencing ART. Some of the adverse drug reactions are mediated through genetic and immunologic factors via the major histocompatibility complex (Chaponda & Pirmohamed, 2011). IgE levels increase with progression of HIV, and altered cytokine profiles are also believed to play a role (Davis & Shearer, 2008). Immune dysregulation in HIV is also thought to make HIV patients more susceptible to reactions to non-ART medications. In addition, ARVs can result in alterations in metabolism of other medications, particularly through the cytochrome P450 pathway, thus increasing their toxicity.

NNRTIS

NNRTIs are the most common ARVs to cause morbilliform skin eruptions, which are usually distributed over the face, trunk, and extremities. Nevirapine is well known for its ability to cause rash, particularly within the first 6 weeks of use. According to the manufacturer, 13% of patients taking nevirapine develop some degree of morbilliform eruption during early treatment; this figure has been reported to be as high as 28% in some populations (Introcaso et al., 2010). Many patients with mild or moderate rash can continue therapy with close monitoring, and the rash will spontaneously resolve. Severe rash is seen in at least 8% of patients, and development of concomitant hepatitis in the drug hypersensitivity syndrome is an indication for immediate discontinuation of nevirapine given the potential for fatal hepatitis. Risk factors for the development of morbilliform eruption with the use of nevirapine include higher CD4$^+$ T-cell count (>250 cells/mm^3 in women and >400 cells/mm^3 in men), lower HIV-1 RNA levels, Chinese ethnicity, and female gender (Davis & Shearer, 2008). In addition, nevirapine can cause the mucocutaneous Stevens–Johnson syndrome at a rate of 0.5% to 1%, although patients with CD4$^+$ T-cell counts of less than 200 cells/mm^3 (i.e., with AIDS) have a 1,000-fold higher risk (Warren et al., 1998). The incidence may be higher in sub-Saharan Africa, where nevirapine is more commonly used in ART. Stevens–Johnson syndrome is characterized by flat, atypical targets or pruritic papules that are widespread or distributed on the trunk first and then spread to the neck, face, and proximal upper extremities. The palms and soles may be early sites of involvement. Bullae developing on the conjunctivae and mucous membranes of the nares, mouth, anorectal junction, vulvovaginal region, and urethral meatus are characteristic, with toxic epidermal necrolysis diagnosed when there is more than 30% body surface area skin detachment (Bolognia et al., 2012). In several studies, the use of prednisone and/or a 2-week lead-in dose of nevirapine 200 mg once daily failed to decrease the occurrence of the nevirapine-associated rash (Knobel et al., 2001); nevertheless, a dose escalation protocol is recommended starting with nevirapine 200 mg/day for 2 weeks, followed by an increase to the standard 400 mg/day dose only if there is no rash or no worsening rash after the trial 2-week period (Anton et al., 1999).

NUCLEOSIDE REVERSE TRANSCRIPTASE INHIBITOR

Abacavir, a nucleoside reverse transcriptase inhibitor, can cause a well-documented, multiorgan, potentially life-threatening hypersensitivity reaction. AHR is seen in 5% to 8% of patients on treatment. Symptoms consist of fever, rash, malaise, fatigue, tachypnea, pharyngitis, cough, wheezing, nausea, vomiting, and diarrhea that commence 9 to 11 days after initiating therapy. Symptoms that become worse with each subsequent dose are a classic characteristic of AHR. Symptoms of AHR recur within 24 hours of rechallenge and can be fatal. Therefore, the use of abacavir in any person suspected to have AHR is contraindicated. Pre-ART genetic testing has shown that the absence of the HLA-B5701 allele dramatically decreases (by 99.9%) the likelihood of developing abacavir hypersensitivity (Mallal et al., 2008). For this reason, the ART guidelines of both the US Department of Health and Human Services (DHHS) and the International Antiviral Society–USA recommend obtaining this test prior to initiation of any abacavir-containing regimen.

PROTEASE INHIBITORS

Protease inhibitors (PIs) are generally associated with lipodystrophy, encompassing peripheral lipoatrophy and central adiposity, which can be an indication for discontinuation. The injectable fillers poly-l-lactic acid and calcium hydroxyapatite are approved for facial fat loss treatment in HIV (Jagdeo et al., 2015). Indinavir has the greatest variety of cutaneous side effects among PIs, including acute porphyria, Stevens–Johnson syndrome, hypersensitivity syndrome, morbilliform drug eruptions, gynecomastia, alopecia, pyogenic granuloma-like lesions, and paronychia (Ward et al., 2002). Ritonavir is a CYP34A inhibitor, and, through this mechanism, it decreases clearance of corticosteroids, thus increasing their levels and the risk of HPA axis dysfunction and Cushing syndrome (Hyle et al., 2013). This should be considered when prescribing systemic steroids, inhaled corticosteroids such as fluticasone, or topical steroids when applied to a large body surface area.

OTHER ARVS

Few other ARVs have a strong association with severe adverse drug reactions. Approximately 6% of persons taking atazanavir, a PI, have reported a typically mild rash not requiring treatment cessation. A hypersensitivity to the fusion inhibitor enfuvirtide has been seen in fewer than 1% of persons taking it. However, 98% of users experience injection site reactions, which are frequently symptomatic (Ball & Kinchelow, 2003). The enfuvirtide injection site reaction is characterized by tender erythema, induration, and nodule or cyst formation. On histology, a palisaded granulomatous response may be seen, with multinucleated cells aggregated around altered collagen, and surrounding eosinophils, histiocytes, lymphocytes, plasma cells, and variable fibrosis. The package insert for raltegravir, an integrase inhibitor, was updated to include dermatologic side effects including Stevens–Johnson syndrome and toxic epidermal necrolysis following postmarketing case reports.

ANTIBIOTICS

Antibiotic drug reactions are seen at a higher rate in PWH than in the general population. Trimethoprim–sulfamethoxazole is a commonly used antibiotic in HIV, especially for the prophylaxis of *Pneumocystis jirovecii* pneumonia (PCP). Given its importance in the prevention of PCP pneumonia, a desensitization schedule has been developed for those patients who have had reactions in the past and would benefit from its use. Desensitization has been successful using the following dosing schedule: an initial dose of trimethoprim 0.4 mg and sulfamethoxazole 2 mg, followed by doubling the dose daily over days 2 to 9 and at 10 days administering the full-strength dose (trimethoprim 160 mg/sulfamethoxazole 800 mg) (Gompels et al., 1999).

RECOMMENDED READING

Hyle EP, Wood BR, Backman ES, et al. High frequency of hypothalamic–pituitary–adrenal axis dysfunction after local corticosteroid injection in HIV-infected patients on protease inhibitor therapy. *J AIDS.* 2013;63(5):602–608.

Introcaso CE, Hines JM, Kovarik CL. Cutaneous toxicities of antiretroviral therapy for HIV: part II. Nonnucleoside reverse transcriptase inhibitors, entry and fusion inhibitors, integrase inhibitors, and immune reconstitution syndrome. *J Am Acad Dermatol.* 2010;63(4):563–570.

CUTANEOUS OIS

LEARNING OBJECTIVE

- Discuss the diagnosis and management of viral, fungal, bacterial, and parasitic OIs occurring in HIV patients

WHAT'S NEW?

The recombinant zoster vaccine (RZV, Shingrix), approved in 2017, shows greater immunogenicity than the live-attenuated zoster vaccine but has yet to be tested in PWH or specifically recommended for PWH by the CDC's Advisory Committee on Immunization Practices (ACIP) (Freedman et al., 2021) or the DHHS.

KEY POINTS

- Cutaneous *Cryptococcus* may manifest before systemic symptoms; therefore, prompt diagnosis and management can prevent fatal outcomes.

- Molluscum, histoplasmosis, and *Cryptococcus* may all present with umbilicated papulonodules; however, there is a central white core to the molluscum lesion, and patients are well as opposed to systemically ill with cryptococcal infection.

- Postherpetic neuralgia is very common in HIV patients who develop herpes zoster, and initiation of gabapentin (Neurontin) along with antiviral therapy at diagnosis may mitigate neuralgia.

- The prozone effect may result in a false-negative syphilis test in HIV patients, and dilution of the assay should be requested when syphilis is suspected.

- The CDC recommends an intensive regimen for the management of crusted scabies as follows: ivermectin dosed at 200 μg/kg taken on days 1, 2, 8, 9, and 15, and, for severe disease, also days 22 and 29, in combination with topical permethrin daily for 7 days and then twice a week until cure.

ONYCHOMYCOSIS

Onychomycosis is reported to affect approximately 2% to 13% of the general population (Rosen et al., 2015) and is very common in PWH. Dermatophytes *Trichophyton mentagrophytes* and *T. rubrum* are responsible for most infections. Proximal subungual onychomycosis is a pattern seen commonly in PWH, especially those with a CD4+ T-cell count of less than 450 cells/mm³, and although it is not considered an AIDS-defining condition, it should prompt testing for HIV infection if not already determined. *T. rubrum* is the offending dermatophyte, although it can also be caused by *T. megninii*. In the general population, superficial white onychomycosis is typically caused by *T. mentagrophytes*, whereas in PWH, *T. rubrum* is the causative agent. The clinical differential includes psoriasis, lichen planus, trauma, and periungual squamous cell carcinoma (SCC). Most topical antifungals do not penetrate the thick nail keratin and thus are ineffective. Efinaconazole is a topical triazole solution for the treatment of onychomycosis; it is applied daily for 48 weeks to affected nails. Localized dermatitis is a potential side effect. In preapproval trials, a modest 15.2% to 17.8% of patients achieved complete cure of onychomycosis. Tavorabole, a boron-based agent that was approved by the US Food and Drug Administration (FDA) for onychomycosis in 2014, had even lower efficacy, with 6.5% to 9.1% of patients achieving clearance (Zeichner, 2015). Terbinafine is considered first-line systemic therapy, dosed at 250 mg/day for

3 or 4 months for toenails and 6 weeks for fingernails (~50% cure rate). Itraconazole may also be effective at 200 mg/day for 3 months for toenails and 6 weeks for fingernails or at 200 mg twice daily for 1 week per month for 3 months for toenails and 2 months for fingernails. The efficacy of fluconazole is lower than that of terbinafine and itraconazole. Patients with active liver disease should not receive terbinafine, and liver function testing at baseline and every 4 to 6 weeks is recommended given the risk of hepatotoxicity. Congestive heart disease is a contraindication to itraconazole use. In addition, itraconazole interacts with more medications compared to terbinafine (de Berker, 2009), particularly with the ART-boosting agents ritonavir and cobicistat. Finally, the causative agent may differ between the general population and PWH, which is relevant when selecting therapy. For example, non-dermatophyte molds, such as *Scytalidium*, *Aspergillus*, and *Fusarium*, and yeast such as *Candida* are implicated in onychomycosis in HIV patients more often than in the general public. Much higher cure rates are achieved with itraconazole than with terbinafine for these organisms, whereas the reverse is true for dermatophytes (Cambuim et al., 2011; Warshaw et al., 2005). For these reasons, and given the potential side effects of systemic therapies, culture of nail clippings involved with onychomycosis is recommended by some dermatologists before initiation of therapy.

CANDIDIASIS

Angular cheilitis is typically caused by *Candida albicans* and presents as fissured white plaques at the angles of the lips. It occurs with some frequency in the elderly, but it may suggest HIV infection in young adults and may warrant testing if there is no other known reason for immunosuppression. Topical antifungal creams are effective and avoid systemic circulation for this focal disease. Associated burning and dysphagia suggest oral candidiasis, with atrophic or removable yellow white pseudomembranous or hyperplastic plaques typically seen on the tongue or dorsal palate. Oral candidiasis is often a harbinger of immunologic failure in patients on ART, although it can also be caused by steroids and antibiotics (Cockerell & Calame, 2013). Nystatin or clotrimazole troches, and oral antifungals such as fluconazole or ketoconazole when there is associated odynophagia, are effective. Ketoconazole should be taken with food and avoided in the setting of malabsorption given the risk of treatment failure.

Candida intertrigo is common in HIV-infected populations, and it can appear as eroded glistening erythematous plaques or as pustules with scale over a macerated erythematous surface within and extending from skin folds. While smaller lesions may be treated with topical antifungals, oral fluconazole or ketoconazole is recommended for larger or extensive plaques.

CUTANEOUS CRYPTOCOCCOSIS

Cryptococcus neoformans causes an AIDS-defining systemic infection, with skin lesions preceding the more common central nervous system and pulmonary involvement in only 10%

of cases. The patient is typically febrile and very ill. Lesions can present as papules that may be umbilicated, nodules, pustules, ulcers, and plaques. A skin biopsy is necessary for diagnosis, revealing round yeast with narrow-based budding and a slimy capsule in a granulomatous or gelatinous background, highlighted by fungal stains. Culture is definitively diagnostic, and treatment is with amphotericin B or fluconazole; adjunctive flucytosine can also be used (Cockerell & Calame, 2013), with close monitoring of renal function for potential flucytosine dose adjustment. ART has decreased the incidence of cryptococcal infection; however, institution of ART in patients with cryptococcal infection can result in fatal IRIS (Lortholary et al., 2005), so ART should not be initiated until 2 to 10 weeks into antifungal therapy (DHHS, 2020). Relapses are not uncommon, and secondary prophylaxis with fluconazole 200 to 400 mg/day for patients with CD4$^+$ T-cell counts of less than 200 cells/mm^3 is recommended.

CUTANEOUS HISTOPLASMOSIS

Histoplasmosis manifests with cutaneous lesions secondary to pulmonary or disseminated disease, as primary cutaneous manifestation is rare. The rash is nonspecific, characterized by diffuse erythematous macules, papules that may be umbilicated, pustules, crusted ulcers, or psoriasiform papules. The face is most often involved, followed by truncal and extremity involvement (Cockerell & Calame, 2013). The differential diagnosis includes molluscum contagiosum and cryptococcosis. HIV patients with cutaneous histoplasmosis may be well appearing on initial presentation; however, prompt diagnosis is important because they can rapidly and fatally decompensate with systemic involvement (Wheat et al., 1990). Diagnosis of cutaneous histoplasmosis requires tissue biopsy, which reveals spores with a pseudocapsule (the fungal wall) parasitizing macrophages. Culture confirms the diagnosis. Mild infection in non-HIV patients is self-limiting and may not require treatment; however, treatment is required in PWH. Treating systemic disease also treats skin involvement and is typically done with itraconazole; amphotericin is reserved for meningitis or other disseminated infection (Hage et al., 2015). Similar to cryptococcosis, relapses can occur, and secondary prophylaxis with itraconazole in AIDS patients is advised.

MOLLUSCUM CONTAGIOSUM

Molluscum is a common viral infection in children and their caregivers, but it warrants testing for HIV in adults with limited exposure to children. Skin-colored discrete umbilicated papules are typical, although giant facial molluscum and extensive beard involvement occur with advanced immunosuppression. While many molluscum lesions will self-resolve with ART, giant molluscum can persist even after immune reconstitution; it is extremely difficult to treat and is stigmatizing. Molluscum is differentiated from cryptococcosis and histoplasmosis, which can also have umbilicated papules, by the presence of a central core in molluscum lesions. Also, patients appear well with molluscum infection, whereas they are systemically ill with cryptococcal and histoplasma

infection. Treatment options include cryotherapy or pulsed dye therapy for smaller lesions and curettage and excision for larger lesions; immune-modulating agents such as topical imiquimod, interferon-alpha, and cimetidine; chemical agents (e.g., cantharidin, KOH, podophyllotoxin, benzoyl peroxide, tretinoin, trichloroacetic acid, lactic acid, glycolic acid, salicylic acid); antivirals (cidofovir); and photodynamic therapy with 5-aminolevulinic acid, which have all shown efficacy in case reports (Drain et al., 2014; Foissac et al., 2014; Leung et al., 2017), although high-quality clinical trial data are lacking.

CONDYLOMATA ACUMINATA

Condylomata acuminata (anogenital warts), which are caused by the human papillomavirus (HPV), are the most common sexually transmitted infection in the US. Warts appear as flesh-colored to gray, rounded to pointy papules, frequently on a short peduncle. Podophyllin, trichloroacetic acid, and cryotherapy are three of the most commonly used treatments for genital warts. Cryotherapy and trichloroacetic acid yield a treatment success rate of 75%, whereas that of podophyllin is reported to be 20% to 50% (Murray et al., 2015). Therapies for recalcitrant anogenital warts include topical 5-fluorouracil, cidofovir, intralesional interferon-α, and surgical excision (Nambudiri et al., 2013). Approximately 5% of men who have sex with men (MSM) and 15% of MSM with HIV have a history of perianal warts. Anogenital warts are more common in women, and women with HIV are five times more likely than their uninfected counterparts to have these warts (Hagensee et al., 2004). In addition, squamous epithelial lesions occur in 79% of women with HIV with anal HPV infection compared to 43% of women without HIV. The frequency of intraepithelial neoplasia within anogenital warts is higher than previously realized, warranting aggressive surveillance and treatment (McCloskey et al., 2007). Although we do not yet have an evidence-based screening and management strategy for such neoplasia, the ANCHOR study aims to do just that for persons with high-grade squamous intraepithelial lesions or worse on anal Pap smears (Atkinson et al., 2019).

HERPES SIMPLEX

Herpes simplex virus (HSV) infection is caused by either HSV-1 or HSV-2 and is a common viral infection in the general population. It presents as grouped vesicles on an erythematous base. In PWH, the infections occur more frequently and are less likely to self-resolve. When CD4$^+$ T cells decrease below 100 cells/mm^3, the incidence of HSV outbreaks reaches 27% (Severson et al., 1999). Recommended treatment for a PWH with recurrent herpes infection is valacyclovir 1 g twice daily for 5 to 10 days or acyclovir 200 mg five times a day for the same period. Acyclovir-resistant HSV has become a problem in patients with AIDS; reported acyclovir resistance in PWH is 10-fold higher than that in immunocompetent counterparts—0.6% and 6%, respectively (Lolis et al., 2008). Resistance to acyclovir also implies resistance to valacyclovir, and, in many cases, famciclovir is also not an effective treatment. Treatment of choice for acyclovir-resistant HSV is intravenous foscarnet or cidofovir. Topical cidofovir and foscarnet have been used as successful treatments as well (Strick et al., 2006).

HERPES ZOSTER

Herpes zoster, also known as shingles, is caused by the reactivation of varicella zoster virus (VZV), which also causes chickenpox. Ten percent to 20% of adults are affected by shingles. As T-cell immunity wanes, with age or immunosuppression, the incidence of infection increases. Therefore, herpes zoster is very common with HIV infection, and it may be the presenting manifestation. In immunocompetent patients, the infection is usually limited to one dermatome. Pain, constitutional symptoms of fever, malaise, and headache may precede the eruptive phase, which consists of clusters of vesicles on an erythematous base within a dermatome. Involvement of multiple dermatomes is common in PWH, and disseminated infection is frequent. Treatment is with acyclovir 800 mg/day for 7 to 10 days, valacyclovir 1 g three times a day, or acyclovir 10 mg/kg when intravenous treatment is warranted. Foscarnet 40 mg/kg three times a day is used for treatment of acyclovir-resistant VZV (Cockerell & Calame, 2013).

Continual pain, referred to as postherpetic neuralgia (PHN), can occur and last months to years. Immunocompromised patients are at a higher risk of developing PHN, and effective, early treatment of pain with gabapentin and/or opioids at presentation along with antivirals can reduce the risk of PHN. Varicella vaccine is recommended in adults without varicella immunity and CD4+ T-cell counts of more than 200 cells/mm³. The live attenuated varicella vaccines (ZVL, Zostavax) should be avoided in PWH with AIDS or manifestations of HIV and CD4+ T-cell counts of less than 200 cells/mm³ or CD4+ T-cell T lymphocytes 15% or less (CDC, ACIP). The newer RZV is more immunogenic than ZVL. It is not a live virus vaccine, and as such it may be safe to give to PWH regardless of their CD4+ T-cell count, but this has yet to be determined in clinical trials, and thus there is no recommendation regarding RZV for PWH in either ACIP or DHHS guidelines.

METHICILLIN-RESISTANT STAPHYLOCOCCUS AUREUS

Staphylococcus aureus has acquired the mecA gene, which makes it less sensitive to many of the antibiotics typically used to treat skin and soft tissue infections. Methicillin-resistant *S. aureus* (MRSA) grew to epidemic proportions during the 2000s, with a higher rate of MRSA infection in PWH. One study reported that the prevalence was 18 times higher in the HIV population compared to the general population (Crum-Cianflone et al., 2007). However, recent data suggest a reduction in MRSA-driven skin and soft tissue infections in PWH from the late 2000s peak (Hemmige et al., 2020).

Incision and drainage is the most important component of treatment for localized skin infections. Many cutaneous MRSA infections are generally sensitive to the antibiotics trimethoprim–sulfamethoxazole, doxycycline, clindamycin, and linezolid. These antibiotics are generally effective against MRSA, and culture and sensitivity data are helpful in guiding treatment. Both skin and nasal colonization are potential reservoirs for reinfection. Studies have indicated that mupirocin can be used to eradicate nasal colonization, whereas chlorhexidine can be used for the skin (Kuehnert et al., 2006).

BACILLARY ANGIOMATOSIS

This infectious disease occurs rarely in PWH, but awareness is important because it is a clinical mimicker of KS that can be treated effectively with erythromycin 500 mg four times a day, yet it is potentially systemic and fatal if untreated. Clinically, purple "grape-like" papules to nodules are seen in a focal or widespread distribution. In contrast to KS, they rarely manifest as patches or plaques. Bacillary angiomatosis can be distinguished from KS on histology, with a lobular capillary proliferation with an edematous stroma and clusters of neutrophils seen throughout the lesion (Cockerell & Calame, 2013). There is often an amorphous material that represents colonies of bacteria, and culture for *Bartonella* speciation has relevance given that *Bartonella quintana* is more frequently associated with neurologic sequelae compared to *B. henselae* (Gasquet et al., 1998).

SYPHILIS

Primary syphilis typically presents with an asymptomatic orogenital ulcer, whereas secondary syphilis is typically papulosquamous to psoriasiform but can mimic many other dermatoses. The color is characteristic, resembling a "clean-cut ham" or having a coppery tint. Palms and soles may present with classic coppery-colored scaly plaques. Temporal, irregular, "moth-eaten" alopecia of the beard, scalp, and eyebrows may occur. Of concern, syphilis has an accelerated rate of progression in HIV, with potential development of neurosyphilis, and can have atypical presentations including multiple chancres and syphilitic vasculitis. Diagnosis can be complicated by the prozone effect, in which a false-negative rapid plasma reagin (RPR) or Venereal Disease Research Laboratory (VDRL) test is achieved due to overwhelming antibody titers interfering with formation of an antigen–antibody lattice network in the test. Dilution of the assay overcomes this false-negative result, and this should be requested when syphilis is suspected and there is a negative result (Smith et al., 2004). Treatment is with penicillin formulations, and better response with decreased progression to neurosyphilis has been noted in PWH on ART (Ghanem et al., 2007).

SCABIES

Scabies is caused by an infestation of the skin by the *Sarcoptes scabiei* mite. The first symptom of scabies is usually pruritus, especially at night. Scabies is a very common infection, with an approximate prevalence of 300 million annual cases (CDC, 2006). Scabies mites cannot jump or fly and therefore require skin-to-skin contact for infection to occur. Scabies mites have not demonstrated the ability to transmit HIV. Diagnosis is made through clinical examination. Burrow scrapings can be examined under a microscope for scabies mites, eggs, and feces; however, the absence of these on microscopic evaluation does not eliminate the possibility of infection. Dermoscopy has been shown to be a valuable tool in the diagnosis of scabies, with a characteristic "delta wing jet" appearance of burrows identified on dermoscopy (Suh et al., 2014).

"Norwegian" or "crusted" scabies is a more florid infection leading to proliferation of heaped-up, crusted burrows teeming with scabies mites. These crusted lesions typically occur in the web spaces of the hands and feet, over the elbows, and on the ears or temples. This typically occurs in highly immunocompromised patients, including PWH with low CD4+ T-cell counts. Norwegian scabies are highly infectious and can be easily spread to healthcare workers by skin-to-skin contact.

Per CDC guidelines, first-line treatment of scabies is either topical permethrin cream or oral ivermectin (Workowski & Bolan, 2015). Permethrin cream is applied below the neck (and above the neck if lesions are evident) and washed off after 8 to 14 hours on days 1 and 14, or ivermectin 200 μg/kg is given on days 1 and 14. The CDC recommendation for treatment of crusted scabies to avoid treatment failure is an intensive regimen of ivermectin dosed at 200 μg/kg taken on days 1, 2, 8, 9, and 15, and, for severe disease, also on days 22 and 29, in combination with topical permethrin daily for 7 days and then twice a week until cure (Ortega-Loayza et al., 2013). Compliance may therefore be a challenge.

AMOEBA

Naegleria fowleri, Balamuthia mandrillaris, and *Acanthamoeba* are free-living protozoa that cause a rapidly progressive fatal infection in the immunocompromised host. *Acanthamoeba* is a recognized pathogen in immunocompromised patients and has been cultured from the cornea, nasal and sinus cavities, ears, throat, lungs, and skin. *Acanthamoeba* can infect the skin directly or can spread to the skin by hematogenous dissemination from primary foci in the lungs or sinuses (Chandrasekar et al., 1997). More frequent sites of cutaneous involvement include the face, trunk, and extremities. The lesions typically present as nonspecific necrotic ulcers or nodules that may be quite tender or asymptomatic. Evaluations should include biopsy with histology showing trophozoites and culture for speciation. The survival rate is poor. Optimal treatment has not been determined; thus, combination therapy is recommended with miltefosine, fluconazole, and pentamidine. Trimethoprim–sulfamethoxazole, metronidazole, and a macrolide can be added to this regime in patients failing therapy (Mayer et al., 2011).

RECOMMENDED READING

Drain PK, Mosam A, Gounder L, et al. Recurrent giant molluscum contagiosum immune reconstitution inflammatory syndrome (IRIS) after initiation of antiretroviral therapy in an HIV-infected man. *Int J STD AIDS*. 2014;25(3):235–238.

McCloskey JC, Metcalf C, French MA, et al. The frequency of high-grade intraepithelial neoplasia in anal/perianal warts is higher than previously recognized. *Int J STD AIDS*. 2007;18(8):538–542.
Smith G, Holman RP. The prozone phenomenon with syphilis and HIV-1 co-infection. *South Med J*. 2004;97(4):379–382.

CUTANEOUS MALIGNANCIES IN HIV

LEARNING OBJECTIVE

- Review the status of cutaneous malignancies in PWH

WHAT'S NEW?

As life expectancy of PWH has increased, cancers have become a more prevalent cause of morbidity and mortality.

KEY POINTS

- In the US, first-line treatment for HIV-associated KS remains ART, with chemotherapy indicated for progressive cutaneous disease or visceral involvement and radiation therapy for bulky obstructive tumors.

- There is an increased risk of metastatic disease in PWH with invasive melanoma, with worse outcomes associated with lower CD4+ T-cell counts.

- There is a three- to fivefold increased risk of developing nonmelanoma skin cancer in HIV, and basal cell cancers (BCCs) and SCCs are more aggressive in PWH.

KAPOSI'S SARCOMA

Prior to the HIV epidemic, KS was rare in the US; it was seen mostly in elderly men from the Mediterranean area or recipients of solid organ transplants. The increasing prevalence of KS in the early HIV years led to the discovery of human herpesvirus-8 (HHV-8), the causative agent of KS. Mucocutaneous violaceous patches, plaques, or nodules may be seen, with biopsy revealing a vascular proliferation on histology with confirmatory HHV-8 immunostaining. First-line treatment for HIV-associated KS is ART. IRIS can result in KS progression during the initiation of ART, and patients on ART can still develop KS (Krown et al., 2008). Chemotherapy is indicated for rapidly progressive cutaneous KS and when there is visceral involvement; radiation may be helpful when bulky plaques cause pain or lymphatic blockage (Murphy et al., 1997). There have been reports of HHV-8 reactivation and development of KS in patients exposed to topical and systemic steroids (Boudhir et al., 2013).

MELANOMA AND NONMELANOMA SKIN CANCERS

The non–AIDS-defining skin cancers in HIV include BCCs, SCCs, and melanomas. Case reports suggest an increased incidence of melanoma in PWH (Wilkins et al., 2006). In addition, PWH are more likely to develop metastases with invasive melanoma, and a lower CD4$^+$ T-cell count is predictive of worse prognosis (Rodrigues et al., 2002). In addition, there is a three- to fivefold increased risk of developing non-melanoma skin cancer in HIV. BCCs are more common than SCCs, as is the case in the general population but in contrast to immunocompromised transplant patients, in whom SCCs are more common. Both BCCs and SCCs are more aggressive in the HIV population (Wilkins et al., 2006). Despite this, screening guidelines for melanoma, BCCs, and SCCs are the same for PWH as those for the general population.

RECOMMENDED READING

Wilkins K, Turner R, Dolev JC, et al. Cutaneous malignancy and human immunodeficiency virus disease. *J Am Acad Dermatol.* 2006;54(2):189–210.

ACKNOWLEDGMENT

The author acknowledges John M. Curtain, PA-C, MPH, the author of this chapter in the previous edition.

REFERENCES

Aboulafia DM, Bundow D, Wilske K, et al. Etanercept for the treatment of human immunodeficiency virus-associated psoriatic arthritis. *Mayo Clin Proc.* 2000;75(10):1093–1098.

Altman K, Vanness E, Westergaard RP. Cutaneous manifestations of human immunodeficiency virus: a clinical update. *Curr Infect Dis Rep.* 2015;17(3):464.

Anton P, Soriano V, Jimenez-Nacher I, et al. Incidence of rash and discontinuation of nevirapine using two different escalating initial doses. *AIDS.* 1999;13(4):524–525.

Atkinson TM, Palefsky J, Li Y, et al.; ANCHOR HRQoL Implementation Group. Reliability and between-group stability of a health-related quality of life symptom index for persons with anal high-grade squamous intraepithelial lesions: an AIDS Malignancy Consortium Study (AMC-A03). *Qual Life Res.* 2019;28(5):1265–1269. doi:10.1007/s11136-018-2089-8

Ball RA, Kinchelow T; ISR Substudy Group. Injection site reactions with the HIV-1 fusion inhibitor enfuvirtide. *J Am Acad Dermatol.* 2003;49(5):826–831.

Bartlett BL, Khambaty M, Mendoza N, et al. Dermatological management of human immunodeficiency virus (HIV). *Skin Therapy Lett.* 2007;12(8):1–3.

Baveewo S, Ssali F, Karamagi C, et al. Validation of World Health Organisation HIV/AIDS clinical staging in predicting initiation of antiretroviral therapy and clinical predictors of low CD4$^+$ T cell count in Uganda. *PLoS One.* 2011;6(5):e19089.

Bellavista S, D'Antuono A, Infusino SD, et al. Pruritic papular eruption in HIV: a case successfully treated with NB-UVB. *Dermatol Ther.* 2013;26(2):173–175.

Bolognia JL, Jorizzo JL, Schaffer J. *Dermatology.* 3rd ed. New York: Elsevier; 2012.

Boonchai W, Laohasrisakul R, Manonukul J, et al. Pruritic papular eruption in HIV seropositive patients: a cutaneous marker for immunosuppression. *Int J Dermatol.* 1999;38(5):348–350.

Boudhir H, Mael-Ainin M, Senouci K, et al. [Kaposi's disease: an unusual side-effect of topical corticosteroids]. *Ann Dermatol Venereol.* 2013;140(6–7):459–461.

Breuer-McHam J, Marshall G, Adu-Oppong A, et al. Alterations in HIV expression in AIDS patients with psoriasis or pruritus treated with phototherapy. *J Am Acad Dermatol.* 1999;40(1):48–60.

Calonje E, Brenn T, Lazar A, et al. *McKee's pathology of the skin.* 4th ed. St. Louis, MO: Saunders; 2012:901.

Cambuim II, Macedo DP, Delgado M, et al. Clinical and mycological evaluation of onychomycosis among Brazilian HIV/AIDS patients [in Portuguese]. *Rev Soc Bras Med Trop.* 2011;44(1):40–42.

Chandrasekar PH, Nandi PS, Fairfax MR, et al. Cutaneous infections due to *Acanthamoeba* in patients with acquired immunodeficiency syndrome. *Arch Intern Med.* 1997;157(5):569–572.

Chaponda M, Pirmohamed M. Hypersensitivity reactions to HIV therapy. *Br J Clin Pharmacol.* 2011;71(5):659–671.

Cockerell C, Calame A. *Cutaneous manifestations of HIV disease.* London: Manson; 2013.

Crum-Cianflone NF, Burgi AA, Hale BR. Increasing rates of community-acquired methicillin-resistant *Staphylococcus aureus* infections among HIV-infected persons. *Int J STD AIDS.* 2007;18(8):521–526.

Davis CM, Shearer WT. Diagnosis and management of HIV drug hypersensitivity. *J Allergy Clin Immunol.* 2008;121(4):826–832, e825.

de Berker D. Clinical practice: fungal nail disease. *N Engl J Med.* 2009;360(20):2108–2116.

de Moraes AP, de Arruda EA, Vitoriano MA, et al. An open-label efficacy pilot study with pimecrolimus cream 1% in adults with facial seborrhoeic dermatitis infected with HIV. *J Eur Acad Dermatol Venereol.* 2007;21(5):596–601.

Department of Health and Human Services. Guidelines for the prevention and treatment of opportunistic enfections in adults and adolescents with HIV. 2020. https://clinicalinfo.hiv.gov/en/guidelines/adult-and-adolescent-opportunistic-infection/cryptococcosis?view=full

Dogra S, Yadav S. Acitretin in psoriasis: an evolving scenario. *Int J Dermatol.* 2014;53(5):525–538.

Dover JS, Johnson RA. Cutaneous manifestations of human immunodeficiency virus infection: part II. *Arch Dermatol.* 1991;127(10):1549–1558.

Drain PK, Mosam A, Gounder L, et al. Recurrent giant molluscum contagiosum immune reconstitution inflammatory syndrome (IRIS) after initiation of antiretroviral therapy in an HIV-infected man. *Int J STD AIDS.* 2014;25(3):235–238.

Duvic M. Immunology of AIDS related to psoriasis. *J Invest Dermatol.* 1990;95(5):38S–40S.

Duvic M, Crane MM, Conant M, et al. Zidovudine improves psoriasis in human immunodeficiency virus-positive males. *Arch Dermatol.* 1994;130(4):447–451.

Eisman S. Pruritic papular eruption in HIV. *Dermatol Clin.* 2006;24(4):449–457.

Farsani TT, Kore S, Nadol P, et al. Etiology and risk factors associated with a pruritic papular eruption in people living with HIV in India. *J Intl AIDS Soc.* 2013;16(1):17325. doi:10.7448/IAS.16.1.17325

Fearfield LA, Rowe A, Francis N, et al. Itchy folliculitis and human immunodeficiency virus infection: clinicopathological and immunological features, pathogenesis and treatment. *Br J Dermatol.* 1999;141(1):3–11.

Foissac M, Goehringer F, Ranaivo IM, et al. Efficacy and safety of intravenous cidofovir in the treatment of giant molluscum contagiosum in an immunosuppressed patient [in French]. *Ann Dermatol Venereol.* 2014;141(10):620–622.

Freedman M, Ault K, Bernstein H. Advisory Committee on Immunization Practices Recommended Immunization Schedule for Adults Aged 19 Years or Older—United States, 2021. *MMWR Morb Mortal Wkly Rep.* 2021;70(6):193–196.

Gasquet S, Maurin M, Brouqui P, et al. Bacillary angiomatosis in immunocompromised patients. *AIDS.* 1998;12(14):1793–1803.

Gelfand JM, Gladman DD, Mease PJ, et al. Epidemiology of psoriatic arthritis in the population of the United States. *J Am Acad Dermatol.* 2005;53(4):573.

Ghanem KG, Erbelding EJ, Wiener ZS, et al. Serological response to syphilis treatment in HIV-positive and HIV-negative patients attending sexually transmitted diseases clinics. *Sex Transm Infect.* 2007;83(2):97–101.

Goldstein B, Berman B, Sukenik E, et al. Correlation of skin disorders with CD4⁺ T cell lymphocyte counts in patients with HIV/AIDS. *J Am Acad Dermatol.* 1997;36(2 Pt 1):262–264.

Gompels MM, Simpson N, Snow M, et al. Desensitization to co-trimoxazole (trimethoprim-sulphamethoxazole) in HIV-infected patients: is patch testing a useful predictor of reaction? *J Infect.* 1999;38:111–115.

Hage CA, Azar MM, Bahr N, et al. Histoplasmosis: up-to-date evidence-based approach to diagnosis and management. *Semin Respir Crit Care Med.* 2015;36(5):729–745.

Hagensee ME, Cameron JE, Leigh JE, et al. Human papillomavirus infection and disease in HIV-infected individuals. *Am J Med Sci.* 2004;328(1):57–63.

Hanifin JM, Reed ML, Eczema P, et al.; Impact Working Group. A population-based survey of eczema prevalence in the United States. *Dermatitis.* 2007;18(2):82–91.

Hemmige V, Arias CA, Pasalar S, et al. Skin and soft tissue infection in people living with human immunodeficiency virus in a large, urban, public healthcare system in Houston, Texas, 2009–2014. *Clin Infect Dis.* 2020;70(9):1985–1992. doi:10.1093/cid/ciz509

Hevia O, Jimenez-Acosta F, Ceballos PI, et al. Pruritic papular eruption of the acquired immunodeficiency syndrome: a clinicopathologic study. *J Am Acad Dermatol.* 1991;24(2 Pt 1):231–235.

Hyle EP, Wood BR, Backman ES, et al. High frequency of hypothalamic-pituitary–adrenal axis dysfunction after local corticosteroid injection in HIV-infected patients on protease inhibitor therapy. *J AIDS.* 2013;63(5):602–608.

Introcaso CE, Hines JM, Kovarik CL. Cutaneous toxicities of antiretroviral therapy for HIV: part II. Nonnucleoside reverse transcriptase inhibitors, entry and fusion inhibitors, integrase inhibitors, and immune reconstitution syndrome. *J Am Acad Dermatol.* 2010;63(4):563–570.

Jagdeo J, Ho D, Lo A, et al. A systematic review of filler agents for aesthetic treatment of HIV facial lipoatrophy (FLA). *J Am Acad Dermatol.* 2015;73(6):1040–1054, e1014.

Kim CM, Vogel J, Jay G, et al. The HIV tat gene transforms human keratinocytes. *Oncogene.* 1992;7(8):1525–1529.

Knobel H, Miro JM, Domingo P, et al. Failure of a short-term prednisone regimen to prevent nevirapine-associated rash: a double-blind placebo-controlled trial: the GESIDA 09/99 study. *J AIDS.* 2001;28(1):14–18.

Krown SE, Lee JY, Dittmer DP; AIDS Malignancy Consortium. More on HIV-associated Kaposi's sarcoma. *N Engl J Med.* 2008;358(5):535–536.

Kuehnert MJ, Kruszon-Moran D, Hill HA, et al. Prevalence of *Staphylococcus aureus* nasal colonization in the United States, 2001–2002. *J Infect Dis.* 2006;193(2):172–179.

Leung AKC, Barankin B, Hon KLE. Molluscum contagiosum: an update. *Recent Pat Inflamm Allergy Drug Discov.* 2017;11(1):22–31. doi:10.2174/1872213X11666170518114456

Lin RY, Lazarus TS. Asthma and related atopic disorders in outpatients attending an urban HIV clinic. *Ann Allergy Asthma Immunol.* 1995;74(6):510–515.

Liu Z, Xie Z, Zhang L, et al. Reliability and validity of dermatology life quality index: assessment of quality of life in human immunodeficiency virus/acquired immunodeficiency syndrome patients with pruritic papular eruption. *J Tradit Chin Med.* 2013;33(5):580–583.

Lolis MS, Gonzalez L, Cohen PJ, et al. Drug-resistant herpes simplex virus in HIV infected patients. *Acta Dermatovenerol Croat.* 2008;16(4):204–208.

Lortholary O, Fontanet A, Memain N, et al.; Cryptococcosis Study Group. Incidence and risk factors of immune reconstitution inflammatory syndrome complicating HIV-associated cryptococcosis in France. *AIDS.* 2005;19(10):1043–1049.

Mallal S, Phillips E, Carosi G, et al. HLA-B*5701 screening for hypersensitivity to abacavir. *N Engl J Med.* 2008;358(6):568–579.

Mallon E, Bunker CB. HIV-associated psoriasis. *AIDS Patient Care STDS.* 2000;14(5):239–246.

Maurer TA. Dermatologic manifestations of HIV infection. *Top HIV Med.* 2005;13(5):149–154.

Mayer PL, Larkin JA, Hennessy JM. Amebic encephalitis. *Surg Neurol Int.* 2011;2:50.

McCloskey JC, Metcalf C, French MA, et al. The frequency of high-grade intraepithelial neoplasia in anal/perianal warts is higher than previously recognized. *Int J STD AIDS.* 2007;18(8):538–542.

Menon K, Van Voorhees AS, Bebo BF, et al. Psoriasis in patients with HIV infection: from the medical board of the National Psoriasis Foundation. *J Am Acad Dermatol.* 2010;62(2):291–299.

Meola T, Soter NA, Ostreicher R, et al. The safety of UVB phototherapy in patients with HIV infection. *J Am Acad Dermatol.* 1993;29(2 Pt 1):216–220.

Mirmirani P, Maurer TA, Berger TG, et al. Skin-related quality of life in HIV-infected patients on highly active antiretroviral therapy. *J Cutan Med Surg.* 2002;6(1):10–15.

Mischo M, von Kobyletzki LB, Bründermann E, et al. Similar appearance, different mechanisms: xerosis in HIV, atopic dermatitis and ageing. *Exp Dermatol.* 2014;23(6):446–448. doi:10.1111/exd.12425

Mohammed S, Vellaisamy SG, Gopalan K, et al. Prevalence of pruritic papular eruption among HIV patients: a cross-sectional study. *Indian J Sex Transm Dis AIDS.* 2019;40(2):146–151. doi:10.4103/ijstd. IJSTD_69_18

Murphy M, Armstrong D, Sepkowitz KA, et al. Regression of AIDS-related Kaposi's sarcoma following treatment with an HIV-1 protease inhibitor. *AIDS.* 1997;11(2):261–262.

Murray H, Barber CJ, Foreman RM, et al.; GBD 2013 DALYs and HALE Collaborators. Global, regional, and national disability-adjusted life years (DALYs) for 306 diseases and injuries and healthy life expectancy (HALE) for 188 countries, 1990–2013: quantifying the epidemiological transition. *Lancet.* 2015;386:2145–2191.

Nakamura M, Abrouk M, Farahnik B, et al. Psoriasis treatment in HIV-positive patients: a systematic review of systemic immunosuppressive therapies. *Cutis.* 2018;101(1):38;42;56. PMID: 29529104

Nambudiri VE, Mutyambizi K, Walls AC, et al. Successful treatment of perianal giant condyloma acuminatum in an immunocompromised host with systemic interleukin 2 and topical cidofovir. *JAMA Dermatol.* 2013;149(9):1068–1070.

Nissen D, Nolte H, Permin H, et al. Evaluation of IgE-sensitization to fungi in HIV-positive patients with eczematous skin reactions. *Ann Allergy Asthma Immunol.* 1999;83(2):153–159.

Nomura T, Katoh M, Yamamoto Y, et al. Eosinophilic pustular folliculitis: a published work-based comprehensive analysis of therapeutic responsiveness. *J Dermatol.* 2016;43(8):919–927. doi:10.1111/1346-8138.13287

Oble DA, Collett E, Hsieh M, et al. A novel T cell receptor transgenic animal model of seborrheic dermatitis-like skin disease. *J Invest Dermatol.* 2005;124(1):151–159.

Obuch ML, Maurer TA, Becker B, et al. Psoriasis and human immunodeficiency virus infection. *J Am Acad Dermatol.* 1992;27(5 Pt 1):667–673.

Okada S, Fujimura T, Furudate S, et al. Immunosuppression-associated eosinophilic pustular folliculitis (IS-EPF) developing after highly active anti-retroviral therapy (HAART): the possible mechanisms through CD163⁺ M2 macrophages. *Eur J Dermatol.* 2013;23(5):713–714.

Ortega-Loayza AG, McCall CO, Nunley JR. Crusted scabies and multiple dosages of ivermectin. *J Drugs Dermatol.* 2013;12(5):584–585.

Osborne GE, Taylor C, Fuller LC. The management of HIV-related skin disease. Part II: neoplasms and inflammatory disorders. *Int J STD AIDS.* 2003;14:235.

Pedrosa AF, Lisboa C, Goncalves Rodrigues A. Malassezia infections: a medical conundrum. *J Am Acad Dermatol.* 2014;71(1):170–176.

Ratnam I, Chiu C, Kandala NB, Easterbrook PJ. Incidence and risk factors for immune reconstitution inflammatory syndrome in an ethnically diverse HIV type 1-infected cohort. *Clin Infect Dis.* 2006;42(3):418–427.

Resneck JS Jr, Van Beek M, Furmanski L, et al. Etiology of pruritic papular eruption with HIV infection in Uganda. *JAMA*. 2004;292(21):2614–2621.

Rigopoulos D, Paparizos V, Katsambas A. Cutaneous markers of HIV infection. *Clin Dermatol*. 2004;22(6):487–498.

Rodrigues LK, Klencke BJ, Vin-Christian K, et al. Altered clinical course of malignant melanoma in HIV-positive patients. *Arch Dermatol*. 2002;138(6):765–770.

Rosen T, Friedlander SF, Kircik L. Onychomycosis: epidemiology, diagnosis, and treatment in a changing landscape. *J Drugs Dermatol*. 2015;14(3):223–233.

Rosenthal D, LeBoit PE, Klumpp L, et al. Human immunodeficiency virus-associated eosinophilic folliculitis. A unique dermatosis associated with advanced human immunodeficiency virus infection. *Arch Dermatol*. 1991;127(2):206–209.

Sadick NS, McNutt NS, Kaplan MH. Papulosquamous dermatoses of AIDS. *J Am Acad Dermatol*. 1990;22(6 Pt 2):1270–1277.

Severson JL, Tyring SK. Relation between herpes simplex viruses and human immunodeficiency virus infections. *Arch Dermatol*. 1999;135(11):1393–1397.

Singh F, Rudikoff D. HIV-associated pruritus: etiology and management. *Am J Clin Dermatol*. 2003;4(3):177–188.

Smith G, Holman RP. The prozone phenomenon with syphilis and HIV-1 co-infection. *South Med J*. 2004;97(4):379–382.

Soeprono FF, Schinella RA, Cockerell CJ, et al. Seborrheic-like dermatitis of acquired immunodeficiency syndrome: a clinicopathologic study. *J Am Acad Dermatol*. 1986;14(2 Pt 1):242–248.

Stanley SK, Folks TM, Fauci AS. Induction of expression of human immunodeficiency virus in a chronically infected promonocytic cell line by ultraviolet irradiation. *AIDS Res Hum Retroviruses*. 1989;5(4):375–384.

Strick LB, Wald A, Celum C. Management of herpes simplex virus type 2 infection in HIV type 1-infected persons. *Clin Infect Dis*. 2006;43(3):347–356.

Suh KS, Han SH, Lee KH, et al. Mites and burrows are frequently found in nodular scabies by dermoscopy and histopathology. *J Am Acad Dermatol*. 2014;71(5):1022–1023.

Toutous-Trellu L, Abraham S, Pechere M, et al. Topical tacrolimus for effective treatment of eosinophilic folliculitis associated with human immunodeficiency virus infection. *Arch Dermatol*. 2005;141(10):1203–1208.

Ward HA, Russo GG, Shrum J. Cutaneous manifestations of antiretroviral therapy. *J Am Acad Dermatol*. 2002;46(2):284–293.

Warren KJ, Boxwell DE, Kim NY, et al. Nevirapine-associated Stevens–Johnson syndrome. *Lancet*. 1998;351(9102):567.

Warshaw EM, Nelson D, Carver SM, et al. A pilot evaluation of pulse itraconazole vs. terbinafine for treatment of *Candida* toenail onychomycosis. *Int J Dermatol*. 2005;44(9):785–788.

Weinberg JL, Kovarik CL. The WHO clinical staging system for HIV/AIDS. *Virtual Mentor*. 2010;12(3):202–206.

Wheat LJ, Connolly-Stringfield PA, Baker RL, et al. Disseminated histoplasmosis in the acquired immune deficiency syndrome: clinical findings, diagnosis and treatment, and review of the literature. *Medicine*. 1990;69(6):361–374.

Wilkins K, Turner R, Dolev JC, et al. Cutaneous malignancy and human immunodeficiency virus disease. *J Am Acad Dermatol*. 2006;54(2):189–210.

Workowski KA, Bolan GA. Sexually transmitted diseases treatment guidelines, 2015. *MMWR Recomm Rep*. 2015;64(RR-03):1–137.

Zancanaro PC, McGirt LY, Mamelak AJ, et al. Cutaneous manifestations of HIV in the era of highly active antiretroviral therapy: an institutional urban clinic experience. *J Am Acad Dermatol*. 2006;54(4):581–588.

Zeichner JA. New topical therapeutic options in the management of superficial fungal infections. *J Drugs Dermatol*. 2015;14(10):s35–s41.

Zheng Y, Niyonsaba F, Ushio H, et al. Cathelicidin LL-37 induces the generation of reactive oxygen species and release of human alpha-defensins from neutrophils. *Br J Dermatol*. 2007;157(6):1124–1131.

31.

ENDOCRINE AND METABOLIC DISORDERS

Rajagopal V. Sekhar

CHAPTER GOALS

Upon completion of this chapter, the reader should be able to:

- Understand the spectrum of endocrine and metabolic complications affecting people with HIV (PWH), and clinical management of these complications

- Understand the mechanism and clinical management of endocrine and metabolic diseases in PWH

INTRODUCTION

With the advent of effective antiretroviral therapies (ART), HIV infection has become a chronic disease. PWH have a longer life expectancy, and we are now able to see the emergence of disorders in such persons who live longer, and these include an increasing prevalence of endocrine and metabolic abnormalities. The underlying etiology of these disorders can be attributed to multiple factors, including the effects of HIV itself, ART, inflammation, endothelial and immune dysfunction, and mitochondrial dysfunction. Since endocrine disorders are often insidious in their development, clinical suspicion and appropriate dynamic testing are necessary for accurate diagnosis and management and should include the participation of an endocrinologist where possible. Since PWH are now living longer, we are witnessing the evolution of HIV as a chronic disease, with new emerging phenotypes that range from an increase in the incidence and prevalence of metabolic diseases such as central obesity, metabolic syndrome, to fatty liver disease. There are also reports of premature or accelerated aging affecting PWH, in which relatively younger PWH develop geriatric complications typically seen in HIV-uninfected people who are 20 to 30 years older. These include physical decline, mitochondrial dysfunction, muscle weakness, inflammation, endothelial dysfunction, insulin resistance, and cognitive decline, but underlying mechanisms are not well understood, and effective interventions are either limited or lacking. This chapter will focus on the historical and the currently evolving perspectives of endocrine and metabolic disorders in HIV infection and will discuss mechanisms, endocrine disorders, emerging complications, and therapeutic strategies.

WHAT'S NEW?

- The emerging phenomenon of premature aging in PWH

- Fatty liver disease, abdominal obesity, and metabolic syndrome, which continue to play a role in PWH

- Endocrine disorders in transgender PWH

- Emerging novel role for glutathione to improve cellular nutrition and cellular health

KEY POINTS

- The endocrine complications of HIV infection are changing, with newer phenomena emerging as PWH continue to live longer.

- Metabolic complications continue to affect an increasing number of PWH.

- HIV infection, ART, and other factors play a role in the development of endocrine disease.

- For endocrine disorders in HIV, early referral to an endocrinologist is suggested.

ENDOCRINE AND METABOLIC DISEASE IN HIV

Although HIV infection has been associated with endocrine and metabolic complications since the 1980s, these complications have been dynamically changing as a result of improvements in pharmacotherapy and increasing lifespan, and other unknown contributors. Of note has been an increase in cardiometabolic complications, premature/accelerated aging, fatty liver disease, and metabolic syndrome, but the underlying mechanisms for many of these disorders are still not completely understood. PWH also continue to have more conventional disorders affecting the endocrine systems involving diabetes, thyroid, adrenal, pituitary, bone, and gonadal systems. This chapter will discuss both existing endocrine and metabolic disease in PWH and emerging new phenomena.

Elevations in inflammation and abnormalities in immune function in PWH could be contributing in part to some of these disorders, and PWH have been described to have elevated proinflammatory cytokines and abnormalities in immune phenomena that affect endocrine function (Merrill et al., 1989; Salim et al., 1988; Tracey & Cerami, 1990). For example, interleukin-1 (IL-1) has been shown to increase adrenocorticotropic hormone (ACTH) in cultured pituitary cells (Meyer et al., 1987; Szebeni et al., 1991). Other pituitary hormones may also be affected; effects include prolactin elevations (Parra et al., 2004) and deficient growth hormone secretion (Koutkia et al., 2004). HIV-positive mononuclear cells can increase interferon-α (Grunfeld et al., 1992) and impair glucocorticoid receptor activity (Norbiato et al., 1996), and abnormalities in IL-1 and tumor necrosis factor (TNF) can affect gonadal function by inhibiting gonadal steroidogenesis (Calkins et al., 1988; Hales et al., 1992; Xiong & Hales, 1993). Interestingly, results from a small pilot study showed that correcting deficiency of the endogenous antioxidant protein glutathione was associated with a striking decline in inflammation with significant decreases in high-sensitivity C-reactive protein (hsCRP) and TNF-α blood levels within 2 weeks (Sekhar et al., 2015), and further studies are needed to confirm and extend these findings.

Another contributor to HIV-related endocrine disease is opportunistic infections. For example, cytomegalovirus (CMV) infection predisposes to an increased risk of developing adrenalitis (Glasgow et al., 1985). Infections caused by mycobacterial pathogens may also affect adrenal function, whereas CMV, cryptococcal, and toxoplasma infections can affect central nervous system (CNS) function and cause retinitis, meningitis, and pituitary disease (Giampalmo et al., 1990). CMV infection has been reported in one instance to cause hypernatremia, likely through a reset osmostat (Keuneke et al., 1999). Thyroid function can be affected by opportunistic pathogens in HIV, including *Pneumocystis jirovecii*, which is a rare cause of thyroiditis (Drucker et al., 1990).

PWH are also experiencing an increase in the incidence and prevalence of metabolic disorders, including centripetal fat accumulation as in the metabolic syndrome, fatty liver disease, and mitochondrial dysfunction. The underlying mechanisms are not well understood, and effective interventions are lacking. There is an urgent need for exploratory studies to guide relevant clinical trials to facilitate identification of mechanisms and develop therapeutic strategies.

The development and clinical use of ART have led to significant benefits for PWH, including decreased early mortality, decreased opportunistic infection, and improved nutritional status. However, these benefits are associated with increases in the incidence and prevalence of endocrine and metabolic complications, most notably dyslipidemia, and changes in body morphology ranging from lipodystrophy (Carr et al., 1998) to central obesity in the context of metabolic syndrome. The roles of antiretroviral drugs (ARVs) are discussed next.

PROTEASE INHIBITORS

The initial use of protease inhibitor (PI) drugs in PWH led to observations of abnormalities in total body fat distribution, most notably an increase in abdominal fat that was initially described by colorful names such as the "protease paunch" (Mishriki et al., 1998) or "Crixivan belly" (Huff et al., 1997–1998). Since then, the PI class of drugs has been linked to the development of abdominal obesity and biochemical abnormalities comprising severe hypertriglyceridemia, dyslipidemia, insulin resistance, and diabetes. Many PIs, including lopinavir/ritonavir, nelfinavir, amprenavir, and saquinavir, are metabolized by the hepatic cytochrome 450 CYP3A4 isoenzyme pathway. PIs have been shown to directly impact insulin resistance. For example, indinavir can inhibit GLUT4 activity and thus impair insulin-stimulated glucose uptake and predispose to hyperglycemia (Caron et al., 2001; Murata et al., 2000). In addition to their permissive role in metabolic and glycemic abnormalities, PIs have also been implicated in the development of prolactin abnormalities (Hutchinson et al., 2000) and in osteomalacia (Cozzolino et al., 2003).

NUCLEOSIDE REVERSE TRANSCRIPTASE INHIBITORS

Nucleoside reverse transcriptase inhibitors (NRTIs) have also been described to induce changes in body morphology. For example, stavudine has been linked to the development of lipoatrophy in HIV (Saint-Marc et al., 1999). These drugs have also been linked to the development of mitochondrial dysfunction (Mallon et al., 2005), which could result in abnormalities of glucose and lipid metabolism (Sekhar et al., 2002; Shikuma et al., 2001).

NONNUCLEOSIDE REVERSE TRANSCRIPTASE INHIBITORS

Nonnucleoside reverse transcriptase inhibitors (NNRTIs) have been linked to dyslipidemia (Padmapriyadarsini et al., 2011) and fat depletion in 3T3-L1 cells (Minami et al., 2011).

INTEGRASE INHIBITORS

Integrase inhibitors have been associated with significant weight gain. The NA-ACCORD, a large observational cohort study in the US and Canada, compared 22,972 adult, ART-naïve PWH initiated with integrase strand transfer inhibitor (INSTI)-, PI-, or NNRTI-based ART and found that compared to PIs and NNRTIs, INSTIs were associated with the highest amount of weight gain, with the highest weight gain being with dolutegravir (+7.2 kg), followed by raltegravir (+5.8 kg) and elvitegravir (+4.1 kg) (Bourgi et al., 2020a). This has also been reported in other studies in PWH on dolutegravir-based regimens (Bourgi et al., 2020b).

ENDOCRINE DISORDERS IN HIV

Any endocrine or metabolic disorder can affect PWH, including metabolic syndrome; disorders of adrenal, thyroid, pituitary, and gonadal function; bone disorders; and dyslipidemia. Bone disorders and dyslipidemia are discussed in chapters 40 and 41, respectively.

DIABETES MELLITUS

The prevalence of diabetes mellitus (DM) is increasing in PWH worldwide (Tzur et al., 2015). Earlier reports such as the Multicenter AIDS Cohort Study (MACS) found that exposure to ART resulted in a 14% incidence of DM in men with HIV (Brown et al., 2005). However, more recent publications have estimated this to be as high as 15.1%, with a relative risk of 2.4 compared to the general population (Duncan et al., 2018). Another study followed PWH for 10 years in Malawi, Africa, and found the prevalence of DM to be higher in every age group (from 30 to 60+) compared to controls (Mathabire et al., 2018). More recently, a study from India found that PWH with lower CD4$^+$ T-cell counts had significantly higher glycemia and insulin resistance (Bajaj et al., 2020). In addition, there are reports suggesting that glycosylated hemoglobin (HbA1c) may underestimate glycemia in PWH (Kim et al., 2009; Slama et al., 2014), which suggests that the magnitude of hyperglycemia in PWH may be even greater. One study examined HbA1c in 1,500 HIV-negative and 1,357 HIV-positive men in the MACS cohort over 13 years and found that HbA1c underestimates glycemia in HIV-positive men (Slama et al., 2014). Another study compared 100 HIV-positive adults with type 2 diabetes to 200 HIV-negative type 2 diabetic participants, found similar results, and linked it to use of abacavir and increased mean corpuscular volume (MCV) (Kim et al., 2009). The reasons for this meteoric rise in the incidence of DM are likely to be multifactorial, but a recent meta-analysis implicated ART as potentially the single most consistent determinant of DM in PWH worldwide (Nduka et al., 2017). Another recent meta-analysis investigated gestational diabetes in pregnant women with HIV and found that the pooled prevalence of gestational diabetes among pregnant women with HIV was high (Biadgo et al., 2019). Collectively, these reports indicate an increase in the incidence and prevalence of DM among PWH and suggest that relying solely on HbA1c could lead to underdiagnosing and undertreating diabetes. The implications are that it is important to carefully screen for hyperglycemia and diabetes in PWH and to correlate HbA1c with other measures of HIV-positive glycemic control, including fasting and prandial home glucose monitoring, for a reliable assessment of glycemic status and control. The overall management of DM in PWH is similar to that in HIV-uninfected persons and requires the combined approach of a team comprising a diabetes educator, dietitian, physician, and diabetes nursing staff and careful attention to the triumvirate of exercise, diet, and pharmacotherapy. Early screening of pregnant women with HIV for gestational diabetes is vital to reduce its complications related to pregnancy. The long-term complications of DM include retinopathy, nephropathy, neuropathy, and coronary artery disease. Interestingly, PWH are at risk of retinitis due to opportunistic infections, to HIV-associated nephropathy (HIVAN), and to neuropathy, and also have an increased risk of cardiovascular disease. The concurrence of these end-organ complications from both HIV infection and DM theoretically suggests that PWH could be at higher risk from the twin burden of two chronic diseases, HIV and DM.

ADRENAL DISORDERS

HIV infection can involve adrenal dysfunction. The incidence of hypoadrenalism is reported to be 20% in PWH (González-González et al., 2001), and postmortem studies have shown that up to two-thirds of people with AIDS may have adrenal involvement (Bricaire et al., 1988). Presentation of adrenal dysfunction may be subtle and escape clinical scrutiny, and it is relatively common in hospitalized PWH (Membreno et al., 1987). The etiology of adrenal hypofunction can range from primary hypoadrenalism involving the adrenal gland, with elevations in adrenocorticotropic hormone (ACTH) levels (Villette et al., 1990), to secondary hypoadrenalism due to pituitary suppression due to inherent pituitary pathology or possibly suppression of the hypothalamic–pituitary–adrenal axis by exogenous steroid use (Danaher et al., 2009; Kaviani et al., 2011). PWH have also been described to develop hyperadrenalism with iatrogenic Cushing syndrome when administered steroids via oral, inhaled, and parenteral routes (Gray et al., 2010; Johnson et al., 2006; Samaras et al., 2005; Yombi et al., 2008).

PWH may also have abnormalities in the mineralocorticoid axis (Stricker, 1999). HIV-positive women with the wasting syndrome may have significant shunting of adrenal steroid metabolism away from androgenic pathways and toward cortisol production (Grinspoon et al., 2001).

THYROID ABNORMALITIES

The clinical presentation of thyroid abnormalities in HIV infection ranges from asymptomatic hypo- or hyperthyroidism to clinically overt disease. The prevalence of thyroid dysfunction appears to be higher in PWH. Although earlier reports suggested that thyroid dysfunction in PWH is generally similar to that seen in HIV-negative populations (Hoffman et al., 2007), recent reports indicate that the prevalence of thyroid dysfunction may be much higher. A recent study evaluated thyroid function in 178 PWH and found that 33% of them had evidence of thyroid dysfunction (Ji et al., 2016). Most of these abnormalities involve hypothyroidism, ranging from an increased prevalence of subclinical hypothyroidism (Madeddu et al., 2006; Silva et al., 2015) to clinical hypothyroidism (Beltran et al., 2003). Factors contributing to thyroid disorders in HIV infection include, but are not limited to, ARVs, infection, and immune factors.

ARVs could play a role in the development of thyroid abnormalities in PWH. For example, HIV-related non-autoimmune primary hypothyroidism and subclinical hypothyroidism have been linked to stavudine, decreased CD4$^+$ T-cell counts, and male gender (Calza et al., 2002; Madeddu et al., 2006; Quirino et al., 2004; Silva et al., 2015).

HIV-related immune and other factors are also linked to the development of abnormal thyroid function tests. For example, CD4$^+$ T-cell counts have been inversely correlated with thyroid binding globulin (Bourdoux et al., 1991), and diminished levels of triiodothyronine (T3) and reverse T3 with increased thyroid binding globulin may be associated with HIV progression. Hyperthyroidism can also occur in

PWH. Autoimmune Graves' disease involves an anti–thyroid-stimulating hormone receptor antibody and can occur after the initiation of ART and after an increase in CD4⁺ T-cell count (Jubault et al., 2000).

Infection as an etiologic factor for thyroid disease was much more prevalent in the pre-ART era and was caused by a wide variety of infectious microorganisms. However, these can still be seen in people not on ART, those with ART drug resistance, or those who are nonadherent to medications.

Although the clinical presentation of thyroid abnormalities ranges from asymptomatic hypo- or hyperthyroidism to clinically overt disease, the diagnostic workup is similar to that in HIV-negative persons and should begin with evaluations of thyroxine and thyrotropin, with additional testing for thyroiditis antibodies where appropriate.

PARATHYROID DISORDERS

Hyperparathyroidism is a condition marked by elevated secretion of parathyroid hormone. It can be primary due to abnormalities within the parathyroid gland itself, most often due to adenoma, and rarely due to cancer. Secondary causes are due to conditions such as renal impairment and vitamin D deficiency. The etiology of primary hyperparathyroidism in the HIV-positive population is similar to the general population and typically presents as hypercalcemia; this should be appropriately investigated, with the final treatment being surgical removal of the parathyroid adenoma. However, vitamin D deficiency is reported to impact a third of PWH (Van den Bout et al., 2008) and is a common cause for secondary hyperparathyroidism (Dao et al., 2011; Mueller et al., 2010) with referrals to endocrinologists. ARVs such as efavirenz have been implicated in the increased prevalence of vitamin D deficiency in PWH (Nylén et al., 2016), but other factors such as CD4⁺ T-cell counts and advanced disease may also play a role (Theodorou et al., 2014). Other ARVs such as tenofovir disoproxil fumarate have also been linked to secondary hyperparathyroidism in PWH (Noe et al., 2018).

GONADAL DYSFUNCTION

Gonadal dysfunction is common in PWH (Crum et al., 2005; Rietschel et al., 2000). In male adults with HIV, decreased levels of testosterone may be associated with fatigue, muscle wasting and sarcopenia, decreased bone density, low libido, weight loss, decreased strength (Grinspoon et al., 1996; Wanke et al., 2000), and impotence (Mylonakis et al., 2001). In a study of 300 PWH, 17% were found to be hypogonadal, and all PWH with low testosterone had secondary hypogonadism. Interestingly, there was no correlation between hypogonadism and erectile dysfunction, but increasing age and a higher body mass index were positively correlated with hypogonadism, whereas smoking was negatively correlated (Crum-Cianflone et al., 2007). Although underlying causes are not fully understood, elevated levels of prolactin have been implicated in the development of male hypogonadism (Collazos et al., 2009). Treatment of PWH with AIDS wasting syndrome with testosterone or placebo was associated with a sustained increase in lean mass only with testosterone after a 6-month period (Grinspoon et al., 1999). Testosterone therapy, especially in older PWH, should involve careful monitoring of prostate-specific antigen levels, liver profiles, and hematocrit levels.

HIV-positive women have increased rates of oligomenorrhea and amenorrhea. HIV has been shown to infect the cervix, uterus, and fallopian tubes (Howell et al., 1997). In one study, 8% of women living with HIV had evidence of early menopause and 48% had anovulatory cycles, whereas women who ovulated had higher CD4⁺ T-cell counts (Chirgwin et al., 1996). In a recent study from Nigeria reporting abnormalities in premenopausal women living with HIV, mean serum levels of the follicle stimulating hormone, luteinizing hormone, progesterone, and estradiol did not differ between the follicular and luteal phase of the menstrual cycle, suggesting loss of hormonal regulation, and the researchers linked these abnormalities to hypothyroidism, which could be corrected with treatment (Ukibe et al., 2017).

Gynecomastia

Males living with HIV have a 2.9% incidence of developing gynecomastia, which is not linked to progression of HIV disease (Biglia et al., 2004) but is linked to hypogonadism, lipoatrophy, hepatitis C (Manfredi et al., 2001), and also lipodystrophy (Biglia et al., 2004). The role of ARVs in the development of gynecomastia is controversial, with no correlation found in some studies (Manfredi et al., 2001), whereas other studies have linked gynecomastia with PI-based ART regimens (Manfredi et al., 2004; Peyriere et al., 1999; Toma & Therrien, 1998). When associated with PI therapy, gynecomastia does not resolve after cessation of ART, and underlying mechanisms are not clear. Treatment of gynecomastia includes removal of any identifiable cause and, in extreme cases, surgical removal.

Pituitary Disease

The pituitary gland is located in the sella turcica and comprises the anterior pituitary (adenohypophysis) and posterior pituitary (neurohypophysis). The adenohypophyseal hormones are intimately involved in controlling thyroid, adrenal, and gonadal function; growth; and milk secretion. The neurohypophysis primarily controls water balance, acting via antidiuretic hormone. Many pituitary hormones are regulated by prohormones secreted by the hypothalamus that are delivered to the pituitary via a portal system through the pituitary stalk (e.g., corticotropin releasing hormone [CRH], growth hormone releasing hormone [GHRH], thyrotropin releasing hormone [TRH], gonadotropin releasing hormone [GnRH], and vasopressin), with the sole exception being prolactin, which is under inhibitory control by dopamine. Therefore, pituitary disease can be caused by pathology at the level of the hypothalamus, pituitary stalk compression, or disease in the pituitary gland itself.

Growth Hormone Disorders

Disorders of growth hormone (GH) are reported in HIV infection. Lipodystrophy in adult PWH is described to have GH deficiency with reduced pulse and amplitude of GH secretion, which may be related to an increased somatostatin tone, decreased ghrelin, and increased circulatory free fatty acid concentrations (Koutkia et al., 2004). HIV-positive children and adults with AIDS wasting syndrome have low levels of insulin-like growth factor-1 (IGF-1) and IGF binding protein 3 and increased concentrations of GH, suggesting resistance to GH (Frost et al., 1996; Pinto et al., 2000; Ratner Kaufman et al., 1997; Rondanelli et al., 2002).

Pituitary Adrenal Disorders

Iatrogenic Cushing syndrome, together with secondary hypoadrenalism, is a frequent observation in PWH who receive steroid therapy (Danaher et al., 2009; Gray et al., 2010; Johnson et al., 2006; Kaviani et al., 2011; Samaras et al., 2005; Yombi et al., 2008). This is likely caused by the effect of several ARVs (almost entirely ritonavir or cobicistat boosting) on the hepatic cytochrome P450 system, which prolongs the half-life of steroids. This results in elevated levels of exogenously administered steroids and suppression of ACTH and thereby of endogenous cortisol production, resulting in iatrogenic Cushing syndrome together with endogenous adrenal insufficiency. Because sudden withdrawal of exogenous steroids in this situation could precipitate a catastrophic adrenal crisis, caution must be exercised while discontinuing steroids, and a gentle taper is recommended.

Prolactin Disorders

PWH have been reported to have disturbances in basal and rhythmic prolactin secretions associated with CD4+ T lymphocytes (Parra et al., 2004). Elevation in serum prolactin is described in PWH (Collazos et al., 2002), and hyperprolactinemia in HIV-positive men has been linked to hypogonadism and gynecomastia (Collazos et al., 2009). Although the etiology of the hyperprolactinemia is unclear, use of PIs has been linked to elevations in prolactin (Ram et al., 2004).

Posterior Pituitary Disorders

Posterior pituitary disorders are caused by excess secretion of antidiuretic hormone (ADH), resulting in hyponatremia, or a paucity of ADH, resulting in diabetes insipidus. In one report, 33% of persons with AIDS were found to have hyponatremia primarily due to the syndrome of inappropriate ADH secretion (Agarwal et al., 1989). PWH may also develop hypernatremia caused by diabetes insipidus due to intracranial pathology; a recently published case report highlights the role of CNS lymphoma in a PWH who presented with diabetes insipidus (Tavares-Bello et al., 2017).

METABOLIC DISORDERS IN HIV

METABOLIC SYNDROME

With increased longevity in PWH, there is also an increasing risk of developing metabolic syndrome, with central obesity, insulin resistance, hypertriglyceridemia, and hypertension, which could predispose to an increased risk of cardiovascular disease (Hadigan et al., 2001). Whereas the prevalence of metabolic syndrome in non-HIV-positive individuals is 3%, PWH taking ART have a prevalence of 16% to 18% (Samaras et al., 2007). HIV-positive women appear to have an even higher burden of metabolic syndrome, with a 33% prevalence compared to 22% for HIV-seronegative women (Sobieszczyk et al., 2008).

Clinically, the previously discussed data translate into PWH having an increased incidence and prevalence of abdominal obesity, insulin resistance, dyslipidemia, and hypertension, all of which contribute to elevated cardiometabolic risk in PWH. Treatment of these disorders involves a combination of patient education; adherence to dietary control; encouragement of physical activity and exercise, where possible; and appropriate pharmacotherapy targeting glycemic control, blood pressure, and lipids.

NONALCOHOLIC FATTY LIVER DISEASE

Liver disease is an important contributor to morbidity and mortality among PWH. Despite the success with therapeutic interventions to cure hepatitis C viral coinfection, there is an increase in the prevalence of nonalcoholic fatty liver disease (NAFLD), defined as liver fat accumulation (causing fatty liver) in the absence of other causes of liver disease such as excess alcohol consumption, viral hepatitis, or any other specific hepatic pathology. NAFLD ranges from simple hepatic steatosis at one end of the spectrum, to nonalcoholic steatohepatitis (NASH) and hepatic fibrosis, which progresses to cirrhosis and hepatocellular carcinoma on the other end. NASH is now the third most common indication for liver transplantation in the US. The prevalence of NAFLD and NASH is increasing in PWH. A study examining PWH with altered transaminases found a reported prevalence of NASH of up to 55% (Morse et al., 2015). NAFLD in HIV may have a more aggressive progression to NASH: a recently published study examined the clinical and histologic differences between HIV-associated NAFLD and primary NAFLD and reported that HIV-associated NAFLD was associated with increased severity of liver disease and higher prevalence of NASH (Vodkin et al., 2015). Furthermore, the presence of NAFLD is linked to the development of systemic inflammation, insulin resistance, diabetes, and cardiovascular disease. Conversely, NAFLD is a well-recognized complication of type 2 diabetes, with reported prevalence as high as 80% to 85%, and, given the rising incidence and prevalence of type 2 diabetes in PWH, NAFLD and NASH could soon become the most significant metabolic complication of HIV infection. Thus, the combination of high prevalence of NAFLD/NASH in PWH with increased severity of NASH makes it an extremely urgent public health concern, especially since mechanisms are not well understood and effective interventions are lacking.

HIV AND MITOCHONDRIAL IMPAIRMENT

PWH are well described to have an impairment in mitochondrial fat oxidation. Mitochondrial impairment is also well described in non-HIV-associated conditions that include type 2 diabetes, obesity, and aging, but underlying mechanisms are unclear and currently there are no viable or effective interventions to reverse mitochondrial dysfunction in any human condition. It is from this perspective that the results of a small pilot study that investigated mechanisms and reported reversibility of mitochondrial impairment are relevant (Nguyen et al., 2014). Based on their discoveries in rodents and older humans (Nguyen et al., 2013) that adequate availability of the endogenous antioxidant protein glutathione is critical for optimal mitochondrial fatty acid oxidation, the investigators evaluated and found that PWH with impaired mitochondrial fat oxidation and oxidative stress had severe deficiency of glutathione, which, in turn, was caused by deficient synthesis due to decreased availability of two of its precursor amino acids, cysteine and glycine. When these amino acids were supplemented in the diet for 2 weeks, it corrected their deficiency, restored glutathione synthesis rates, increased glutathione concentrations, and lowered oxidative stress. This was associated with a significant improvement of mitochondrial fuel oxidation in the fasted and fed states, together with a 31% decrease in insulin resistance, a decrease in total body fat and waist circumference (Nguyen et al., 2014), and a decrease in inflammation (Sekhar et al., 2015). Further large trials are needed to confirm and extend these results. If true, this discovery could have profound implications for improving the metabolic health of PWH by using nutritional supplementation of oral cysteine and glycine to correct glutathione deficiency.

PREMATURE AGING IN PWH

Effective ART has improved the health and life expectancy of PWH (Mack et al., 2003; Palella et al., 1998). However, emerging evidence suggests that PWH are developing premature aging, where complications typically associated with a geriatric age range of 70 to 80 years are being reported in people 10 to 20 years earlier (Bhatia et al., 2012; Guaraldi et al., 2011; Jiminez et al., 2018; Önen & Overton, 2011; Rajasuriar et al., 2017). A recent report where 336 young PWH with a median age of 44 years were compared to uninfected controls matched by age, sex and ethnicity found that PWH had significantly higher manifestation of geriatric conditions, with lower quality-of-life scores, a fivefold higher utilization of healthcare resources, and a fourfold increase in mortality (Rajasuriar et al., 2017). Premature aging in PWH has also been reported to be linked to comorbidities typically associated with a geriatric age, including slower gait speed (Schrack et al., 2015), declining strength and physical function (Khoury et al.,

2017), impaired cognition (Kuhn et al., 2019; Wang et al., 2017), mitochondrial aging (Nguyen et al., 2014; Payne et al., 2011), and elevated inflammation (McDonald et al., 2013; Monczor et al., 2018; Sekhar et al., 2015). These whole-body measures indicative of premature aging in PWH are also supported by cellular findings in corneal epithelial cells, monocyte and immune dysfunction, and the emergence of frailty at an earlier age. Although premature aging in PWH is now being recognized as a new, significant public health challenge, there is limited knowledge about underlying causal mechanisms, and effective interventions are lacking (Önen.et al, 2011; Jimenez et al, 2014).

ENDOCRINE AND METABOLIC COMPLICATIONS IN TRANSGENDER PWH

Although transgender PWH usually receive hormonal therapy and could develop endocrine and metabolic complications, carefully conducted studies are limited. A recent matched case–control study of metabolic syndrome and thyroid and adrenal function compared transgender women (cases) to cisgender HIV-positive men (controls) and found no differences between the two groups in terms of metabolic syndrome, but there was a higher frequency of subclinical hypothyroidism (median TSH 1.6-fold higher), which was associated with a higher body mass index and use of steroids, and also adrenal insufficiency found in transgender women (Pommier et al., 2019). Additional studies are needed to further understand and define the endocrine and metabolic complications in transgender PWH.

CONCLUSION

PWH can be affected by endocrine and metabolic abnormalities. Although the more common disorders are dyslipidemia, diabetes, metabolic syndrome, and insulin resistance, other disorders affecting bone, adrenal glands, pituitary, and thyroid function may also be present. For rapid diagnosis and treatment of endocrine disorders in PWH, early referral to an endocrinologist is highly recommended.

REFERENCES

Agarwal A, Soni A, Ciechanowsky M, et al. Hyponatremia in patients with the acquired immunodeficiency syndrome. *Nephron.* 1989;53:317–321.

Bajaj S, Sonkar KK, Verma S, et al. Assessment of glycemic status, insulin resistance and hypogonadism in HIV-infected male patients. *J Assoc Physicians India.* 2020;68(8):43–46.

Beltran S, Lescure FX, Desailloud R, et al. Increased prevalence of hypothyroidism among human immunodeficiency virus-infected patients: a need for screening. *Clin Infect Dis.* 2003;37:579–583.

Bhatia R, Ryscavage P, Taiwo B. Accelerated aging and human immunodeficiency virus infection: emerging challenges of growing older in the era of successful antiretroviral therapy. *J Neurovirol.* 2012;18(4):247–255.

Biadgo B, Ambachew S, Abebe M et al. Gestational diabetes mellitus in HIV-infected pregnant women: a systematic review and meta-analysis. *Diabetes Res Clin Pract*. 2019;155:107800.

Biglia A, Blanco JL, Martínez E, et al. Gynecomastia among HIV-positive patients is associated with hypogonadism: a case–control study. *Clin Infect Dis*. 2004;39(10):1514–1519.

Bourdoux PP, De Wit SA, Servais GM, et al. Biochemical thyroid profile in patients infected with human immunodeficiency virus. *Thyroid*. 1991;1:147–149.

Bourgi K, Jenkins CA, Rebeiro PF et al. Weight gain among treatment-naïve persons with HIV starting integrase inhibitors compared to non-nucleoside reverse transcriptase inhibitors or protease inhibitors in a large observational cohort in the United States and Canada. *J Int AIDS Soc*. 2020a;23(4):325484.

Bourgi K, Rebeiro PF, Turner M, et al. Greater weight gain in treatment-naive persons starting dolutegravir-based antiretroviral therapy. *Clin Infect Dis*. 2020b;17;70(7):1267–1274.

Bricaire F, Marche C, Zoubi D, et al. Adrenocortical lesions and AIDS. *Lancet*. 1988;1:881.

Brown TT, Cole SR, Li X, et al. Antiretroviral therapy and the prevalence and incidence of diabetes mellitus in the Multicenter AIDS Cohort Study. *Arch Intern Med*. 2005;165:1179–1184.

Calkins JH, Siegel MM, Nankin HR, et al. Interleukin-1 inhibits Leydig cell steroidogenesis in primary cell culture. *J Clin Endocrinol Metab*. 1988;123:1605–1610.

Calza L, Manfredi R, Chiodo F. Subclinical hypothyroidism in HIV-positive patients receiving highly active antiretroviral therapy. *J AIDS*. 2002;31:361–363.

Caron M, Auclair M, Vigouroux C, et al. The HIV protease inhibitor indinavir impairs sterol regulatory element-binding protein-1 intranuclear localization, inhibits preadipocyte differentiation, and induces insulin resistance. *Diabetes*. 2001;50:1378–1388.

Carr A, Samaras K, Burton S, et al. A syndrome of peripheral lipodystrophy, hyperlipidaemia and insulin resistance in patients receiving HIV protease inhibitors. *AIDS*. 1998;12(7):F51–F58.

Chirgwin KD, Feldman J, Muneyyirci-Delale O, et al. Menstrual function in human immunodeficiency virus-infected women without acquired immunodeficiency syndrome. *J AIDS Hum Retrovirol*. 1996;12:489–494.

Collazos J, Esteban M. Has prolactin a role in the hypogonadal status of HIV-positive patients? *J Int Assoc Physicians AIDS Care*. 2009;8(1):43–46.

Collazos J, Ibarra S, Martinez E, et al. Serum prolactin concentrations in patients infected with HIV. *HIV Clin Trials*. 2002;3:133–138.

Cozzolino M, Vidal M, Arcidiacono MV, et al. HIV-protease inhibitors impair vitamin D bioactivation to 1,25-dihydroxyvitamin D. *AIDS*. 2003;17:513–520.

Crum NF, Furtek KJ, Olson PE, et al. A review of hypogonadism and erectile dysfunction among HIV-infected men during the pre- and post-HAART eras: diagnosis, pathogenesis, and management. *AIDS Patient Care STDs*. 2005;19(10):655–671.

Crum-Cianflone NF, Bavaro M, Hale B, et al. Erectile dysfunction and hypogonadism among men with HIV. *AIDS Patient Care STDs*. 2007;21:9–19.

Danaher PJ, Salsbury TL, Delmar JA. Metabolic derangement after injection of triamcinolone into the hip of an HIV-infected patient receiving ritonavir. *Orthopedics*. 2009;32(6):450.

Dao CN, Patel P, Overton ET, et al. Low vitamin D among HIV-infected adults: prevalence of and risk factors for low vitamin D Levels in a cohort of HIV-infected adults and comparison to prevalence among adults in the US general population. *Clin Infect Dis*. 2011;52:396.

Drucker DJ, Bailey D, Rotstein L. Thyroiditis as the presenting manifestation of disseminated extrapulmonary *Pneumocystis carinii* infection. *J Clin Endocrinol Metab*. 1990;71:1663–1665.

Duncan AD, Goff LM, Peters BS. Type 2 diabetes prevalence and its risk factors in HIV: a cross-sectional study. *PLOS One*. 2018;13(3):e0194199.

Frost RA, Fuhrer J, Steigbigel R. Wasting in the acquired immune deficiency syndrome is associated with multiple defects in the serum insulin-like growth factor system. *Clin Endocrinol*. 1996;44:501.

Giampalmo A, Buffa D, Quaglia AC. AIDS pathology: various critical considerations (especially regarding the brain, the heart, the lungs, the hypophysis and the adrenal glands). *Pathologica*. 1990;82(1982):663–677.

Glasgow BJ, Steinsapir KD, Anders K, et al. Adrenal pathology in the acquired immune deficiency syndrome. *Am J Clin Pathol*. 1985;84:594–597.

González-González JG, de la Garza-Hernández NE, Garza-Morán RA, et al. Prevalence of abnormal adrenocortical function in human immunodeficiency virus infection by low-dose cosyntropin test. *Int J STD AIDS*. 2001;12(12):804–810.

Gray D, Roux P, Carrihill M, et al. Adrenal suppression and Cushing's syndrome secondary to ritonavir and budesonide. *S Afr Med J*. 2010;100(5):296–297

Grinspoon S, Corcoran C, Anderson E, et al. Sustained anabolic effects of long-term androgen administration in men with AIDS and wasting. *Clin Infect Dis*. 1999;28:634–636.

Grinspoon S, Corcoran C, Lee K, et al. Loss of lean body and muscle mass correlates with androgen levels in hypogonadal men with acquired immunodeficiency syndrome and wasting. *J Clin Endocrinol Metab*. 1996;81:4051–4058.

Grinspoon S, Corcoran C, Stanley T, et al. Mechanisms of androgen deficiency in human immunodeficiency virus-infected women with the wasting syndrome. *J Clin Endocrinol Metab*. 2001;86:4120–4126.

Grunfeld C, Pang M, Doerrler W, et al. Lipids, lipoproteins, triglyceride clearance, and cytokines in human immunodeficiency virus infection and the acquired immunodeficiency syndrome. *J Clin Endocrinol Metab*. 1992;74:1045–1052.

Guaraldi G, Orlando G, Zona S, et al. Premature age-related comorbidities among HIV-infected persons compared with the general population. *Clin Infect Dis*. 2011;53:1120–1126.

Hadigan C, Meigs JB, Corcoran C, et al. Metabolic abnormalities and cardiovascular disease risk factors in adults with human immunodeficiency virus infection and lipodystrophy. *Clin Infect Dis*. 2001;32(1):130–139.

Hales DB. Interleukin 1 inhibits Leydig cell steroidogenesis primarily by decreasing 17α-hydroxylase/C17–20 lyase cytochrome P450 expression. *Endocrinology*. 1992;131:2165–2172.

Hoffman CJ, Brown TT. Thyroid function abnormalities in HIV infected patients. *Clin Infect Dis*. 2007;45:488–494.

Howell AL, Edkins RD, Rier SE, et al. Human immunodeficiency virus type 1 infection of cells and tissues from the upper and lower human female reproductive tract. *J Virol*. 1997;71:3498–3506.

Huff A. Protease inhibitor side effects take people by surprise. *GMHC Treat Issues*. 1997–1998;12(1):25–27.

Hutchinson J, Murphy M, Harries R, et al. Galactorrhoea and hyper-prolactinoma associated with protease inhibitors. *Lancet*. 2000;356:1003–1004.

Ji S, Jin C, Hoxtermann S, et al. Prevalence and influencing factors of thyroid dysfunction in HIV-positive patients. *Biomed Res Int*. 2016;3874257.

Jiménez Z, Sánchez-Conde M, Brañas F. HIV infection as a cause of accelerated aging and frailty. *Rev Esp Geriatr Gerontol*. 2018;53(2):105–110.

Johnson SR, Marion AA, Vrchoticky T, et al. Cushing syndrome with secondary adrenal insufficiency from concomitant therapy with ritonavir and fluticasone. *J Pediatr*. 2006;148(3):386–388.

Jubault V, Penformin F, Schillo F, et al. Sequential occurrence of thyroid autoantibodies and Graves' disease after immune restoration in severely immunocompromised human immunodeficiency virus-1 infected patients. *J Clin Endocrinol Metab*. 2000;85:4254–4257.

Kaviani N, Bukberg P, Manessis A, et al. Iatrogenic osteoporosis, bilateral HIP osteonecrosis, and secondary adrenal suppression in an HIV-positive man receiving inhaled corticosteroids and ritonavir-boosted highly active antiretroviral therapy. *Endocr Pract*. 2011;17(1):74–78.

Keuneke C, Anders HJ, Schlöndorff D. Adipsic hypernatremia in two patients with AIDS and cytomegalovirus encephalitis. *Am J Kidney Dis*. 1999;33(2):379–382.

Khoury AL, Morey MC, Wong TC et al. Diminished physical function in older HIV-infected adults in the Southeastern U.S. despite successful antiretroviral therapy. *PloS One*. 2017;12(6):e0179874.

Kim PS, Woods C, Georgoff P, et al. A1c underestimates glycemia in HIV infection. *Diabetes Care*. 2009;32(9):1591–1593.

Koutkia P, Meininger G, Canavan B, et al. Metabolic regulation of growth hormone by free fatty acids, somatostatin, and ghrelin in HIV-lipodystrophy. *Am J Physiol Endocrinol Metab*. 2004;286(2):E296–E303.

Kuhn T, Jin Y, Huang C, et al. The joint effect of aging and HIV infection on microstructure of white matter bundles. *Hum Brain Mapp*. 2019;40(15):4370–4380.

Mack KA, Ory MG. AIDS and older Americans at the end of the twentieth century. *J AIDS*. 2003;33(Suppl 2):S68–S75.

Madeddu G, Spanu A, Chessa F, et al. Thyroid function in human immunodeficiency virus patients treated with highly active antiretroviral therapy (HAART): a longitudinal study. *Clin Endocrinol*. 2006;64(4):375–383.

Mallon PW, Unemori P, Sedwell R, et al. In vivo, nucleoside reverse-transcriptase inhibitors alter expression of both mitochondrial and lipid metabolism genes in the absence of depletion of mitochondrial DNA. *J Infect Dis*. 2005;191(10):1686–1696.

Manfredi R, Calza L, Chiodo F. Gynecomastia associated with highly active antiretroviral therapy. *Ann Pharmacother*. 2001;35(4):438–439.

Manfredi R, Calza L, Chiodo F. Another emerging event occurring during HIV infection treated with any antiretroviral therapy: frequency and role of gynecomastia. *Infez Med*. 2004;12(1):51–59.

Mathabire Rücker SC, Tayea A, Bitilinyu-Bangoh J, et al. High rates of hypertension, diabetes, elevated low-density lipoprotein cholesterol, and cardiovascular disease risk factors in HIV-positive patients in Malawi. *AIDS*. 2018;32(2):253–260.

McDonald P, Moyo S, Gabaitiri L, et al. Persistently elevated serum interleukin-6 predicts mortality among adults receiving combination antiretroviral therapy in Botswana: results from a clinical trial. *AIDS Res Hum Retroviruses*. 2013;29(7):993–999.

Membreno L, Irony I, Dere W, et al. Adrenocortical function in acquired immunodeficiency syndrome. *J Clin Endocrinol Metab*. 1987;65:482–487.

Merrill JE, Koyanagi Y, Chen ISY. Interleukin-1 and tumor necrosis factor α can be induced from mononuclear phagocytes by human immunodeficiency virus type 1 binding to the CD4 receptor. *J Virol*. 1989;63:4404–4408.

Meyer WJ, Smith EM, Richards GE, et al. In vivo immunoreactive adrenocorticotropin (ACTH) production by human mononuclear leukocytes from normal and ACTH-deficient individuals. *J Clin Endocrinol Metab*. 1987;64:98–105.

Minami R, Yamamoto M, Takahama S, et al. Comparison of the influence of four classes of HIV antiretrovirals on adipogenic differentiation: the minimal effect of raltegravir and atazanavir. *J Infect Chemother*. 2011;17(2):183–188.

Mishriki YY. A baffling case of bulging belly: protease paunch. *Postgrad Med*. 1998;104(3):45–46.

Monczor AN, Li X, Palella FJ Jr, et al. Systemic inflammation characterizes lack of metabolic health in nonobese HIV-infected men. *Mediators Inflamm*. 2018;2018:5327361.

Morse CG, McLaughlin M, Matthews L, et al. Nonalcoholic steatohepatitis and hepatic fibrosis in HIV-1-monoinfected adults with elevated aminotransferase levels on antiretroviral therapy. *Clin Infect Dis*. 2015;60(10):1569–1578.

Mueller NJ, Fux CA, Ledergerber B, et al. High prevalence of severe vitamin D deficiency in combined antiretroviral therapy-naive and successfully treated Swiss HIV patients. *AIDS*. 2010;24:1127.

Murata H, Hruz PW, Mueckler M. The mechanism of insulin resistance caused by HIV protease inhibitor therapy. *J Biol Chem*. 2000;275:20251–20254.

Mylonakis E, Koutkia P, Grinspoon S. Diagnosis and treatment of androgen deficiency in human immunodeficiency virus-infected men and women. *Clin Infect Dis*. 2001;33:857–864.

Nduka CU, Stranges S, Kimani PK, et al. Is there sufficient evidence for a causal association between antiretroviral therapy and diabetes in HIV patients? A meta-analysis. *Diabetes Metab Res Rev*. 2017;33(6):e2902.

Nguyen D, Hsu JW, Jahoor F, et al. Effect of increasing glutathione with cysteine and glycine supplementation on mitochondrial fuel oxidation, insulin sensitivity, and body composition in older HIV-infected patients. *J Clin Endocrinol Metab*. 2014;99(1):169–177.

Nguyen D, Samson SL, Reddy VT, et al. Impaired mitochondrial fatty acid oxidation and insulin resistance in aging: a novel protective role of glutathione. *Aging Cell*. 2013;12(3):415–425.

Noe S, Oldenbuettel C, Heldwein S, et al. Secondary hyperparathyroidism in patients in Central Europe. *Horm Metab Res*. 2018;50(4):317–324.

Norbiato G, Bevilacqua M, Vago T, et al. Glucocorticoids and interferon-alpha in the acquired immunodeficiency syndrome. *J Clin Endocrinol Metab*. 1996;81:2601–2606.

Nylén H, Habtewold A, Makonnen E, et al. Prevalence and risk factors for efavirenz-based antiretroviral treatment-associated severe vitamin D deficiency: a prospective cohort study. *Medicine*. 2016;95(34):e4631.

Önen NF, Overton ET. A review of premature frailty in HIV-infected persons; another manifestation of HIV-related accelerated aging. *Curr Aging Sci*. 2011;4(1):33–41.

Padmapriyadarsini C, Ramesh Kumar S, Terrin N, et al. Dyslipidemia among HIV-infected patients with tuberculosis taking once-daily nonnucleoside reverse-transcriptase inhibitor-based antiretroviral therapy in India. *Clin Infect Dis*. 2011;52(4):540–546.

Palella FJ Jr., Delaney KM, Moorman AC, et al. Declining morbidity and mortality among patients with advanced human immunodeficiency virus infection. HIV Outpatient Study Investigators. *N Engl J Med*. 1998;338:853–860.

Parra A, Reyes-Terán G, Ramírez-Peredo J, et al. Differences in nocturnal basal and rhythmic prolactin secretion in untreated compared to treated HIV-infected men are associated with CD4+ T-lymphocytes. *Immunol Cell Biol*. 2004;82(1):24–31.

Payne BA, Wilson IJ, Hateley CA, et al. Mitochondrial aging is accelerated by anti-retroviral therapy through the clonal expansion of mtDNA mutations. *Nat Genet*. 2011;43(8):806–810.

Peyriere H, Mauboussin JM, Rouanet I, et al. Report of gynecomastia in five male patients during antiretroviral therapy for HIV infection. *AIDS*. 1999;13:2167–2169.

Pinto G, Blanche S, Thiriet I, et al. Growth hormone treatment of children with human immunodeficiency virus-associated growth failure. *Eur J Pediatr*. 2000;159:937–938.

Pommier JD, Laouenan C, Michard F, et al. Metabolic syndrome and endocrine status in HIV-infected transwomen. *AIDS*. 2019;33(5):855–865.

Quirino T, Bongiovanni M, Ricci E, et al. Hypothyroidism in HIV-infected patients who have or have not received HAART. *Clin Infect Dis*. 2004;38:596–597.

Rajasuriar R, Chong ML, Ahmad Bashah NS, et al. Major health impact of accelerated aging in young HIV-infected individuals on antiretroviral therapy. *AIDS*. 2017, 31(10):1393–1403.

Ram S, Acharya S, Fernando JJ, et al. Serum prolactin in HIV infection. *Clin Lab*. 2004;50:617–620.

Ratner Kaufman F, Gertner JM, Sleeper LA, et al. Growth hormone secretion in HIV-positive versus HIV-negative hemophilic males with abnormal growth and pubertal development. The Hemophilia Growth and Development Study. *J AIDS Hum Retrovirol*. 1997;15:137–144.

Rietschel P, Corcoran C, Stanley T, et al. Prevalence of hypogonadism among men with weight loss related to human immunodeficiency virus infection who were receiving highly active antiretroviral therapy. *Clin Infect Dis*. 2000;31:1240–1244.

Rondanelli M, Caselli D, Arico M, et al. Insulin-like growth factor 1 (IGF-1) and IGF-binding protein 3 response to growth hormone is impaired in HIV-infected children. *AIDS Res Hum Retroviruses*. 2002;18:331–339.

Saint-Marc T, Partisani M, Poizot-Martin I, et al. A syndrome of peripheral fat wasting (lipodystrophy) in patients receiving long-term nucleoside analogue therapy. *AIDS*. 1999;13(13):1659–1667.

Salim YS, Faber V, Wiik A, et al. Anticorticosteroid antibodies in AIDS patients. *APMIS*. 1988;96:889–894.

Samaras K, Pett S, Gowers A, et al. Iatrogenic Cushing's syndrome with osteoporosis and secondary adrenal failure in human immunodeficiency virus-infected patients receiving inhaled corticosteroids and ritonavir-boosted protease inhibitors: six cases. *J Clin Endocrinol Metab*. 2005;90(7):4394–4398.

Samaras K, Wand H, Law M, et al. Prevalence of metabolic syndrome in HIV infected using International Diabetes Foundation and Adult Treatment Panel III criteria: associations with insulin resistance, disturbed body fat compartmentalization, elevated C-reactive protein, and hypoadiponectinemia. *Diabetes Care*. 2007;30:113–119.

Schrack JA, Althoff KN, Jacobson LP et al. Accelerated gait speed decline in HIV-infected men. *J AIDS*. 2015;70(4):370–376.

Sekhar RV, Jahoor F, White AC, et al. Metabolic basis of HIV-lipodystrophy syndrome. *Am J Physiol Endocrinol Metab*. 2002;283(2):E332–E337.

Sekhar RV, Liu CW, Rice S. Increasing glutathione concentrations with cysteine and glycine supplementation lowers inflammation in HIV patients. *AIDS*. 2015;29(14):1899–1900.

Shikuma CM, Hu N, Milne C, et al. Mitochondrial DNA decrease in subcutaneous adipose tissue of HIV-infected individuals with peripheral lipoatrophy. *AIDS*. 2001;15:1801–1809.

Silva GA, Andrade MC, Sugui Dde A, et al. Association between antiretrovirals and thyroid diseases: a cross-sectional study. *Arch Endocrinol Metab*. 2015;59(2):116–122.

Slama L, Palella FJ, Abraham AG, et al. Inaccuracy of haemoglobin A1c among HIV-infected men: effects of CD4 cell count, antiretroviral therapies and haematological parameters. *J Antimicrob Chemother*. 2014;69(12):2260–2267.

Sobieszczyk ME, Hoover DR, Anastos K, et al. Prevalence and predictors of metabolic syndrome among HIV-infected and HIV-uninfected women in the Women's Interagency HIV Study. *J AIDS*. 2008;48:272–280.

Stricker RB, Goldberg DA, Hu C, et al. A syndrome resembling primary aldosteronism (Conn syndrome) in untreated HIV disease. *AIDS*. 1999;13:1791–1792.

Szebeni J, Dieffenbach C, Wahl SM, et al. Induction of alpha interferon by human immunodeficiency virus type 1 in human monocyte–macrophage cultures. *J Virol*. 1991;65:6362–6364.

Tavares-Bello C, Sousa Santos F, Sequiera Duarte J, et al. Diabetes insipidus and hypopituitarism in HIV: an unexpected cause. *Endocrinol Diabetes Metab Case Rep*. 2017;2017:17–0024.

Theodorou M, Serté T, Van Gossum M, et al. Factors associated with vitamin D deficiency in a population of 2044 HIV-infected patients. *Clin Nutr*. 2014;33(2):274–279.

Toma E, Therrien R. Gynecomastia during indinavir antiretroviral therapy in HIV infection. *AIDS*. 1998;12:681–682.

Tracey KJ, Cerami A. Metabolic responses to cachectin/TNF: a brief review. *Ann N Y Acad Sci*. 1990;587:325–331.

Tzur F, Chowers M, Agmon-Levin N, et al. Increased prevalence of diabetes mellitus in a non-obese adult population: HIV-infected Ethiopians. *Isr Med Assoc J*. 2015;17(10):620–623.

Ukibe NR, Ukibe SN, Emelumadu OF, et al. Impact of thyroid function abnormalities on reproductive hormones during menstrual cycle in premenopausal HIV infected females at NAUTH, Nnewi, Nigeria. *PLoS One*. 2017;12(7):e0176361.

Van den Bout-Van Den Beukel C, Fievez L, Michels M, et al. Vitamin D deficiency among HIV type 1-infected individuals in the Netherlands: effects of antiretroviral therapy. *AIDS Res Hum Retrovir*. 2008;24:1375–1382.

Villette JM, Bourin P, Doinel C, et al. Circadian variations in plasma levels of hypophyseal, adrenocortical and testicular hormones in men infected with human immunodeficiency virus. *J Clin Endocrinol Metab*. 1990;70:572–577.

Vodkin I, Valasek MA, Bettencourt R, et al. Clinical, biochemical and histological differences between HIV-associated NAFLD and primary NAFLD: a case-control study. *Aliment Pharmacol Ther*. 2015;41(4):368–378.

Wang Y, Santerre M, Tempera I, et al. HIV-1 Vpr disrupts mitochondria axonal transport and accelerates neuronal aging. *Neuropharmacology*. 2017, 117:364–375.

Wanke CA, Silva M, Knox TA, et al. Weight loss and wasting remain common complications in individuals infected with human immunodeficiency virus in the era of highly active antiretroviral therapy. *Clin Infect Dis*. 2000;31:803.

Xiong Y, Hales DB. The role of the tumor necrosis factor-alpha in the regulation of mouse Leydig cell steroidogenesis. *Endocrinology*. 1993;132:2438–2444.

Yombi JC, Maiter D, Belkhir L, et al. Cushing's syndrome and secondary adrenal insufficiency after a single intra-articular administration of triamcinolone acetonide in HIV-infected patients treated with ritonavir. *Clin Rheumatol*. 2008;27(Suppl 2):S79–S82.

32.

NON-OPPORTUNISTIC INFECTIONS
RESPIRATORY COMPLICATIONS

Priyanka Chakrabarti

CHAPTER GOAL

Upon completion of this chapter, the reader should be able to:

- Demonstrate knowledge regarding the diagnosis and treatment of respiratory complications in people with HIV (PWH)

LEARNING OBJECTIVE

- Review and characterize the respiratory complications related to HIV infection to provide early and accurate diagnosis and treatment

KEY POINTS

NONSPECIFIC INTERSTITIAL PNEUMONITIS

- Nonspecific interstitial pneumonitis (NSIP) encompasses several lymphocytic pulmonary syndromes, including follicular bronchiolitis, lymphocytic bronchiolitis, lymphocytic interstitial pneumonitis (LIP), and diffuse infiltrative CD8+ lymphocytosis syndrome (DILS).
- PWH may be asymptomatic or present with dyspnea, nonproductive cough, and fever in a patient with CD4+ T-cell counts greater than 200 cells/mm³. X-ray findings are nonspecific but characteristically show bilateral reticulonodular "interstitial" infiltrates.
- The diagnosis of NSIP requires histologic confirmation by biopsy. The optimal treatment remains unclear.

LYMPHOCYTIC INTERSTITIAL PNEUMONITIS

- LIP is a common respiratory complication of HIV infection in children but a rare complication in adults with HIV.
- It presents with slowly progressive dyspnea and nonproductive cough. X-ray findings are nonspecific but characteristically show bilateral reticulonodular "interstitial" infiltrates with a basal lung predominance.
- The diagnosis requires histologic confirmation by biopsy. Antiretroviral therapy (ART) has been used with success for treatment.

PULMONARY ARTERIAL HYPERTENSION

- The prevalence of pulmonary arterial hypertension (PAH) is higher in PWH compared to the general population.
- The clinical presentation is like that in the general population, with progressive dyspnea, nonproductive cough, chest pain, and sometimes syncope or presyncope. These symptoms should prompt an evaluation for early diagnosis.
- The diagnosis is first suggested by a chest radiograph revealing prominent pulmonary arteries or by electrocardiography. Right heart catheterization is the standard of diagnosis.
- Potential therapies for HIV-associated PAH include ART, oxygen, diuretics, and directed therapy. Prostanoids (epoprostenol, treprostinil, and iloprost), endothelin receptor antagonists (bosentan), and phosphodiesterase-5 inhibitors (sildenafil) are used in persons with HIV-associated PAH and have improved mortality.

NONSPECIFIC INTERSTITIAL PNEUMONITIS

The prevalence of NSIP is unknown. It was found in 48% of asymptomatic PWH in the 1980s (Ognibene et al., 1988) and in 38% of PWH who had pulmonary symptoms or abnormal imaging studies (Suffredini et al., 1987). Different from LIP, it has been characterized only in adults and not in children.

The etiology of NSIP is unknown. Evidence suggests immune dysregulation may contribute, and thus the prevalence of NISP has declined with the use of combination ART (Collins et al., 2019). NISP encompasses several lymphocytic pulmonary syndromes in PWH: follicular bronchiolitis, lymphocytic bronchiolitis, LIP, and DILS. Histologically, it is characterized by the presence of perivascular and peribronchial interstitial lymphocytes, plasma cells, and macrophages; however, these are also found along the pleura and interlobar fibrous septa (Travis et al., 1992).

Clinical symptoms are minimal or nonexistent; dyspnea, nonproductive cough, and fever have been reported (Suffredini et al., 1987). Physical exam may reveal crackles. Imaging studies may be normal or may show diffuse interstitial infiltrates (reticular, reticulonodular, or alveolar). Pleural effusions may also be seen. High-resolution computed tomography (CT) is also unspecific. Ground-glass pattern, consolidations, and honeycombing have been described. Similar to LIP, spirometry typically shows decreased diffusing capacity. Definitive diagnosis is made by histologic confirmation. The treatment is unclear. It can remain stable for many years or regress on its own. Theoretically, ART may improve its symptoms, but there is no pathologic evidence to support this theory.

HIV LYMPHOCYTIC INTERSTITIAL PNEUMONITIS

LIP is a rare histopathologic disease that accounts for 40% of lung diseases in children with AIDS but only 1% or 2% of lung diseases in HIV-infected adults (Anderson & Lee, 1988; Stover et al., 1985).

Histologically, LIP is characterized by diffuse infiltration with polyclonal lymphocytes and occasionally plasma cells and histiocytes into the alveolar septa and along lymphatic vessels (Halprin et al., 1972). Type II pneumocyte hyperplasia and germinal centers within lymphoid follicles are commonly found. Biopsies show predominance of CD8$^+$ and CD20$^+$ cells. Fibrosis may develop in advanced cases.

Although the etiology of LIP is not clear, it has been suggested that Epstein–Barr virus (EBV) may play a role. EBV DNA samples have been found in fragments of lung tissues taken from children with LIP (Reddy et al., 1988). However, other studies have not shown any difference in the frequency of EBV in lung biopsies when comparing adult PWH with LIP and control groups (van Zyl-Smit et al., 2015). HIV itself may play a role in the pathology of LIP, as has been demonstrated in a transgenic mouse model in which HIV induced an LIP syndrome (Hanna et al., 1998). HIV RNA copies have been obtained in lung biopsy samples of PWH with LIP, and HIV-specific IgG is frequently present in the bronchoalveolar lavage fluid (Resnick et al., 1987). A predominant CD8$^+$ T-cell infiltrate was found on histology in PWH who had LIP (van Zyl-Smit et al., 2015). Human T-lymphotropic virus type I (HTLV-I) has been linked to LIP in Japan (Setoguchi et al., 1991).

The clinical presentation of LIP is similar in adults and children. Cough is the predominant symptom associated with slowly progressive dyspnea. Symptoms are usually present for several months. Fever, chest pain, weight loss, and arthralgias have also been reported. Physical exam may be completely normal or may reveal crackles. Children may have clubbing, salivary gland enlargement, lymphadenopathy, and hepatosplenomegaly.

Chest x-rays are normal or show bilateral reticular or nodular opacities. Focal areas of confluent pulmonary opacifications have been described as well as pulmonary cysts and patchy consolidations, the latter being less common. Chest CT shows diffuse ground-glass opacities with small nodules (2–3 mm) in a peribronchovascular distribution (Pitcher et al., 2010). Like other diffuse interstitial lung diseases, spirometry typically shows decreased total lung capacity and decreased diffusing capacity.

There is no consensus regarding the optimal treatment for LIP in PWH. Corticosteroids at a dosage of 1 mg/kg/day are recommended. However, in several case reports, ART has been demonstrated to be effective by itself (Garcia Lujan et al., 2004; Innes et al., 2004; Ripamonti et al., 2003).

DIFFUSE INFILTRATIVE CD8$^+$ LYMPHOCYTE SYNDROME

DILS is a rare multisystemic syndrome characterized by CD8$^+$ T-cell lymphocytosis associated with a CD8$^+$ T-cell infiltration of multiple organs. It is primarily characterized by parotid gland enlargement, xerophthalmia, xerostomia, and interstitial pneumonitis. Respiratory clinical manifestations include nonproductive cough and dyspnea. Diffuse lymphadenopathy, hepatosplenomegaly, lymphocytic gastritis, and seventh cranial nerve palsy have also been described.

Histologic examination demonstrates visceral lymphocytic infiltration that could be a direct consequence of the large amount of CD8$^+$ T cells. Lymphoid follicles with CD8$^+$ germinal centers are seen in salivary and parotid gland biopsies. HIV has been detected in macrophages within the germinal center of lymphoid tissues; therefore, ART plays a major role in treatment. Immunosuppression with steroids is also recommended,

PULMONARY ARTERIAL HYPERTENSION

PAH has a higher prevalence among PWH compared to the general population. It was reported to be 0.5% in 1991 (Speich et al., 1991) and remains the same in the combination ART era (Opravil & Sereni, 2008; Sitbon et al., 2008; Zuber et al., 2004).

The occurrence of PAH in PWH is not related to the CD4$^+$ T-cell count. No risk factors have been found. However, a small study reported that chronic hepatitis C, drug addiction, and female sex tripled the risk of developing PAH (Quezada et al., 2012). In a series that compared PAH in PWH and PAH in non–HIV-infected participants, PWH were significantly younger and had milder disease (50% vs. 75% had New York Heart Association functional class III or IV, respectively) (Petipretz et al., 1994).

The clinical presentation of PAH in PWH is similar to that of uninfected patients. PWH experience symptoms related to right heart dysfunction, such as progressive shortness of breath, pedal edema, nonproductive cough, fatigue, syncope, and chest pain. Physical exam may reveal increased intensity of the pulmonary second heart sound, third and fourth sound gallop, tricuspid and pulmonary regurgitation murmurs, elevated jugular venous pressure, and peripheral edema.

The diagnosis is usually made 6 months after the development of symptoms. Chest x-rays may show cardiomegaly and enlarged pulmonary artery, but clear lung fields. Transthoracic Doppler echocardiogram shows systolic flattening of the interventricular septum, enlargement of the right atrium and the right ventricle, and a reduction in both left ventricular systolic and left ventricular diastolic dimensions. It is important to note that a thorough evaluation should be done to exclude other causes of pulmonary hypertension.

Right heart catheterization is still the standard for diagnosing PAH and for assessing its severity and response to treatment. PAH is defined by an mean pulmonary arterial pressure (mPAP) of 25 mmHg or higher, a mean pulmonary capillary wedge pressure of 15 mmHg or less, and a normal or reduced cardiac output (Galie et al., 2009).

Treatment of HIV-associated PAH is similar to that of PAH in non–HIV-infected patients. Supportive therapy includes exercise, oxygen administration, diuretics, and digoxin. Oxygen is recommended if arterial blood oxygen pressure is 60 mmHg or less. Diuretics reduce the right ventricular preload and are recommended in PWH with right ventricular failure. The role of digoxin is controversial; however, it has been shown to improve cardiac output in PWH with acute right ventricular dysfunction attributable to PAH. PWH should be counseled against smoking and pregnancy. Anticoagulation is not routinely recommended in PWH as there is no direct evidence of its benefit. Similarly, calcium channel blockers are of limited efficacy as vasoreactivity has been shown in only a small number of persons. Although there is no conclusive evidence of the effect of ART on the progression of HIV-associated PAH, it is recommended to start ART in all PWH with PAH regardless of the CD4$^+$ T-cell count, as supported by current guidelines. ART has been demonstrated to cause improvements in pressure gradient over time and to significantly reduce the risk of death in HIV-associated PAH.

Specific therapy for PAH has also been evaluated in HIV-associated PAH. Although there are no controlled clinical trials, prostanoids (epoprostenol, treprostinil, and iloprost), endothelin receptor antagonists (bosentan), and phosphodiesterase-5 inhibitors (sildenafil) have been used in PWH with PAH and have been shown to improve symptoms and hemodynamic parameters. Caution should be taken with the use of these medications due to possible severe drug interactions, particularly with protease inhibitors and cobicistat.

PAH is an independent risk factor for death among PWH (Opravil & Sereni, 2008). However, with the advent of ART and the new treatment modalities, the overall survival rate is 88% at 1 year and 72% at 3 years (Degano et al., 2010).

REFERENCES

Anderson V, Lee H. Lymphocytic interstitial pneumonitis in pediatric AIDS. *Pediatr Pathol.* 1988;8:417–421.

Collins B, Mulhall P, Travaline J. Nonspecific interstitial pneumonia in a patient with HIV. *SN Comprehensive Clin Med.* 2019;1:203–204.

Degano B, Guillaume M, Savale L, et al. HIV-associated pulmonary arterial hypertension: survival and prognostic factors in the modern therapeutic era. *AIDS.* 2010;24:67–75

Galie N, Hoeper M, Humbert M. Guidelines for the diagnosis and treatment of pulmonary hypertension. *Eur Heart J.* 2009;30:2493–2537.

Garcia Lujan R, Echave-Sustaeta J, Garcia Quero C, et al. Lymphoid interstitial pneumonia resolved through antiretroviral therapy in an adult infected by human immunodeficiency virus. *Arch Bronconeumol.* 2004;40:537–539.

Halprin G, Ramirez J, Pratt O. Lymphoid interstitial pneumonia. *Chest.* 1972;62:418–423.

Hanna Z, Kay DG, Cool M, et al. Transgenic mice expressing human immunodeficiency virus type 1 in immune cells develop a severe AIDS-like disease. *J Virol.* 1998;72:121–132.

Innes A, Huang L, Nishimura S. Resolution of lymphocytic interstitial pneumonitis in an HIV infected adult after treatment with HAART. *Sex Transm Infect.* 2004;80:417–418.

Ognibene F, Masur H, Rogers P, et al. Nonspecific interstitial pneumonitis without evidence of *Pneumocystis carinii* in asymptomatic patients infected with human immunodeficiency virus (HIV). *Ann Intern Med.* 1988;109:874–879.

Opravil M, Sereni D. Natural history of HIV-associated pulmonary arterial hypertension: trends in the HAART era. *AIDS.* 2008;22:35–40.

Petipretz P, Brenot F, Azarian R. Pulmonary hypertension in patients with human immunodeficiency virus infection: comparison with primary pulmonary hypertension. *Circulation.* 1994;89:2722–2727.

Pitcher R, Beningfield S, Zar H. Chest radiographic features of lymphocytic pneumonitis in HIV-infected children. *Clin Radiol.* 2010;65:150–154.

Quezada M, Martin-Carbonero L, Soriano V, et al. Prevalence and risk factors associated with pulmonary hypertension in HIV-infected patients on regular follow-up. *AIDS.* 2012;26:1387–1392.

Reddy A, Lyall E, Crawford D. Epstein–Barr virus and lymphoid interstitial pneumonitis: an association revisited. *Pediatr Infect Dis J.* 1998;17:82–83.

Resnick L, Pitchenik A, Fisher E, et al. Detection of HTLVIII/LAV specific IgG and antigen in bronchoalveolar lavage fluid from two patients with lymphocytic interstitial pneumonitis associated with AIDS related complex. *Am J Med.* 1987;82:553–556.

Ripamonti D, Rizzi M, Maggiolo F, et al. Resolution of lymphocytic interstitial pneumonia in a human immunodeficiency virus infected adult following the start of highly antiretroviral therapy. *Scand J Infect Dis.* 2003;35:348–351.

Setoguchi Y, Takahashi S, Nukiwa T, et al. Detection of human T-cell lymphotropic virus type I-related antibodies in patients with lymphocytic interstitial pneumonia. *Am Rev Respir Dis.* 1991;144:1361–1365.

Sitbon O, Lascoux-Combe C, Delfraissy JF, et al. Prevalence of HIV-related pulmonary arterial hypertension in the current antiretroviral therapy era. *Am J Respir Crit Care Med.* 2008;177:108–113.

Speich R, Jenni R, Opravil M, et al. Primary pulmonary hypertension in HIV infection. *Chest.* 1991;100:1268–1271.

Stover D, White D, Romano P, et al. Spectrum of pulmonary diseases associated with the acquired immune deficiency syndrome. *Am J Med.* 1985;78:429–437.

Suffredini A, Ognibene F, Lack E, et al. Nonspecific interstitial pneumonitis: a common cause of pulmonary disease in the acquired immunodeficiency syndrome. *Ann Intern Med.* 1987;107:7–13.

Travis W, Fox C, Devaney K. Lymphoid pneumonitis in 50 adult patients infected with the human immunodeficiency virus: lymphocytic interstitial pneumonitis versus nonspecific interstitial pneumonitis. *Hum Pathol.* 1992;23:529–541.

van Zyl-Smit RN, Naidoo J, Wainwright H, et al. HIV-associated lymphocytic interstitial pneumonia: a clinical, histological and radiographic study from an HIV endemic resource-poor setting. *BMC Pulm Med.* 2015;15:38–44.

Zuber J, Calmy A, Evison J. Pulmonary arterial hypertension related to HIV infection improved hemodynamics and survival associated with antiretroviral therapy. *Clin Infect Dis.* 2004;38:1178–1185.

33.

PSYCHIATRIC ILLNESS AND TREATMENT IN HIV POPULATIONS

Elizabeth H. David and Erica Taylor

CHAPTER GOAL

Upon completion of this chapter, the reader should be able to:

- Discuss the psychiatric concomitants of HIV illness and the role of psychiatric care in the overall treatment of HIV populations

---

INTRODUCTION

From the earliest recognized AIDS deaths in 1981 to the commencement of combination antiretroviral therapy (ART) in the mid-1990s and the simpler combination ART regimens now available, HIV has remained a disease and an epidemic in constant evolution. For many years a near-certain death sentence, it has become a treatable chronic condition, with issues of HIV-associated dementia and rapid death by opportunistic infection generally replaced by treatment of "premature" aging and slow neurologic decline and questions of maximizing adherence to treatment. Issues that have not changed include the tremendous psychosocial burden to the individual and family and the economic cost to persons with HIV (PWH) and society, as well as factors of stigmatization and marginalization of HIV populations. Many HIV-positive individuals were already stigmatized before contracting this illness. The prevalence of HIV infection is much higher in gay/bi/transsexual populations, in people of color, in substance abusers, in prison populations, in the homeless, in individuals with histories of physical and emotional trauma, and in people with mental illness (Whetten et al., 2008). HIV infection then adds to the burden through the psychological manifestations it causes (demoralization, depression, mania, anxiety, insomnia, and neurocognitive deficits), through disturbances in appearance (wasting, lipodystrophy, and Kaposi's sarcoma) and function (kidney disease, diabetes, sexual dysfunction, and chronic pain), and through tremendous losses (people, independence, health, employment, and sense of control). From the earliest days of the epidemic, it has been recognized that mental illness and HIV infection are closely related (Hoffman, 1984), with some estimates of comorbidity as high as 50% to 70% (Blashill et al., 2011; Gaynes et al., 2008). Psychiatric illnesses are in and of themselves potentially lethal conditions, with increased rates of suicide and increased rates of illness and death from other conditions, including cancer, diabetes, and cardiovascular and cerebrovascular disease. They are associated with tremendous costs in terms of quality of life, lost productivity, and treatment. In combination with HIV-related illness, these issues are magnified.

Addressing these complex mental health issues is central to prevention, diagnosis, and treatment of HIV-related illness. Psychiatric illness is both a risk factor for disease and a barrier to adequate treatment. Substance abuse and "triple diagnosis" individuals (HIV, substance abuse, and mental illness) have been particularly problematic (see Chapter 26). The chronically mentally ill are both overrepresented in this population and more difficult to reach and treat due to homelessness, distrust, and the unstructured nature of their lives. Survivors of physical and emotional trauma are a group increasingly recognized as both vulnerable to HIV infection and difficult to treat. They are prone to risk behaviors but slow to establish trusting relationships with treaters. In addition to these issues of primary mental illness is the factor of secondary mental health problems—those caused by the virus and/or its treatment.

LEARNING OBJECTIVES

- Discuss the bidirectional causes of the close association between HIV infection and psychiatric illness/symptoms

- Recognize symptoms suggesting the presence of a psychiatric component to the clinical picture

- Describe general principles of treatment and when specific intervention by mental health professionals is advised

WHAT'S NEW?

This chapter has been updated to reflect terminology from the fifth edition of the *Diagnostic and Statistical Manual of Mental Disorders* (DSM-5; American Psychiatric Association, 2013), and additional recommendations regarding in- and outpatient psychiatric consultation have been added. This chapter includes a section addressing PWH living through the COVID-19 pandemic.

MENTAL ILLNESS AND HIV INFECTION

The interaction between HIV and mental illness is complex. For many individuals, the psychiatric condition is a preexisting one, predisposing to HIV infection through behavioral factors and risk environment (Meade 2012; Prince et al., 2012; Rhodes, 2002). The risk factors for HIV are well established and involve blood/bodily fluid contact with infected individuals through unprotected sexual behaviors, needle sharing, multiple sexual partners, and fetal/natal exposure. Individuals with preexisting psychiatric illness often engage in risky behaviors with little thought or fear of consequences. This relates to increased emotional immaturity and impulsivity (bipolar disorder, personality disorders, anxiety conditions, and posttraumatic stress disorder [PTSD]), poor contact with reality (schizophrenia and other psychotic conditions), denial and disinhibition (substance use disorders), cognitive dysfunction (major neurocognitive disorders and dementia), active thoughts of self-harm (depression), and victimization or impaired judgment (Kent et al., 2011; Owe-Larssom et al., 2009). Barriers to treatment, such as distrust of authority (including fear of legal consequences), poor communication skills, limited access (financial and transportation), lack of motivation, and unstructured lifestyle, all result in poor overall health care and delayed diagnosis of all health issues. Diagnosis of mental health issues is frequently challenging, and adherence to treatment is frequently impacted by these same factors.

Even for PWH without psychiatric illness, the diagnosis of serious medical illness is a significant emotional blow. Freud (1910) stated that emotional health involves the ability to integrate and balance aspects of love, work, and play. What could more thoroughly disrupt this balance and integration than an illness such as HIV, with so many devastating consequences, such as a complex regimen of treatment and so many far-reaching biological, psychological, and social consequences? Every day, every pill, every medical visit, and every secret kept from family, friends, and coworkers is a reminder that one is compromised, vulnerable, damaged, not normal. In her landmark work, Kubler-Ross (1969) discussed this trauma and the individual's response to it through repetitive processes of denial, anger, bargaining, and depression before (ideally) reaching a degree of acceptance. Treaters see the negative aspect of this emotional upheaval in its behavioral correlates: unrealistic anger at medical staff, equally unrealistic expectations of outcomes, guilt, fear, increased substance use, demoralization/hopelessness/amotivation, poor adherence to treatment, suicidal thoughts/suicide, and helplessness/neediness. We can help through building a positive and supportive treatment alliance that facilitates communication, acknowledges the huge cost to the individual, tolerates some of the stress behaviors, and does not take these behaviors personally but also sets limits of appropriateness. Timely referral to a psychiatrist or a psychotherapist is essential when stress becomes distress and behavior goes beyond those limits of appropriateness or when the person becomes dangerous to him- or herself or others.

HIV enters the central nervous system (CNS) very early in the course of systemic infection, and the brain becomes an important site of damage in PWH (Ho et al., 1985). This causes many of those infected to develop neurologic and psychological symptoms with etiology posited to relate to functional disturbances in inflammatory processes. Activated circulating monocytes introduce the virus across the blood–brain barrier, and CNS macrophages, microglia, and astrocytes each become infected, releasing cytokines and chemokines that lead to neuronal cell damage (Williams et al., 2014). Evidence also suggests a disturbance in glutamate functioning within the CNS, with increased extracellular glutamate leading to excitotoxicity (Vazquez-Santiago et al., 2014). Accelerated aging from HIV infection and HIV treatments, damage caused by opportunistic infections or comorbid medical conditions (e.g., hepatitis C virus), and concomitant use of drugs of abuse (Gannon et al., 2011) also play important roles. AIDS mania and a continuum of neurocognitive deficits from very subtle to frank and debilitating dementia are well-defined psychiatric syndromes directly related to the presence of virus, but depression, insomnia, and anxiety are also among the mental health symptoms that result from the infection itself. This part of disease progression seems to be less amenable to ART compared to the more peripheral manifestations (Heaton et al., 2010), although antiretrovirals (ARVs) with higher levels of CNS penetration may promote improvement in some functions (Cysique et al., 2004). Unfortunately, those agents capable of crossing the blood–brain barrier are also the medications most likely to have psychiatric symptomatology as a side effect of use—a Pyrrhic victory in many ways.

Regardless of etiology, the presence of psychiatric symptoms and substance abuse is associated with poorer outcomes in HIV illness—lower levels of treatment adherence, slower virologic suppression, decreased subjective quality of life, increased morbidity and mortality, and increased utilization of medical services (Blashill et al., 2011; Carrico et al., 2011; Leserman, 2008; Nel & Kagee, 2011; Pence et al., 2007). Adequate treatment of the psychiatric illness, however, improves outcome across all categories (Cook et al., 2006; Horberg et al., 2008; Mellins et al., 2009; Walkup et al., 2008). Although most of the literature cited in this chapter relates to adult PWH, the diagnostic descriptions and treatments can, for the most part, be applied to adolescents and children (Benton, 2010; Rao et al., 2007).

PSYCHIATRIC DISORDERS AND TREATMENT

Careful diagnosis is essential given the complex interaction among psychiatric illness, HIV infection, substance abuse, comorbid medical conditions, and side effects of medications. Psychiatric illness cannot be diagnosed if these other medical factors play the primary role in causing symptoms (i.e., delirium), and psychiatric medications will seldom be of benefit in those cases. The following brief descriptions are based on the criteria from DSM-5 (American Psychiatric Association, 2013). The context of HIV infection results in no appreciable changes from the usual clinical manifestations of psychiatric disorders, with the possible exception of AIDS mania. Equally, pharmacologic and nonpharmacologic approaches to the treatment of psychiatric illness in the context of HIV illness are not radically different from those in HIV-negative populations. PWH do seem to have some increased sensitivity to the side effects of antipsychotic drugs, even absent of ART (Hriso et al., 1991; Kelly et al., 2002; Ramachandran et al., 1997). Because many psychopharmacologic agents are metabolized by the same elements of the cytochrome P450 isoenzyme system that metabolize protease inhibitors (PIs) and nonnucleoside/nucleotide reverse transcriptase inhibitors (NNRTIs), there were many fears early on that they could not be used concomitantly. In fact, however, there are surprisingly few clinically significant interactions except as specifically noted in the following sections. As in all clinical situations, however, a "start low and go slow" philosophy is warranted, and the relative risks and benefits of treatment must be carefully weighed.

STRESS AND ADJUSTMENT DISORDERS

There are multiple stressors associated with living with a serious and debilitating illness. Some kinds of emotional and behavioral reactions to this stress are normal and short-lived and do not require treatment beyond support, reassurance, education, and therapeutic optimism. Assistance with access to resources and support networks or with informing family or significant others of the diagnosis can be "curative." Such reactions typically occur immediately after diagnosis and at periods of acute change in the illness (opportunistic infections, deteriorating CD4+/viral load indices, initiation of ART, and onset of other comorbid medical complications) or in social circumstances (loss and financial problems). Typically, individuals with these acute stress reactions are able to attribute the onset and nature of their symptoms to specific life events. They can also be distracted from their emotions and symptoms and are capable of feeling pleasure and interest in other things. *Adjustment reactions* (normal responses to stressful circumstances) are typically treated with supportive counseling and psychotherapy. It is only when stress reactions—anger, worry, guilt, sadness, and insomnia—are sustained for months, reach a point that they interfere with normal life functioning, or actually threaten survival (substance abuse, high-risk activities, and self-destructive thoughts/behaviors) that they require intervention. *Adjustment disorders* may also respond to support and psychotherapy, but they may necessitate psychiatric medications and/or hospital admission. The specific medication used depends on the symptoms being manifested. A complex of sadness, guilt, and insomnia frequently responds to use of antidepressants, particularly the more sedating ones (sertraline and mirtazapine). Symptoms on the anxiety continuum may benefit from use of almost any medication with a sedating side effect. Low-dose trazodone or antihistamine (hydroxyzine or diphenhydramine are commonly used) can be helpful, although caution must be used because these agents tend to cause drying of mucous membranes, which can exacerbate oral thrush. Antihistamines

should be used in caution in elderly PWH and those with dementia as these medications can increase the risk of delirium in these populations. The use of benzodiazepines is rarely indicated (see later discussion). Because of the known relationship between stress and compromised immune function, early appropriate intervention is important (Leserman, 2008).

ANXIETY DISORDERS AND PTSD

This group of illnesses includes generalized anxiety disorder (persistent feelings of anxiety), the phobias (irrational fear of a particular thing or behavior), panic disorder (spontaneous attacks of intense anxiety), and obsessive–compulsive disorder (intrusive anxiety-provoking thoughts that compel ritualized behaviors thought to alleviate that anxiety). PTSD (anxiety-related thoughts and behaviors connected to memories of past traumatic life experiences) was formerly included in this group, but it has been separated into its own category in DMS-5. All involve activation of the sympathetic nervous system (psychological and physiologic fight–flight–freeze responses) in situationally inappropriate circumstances because there is no current emergency. Careful diagnosis requires that endocrine disorders (especially thyroid-related), substance use (including caffeine, steroids, and psychostimulants), agitated depression, dementia, and delirium be eliminated as primary etiologic factors. PWH have rates of anxiety disorders greater than those of the general population (Gaynes et al., 2008; Klinkenberg & Dacks, 2004; Martinez et al., 2002) as well as an increased incidence of past traumatic experiences (Pence et al., 2009). Treatment ideally consists of a combination of psychotherapy (supportive, interpersonal, mindfulness, cognitive–behavioral, biofeedback, exposure and response prevention, flooding, etc.) and psychopharmacotherapy with antidepressants and/or anti-anxiety agents. Because therapeutic benefit with antidepressants is delayed in onset, it may be useful to supplement early treatment with low-dose benzodiazepine—lorazepam or another short-acting agent for panic disorder or phobias (used as needed at onset of panic attack or exposure to phobic object, but no more than three or four times a day) and clonazepam or another long-acting medication for generalized anxiety. Benzodiazepines are rarely the regimen of choice for more than the first 2 to 4 weeks, however, and should be discontinued at the earliest time practical. Some alternative treatments have also been shown to be effective, including relaxation/meditation, breath training, acupuncture, and guided imagery. All of the antidepressants except bupropion have efficacy in anxiety disorders, and selection of a specific medication should be based on safety (the serotonin and serotonin/norepinephrine reuptake inhibitors [SNRIs] are overall much safer than tricyclics or monoamine oxidase inhibitors [MAOIs]), side-effect profile (relative sedation vs. excitation, potential for gastric symptoms, appetite stimulation vs. suppression, anticholinergic effects, concerns for liver function, assistance with pain control, etc.), and past response to medications in the PWH or a family member. The selective serotonin reuptake inhibitors (SSRIs) can increase dream and flashback symptoms in individuals with past traumatic experiences, although small doses of prazosin can mitigate this effect. As noted previously, antianxiety agents include benzodiazepines, antihistamines, buspirone, and small doses of antidepressants (e.g., trazodone) or atypical antipsychotics (e.g., quetiapine [Seroquel]—an off-label use). All except buspirone work by sedating the individual, and they can be taken at the onset of anxiety symptoms. (Buspirone, like the antidepressants, must be taken on a regular basis to be effective.) The benzodiazepines also disinhibit behaviors, cause various degrees of cognitive impairment including amnesia and motor slowing/incoordination (a serious issue in a population already at risk for neurocognitive impairment), increase the risk of falls, and can trigger relapse or increased substance use in individuals with substance abuse problems. They are meant for temporary use only and can usually be discontinued when the antidepressants have become effective (2–4 weeks). A consensus survey of psychiatrists treating PWH revealed clonazepam to be the most frequently used benzodiazepine, followed by lorazepam (Freudenreich et al., 2010). Alprazolam, midazolam, and triazolam should be avoided due to their high potential for addiction and their adverse interactions with ARVs. Again, the byword for concomitant use of any psychopharmacologic agent with an ARV is "start low and go slow."

AFFECTIVE DISORDERS

Disorders of mood, particularly depression, are the most common psychiatric manifestations of HIV disease, with rates much higher in PWH than in the general population (Berger-Greenstein et al., 2007; Gaynes et al., 2011; Treisman & Angelinno, 2007) and increasing frequency with advancing disease (Atkinson et al., 2008). Depression hinders treatment of PWH, thus increasing risk of disease progression and spread (Benton, 2008; Villes et al., 2007), and it may have direct effects on immune responses (Alciati et al., 2007). Risk of suicidal ideation and attempts is significantly increased (Fermamdez et al., 2006), as is successful suicide (Carrico, 2010). Adequate treatment, however, reverses all these trends for both depression (Horberg et al., 2008; Mellins et al., 2009; Walkup et al., 2008) and bipolar disorder (Walkup et al., 2011).

Major depression consists of a constellation of symptoms related to persistent low mood (crying spells, guilt, low self-esteem, negative ruminations, social isolation, and loss of pleasure and interest), mental slowing (poor attention, concentration, memory, and energy; loss of libido; and motor retardation), and changes in behavior (increased or decreased sleep or appetite). Those with severe illness may also have psychotic symptoms (hallucinations and delusions), usually with depressive content. Careful diagnosis is essential because many of these symptoms might also be caused by serious medical illness, major neurocognitive impairment (dementia and delirium), side effects of medications, substance abuse, or grief and loss. Unlike adjustment disorders, individuals with major depression generally cannot cite a precipitating event nor be distracted from their negative emotions. It is the relentless nature of the symptoms that results in a sense of hopelessness and despair, with a progressive narrowing of emotional focus until it may seem that death (suicide) is the only way out.

Treatment ideally consists of combined psychotherapy and psychopharmacology with antidepressant medications, sometimes adding augmenting agents (a second antidepressant from another class, lithium, testosterone, thyroid medications, psychostimulants, and mood stabilizers). Low doses of antipsychotics are indicated on a temporary basis if psychotic features are present. Ketamine in very low doses is being used in some centers, but it must be used with extreme caution in PWH on ART. Replicated evidence has shown psychotherapeutic interventions (such as cognitive–behavioral therapy, stress management interventions and supportive therapy) have moderate antidepressant effects on PWH (van Luenen et al., 2018). Alternative treatments including exercise, meditation/relaxation, acupuncture, and herbal medications have been found to be helpful. Individuals on St. John's wort should be cautioned, however, because this popular herbal antidepressant has significant adverse clinical interactions with multiple ARVs, anticancer drugs, anti-inflammatory agents, antibiotics, psychopharmacologic agents, cardiovascular drugs, anti-hypoglycemics, oral contraceptives, proton pump inhibitors, statins, and anti-asthmatic medications (Nicolussi et al., 2019). All of the normal antidepressant drugs show efficacy in the HIV-positive population, and choice of a particular medication should be based on safety (Watkins et al., 2011), side-effect profile, and past response to medications in the PWH or a family member. A consensus study revealed that the SSRIs are the most common first-line drugs, with citalopram the number-one choice (Freudenreich et al., 2010), although this may be changing with newer US Food and Drug Administration (FDA) warnings about QT prolongation caused by this medication in higher doses. The SSRIs do have an anticoagulant effect, and used in the long term they can result in significant decreases in bone density. They can also cause bruxism and extrapyramidal side effects as well as sexual dysfunction. Switching drugs within a pharmacologic class is of benefit if individuals find specific side effects intolerable. If a medication in any given class of antidepressants fails to show therapeutic benefit (8- to 12-week trial of adequate doses), a switch to another class of drugs is advised because agents within any given class have similar efficacy (Warden & Rush, 2007), so a switch to an SNRI (venlafaxine and duloxetine) and then to bupropion is a useful algorithm when there is treatment failure (Freudenreich et al., 2010). Particular caution is suggested in using bupropion (either as an antidepressant or in smoking cessation) in combination with the PIs (especially saquinavir or indinavir) or NNRTIs (especially efavirenz) because metabolism of bupropion can be inhibited, thus increasing the risk of seizures. Lopinavir/ ritonavir, on the other hand, increases metabolism of bupropion, so bupropion doses must be increased when used with this ARV combination (Hogeland et al., 2007). Mirtazapine can be particularly useful for those with chronic pain, weight loss, nausea, and vomiting (especially from chemotherapy regimens). MAOIs are not generally used in this population, and they are contraindicated for concomitant use with other antidepressants and most antipsychotics. Of note, the antibiotic linezolid is also an MAOI.

All antidepressant regimens take several weeks to have therapeutic benefit, and the symptoms may not all resolve simultaneously. For this reason, particular caution and close observation are warranted in the early weeks of treatment: if energy, motivation, and a sense of agency return before suicidal thoughts and impulses disappear, a person who has had suicidal thoughts but insufficient energy to act on them may suddenly find the energy to act. The use of antidepressants in children and younger adolescents is particularly fraught with the danger of suicide, and most antidepressant medications now carry a "black box" warning for this population. Inpatient psychiatric treatment is necessary if there are questions of safety, and this is obviously a situation in which it is best to err on the side of caution. Duration of treatment is a significant question. In the general population, an individual with a single episode of depression is generally treated for 4 to 6 months, whereas individuals with more than two episodes receive protracted therapy with antidepressants. Because of concurrent medical illnesses, stress, and the propensity for HIV virus to cause/exacerbate affective symptoms, long-term use of antidepressants is frequently necessary.

Bipolar disorder is defined by intermittent episodes of low (depressive) and high (hypomanic or manic) moods, each lasting days, weeks, or months and in a continuum of severity from mild to disabling. These mood swings are not a reaction to life events. The lows are identical to the depressive episodes described previously. The high episodes consist of persistent elevated mood tone (euphoric or irritable), increased energy (racing thoughts that bounce from topic to topic, little need for sleep, rapid speech, and increased libido), and an inflated sense of self-worth, and they often lead to engaging in risky behaviors. In mania, there can be frank psychosis, with delusions (usually grandiose), disorganized thinking, and hallucinations leading to severe impairment in functioning and judgment. Bipolar disorder occurs at higher rates among PWH than in the general population (DeSousa Gurgel et al., 2013). Psychopharmacologic treatment consists of mood stabilizer medications (lithium, valproic acid, carbamazepine, lamotrigine, and "second-generation" antipsychotic medications), with antidepressants and antipsychotics added if these symptoms are prominent. Some clinicians believe that a long-acting benzodiazepine can be helpful in the first days of treatment for active mania, but these agents can further disinhibit and should be used only on a short-term basis. All of these medications are effective and reasonably safe in HIV populations. Lithium has a very narrow window of safety, and it is eliminated by the kidney. Particular caution is necessary in individuals with kidney dysfunction, diarrhea, electrolyte disturbances, or cognitive impairment, but there are no specific interactions with ARVs. Lithium can cause or exacerbate thyroid dysfunction, tremor, acne, and psoriasis. Valproic acid appears to have few clinically significant drug interactions with ARVs. However, it is metabolized by the liver, and it can increase liver enzymes and cause ammonemia. In addition, there is risk of severe hepatitis, weight gain, thrombocytopenia, nystagmus, and tremor. The use of carbamazepine is more complicated: it is metabolized by the cytochrome P450 system, and it induces its own metabolism. There have been reports of clinically significant carbamazepine toxicity when used in combination with ritonavir and other potent CYP3A4 inhibitors and also of virologic failure caused by enzyme induction (Liedtke et al., 2004). In addition, carbamazepine causes a significant risk for bone marrow suppression. Lamotrigine is effective particularly for depressive symptoms and appears to be safe when used in combination with ART. Initiation and discontinuation of this agent must be managed very carefully due to the risk of life-threatening Stevens–Johnson syndrome. It should be remembered that use of antidepressants without a mood stabilizer in a bipolar person can trigger a manic episode.

AIDS mania is a specific manifestation of late-stage HIV infection, rarely seen in the combination ART era. The mood is more likely to be irritable, sullen, and withdrawn than euphoric and hypertalkative, and there is frequently no prior personal or family history of psychiatric illness. Otherwise, the symptoms are typical of mania. Episodes, however, tend to be protracted, frequently with a prodrome of progressive cognitive decline. Symptoms do not usually respond to the usual psychopharmacologic approaches, nor is there spontaneous remission if the condition is left untreated. The treatment of choice is initiation of aggressive ART.

PSYCHOTIC DISORDERS

The psychotic disorders are defined by loss of contact with reality (hallucinations and delusions) as well as by varying degrees of disorganized thinking and behavior. Insight and judgment are often compromised, and it is frequently difficult to communicate clearly with these individuals because they can seem lost in their own, sometimes quite bizarre, world. Symptoms can be present on a temporary/episodic basis (brief psychotic episode and schizophreniform disorder) or may be more chronic (schizophrenia). Although disruptions of thinking and behavior are most typical, any psychotic illnesses may involve some affective symptoms, even if only because the person recognizes that they are somehow different from others. When symptoms of an emotional nature (depression or excitation) are a prominent and invariant part of the psychosis, schizoaffective disorder must be considered. Differential diagnosis includes affective disorder with psychotic features, medical illness (psychosis secondary to a medical condition such as HIV), side effects of medications, delirium/dementia, and substance abuse. Initial medical workup of anyone with a new-onset psychosis should probably include a urine drug screen (although many of the newer synthetic substances do not appear on standard tests), serology, endocrine screen, liver function tests, and computed tomography and/or magnetic resonance imaging of the brain. Visual hallucinations are rare in primary psychiatric illness, and they should also prompt a more complete medical evaluation. The chronically mentally ill are at increased risk of exposure to HIV due to factors such as homelessness, poor insight/judgment, lack of knowledge, victimization, and increased rates of substance abuse and other high-risk behaviors (Prince et al., 2012). Without adequate psychiatric treatment, their psychosis is a serious barrier to medical treatment due to poor adherence, difficulties communicating with providers, and unstable lifestyle (Carrico et al., 2011).

Treatment consists of control of symptoms with medications along with psychosocial support. All the antipsychotic medications work in PWH. As previously noted, PWH, even without ART, seem to be somewhat more sensitive to the dopamine-mediated extrapyramidal side effects of these drugs. These side effects are most common with the high-potency first-generation antipsychotics (i.e., haloperidol and fluphenazine). Both the first-generation and newer antipsychotics have significant risk for metabolic, cardiac (prolonged QT intervals), and endocrine side effects, and all are metabolized by the liver. They do not seem to have clinically significant interactions with ARVs, with the possible exception of lurasidone, but the issue of QT prolongation should be closely monitored because some of the ARVs also have this side effect. In the consensus survey, quetiapine was the most used agent for psychosis, perhaps because it is also useful in mood stabilization and sedation (Freudenreich et al., 2010). A recent meta-analysis also revealed that quetiapine is the safest of the antipsychotic drugs to use for psychosis and behavioral control in individuals with dementia (Kales et al., 2012). Clozapine and the low-potency first-generation medications (chlorpromazine and thioridazine) are seldom used (Freudenreich et al., 2010), although certainly not contraindicated. Use of depot injections tends to result in fewer side effects than seen with daily oral formulations and can be particularly useful in individuals for whom compliance with antipsychotic medication is problematic. It is safest, however, to initiate treatment with oral medication and then switch to the long-acting forms later.

PERSONALITY DISORDERS AND THE DIFFICULT-TO-TREAT PWH

Personality can be thought of as enduring patterns of behavior, and this is partly what we refer to when we say we "know" a person—he or she has somewhat predictable responses to given circumstances, a familiar emotional tone, consistent belief systems, and a well-formed sense of identity and agency. When these patterns are stable and healthy, one's responses to adversity (coping techniques) help to mitigate stress, and one can modulate emotional responses to fit the circumstances, thus maintaining a stable sense of self and other and control over one's world. In personality disorders, an individual is stuck in repetitive patterns that do not work: coping techniques that actually escalate stressful situations, relationship paradigms that result in little perceived support and an increasing sense of frustration by and with others, spiraling loss of emotional control, and, ultimately, the fearful recognition that one is out of control of both internal and external worlds. Borderline and antisocial personality disorders are common in HIV-positive populations because these individuals tend to engage in high-risk behaviors that expose them to contracting the virus. The presence of these character pathologies also complicates treatment adherence (Gilchrist et al.,

2011; Hansen et al., 2009). They tend to be easily frustrated, to expect immediate gratification, to want sure-fire/magical interventions, and to demand "special" treatment from everybody. They also challenge authority and have limited ability to structure their own lives adequately and consistently. As difficult and challenging as it can be to work with these individuals, it is important to remember that their behavior is not intentional—it is their best effort to adjust to and control their chaotic world (Groves, 1978). Frequently, the emotions they engender in others are only reflections of the emotional turmoil within themselves.

These are individuals for whom referral to psychotherapy and the presence of a strong, consistent treatment team with a clearly delineated treatment contract are essential to preserve coherent participation in medical care. Because their psychological symptoms tend to be so reactive to events in the environment, switching rapidly and wildly, caution should be used in initiating medications. Although consistent use of an SSRI or a mood stabilizer may be useful, chasing symptoms with medications is contraindicated. It is generally much more useful to help these individuals understand that their problems may be related to their own patterns of response and poor behavioral choices than to teach them that medication is going to provide them with internal peace or a sense of purpose, meaning, security, and attachment.

SUBSTANCE USE DISORDERS

For a full discussion of this topic, see Chapter 26. Suffice it to say here that concurrent substance abuse complicates diagnosis and treatment of all other psychiatric conditions as well as HIV-related illnesses. These complications, as well as problems with adherence to treatment and overall morbidity and mortality, are additive in nature. It is essential to good treatment of HIV illness that clinicians screen for substance abuse and address it consistently and aggressively.

MAJOR NEUROCOGNITIVE DISORDERS (DELIRIUM AND DEMENTIA)

HIV infection is associated with a number of CNS complications that may be temporary (delirium) or permanent (the continuum of neurocognitive deficits from asymptomatic to frank dementia).

Dementia is a common manifestation of HIV illness, and it is discussed in Chapter 34.

Delirium is a potentially life-threatening medical condition, generally of sudden and rapid onset and pursuing a waxing-and-waning course. Also referred to as *encephalopathy*, delirium is the most common neuropsychiatric diagnosis in hospitalized or critically ill PWH, with an estimated frequency of 40% to 65% (Gallago et al., 2011). It can manifest with any psychiatric symptom (anxiety, depression, mania, and psychosis) but most frequently includes disturbances in orientation, awareness/alertness, reality testing (hallucinations, including visual—which are very unusual in primary psychiatric conditions), communication (mumbled, incoherent speech), and motor behavior (lethargy, agitation, and picking at skin/clothing/intravenous lines). Several screening tools are used to diagnose delirium, of which the Cognitive Assessment Measurement Scale (CAMS and CAMS-ICU) is probably the most thoroughly researched. Definitive treatment involves correction of the underlying medical condition (infection, electrolyte disturbance, medication side effect, endocrine imbalance, intoxication, etc.). *Temporary* use of low-dose antipsychotic medications can be helpful, but they should be tapered and discontinued as the delirium resolves. Avoid the use of any anticholinergic agents (particularly diphenhydramine and other antihistamines) and of antipsychotics with high anticholinergic side effects (chlorpromazine [Thorazine] and thioridazine). Olanzapine, a sedating antipsychotic, may help with agitation but has been reported to cause, exacerbate, and/or prolong delirium in some cases. Use of benzodiazepines is also generally counterproductive, with the obvious exception of delirium caused by alcohol or benzodiazepine withdrawal. Measures that improve the individual's connection with reality can be very helpful. These include constant soft lighting (shadows are often misperceived), quiet and soothing background noise, a visible clock and/or calendar in the room, a written list of names of nursing staff and others, and repeated self-introduction of caregivers and visitors.

SEXUAL DYSFUNCTION

Sexual dysfunctions are very common in HIV illness. Disorders of desire (hypoactive sexual desire disorder) may be almost universal in PWH and erectile dysfunction is very common in men with AIDS (Shindel et al., 2011). Although certainly related to stress, depression, and uncertainties about spreading the disease to sexual partners, it also seems that the virus itself, the myriad comorbid conditions (including hypogonadism, diabetes, and peripheral neuropathy), and the multiple medications used to treat all these conditions play a role (Collazos, 2007; Huntingdon et al., 2020; Moreno-Pérez et al., 2010; Scanavino, 2011).

Treatment, therefore, is obviously complex. To the degree that these disorders are due to secondary issues, efforts can be made to change those conditions. Depression, stress, and comorbid conditions can be treated, and sometimes medications can be changed, or doses modified, to minimize sexual side effects. Sexual counseling and therapy are helpful in teaching the PWH that sexual behavior and loving are not always about intercourse. Medications for erectile dysfunction (sildenafil, vardenafil, and tadalafil) can be used in this population, but doses must be reduced when given in the context of ART because metabolism is delayed. This obviously increases the probability of adverse side effects from the erectile dysfunction drugs, including visual changes, priapism, hypotension, and myocardial infarct. As with all medications, risks and benefits must be carefully weighed by the PWH and the clinician.

SLEEP DISTURBANCE

Insomnia is defined as difficulty initiating and/or maintaining sleep or overall non-restful sleep. It tends to impair daytime function, and it is even more common in PWH than in the general population. This condition has been linked to poor quality of life and nonadherence to treatment (Saberi et al., 2011). Stress and depression play a role in etiology, and some ARVs disrupt sleep continuity. Efavirenz, a medication from the NNRTI class, is most consistently associated with sleep disturbances, including delayed sleep initiation, impaired sleep maintenance, and vivid nightmares. However, it appears that insomnia may be a primary symptom of viral presence, with changes in sleep architecture and decreased sleep efficiency noted even prior to onset of any symptoms of HIV/AIDS (Norman et al., 1992).

Pharmacologic treatment of insomnia includes the use of benzodiazepines, nonbenzodiazepine hypnotics, antihistamines, antidepressants, and antipsychotics. Of the benzodiazepines, clonazepam, lorazepam, oxazepam, and temazepam are relatively safe, although, as previously noted, their use in individuals with current or past substance abuse is problematic. Use of alprazolam, flurazepam, quazepam, and triazolam is contraindicated with ARVs and ketoconazole and also in those with kidney or hepatic disease. Sustained use of benzodiazepine medications is rarely, if ever, indicated. All of the nonbenzodiazepine hypnotics (eszopiclone, zaleplon, and zolpidem) are relatively safe in HIV populations, although dosages of zolpidem should be reduced if used with PIs, even in boosting dosages. Dosages of all nonbenzodiazepine hypnotics should also be reduced in those with hepatic disease. Antihistamines (especially diphenhydramine and hydroxyzine) are typically effective, and they are safe in PWH. However, it should be remembered that some individuals have paradoxical excitatory responses to these medications. Sleep induction is an off-label use for any antidepressant or antipsychotic. Nonetheless, low-dose tricyclics (especially doxepin and amitriptyline) and mirtazapine can be very useful in this regard. They can also help with control of neuropathic pain, which can improve sleep quality. In higher doses, all are associated with weight gain, which can be beneficial in some cases. Trazodone is frequently used to induce and maintain sleep in normal populations, but its use in PWH on ART is problematic because final metabolism of the trazodone is slowed and untoward side effects (sleep disruption, vivid dreams, increased sedation, anxiety, and hypotension) occur. Of the antipsychotics, quetiapine and olanzapine are frequently used, although again this is an off-label usage. As previously noted, PWH are much more sensitive to the extrapyramidal side effects of these medications. They also cause endocrine disturbances (prolactinemia) and metabolic side effects that may be cumulative with those of ART, such as lipodystrophy, hyperlipidemia, and insulin resistance (Omonuwa et al., 2009). Brief behavioral treatment for insomnia, a psychological treatment modality, has also been shown to improve the sleep outcomes of PWH and insomnia (Buchanan et al., 2018).

PSYCHIATRIC EFFECTS OF ART

Many of the ARV agents have prominent psychiatric side effects that have been discussed previously. The most prominent of these psychiatric symptoms is vivid dreams and nightmares (Abers et al., 2014). Unfortunately, these issues seem to be more common, problematic, and sustained in individuals who are already vulnerable to or experiencing psychiatric symptoms—that is, those with chronic mental illness. The vivid dreams and nightmares can be especially troubling for individuals with PTSD or past traumatic experiences. Although psychiatric diagnoses should not be a contraindication for use of these agents when indicated, special caution and close follow-up are certainly warranted. As with PTSD, low-dose prazosin can sometimes ameliorate the sleep disturbance experienced.

USE OF PSYCHIATRIC CONSULTATION

Mental health issues in PWH are very common (Bing et al., 2001; Robertson et al., 2014). In an ideal world, mental health professionals would be integrated into every HIV treatment setting, and individuals suspected of having significant illness or distress could be seen rapidly and frequently after referral. In reality, this is rarely the case, and even when psychiatrists and other mental health providers are onsite, visits are commonly delayed due to the sheer number of those needing care.

So, when is referral most warranted and useful? First and foremost, the individual must be aware of and agree to mental health evaluation. Exceptions to this relate to those individuals who are incapable of understanding the need for assessment and treatment, who are imminently dangerous to self or others, or who are systematically destroying themselves and their treatment/treatment team by their behavior. Beyond that, the first part of a decision for referral rests on the primary problem and referring to the correct person. Certain individuals will benefit most from referral to support groups of like-minded people with similar problems, and many actually prefer this form of treatment. Although there are certainly exceptions, most psychiatrists are not the primary resource for either substance abuse counseling or for individual/marital/group psychotherapy. The first task is handled, in general, by specific substance abuse counselors and by self-help groups (Alcoholics Anonymous, Narcotics Anonymous, etc.). Psychotherapy is also more frequently done by behavioral specialists other than psychiatrists (psychologists, social workers, licensed counselors, etc.). Pain management and medical management of substance detoxification and sobriety are also frequently handled by other caregivers. In most settings, it is possible to refer directly to these providers, who can then screen for cases requiring specific psychiatric intervention. Psychologists are specifically trained in diagnostic processes (including psychological and neuropsychological testing and screening) and in psychotherapeutic interventions. Psychiatrists, although trained in behavioral interventions and therapy techniques, are medical doctors, and they are the first-line resource for evaluation of individuals with complex psychiatric/medical issues, those who will probably require psychotropic medications, and those who have not responded to conventional psychotropic medications.

Although psychiatrists can be helpful in diagnosing delirium and can assist in behavioral management of symptoms, the presence of these major neurocognitive disorders (including acute intoxication) generally makes it impossible to ascertain if there is true psychiatric illness underlying the current medical process. The final caveat is this: When in doubt, consult. I know I would much rather be included when I am not needed than absent when I could be of help, and I think most psychiatrists feel the same.

CULTURAL CONSIDERATIONS IN TREATING COMORBID HIV AND PSYCHIATRIC ILLNESS

The stigma associated with living with HIV is very well known, as is the stigma associated with psychiatric illness, but when the two are combined the consequences can be multiplicative and mutually reinforcing. Often it is fear of marginalization and/or discrimination that causes individuals to avoid HIV and mental health screenings and to be poorly adherent to treatment once diagnoses are made. These obstacles are further magnified when the individuals impacted by comorbid HIV and psychiatric illness belong to historically marginalized demographic groups. Whether it is because of their gender, ethnicity, or sexual orientation, individuals may encounter challenges in both navigating the healthcare system and receiving care that is uniquely suited to their needs. For instance, African and Caribbean Black women have been found to experience higher rates of HIV-related stigma and are more likely to report being marginalized or discriminated against based on racist and sexist stereotypes (Loutfy et al., 2012). This finding is of particular concern and importance in the US, as African American women continue to be disproportionately represented among new HIV cases (Centers for Disease Control and Prevention [CDC], 2014). Despite these statistics and the best efforts of public health clinicians, many HIV/mental health interventions lack sufficient cultural sensitivity and are therefore less likely to be effective across different demographic groups. A 2016 cohort study of 31,000 HIV-infected individuals found that while 47% of respondents had an indication for antidepressant treatment, Black non-Hispanics, Hispanics, and other non-White ethnicities were significantly less likely to initiate antidepressant treatment than their White non-Hispanic peers (Bengtson et al., 2016). These findings suggest a strong cultural component to acceptance of mental health treatment, one that may be mediated by historical mistrust of the healthcare system and/or a reliance on alternative methods of emotional support. In 2016, respondents in a qualitative study of primary care providers who treat African American PWH reported that their patients were more likely to seek emotional support from family or their spiritual community rather than seeking formal mental health treatment (Le et al., 2016). Accordingly, interventions aimed at identifying and preventing adverse HIV and mental health outcomes in these vulnerable groups should be tailored to address these pervasive cultural stigmas and norms. Neither HIV treatment nor mental health treatment is a one-size-fits-all endeavor, and clinicians should continue to enlist the input of PWH, families, and spiritual and community leaders to develop programs that suit the diversity and cultural sensitivities of the people they seek to help and heal.

PSYCHOSOCIAL CONSIDERTATION DURING THE COVID-19 PANDEMIC

The emergence of the novel coronavirus disease known as COVID-19 and subsequent declaration of a pandemic with CDC recommendations for physical distancing and social isolation may disproportionally impact the psychological health of PWH. Older PWH are known to experience increased rates of loneliness and social isolation (Halkitis et al., 2017). This fact and the public health recommendations to reduce risk of transmission of COVID-19 are likely leading to a unique experience of stress in PWH.

For PWH who lived through the 1980s and 1990s prior to the development and FDA approval of combination ART, the COVID-19 pandemic may be a traumatic reminder of the early HIV pandemic. There are fears of a viral infection spreading among the community, with no known cure or treatment, and health agencies are urging behavioral change to reduce spread of illness. Having emerged from East Asia, COVID-19 has sparked racist belief among communities just as HIV sparked homophobia. A lack of knowledge and understanding about COVID-19, like HIV in the early years, has led to conspiracy theories and disbelief. These recurring themes of large-scale infectious diseases can retrigger memories of death, fear, and uncertainty.

Thus, PWH represent a population that is uniquely impacted by the COVID-19 pandemic, whether they contract the coronavirus or not. As such, all providers should strive to pay particular attention to their patients with HIV as we move through the COVID-19 pandemic.

CONCLUSION

From the earliest days of the AIDS epidemic, it has been apparent that large numbers of PWH also have psychiatric illness. This, of course, raises the question of the direction of relatedness: Is psychiatric illness a risk factor for HIV infection, or does the HIV virus cause or predispose to psychiatric symptoms? The answer seems to be "yes"—the association goes both ways. Individuals with psychiatric illness (depression, bipolar disorders, anxiety disorders, PTSD, schizophrenia, dementia, and substance use disorders) tend to engage in behaviors that place them at increased risk for exposure to the HIV virus. Contracting HIV infection results in numerous psychosocial stressors that trigger or exacerbate expression of psychological symptoms in vulnerable individuals. The virus itself precipitates changes in the CNS that cause psychiatric manifestations. Finally, treatment with certain of the current ARVs can result in psychiatric/behavioral symptoms. In turn, the presence of these psychiatric symptoms creates additional problems with diagnosis and treatment of HIV-related illnesses.

All PWH should be screened for the presence of psychiatric illness. Fortunately, PWH respond well to traditional psychopharmacologic and psychotherapeutic approaches to mental distress and illness, and, with adequate psychiatric treatment, they have good adherence and response to HIV treatment. Psychiatric illness alone is no longer considered to be a contraindication to full treatment of HIV or AIDS.

REFERENCES

Abers MS, Shandera WX, Kass JS. Neurological and psychiatric adverse effects of antiretroviral drugs. *CNS Drugs*. 2014;28(2):131–145.

Alciati A, Gallo L, Monforte AD, et al. Major depression-related immunological changes and combination antiretroviral therapy in HIV-seropositive patients. *Hum Psychopharmacol*. 2007;22(1):33–40.

American Psychiatric Association. *Diagnostic and statistical manual of mental disorders*. 5th ed. Arlington, VA: American Psychiatric Publishing; 2013.

Atkinson JH, Heaeton RK, Patterson TL, et al. Two-year prospective study of major depressive disorder in HIV-positive men. *J Affect Disord*. 2008;108:225–233.

Bengtson AM, Pence BW, Crane HM, et al. Disparities in depressive symptoms and antidepressant treatment by gender and race/ethnicity among people living with HIV in the United States. *PLoS One*. 2016;11(8):e0160738.

Benton TD. Depression and HIV/AIDS. *Curr Psychiatry Rep*. 2008;10(3):280–285.

Benton TD. Psychiatric considerations in children and adolescents with HIV/AIDS. *Child Adolesc Psychiatr Clin North Am*. 2010;19(2):387–400.

Berger-Greenstein JA, Cuevas CA, Brady SM, et al. Major depression in patients with HIV/AIDS and substance abuse. *AIDS Patient Care STDS*. 2007;21:942–949.

Bing EG, Burnam MA, Longshore D, et al. Psychiatric disorders and drug use among human immunodeficiency virus-infected adults in the United States. *Arch Gen Psychiatry*. 2001;58:721–728.

Blashill AJ, Perry N, Safren SA. Mental health: a focus on stress, coping, and mental illness as it relates to treatment retention, adherence, and other health outcomes. *Curr HIV/AIDS Rep*. 2011;8(4):215–222.

Buchanan DT, McCurry SM, Eilers K, et al. Brief behavioral treatment for insomnia in persons living with HIV. *Behav Sleep Med*. 2018;16(3):244–258. doi:10.1080/15402002.2016.1188392

Carrico A. Elevated suicide rate among HIV-positive persons despite benefits of antiretroviral therapy: implications for a stress and coping model of suicide. *Am J Psychiatry*. 2010;167:117–119.

Carrico AW, Bangsberg DR, Weisner SD, et al. Psychiatric correlates of HAART utilization and viral load among HIV-positive impoverished persons. *AIDS*. 2011;25(8):1113–1118.

Centers for Disease Control and Prevention. HIV among African Americans. 2014. http://www.cdc.gov/hiv/group/racialethnic/africanamericans/index.html

Collazos J. Sexual dysfunction in the highly active antiretroviral therapy era. *AIDS Rev*. 2007;9:237–245.

Cook JA, Burke-Miller J, Anastos K, et al. Effects of treated and untreated depressive symptoms on highly active antiretroviral therapy use in a US multi-site cohort of HIV-positive women. *AIDS Care*. 2006;18(2):3–100.

Cysique LA, Maruff P, Brew BJ. Prevalence and pattern of neuropsychological impairment in human immunodeficiency virus-infected/acquired immunodeficiency syndrome (HIV/AIDS) patients across pre- and post-highly active antiretroviral therapy eras: a combined study of two cohorts. *J Neurovirol*. 2004;10(6):350–357.

de Sousa Gurgel W, da Silva Carneiro AH, Barreto Reboucas D, et al. Affective Disorders Study Group (GETA): prevalence of bipolar disorder in a HIV-infected outpatient population. *AIDS Care.* 2013;25(12):1499–1503.

Freudenreich O, Goforth HW, Cozza KL, et al. Psychiatric treatment of persons with HIV/AIDS: an HIV psychiatry consensus survey of current practices. *Psychosomatics.* 2010;51:480–488.

Gallego L, Barreiro P, Lopez-Ibor JJ. Diagnosis and clinical features of major neuropsychiatric disorders in HIV infection. *AIDS Rev.* 2011;13:171–179.

Gannon P, Khan MZ, Kolson DL. Current understanding of HIV-associated neurocognitive disorders pathogenesis. *Curr Opin Neurol.* 2011;24(3):275–283.

Gaynes BN, Farley JF, Dusetzina SB, et al. Does the presence of accompanying symptom clusters differentiate the comparative effectiveness of second-line medication strategies for treating depression? *Depress Anxiety.* 2011;28(11):989–998.

Gaynes BN, Pence BW, Eron JJ Jr, et al. Prevalence and comorbidity of psychiatric diagnoses based on reference standard in an HIV+ population. *Psychosom Med.* 2008;70:505–511.

Gilchrist G, Blazquez A, Torrens M. Psychiatric, behavioral and social risk factors for HIV infection among female drug users. *AIDS Behav.* 2011;15(8):1834–1843.

Groves JE. Taking care of the hateful patient. *N Engl J Med.* 1978;298:883–887.

Halkitis PN, Krause KD, Vieira DL. Mental health, psychosocial challenges and resilience in older adults living with HIV. *Interdiscip Top Gerontol Geriatr.* 2017;42:187–203.

Hansen N, Vaughan E, Cavanaugh C, et al. Health-related quality of life in bereaved HIV-positive adults: relationships between HIV symptoms, grief, social support, and axis II indication. *Health Psychol.* 2009;28:249–257.

Heaton RK, Clifford DB, Franklin DR, et al. HIV-associated neurocognitive disorders persist in the era of potent antiretroviral therapy: CHARTER study. *Neurology.* 2010;75(23):2087–2096.

Ho D, Tota TR, Schooley RT, et al. Isolation of HTV-III from cerebrospinal fluid and neural tissues of patients with neurologic syndromes relate to the acquired immunodeficiency syndrome. *N Engl J Med.* 1985;313(24):1493–1497.

Hoffman RS. Neuropsychiatric complications of AIDS. *Psychosomatics.* 1984;25:393–395.

Hogeland GW, Swindells S, McNabb JC, et al. Lopinavir/ritonavir reduces bupropion plasma concentrations in healthy subjects. *Clin Pharmacol Ther.* 2007;81(1):69–75.

Horberg MA, Silverberg MJ, Hurley LB, et al. Effects of depression and selective serotonin reuptake inhibitor use on adherence to highly active antiretroviral therapy and on clinical outcomes in HIV-positive patients. *J AIDS.* 2008;7(3):384–390.

Hriso E, Kuhn T, Masdeu JC, Grundman M. Extrapyramidal symptoms due to dopamine-blocking agents in patients with AIDS encephalopathy. *J Psychiatry.* 1991 Nov;148(11):1558–1561.

Huntingdon B, Muscat DM, de Wit J, et al. Factors associated with general sexual functioning and sexual satisfaction among people living with HIV: a systematic review. *J Sex Res.* 2020;57(7):824–835. doi:10.1080/00224499.2019.1689379

Kales HC, Kim HM, Zivin K, et al. Risk of mortality among individual antipsychotics in patients with dementia. 2012;169:71–79.

Kelly DV, Beique LC, Bowmer MI. Extrapyramidal symptoms with ritonavir/indinavir plus risperdone. *Ann Pharmacother.* 2002;36(5):827–830.

Kent LK, Blumenfield M. Psychodynamic psychiatry in the general medical setting. *J Am Acad Psychoanal Dyn Psychiatry.* 2011;9(1):41–62.

Klinkenberg WD, Dacks SL; HIV/AIDS Treatment Adherence, Health Outcomes and Cost Study Group. Mental disorders and drug abuse in persons living with HIV/AIDS. *AIDS Care.* 2004;16(Suppl 1):S22–S42.

Kubler-Ross E. *On death and dying.* New York: Macmillan; 1969.

Le H-N, Hipolito MMS, Lambert S, et al. Culturally sensitive approaches to identification and treatment of depression among HIV infected African American adults: a qualitative study of primary care providers' perspectives. *J Depress Anxiety.* 2016;5(2):223.

Leserman J. Role of depression, stress and trauma in HIV disease progression in HIV. *Psychosom Med.* 2008;70:539–545.

Liedtke MD, Lockhart SM, Rathbun RC. Anticonvulsant and antiretroviral interactions. *Ann Pharmacother.* 2004;38(3):482–489. doi:10.1345/aph.1D309

Loutfy MR, Logie CH, Zhang Y, et al. Gender and ethnicity differences in HIV-related stigma experienced by people living with HIV in Ontario, Canada. *PLoS One.* 2012;7(12): e48168.

Martinez A, Israelski BS, Walker C, et al. Posttraumatic stress disorder in women attending human immunodeficiency virus outpatient clinics. *AIDS Patient Care STDs.* 2002;98:9–17.

Meade CS, Bevilacqua LA, Key MD. Bipolar disorder is associated with HIV transmission risk behavior among patients in treatment for HIV. *AIDS Behav.* 2012;16(8):2267–2271.

Mellins CA, Havens JF, McDonnell C, et al. Adherence to antiretroviral medications and medical care in HIV-positive adults diagnosed with mental and substance abuse disorders. *AIDS Care.* 2009;21(2):168–177.

Moreno-Pérez O, Escoín C, Serna-Candel C. Risk factors for sexual and erectile dysfunction in HIV-infected men: the role of protease inhibitors. *AIDS.* 2010;24:255–264.

Nel A, Kagee A. Common mental health problems and antiretroviral therapy adherence. *AIDS Care.* 2011;23(11):1360–1365.

Nicolussi S, Drewe J, Butterweck V, et al. Clinical relevance of St. John's wort drug interactions revisited. *Br J Pharm.* 2019;177(6):1212–1226.

Norman SE, Cheick AD, Freeman C, et al. Sleep disturbances in men with asymptomatic human immunodeficiency (HIV) infection. *Sleep.* 1992;15:150–155.

Omonuwa TS, Goforth HW, Preud'homme X, et al. The pharmacologic management of insomnia in patients with HIV. *J Clin Sleep Med.* 2009;5(3):251–262.

Owe-Larssom B, Sall L, Allgulander C. HIV infection and psychiatric illness. *Afr J Psychiatry.* 2009;115–128.

Pence BW. The impact of mental health and traumatic life experiences on antiretroviral treatment outcomes for people living with HIV/AIDS. *J Antimicrob Chemother.* 2009;63(4):636–640.

Pence BW, Miller WC, Gaynes BN, et al. Psychiatric illness and virologic response in patients initiating highly active antiretroviral therapy. *J AIDS.* 2007;44(2):159–165.

Prince JD, Walkup J, Akincigil A, et al. Serious mental illness and risk of new HIV/AIDS diagnosis: an analysis of Medicaid beneficiaries in eight states. *Psych Serv.* 2012;63(10):1032–1038.

Ramachandran G, Glickman L, Levenson J, et al. Incidence of extrapyramidal syndromes in AIDS patients and a comparison group of medically ill inpatients. *J Neuropsych Clin Neurosci* 1997;9:579–583.

Rao R, Sagar R, Kabra SK, et al. Psychiatric morbidity in HIV-positive children. *AIDS Care.* 2007;19(6):828–833.

Rhodes T. The "risk environment": a framework for understanding and reducing drug-related harm. *Int J Drug Policy.* 2002;13:85–94.

Robertson K, Bayon C, Molina JM, et al. Screening for neurocognitive impairment, depression, and anxiety in HIV-infected patients in Western Europe and Canada. *AIDS Care.* 2014;26(12):1555–1561.

Saberi P, Neilands TB, Johnson MO. Quality of sleep: associations with antiretroviral nonadherence. *AIDS Patient Care STDs.* 2011;26(9):517–524.

Scanavino M de T. Sexual dysfunctions of HIV-positive men: associated factors, pathophysiology issues, and clinical management. *Adv Urol.* 2011;2011:854792.

Shindel A, Horberg M Smith J, et al. Sexual dysfunction, HIV, and AIDS in men who have sex with men. *AIDS Patient Care STDs.* 2011;25:41–49.

Treisman G, Angelinno A. Interrelation between psychiatric disorders and the prevention and treatment of HIV infection. *Clin Infect Dis.* 2007;45(Suppl 4):S313–S317.

van Luenen S, Garnefski N, Spinhoven P, et al. The benefits of psychosocial interventions for mental health in people living with HIV: a systemic review and meta-analysis. *AIDS Behav.* 2018;22:9–42.

Vazquez-Santiago FJ, Noel RJ Jr, Porter JT, et al. Glutamate metabolism and HIV-associated neurocognitive disorders. *J Neurovirol.* 2014;20(4):31–331.

Villes V, Spire B, Lewden C, et al. The effect of depressive symptoms at ART initiation on HIV clinical progression and mortality: implications in clinical practice. *Antivir Ther.* 2007;12:1067–1071.

Walkup J, Akincigil A, Chakravarty S, et al. Bipolar medication use and adherence to antiretroviral therapy among patients with HIV-AIDS and bipolar disorder. *Psychiatr Serv.* 2011;62(3):313–316.

Walkup J, Wei W, Sambamoorthi U, et al. Antidepressant treatment and adherence to combination antiretroviral therapy among patients with AIDS and diagnosed depression. *Psychiatr Q.* 2008;79(1):43.

Warden D, Rush AJ. The STAR*D project results: a comprehensive review of findings. *Curr Psychiatry Rep.* 2007;9(6):449–459.

Watkins CC, Pieper AA, Treisman GJ. Safety considerations in drug treatment of depression in HIV-positive patients: an updated review. *Drug Saf.* 2011;34(8):623–639.

Whetten K, Reif S, Whetten R, et al. Trauma, mental health, distrust and stigma among HIV-positive persons: implications for effective care. *Psychosom Med.* 2008;70(5):531–538.

Williams DW, Veenstra M, Gaskill PJ, et al. Monocyte mediated HIV neuropathogenesis: mechanisms that contribute to HIV associated neurocognitive disorders. *Curr HIV Res.* 2014;12(2): 85096.

34.

NEUROLOGIC EFFECTS OF HIV INFECTION

Rodrigo Hasbun and Joseph S. Kass

HIV-ASSOCIATED NEUROCOGNITIVE DISORDERS

LEARNING OBJECTIVE

- Discuss the clinical features, differential diagnosis, and management of HIV-associated neurocognitive disorders

WHAT'S NEW?

- CD8+ T-cell encephalitis has been described as a severe form of HIV-associated neurocognitive disorder (HAND).

- The central nervous system (CNS) penetration-effectiveness score has been correlated with cerebrospinal fluid (CSF) viral escape.

- CSF viral escape occurred in 7.2% of 1,063 patients, with the most important predictor being a regimen composed of protease inhibitors (PIs) (especially atazanavir) and nucleoside reverse transcriptase inhibitors (NRTIs). Neurocognitive impairment has been associated with lack of retention-in-care in older adults and with virologic failure. When coupled with frailty, it is associated with greater risk for falls, disability, and death.

- The impact of the CNS-targeted combination antiretroviral therapy (ART) on HAND is currently being explored.

KEY POINTS

- There is a high prevalence of HAND in ART-naïve patients and in patients treated with ART with virologic suppression.

- Rapid screening tools such as the Montreal Cognitive Assessment test and the Frontal Assessment Battery test have been evaluated for their use in diagnosing HAND in the clinic.

- HAND is associated with significant cognitive, behavioral, and motor abnormalities that can impact ART adherence, retention-in-care in older individuals, virologic success, and quality of life.

- CNS-targeted ART can be considered in patients with HAND, and corticosteroids can be considered in patients with CD8+ T-cell encephalitis.

Despite the use of combination ART with suppressed viremia, up to 39% of patients currently have neurocognitive impairment (Metra et al., 2020) and up to 42% of patients have at least 1 copy/mL of HIV-1 RNA in the CSF (Anderson et al., 2017). It is unclear if inadequate CSF penetration by some of the antiretroviral agents (ARVs) accounts for this high prevalence and whether CNS-active ART improves cognitive impairment. However, higher CSF penetration scores have been correlated with a lower probability of detectable CSF HIV RNA levels (Anderson et al., 2017; Hammond et al., 2014). A recent study documented that CSF viral escape occurred in 7.2% of 1,063 patients, with the most important predictor being a regimen composed of PIs (especially atazanavir) and NRTIs (Mukerji et al., 2018). CSF viral escape may be either symptomatic or asymptomatic (Patel et al., 2018). Integrase inhibitors such as bictegravir attain adequate CSF levels and could account for the paucity of symptomatic CSF viral escape cases that are currently being reported (Tiraboshi et al., 2019).

HIV causes a chronic form of encephalitis (HIVE) that is clinically characterized by either dementia or mild neurocognitive impairment. Since the introduction of combination ART in 1996, the incidence of HIV dementia has decreased by 50% (McArthur et al., 2005), but the prevalence of mild neurocognitive disorder has increased up to 39% (Robertson et al., 2007). HIVE is the result of direct microglial infection or interruption of trophic factors or caused by inflammatory cytokines (Boisse et al., 2008). HIV enters the brain primarily by the "Trojan horse mechanism": it is carried by monocytes and lymphocytes that cross the blood–brain barrier. HIV has a predilection for the basal ganglia, deep white matter, and hippocampus, resulting in a subcortical dementia. Brain computed tomography (CT) scanning or magnetic resonance imaging (MRI) typically shows cerebral atrophy and symmetrical white matter lesions. HIV dementia is a diagnosis of exclusion; other coinfections (e.g., JC virus-associated progressive multifocal leukoencephalopathy [PML], hepatitis C, neurosyphilis, and cryptococcal meningitis), cerebrovascular disease, malnutrition, and drug abuse should be ruled out before making the diagnosis. In persons with HIV

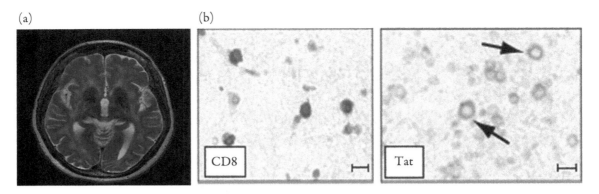

Figure 34.1 (A) Magnetic resonance imaging of a PWH with virologic suppression for 4 years with biopsy-proven CD8⁺ T-cell encephalitis. (B) The presence of CD8⁺ T cells and HIV Tat antigens on brain biopsy and arrows point to stained HIV Tat antigens. SOURCE: Johnson TP, et al. *PNAS*. 2013.13;110(33):13588–13593.

(PWH) receiving ART with immunologic response, a severe manifestation of symptomatic CSF viral escape called CD8⁺ T-cell encephalitis has been described (Lescure et al., 2013). Patients can present with neurocognitive impairment, headache, focal neurologic deficits, and seizures, with MRI of the brain showing bilateral white matter lesions. CSF usually shows a lymphocytic pleocytosis with CD8⁺ T cells greater than 65%. A brain biopsy, if performed, shows pronounced CD8⁺ T-cell infiltration with the presence of scant HIV antigens (Figure 34.1) (Johnson et al., 2013). Patients improve dramatically with corticosteroids and with improved CNS penetration of their ART regimen. The optimal dose and duration of corticosteroids are currently unknown.

Neuropsychological impairment is a surrogate marker for the presence of HIVE on autopsy (Cherner et al., 2002). Cognitive impairment has also been associated with ART nonadherence (Maggiolo et al., 2007), lack of retention-in-care in older adults (Jacks et al., 2015), and a negative impact on quality of life. In the pre-ART era, it was shown to be an independent predictor of death (Ellis et al., 1997). Furthermore, CSF HIV RNA levels are increased in PWH with neurocognitive impairment, as are several CSF biomarker levels, such as tumor necrosis-α, neurofilament light, neopterin, β2 microglobulin, and monocyte chemotactic protein-1 (Boisse et al., 2008). A recent clinical model identified the following variables as associated with detectable CSF viral load: detectable serum HIV-1 RNA on polymerase chain reaction (PCR), a CNS penetration score lower than 9, non-Caucasian race, less than 95% ART adherence, depression, and less than 36 months of ART duration (Hammond et al., 2014).

CLINICAL MANIFESTATIONS OF HAND

The clinical features of HAND are related to the involvement of HIV in the subcortical structures. The following can occur: slowing of processing speed; motor and psychomotor abnormalities; and executive, planning, or multitasking dysfunction (Valcour et al., 2011c). HAND affects the following three areas:

- Cognitive: Memory, concentration, mental processing speed, and comprehension

- Behavioral: Apathy, depression, agitation, and sometimes mania

- Motor function: Unsteady gait, poor coordination, abnormal tone, and tremors

In addition, patients with CD8⁺ T-cell encephalitis can also manifest with new-onset seizures, status epilepticus, and altered mental status. Furthermore, HAND is associated with virologic failure (Shahani et al., 2018), and, when combined with frailty, it is associated with greater risk for falls, disability, and death (Erlandson et al., 2019).

RISK FACTORS

Several studies have documented host genetic factors (polymorphisms in apolipoprotein E4, chemokine receptor CCR2, and monocyte chemoattractant protein-1), HIV-specific disease factors (history of AIDS-defining illness or low CD4⁺ T-cell nadir, particular HIV variants, HIV RNA levels in CSF, duration of HIV infection, and older age at conversion), and comorbidities (>50 years of age, anemia, vascular disease, metabolic abnormalities, and hepatitis C coinfection) associated with HAND (Alfahad & Nath, 2013).

SCREENING TOOLS FOR COGNITIVE IMPAIRMENT

Despite the high prevalence of HAND in HIV clinics, it has not become routine to screen patients for cognitive impairment or to consider more CNS-active ART for those affected, even though there are now recommendations from an international consortium to do so (Mind Exchange Working Group, 2013). Screening tools that have been evaluated in HAND include several versions of the HIV dementia scale, the Mini Mental Status Exam (MMSE), standardized questionnaires that assess symptoms such as the Medical Outcomes survey, and the Montreal Cognitive Assessment (MoCA) and Frontal Assessment Battery test. The dementia scales are reliable but only in severe cases of HAND, the MMSE is not sensitive enough to detect HAND, and the subjective reporting of cognitive symptoms will miss patients due to poor insight or due to mood disturbances (Valcour, 2011a; Valcour et al., 2011b). The MMSE is now proprietary. Studies have shown that the MoCA is a rapid, reliable, and sensitive test to detect cognitive impairment in PWH (Hasbun et al., 2012; Rosca et al., 2019). A recent large study comparing different screening tools for HAND showed the Frontal Assessment Battery test had the highest correct classification rate (Triunfo et al., 2018).

DEFINITIONS OF NEUROCOGNITIVE DISORDERS

In 2007, the diagnostic criteria for HIV-associated neurocognitive disorders were revised (Antinori et al., 2007). Three HANDs were defined in these new criteria: asymptomatic neurocognitive impairment, mild neurocognitive disorder, and HIV-associated dementia. Asymptomatic neurocognitive impairment was defined as having a combination of the following: (1) an acquired mild to moderate impairment in cognitive function documented by a score of at least one standard deviation below demographically corrected norms on tests on at least two different cognitive domains, (2) the functional impairment has been seen for more than 1 month, (3) the impairment does not meet criteria for delirium or dementia, and (4) the cognitive impairment is not fully explained by comorbid conditions. The definition of mild neurocognitive disorder is identical to that of asymptomatic neurocognitive impairment, but it also includes interference with activities of daily living. The diagnosis of HIV-associated dementia includes a marked impairment of cognitive impairment. Another approach to define neurocognitive impairment is the utilization of the Global Deficit Score (Jacks et al., 2015) that considers both the number and severity of the individual's performance deficits on the battery of standardized tests.

CSF ACTIVITY OF ARVS

There are currently more than 30 US Food and Drug Administration (FDA)-approved ARVs or combinations in six mechanical classes for treatment of HIV infection, but only some have adequate CSF penetration (US Department of Health and Human Services [DHHS], 2020a). The CNS penetration-effectiveness score has been designed to classify the different ARVs on the basis of their capability of lowering CSF RNA levels (Letendre, 2011). ARVs were assigned a score from 1 to 4 based on their chemical properties, CSF penetration, and/or effectiveness in CNS studies (Table 34.1). A higher CNS penetration score was associated with higher virologic suppression in the CSF (Letendre et al., 2010). Furthermore, a study showed that 10% of patients with virologic suppression in the serum had viral escape (detectable CSF viral loads) (Edén et al., 2010). In addition, a higher CSF penetration score is associated with a lower rate of neurocognitive impairment (Carvalhal et al., 2016).

Very few randomized studies have evaluated the impact of CNS-active ARVs in HAND. In the pre-ART era, zidovudine (AZT) demonstrated efficacy in the treatment of HIV-associated dementia in a randomized clinical trial. The AIDS Clinical Trial Group Study 005 randomized HIV patients with dementia to 2,000 mg/day AZT, 1,000 mg/day AZT, or placebo (Sidtis et al., 1993). The greatest neuropsychological improvement was seen in patients treated with high-dose AZT. In the ART era, a trial involving 49 patients found no neurocognitive benefit of CNS-targeted ART (Ellis et al., 2014). Additionally, a recent prospective study of 981 adults enrolled in the Swiss HIV Cohort Study found no correlation between a newly updated CNS penetration-effectiveness score and HAND as defined by the Frascati criteria (Santos et al., 2019).

RECOMMENDED READING

Calcagno A, Di Perri G, Bonora S. Pharmacokinetics and pharmacodynamics of antiretrovirals in the central nervous system. *Clin Pharmacokinet*. 2014;53(10):891–906. https://www.ncbi.nlm.nih.gov/pubmed/25200312

Table 34.1 CNS PENETRATION-EFFECTIVENESS (CPE) SCORE OF DIFFERENT ARVS

DRUG CLASS	4	3	2	1
NRTIs	Zidovudine	Abacavir Emtricitabine	Didanosine Lamivudine Stavudine	Tenofovir Zalcitabine
NNRTIs	Nevirapine	Delavirdine Efavirenz	Etravirine	
PIs	Indinavir	Darunavir/ritonavir Fosamprenavir/ritonavir Indinavir/itonavir Lopinavir/ritonavir	Atazanavir Atazanavir/r Fosamprenavir	Nelfinavir Ritonavir Saquinavir Saquinavir/ritonavir
Entry/fusion inhibitors		Maraviroc		Enfuvirtide
Integrase inhibitors		Raltegravir Dolutegravir		

Adapted from Letendre et al. *Top Antivir Med*. 2011;19(4):137–142.

Letendre SL, Mills AM, Tashima KT, et al. ING116070: a study of the pharmacokinetics and antiviral activity of dolutegravir in cerebrospinal fluid in HIV-1-infected, antiretroviral therapy-naïve subjects. *Clin Infect Dis.* 2014;59(7):1032–1037. https://www.ncbi.nlm.nih.gov/pubmed/24944232

MYELOPATHY

LEARNING OBJECTIVE

Discuss the clinical presentation, differential diagnosis, and management of HIV-associated vacuolar myelopathy in PWH.

WHAT'S NEW?

The incidence of vacuolar myelopathy has been reduced significantly. It remains a cause of disability in end-stage HIV and has a poor prognosis.

KEY POINTS

- Vacuolar myelopathy is an uncommon complication of HIV infection and tends to occur in the late stages of HIV infection.

- Acute transverse myelitis and inflammatory CSF are unlikely to be vacuolar myelopathy.

- Human T-cell lymphotropic virus type 1 (HTLV-1) infection is another infectious cause of myelopathy, and it should be considered in endemic geographic areas and in cases of coinfection with HIV.

- HIV and HTLV-1 can both cause a chronic myelopathy involving dorsal and lateral columns.

- The workup for a myelopathic patient includes MRI of the spine with and without contrast and may include CSF analysis and investigations for nutritional deficiencies and toxic agents.

HIV-ASSOCIATED VACUOLAR MYELOPATHY

PWH may develop myelopathy for many reasons. At the time of seroconversion, an acute transverse myelitis may develop, whereas those with severe immunosuppression are at risk of developing HIV-associated vacuolar myelopathy or a secondary process such as opportunistic infection or neoplasm that either invades or compresses the spinal cord. PWH may also develop myelopathy from causes typical of the general population without HIV, such as spondylosis with spinal stenosis.

Primary HIV-associated acute transverse myelitis is a rare inflammatory myelopathy resulting from immune activation, and it typically develops within days to weeks of acute HIV seroconversion. Presentation is of an acute myelopathy, with weakness, numbness with typically with a thoracic sensory level, sphincter dysfunction, hyperreflexia, and spasticity. CSF is typically inflammatory with a lymphocytic pleocytosis. This acute transverse myelitis tends to respond well to steroids, intravenous immunoglobulin (IVIG), and ART (Hamada et al., 2011).

In contrast, vacuolar myelopathy is a chronic myelopathy seen in the late stages of HIV infection and affects 10% to 15% of untreated people with an AIDS diagnosis. PWH typically experience a slow, painless progression of neurologic symptoms over several months, most commonly lower extremity weakness and spasticity (Di Rocco et al., 1999). Patients typically complain of progressive weakness or clumsiness in the lower extremities, as well as leg cramps and difficulty walking. Urinary symptoms such as frequency and urgency, along with erectile dysfunction, are also common. Sensation in the legs, particularly proprioception and vibratory sense, is usually impaired, but a clear sensory level on the trunk is unusual. Arms are typically spared until advanced-stage disease. Localized back pain is not a common feature. Individuals are also typically hyperreflexic in the lower extremities (hyperreflexia may spread to the upper extremities if the cervical cord is involved) and exhibit extensor plantar responses. PWH with vacuolar myelopathy present very similarly to persons with subacute combined degeneration due to vitamin B12 deficiency. Acute transverse myelitis, a prominent sensory level, or high numbers of inflammatory cells in the CSF should suggest another diagnosis. Although new HIV infections have been associated with acute myelopathy, this acute inflammatory process is a different entity from vacuolar myelopathy. Acute transverse myelitis associated with HIV seroconversion may respond well to steroids, IVIG, and ART (Hamada et al., 2011).

Vacuolar myelopathy is the result of a chronic inflammatory degeneration with vacuolization and myelin pallor of the lateral and posterior tracts, typically affecting the thoracic cord most severely. On histologic examination, the lateral and dorsal columns demonstrate axonal injury and macrophage infiltration with lipid-laden macrophages and microglia infected with HIV (Dal Pan et al., 1997; Petito et al., 1994; Tyor et al., 1993). As many as 20% to 50% of individuals with AIDS may have pathologic evidence of vacuolar myelopathy at autopsy (Dal Pan & Berger, 1994; Di Rocco & Simpson, 1998; McArthur et al., 2005), yet it manifests clinically in only 6.5% to 10% of individuals with an AIDS diagnosis (Cho & Vaitkevicius, 2012).

There is no effective treatment for vacuolar myelopathy. Patients with vacuolar myelopathy often have coexisting HIV-associated dementia and peripheral neuropathies. Rehabilitation is helpful to maximize physical capacity. ART does not appear to alter the natural history of the disease (Banks et al., 2002). Antispasmodic agents such as baclofen, tizanidine, and botulinum toxin can be used for symptomatic relief.

The differential diagnosis for myelopathy in an HIV patient is broad and includes the following categories: (1) infections, including HTLV-1-associated myelopathy/tropical spastic paraparesis (HAM/TSP; discussed later), tuberculosis (TB) spondylitis or meningomyelitis, cytomegalovirus (CMV) radiculomyelitis, varicella zoster myelitis, toxoplasma myelopathy, neurosyphilis with tabes dorsalis, and bacterial epidural abscess (particularly among intravenous drug users); (2) neoplastic diseases, especially lymphoma and spinal metastases from systemic neoplasms; (3) nutritional deficiencies such as B12, folate, copper, thiamine (presenting as beriberi), and vitamin E; and (4) toxic etiologies such as lathyrism (Di Rocco et al., 1998). Thus, an MRI of the spinal cord with and without contrast, lumbar puncture with CSF analysis, and serum analysis for vitamin and mineral deficiencies will be needed to evaluate for these etiologies (Chong et al., 1999).

Clinicians should consider common infectious causes initially. One study from Cape Town, Africa—an area known for a high prevalence of TB and HIV—reviewed 216 cases of myelopathy and cauda equina syndrome in HIV-positive patients (median CD4+ count 185 cells/mm³). Investigators found that 68% of myelopathy cases were due to TB (Candy et al., 2014). This large number of TB-related myelopathy cases in HIV patients has also been seen in other small studies in Africa (Bhigjee et al., 2001; Modi et al., 2011). TB spondylitis could be diagnosed radiographically with a high degree of certainty using MRI, and the diagnosis was confirmed with either CSF analysis or open biopsy.

HTLV-1–ASSOCIATED MYELOPATHY/TROPICAL SPASTIC PARAPARESIS

HTLV-1 is a retrovirus that is T cell-tropic and causes a proliferation of T cells (Manns et al., 1999). Although its full disease spectrum remains unknown, this virus is associated with adult T-cell leukemia/lymphoma, uveitis, and HAM, which is also referred to as TSP. The prevalence of HTLV-1 infection increases with age, and it is more common in women than in men. It is also geographically clustered, with high rates in southern Japan, the Caribbean, areas of Africa, the Middle East, South America, the Pacific Melanesian Islands, and Papua New Guinea. Among low-risk groups in the US and Europe, seroprevalence is approximately 1%. The majority of these patients remain asymptomatic during their lifetime. Approximately 1% of these HTLV-positive patients develop a myelopathy (Pillat et al., 2011). Given the overlapping risk factors for both HIV infection and HTLV-1 infection, it is important to consider HIV and HTLV-1 coinfection in HIV patients presenting with a slowly progressive myelopathy.

HAM patients present with progressive muscle weakness in the legs, hyperreflexia, clonus, extensor plantar responses, sensory disturbances, urinary incontinence, impotence, and lower back pain. HTLV-1 antibodies are present in both plasma and the CSF, as well as in brain and spinal cord tissue.

The diagnostic approach to HAM/TSP is similar to that outlined previously for vacuolar myelopathy, including MRI of the spine with and without contrast, lumbar puncture, and an investigation for nutritional deficiencies and toxic exposures. Definitive diagnosis requires an assay to detect HTLV-1 antibodies in plasma and CSF, including an assay capable of distinguishing between HTLV-1 and HTLV-2.

There is evidence that immune-modulating therapy, such as corticosteroids and IVIG, may be beneficial in the treatment of HTLV-1 myelopathy. Research is under way to develop new therapies in addition to preventive and therapeutic vaccines for HTLV-1 (Martin & Taylor, 2011), but currently prevention education, particularly regarding breastfeeding and sexual behavior, is the only known method of reducing incidence.

MRI IN HIV-ASSOCIATED VACUOLAR MYELOPATHY

MRI of the spinal cord in vacuolar myelopathy is nonspecific and thus lacks pathognomonic features to differentiate it from non–HIV-related spinal cord disease. The spinal cord may appear normal, but the most affected spinal cords appear atrophic with or without hyperintensities on T2-weighted images (Chong et al., 1999; Yousem & Grossman, 2010).

RECOMMENDED READING

Di Rocco A. Diseases of the spinal cord in human immunodeficiency virus infection. *Semin Neurol*. 1999;19:151–155.

Manns A, Hisada M, La Grenade L. Human T-lymphotropic virus type I infection. *Lancet*. 1999;353:1951–1958.

MENINGITIS

LEARNING OBJECTIVE

- Review the differential diagnosis and clinical management of meningitis in PWH

WHAT'S NEW?

- ART initiation should be deferred in cryptococcal meningitis.

- HIV testing is done in only 50% of CNS infections even though the Centers for Disease Control and Prevention (CDC) recommends universal testing.

- Meningococcal A vaccine has decreased the burden of meningococcal meningitis serogroup A in Africa, but outbreaks remain with non-A serogroup meningococcal or non-meningococcal meningitis isolates.

KEY POINTS

- The differential diagnosis of meningitis in PWH is broad (viral, bacterial, fungal, mycobacterial, lymphomatous, etc.) (Table 34.2).

- All adults with meningitis should be tested for HIV.

- Meningitis in PWH is usually treatable, and a cause should be investigated.

- A meta-analysis of studies of meningitis in PWH in Africa documented that the three most common causes were *Cryptococcus neoformans*, *Mycobacterium tuberculosis*, and bacterial meningitis.

Table 34.2 CAUSES OF MENINGITIS IN PWH

Viral	Acute HIV seroconversion, CD8⁺ T-cell encephalitis, enterovirus, herpes simplex virus, arboviruses (West Nile virus, St. Louis encephalitis), CMV, varicella zoster virus, influenza virus, EBV, lymphocytic choriomeningitis virus, mumps
Bacterial	Bacterial meningitis, endocarditis, parameningeal focus (e.g., epidural abscess and mastoiditis), syphilis, Lyme disease, *Mycoplasma pneumoniae*, *Bartonella henselae*, *Brucella* species, *Ehrlichia*, *Rickettsia*, leptospirosis, *Mycobacterium tuberculosis*
Fungal	*Cryptococcus neoformans*, *Coccidioides immitis*, *Histoplasma capsulatum*, *Aspergillus* species, zygomycosis
Parasitic	*Naegleria/Acanthamoeba*, *Taenia solium*, *Angiostrongylus cantonensis*, *Toxoplasma gondii*
Noninfectious	Medications (e.g., antibiotics and nonsteroidal anti-inflammatory drugs), meningeal carcinomatosis (lymphoma and leukemia), vasculitis, chemical meningitis (intrathecal injections and spinal anesthesia), seizures

NEUROLOGIC EVENTS IN EARLY STAGE HIV INFECTION

Acute HIV infection may manifest as an "aseptic meningitis" presentation, but this is most likely underdiagnosed as less than 50% of adults with meningitis are tested for HIV and only 1% are tested for HIV-1 RNA levels to rule out HIV seroconversion syndrome (Ma et al., 2020). Individuals with HIV exposure and infection may present with severe headache, stiff neck, diffuse macular rash, photophobia, and a lymphocytic pleocytosis in the CSF. Patients typically have positive HIV RNA levels and/or a positive HIV p24 antigen.

Approximately one-third of PWH who present with meningitis do so during the early stages of the HIV disease (i.e., CD4⁺ T-cell count >200 cells/mm³) (Vigil et al., 2018). The most common causes of meningitis in these patients are herpes simplex type 2, varicella zoster virus (VZV), and arboviruses (West Nile, St. Louis encephalitis). Herpes simplex type 2 can present with the initial genital outbreak of herpes or in patients with recurrent episodes of aseptic meningitis (Mollaret's meningitis). Arboviruses should be suspected in the summer and fall in patients with fever and recent mosquito bites. Unfortunately, viral PCR and arboviral serologies are obtained in the minority of patients with meningitis (Nesher et al., 2016; Shukla et al., 2017). Other less common causes of meningitis in PWH include VZV, syphilis, and bacterial meningitis. VZV can present with a dermatomal vesicular rash and an aseptic meningitis presentation, and the diagnosis of VZV meningitis should prompt screening for HIV. In more advanced stages of HIV infection, VZV can present as disseminated disease. It can also present without a rash (zoster sine herpete); with the Ramsay–Hunt syndrome; or with stroke, myelopathy, retinitis, or encephalitis.

The diagnosis is made by a CSF VZV PCR or by a CSF anti-VZV antibody or presumptively from a VZV PCR of a vesicular lesion in patient presenting with a CNS infection. CSF VZV PCR has a specificity of greater than 95% but a sensitivity of only 30%. A positive VZV PCR confirms the diagnosis, but a negative test does not rule out the diagnosis. CSF anti-VZV antibody is the more sensitive test, with a 98% sensitivity (Aberle et al., 2005; DeBiasi et al., 2004; Nagel et al., 2007; Osiro & Salomon, 2017). Treatment is with high-dose intravenous acyclovir.

Syphilis can also present as an aseptic meningitis syndrome in patients with a diffuse rash that involves the palms and soles. A serum rapid plasma reagin (RPR) of greater than 1:32 and a CD4⁺ T-cell count of less than 350 cells/mm³ are associated with neurosyphilis and should prompt the performance of a lumbar puncture (Marra et al., 2004). Bacterial meningitis represents a diagnostic consideration in all stages of HIV, but its incidence has decreased with the advent of the conjugate vaccines (Lopez Castelblanco et al., 2014). If bacterial meningitis is suspected, intravenous dexamethasone and antibiotic therapy with vancomycin, ceftriaxone, and ampicillin should be initiated to cover for *Streptococcus pneumoniae*, *Neisseria meningitides*, and *Listeria monocytogenes* until CSF cultures are negative (Tunkel et al., 2004). If the patient has *L. monocytogenes* or *C. neoformans* meningitis, dexamethasone should be discontinued as its use has been associated with higher mortality or morbidity, respectively (Beardsley et al., 2016; Charlier et al., 2017). Furthermore, delayed cerebral injury has been documented in 4% of patients with bacterial meningitis with an association with the use of steroids (Gallegos et al., 2018). Despite this, dexamethasone should continue to be used in pneumococcal meningitis, where it is associated with a decrease in mortality (Hasbun et al., 2017).

NEUROLOGIC EVENTS IN LATE-STAGE HIV INFECTION

The most common cause of meningitis in patients with advanced immunosuppression (CD4⁺ T-cell count <200 cells/mm³) is *C. neoformans*, TB, CMV, and toxoplasmosis. In cryptococcal meningitis, the CSF examination typically shows a lymphocytic pleocytosis, but inflammation may be absent. CSF India ink examination is positive in up to 50% of cases, and the CSF cryptococcal antigen test is positive in approximately 90% of cases. The Film array multiplex meningitis encephalitis PCR panel that includes *C. neoformans* or *C. gattii* can be falsely negative in up to 50% of cryptococcal isolates, and testing should be combined with a cryptococcal antigen (Leisman et al., 2018). An opening pressure should be documented since elevated opening pressure is associated with higher CSF fungal burden and higher neurologic morbidity and mortality (Gambarin & Hamill, 2002). The preferred therapy for cryptococcal meningitis is a combination of intravenous amphotericin B deoxycholate at 0.7 to 1 mg/kg/day plus flucytosine 100 mg/kg/day divided in four doses for 2 weeks followed by oral fluconazole 400 mg/day. Daily CSF drainage is necessary to decrease the intracranial hypertension (i.e., >25 cmH$_2$O) by repeat lumbar punctures. Temporary percutaneous lumbar drains or ventriculostomy may be required if persistent elevations in intracranial pressure occur, as measured by lumbar puncture (Perfect et al., 2012). If flucytosine is not available or the patient experiences drug toxicity, the treatment regimen can be switched to a combination of amphotericin B with fluconazole either 400 mg or 800 mg once daily for 14 days. A repeat lumbar puncture should be done at the end of the 2-week period to document a negative CSF fungal culture. Intravenous amphotericin B should be continued if the patient has persistently positive CSF cultures, is clinically deteriorating or comatose, or has persistently elevated and symptomatic intracranial pressures (Perfect et al., 2012). A therapeutic lumbar puncture to decrease intracranial pressure was associated with a reduced risk of death in a study performed in Africa (Rolfes et al., 2014). It was also documented that ART should be delayed until 5 weeks after initial presentation to avoid an increase in mortality in this same study cohort (Boulware et al., 2014).

CMV can cause meningitis, ventriculitis, polyradiculitis, polyradiculomyelopathy, retinitis, esophagitis, and colitis in patients with advanced HIV disease (CD4$^+$ T-cell count <50 cells/mm^3). CMV infection of the nervous system accounts for fewer than 1% of CMV infections in PWH (McCutchan, 1995) and often develops concurrently with other, more common CMV extraneural disease such as retinitis or gastrointestinal involvement even while individuals are on treatment with ganciclovir for extra-CNS disease (Bermann & Kim, 1994). CMV encephalitis is the most common manifestation of CNS infection due to CMV. Clinically, infection can present as diffuse encephalitis, ventriculoencephalitis, or focal encephalitis. Diffuse encephalitis develops over several weeks and thus presents subacutely with memory loss, attention and concentration difficulties, and delirium. Focal neurologic deficits may also be seen. Pathologically, microglial nodules may be found in the cortex, brainstem, cerebellum, and basal ganglia, occurring most commonly in gray matter (Morgello et al., 1987). On neuroimaging, MRI may show a variety of patterns. The brain may appear normal, or it may show hyperintense T2 lesions in the areas described previously and nodular lesions with or without enhancement on T1 postcontrast images (Maschke et al., 2002).

Ventriculoencephalitis presents with lethargy, confusion, cranial nerve deficits, ataxia, and focal neurologic deficits, and it sometimes occurs concomitantly with CMV polyradiculitis. Ventriculoencephalitis may be more insidious in onset and have a poorer prognosis (Maschke et al., 2002). Pathologically, necrotizing lesions are seen in the ventricular system, and imaging shows periventricular enhancement with or without ventriculomegaly. The third and less common type of CMV encephalitis, focal encephalitis, presents with focal neurologic deficits corresponding to a cerebral mass lesion. MRI will show ring-enhancing lesions with surrounding edema.

CSF PCR for CMV DNA confirms the diagnosis of CMV encephalitis. The CSF may also show pleocytosis with either a polymorphonuclear or a mononuclear predominance, along with elevated protein and decreased glucose levels. Viral culture is rarely positive. The detection of other viruses often confounds the diagnosis; thus, the index of suspicion must be based on the presentation and imaging findings in the context of profound immunosuppression. The differential diagnosis for CMV encephalitis must include HIV encephalitis, PML, and neurosyphilis. When CMV encephalitis presents as a ring-enhancing lesion, the differential diagnosis expands to other etiologies known to present similarly, such as toxoplasmosis, primary CNS lymphoma, and tuberculous meningitis with tuberculomas (Offiah & Turnbull, 2006).

CMV is treated initially with intravenous ganciclovir 5 mg/kg every 12 hours, and then the patient is switched to oral valganciclovir when stable (DHHS, 2020b). Sometimes in severe encephalitis cases, combination treatment with both ganciclovir and foscarnet has been used (Portegies et al., 2004; Silva et al., 2010). Cidofovir can be used as an alternative treatment option. Empiric treatment of CMV infection is often advised because CSF results may be delayed.

Mycobacterial TB can occur at any stage of the HIV illness, but extrapulmonary disease (e.g., meningitis, lymphadenitis, pleuritis, and pericarditis) occurs more frequently in patients with CD4$^+$ T-cell counts of less than 200 cells/mm^3. The incidence of TB has declined in the US, and there are fewer than 1,000 cases of coinfection reported annually (DHHS, 2020b). TB and HIV must be treated together rather than sequentially, particularly in patients with CD4$^+$ T-cell counts less than 50 cells/mm^3. Tuberculous meningitis usually has a subacute to chronic presentation, lymphocytic pleocytosis, a low CSF glucose, and basilar involvement with cranial nerve palsies and altered mental status. A Thwaites diagnostic score of less than 4 (5 parameters—age, duration of illness, white blood cell count, total CSF white blood cell count, and percentage of CSF neutrophils) or a Lancet consensus score of greater than 6 (20 parameters divided into four categories: clinical, CSF, CNS imaging, and evidence of TB elsewhere) indicate possible TB meningitis, and patients with these scores should be considered for empiric therapy. The CSF acid-fast bacilli smear is insensitive, and CSF cultures are positive in only 38% to 88% of cases (Thwaites, 2012). Caution should be used in areas with neurobrucellosis as patients may also have suggestive scores for TB meningitis (Erdem et al., 2015). A CSF *M. tuberculosis* PCR and an adenosine deaminase level can also aid in the diagnosis. Duration of treatment is 1 year. The mortality is higher for PWH than those without HIV and TB meningitis (51.3% vs. 23%; Thao et al., 2013). Prognostic factors for death in HIV-coinfected patients include severity of illness, lower CSF pleocytosis, lower weight, lower CD4$^+$ T-cell counts, and abnormal sodium levels (Thao et al., 2018).

Finally, toxoplasmosis may also present with a meningitis/encephalitis presentation in patients with advanced AIDS (Opintan et al., 2017). Toxoplasmosis classically presents with fever, focal neurologic signs, seizures, and headaches, with MRI of the brain showing multiple ring-enhancing lesions.

Toxoplasmosis is a very unlikely cause of disease if the serum toxoplasma IgG is negative (Rosenow & Hirschfeld, 2007). If the serology is negative or the neuroimaging is not suggestive of toxoplasmosis, an early brain biopsy is advocated (Rosenow & Hirschfeld, 2007).

MENINGITIS IN HIV-POSITIVE VERSUS HIV-NEGATIVE PATIENTS

A recent study of 549 adults with community-acquired meningitis who were tested for HIV revealed that 25% were infected (Vigil et al., 2018). PWH presented with fewer meningeal symptoms (headache, neck stiffness, and Kernig's sign) but with higher rates of hypoglycorrhachia, elevated CSF protein, and abnormal cranial imaging. PWH also were more likely to have cryptococcal meningitis, neurosyphilis, and VZV than those without HIV. PWH were also more likely to have a pathogen identified (57%) than those without HIV (31%). An adverse clinical outcome was seen in approximately 25% of patients, with abnormal neurologic exam and hypoglycorrhachia being identified as predictors. HIV coinfection was not associated with an adverse outcome.

IMMUNE RECONSTITUTION SYNDROME IN HIV

Immune reconstitution inflammatory syndrome (IRIS) occurs after the initiation of combination ART and either "unmasks" a previous subclinical infection or worsens a known infection despite appropriate therapy (paradoxical reaction). In the CNS, IRIS can develop with many opportunistic processes, most commonly cryptococcal meningitis, TB meningitis, and PML (Huis in't Veld et al., 2012). The two most common and serious CNS IRIS events are cryptococcal and tuberculous meningitis. TB IRIS usually presents between a few weeks and 3 months after the initiation of ART, and it can present with meningitis or tuberculomas or both. Risk factors include low $CD4^+$ T-cell counts, disseminated TB, and extrapulmonary TB. Treatment should consist of adjunctive steroids. CSF acid-fast bacilli cultures are typically negative. Cryptococcal IRIS can develop between 1 and 10 months after initiating ART and can present as culture-negative meningitis, cryptococcomas, pneumonitis, and/or lymphadenopathy. Adjunctive steroids should be considered. Additionally, $CD8^+$ T-cell encephalitis syndrome has been described in patients receiving ART with low or undetectable serum HIV RNA levels (Lescure et al., 2013). These patients usually have a low $CD4^+$ T-cell count nadir and a history of opportunistic infections, and they usually present with high $CD4^+$ T-cell counts. They can present with memory disturbances, headaches, diplopia, ataxia, and, sometimes, seizures. MRI of the brain shows bilateral white matter lesions, and CSF shows lymphocytic pleocytosis with detectable CSF HIV RNA. The treatment is corticosteroids and optimizing the CNS penetration of ART.

MENINGITIS IN RESOURCE-LIMITED COUNTRIES

A review of 1,303 episodes of meningitis with confirmed etiologies among PWH in sub-Saharan Africa showed that 52% had cryptococcal meningitis, 19.6% had TB, 14.2% had bacterial meningitis, and 14.2% had other etiologies (Veltman et al., 2014). Mortality rates were high, ranging from 25% to 68% in the different studies. A recent clinical trial done in Africa concluded that a 1-week course of amphotericin B plus flucytosine or a 2-week course of fluconazole plus flucytosine is an effective option in resource-limited settings (Molloy et al., 2018).

DISTAL SYMMETRIC POLYNEUROPATHY

WHAT'S NEW?

A high-concentration capsaicin dermal patch has shown efficacy in patients with painful HIV distal symmetric polyneuropathy (DSPN) and in one study produced a sustained reduction in pain over 12 weeks.

KEY POINTS

- DSPN is the most common neurologic complication of HIV infection, occurring in 30% to 60% of patients.

- ARV toxic neuropathy is associated with use of older NRTI therapy, especially didanosine and stavudine.

- Treatment includes removal of neurotoxins and management of pain/discomfort.

DSPN occurs in 30% to 60% of all PWH (Ellis et al., 2010; Evans et al., 2011), making it the most common neurologic complication in HIV disease. Its incidence increases to as high as 62% in advanced HIV/AIDS (Schifitto et al., 2002; Simpson et al., 2006). DSPN may develop at any time after the onset of HIV infection, with a mean time to developing neuropathy of 9.5 years after HIV diagnosis (Robinson-Papp et al., 2009b). However, a smaller study suggested that signs of neuropathy may be detected in as many as 35% of PWH a median of only 3.5 months after HIV transmission (Wang et al., 2014). Although the etiology is still under investigation, it is most likely an indirect result of HIV infection, probably through immune-mediated mechanisms (Pardo et al., 2001).

Advanced immunosuppression was the major risk factor for developing DSPN before the advent of ART (Childs, 1999); it remains a risk factor in untreated individuals (Vecchio et al., 2020). Risk factors for developing DSPN among ART-treated individuals include older age, Caucasian race, lower hemoglobin levels, hypertriglyceridemia, lower $CD4^+$ cell count nadir, current combination ART use, and past use of the dideoxynucleoside drugs (didanosine, stavudine, and zalcitabine [D-drugs]) (Banerjee et al., 2011; Ellis et al., 2010; Simpson et al.,

2006; Tagliati et al., 1999). Although the prevalence of DSPN appears to decline with ART initiation and effective viral suppression and immune recovery (Ellis et al., 2010; Vecchio et al., 2020), even ART-treated individuals with undetectable viral loads and higher CD4+ cell counts may develop DSPN (Verma et al., 2004). Virologically suppressed individuals who initiate ART after CD4+ T-cell counts fall below 350/mm³ appear to be at increased risk of DSPN compared to those who never achieve that degree of immunosuppression. This correlation holds true even after adjusting for age, duration of HIV infection, and use of D-drugs. It also suggests that earlier initiation of ART may help reduce the risk of DSPN, but the elevated risk of DSPN in individuals who experience a low CD4 nadir is independent of the eventual success of ART therapy in achieving virologic suppression (Ellis et al., 2010).

Neuropathy associated with D-drugs (the NRTIs, especially didanosine, stavudine, and zalcitabine) is the only neurologic complication of HIV that has increased since the introduction of ART (Keswani et al., 2002). The risk of ARV toxic neuropathy (ATN) appears to be substantially higher when didanosine and stavudine are used together, especially when combined with hydroxyurea (Moore et al., 2000). DSPN and ATN are clinically very similar, although ATN often has a more acute onset with more rapid progression (Pardo et al., 2001; Price et al., 1999). A current hypothesis is that mitochondrial dysfunction mediates NRTI toxicity (Kallianpur & Hulgan, 2009).

Patients with DSPN typically come to medical attention when they experience symmetric spontaneous and evoked pains predominantly in the feet and progressing to the upper extremities, along with tingling, numbness, stabbing sensations, and burning (Figure 34.2) (Cornblath & McArthur, 1988; DeVivo et al., 2000; Price et al., 1999; Wulff & Simpson, 1999a). In research cohorts, DPSN may be detected in the absence of clinical symptoms if one of the following signs manifests bilaterally: diminished ability to recognize vibration and reduced sharp/dull discrimination in the feet and toes or reduced ankle reflexes. Not all DSPN patients experience neuropathic pain. For example, although 57% of the over 1,500 CHARTER cohort subjects were diagnosed with DSPN, only 38% reported neuropathic symptoms (Ellis et al., 2010). Risk factors for neuropathic pain differed from risk factors for DSPN itself and included past D-drug use (didanosine, stavudine, zalcitabine) and higher rather than lower CD4+ T-cell nadir (Ellis et al., 2010).

DSPN is the result of damage to and loss of both large- and small-caliber sensory nerve fibers, with macrophage infiltration in the dorsal root ganglia and along the nerve trunks (Keswani et al., 2002). Activation of macrophages and production of proinflammatory cytokines appear to play a significant role in the neuropathogenesis of DSPN (Pardo et al., 2001). Secreted viral proteins such as the envelope glycoprotein gp120 may also contribute to HIV-induced neurotoxicity (Keswani et al., 2003). DNA damage in the mitochondria of distal axons may add to the distal degeneration of sensory nerve fibers (Lehmann et al., 2011). Sural nerve biopsies obtained from patients with ARV toxic neuropathy have shown severe axonal destruction, prominent in unmyelinated fibers (Dalakas & Cupler, 1996). Prominent mitochondrial abnormalities have more significantly been noted in association with NRTIs, supporting the suggestion that neuronal mitochondrial damage underlies ATN (Chen et al., 1991). Further support for this concept is derived from in vitro observations of graded inhibition of γ-DNA polymerase by different NRTIs (Martin et al., 1994). The D-drugs are the most potent inhibitors of this enzyme in vitro (Martin et al., 1994), whereas zidovudine, lamivudine, abacavir, emtricitabine, and tenofovir have only minimal effects. Mitochondrial DNA content in lymphocytes, however, does not correlate with the presence of ATN (Simpson et al., 2006).

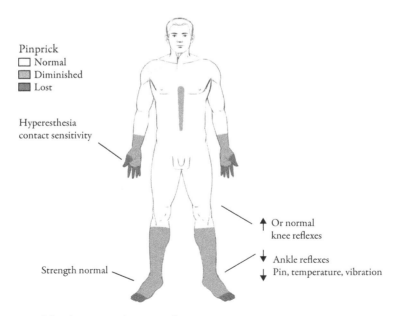

Pinprick
□ Normal
▨ Diminished
■ Lost

Hyperesthesia contact sensitivity

↑ Or normal knee reflexes

↓ Ankle reflexes
↓ Pin, temperature, vibration

Strength normal

Figure 34.2 Typical signs and symptoms of distal sensory polyneuropathy

The differential diagnosis of DSPN/ATN includes other toxic neuropathies, including those caused by other medications commonly used in HIV/AIDS patients such as metronidazole, dapsone, vincristine, isoniazid (DeVivo et al., 2000), and fluoroquinolones (Cohen et al., 2001), as well as diabetes mellitus, vitamin B12 deficiency, diffuse infiltrative lymphocytosis syndrome, alcohol abuse, hepatitis C, and uremia (DeVivo et al., 2000; Williams et al., 2002).

Both DSPN and ATN are usually diagnosed on clinical grounds. Marra et al. (1998) reported that a brief screening examination, performed at a single center by trained nonphysicians, correlated well with the diagnosis of DSPN as made by an experienced AIDS neurologist. In a multicenter study, however, nonphysician neurologic findings were less reliable (Simpson et al., 2006). Nerve conduction studies can be useful, typically showing axonal neuropathy with absent or reduced sensory nerve action potentials, although they might be normal in either mild cases or when the neuropathy is restricted to small fibers (DeVivo et al., 2000). Punch skin biopsies have been used to identify reduced densities of unmyelinated nerve fibers in HIV-associated sensory neuropathies. Skin biopsy analysis is now available in some settings, and it is particularly helpful either when symptoms of burning pain are more prominent than actual neurologic signs or when a nonorganic cause of sensory symptoms is suspected (Polydefkis et al., 2002). Quantitative sudomotor axon reflex test may also be performed to document small-fiber neuropathy. In a study of 102 patients with HIV, autonomic dysfunction was present in 62% of participants (Robinson-Papp et al., 2013). Sural nerve biopsy is rarely indicated except when mononeuritis multiplex is present, because this entity raises the specter of vasculitis.

Diagnosis of neurotoxic neuropathy can be confirmed by withdrawal of the suspected neurotoxin and monitoring for attenuation of symptoms. Symptoms typically improve or resolve over 2 to 10 weeks in approximately two-thirds of patients (Blum et al., 1996). When ARV alternatives are not available, one can "treat through" by maintaining the ART regimen and adding adjuvant pain-modifying agents. If the ART regimen must be switched to remove the offending agent, this is usually feasible except in heavily treated patients. Symptoms may not always subside upon stopping the offending agent—or if they do, recovery may be only partial (Price et al., 1999; Wulff & Simpson, 1999a).

Treatment of HIV sensory neuropathies focuses on removing neurotoxins and managing pain and discomfort. One study showed that 40% of PWH have severe pain, with a numeric pain rating scale of 5 or greater out of 10, and 90% experience some pain (Smyth et al., 2007). Experiencing neuropathic pain appears to increase the risk of both being unemployed and experiencing dependence in instrumental activities of daily living (IADLS) (Ellis et al., 2010). In addition, neuropathic pain itself, but not its severity, is associated with current major depressive disorder and greater severity of depressive symptoms (Ellis et al., 2010).

Although there is no FDA-approved treatment for the pain often associated with DSPN caused by HIV, various pain-modifying agents have been used for HIV sensory neuropathies, as they have for diabetic polyneuropathy, including antidepressants, anticonvulsants, and narcotics. In mild neuropathies, over-the-counter treatments such as acetaminophen can be helpful (DeVivo et al., 2000; Wulff & Simpson, 1999a). One randomized controlled study demonstrated evidence of efficacy for topical capsaicin 8% (Simpson et al., 2008). Night splints may also be useful in the management of neuropathic pain with improvement of sleep (Sandoval et al., 2010). Although pain-modifying anticonvulsants and antidepressants have been useful clinically (DeVivo et al., 2000; Wulff & Simpson, 1999a) and can improve quality of life and function for many patients with HIV sensory neuropathies (Simpson, 2003), placebo-controlled trials on neuropathic pain have shown no significant benefit from amitriptyline, low-dose topical capsaicin, pregabalin, gabapentin, subcutaneous recombinant human nerve growth factor, subcutaneous prosaptide, intranasal peptide T, or lamotrigine (Phillips et al., 2010). Lamotrigine did show some superiority to placebo in the neurotoxic ARV-exposed stratum as a secondary outcome measure of the study. Although placebo-controlled trials have been negative, tricyclic antidepressants (e.g., desipramine and amitriptyline) occasionally can be useful. Sedation is common with some, particularly amitriptyline, so these are more useful for control of nighttime neuropathic pain. Daytime sedation can generally be avoided by using small doses and escalating slowly. Pain-modifying anticonvulsants have also been useful clinically (DeVivo et al., 2000; Wulff & Simpson, 1999a) and can improve quality of life and function for many patients with HIV sensory neuropathies (Simpson, 2003). Use of opiate medication must be approached with caution due to the prevalence of risk factors for aberrant prescription opiate use that is often found in this population (Chou et al., 2009). Alternative treatments include acupuncture and hypnosis (Dorfman et al., 2013). Further management details are provided by Verma et al. (2004).

CONSIDERATIONS FOR RESOURCE-LIMITED SETTINGS

A recent study of DSPN in seven resource-limited settings estimated DSPN incidence in PWH who were ART-naive and had a CD4+ T-cell count of less than 300 cells/mm³ compared to people without HIV and PWH virally suppressed on one of three ART regimens. A total of 860 PWH were enrolled from Brazil, India, Malawi, Peru, South Africa, Thailand, and Zimbabwe. Before initiating combination ART, 21.3% of PWH had DSPN compared with 8.5% of people without HIV. PWH with DSPN were more likely to report inability to work and depression than PWH without DSPN. Overall prevalence of DSPN among those virally suppressed on ART decreased from 20.3% at week 48 to 15.3% at week 144 and finally to 10.3% at week 192. Incident DSPN was seen in 127 PWH. Longitudinally, DSPN was more likely in older individuals and PWH with less education ($p = 0.03$). There was no significant association between ART regimen and DSPN (Vecchio et al., 2020).

INFLAMMATORY DEMYELINATING POLYNEUROPATHY

LEARNING OBJECTIVE

- Discuss the clinical features, differential diagnosis, and management of acute inflammatory demyelinating polyneuropathy (AIDP) and chronic inflammatory demyelinating polyneuropathy (CIDP) in PWH

WHAT'S NEW?

The differential diagnosis of AIDP includes disorders of the spinal cord such as transverse myelitis, acute spinal cord compression, and acute infarction of the spinal cord; disorders affecting anterior horn cells, including poliomyelitis and West Nile virus; acute peripheral neuropathies such as tick paralysis, porphyria, Lyme disease, and lead or arsenic poisoning; and neuromuscular junction disorders such as botulism, myasthenia gravis, or Lambert–Eaton myasthenic syndrome.

KEY POINTS

- AIDP and CIDP are not common HIV-associated peripheral neuropathies. Their cause is autoimmune-induced inflammation and breakdown of peripheral nerve myelin.

- AIDP has rapid onset and progression and often develops during HIV seroconversion or before immunosuppression has evolved.

- AIDP and CIDP in PWH are not associated with the classic CSF albuminocytological dissociation expected in people without HIV. PWH often have a CSF lymphocytic pleocytosis.

- AIDP is treated with either plasmapheresis or IVIG and with ganciclovir/foscarnet/cidofovir if CMV is detected as a causative agent.

- CIDP is treated with corticosteroids or intermittent courses of either plasmapheresis or IVIG that may be continued long term until therapeutic response.

Peripheral neuropathy is the most common neurologic manifestation in patients with HIV/AIDS and can manifest in a number of ways: DPSN, AIDP and CIDP, mononeuritis multiplex, autonomic neuropathy, and progressive polyradiculopathy (Wulff & Simpson, 1999b; Wulff et al., 2000). Whereas DSPN is the most common presentation and can occur secondary to direct HIV infection or as a side effect of NRTIs (Parry et al., 1997; Wulff et al., 2000), inflammatory demyelinating neuropathies in patients with HIV are much less common (Leger et al., 1989).

Inflammatory demyelinating polyradiculopathies are classified as either acute or chronic based on the duration of symptom progression. AIDP, also known as Guillain–Barré syndrome (GBS), is defined as progressive, usually ascending weakness and sensory symptoms with symptom nadir by 4 weeks. In contrast, CIDP is classified by progressive proximal and distal weakness and sensory loss with symptom progression for longer than 8 weeks.

The association between inflammatory polyneuropathies and HIV was first reported in 1985 by Lipkin et al. AIDP typically occurs in the early stages of HIV infection during the seroconversion stage or during early HIV infection before seroconversion has evolved (Markarian et al., 1998; Mishra et al., 1985; Wulff & Simpson, 1999b). In patients with relatively intact immune function, AIDP may be the first clinical manifestation of HIV infection (Parry et al., 1997). Miller–Fischer/GBS overlap syndrome has been reported in advanced AIDS, with elevated anti-GQ1b antibody titer despite severe immunosuppression (Hiraga et al., 2007). GBS has also been reported as an manifestation of IRIS in patients treated with combination ART and a dramatic increase in CD4[+] T-cell counts (Piliero et al., 2003; Rauschkaa et al., 2003). CIDP generally occurs later during the advanced stage of HIV infection (Verma, 2001; Verma & Bradley, 2000).

PATHOGENESIS

Both AIDP and CIDP are thought to be due to an underlying autoimmune inflammatory response against peripheral nerve myelin-associated antigens, resulting in breakdown of peripheral nerve myelin (Radziwill et al., 2002). Rarely, HIV infection has been reported in association with an acute axonal motor neuropathy, where the pathology is thought to be associated with an immune response against the peripheral nerve axon (Dardis et al., 2015; Goldstein et al., 2013; Jadhav et al., 2014; Wagner & Bromber, 2007).

CLINICAL FEATURES

AIDP is frequently associated with a preceding illness, such as upper respiratory infection or acute enterocolitis. AIDP commonly presents with paresthesias, followed by back pain, ascending symmetric numbness and weakness, and absent reflexes. Patients may also experience facial weakness, ophthalmoplegia, and autonomic dysfunction (commonly labile blood pressures and tachycardia).

CIDP can present with progressive or relapsing proximal and distal weakness, sensory loss, and absent reflexes. Pain is a less common presentation (Dimachkie & Barohn, 2014).

CSF ANALYSIS

CSF is characteristically acellular in AIDP in persons without HIV. Protein levels may be normal during the first week of the illness but will increase within 2 or 3 weeks after symptom onset. Elevated CSF protein has been associated mainly with increased permeability of the blood–CSF barrier (Winer, 2001). On the other hand, AIDP seen with HIV infection may be associated with lymphocytic pleocytosis. In a study of 10 patients with HIV-associated AIDP, CSF white blood cell count ranged from 2 to 17 cells/mm³ (Brannagan & Zhou, 2003). The presence of increased protein in the CSF is useful for the diagnosis, and a lymphocytic CSF pleocytosis (10–50 cells/mm³) distinguishes HIV-associated inflammatory demyelinating neuropathies from those without HIV infection (Wulff & Simpson, 1999b). However, the absence of CSF pleocytosis does not rule out HIV infection and hence warrants testing HIV in all patients with AIDP (Brannagan & Zhou, 2003). In addition, either elevated CSF protein or elevated white blood cell counts may be found in people with HIV (Marshall et al., 1988). Generally, CSF pleocytosis is suggestive of either inflammatory/infectious etiology or underlying malignancy. Markedly elevated cell counts or the presence of CSF polymorphonuclear granulocytes in a patient whose clinical presentation appears typical of either AIDP or CIDP should alert the physician to seriously consider alternative diagnoses (Hughes et al., 1991). Enterovirus myelitis, West Nile myelitis, European tick-borne encephalitis virus, and herpes virus infection (CMV, VZV, EBV, and HSV-1 and -2) may show an initial polymorphonuclear pleocytosis. Lyme disease and HIV infection need to be considered with a lymphocytic pleocytosis (Rauschkaa et al., 2003).

Brannagan and Zhou (2003) reported that the mean CD4⁺ T-cell count was 367 cells/mm³ (range, 55–800 cells/mm³) in a series of 10 HIV-positive patients with GBS. An acute polyradiculopathy in patients with CD4⁺ T-cell count of less than 50 cells/mm³ may be secondary to CMV infection, and empiric ganciclovir is indicated (Brannagan & Zhou, 2003).

ELECTROPHYSIOLOGY

Diagnosis is aided by nerve conduction studies showing features of demyelination—that is, slowing of nerve conduction velocities, prolonged distal latencies, temporal dispersion, conduction block, and prolonged F-wave latencies.

BIOPSY

Nerve biopsies are rarely performed to diagnose either AIDP or CIDP, but biopsy may be considered if the clinical or physiologic picture is atypical. Pathology includes macrophage-mediated segmental demyelination and an inflammatory infiltrate (Cornblath et al., 1987).

DIFFERENTIAL DIAGNOSIS

The differential diagnosis of AIDP includes disorders of the spinal cord such as transverse myelitis, acute spinal cord compression, and acute infarction of the spinal cord (which in the initial phases may present with flaccid areflexia below the level of the lesion due to spinal shock); disorders affecting anterior horn cells, including poliomyelitis and West Nile virus; acute peripheral neuropathies such as tick paralysis, porphyria, Lyme disease, and lead or arsenic poisoning; and neuromuscular junction disorders such as botulism, myasthenia gravis, or Lambert–Eaton myasthenic syndrome (Wakerly & Yuki, 2015). TB, toxoplasmosis, and HSV-2, syphilis, and lymphoma can also present with signs and symptoms of polyradiculitis.

In patients with subacute/chronic neuropathy and HIV infection with CD4⁺ T-cell counts of less than 50 cells/mm³, mononeuritis multiplex, DSPN, and CMV-related polyradiculomyelitis or polyradiculitis need to be considered in the differential diagnosis. CMV polyradiculitis (or polyradiculomyelitis if the infection involves not only the nerve roots but also the spinal cord) typically presents as an ascending weakness beginning in the lower extremities with areflexia, sensory loss, and weakness. Patients typically experience urinary retention and decreased anal sphincter tone. MRI of the spine with contrast demonstrates enhancement of the nerve roots, typically involving the cauda equina. Nerve conduction studies will show low compound muscle action potentials and mildly slowed conduction velocity corresponding to axonal involvement. Electromyography will show acute denervation with spontaneous activity and decreased recruitment. CSF studies in CMV polyradiculitis usually reveal a polymorphonuclear-predominant pleocytosis, elevated protein, and decreased glucose levels. CSF PCR for CMV DNA can confirm the diagnosis.

CMV infection of the peripheral nervous system may also manifest as an asymmetric multifocal neuropathy, observed in HIV patients with low CD4⁺ T-cell counts. Infection affects individual peripheral nerves, with the radial, ulnar, peroneal, and lateral cutaneous nerves of the thigh being most commonly involved (Anders & Goebel, 1999). Rapid progression has been reported and can become confluent (Robinson-Papp et al., 2009b), mimicking an acute/subacute polyneuropathy. Electrodiagnostic studies of the nerves show multifocal sensory and motor nerve dysfunction in an axonal pattern with acute denervation. CSF studies may or may not be positive for CMV PCR, and nerve biopsy may also fail to reveal CMV. Empiric treatment is warranted when clinical suspicion is high, especially in the setting of concomitant CMV infection affecting other organs. Treatment is also with either ganciclovir or foscarnet as the first-line option. The differential diagnosis should include mononeuritis multiplex in PWH with high CD4⁺ T-cell counts, hepatitis C with cryoglobulinemia, mononeuritis multiplex due to vasculitis in association with B-cell lymphoma, and DSPN associated with either HIV or ART with D-drugs.

TREATMENT

AIDP is treated with either high-dose IVIG therapy or plasmapheresis. These treatments enhance recovery and arrest clinical progression (Cornblath et al., 1987; Hadden et al., 1998; Plasma Exchange/Sandoglobulin Guillain–Barré Syndrome Trial Group, 1997). IVIG and plasma exchange have been shown to be equally effective in treating HIV-negative AIDP (Plasma Exchange/Sandoglobulin Guillain–Barré Trial Group, 1997; van der Meche, 1992). In 2015, Rosca et al. reported improvement in CD4⁺ and CD8⁺ T-cell counts and HIV-1 RNA levels in their patient treated with IVIG for HIV-associated GBS. Due to the possibility of CMV polyradiculomyelitis or polyradiculitis, patients with severe immunosuppression (CD4⁺ T-cell counts <50 cells/mm³) should be treated with intravenous ganciclovir, foscarnet, or cidofovir or a combination of these, in addition to the standard treatment. CIDP is treated with oral prednisone, pulse intravenous high-dose methylprednisolone or dexamethasone, or intermittent courses of plasmapheresis or IVIG. A randomized controlled study confirmed the benefit of prednisone in HIV-related CIDP, although this treatment approach may worsen immunosuppression (Lindenbaum et al., 2001). Acute relapses in CIDP are treated with either IVIG or plasmapheresis.

PROGNOSIS

Initial clinical course and response to pharmacologic treatment in AIDP is similar in HIV-seropositive and -seronegative patients (Verma, 2001). Schreiber et al. (2011) reported on a patient with GBS as the initial presentation of HIV infection who recovered fully using IVIG and rehabilitation without initiation of ART, suggesting that patients with GBS early in the course of HIV infection may behave like those with GBS without HIV infection. Compared to HIV-negative patients, HIV-associated GBS patients may experience relapses and may be more likely to develop CIDP (Brannagan & Zhou, 2003). With CIDP, although treatment can halt the progression of the disease and remyelination of the peripheral nerves can occur, there is evidence that unrecoverable secondary axonal damage can occur in some cases (Hughes et al., 1991).

NEUROLOGIC COMPLICATIONS OF HIV PATIENTS WITH CMV INFECTION

LEARNING OBJECTIVE

- Discuss the clinical syndromes, differential diagnosis, and management of neurologic complications of CMV infection in HIV-positive patients

KEY POINTS

- CMV CNS disease occurs late in the course of HIV and may involve different parts of the CNS.

- Diagnosis is based on the clinical findings, results of imaging, and virologic markers.

- The treatment should be started empirically while awaiting the CSF PCR results.

CMV, a member of the herpesvirus family, is a frequent opportunistic viral infection in PWH and occurs when the $CD4^+$ T-cell count is less than 100 cells/mm^3 due to reactivation of latent infection. CMV infection of the nervous system accounts for fewer than 1% of CMV infections in PWH (McCutchan, 1995) and often develops concurrently with other, more common CMV extraneural diseases such as retinitis or gastrointestinal involvement. Clinical syndromes of CMV infection in the nervous system include encephalitis, polyradiculomyelitis, polyradiculitis, and multifocal neuropathy (Anders & Goebel, 1999). Although these syndromes are uncommon, recognition, treatment with antivirals, and restoration of immune response are paramount to reduce the risk of death.

CMV encephalitis is the most common manifestation of CNS infection due to CMV. Clinically, infection can present as diffuse encephalitis, ventriculoencephalitis, or focal encephalitis. Diffuse encephalitis develops over several weeks and thus presents subacutely with memory loss, attention and concentration difficulties, and delirium. Focal neurologic deficits may also be seen. Pathologically, microglial nodules may be found in the cortex, brainstem, cerebellum, and basal ganglia, occurring most commonly in gray matter (Morgello et al., 1987). On neuroimaging, MRI may show a variety of patterns. The brain may appear normal, or it may show hyperintense T2 lesions in the areas described previously and nodular lesions with or without enhancement on T1 postcontrast images (Maschke et al., 2002).

Ventriculoencephalitis presents with lethargy, confusion, cranial nerve deficits, ataxia, and focal neurologic deficits, and it sometimes occurs concomitantly with CMV polyradiculitis. Ventriculoencephalitis may be more insidious in onset and have a poorer prognosis (Maschke et al., 2002). CMV encephalitis has been reported to occur even while patients are on treatment with ganciclovir for extra-CNS disease (Bermann & Kim, 1994). Pathologically, necrotizing lesions are seen in the ventricular system, and imaging shows periventricular enhancement with or without ventriculomegaly. The third and less common type of CMV encephalitis, focal encephalitis, presents with focal neurologic deficits corresponding to a cerebral mass lesion. MRI will show ring-enhancing lesions with surrounding edema.

CSF PCR for CMV DNA confirms the diagnosis of CMV encephalitis. The CSF may also show pleocytosis with either a polymorphonuclear or a mononuclear predominance, along with elevated protein and decreased glucose levels. Viral culture is rarely positive. The detection of other viruses often confounds the diagnosis; thus, the index of suspicion must be based on the presentation and imaging findings in the context of profound immunosuppression. The differential diagnosis for CMV encephalitis must include HIV encephalitis, PML, and neurosyphilis. When CMV encephalitis presents as a ring-enhancing lesion, the differential diagnosis expands to other etiologies known to present similarly, such as toxoplasmosis, primary CNS lymphoma, and tuberculous meningitis with tuberculomas (Offiah & Turnbull, 2006).

CMV polyradiculitis (or polyradiculomyelitis if the infection involves not only the nerve roots but also the spinal cord) typically presents as an ascending weakness beginning in the lower extremities with areflexia, sensory loss, and weakness. Patients typically experience urinary retention and decreased anal sphincter tone. MRI of the spine with contrast demonstrates enhancement of the nerve roots, typically involving the cauda equina. Nerve conduction studies will show low compound muscle action potentials and mildly slowed conduction velocity corresponding to axonal involvement. Electromyography will show acute denervation with spontaneous activity and decreased recruitment. CSF studies in CMV polyradiculitis usually reveal a polymorphonuclear-predominant pleocytosis, elevated protein, and decreased glucose levels. CSF PCR for CMV DNA can confirm the diagnosis.

The differential diagnosis of CMV polyradiculitis includes GBS, which may be clinically indistinguishable and only differentiated on nerve conduction studies showing a more demyelinating pattern (Corral et al., 1997). Other opportunistic infections, including TB, toxoplasmosis, and HSV-2, can present in a similar manner. Syphilis and lymphoma can also cause polyradiculitis.

Treatment for both CMV encephalitis and CMV polyradiculitis/polyradiculomyelitis is similar. Induction treatment with either intravenous ganciclovir or foscarnet is the usual first-line treatment option. Sometimes in severe encephalitis cases, combination treatment with both ganciclovir and foscarnet has been used (Portegies et al., 2004; Silva et al., 2010). Cidofovir can be used as an alternative treatment option. Empiric treatment of CMV infection is often advised because CSF results may be delayed. Maintenance treatment with ganciclovir has been recommended, but the duration of treatment has not been well studied. Of note, patients with CMV polyradiculitis/polyradiculomyelitis have been shown to be more responsive to treatment compared to CMV encephalitis patients (Cinque et al., 1998).

The best-described CMV infection of the peripheral nervous system is an asymmetric multifocal neuropathy, observed in HIV patients with low CD4+ counts. Infection affects individual peripheral nerves, with the radial, ulnar, peroneal, and lateral cutaneous nerves of the thigh being most commonly involved (Anders & Goebel, 1999). Rapid progression has been reported and can become confluent (Robinson-Papp et al., 2009a). Electrodiagnostic studies of the nerves show multifocal sensory and motor nerve dysfunction in an axonal pattern with acute denervation. CSF studies may or may not be positive for CMV PCR, and nerve biopsy may also fail to reveal CMV. Empiric treatment is warranted when clinical suspicion is high, especially in the setting of concomitant CMV infection affecting other organs. Treatment is also with either ganciclovir or foscarnet as the first-line option. The differential diagnosis should include mononeuropathy multiplex in HIV patients with high CD4+ T-cell counts, hepatitis C with cryoglobulinemia, mononeuropathy multiplex due to vasculitis in association with B-cell lymphoma, and distal sensory polyneuropathy associated with either HIV or ART with dideoxynucleoside reverse transcriptase inhibitors.

INTRACRANIAL LESIONS

LEARNING OBJECTIVE

- Discuss the clinical presentation, differential diagnosis, and treatment of intracranial lesions in PWH

WHAT'S NEW?

Due to concern for drug–drug interactions, particularly in patients receiving ART, most clinicians favor levetiracetam as the first-line treatment for managing seizures. In the setting of status epilepticus, fosphenytoin, levetiracetam, and valproate appear to have equal efficacy. Enzyme-inducing antiepileptic drugs should be avoided in people on ART regimens that include PIs or NNRTIs.

KEY POINTS

- Intracranial focal lesions in HIV specifically occur in PWH with CD4+ T-cell counts less than 200 cell/mm³.

- The most common focal mass lesion is toxoplasmosis. The use of prophylactic agents such as trimethoprim–sulfamethoxazole can decrease the incidence of toxoplasmosis.

- Primary central nervous system lymphoma (PCNSL) is the most common brain neoplasm seen in PWH. On imaging studies, it is usually a solitary intracranial mass lesion in the setting of a negative toxoplasmosis serology.

- PML on neuroimaging is a nonenhancing lesion of the white matter involving the subcortical U-fibers without edema or mass effect.

Intracranial mass lesions are common neurologic findings and account for as many as half of the neurologic disorders seen in PWH. Although intracranial mass lesions typically occur in PWH with advanced immunosuppression (CD4+ counts <200 cells/mm³), an intracranial lesion can occasionally be the initial presenting symptom of AIDS. Intracranial lesions in PWH can be broadly categorized into three groups: opportunistic infections, neoplasms, and cerebrovascular disease (American Academy of Neurology [AAN], 1998).

The clinical presentation of intracranial lesions varies depending on the underlying etiology. Typical presenting clinical symptoms include alteration in level of awareness and consciousness as well as focal neurologic deficits. In developed countries such as the US, the most common etiologies include toxoplasmosis, PCNSL, bacterial and fungal abscesses, and PML. Additional entities on the differential diagnosis include primary brain tumor, brain metastasis from systemic cancer, tuberculoma, and lesions of fungal origin. Differentiating among this large differential diagnosis of intracranial lesions can be challenging, especially with regard to use of biopsy for establishing the diagnosis. However, in patients with large lesions with mass effect and impending herniation, open biopsy with decompression is recommended. The correct diagnosis is paramount to effectively managing the causal pathogen in a timely manner. Achieving this goal requires a knowledge-based diagnostic algorithm that accounts for the relative frequency of various types of intracranial lesions. Figure 34.3 provides a useful process of differential considerations based on level of immunosuppression, typical clinical and radiographic presentations, management options, and prognosis with or without empirical treatment (AAN, 1998).

Cerebral toxoplasmosis is the most common cause of space-occupying intracranial focal mass lesions in PWH and typically results from reactivation of latent infection of *Toxoplasma gondii*, an obligate intracellular parasite (AAN,

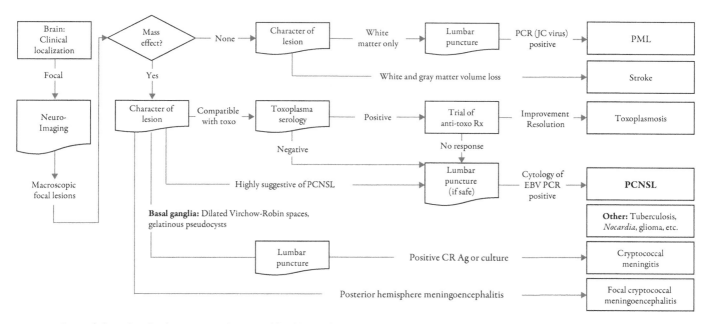

Figure 34.3 General algorithm for diagnostic evaluation of focal brain disease   SOURCE: Adapted from American Academy of Neurology (AAN). *Neurology.* 1998;50:21–26.

2000a). In the US, there has been a decline in the incidence of cerebral toxoplasmosis due to widespread use of prophylactic agents such as trimethoprim–sulfamethoxazole and ART in PWH (AAN, 1998).

Toxoplasmosis often presents with subacute changes in level of consciousness, fever, headaches, seizures, and focal neurologic deficit. It should be suspected in any HIV patient with an intracranial mass lesion, especially if the patient has a CD4+ T-cell count of less than 100 cells/mm³, is not receiving toxoplasmosis prophylaxis, and has immunoglobulin G antibodies to *T. gondii* (AAN, 2000a). Investigative studies such as CSF analysis, toxoplasma serology, or imaging studies do not always provide a definitive diagnosis. In this patient population, lumbar puncture is often contraindicated due to the presence of lesions with mass effect and increased risk of herniation. If CSF is obtained, analysis frequently shows nonspecific mild mononuclear pleocytosis with elevated protein. PCR can increase the utility of CSF analysis. PCR can detect *T. gondii* with high specificity (100%) but variable sensitivity (30–50%) (AAN, 2002). Consequently, whereas a positive PCR result is highly suggestive of the diagnosis, a negative result does not exclude it.

Imaging studies can also provide supportive information. MRI with and without contrast has greater sensitivity than contrast-enhanced CT, especially for detecting multiple lesions, subcortical lesions, and posterior fossa involvement. However, neither imaging modality alone is sufficient to make a diagnosis because there is no pathognomonic radiographically distinguishing feature of toxoplasmosis compared to PCNSL. Toxoplasmosis typically presents as multiple, homogeneous, ring-enhancing lesions with cerebral edema and mass effect. It has a predilection for the basal ganglia and corticomedullary junction, with involvement of both white and gray matter (AAN, 2000a). Although a solitary mass lesion with edema is often observed in PCNSL, it can also be

seen in toxoplasmosis (AAN, 2000a). Thallium single-photon emission computed tomography (SPECT) and positron emission tomography (PET) can be useful in distinguishing toxoplasmosis from lymphoma. Lymphoma has increased thallium uptake on SPECT and hypermetabolism of glucose and methionine on PET. Toxoplasma is hypometabolic on PET and does not show uptake of thallium (AAN, 2000a). As a result of the limitation of the investigative modalities mentioned previously, diagnosis of toxoplasmosis is often presumptive and based on clinical and radiographic findings, as well as clinical and radiographic response to empiric treatment within the first 2 weeks. Open or stereotactic brain biopsy can yield a definitive diagnosis; however, there is morbidity and even mortality associated with the procedure due to subsequent intracranial hemorrhage. Biopsy is often pursued as a last resort in patients who do not improve with empiric management, have large mass effect with impending herniation, and require a rapid definitive diagnosis.

Empirical anti-toxoplasma therapy is usually started once toxoplasmosis is suspected. First-line treatment includes the use of sulfadiazine, pyrimethamine, and folinic acid (leucovorin) (AAN, 2000a). Folinic acid must be given to counteract myelosuppression from use of pyrimethamine. Treatment duration is at least 6 weeks before beginning secondary prophylaxis with pyrimethamine alone or pyrimethamine and a sulfonamide. Recrudescence occurs in up to 30% of patients, usually due to poor adherence to secondary prophylaxis; however, it can occur despite good adherence to the treatment plan (AAN, 2000a). In patients with sulfa allergy or intolerance, clindamycin is an alternative to sulfadiazine; however, use of clindamycin is associated with a slightly increased incidence of recrudescence. If the patient is intolerant to both sulfadiazine and clindamycin, alternatives include high-dose trimethoprim–sulfamethoxazole, azithromycin, and atovaquone. Atovaquone is less well tolerated due to gastrointestinal side effects. There is usually clinical improvement within the first 10 to 14 days of treatment. Clinical improvement occurs prior to radiographic evidence of improvement, which may be noted within 2 or 3 weeks. Lack of improvement within the first 2 weeks should raise suspicion for an alternative diagnosis.

The use of adjunctive corticosteroids, such as dexamethasone, should be brief and implemented only in very particular circumstances, such as when there is clinical evidence of midline shift or impending herniation, signs of critically elevated intracranial pressure, or clinical deterioration within the first 48 hours of therapy. Under these circumstances, the benefits of steroids outweigh the many risks of steroid administration. Steroids may serve to confound the diagnosis for several reasons. Steroids can improve the clinical presentation, making it difficult to distinguish between the anti-inflammatory effects of the steroids and the therapeutic effectiveness of empiric anti-toxoplasmosis treatment. In addition, steroid's anti-inflammatory actions affect the radiographic presentation by decreasing the intensity of contrast enhancement and surrounding edema, thus interfering with reliable comparative interpretation of subsequent radiographic images. Steroids can also complicate the pathologic diagnosis of PCNSL if a biopsy is needed, rendering the biopsy falsely negative for the presence of lymphoma. Aside from more acute steroid complications such as avascular necrosis, hyperglycemia, and psychiatric symptoms, the prolonged use of steroids can also make the patient susceptible to other opportunistic infections.

An important differential diagnosis is PCNSL. It is one of the four AIDS-defining neoplasms (the others are systemic non-Hodgkin's lymphoma, Kaposi's sarcoma, and invasive cervical carcinoma). PCNSL is commonly seen in HIV patients with CD4+ T-cell counts of less than 50 cells/mm³ and is rarely the initial presenting symptom of AIDS. The pathogenesis is also strongly related to reactivation of latent EBV infection. The clinical presentation is very similar to that of toxoplasmosis, with alteration of the level of consciousness, impaired cognitive function, seizures, and focal neurologic deficits such as aphasia and hemiparesis. Investigative studies such as CSF analysis and imaging are often utilized. Lumbar puncture should be obtained only if there are no contraindications, such as risk of herniation. CSF analysis, particularly cytology, can be helpful, but it has a very low sensitivity. PCR assay of CSF for EBV DNA can be diagnostic. PCR for EBV has a sensitivity greater than 80% and a specificity greater than 95%. As with toxoplasmosis, MRI often provides a higher diagnostic yield than CT scan, but CT with contrast remains useful, particularly in patients who have a contraindication to MRI. PCNSL can present with single or multiple well-defined, ring or patchy enhancing lesions with edema and mass effect. It often involves supratentorial regions such as the corpus callosum and periventricular or periependymal areas (PCNSL in AIDS) (AAN, 2000b). As previously mentioned, SPECT and PET can be useful in differentiating lymphoma from other etiologies, including toxoplasmosis. Although PET and SPECT have limited sensitivity, they have high specificity. A diagnosis is often made using a combination of CSF cytology, toxoplasmosis serologic testing,

failure of a trial of empiric antibiotics usually for treatment of toxoplasmosis, and positive CSF PCR for EBV; if necessary, a brain biopsy may be obtained (AAN, 2000b). Open or stereotactic brain biopsy is typically required prior to whole-brain irradiation, which is the current mainstay treatment for PCNSL. Whole-brain radiation appears to be able to prevent further neurologic progression or produce reversal of deficits. However, the treatment plan is based on the patient's overall health status. There can be spread of lymphoma with involvement of the eyes; therefore, a complete ophthalmologic examination including a slit-lamp examination should be performed (AAN, 2000b).

Other etiologies of intracranial mass lesions include other neoplasms, cerebrovascular disease, and opportunistic infections. Kaposi's sarcoma may rarely manifest as an intracranial lesion. Furthermore, patients with HIV may also develop brain lesions unrelated to immunocompromised status, such as glioma or metastatic disease.

In addition to toxoplasmosis, patients with HIV may develop parasitic, fungal, or bacterial infections that present as a mass lesion. Most of these opportunistic infections present with meningitis and focal neurologic signs and symptoms related to the presence of a mass lesion. Although neurocysticercosis (NCC) is not more common in patients with HIV, the incidence of HIV infection is growing in countries where NCC is endemic. Coinfection has been rarely reported, but reports of concomitant infection with HIV, NCC, and an additional pathogen have been reported. Furthermore, in the setting of immunocompromise, interpretation of imaging findings may be particularly difficult. On imaging studies, the appearance of NCC varies depending on the stage of infection. MRI is favored over CT scan, especially for evaluation of intraventricular and cisternal/subarachnoid cysts as well as cystic degeneration and pericystic inflammatory reaction (Serpa et al., 2007).

Common bacterial mass lesions include abscess from *Mycobacterium tuberculosis, Nocardia, Listeria monocytogenes,* and *Treponema pallidum.* In developing countries, particularly in highly endemic areas such as Southeast Asia and Africa, tuberculous meningitis is common. Due to its proclivity for the basal meninges, tuberculous meningitis often presents clinically with multiple cranial neuropathies and hydrocephalus (AAN, 2000a). Neuroimaging may show masses, which are often tuberculomas. Intracranial tuberculomas can be seen on MRI as hypointense or isointense due to varying amounts of caseous necrosis. This variable appearance of intracranial tuberculoma is attributed to the changing nature of the granulomatous lesion (Park & Song, 2008). The diagnosis of tuberculous meningitis can be challenging and requires a combination of CSF analysis including culture for TB, acid-fast bacilli stain, and TB PCR along with a clinical evaluation for systemic TB.

Common etiologies of fungal abscesses include *Cryptococcus neoformans, Candida albicans,* aspergillosis, mucormycosis histoplasmosis, and coccidioidomycosis. Of these fungi, cryptococcosis is the most common opportunistic fungal infection in PWH and arises from an acquired infection from *C. neoformans,* an encapsulated yeast. The widespread use of fluconazole as prophylaxis has resulted in a decrease in incidence. Neuroimaging, usually a contrast-enhanced brain MRI, may show cryptococcomas—multiple enhancing lesions of various sizes most often seen within perivascular spaces. These lesions usually resolve with treatment. A definitive diagnosis is made by a positive CSF culture for *C. neoformans*, a positive CSF India ink stain, or a reactive CSF cryptococcal antigen test. For additional information, see Chapter 28.

PML is characterized by multifocal areas of demyelination, often in subcortical and periventricular areas. The pathogenesis is reactivation of JC virus infecting oligodendroglia in the setting of advanced immunosuppression. On imaging studies, the lesions do not enhance with contrast and do not produce any edema or mass effect. The subcortical U-fibers are involved. However, in the setting of IRIS, on MRI with contrast, PML can present with contrast enhancement, focal edema, and mass effect (Tan & Roda, 2009).

PWH with intracranial lesions are at heightened risk for developing seizures. Antiepileptic drugs (AEDs) should not be given for routine prophylaxis to patients with a CNS mass lesion because not all individuals with CNS lesions will develop seizures. However, once the patient experiences a seizure, chronic AED administration is appropriate. In 2012, the AAN issued an evidence-based guideline for clinicians about AED selection for people with HIV/AIDS (Birbeck et al., 2012). The guideline describes the strength of evidence for each of its recommendations based on the quality of evidence available from clinical investigations. The vast majority of the recommendations in this guideline were rated as having weak evidence.

The AAN guideline states that it may be important to avoid enzyme-inducing AEDs in people on ART regimens that include PIs or NNRTIs because pharmacokinetic interactions may result in virologic failure (Birbeck et al., 2012). Phenobarbital, phenytoin, and carbamazepine are commonly used enzyme-inducing AEDs, and phenobarbital, although rarely used in high-resource countries, is the mainstay of seizure management in low-resource countries where HIV is highly prevalent. The guideline identifies circumstances in which specific dose adjustments to the ART regimen should be made when certain AEDs are used concomitantly. For example, patients concurrently on phenytoin and lopinavir/ritonavir may need a 50% dosage increase in lopinavir/ritonavir to maintain adequate serum levels of the PI to ensure virologic control. Patients taking both atazanavir/ritonavir and lamotrigine may require a 50% increase in the lamotrigine dose to maintain adequate serum levels of the AED and thereby seizure control. Patients taking both zidovudine and the P450 inhibitor valproic acid may require a zidovudine dose reduction to maintain unchanged zidovudine levels (Birbeck et al., 2012). Although not specifically recommended in the guideline, renally excreted medications such as levetiracetam are often favored for patients on ART given their lack of drug–drug interactions. Although previously either intravenous phenytoin or fosphenytoin was the recommended treatment for status epilepticus, a recent study comparing three intravenous AEDs—levetiracetam (60 mg/kg), fosphenytoin (20 mg/kg), and valproic acid (40 mg/kg)—for the treatment of benzodiazepine-refractory status epilepticus in both children and adults determined that each medication had similar efficacy (Kapur et al., 2019). Although this study was not specific for PWH and the etiologies of status epilepticus varied, the results of this study should be applicable to PWH presenting with a mass lesion causing status epilepticus.

Using the approach discussed in this chapter, common etiologies of intracranial mass lesion can be systemically evaluated in order to make a diagnosis and institute therapy. In settings with limited resources such as sophisticated neuroimaging, CSF PCR, and biopsy, clinical findings on the history and physical exam combined with the prevalence of infectious etiologies should guide the diagnosis and subsequent empiric therapeutic intervention.

REFERENCES

Aberle SW, Aberle JH, Steininger C, et al. Quantitative real time PCR detection of varicella-zoster virus DNA in cerebrospinal fluid in patients with neurological disease. *Med Microbiol Immunol.* 2005;194:7–12.

Alfahad T, Nath A. Update on HIV-associated neurocognitive disorders. *Curr Neurol Neurosci Rep.* 2013;13:387.

American Academy of Neurology. Evaluation and management of intracranial mass lesions in AIDS: report of the Quality Standards Subcommittee of the American Academy of Neurology. *Neurology.* 1998;50:21–26.

American Academy of Neurology. Opportunistic infections: toxoplasmosis. The neurologic complications of AIDS. *Neurol Continuum.* 2000a;6(5):128–149.

American Academy of Neurology. Primary central nervous system lymphoma in AIDS. The neurologic complications of AIDS. *Neurol Continuum.* 2000b;6(5):177–185.

American Academy of Neurology. Opportunistic and fungal infections of the central nervous system. *Neurol Continuum.* 2002;8(3):125.

Anders HJ, Goebel FD. Neurological manifestations of cytomegalovirus infection in the acquired immunodeficiency syndrome. *Int J STD AIDS.* 1999;10:151–161.

Anderson AM, Muñoz-Moreno JA, McClernon DR, et al. Prevalence and correlates of persistent HIV-1 RNA in cerebrospinal fluid during antiretroviral therapy. *J Infect Dis.* 2017;215(1):105–113.

Antinori A, Arendt G, Becker JT, et al. Updated research nosology for HIV-associated neurocognitive disorders. *Neurology.* 2007;69(18):1789–1799.

Banerjee S, McCutchan JA, Ances BM, et al. Hypertriglyceridemia in combination antiretroviral-treated HIV-positive individuals: potential impact on HIV sensory polyneuropathy. *AIDS.* 2011;25(2):F1–F6.

Banks LT, Geraci A, Liu M, et al. A natural history of HIV myelopathy in the HAART era. *Neurology.* 2002;58:A441.

Beardsley J, Wolbers M, Kibengo FM, et al. Adjunctive dexamethasone in HIV-associated cryptococcal meningitis. *N Engl J Med.* 2016;374(6):542–54.

Bermann SM, Kim RC. The development of cytomegalovirus encephalitis in AIDS patients receiving ganciclovir. *Am J Med.* 1994;96:415–419.

Bhigjee AI, Madurai S, Bill PL, et al. Spectrum of myelopathies in HIV seropositive South African patients. *Neurology.* 2001;57:348–351.

Birbeck G, French J, Perucca E, et al. Evidence-based guideline: antiepileptic drug selection for people with HIV/AIDS: report of the Quality Standards Subcommittee of the American Academy of Neurology and the Ad Hoc Task Force of the Commission on Therapeutic Strategies of the International League Against Epilepsy. *Neurology.* 2012;78(2):139–145.

Blum AS, Dal Pan GJ, Feinberg J, et al. Low-dose zalcitabine-related toxic neuropathy: frequency, natural history, and risk factors. *Neurology*. 1996;46(4):999–1003.

Boisse L, Gill MJ, Power C. HIV infection of the central nervous system: clinical features and neuropathogenesis. *Neurol Clin*. 2008;26:799–819.

Boulware DR, Meya DB, Muzoora C, et al. Timing of antiretroviral therapy after diagnosis of cryptococcal meningitis. *N Engl J Med*. 2014;370:2487–2498.

Brannagan TH 3rd, Zhou Y. HIV associated Guillain–Barré syndrome. *J Neurol Sci*. 2003;208(1–2):39–42.

Candy S, Chang G, Andronikous S. Acute myelopathy or cauda equine syndrome in HIV positive adults in a tuberculosis endemic setting: MRI, clinical, and pathologic findings. *AJNR*. 2014;35(8):1634–1641.

Carvalhal A, Gill MJ, Letendre SL, et al. Central nervous system penetration effectiveness of antiretroviral drugs and neuropsychological impairment in the Ontario HIV Treatment Network Cohort Study. *J Neurovirol*. 2016;22(3):349–357.

Charlier C, Perrodeau E, Leclercq A, et al. Clinical features and prognostic factors of listeriosis: the MONALISA national prospective cohort study. *Lancet Infect Dis*. 2017;17(5):510–519.

Chen CH, Vazquez-Padua M, Cheng YC. Effect of anti-human immunodeficiency virus nucleoside analogs on mitochondrial DNA and its implication for delayed toxicity. *Mol Pharmacol*. 1991;39(5):625–628.

Cherner M, Masliah E, Ellis RJ, et al. Neurocognitive dysfunction predicts postmortem findings of HIV encephalitis. *Neurology*. 2002;59(10):1563–1567.

Cherry CL, Wesselingh SL, Lal L, et al. Evaluation of a clinical screening tool for HIV-associated sensory neuropathies. *Neurology*. 2005;65(11):1778–1781.

Childs E, Lyles R, Selnes OA, et al. Plasma viral load and CD4+ lymphocytes predict HIV-associated dementia and sensory neurology. *Neurology*. 1999;52:607–613.

Cho T, Vaitkevicius H. Infectious myelopathies. *Continuum*. 2012;18(6):1351–1373.

Chong J, Di Rocco A, Tagliati M, et al. MR findings in AIDS-associated myelopathy. *Am J Neuroradiol*. 1999;20(8):1412–1416.

Chou R, Fanciullo GJ, Fine PG, et al. Opioids for chronic noncancer pain: prediction and identification of aberrant drug-related behaviors: a review of the evidence for an American Pain Society and American Academy of Pain Medicine clinical practice guideline. *J Pain*. 2009;10(2):131–146.

Cinque P, Cleator GM, Weber T, et al. Clinical review diagnosis and clinical management of neurological disorders caused by cytomegalovirus in AIDS patients. *J Neurovirol*. 1998;4:120–132.

Cohen JS. Peripheral neuropathy associated with fluoroquinolones. *Ann Pharmacother*. 2001;35(12):1540–1547.

Cornblath DR, McArthur JC. Predominantly sensory neuropathy in patients with AIDS and AIDS-related complex. *Neurology*. 1988;38(5):794–796.

Cornblath DR, McArthur JC, Kennedy PGE, et al. Inflammatory demyelinating peripheral neuropathies associated with human T-cell lymphotropic virus type III infection. *Ann Neurol*. 1987;21:32040.

Corral I, Quereda C, Casado JL, et al. Acute polyradiculopathies in HIV-positive patients. *J Neurol*. 1997;244:499–504.

Dalakas MC, Cupler EJ. Neuropathies in HIV infection. *Baillieres Clin Neurol*. 1996;5(1):199–218.

Dal Pan GJ, Berger JR. Spinal cord disease in human immunodeficiency virus infection. In: Berger JR, Levy RM, eds. *AIDS and the nervous system*. 2nd ed. Philadelphia: Lippincott-Raven; 1997:173–187.

Dal Pan GJ, Glass JD, McArthur JC. Clinicopathologic correlations of HIV-1-associated vacuolar myelopathy: an autopsy-based case-control study. *Neurology*. 1994;44(11):2159–2164.

Dardis C. Acute motor axonal neuropathy in a patient with prolonged CD4 depletion due to HIV: a local variant of macrophage activation syndrome? *Oxford Med Case Rep*. 2015;2:200–2002.

DeBiasi RL, Tyler KL. Molecular methods diagnosis of viral encephalitis. *Clin Microbiol Rev*. 2004;17(4):903–925.

Department of Health and Human Services, Panel on Antiretroviral Guidelines for Adults and Adolescents. Guidelines for the use of antiretroviral agents in HIV-1-infected adults and adolescents. 2020a. https://clinicalinfo.hiv.gov/sites/default/files/inline-files/AdultandAdolescentGL.pdf

Department of Health and Human Services, Panel on Opportunistic Infections in HIV-Positive Adults and Adolescents. Guidelines for the prevention and treatment of opportunistic infections in HIV-positive adults and adolescents: recommendations from the Centers for Disease Control and Prevention, the National Institutes of Health, and the HIV Medicine Association of the Infectious Diseases Society of America. 2020b. https://clinicalinfo.hiv.gov/sites/default/files/inline-files/adult_oi.pdf

DeVivo DC, Percy AK, Chiriboga CA, et al. Neuromuscular disorders in HIV-1 infection. *Continuum*. 2000;6:73–76.

Dimachkie MM, Barohn RJ. Distal myopathies. *Neurol Clin*. 2014;32(3):817–842.

Di Rocco A. Diseases of the spinal cord in human immunodeficiency virus infection. *Semin Neurol*. 1999;19:151–155.

Di Rocco A, Simpson DM. AIDS-associated vacuolar myelopathy. *AIDS Patient Care STDs*. 1998;12(6):457–461.

Dorfman D, George MC, Schnur J, et al. Hypnosis for treatment of HIV neuropathic pain: a preliminary report. *Pain Med*. 2013;14:1048–1056.

Edén A, Fuchs D, Hagberg L, et al. HIV-1 viral escape in cerebrospinal fluid of subjects on suppressive treatment. *J Infect Dis*. 2010;202(12):1819–1825.

Ellis R, Deutsch R, Heaton RK, et al. Neurocognitive impairment is an independent risk factor for death in HIV infection: San Diego HIV Neurobehavioral Research Center Group. *Arch Neurol*. 1997;54(4):416–424.

Ellis RJ, Letendre SL, Vaida F, et al. Randomized trial of central nervous system targeted antiretrovirals for HIV-associated neurocognitive disorder. *Clin Infect Dis*. 2014;58(7):1015–1022.

Ellis RJ, Rosario D, Clifford DB, et al. Continued high prevalence and adverse clinical impact of human immunodeficiency virus-associated sensory neuropathy in the era of combination antiretroviral therapy: the CHARTER Study. *Arch Neurol*. 2010;67(5):552–558.

Erdem H, Senbayrak S, Gencer S, et al. Tuberculosis and brucellosis meningitis differential diagnosis. *Travel Med Infect Dis*. 2015;13(2):185–191.

Erlandson KM, Perez J, Abdo M, et al. Frailty, neurocognitive impairment, or both in predicting poor health outcomes among adults living with human immunodeficiency virus. *Clin Infect Dis*. 2019;68(1):131–138.

Evans SR, Ellis RJ, Chen H, et al. Peripheral neuropathy in HIV: prevalence and risk factors. *AIDS*. 2011;25(7):919–928.

Gallegos, C, Tobolowsky F, Nigo M, Hasbun R. Delayed cerebral thrombosis in adults with bacterial meningitis: a novel complication of adjunctive steroids? *Crit Care Med*. 2018;46(8):e 811–e814.

Gambarin KH, Hamill RJ. Management of increased intracranial pressure in cryptococcal meningitis. *Curr Infect Dis Rep*. 2002;4(4):332–338.

Goldstein JM, Azizi SA, Booss J, et al. Human immunodeficiency virus-associated motor axonal polyradiculoneuropathy. *Arch Neurol*. 1993;50:1316–1319.

Hadden RD, Cornblath DR, Hughes RA, et al.; Plasma Exchange/Sandoglobulin Guillain–Barré Syndrome Trial Group. Electrophysiological classification of Guillain–Barré syndrome: clinical associations and outcome. *Ann Neurol*. 1998;44(5):780–788.

Hamada Y, Watanabe K, Aoki T, et al. Primary HIV infection with acute transverse myelitis. *Intern Med*. 2011;50:1615–1617.

Hammond ER, Crum RM, Treisman GJ, et al. The cerebrospinal fluid HIV risk score for assessing central nervous system activity in persons with HIV. *Am J Epidemiol*. 2014;180(3):297–307.

Hasbun R, Eraso J, Ramireddy S, et al. Screening for neurocognitive impairment in HIV individuals: the utility of the Montreal Cognitive Assessment Test. *J AIDS Clinic Res*. 2012;3:10.

Hasbun R, Rosenthal N, Balada-Llasat JM, et al. Epidemiology of meningitis and encephalitis in the United States, 2011–2014. *Clin Infect Dis*. 2017;65(3):359–363.

Hiraga A, Kuwabara S, Nakamura A, et al. Fisher/Guillain–Barré overlap syndrome in advanced AIDS. *J Neurol Sci*. 2007;258(1–2):148–150.

Hughes RA. Inflammatory neuropathy: sixth meeting of the Peripheral Neuropathy Association. St. Catherine's College, Oxford, England, August 14–18, 1990. *Neurology*. 1991;41(5):758–759.

Huis in't Veld D, Sun HY, Hung CC, et al. The immune reconstitution inflammatory syndrome related to HIV co-infections: a review. *Eur J Clin Microbiol Infect Dis*. 2012;31(6):919–927.

Jacks A, Wainwright D, Salazar L, et al. Neurocognitive deficits increase lack of retention-in-care among older with newly diagnosed HIV infection. *AIDS*. 2015;29(13):1711–1714.

Jadhav S, Agrawal M, Rathi S. Acute motor axonal neuropathy in HIV infection. *Indian J Pediatr*. 2014;81:193.

Johnson TP, Patel K, Johnson KR, et al. Induction of IL-17 and nonclassical T-cell activation by HIV-Tat protein. *Proc Natl Acad Sci USA*. 2013;110:13588–13593.

Kallianpur AR, Hulgan T. Pharmacogenetics of nucleoside reverse-transcriptase inhibitor-associated peripheral neuropathy. *Pharmacogenomics*. 2009;10(4):623–637.

Kapur J, Elm J, Chamberlain JM, et al. Randomized trial of three anticonvulsant medications for status epilepticus. *N Engl J Med*. 2019;381:2103–2113.

Keswani SC, Pardo CA, Cherry CL, et al. HIV-associated sensory neuropathies. *AIDS*. 2002;16(16):2105–2117.

Keswani SC, Polley M, Pardo CA, et al. Schwann cell chemokine receptors mediate HIV-1 gp120 toxicity to sensory neurons. *Arch Neurol*. 2003;54(3):287–296.

Leger JM, Bouche P, Bolgert F, et al. The spectrum of polyneuropathies in patients infected with HIV. *J Neurol Neurosurg Psychiatry*. 1989;52(12):1369–1374.

Lehmann HC, Chen W, Borzan J, et al. Mitochondrial dysfunction in distal axons contributes to human immunodeficiency virus sensory neuropathy. *Arch Neurol*. 2011;69(1):100–110.

Leisman RM, Strasburg AP, Heitman AK, et al. Evaluation of a commercial multiplex molecular panel for diagnosis of infectious meningitis and encephalitis. *J Clin Microb*. 2018;56 (4):1927–1937.

Lescure FX, Moulignier A, Savatovsky J, et al. CD8 encephalitis in HIV-positive patients receiving cART: a treatable entity. *Clin Infect Dis*. 2013;57(1):101–108.

Letendre S. Central nervous system complications in HIV disease: HIV-associated neurocognitive disorder. *Top Antivir Med*. 2011;19(4):137–142.

Letendre S, Fitzsimons C, Ellis R, et al. Correlates of CSF viral loads in 1221 volunteers of the CHARTER Cohort [Abstract 172]. Paper presented at the 17th Conference on Retrovirus and Opportunistic Infections, San Francisco, February 16–19, 2010.

Lindenbaum Y, Kissel JT, Mendell JR. Treatment approaches for Guillain–Barré syndrome and chronic inflammatory demyelinating polyradiculopathy. *Neurol Clin*. 2001;19(1):187–204.

Lipkin WI, Parry G, Kiprov D, et al. Inflammatory neuropathy in homosexual men with lymphadenopathy. *Neurology*. 1985;35(10):1479–1483.

Lopez Castelblanco R, Lee M, Hasbun R. Epidemiology of bacterial meningitis in the US: a population-based study. *Lancet Infect Dis*. 2014;14:813–819.

Ma B, Vigil K, Hasbun R. HIV testing in adults presenting with CNS infections. *Open Forum Infect Dis*. 2020; Jun; 7(6): ofaa217

Maggiolo F, Airoldi M, Kleinloog HD, et al. Effect of adherence to HAART on virologic outcome and on the selection of resistance-conferring mutations in NNRTI- or PI-treated patients. *HIV Clin Trials*. 2007;8(5):282–292.

Manns A, Hisada M, La Grenade L. Human T-lymphotropic virus type I infection. *Lancet*. 1999;353(9168):1951–1958.

Markarian Y, Wulff EA, Simpson DM. Peripheral neuropathy in HIV disease. *AIDS Clin Care*. 1998;10(12):89–91, 93, 98.

Marra C, Boutin P, Collier AC. Screening for distal sensory peripheral neuropathy in HIV-positive persons in research and clinical settings. *Neurology*. 1998;51(6):1678–1681.

Marra C, Maxwell CL, Smith SL, et al. Cerebrospinal fluid abnormalities in patients with syphilis: association with clinical and laboratory features. *J Infect Dis*. 2004;189(3):369–376.

Marshall DW, Brey RL, Cahill WT, et al. Spectrum of cerebrospinal fluid findings in various stages of human immunodeficiency virus infection. *Arch Neurol*. 1988;45:954–958.

Martin F, Taylor GP. Prospects for the management of human T-cell lymphotropic virus type 1-associated myelopathy. *AIDS Rev*. 2011;13(3):161–170.

Martin JL, Brown CE, Matthews-Davis N, et al. Effects of antiviral nucleoside analogs on human DNA polymerases and mitochondrial DNA synthesis. *Antimicrob Agents Chemother*. 1994;38(12):2743–2749.

Maschke M, Kastrup O, Diener HC. CNS manifestations of cytomegalovirus infections diagnosis and treatment. *CNS Drugs*. 2002;16(5):303–315.

McArthur JC, Brew BJ, Nath A. Neurological complications of HIV infection. *Lancet Neurol*. 2005;4(9):543–555.

McCutchan JA. Cytomegalovirus infections of the nervous system in patients with AIDS. *Clin Infect Dis*. 1995;20(4):747–754.

Métral M, Darling K, Locatelli I, et al. The Neurocognitive Assessment in the Metabolic and Aging Cohort (NAMACO) study: baseline participant profile. *HIV Med*. 2020;21(1):30–42

Mind Exchange Working Group. Assessment, diagnosis, and treatment of HIV-associated neurocognitive disorder: a consensus report of the Mind Exchange Program. *Clin Infect Dis*. 2013;56(7):1004–1017.

Mishra BB, Sommers W, Koski CL, et al. Acute inflammatory demyelinating polyneuropathy in the acquired immune deficiency syndrome. *Ann Neurol*. 1985;18:131–132.

Modi G, Ranchhod J, Hari K, et al. Non-traumatic myelopathy at the Chris Hani Baragwanath Hospital, South Africa—the influence of HIV. *QJM*. 2011: 104:697–703.

Molloy S, Kanyama C, Heyderman RS, et al. Antifungal combinations for treatment of cryptococcal meningitis. *N Engl J Med*. 2018; 378 (11): 1004–1017.

Moore RD, Wong WM, Keruly JC, et al. Incidence of neuropathy in HIV-positive patients on monotherapy versus those on combination therapy with didanosine, stavudine and hydroxyurea. *AIDS*. 2000;14(3):273–278.

Morgello S, Cho ES, Nielsen S, et al. Cytomegalovirus encephalitis in patients with acquired immunodeficiency syndrome: an autopsy study of 30 cases and a review of the literature. *Hum Pathol*. 1987;18:289–297.

Mukerji SS, Misra V, Lorenz D, et al. Impact of antiretroviral regimens on cerebrospinal fluid viral escape in a prospective multicohort study of antiretroviral therapy-experienced human immunodeficiency virus-1- infected adults in the United States. *Clin Infect Dis*. 2018;67(8):1182–1190.

Nagel MA, Forghani B, Mahalingam R, et al. The value of detecting anti-VZV IgG antibody in CSF to diagnose VZV vasculopathy. *Neurology*. 2007;68(13):1069–1073.

Nesher L, Hadi CM, Salazar L, et al. Epidemiology of meningitis with a negative CSF Gram-stain: underutilization of available diagnostic tests. *Epidemiol Infect*. 2016; 144(1):189–197.

Offiah CE, Turnbull IW. The imaging appearances of intracranial CNS infections in adult HIV and AIDS patients. *Clin Radiol*. 2006;61:393–401.

Opintan JA, Awadzi BK, Biney IJK, et al. High rates of cerebral toxoplasmosis in HIV patients presenting with meningitis in Accra, Ghana. *Trans R Soc Trop Med Hyg*. 2017;111(10):464–471.

Osiro S, Salomon N. Varicella-zoster (VZV) multifocal vasculopathy in a patient with systemic lupus erythematosus—a diagnostic and treatment dilemma. *IDCases*. 2007;81–83.

Pardo CA, McArthur JC, Griffin JW. HIV neuropathy: insights in the pathology of HIV peripheral nerve disease. *J Peripheral Nerv Syst*. 2001;6(1):21–27.

Park H, Song Y. Multiple tuberculoma involving the brain and spinal cord in a patient with miliary pulmonary tuberculosis. *J Korean Neurosurg Soc.* 2008;44(1):36–39.

Parry O, Mielke J, Latif AS, et al. Peripheral neuropathy in individuals with HIV infection in Zimbabwe. *Acta Neurol Scand.* 1997;96(4):218–222.

Patel AK, Patel KK, Gohel S, et al. Incidence of symptomatic CSF viral escape in HIV infected patients receiving atazanavir/ritonavir-containing ART: a tertiary care cohort in western India. *J Neurovirol* 2018;24(4):498–505.

Perfect JR, Dismukes WE, Dromer F, et al. Clinical practice guidelines for the treatment of cryptococcal disease: 2010 update from the Infectious Diseases Society of America. *Clin Infect Dis.* 2012;50:291–322.

Petito CK, Vecchio D, Chen YT. HIV antigen and DNA in AIDS spinal cords correlate with macrophage infiltration but not with vacuolar myelopathy. *J Neuropathol Exp Neurol.* 1994;53(1):86–94.

Phillips TJ, Cherry CL, Cox S, et al. Pharmacological treatment of painful HIV-associated sensory neuropathy: a systematic review and meta-analysis of randomised controlled trials. *PLoS One.* 2010;5(12):e14433.

Piliero PJ, Fish DG, Preston S, et al. Guillain–Barré syndrome associated with immune reconstitution. *Clin Infect Dis.* 2003;36(9):e111–e114.

Pillat MM, Bauer ME, de Oliveira AC, et al. HTLV-1-associated myelopathy/tropical spastic paraparesis (HAM/TSP): still an obscure disease. *Cent Nerv Syst Agents Med Chem.* 2011;11(4):239–245.

Plasma Exchange/Sandoglobulin Guillain–Barré Syndrome Trial Group. Randomised trial of plasma exchange, intravenous immunoglobulin, and combined treatments in Guillain–Barré syndrome. *Lancet.* 1997;349:225–230.

Polydefkis M, Yiannoutsos CT, Cohen BA, et al. Reduced intraepidermal nerve fiber density in HIV-associated sensory neuropathy. *Neurology.* 2002;58(1):115–119.

Portegies P, Solod L, Cinque P, et al. EFNS Task Force guidelines for the diagnosis and management of neurological complications of HIV infection. *Eur J Neurol.* 2004;11:297–304.

Price RW, Yiannoutsos CT, Clifford DB, et al. Neurological outcomes in late HIV infection: adverse impact of neurological impairment on survival and protective effect of antiviral therapy. AIDS Clinical Trial Group and Neurological AIDS Research Consortium Study Team. *AIDS.* 1999;13(13):1677–1685.

Radziwill AJ, Kuntzer T, Steck AJ. Immunopathology and treatments of Guillain–Barré syndrome and of chronic inflammatory demyelinating polyneuropathy. *Rev Neurol.* 2002;158(3):301–310.

Rauschkaa H, Jellingerb K, Lassmannc H, et al. Guillain–Barré syndrome with marked pleocytosis or a significant proportion of polymorphonuclear granulocytes in the cerebrospinal fluid: neuropathological investigation of five cases and review of differential diagnoses. *Eur J Neurol.* 2003;10:479–486.

Robertson KR, Smurzynski M, Parsons TD, et al. The prevalence and incidence of neurocognitive impairment in the HAART era. *AIDS.* 2007;21:1915–1921.

Robinson-Papp J, Gonzalez-Duarte A, Simpson DM, et al. The roles of ethnicity and antiretrovirals in HIV-associated polyneuropathy: a pilot study. *J AIDS.* 2009a;51(5):569–573.

Robinson-Papp J, Sharma S, Simpson DM, et al. Autonomic dysfunction is common in HIV and associated with distal symmetric polyneuropathy. *J Neurovirol.* 2013;19:172–180.

Robinson-Papp J, Simpson DM. Neuromuscular diseases associated with HIV-1 infection. *Muscle Nerve.* 2009b;40(6):1043–1053.

Rolfes MA, Hullsiek KH, Rhein J, et al. The effect of therapeutic lumbar punctures on acute mortality from cryptococcal meningitis. *Clin Infect Dis.* 2014;59(11):1607–1614.

Rosca EC, Albarqouni L, Simu M. Montreal cognitive assessment (MoCA) for HIV-associated neurocognitive disorders. *Neuropsychol Rev.* 2019;29(3):313–327.

Rosca EC, Rosca O, Simu M. Intravenous immunoglobulin treatment in a HIV-1 positive patient with Guillain–Barré syndrome. *Int Immunopharmacol.* 2015;29(2):964–965.

Rosenow JM, Hirschfeld A. Utility of brain biopsy in patient with acquired immunodeficiency syndrome before and after introduction of highly active antiretroviral therapy, *Neurosurgery.* 2007;61(1):130–141.

Sandoval R, Runft B, Roddey T. Pilot study: does lower extremity night splinting assist in the management of painful peripheral neuropathy in the HIV/AIDS population? *J Int Assoc Phys AIDS Care.* 2010;9(6):368–381.

Santos AM, Locatelli I, Metral M, et al. Cross-sectional and cumulative longitudinal central nervous system effectiveness scores are not associated with neurocognitive impairment in a well-treated aging HIV-positive population in Switzerland. *Open Forum Infect Dis.* 2019;6(7):ofz277.

Schifitto G, McDermott MP, McArthur JC, et al.; Dana Consortium on the Therapy of HIV Dementia and Related Cognitive Disorders. Incidence of and risk factors for HIV-associated distal sensory polyneuropathy. *Neurology.* 2002;58(12):1764–1768.

Schreiber AL, Norbury JW, DeSousa EA. Functional recovery of untreated human immunodeficiency virus-associated Guillain–Barré syndrome: a case report. *Ann Phys Rehabil Med.* 2011;54:519–524.

Serpa JA, Moran A, Goodman JC, et al. Neurocysticercosis in the HIV era: a case report and review of the literature. *Am J Trop Med Hyg.* 2007;77(1):113–117.

Shahani L, Salazar L, Woods SP, et al. Baseline neurocognitive functioning predicts viral load suppression at 1-year follow-up among newly diagnosed HIV infected patients. *AIDS Behav.* 2018;22(10):3209–3213.

Shukla B, Aguilera EA, Salazar L, et al. Aseptic meningitis in adults and children: diagnostic and management challenges. *J Clin Virol.* 2017;94:110–114.

Sidtis JJ, Gatsonis C, Price RW, et al.; AIDS Clinical Trials Group. Zidovudine treatment of the AIDS dementia complex: results of a placebo-controlled trial. *Ann Neurol.* 1993;33:343–349.

Silva CA, Penalva de Oliveira AC, Vilas-Boas L, et al. Neurologic cytomegalovirus complications in patients with AIDS: retrospective review of 13 cases and review of the literature. *Rev Inst Med Trop Sao Paulo.* 2010;52(6):305–310.

Simpson DM, Brown S, Tobias J; NGX-4010 C107 Study Group. Controlled trial of high-concentration capsaicin patch for treatment of painful HIV neuropathy. *Neurology.* 2008;70:2305–2313.

Simpson DM, Kitch D, Evans SR, et al.; ACTG A5117 Study Group. HIV neuropathy natural history cohort study: assessment measures and risk factors. *Neurology.* 2006;66(11):1679–1687.

Simpson JK 3rd. Chronic neuropathic pain. *N Engl J Med.* 2003;348(26):2688–2689.

Smyth K, Affandi JS, McArthur JC, et al. Prevalence of and risk factors for HIV-associated neuropathy in Melbourne, Australia 1993–2006. *HIV Med.* 2007;8:367–373.

Tagliati M, Grinnell J, Godbold J, et al. Peripheral nerve function in HIV infection: clinical, electrophysiologic, and laboratory findings. *Arch Neurol.* 1999;56(1):84–89.

Tan K, Roda R, Ostrow L, et al. PML-IRIS in patients with HIV infection: clinical manifestations and treatment with steroids. *Neurology.* 2009;72(17):1458–1464.

Thao LTP, Heemskerk AD, Geskus RB, et al. Prognostic models for 9-month mortality in tuberculous meningitis. *Clin Infect Dis.* 2018;66(4):523–532.

Thwaites GE. The management of suspected encephalitis. *BMJ.* 2012;344.

Tirbaboshi J, Arkaitz I, Saye H., et al. Total and unbound bictegravir concentrations and viral suppression in cerebrospinal fluid of human immunodeficiency virus-infected patients. *J Infect Dis.* 2019;221(9):1425–1428.

Triunfo M, Vai D, Montrucchio C, et al. Diagnostic accuracy of new and old cognitive screening tools for HIV-associated neurocognitive disorders. *HIV Med.* 2018;19:455–464.

Tunkel AR, Glaser CA, Bloch KC, et al. The management of encephalitis: clinical practice guidelines by the Infectious Diseases Society of America. *Clin Infect Dis.* 2004;47(3):303–327.

Tyor WR, Glass JD, Baumrind N, et al. Cytokine expression of macrophages in HIV-1-associated vacuolar myelopathy. *Neurology*. 1993;43(5):1002–1009.

Valcour V. Evaluating cognitive impairment in the clinical setting: practical screening and assessment tools. *Top Antivir Med*. 2011;19(5):175–180.

Valcour V, Paul R, Chiao S, et al. Screening for cognitive impairment in human immunodeficiency virus. *Clin Infect Dis*. 2011a;53(8):836–842.

Valcour V, Sithinamsuwan P, Letendre S, et al. Pathogenesis of HIV in the central nervous system. *Curr HIV/AIDS Rep*. 2011b;8(1):54–61.

Van der Meche FG, Schitz PI; Dutch Guillain–Barré Study Group. A randomized trial comparing intravenous immune globulin and plasma exchange in Guillain–Barré syndrome. *N Engl J Med*. 1992;326(17):1123–1129.

Vecchio AC, Marra CM, Schouten J, et al. Distal sensory peripheral neurology in human immunodeficiency virus type 1-positive individuals before and after antiretroviral therapy initiative in diverse resource-limited settings. *Clin Infect Dis*. 2020;71(1):158–165.

Veltman JA, Bristow CC, Klausner JD. Meningitis in HIV-positive patients in sub-Saharan Africa: a review. *J Int AIDS Soc*. 2014;17:19184.

Verma A. Epidemiology and clinical features: HIV-1 associated neuropathies. *J Peripheral Nerv Syst*. 2001;6(1):8–13.

Verma A, Bradley WG. HIV-1 associated neuropathies. *CNS Spectrums*. 2000;5(5):66–67.

Verma S, Estanislao L, Mintz L, et al. Controlling neuropathic pain in HIV. *Curr HIV/AIDS Rep*. 2004;1(3):136–141.

Vigil KJ, Salazar L, Hasbun R. Community-acquired meningitis in HIV-infected patients in the United States. *AIDS Patient Care STDs*. 2018;32(2):42–47.

Wagner JC, Bromber MB. HIV infection presenting with motor axonal variant of Guillain–Barré syndrome. *J Clin Neuromusc Disord*. 2007;9:303–305.

Wakerly BR, Yuki N. Mimics and chameleons in Guillain–Barré and Miller–Fisher syndromes. *Practical Neurol*. 2015;15:90–99.

Wang SX, Ho EL, Grill M, et al. Peripheral neuropathy in primary HIV infection associates with systemic and CNS immune activation. *J AIDS*. 2014;66(3):303–310.

Williams D, Geraci A, Simpson DM. AIDS and AIDS-treatment neuropathies. *Curr Headache Rep*. 2002;6(2):125–130.

Winer JB. Guillain–Barré syndrome. J Clin Pathol. 2001;54:381–385.

Wulff EA, Simpson DM. Neuromuscular complications of the human immunodeficiency virus type 1 infection. Semin Neurol. 1999a;19(2):157–164.

Wulff EA, Simpson DM. Neuromuscular complications of HIV-1 infection. Curr Infect Dis Rep. 1999b;1(2):192–197.

Wulff EA, Wang AK, Simpson DM. HIV-associated peripheral neuropathy: epidemiology, pathophysiology and treatment. *Drugs*. 2000;59(6):1251–1260.

Yousem DM, Grossman RI. *The requisites: neuroradiology*. 3rd ed. Philadelphia: Mosby; 2010:209.

35.

HIV AND HEPATITIS COINFECTION

Karen J. Vigil

CHAPTER GOAL

Upon completion of this chapter, the reader should be able to:

- Discuss the epidemiology, clinical presentation, diagnosis, treatment, and complications of hepatitis B and hepatitis C in people with HIV (PWH)

INTRODUCTION

Hepatitis B virus (HBV) and hepatitis C virus (HCV) are the leading causes of cirrhosis and hepatocellular carcinoma (HCC) worldwide. They are transmitted perinatally or through early childhood exposure, sexual contact, and injection drug use. Approximately 10% of PWH also have chronic HBV infection, and up to 30% have coinfection with HCV.

HIV AND HEPATITIS B COINFECTION

LEARNING OBJECTIVE

- Discuss the clinical presentation, diagnosis, treatment, and treatment complications of HBV in PWH

WHAT'S NEW?

- Heplisav-B® is a CpG conjugated hepatitis B vaccine that only requires two doses (0 and 1 month).

- Tenofovir alafenamide (TAF) demonstrated similar efficacy in HBeAg-positive and HBeAg-negative people and less bone density and renal function decline than tenofovir disoproxil fumarate (TDF) in two large phase 3 clinical trials among HIV-negative persons with chronic HBV infection.

KEY POINTS

- All PWH should have a complete evaluation for HBV infection.

- People without evidence of prior immunity or current HBV infection should be vaccinated against HBV.

- All PWH and HBV coinfection should receive treatment for both viruses, regardless of CD4+ T-cell count or independent need for HBV treatment.

- HBV treatment in persons coinfected with HIV and HBV should include two active agents against HBV, in the context of fully suppressive antiretroviral therapy (ART) against HIV.

CLINICAL PRESENTATION

Acute hepatitis B occurs 1 to 4 months after exposure. Approximately 30% of persons will present with icteric hepatitis and symptoms of fatigue, fever, right upper quadrant pain, and nausea, while the majority will have a subclinical presentation. Fulminant hepatitis is uncommon and develops in less than 0.5% of people.

Around 20% of PWH will progress to chronic HBV, compared to less than 10% of HIV-negative people. Of those, 15% to 40% will progress to end-stage liver disease or HCC and 25% will die due to complications of HBV.

DIAGNOSIS AND EVALUATION

Initial testing for HBV should include serologic testing for surface antigen (HBsAg), core antibody (anti-HBc total), and surface antibody (anti-HBs). HBsAg can usually be detected approximately 4 weeks after exposure. Resolution of acute HBV is characterized by negative HBsAg and the presence of anti-HBs and anti-HBc, but reactivation may recur with severe immunosuppression. Chronic HBV is defined as the presence of HBsAg detected in two occasions at least 6 months apart. Occult HBV, defined as the presence of anti-HBc alone with HBV DNA viremia, has been found in approximately 5% of persons with isolated anti-HBc. Other possible causes of isolated anti-HBc are the "window phase" of acute HBV infection (between loss of HBsAg and emergence of anti-HBs), resolved hepatitis B infection, or a false-positive test. Individuals with occult HBV are also at increased risk of HBV reactivation and of HCC (Shire et al., 2004).

Persons with chronic HBV should be tested for HBe antigen (HBeAg), antibody (anti-HBe), and HBV DNA. Individuals with HBeAg usually have high HBV DNA and elevated alanine aminotransferase (ALT) levels and are at high risk of future liver complications. A conversion from HBeAg to anti-HBe can imply a transition from active disease to an inactive carrier state, but this occurs less commonly in people coinfected with HIV and HBV. This inactive carrier state is also characterized by HBV DNA of less than 2,000 IU/mL and normal ALT. These persons do remain at risk for reactivation of HBV and liver disease progression, but at a lower rate than in individuals with active disease. Finally, there also exists a state of HBeAg-negative active hepatitis, which is a result of mutations in the pre-core and core promoter regions. These individuals are at significant risk of progressive liver disease, and HBV DNA levels should be monitored regularly, with treatment instituted as recommended (Hadziyannis & Papatheodoridis, 2006).

Elevations of hepatic transaminases are suggestive of inflammation, and hepatic synthetic function is measured by serum albumin and coagulation factors. An assessment of the degree of liver fibrosis is important, and options for this include liver biopsy or noninvasive testing such as transient elastography or an increasing array of serum biomarker tests. Persons with cirrhosis should have HCC screening by ultrasound every 6 to 12 months, and all persons with cirrhosis should be comanaged with a hepatologist (Lok & McMahon, 2009).

Current HIV guidelines recommend ART for all PWH; persons with HIV-HBV should be a priority group for HIV treatment. ART must include two drugs with activity against HBV, such as TAF or TDF plus emtricitabine (FTC) or lamivudine, regardless of the exact stage of HBV or degree of liver fibrosis (Terrault et al., 2018).

COINFECTION CONSIDERATIONS

In general terms, the presence of HIV coinfection worsens outcomes related to HBV. PWH are less likely to resolve acute HBV exposure and have higher levels of HBV DNA levels compared to those without HIV (Colin et al., 1999). Coinfection with HIV and HBV is associated with more rapid progression of HBV-related cirrhosis, HCC, and fatal hepatic failure (Thio et al., 2002). Indeed, HBV infection was associated with a relative risk of 3.73 for liver-related deaths in participants who were coinfected with HIV and HBV in the Data Collection on Adverse Events of Anti-HIV Drugs (D:A:D) study (Weber et al., 2006).

Because the immune response plays a key role in both HBV clearance and the immune damage associated with chronic HBV infection, coinfection with HIV and HBV impacts the course of HBV infection. HIV-induced immunosuppression increases the risk of reactivation of quiescent HBV, and initiation of ART may result in exacerbation of HBV liver disease (hepatitis flares) or fulminant hepatitis (Sulkowski et al., 2001).

Stopping antiretroviral agents (ARVs) with activity against HBV (lamivudine, FTC, and TDF or TAF) may lead to frequent HBV rebound, sometimes accompanied by a severe flare of HBV and hepatocellular damage (Dore et al., 2010). Thus, when persons coinfected with HIV and HBV change ART regimens, it is crucial to maintain agents with anti-HBV activity. If anti-HBV treatment is discontinued, serum transaminase levels should be monitored regularly; if a hepatic flare occurs, then HBV therapy should be restarted immediately because this could be life-saving (US Department of Health and Human Services [DHHS], Panel on Guidelines for the Prevention and Treatment of Opportunistic Infections, 2020).

HBV PREVENTION

People with HIV should be counseled about transmission risks for HBV, including sexual transmission, sharing of needles and syringes, and tattooing or body piercing. People at risk for HBV should be advised to avoid these behaviors associated with transmission (DHHS, 2020b).

HBV vaccination is the most effective way to prevent HBV infection. If there is no evidence of chronic infection or previous vaccination (anti-HBs <10 IU/mL), then a hepatitis B vaccination series should be administered (DHHS, 2020b). Individuals who are positive for anti-HBs and anti-HBc have a resolved infection and do not require vaccination. Individuals with "isolated anti-HBc" (see previous description) who have an undetectable HBV DNA level should receive a complete HBV vaccine series.

Unfortunately, the preventive HBV vaccination is less effective in PWH, with efficacy rates in this population of approximately 65%, and those with a CD4$^+$ T-cell count of less than 350 cells/mm^3 have even lower response rates. HBV vaccination of all nonimmune PWH is currently recommended regardless of CD4$^+$ T-cell count, and vaccination should not be deferred in persons with CD4$^+$ T-cell counts of less than 350 cells/mm^3 (DHHS, 2020b). Various revaccination strategies are available for persons who do not respond to an initial series, and research attempting to determine the optimal vaccine series for initial vaccination to improve response rates is ongoing (Launay et al., 2011). A repeat three-dose vaccination series or a double dose of vaccine is recommended in PWH not responding to a complete vaccination (Terrault et al., 2018).

The use of HBV-active ARVs to prevent acquisition of HBV in PWH who have not responded to a vaccine series is an emerging idea. In one study, tenofovir use was particularly protective against acquisition of primary HBV infection in PWH (Heuft et al., 2014).

Persons coinfected with HIV and HBV should also be vaccinated against hepatitis A if susceptible, and they should avoid alcohol consumption.

GOALS OF TREATMENT

The goals of treatment for HBV infection are to achieve sustained suppression of viral replication (SVR) to below detectable levels and to improve or stabilize the degree of liver disease in order to prevent cirrhosis, hepatic failure, and HCC. Measurements of response to therapy include the decline in HBV DNA to undetectable levels, loss of HBeAg or gain of anti-HBe antibody (termed seroconversion), normalization of serum ALT, and improvement in liver histology.

Functional cure is represented by an undetectable HBsAg, which may reduce progression to cirrhosis and liver cancer (Sherman, 2015).

HIV TREATMENT RECOMMENDATIONS IN THE SETTING OF HBV COINFECTION

Because coinfection with HIV is associated with more rapid progression of HBV-related liver disease and there is evidence that earlier treatment of HIV may slow the development of liver disease by improving immune function and reducing HIV-related inflammation and immune activation, current HIV treatment guidelines recommend that all persons coinfected with HIV and HBV start ART and that the ART regimen include drugs with activity against both viruses (DHHS, 2020a).

The Opportunistic Infections Working Group makes the following recommendations for persons coinfected with HIV and HBV (American Association for the Study of Liver Disease/Infectious Diseases Society of America, 2018; DHHS, 2020b; Terrault et al., 2018):

- Regardless of the CD4+ T-cell count or the need for HBV treatment, ART that includes agents active against both HIV and HBV is recommended for all persons coinfected with HIV and HBV.

- ART must include two drugs active against HBV, preferably TDF or TAF and FTC or lamivudine, regardless of the level of HBV DNA.

- If the individual refuses HIV treatment, then there are few options available to treat HBV because entecavir (ETV) given without suppressive ART may result in HIV resistance, and telbivudine and adefovir are not recommended. A 48-week course of pegylated (Peg) interferon (IFN)-α-2a can be considered in such circumstances (Terrault et al., 2018).

- If tenofovir use is not acceptable as part of the ART regimen, the alternative recommendation is to use ETV in addition to a fully suppressive ART.

- Chronic use of lamivudine or FTC as the single active agent against HBV should be avoided because of the high rate of subsequent HBV resistance.

Individuals being treated for HBV should have HBV DNA measured every 12 to 24 weeks. If the HBV DNA is greater than 1,000 IU/mL after 1 year, then adherence to medication should be assessed and HBV resistance testing considered. Viral failure and resistance are more common in PWH with HBV, especially when lamivudine is used alone for treatment. The risk of resistance has declined with the use of more potent drugs such as tenofovir and ETV (Luetkemeyer et al., 2011). Unfortunately, even with long-term suppression of HBV DNA, the loss of HBsAg (functional cure) of HBV is not common in PWH coinfection (Sherman, 2015), and indefinite treatment is usually recommended.

SPECIAL CONSIDERATIONS
IMMUNE RECONSTITUTION INFLAMMATORY SYNDROME

Immune reconstitution during the course of treatment for coinfection with HIV and HBV can lead to a severe flare of chronic HBV infection, with significant increases in hepatic transaminases, perhaps due to enhanced host immune responses against HBV. HBV-associated immune reconstitution inflammatory syndrome (IRIS) is most likely to occur during the first few weeks after starting ART and can present as acute hepatitis. Careful monitoring of hepatic transaminases after the initiation of ART is helpful (Audsley et al., 2011). Development of signs of hepatic synthetic dysfunction, such as elevated prothrombin time or low albumin, should prompt evaluation by a hepatologist. Distinguishing between HBV-related IRIS and drug-induced liver toxicity can be challenging and may require examination of liver histology and consultation with a hepatologist. Very little information is available regarding the best treatment for HBV-related IRIS, and the decision regarding whether to continue, modify, or interrupt therapy should be individualized based on the severity of hepatic injury.

TREATMENT INTERRUPTIONS

Due to the overlap in anti-HIV and HBV activity of FTC, lamivudine, and tenofovir, interruption of treatment should be avoided in patients coinfected with HIV and HBV to avoid potentially severe flares of HBV with hepatic inflammation and necrosis. In particular, when there is a need to discontinue one of the HBV-active drugs in the HIV treatment regimen, careful follow-up of liver function tests is required, and addition of a second agent with anti-HBV activity should be considered. If there is a need to change ART due to HIV resistance and HBV suppression is maintained despite HIV treatment failure, the ARVs with activity against HBV should be continued for HBV treatment in addition to other appropriate ARVs.

TREATMENT OPTIONS FOR HEPATITIS B INFECTION

It is currently recommended to start all ART in all PWH. The preferred treatment regimen for people with HIV/HBV coinfection is ART with the backbone regimen of TAF or TDF with lamivudine or FTC. Both TDF and TAF have a high genetic barrier of resistance. Monotherapy with lamivudine or FTC is not recommended due to the increased possibility to develop resistance. Treatment is recommended lifelong. Discontinuation of treatment has been associated with hepatitis flares. Treatment of HBV alone is not recommended.

SUMMARY

Hepatitis B infection is a common and potentially severe comorbidity for PWH. Screening for HBV infection, vaccination, and careful assessment of chronic HBV infection are important components of HIV care. Consideration of chronic HBV status when selecting HIV treatment regimens is essential in optimizing management of both infections. Monitoring for response to treatment for HBV and screening for complications such as cirrhosis or HCC are part of the ongoing care of persons with HIV/HBV.

HIV AND HEPATITIS C COINFECTION

LEARNING OBJECTIVE

- Discuss the clinical presentation, diagnosis, and treatment of HCV in PWH

WHAT'S NEW?

- The treatment of HCV has changed dramatically during the past few years. The emergence of new interferon-free, oral, direct-acting antivirals (DAAs) achieves a cure rate of greater than 90% of persons with chronic HCV infections.

- Individuals who developed acute HCV should be treated immediately and not wait for spontaneous resolution to decrease the incidence of new cases in the general population.

KEY POINTS

- The coinfection epidemic is evolving. The Swiss HIV Cohort Study group has observed an 18-fold increase in HIV/HCV coinfection in men who have sex with men (MSM) from 1998 to 2011, in association with a history of unsafe sex, a past syphilis history, and chronic HBV.

- Because ART may slow the progression of HCV-related liver disease, it should be considered for all persons coinfected with HIV and HCV, regardless of CD4+ T-cell count. If treatment with the new DAAs is planned, the ART regimen may need to be modified to reduce the potential for drug–drug interactions and/or drug toxicities that may develop during the period of concurrent HIV and HCV treatment.

- Although HCV treatment regimens are now much simpler and all oral, factors such as renal disease, drug–drug interactions, disease severity, and especially cost considerations remain.

EPIDEMIOLOGY

With many of the 1.2 million Americans with HIV already in care for their HIV, HIV providers are in a unique position to treat and likely cure HCV in those persons coinfected with HIV and HCV. Rapid progress in HCV therapeutics has benefited greatly from the framework that previous HIV research laid down during the past 30 years, rocketing along at breakneck speed and condensing into years what previously would have taken decades. HIV providers, with their intimate knowledge of virology, resistance, drug–drug interactions, and the psychosocial needs of this population, stand in unique stead to treat HCV.

As ART continues to extend the lifespan of PWH by decades, HCV coinfection has become an increasingly important cause of both morbidity and mortality. Liver disease has emerged as the leading cause of non–AIDS-related deaths in PWH with HCV or HBV (Centers for Disease Control and Prevention, 2020). HCV coinfection places a growing burden on the HIV healthcare delivery system, as evidenced by an analysis conducted by the AIDS Clinical Trials Group (ACTG) Longitudinal Linked Randomized Trials cohort. When controlling for age, race, sex, history of AIDS-defining events, and current CD4+ T-cell count and HIV RNA levels, the relative risk of hospitalization, emergency department visits, and disability days for persons coinfected with HIV and HCV versus HIV mono-infected participants was 1.8 (95% confidence interval [CI], 1.3–2.5), 1.7 (95% CI, 1.4–2.1), and 1.6 (95% CI, 1.3–1.9), respectively. Based on the ACTG's study findings, programs serving persons coinfected with HIV and HCV can expect to experience an almost 70% higher rate of utilization for this group (Linas et al., 2011). A study from the New York City Department of Health and Mental Hygiene using death certificate data showed persons coinfected with HIV and HCV to be at exceptionally high risk for premature death (median age, 52.0 years) compared to those with HCV alone (median age, 60.0 years) or those with neither virus (median age, 78.0 years). Decedents had an odds ratio of 2.2 for death from liver cancer and 3.1 for drug-related causes, with 53.6% of deaths attributed to HIV/AIDS and 94% occurring prematurely (defined as younger than age 65 years) (Pinchoff et al., 2014).

HCV is a single-stranded RNA virus transmitted primarily through blood exposure and, less commonly, through sexual or vertical transmission. Because HIV and HCV share similar routes of transmission, approximately one-fifth of all PWH in the US are also infected with HCV. This percentage increases to 80% for people who inject drugs (PWID) (Centers for Disease Control and Prevention, 2014). Heterosexual transmission risk is low and generally quoted as less than 1% per year, although high-risk sex practices such as aggressive anal intercourse and multiple sex partners increase transmission risk. Vertical transmission is possible, with pregnant women coinfected with HIV and HCV having a 15% to 20% chance of passing HCV to their infants compared to the 5% to 15% rate in infants born to HCV mono-infected mothers (Bevilacqua et al., 2009; Mast et al., 2005). Most studies to date do not support elective cesarean delivery for HCV-positive women. Breastfeeding is not known to transmit HCV, but because breastfeeding may transmit HIV, it is contraindicated for mothers coinfected with HIV and HCV in the US.

In recent years, coinfection has been a changing epidemic, as evidenced by data from the Swiss Cohort Study. What was once a disease of PWID and hemophiliacs has become a sexually transmitted disease of MSM. The 4.1 cases per 100 person-years seen in MSM in 2011 in the Swiss Cohort Study represented an 18-fold increase from 1998, with HCV seen in association with a history of unsafe anal sex, a past syphilis history, and chronic HBV (Wandeler et al., 2012). In 2011, a report was published that included 5-year data from 74 MSM with HIV who had no history of injectable drug use (IDU) and had newly elevated ALT levels with a positive HCV antibody test (Fierer et al., 2012). This matched case–control study was conducted beginning in July 2007 and examined men who were within 12 months of the clinical onset of HIV infection and who had no IDU history. MSM with HIV newly infected with HCV were significantly more likely to have had receptive anal intercourse (matched odds ratio [mOR], 24.87) or insertive anal intercourse (mOR, 2.62) with no condom use and with ejaculation, engaged in group sex (mOR, 19.2), engaged in sex while high on drugs (mOR, 11.37), previously had syphilis (mOR, 8.8), and had sex while using crystal methamphetamine (mOR, 26.8). HIV coinfection results in increased HCV RNA levels, which are thought to increase the infectiousness of HCV acquired through sexual contact. People with HIV should be counseled that unprotected sex can transmit other infections, including HCV.

The connection between prescription narcotic abuse, HIV, and HCV was highlighted by a community outbreak of HIV linked to IDU of oxymorphone in a rural county of Indiana. Prior to this investigation, only 5 HIV cases per year were reported. As of April 21, 2015, 135 persons had confirmed or probable HIV infection in a community of 4,200 persons. Mean age was 35 years, with 54.8% being males, 80% reporting IDU, and 17% who had not yet been interviewed. All reported their drug of choice was injectable crushed oxymorphone, sometimes with other illicit drugs. Of these, 7.4% were female commercial sex workers. Strikingly, coinfection with HCV was found in 84.4% of individuals (Conrad et al., 2015). Those interviewed reported an average of 9 syringe-sharing or sex partners and social contacts who may be at risk. Of the 230 contacts tested, 109 (47.4%) were positive for HIV. IDU in this community is multigenerational, with the crushed oxymorphone (40-mg tablets are not designed to resist crushing) dissolved in nonsterile water and injected via insulin syringes, with the syringes often shared. This outbreak highlights the vulnerability of many resource-poor rural communities that traditionally have low rates of HIV and HCV and the need for community interventions at multiple levels. This is a reminder of how often concomitant transmission of the two viruses continues to occur, particularly in vulnerable PWID and MSM.

CLINICAL COURSE

The most striking feature of HCV when acquired by a person with HIV is its ability to cause chronic hepatitis in up to 90% of persons within 6 months. This occurs due to the lack of CD4+ T-cell responses and significantly reduced IFN-γ ELISpot responses against HCV (Elliott et al., 2006). Between 60% and 70% of chronically infected persons will have fluctuating serum ALT levels because this is the enzyme most associated with liver cell injury in HCV. Less than 20%

have nonspecific symptoms, including fatigue and generalized weakness. There are significant similarities and differences between HIV and HCV. Both are RNA viruses with rapid replication rates (10 trillion HCV virions vs. 10 billion HIV virions produced daily). Both are prone to frequent mutations and exist as heterogeneous quasi-species to avoid the immune system. Both viruses incite abundant but ineffective antibody responses. Although both have many reservoirs in the human body, HCV exists primarily in the cytoplasm of hepatocytes and can be eradicated from the body. HIV is integrated into the nuclei of CD4+ T lymphocytes and long-lived memory T-cell reservoirs and therefore cannot be eradicated with current ART. HCV RNA levels are only broadly predictive of long-term prognosis, whereas HIV RNA is very predictive of clinical events in untreated persons.

There are six different HCV genotypes (1–6) at various prevalence rates throughout the world. In the US, genotype (GT) 1 accounts for two-thirds of cases, with GTs 2 through 4 occurring less commonly.

DIAGNOSIS

HCV may be diagnosed earlier in asymptomatic PWH with elevated ALT/AST levels due to greater frequency of lab monitoring (Mohsen & Easterbrook, 2003). Coinfection with HIV greatly impacts the natural history of HCV infection. Individuals coinfected with HIV and HCV are less likely to spontaneously clear HCV, have increased HCV RNA, and progress more rapidly to cirrhosis and end-stage liver disease (Asselah et al., 2006). Predictors of severe liver fibrosis include age older than 40 years at time of infection, alcohol consumption of more than 50 g/day, daily marijuana use, high body mass index, male gender, postmenopausal status, and longer duration of infection (Poynard et al., 1997). Although ART may slow this rate, it continues to exceed that seen in persons with HCV mono-infection. Low CD4+ T-cell counts also appear to magnify the progression. A meta-analysis of eight studies that examined the role of HIV with HCV found that persons coinfected with HIV and HCV had approximately twice the risk of cirrhosis on liver biopsy and six times the risk of decompensated liver disease with ascites, varices, or encephalopathy compared to HCV mono-infected individuals (Poynard et al., 1997). A Veterans Health Administration study examined 4,820 persons coinfected with HIV and HCV and 6,079 persons with HCV in care from 1997 to 2010. All had detectable HCV RNA levels and were HCV treatment naive. Hepatic decompensation was significantly greater at 10 years in the HIV/HCV group (7.4% vs. 4.8%; p < 0.001) (Lo et al., 2014). Persons coinfected with HIV and HCV had a higher rate of hepatic decompensation (hazard ratio [HR], 1.56 when accounting for competing risks), even when HIV RNA levels were maintained under 1,000 copies/mL (HR, 1.44). Approximately one-third of persons with chronic HCV will progress to cirrhosis at a median time of less than 20 years (Thomas et al., 2000). Once cirrhosis has developed, 50% will decompensate within the first 5 years, with ascites being the usual first sign. Approximately 1% to 4% of cirrhotic individuals per year will develop HCC.

Median survival time is 35 months versus 65 months for those without HIV (Beretta et al., 2011).

Although the average time from infection to fibrosis is shortened from 35 to 25 years in persons coinfected with HIV and HCV, Fierer's group at Mt. Sinai School of Medicine (New York City) found that MSM with HIV who developed HCV had a much more rapid onset of fibrosis. In a 2008 analysis, 9 of 11 (82%) men had stage 2 (moderate) fibrosis at a median of only 4 months after diagnosis (Fierer et al., 2012). In 2013, Fierer et al. reported on four individuals who developed decompensated cirrhosis and death within 2 to 8 years after HCV infection. The authors noted that the order in which the infections are acquired is important. When HCV is acquired after HIV, there is accelerated progression to fibrosis that may be proportional to the degree of immunosuppression. However, not all studies have seen such rapid progression. The European NEAT cohort evaluated fibrosis rates in 41 PWH who subsequently developed HCV. Most were MSM on ART with a mean CD4$^+$ T-cell count of 500 cells/mm^3. FibroScan transient elastometry (used to assess liver stiffness) over a maximum follow-up of 8 years found no significant hepatic changes (Boesecke et al., 2014).

Deferring HCV treatment in the age of DAAs may lead to increased rates of HCC and death. Data from the Swiss HIV Cohort Study and published HCV data were used for mathematical modeling to predict the decrease in progression to cirrhosis, HCC, and death in persons coinfected with HIV and HCV. If therapy was initiated during stage F0 or F1, the percentage of liver-related deaths was 2%. However, if treatment was deferred until the F3 or F4 stage, mortality increased to 7% and 22%, respectively. If individuals are not treated immediately, they remain infectious. Important from a public health perspective, those treated between 1 month and 1 year after diagnosis remained infectious from a HCV standpoint for approximately 5 years, compared to 12 years for stage 2, 15 years for stage 3, and nearly 20 years for stage 4 (Zahnd et al., 2016).

DECISION TO TREAT

According to the Infectious Disease Society of America's "Primary Care Guidelines for HIV," all PWH should be screened for HCV with antibody testing upon entry into care and annually thereafter for those at risk and whenever HCV infection is suspected (Aberg et al., 2014). HCV RNA levels should be tested in all those with a positive antibody test to assess for active disease because antibodies persist for a lifetime even in persons who have cleared the virus. Infants born to mothers coinfected with HIV and HCV should also have antibody testing performed. Seronegative at-risk individuals, along with those with evidence of past HCV infection, should undergo annual screening. HCV transmission may be facilitated by the presence of genital erosions related to sexually transmitted diseases. Reinfection with HCV can occur, so individuals should be aware that high-risk behaviors put them at risk for reinfection (Danta & Dusheiko, 2008). Persons with HCV/HIV coinfection should be advised to avoid alcohol consumption and to avoid sharing razors, toothbrushes, syringes, and so on to prevent spread of infection to others. Those who are susceptible to hepatitis A or hepatitis B should be vaccinated against these viruses because dual or triple infections are typically more severe (Low et al., 2008).

Although the increased likelihood of ART-associated liver toxicity with underlying HCV infection may complicate HIV treatment, this must be balanced against the increased risk of fibrosis with lower CD4$^+$ T-cell counts (Sulkowski et al., 2000). It should not discourage HIV providers from following DHHS treatment guidelines, given the improved survival of individuals coinfected with HIV and HCV on ART and the fact that newer ARVs are much less likely to cause hepatotoxicity. The benefit of HIV treatment on HCV was noted in 10,900 ART-naive persons coinfected with HIV and HCV in the Veterans Aging Cohort Study's Virtual Cohort (Anderson et al., 2014). This study examined incident or new cases of liver decompensation occurring from 1996 to 2010. The cohort was 60% Black, median age was 47 years, and one-third had baseline CD4$^+$ T-cell counts of less than 200 cells/mm^3. During a median 3.1 years of follow-up, 69% initiated ART and 36% started IFN-based HCV treatment. During the 46,444 person-years of follow-up, 645 liver decompensation events occurred in 6% of participants. Those starting ART by prescription refill history had a significantly lower rate of liver decompensation (HR, 0.72, or 28% risk reduction). When examining those with HIV RNA of more than 400 copies/mL at baseline (making the assumption that those with lower HIV RNA were on unreported ART), the risk reduction was even more dramatic (HR, 0.59, or 41% risk reduction). The study authors concluded that all persons coinfected with HIV and HCV should receive ART to lower the risk of end-stage liver disease. This is in keeping with current DHHS treatment guidelines for ART in HIV infection.

The provider and individual must weigh many variables when deciding to treat HCV, including disease severity, extrahepatic manifestations, risk of side effects, comorbid conditions such as renal disease, and likelihood of cure with the availability of more effective and well-tolerated DAA HCV regimens. Treatment goals should include viral eradication, prevention of disease progression, improved quality of life, increased rates of survival, decreased risk of cirrhosis and HCC, and normalization of liver enzymes to simplify chronic ART. For most persons coinfected with HIV and HCV, even those with cirrhosis, the potential for preservation of immune function, reduction of immune activation and inflammation, and slowing progression of liver disease outweighs the risk of drug-induced liver injury, so ART should always be considered regardless of the CD4$^+$ T-cell count. If the CD4$^+$ T-cell count is less than 200 cells/mm^3, HIV treatment to improve the immune status must take precedence. Initial ART regimens for people coinfected with HIV and HCV are similar to those for PWH without HCV infection. However, drug–drug interactions between ARVs and direct acting antivirals (DAA's) should be considered when choosing the initial therapy or when switching a suppressive ART regimen in order to start treatment for HCV.

Testing for HCV RNA by polymerase chain reaction is the only reliable way to diagnose acute HCV infection because approximately 30% of individuals do not have detectable antibodies at the onset of symptoms. A positive HCV antibody test with history of a prior negative HCV antibody test is also indicative of recent seroconversion. More than 90% will have antibodies by 3 months after exposure, with less than 5% of persons coinfected with HIV and HCV (usually those with advanced immunosuppression) failing to produce detectable HCV antibodies. Acute HCV is asymptomatic in 70% to 80% of cases, but cure rates are significantly higher with acute disease. It is therefore important to routinely screen at-risk individuals and promptly investigate elevated hepatic transaminase levels. Acutely infected HCV persons who are symptomatic have a higher likelihood of spontaneous viral clearance, so they should be monitored for 12 weeks before initiating HCV therapy. Asymptomatic individuals have a lower rate of spontaneous clearance, so they may benefit from early therapy. If HCV RNA remains elevated at 12 weeks after seroconversion, treatment should be strongly considered. If RNA is still present at 6 months, spontaneous clearance is unlikely, and the infection is considered chronic. Due to high efficacy and safety, the same DAA regimens used to treat chronic HCV may now be used to treat acute HCV. Acute HCV infection may present with flu-like symptoms, nausea, abdominal pain, and jaundice. Infrequently, severe hepatic dysfunction with transaminases up to 10 times normal is seen, but fulminant hepatitis is rare (DHHS, 2020c).

Prior to initiating HCV treatment in persons coinfected with HIV and HCV, specific baseline lab tests should be conducted. These include a complete blood count (CBC) with platelets, hepatic function panel including ALT, AST, alkaline phosphatase, albumin, and total bilirubin, prothrombin time/international normalized ratio (PT/INR), calculated glomerular filtration rate (eGFR), HIV and HCV RNA, CD4+ T-cell count, and HCV genotype and subtype. A pregnancy test is recommended for all females of childbearing potential if ribavirin (RBV) use is planned because RBV is a known teratogen. Counseling against alcohol consumption is key because this can rapidly worsen fibrosis. HBV and hepatitis A virus vaccination should be offered to all people without evidence of exposure to these infections.

A screening ultrasound is recommended to rule out cirrhosis and HCC in those with laboratory or clinical evidence of significant fibrosis or cirrhosis. Conventional computed tomography, magnetic resonance imaging, or single-photon emission computed tomography (SPECT) may be used, but these are generally reserved for evaluation of liver masses or screening individuals with more advanced fibrosis/cirrhosis. Although liver biopsy has been considered the gold standard in assessing disease stage, it is invasive and uncomfortable and has a bleeding risk (1/10,000 experience severe bleeding or fatality). Biopsies are generally scored from 0 to 4 based on degree of inflammation (grade) and degree of fibrosis (stage). Metavir scoring is one of the most common systems for interpreting a liver biopsy (Figure 35.1).

Because of the risks associated with biopsy, alternatives such as FibroScan and FibroSURE have rapidly risen in popularity and acceptance in clinical practice. FibroScan utilizes a mild-amplitude, low-frequency vibration transmitted through the liver to measure tissue "stiffness." This noninvasive and less expensive monitoring tool has been used in Europe for more than a decade and has been approved in the US since 2013 for clinical use. FibroSURE uses six blood serum tests (α_2-macroglobulin, haptoglobin, apolipoprotein A1, γ-glutamyl transferase, ALT, and total bilirubin) along with age and gender to generate a score that correlates with degree of liver disease. Other noninvasive biomarker formulas, such as APRI, which incorporates platelet counts with tests of coagulation and transaminases, and fibrosis-4 (FIB-4) may also be used to evaluate degree of fibrosis. APRI and FibroSURE have been validated in coinfection and predict

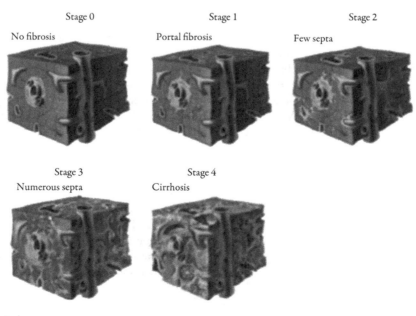

Stage 0
No fibrosis

Stage 1
Portal fibrosis

Stage 2
Few septa

Stage 3
Numerous septa

Stage 4
Cirrhosis

Figure 35.1 Metavir histologic staging

no disease versus cirrhosis accurately but are not as accurate in the midrange of the disease spectrum (Rallon et al., 2011; Schneider & Sarrazin, 2014).

Several formulas are used to assess the degree of cirrhosis. The Child–Turcotte–Pugh score uses encephalopathy, ascites, bilirubin, albumin, and PT or INR to classify severity of cirrhosis (class A, 5 or 6 points; class B, 7–9 points; and class C, 10–15 points). The Model for End-Stage Liver Disease (MELD) score uses serum creatinine, bilirubin, and INR and two or more dialysis sessions within the previous week to predict probability of survival for persons with end-stage liver disease. This is the formula currently used for liver allocation by the United Network of Organ Sharing and predicts the 3-month mortality rate. A MELD calculator is provided on the Mayo Clinic website (http://www.mayoclinic.org/medical-professionals/model-end-stage-liver-disease/meld-model). The HALT-C formula for predicting cirrhosis uses platelet count, INR, AST, and ALT to predict the probability of a biopsy demonstrating cirrhosis (Lok & McMahon, 2009).

THERAPEUTIC MODALITIES

Multiple, all-oral combinations of DAAs are now available as the recommended regimens for treatment (Table 35.1). Peg-IFN-α-2a or -2b and RBV had a cure rate of approximately 50% and had severe side effects that will usually preclude treatment completion. These injectable Peg-IFNs have been fully replaced by safer, more efficacious, and much better tolerated all-oral combinations, with guidelines no longer recommending their use. Evidence supports treating all people with HCV unless their life expectancy is less than 12 months because of a non–liver-related condition. As such, current guidelines places PWH in the "high priority" for treatment category given the increased risk of fibrosis and HCC. Treatment response is similar in persons coinfected with HIV and HCV compared with persons with only HCV.

Monitoring of HCV RNA during treatment is not recommended. No data support discontinuing treatment if the person is viremic. HCV RNA should be obtained at 12 weeks after treatment to determine cure (SVR12).

Drug–drug interactions increase the complexity of treating HCV in PWH on ART, as does the issue of renal function. Based on current evidence, the preferred treatment for persons with chronic kidney disease (CKD) stage 4 or 5 (eGFR <30 mL/min or end-stage renal disease) is either sofosbuvir (SOF; 400 mg)/velpatasvir (VEL; 100 mg) or glecaprevir (GLE; 300 mg)/pibrentasvir (PIB; 120 mg). ART switches may need to occur prior to treatment for HCV. Individuals may return to their prior regimen after treatment is completed. Although choosing a regimen to avoid drug interactions may seem daunting, interrupting ART while on HCV treatment is not recommended. Treatment interruption is associated with increased cardiovascular events as well as fibrosis progression and liver-related events. Because this area is in constant flux, see "Guidelines for the Use of Antiretroviral Agents in Adults and Adolescents with HIV" (DHHS, 2020a), under the HIV/HCV coinfection section, and "HCV Guidance: Recommendations for Testing, Managing, and Treating Hepatitis C" (American Association for the Study of Liver Disease/Infectious Diseases Society of America, 2018), under the Management of Unique Populations section, for current advice on ART for HIV when treating HCV.

The standard of care for hepatitis C now are the oral DAAs. They are engineered to work at multiple HCV-specific sites,

Table 35.1 CURRENT DAAS FOR HEPATITIS C

AGENT	GENOTYPES TREATED	CLASS	GFR	COMMENTS
Elbasvir/grazoprevir (Zepatier)	1 and 4	NS5A inhibitor ± NS3/4A protease inhibitor	No dose adjustment in patients with renal impairment, including those on hemodialysis	NS5A testing required in patients with GT 1a
Ledipasvir/sofosbuvir (Harvoni)	1–6	NS5A inhibitor ± nucleotide polymerase inhibitor (NS5B)	No dosage recommendation for patients with GFR < 30	First fixed oral combination
Sofosbuvir/ velpatasvir (Epclusa)	1–6	Nucleotide polymerase inhibitor (NS5B) ± NS5A inhibitor	No dosage recommendation for patients with GFR < 30	
Sofosbuvir/ velpatasvir/ voxilapresvir (Vosevi)	1–6	Nucleotide polymerase inhibitor (NS5B) ± NS5A inhibitor ± NS3/4A protease inhibitor	No dosage recommendation for patients with GFR < 30	For patients who have failed therapy with a NS5A inhibitor-containing regimen
Glecaprevir/ pibrentasvir (Mavyret)	1–6	HCV NS3/4A protease inhibitor ± HCV NS5A inhibitor	No dose adjustment in patients with renal impairment, including those on hemodialysis	
Daclatasvir (Daklinza)* ± Sofosbuvir (Sovaldi*) (alternative regimen)	1 and 3	NS5A inhibitor ± nucleotide polymerase inhibitor (NS5B)	No dosage adjustment required for patients with any degree of renal impairment	Several drug interactions with ARVs

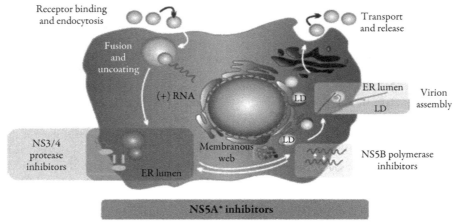

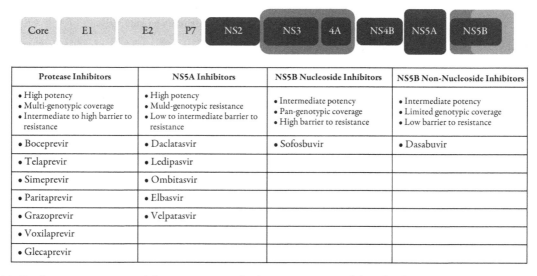

Figure 35.2 HCV life cycle and antiviral therapy for people with HCV. ER = endoplasmic reticulum; LD = luminal domain.

such as the protease and polymerase enzymes (Figure 35.2). The first-generation agents, boceprevir and telaprevir, were NS3/4A protease inhibitors (PIs). Although they were briefly "state of the art" between their licensure in 2010 and 2012, they are no longer recommended in the US because more efficacious and less toxic drugs have been developed. The agents in the second wave of HCV therapies have simple rules for use, shorter duration of therapy, and fewer drug–drug interactions and side effects, and they are highly effective in both persons with only HCV infection and persons coinfected with both HIV and HCV. The results in persons coinfected with HIV and HCV have been so impressive and so similar to those seen in mono-infection that many researchers are calling for a halt to separate trials in PWH.

DIRECT-ACTING AGENTS

The HCV genome encodes 10 polyproteins, 7 nonstructural proteins, and 3 structural proteins (NS3/4A, NS5A, NS5B) that play an important role in HCV replication and are the target of current DAAs (Figure 35.3). SOF and simeprevir were the initial second-generation DAAs approved in the US. Simeprevir was discontinued in May 2018 due to decreased utilization. However, SOF has become the cornerstone of most of the current combination treatments for hepatitis C.

NS5B POLYMERASE INHIBITOR(S)

NS5B polymerase is required for viral replication, acting as a chain terminator. SOF is a nucleotide analog inhibitor of this enzyme. The NS5B site is highly conserved among all genotypes; SOF is pan-genotypic. It is given as 400 mg once daily. It is not metabolized by the CYP450 enzyme complex and thus is an ideal candidate for use in HIV/HCV coinfection.

The nonnucleoside polymerase inhibitor dasavuvir was coformulated with ombitasvir, paritaprevir, and ritonavir (RTV) as a fixed-dose combination. It had a lower genetic barrier of resistance and is no longer available on the market.

Core	E1	E2	P7	NS2	NS3	4A	NS4B	NS5A	NS5B

Protease Inhibitors	NS5A Inhibitors	NS5B Nucleoside Inhibitors	NS5B Non-Nucleoside Inhibitors
• High potency • Multi-genotypic coverage • Intermediate to high barrier to resistance	• High potency • Muld-genotypic resistance • Low to intermediate barrier to resistance	• Intermediate potency • Pan-genotypic coverage • High barrier to resistance	• Intermediate potency • Limited genotypic coverage • Low barrier to resistance
• Boceprevir	• Daclatasvir	• Sofosbuvir	• Dasabuvir
• Telaprevir	• Ledipasvir		
• Simeprevir	• Ombitasvir		
• Paritaprevir	• Elbasvir		
• Grazoprevir	• Velpatasvir		
• Voxilaprevir			
• Glecaprevir			

Figure 35.3 Hepatitis C polyprotein structure and therapeutic targets for direct-acting antiviral drug development Adapted from Poordad F and Chee GM. *Curr Gastroenterol Rep.* 2012;14(1):74–77.

NS3/4A PROTEASE INHIBITORS

GLE, grazoprevir (GRZ), paritaprevir, and voxilaprevir (VOX) are the current DAAs available in this class. They are noncovalent inhibitors of the NS3/4A serine protease of HCV.

NS5A INHIBITORS

The exact mechanism of action of the NS5A inhibitors is not completely understood. However, some studies showed that they bind to the N-terminal domain of NS5A, causing structural distortion and inhibiting both viral RNA replication and virion assembly at an early stage. Daclatasvir, elbasvir (ELB), ledipasvir (LDV), ombitasvir, PIB, and VEL are antivirals in this class. Daclatasvir is no longer on the market. All others are coformulated in fixed-dose combinations.

FIXED-DOSE COMBINATIONS
LEDIPASVIR/SOFOSBUVIR

LDV/SOF (trade name Harvoni®; LDV 90 mg/SOF 400 mg) was the first IFN- and RBV-free once-daily, single-tablet regimen for HCV approved by the US Food and Drug Administration (on October 14, 2014).

The ION-4 study was a phase 3, multicenter, open-label trial of 335 persons coinfected with HIV and HCV. Enrolled participants had GT 1 and 4 (75% GT 1a, 23% GT 1b, and 2% GT 4), 20% had compensated cirrhosis, and 55% were treatment experienced. Based on drug–drug interaction data available at the beginning of the trial, ARTs allowed in study were FTC/TDF with efavirenz (EFV), RPV, or raltegravir (RAL). The primary endpoint was SVR12 after treatment, with SVR24 as the secondary endpoint.

No difference in response rates at week 12 of treatment was seen with GT 1a versus GT 1b based on sex, treatment history, concomitant ART, or cirrhosis status. Thirteen individuals (4%) did not achieve SVR. One person died at week 4 of treatment, 2 had breakthrough on treatment that was believed to likely be related to poor adherence by treating physicians, and 10 relapsed after treatment. All 10 relapsers were Black, with 7 having the TT allele in the gene encoding IL28B (which confers an increased risk of failure with IFN-containing regimens). Black race and the presence of the TT allele were found as a significant association in the univariate analysis. Black race alone in the multivariate analysis was significantly associated with relapse. The association of lower SVR with Black race (Blacks made up 34% of the study population) was not seen in the studies of LDV/SOB in persons infected with HCV only and was not related to the CYP2B6 polymorphism, which is more common in Blacks and results in increased EFV levels (Naggie et al., 2015).

LDV/SOF increases exposure to TDF by approximately 40%. Individuals on RTV-containing regimens may experience a relative increase of 30% to 60% in TDF exposure and so were excluded from the trial, along with those on cobicistat-containing combinations. Although 77% of persons had an adverse event, these were usually mild to moderate and resulted in no premature study discontinuations. Headache (25%), fatigue (21%), and diarrhea (11%) were the most common adverse events. Eight individuals experienced 15 serious adverse events, with HCC in two persons and portal vein thrombosis in two persons—all being reported in participants with cirrhosis. Three persons experienced serious infections. Grade 3 laboratory abnormalities occurred in 9% and grade 4 laboratory abnormalities in 2% of individuals, with elevations in lipase, creatinine phosphokinase, and serum glucose being most common.

ELBASVIR/GRAZOPREVIR

ELB/GRZ (trade name Zepatier®) is a fixed-dose combination of 50 mg ELB, an NS5A inhibitor, and 100 mg GRZ, an NS3/4A protease inhibitor, taken once a day with or without food for the treatment of chronic HCV GT 1 or 4 infection in adults. Treatment is typically 12 weeks. RBV is added and treatment extended to 16 weeks if baseline NS5A polymorphisms are found in a GT 1a person. RBV may be added in GT 1a or 1b persons who are Peg/RBV/PI experienced. GT 4 persons who are Peg/IFN/RBV experienced also receive 16 weeks of treatment. RBV is given as two daily doses depending on baseline NS5A polymorphisms and treatment experience. No dosage adjustment for ELB/GRZ is needed for renal impairment, including those on hemodialysis, although the RBV may need adjustment per guidelines. It is contraindicated in those with Child–Pugh B or C disease. ELB/GRZ is contraindicated with OATP1B1/3 inhibitors and strong CYP3A inducers such as EFV. Other contraindicated drugs include phenytoin and carbamazepine, rifampin, and St. John's wort. Coadministration with nafcillin, ketoconazole, bosentan, modafinil, ETV, and cobicistat-containing compounds is not recommended. The risk of ALT elevations may be elevated with zidovudine (ATZ), DRV, lopinavir (LPV), and cyclosporine. Statins also interact with ELB/GRZ. Thus, atorvastatin should not exceed 20 mg; rosuvastatin should not exceed 10 mg; and the lowest possible dose of fluvastatin, lovastatin, and simvastatin should be used. Tacrolimus levels may be increased by ELB/GRZ.

ELB/GRZ was approved for the treatment of GT 1 and 4 only based on results from the C-EDGE study. A total of 299 individuals were enrolled with GT 1, 4, and 6. The SVR12 was only 92% in persons with GT 1a, but it was 99% in persons with GT 1b and 100% in GT 4. Further analysis demonstrated lower SVR12 rates in persons with baseline NS5A resistance-associated variants (at positions 28, 30, 31, and 93) associated with more than fivefold loss in ELB susceptibility. Therefore, a baseline resistance test is recommended in people with GT 1a. If baseline resistance mutations are found, treatment should be extended for 16 weeks and RBV should be added.

In the C-EDGE Coinfection trial—a phase 3, open-label trial involving 218 HCV treatment-naive HCV/HIV coinfected individuals who received ELB/GRZ one tablet daily for 12 weeks—95.0% of individuals achieved a cure, with six relapses and one reinfection. The drug worked equally well in GT 1a or 1b and GT 4. Seven percent of participants reported fatigue, 7% headache, 5% nausea, 5% insomnia, and 5% diarrhea. No serious adverse events occurred (Rockstroh et al., 2015).

It should be noted that the Food and Drug Administration has issued a "black box" warning that ELB/GRZ could cause liver function test elevations of more than five times the upper limit of normal. Therefore, it is recommended to monitor liver function tests while on treatment.

SOFOSBUVIR/VELPATASVIR

SOF/VEL (trade name Epclusa®) is a pan-genotypic regimen approved on June 28, 2016, to be given as a once-daily fixed-dose combination tablet for 12 weeks in persons without cirrhosis or with compensated cirrhosis. In individuals with decompensated cirrhosis it must be used with RBV. VEL is a HCV NS5A inhibitor required for viral replication.

The ASTRAL-1 study was a randomized, double-blind, placebo-controlled study that evaluated 12 weeks of treatment with SOF/VEL compared to placebo in treatment-naive and Peg-IFN treatment-experienced individuals without cirrhosis or with compensated cirrhosis. Persons with all genotypes were included. Of 328 persons with GT 1, 98% achieved SVR12. Rates were similar in persons with compensated cirrhosis. Even in previously treatment-experienced persons with IFN-based regimens and first-generation protease inhibitors, this combination achieved more than 96% efficacy (Pianko et al., 2015).

In the ASTRAL-5 study, VEL/SOF was given to 106 people with HIV/HCV coinfection, virally suppressed on ART containing RAL, rilpivirine, or RTV-boosted protease inhibitors either with tenofovir or abacavir. Genotypes 1 to 4 were included; 18% of participants had compensated cirrhosis. SVR12 was achieved in 95% of the individuals, and it was well tolerated: the most commonly reported side effects were fatigue, headaches, nausea, and insomnia.

GLECAPREVIR/PIBRENTASVIR

GLE (200 mg)/PIB (120 mg) comes as three tablets to be taken once a day (trade name Mavyret®). This combination has several advantages compared to others. Not only is it pan-genotypic, but it could also be used in persons with chronic kidney disease and is approved for 8 weeks in treatment-naive individuals with no cirrhosis based on data from the ENDURANCE-1 and ENDURANCE-3 studies.

In the ENDURANCE-1 and ENDURANCE-3 trials, out of 1,208 persons with GT 1 and 3 treated for 8 weeks, 99.1% (95% CI, 98–100%) of people with GT 1 and 95% (95% CI, 91–98; 149 of 157 persons) of persons with GT 3 achieved SVR12 (Zeuzem et al., 2018). It is also approved for use in treatment-experienced persons for a total of 8 to 16 weeks based on cirrhosis stage and previously used DAA. Of note, this combination is contraindicated in individuals with advanced cirrhosis (Child–Pugh B or C).

The EXPEDITION-2 study evaluated 8 weeks of GLE/PIB in persons coinfected with HIV and HCV. Overall SVR12 rate was 98%.

SOFOSBUVIR/VELPATASVIR/VOXILAPREVIR

SOF/VEL/VOX (trade name Vosevi®) is a 12-week pan-genotypic, single-tablet, fixed-dose DAA indicated in persons with HCV GT 1a who have failed therapy with a NS5A inhibitor-containing regimen. VOX is a reversible potent inhibitor of the NS3/4A protease required for the cleavage of the HCV encoded polyprotein. The single-tablet regimen consists of 400 mg SOF, 100 mg VEL, and 100 mg VOX. It is administered once daily with food. Persons with advanced liver disease (Child–Pugh B and C) should not take this regimen.

POLARIS-1 and POLARIS-4 assessed the efficacy and safety of SOF/VEL/VOX for 12 weeks in persons with HCV infection who had previously received unsuccessful treatment with DAA-based regimens. All HCV genotypes were included; 46% of individuals had cirrhosis. The most common NS5A inhibitors used in previous unsuccessful treatment were LDV (55% of persons), daclatasvir (23%), and ombitasvir (13%) in POLARIS-1, while in POLARIS-4, the most common agent given was SOF (85%). SVR rates were 96% and 100% for GT 1a ($n = 101$) and GT 1b ($n = 45$), respectively. In POLARIS-1 and POLARIS-4, 83% and 49% of participants had baseline viral substitutions associated with resistance to NS3 inhibitors or NS5A inhibitors. SVR12 was achieved in 97% (199 of 205) of participants in POLARIS-1 and 100% (83 of 83) in POLARIS-4.

In a phase 2, open-label study, 49 persons with HCV GT 1 infection who previously failed to achieve SVR on a DAA-based regimen were randomized to receive SOF/VEL/VOX with or without RBV for 12 weeks. The primary efficacy endpoint was the proportion of individuals who achieved SVR12. SVR12 was achieved by 24 of 24 persons (100%; 95% CI, 86–100%) receiving SOF/VEL/VOX alone and 24 of 25 (96%; 95% CI, 80–100%) receiving the same treatment with RBV. Virologic response was achieved by 13 of 13 (100%) persons without baseline resistance-associated substitutions (RASs) and by 34 of 35 (97%) with baseline RASs. No large, randomized, controlled studies in persons coinfected with HIV/HCV have been done.

TREATMENT FAILURES

For those who fail HCV treatment, assessment for disease progression should be done every 6 to 12 months with a hepatic function panel, CBC, and INR. For patients with F3 or F4 disease, HCC surveillance every 6 months with ultrasound is advised. Cirrhotic patients should be referred to a hepatologist and have endoscopic evaluation for varices. Retreatment depends on GT, initial treatment, and reason for failure and is outside the scope of this chapter.

Liver transplantation is a possibility in persons in whom HCV therapy is contraindicated due to decompensated cirrhosis. As long as the CD4+ T-cell count is greater than 100 cells/mm^3 and HIV RNA levels are less than 400 copies/mL and without other contraindications (e.g., metastatic disease, ongoing alcohol or drug abuse, and active opportunistic infection), PWH may be appropriate for referral to a transplant center for evaluation. Studies have shown higher rates of waitlist mortality and posttransplant mortality, as well as more severe recurrent HCV disease (Terrault et al., 2012). Data from a prospective multicenter trial showed lower 3-year survival (60% vs. 79%; $p < 0.001$) in persons coinfected with HIV and HCV versus those with only HCV, as well as lower graft survival (53% vs. 74%; $p < 0.001$). Graft rejection was more common in those with coinfection (35% vs. 18%), likely related to the difficulties of managing immunosuppressive drugs in this population (Zahnd et al., 2015). New DAA drug therapy in HCV mono-infected persons and those coinfected with HIV and HCV has shown pretransplant and posttransplant virologic responses of 70% to 93% in some trials.

SUMMARY

The world of HIV/HCV coinfection is in rapid flux. Similar to HIV treatment, a combination of oral agents that disrupt the HCV virus at various sites of the life cycle has the best chance for decreasing viral replication in the long term and curing infection. Questions regarding optimal combinations as well as drug access and costs will need to be addressed in the next several years if the majority of persons coinfected with HIV and HCV are to be effectively treated.

ACKNOWLEDGMENT

The authors acknowledge Aimee Wilkin, MD, MPH, the author of the first section of this chapter in the previous edition.

REFERENCES

Aberg JA, Gallant JE, Ghanem KG, et al. Primary care guidelines for the management of persons infected with HIV: 2013 update by the HIV Medicine Association of the Infectious Diseases Society of America. *Clin Infect Dis.* 2014;58(1):e1–e34.

American Association for the Study of Liver Disease/Infectious Diseases Society of America. HCV guidance: recommendations for testing, managing, and treating hepatitis C. 2018. http://www.hcvguide-lines.org

Anderson JP, Tchetgen EJ, Lo R, et al. Antiretroviral therapy reduces the rate of hepatic decompensation among HIV and hepatitis C virus-coinfected veterans. *Clin Infect Dis.* 2014;58(5):719–727.

Asselah T, Rubbia-Brandt L, Marcellin P, et al. Steatosis in chronic hepatitis C: why does it really matter? *Gut.* 2006;55(1):123–130.

Audsley J, Seaberg E, Sasadeusz J, et al. Factors associated with elevated ALT in an international HIV/HBV coinfected cohort on long-term HAART. *PLoS One.* 2011;6(11):e26482.

Beretta M, Garlassi E, Cacopardo B, et al. Hepatocellular carcinoma in HIV-infected patients: check early, treat hard. *Oncologist.* 2011;16(9):1258–1269.

Bevilacqua E, Fabris A, Floreano P, et al. Genetic factors in mother-to-child transmission of HCV infection. *Virology.* 2009;390(1):64–70.

Boesecke C, Ingiliz P, Mandoerfer M, et al.; the NEAT Study Group. Is there long-term evidence of advanced liver fibrosis after acute hepatitis C in HIV coinfection? [Abstract 644]. Paper presented at the 21st Conference on Retroviruses and Opportunistic Infections, Boston, March 3–6, 2014.

Centers for Disease Control and Prevention. HIV/AIDS and viral hepatitis fact sheet. 2020. http://www.cdc.gov/hepatitis/populations/hiv.htm

Colin J, Cazals-Hatem D, Loriot M, et al. Influence of human immunodeficiency virus infection on chronic hepatitis B in homosexual men. *Hepatology.* 1999;29(4):1306–1310.

Conrad C, Bradley H, Broz D, et al. Community outbreak of HIV infection linked to injection drug use of oxymorphone—Indiana, 2015. *MMWR.* 2015;64(16):443–444.

Danta M, Dusheiko GM. Acute HCV in HIV-positive individuals—a review. *Curr Pharm Des.* 2008;14(17):1690–1697.

Department of Health and Human Services, Panel on Antiretroviral Guidelines for Adults and Adolescents. Guidelines for the use of antiretroviral agents in adults and adolescents with HIV. 2020a. https://clinicalinfo.hiv.gov/sites/default/files/inline-files/AdultandAdolescentGL.pdf

Department of Health and Human Services, Panel on Guidelines for the Prevention and Treatment of Opportunistic Infections in Adults and Adolescents with HIV. Guidelines for the prevention and treatment of opportunistic infections in HIV-infected adults and adolescents: recommendations from the Centers for Disease Control and Prevention, the National Institutes of Health, and the HIV Medicine Association of the Infectious Diseases Society of America. 2020b.https://clinicalinfo.hiv.gov/sites/default/files/inline-files/adult_oi.pdf

Dore G, Soriano V, Rockstroh J, et al. Frequent hepatitis B virus rebound among HIV-hepatitis B virus coinfected patients following antiretroviral therapy interruption. *AIDS.* 2010;24(6):857–865.

Elliott LN, Lloyd A, Ziegler JB, et al. Protective immunity against hepatitis C virus infection. *Immunol Cell Biol.* 2006;84:239–249.

Fierer DS, Dieterich DT, Fiel MI, et al. Rapid progression to decompensated cirrhosis, liver transplant, and death in HIV-infected men after primary hepatitis C virus infection. *Clin Infect Dis.* 2013;56(7):1038–1043.

Fierer DS, Mullen MP, Dieterich DT, et al. Early-onset liver fibrosis due to primary hepatitis C virus infection is higher over time in HIV-infected men. *Clin Infect Dis.* 2012;55(6):887–889.

Hadziyannis S, Papatheodoridis G. Hepatitis B e antigen-negative chronic hepatitis B: natural history and treatment. *Semin Liver Dis.* 2006;26:130–141.

Heuft M, Houba S, van den Berk G, et al. Protective effect of hepatitis B virus-active antiretroviral therapy against primary hepatitis B virus infection. *AIDS.* 2014;28(7):999–1005.

Launay O, Van der Vliet D, Rosenberg A, et al. Safety and immunogenicity of 4 intramuscular double doses and 4 intradermal low doses vs. standard hepatitis B vaccine regimen in adults with HIV-1: a randomized controlled trial. *JAMA.* 2011;305(14):1432–1440.

Linas BP, Wang B, Smurzynski M, et al. The impact of HIV/HCV coinfection on health care utilization and disability: results of the ACTG Longitudinal Linked Randomized Trials (ALLRT) Cohort. *J Viral Hepat.* 2011;18(7):506–512.

Lo Re III V, Kallan M, Tate J, et al. Hepatic decompensation in antiretroviral-treated patients coinfected with HIV and hepatitis C virus compared with hepatitis C virus-monoinfected patients: a cohort study. *Ann Intern Med.* 2014;160(6):369–379.

Lok AS, McMahon BJ. Chronic hepatitis B: update 2009. *Hepatology.* 2009;50(3):661–662.

Low E, Vogel M, Rockstroh J, et al. Acute hepatitis C in HIV-positive individuals. *AIDS Rev.* 2008;10(4):245–253.

Luetkemeyer A, Charlebois E, Hare C, et al. Resistance patterns and response to entecavir intensification among HIV–HBV-coinfected adults with persistent HBV viremia. *J AIDS.* 2011;58(3):e96–e99.

Mast EE, Hwang LY, Seto DS, et al. Risk factors for perinatal transmission of hepatitis C virus (HCV) and the natural history of HCV infection acquired in infancy. *J Infect Dis.* 2005;192(11):1880–1889.

Mohsen AH, Easterbrook P. Hepatitis C testing in HIV infected patients. *Sex Transm Infect.* 2003;79(1):76.

Naggie S, Cooper C, Saag M, et al. Ledipasvir and sofosbuvir for HCV in patients coinfected with HIV-1. *N Engl J Med.* 2015;373(8):705–713.

Pianko S, Flamm SL, Shiffman ML, et al. Sofosbuvir plus velpatasvir combination therapy for treatment-experienced patients with genotype 1 or 3 hepatitis C virus infection: a randomized trial. *Ann Intern Med*. 2015;163(11):809–817.

Pinchoff J, Drobnik A, Bornschlegel K, et al. Deaths among people with hepatitis C in New York City, 2000–2011. *Clin Infect Dis*. 2014;58(8):1047–1054.

Poynard T, Bedossa P, Opolon P. Natural history of liver fibrosis progression in patients with chronic hepatitis C. The OBSVIRC, METAVIR, CLINIVIR, and DOSVIRC groups. *Lancet*. 1997;349(9055):825–832.

Rallon NI, Soriano V, Naggie S, et al. IL28B gene polymorphism and viral kinetics in HIV. HCV coinfected patients treated with pegylated interferon and ribavirin. *AIDS*. 2011;25(8):1025–1033.

Rockstroh JK, Nelson M, Katlama C, et al. Efficacy and safety of grazoprevir (MK-5172) and elbasvir (MK-8742) in patients with hepatitis C virus and HIV coinfection (C-EDGE COINFECTION): a nonrandomised, open-label trial. *Lancet HIV*. 2015;2(8):e319–e327.

Schneider MD, Sarrazin C. Commentary: antiviral therapy of hepatitis C in 2014: do we need resistance testing? *Antivir Res*. 2014;105:64–71.

Sherman K. Management of the hepatitis B virus/HIV-coinfected patient. *Top Antivir Med*. 2015;23(3):111–114.

Shire N, Rouster S, Rajicic N, et al. Occult hepatitis B in HIV-infected patients. *J AIDS*. 2004;36(3):869–875.

Sulkowski M, Mast EE, Seeff LB, et al. Hepatitis C virus infection as an opportunistic disease in persons infected with human immunodeficiency virus. *Clin Infect Dis*. 2000;30(Suppl 1):S77–S84.

Sulkowski M, Thomas DL, Chaisson RE, et al. Hepatotoxicity associated with antiretrovirals in adults infected with HIV and the role of hepatitis C or B infection. *JAMA*. 2000;283:74–80.

Sulkowski M, Thomas D, Chaisson R, et al. Reactivation of hepatitis B virus replication accompanied by acute hepatitis in patients receiving highly active antiretroviral therapy. *Clin Infect Dis*. 2001;32(1):144–148.

Terrault N, Lok A, McMahon B, et al. Update on prevention, diagnosis, and treatment of chronic hepatitis B: AASLD 2018 Hepatitis B Guidance. *Hepatology*. 2018;67:1560–1599.

Thio C, Seaberg E, Skolasky R Jr, et al. HIV-1, hepatitis B virus, and risk of liver-related mortality in the Multicenter Cohort Study (MACS). *Lancet*. 2002;360(9349):1921–1926.

Thomas DL, Strathdee SA, Vlahov D. Long-term prognosis of hepatitis C virus infection. *JAMA*. 2000;284(20):2592.

Wandeler G, Gsponer T, Bregenzer A, et al. Hepatitis C virus infections in the Swiss HIV Cohort Study: a rapidly evolving epidemic. *Clin Infect Dis*. 2012;55(10):1408–1416.

Weber R, Sabin CA, Friis-Moller N, et al. Liver-related deaths in persons infected with the human immunodeficiency virus: the D:A:D study. *Arch Intern Med*. 2006;166(15):1632–1641.

Zahnd C, Salazar-Vizcaya L, Dufour JF, et al. Modelling the impact of deferring HCV treatment on liver-related complications in HIV coinfected men who have sex with men. *J Hepatol*. 2016;65(1):26–32.

Zeuzem S, Foster GR, Wwang S, et al. Glecaprevir–pibrentasvir for 8 or 12 weeks in HCV genotype 1 or 3 infection. *N Engl J Med*. 2018;378(4):354.

36.

THE COVID-19 PANDEMIC AND HIV

Richard C. Prokesch

LEARNING OBJECTIVES

- Provide a brief overview of the COVID-19 pandemic and how it impacts persons with HIV (PWH), with special considerations for healthcare providers

- Summarize findings of investigations designed to determine whether PWH are more likely to acquire COVID-19 compared to people without HIV infection

- Discuss guidance and best practices directing the delivery of healthcare during a pandemic

KEY POINTS

- SARS-CoV-2 infection has been rampant around the world and especially in the US; the pandemic has impacted the overall global economy as well as activities of daily living and has stressed healthcare systems.

- HIV does not appear to be an independent risk factor for developing COVID-19; PWH who are taking effective antiretroviral therapy (ART) have no greater risk of contracting or developing severe COVID-19 than individuals without HIV infection.

- With approximately half of the US population of PWH over 50 years old, and many experiencing multiple comorbidities of aging (e.g., diabetes mellitus, hypertension, cardiopulmonary disease), these persons are at increased risk of serious COVID-19 disease.

- All PWH should be up to date with their immunizations, especially for seasonal influenza and pneumococcal pneumonia.

INTRODUCTION

On New Years' Eve 2019, the World Health Organization (WHO) China Country Office was notified about cases of pneumonia with unknown etiology in Wuhan City in Hubei Province of central China (WHO, 2020). Over the next few weeks, the number of cases rapidly increased and the etiology was eventually determined to be a novel coronavirus, SARS-CoV-2; the disease syndrome became known as COVID-19.

The virus likely was a zoonotic transmission from bats to an intermediate host thought to be a pangolin (a type of nocturnal anteater) and then to humans. Since it was a novel virus, the global population had little underlying immunity and thus it spread prolifically, with devastating worldwide consequences.

The majority of people infected with COVID-19 are asymptomatic or only have mild symptoms, and thus "silent" transmission has been a major contributor to the growth of the pandemic. As of late October 2020, WHO surveillance data (available at covid19.who.int) indicate there have been over 46,400,000 confirmed COVID-19 cases worldwide and over 1,200,000 deaths. Despite initially involving primarily China and Italy, the US has thus far had the most cases: over 9,280,000 confirmed cases and over 230,000 deaths. Control of the pandemic in the US has been hampered by variable uptake of established prevention measures, lack of adequate testing (and limited access to testing in some areas), insufficient case tracking, as well as politicization. The infection has also disproportionally affected communities of color and populations in congregate settings (e.g., nursing homes, correctional facilities, shelters).

CLINICAL PRESENTATION AND TREATMENT

As mentioned, many individuals with COVID-19 have no or mild symptoms. Those who become symptomatic often have a flu-like prodrome with fevers, myalgias, and fatigue followed by respiratory symptoms including shortness of breath, dyspnea on exertion, nonproductive cough, and hypoxemia. Some people lose the sensations of smell and taste. Gastrointestinal symptoms including diarrhea and abdominal pain are also relatively common. Individuals who require hospitalization may progress to severe respiratory failure and "cytokine storm" may ensue from an overzealous and unregulated immune response, leading to acute respiratory distress syndrome, renal failure, thromboembolic events, and death.

The antiviral remdesivir, a nucleotide RNA polymerase inhibitor active in vitro against SARS-CoV-2, was found in two studies to reduce time to recovery (especially if given early in the disease course). Overall, evidence for clinical benefit with remdesivir is strongest in patients with COVID-19 pneumonia who require hospitalization and supplemental oxygen or ventilator support (Beigel et al., 2020; Wang et al., 2020). Additionally, for patients with severe COVID-19, dexamethasone has been shown to have a survival advantage compared to standard-of-care (no dexamethasone). In one meta-analysis of over 1,700 critically ill patients, glucocorticoids reduced 28-day mortality (Sterne et al., 2020). Data on other therapies (e.g., convalescent plasma, IL-6 pathway inhibitors, other antiviral agents) are limited at this time (Bhimraj et al., 2020).

HIV/COVID-19 COINFECTION

Based on available evidence to date, PWH on effective ART do not appear to have increased risk for acquiring SARS-CoV-2 infection and do not appear to experience worse COVID-19 outcomes compared to individuals without HIV. Various European and US studies of hospitalized PWH suggest that PWH have infection rates similar to those of individuals without HIV infection; clinical, radiographic, and laboratory features are also similar (Del Amo et al., 2020; Park et al., 2020; Vizcarra et al., 2020). A multicenter research network study in the US found no difference in mortality by HIV status (Hadi et al., 2020). Although PWH with low CD4$^+$ T-cell counts or those who are not taking ART might theoretically be at higher risk of acquiring SARS-CoV-2 infection and/or at higher risk for severe COVID-19 disease, this has not generally been demonstrated in high-income countries, although data are limited. Two studies from New York showed that hospitalized PWH did not have significantly different outcomes (e.g., intubation, length of stay, mortality) compared to individuals without HIV (Patel et al., 2020; Sigel et al., 2020). Although sample size was small, in one study (Sigel et al., 2020) it appeared that subjects with HIV who died in the hospital had overall lower CD4$^+$ T-cell counts compared to subjects with HIV who did not die. A second multicenter, registry-based US study found that although severe clinical outcomes occurred fairly commonly in PWH with COVID-19, this risk was primarily driven by age, comorbidity, and lower CD4$^+$ T-cell counts (despite HIV viral suppression) (Dandachi et al., 2020).

In general, serious COVID-19 disease is seen more frequently in older persons, especially those over 60 (CDC COVID-19 Response Team, 2020). Importantly, approximately half of all PWH in the US are 50 years of age or older. Further, underlying medical conditions that have been shown to increase the risk of severe illness from COVID-19 include hypertension, obesity (body mass index ≥ 30), chronic kidney disease, type 2 diabetes, cancer, serious heart conditions, and chronic obstructive pulmonary disease (Chen et al., 2020; Fung & Babik, 2020; Lighter et al., 2020; Lippi & Henry, 2020; Petrilli et al., 2020; Richardson et al., 2020; Yang et al., 2020). Therefore, PWH—and especially older PWH—who also have any of these comorbidities are at increased risk for severe COVID-19 infection. It is therefore especially critical that all PWH receive effective ART and adhere to their medications, in order to achieve/maintain viral load suppression and maintain immune competence.

COVID-19 AND HIV CARE

The COVID-19 pandemic has greatly impacted and complicated many aspects of care for PWH. Fortunately, a supply chain shortage of ART medications has not been observed to date, although some other medication-related factors have affected access to ART for some patients (e.g., changes in insurance status, modified pharmacy hours, delays in communications regarding refills). With rapid spread of the virus in March and April 2020, many clinical practices were shuttered and hospital systems quickly became overwhelmed. Over subsequent months, remote ("virtual") visits became increasingly utilized by providers/patients who had access to secure telemedicine platforms. Telemedicine and virtual visits also increased. For some practices that were already facing challenges with ensuring high levels of ongoing engagement/retention in care and ART adherence, such changes in service delivery created new stressors.

Modifications in care spurred by the pandemic include increasing prescription quantities to 90 days or longer to reduce frequency of travel to pharmacies (sometimes this practice was also extended to patients who had not attended a recent medical appointment); less frequent HIV-related laboratory monitoring for clinically stable patients (to reduce travel for separate phlebotomy services); and extended enrollment periods or flexibility with regard to medical insurance coverage. For many clinical practices that were able to resume in-person care, personal protective equipment and mask requirements were instituted along with physical/social distancing and previsit screening measures.

Overall, health care utilization for non-COVID-19-related illnesses has been greatly affected by the pandemic (Lange et al., 2020). Importantly, PWH may be hesitant to seek medical care (or delay seeking care) due to fears of exposure in clinical settings. Further, as the attention of many providers has been largely diverted to COVID-19 responses and recognition (especially in acute-care settings), other important diagnoses with similar presentation, such as *Pneumocystis jirovecii* pneumonia, may be overlooked (Coleman et al., 2020). More important than ever, providers should ensure that PWH are up to date with immunizations, including seasonal influenza and pneumococcal vaccines. The overlap of COVID-19 and influenza during the winter season is of particular concern. Box 36.1 includes key recommendations regarding COVID-19 and special considerations for the care of persons with HIV.

ART provision and monitoring of PWH are not the only aspects of HIV care that have been significantly affected by the pandemic. HIV prevention services, including preexposure prophylaxis (PrEP) care and screening for HIV and sexually transmitted infections, have also been markedly interrupted. Some individuals on PrEP have discontinued medications and/or have been unable to undergo regular lab monitoring because of decreased access to care providers (Stephenson et al., 2020). Providers should maintain contact with individuals who are at risk for HIV acquisition and attempt to address PrEP barriers to help ensure access to effective HIV prevention interventions.

REFERENCES

Beigel JH, Tomashek KM, Dodd LE, et al.; ACTT-1 Study Group Members. Remdesivir for the treatment of COVID-19: preliminary report. *N Engl J Med*. 2020;383(19):1813–1826. doi:10.1056/NEJMoa2007764

Bhimraj A, Morgan RL, Shumaker AH, et al. Infectious Diseases Society of America guidelines on the treatment and management of patients with COVID-19. 2020. www.idsociety.org/COVID19guidelines

CDC COVID-19 Response Team. Severe outcomes among patients with coronavirus disease 2019 (COVID-19)—United States, February 12–March 16, 2020. *MMWR Morb Mortal Wkly Rep*. 2020;69:343–346. doi:http://dx.doi.org/10.15585.mmwr.mm6912e2

Chen R, Liang W, Jiang M, et al. Risk factors of fatal outcome in hospitalized subjects with coronavirus disease 2019 from a nationwide analysis in China. *Chest*. 2020;158(1):97–105.

Coleman H, Snell LB, Simons R, et al. Coronavirus disease 2019 and *Pneumocystis jirovecii* pneumonia: a diagnostic dilemma in HIV. *AIDS*. 2020;34(8):1258–1260.

Dandachi D, Geiger G, Montgomery MW, et al.; HIV-COVID-19 Consortium. Characteristics, comorbidities, and outcomes in a multicenter registry of patients with HIV and coronavirus disease-19. *Clin Infect Dis*. 2020;ciaa1339 [E-pub before print]. doi:10.1093/cid/ciaa1339

Del Amo J, Polo R, Moreno S, et al. Incidence and severity of COVID-19 in HIV-positive persons receiving antiretroviral therapy: a cohort study. *Ann Intern Med*. 2020;173(7):536–541.

Fung M, Babik JM. COVID-19 in immunocompromised hosts: what we know so far. *Clin Infect Dis*. 2020:ciaa863 [E-pub before print].

Hadi YB, Naqvi SFZ, Kupec JT, et al. Characteristics and outcomes of COVID-19 in patients with HIV: a multi-center research network study. *AIDS*. 2020;34(13):F3–F8.

Lange SJ, Ritchey MD, Goodman AB, et al. Potential indirect effects of the COVID-19 pandemic on use of emergency departments for acute life-threatening conditions—United States, January–May 2020. *MMWR Morb Mortal Wkly Rep*. 2020;69(25):795–800. doi:10.15585/mmwr.mm6925e2

Lighter J, Phillips M, Hochman S, et al. Obesity in patients younger than 60 years is a risk factor for COVID-19 hospital admission. *Clin Infect Dis*. 2020;71(15):896–897.

Lippi G, Henry BM. Chronic obstructive pulmonary disease is associated with severe coronavirus disease 2019 (COVID-19). *Respir Med*. 2020;167:105941.

Park LS, Rentsch CT, Sigel K, et al. COVID-19 in the largest US HIV cohort [Abstract LBPEC23]. AIDS2020: 23rd International AIDS Conference [Virtual], July 6–10, 2020.

Patel VV, Felsen UR, Fisher M, et al. Clinical outcomes by HIV serostatus, CD4 count, and viral suppression among people hospitalized with COVID-19 in the Bronx, New York [Abstract OABLB0102]. 23rd International AIDS Conference, 2020.

Petrilli CM, Jones SA, Yang J, et al. Factors associated with hospital admission and critical illness among 5279 people with coronavirus disease 2019 in New York City: prospective cohort study. *BMJ*. 2020;369:m1966. doi:10.1136/bmj.m1966

Richardson S, Hirsch JS, Narasimhan M, et al. Presenting characteristics, comorbidities, and outcomes among 5700 patients hospitalized with COVID-19 in the New York City area. *JAMA*. 2020;323(20):2052–2059.

Sigel K, Swartz T, Golden E, et al. COVID-19 and people with HIV infection: outcomes for hospitalized patients in New York City. *Clin Infect Dis*. 2020;71(11):2933–2938. doi:10.1093/cid/ciaa880

Sterne JA, Murthy S, Diaz JV, et al.; WHO Rapid Evidence Appraisal for COVID-19 Therapies (REACT) Working Group. Association between administration of systemic corticosteroids and mortality among critically ill patients with COVID-19: a meta-analysis. *JAMA*. 2020;324(13):1330–1341. doi:10.1001/jama.2020.17023

Stephenson R, Chavanduka TMD, Rosso MT, et al. Sex in the time of COVID-19: results of an online survey of gay, bisexual and other men who have sex with men's experience of sex and HIV prevention during the US COVID-19 epidemic. *AIDS Behav.* 2020 [E-pub ahead of print]. doi:10.1007/s10461-020-03024-8

Vizcarra P, Perez-Elias MJ, Quereda C, et al. Description of COVID-19 in HIV-infected individuals: a single-centre, prospective cohort. *Lancet HIV.* 2020;7(8):e554–e564.

Wang Y, Zhand D, Du G, et al. Remdesivir in adults with severe COVID-19: a randomized, double-blind, placebo-controlled, multicenter trial. *Lancet.* 2020;395(10236):1569–1578.

World Health Organization. Situation Report 1: novel coronavirus (2018-nCoV). January 21, 2020. https://www.who.int/docs/default-source/coronaviruse/situation-reports/20200121-sitrep-1-2019-ncov.pdf

Yang J, Zheng Y, Gou X, et al. Prevalence of comorbidities and its effects in patients infected with SARS-CoV-2: a systematic review and meta-analysis. *Int J Infect Dis.* 2020;94:91–95.

37.

SEXUALLY TRANSMITTED DISEASES

Karen J. Vigil

LEARNING OBJECTIVE

Upon completion of this chapter, the reader should be able to:

- Demonstrate knowledge about established and evolving science regarding the diagnosis and treatment of the most prevalent sexually transmitted diseases (STDs) in patients with HIV infection (PWH), in order to decrease the rate of transmission.

STDs are common in PWH. Education and counseling on changes in sexual behaviors of patients with STDs and their sexual partners, identification of asymptomatic infection, and effective diagnosis and treatment represent the cornerstone for prevention.

GENITAL ULCERS

In the US, most young, sexually active patients who have genital, anal, or perianal ulcers have either genital herpes or syphilis, herpes being the more prevalent. Less common causes include chancroid and donovanosis.

SYPHILIS

WHAT'S NEW?

Syphilis incidence continues to increase and is more prevalent in PWH and men who have sex with men (MSM). PWH with syphilis should have a detailed neurologic examination. Patients with abnormal signs or symptoms should undergo cerebrospinal fluid (CSF) analysis.

KEY POINTS

- Syphilis incidence continues to increase and is more prevalent in PWH and MSM.

- Clinical manifestations are similar to the general population, but complications may be more common (condyloma lata and lues maligna).

- Special attention to neurologic site involvement is required, as laboratory-defined neurosyphilis may be more common among PWH.

- Although CSF abnormalities are more likely in PWH with a CD4+ cell count of 350 cells/mm^3 or less and a rapid plasma reagin (RPR) titer of 1:32 or more, lumbar puncture is recommended only if there any sign or symptom of neurologic involvement.

- Penicillin is the treatment of choice for syphilis; alternatives have not been well studied in PWH.

Syphilis is a systemic disease caused by *Treponema pallidum*. Between 2005 and 2013, the number of reported cases of primary and secondary syphilis nearly doubled. The annual rate increased from 2.9 to 5.3 cases per 100,000 population (Patton et al., 2014). In 2012, MSM accounted for 83.9% of cases. Coinfection with HIV has been reported to be as much as 50% to 70% among MSM, with a high HIV seroconversion rate in patients with primary and secondary syphilis (Su & Weinstock, 2011).

PRIMARY SYPHILIS

Primary syphilis refers to the chancre: a single, painless lesion with a clean base and indurated, raised borders. Chancres appear 1 week to 1 month after exposure. They are usually in the genital area but can occur anywhere on the body, including the oral cavity.

SECONDARY SYPHILIS

Secondary syphilis is characterized by a maculopapular erythematous rash that may involve the palms and soles. It typically occurs 3 weeks to 3 months after exposure. In PWH, rash could present with other several forms, including papulosquamous, vesicular, and pustular forms. Condylomata lata (broad-based, fleshy wart-like lesions that occur in moist, warm body areas) and lues maligna (pustular ulceronodular syphilides) are complications of secondary syphilis and are more frequent in PWH.

LATENT SYPHILIS

Latent syphilis is defined by a positive serologic test in the absence of any clinical signs or symptoms of syphilis. Early latent syphilis is defined as one acquired within the preceding year. All other forms are either late latent syphilis or latent syphilis of unknown duration. The importance of this classification is secondary to transmission, which is possible in any of the stages until early latent syphilis.

NEUROSYPHILIS

Central nervous system (CNS) involvement may occur at any stage of syphilis. CSF laboratory abnormalities are common in persons with early syphilis, even in the absence of neurologic signs or symptoms. No evidence exists to support variation from recommended treatment for early syphilis for patients found to have such abnormalities. If clinical evidence of neurologic involvement is observed, a CSF examination should be performed.

Neurosyphilis can take any of several other forms, including uveitis, retinitis, sensorineural hearing loss (otosyphilis), or CNS vasculitis. A lumbar puncture and CSF examination should be performed for all patients with syphilitic eye disease to identify those with abnormalities; patients found to have abnormal CSF test results should be provided follow-up CSF examinations to assess treatment response.

The 2015 Centers for Disease Control and Prevention (CDC) treatment guidelines (Workowski et al., 2015) recommend CSF examination:

- If there is evidence of neurologic symptoms
- If there are ophthalmologic or auditory signs or symptoms
- In patients with clinical presentation of tertiary syphilis (e.g., aortitis or gumma)
- In patients with treatment failure

CSF abnormalities are most likely in PWH with syphilis of any stage when the CD4$^+$ cell count is 350 cells/mm^3 or less and a serum RPR titer exceeds 1:32 (Libois et al., 2007; Marra et al., 2004). However, CSF examination has not been associated with improved clinical outcomes in the absence of neurologic signs and symptoms.

Other presentation of tertiary syphilis includes cardiovascular syphilis and gummatous syphilis. Cases of rapid progression after initial infection have been reported with both entities (Maharajan & Sampath Kumaar, 2005; Weinert et al., 2008).

DIAGNOSIS

Primary chancre could be diagnosed by visualization of spirochetes under darkfield microscopic examination. This applies to genital lesions and not oral lesions because of the presence of nonpathogenic spirochetes in the mouth.

Non-treponemal antigen tests (Venereal Disease Research Laboratory [VDRL] and RPR) detect antibodies to antigens in the host after modification by *T. pallidum*. They become positive 4 to 6 weeks after infection or 1 to 3 weeks after the appearance of a primary lesion.

Treponemal tests (TPHA, TPPA, and FTA-ABS) detect antibodies that react with *T. pallidum* antigens. They are confirmatory for syphilis.

Making the diagnosis of neurosyphilis in PWH is difficult since HIV itself cause CSF abnormalities. Classic CSF findings in neurosyphilis are lymphocytic pleocytosis, total protein elevation, and a positive VDRL test. CSF VDRL results may be falsely negative in 30% to 70% of cases of neurosyphilis.

TREATMENT

PWH who have early syphilis might be at increased risk for neurologic complications (Lee et al., 2007) and might have higher rates of serologic treatment failure with currently recommended regimens than people without HIV. No treatment regimens for syphilis have been demonstrated to be more effective in preventing neurosyphilis in PWH than the syphilis regimens recommended for HIV-negative patients (Rolfs et al., 1997). Careful follow-up after therapy is essential. The recommended and alternative treatment regimens for syphilis (Workowski et al., 2015) in PWH are summarized in Table 37.1.

FOLLOW-UP

PWH should be evaluated clinically and serologically for treatment failure at 3, 6, 9, 12, and 24 months after therapy. If the patient meets criteria for treatment failure (signs or symptoms that persist or recur or a sustained fourfold increase in non-treponemal test titer), a new lumbar puncture with CSF examination should be performed and new

Table 37.1 RECOMMENDED AND ALTERNATIVE TREATMENT REGIMENS FOR SYPHILIS IN PWH

	RECOMMENDED REGIMEN	ALTERNATIVE REGIMEN
Primary, secondary, and early latent syphilis	Benzathine penicillin G, 2.4 MU IM in a single dose	
Late latent syphilis or syphilis of unknown duration	Benzathine penicillin G, at weekly doses of 2.4 MU for 3 weeks	
Neurosyphilis	Aqueous crystalline penicillin G 18–24 MU/day, administered as 3–4 MU IV every 4 hours or continuous infusion, for 10–14 days	Procaine penicillin 2.4 MU IM once daily *PLUS* Probenecid 500 mg orally 4 times a day, both for 10–14 days

MU, million units; IM, intramuscularly; IV, intravenously

treatment should be initiated. CSF examination and retreatment also should be strongly considered for PWH whose non-treponemal test titers do not decrease fourfold within 6 to 12 months of therapy. If CSF examination is normal, treatment with benzathine penicillin G administered as 2.4 million units given intramuscularly at weekly intervals for 3 weeks is recommended.

For neurosyphilis, if CSF pleocytosis was present initially, a CSF examination should be repeated every 6 months until the cell count is normal. Research studies suggest that CSF improvement might occur much slower in PWH, especially those with more advanced immunosuppression. If the cell count has not decreased after 6 months or if the CSF is not normal after 2 years, retreatment should be considered.

GONORRHEA

WHAT'S NEW?

Dual therapy for gonorrhea with ceftriaxone and azithromycin is recommended to hinder the development of antimicrobial-resistant *Neisseria gonorrhoeae* and to treat possible coinfection with *Chlamydia trachomatis*.

KEY POINTS

- Gonococcal infection remains an important cause of urethritis, cervicitis, pharyngitis, and proctitis in sexually active PWH.

- Asymptomatic infection with gonorrhea and chlamydia is common at the female cervical site and at male pharyngeal and rectal sites, such that routine, periodic screening for this STD is required to detect such cases.

- Nucleic acid–based testing offers high sensitivity, ease of sample collection, and use of noninvasively acquired specimens (i.e., urine), though such tests are not cleared by the US Food and Drug Administration (FDA) for use with all specimen types.

- Antimicrobial resistance to fluoroquinolone and oral cephalosporins has been reported.

- Recommended treatment for gonorrhea is Ceftriaxone 500mg IM single dose. If Chlamydia has not been excluded, doxycycline 100mg BID for 7 days should be given.

Gonorrhea is caused by *N. gonorrhoeae*. In 2018, 583,405 cases of gonorrhea were reported to the CDC (Gonorrhea—CDC Fact Sheet, 2021), representing a 5% increased rate from the previous year and an 82% increase since 2009. PWH are significantly more likely to have gonorrhea than HIV-uninfected men (Kent et al., 2005).

CLINICAL PRESENTATION

Acute urethritis is the main manifestation of gonorrhea. In men, urethral discharge—initially scant and later purulent—and dysuria are the major symptoms. The incubation period ranges from 1 to 10 days. Local complications include acute epididymitis, penile edema, penile lymphangitis, periurethral abscess, acute prostatitis, seminal vesiculitis, or infections of Tyson's and Cowper's glands. In women, gonorrhea presents as cervicitis and/or asymptomatic urethritis. However, physical exam may show purulent or mucopurulent cervical exudates.

N. gonorrhoeae may also cause rectal infection that could be asymptomatic or manifest as proctitis. Up to one-third of MSM who have gonorrhea have positive rectal cultures (Handsfield et al., 1980). Pharyngeal infection has also been reported but is usually asymptomatic.

Disseminated gonococcal infection results from bacteremic dissemination of *N. gonorrhoeae*. It can cause arthritis that primarily involves an asymmetric distribution in the knees, elbows, and more distal joints. A dermatitis picture with multiple discrete papules and pustules, often with a hemorrhagic component, is present in approximately 75% of patients.

DIAGNOSIS

Gram stain of urethral discharge reveals gram-negative diplococci during the first week after onset in men. In women this is less common. Although cultures represent the gold standard for diagnosis, nucleic acid amplification tests (NAATs) in cervical swab, urethral swab, or urine have excellent sensitivity and specificity.

TREATMENT

Quinolone-resistant *N. gonorrhoeae* strains are widely disseminated throughout the US and the world. Treatment failure to oral cephalosporins has been reported in Asia, Europe, Africa, and Canada (Lewis et al., 2013; Unemo et al., 2012). Therefore, quinolones and oral cephalosporins are no longer recommended for the treatment of gonorrhea in the US. Recommended regimens (St Cyr et al., 2020) in PWH are summarized in Table 37.2. There are limited data on alternative treatments for people with cephalosporin or IgE-mediated penicillin allergy. Options include either gentamicin (240 mg) or gemifloxacin (320 mg) plus 2 grams azithromycin. However, consultation with an infectious disease specialist is recommended (Kirkcaldy et al., 2014).

FOLLOW-UP

If failure to ceftriaxone is suspected, patients should be retreated with at least 250 mg ceftriaxone given intramuscularly or intravenously. Partner treatment should be ensured and the situation should be reported to the CDC.

Table 37.2 RECOMMENDED TREATMENT REGIMENS FOR GONORRHEA INFECTION IN PWH

	RECOMMENDED REGIMEN
Uncomplicated gonococcal infections of the pharynx, cervix, urethra, and rectum	Ceftriaxone 500 mg Im in a single dose (for persons weighing <150 kg) Ceftriaxone 1 gram Im in a single dose (for persons weighing 150 kg or more)
Disseminated gonococcal infection	Ceftriaxone 1 gram Im or IV daily
Gonococcal meningitis and endocarditis	Ceftriaxone 1–2 grams IV every 12 hours for 10–14 days for meningitis and for at least 4 weeks for endocarditis

IM, intramuscularly; IV, intravenously; PO, orally

CHLAMYDIA INFECTIONS

WHAT'S NEW?

Due to the high prevalence of *C. trachomatis* infection in women and men who were treated for chlamydial infection during the preceding several months, chlamydia-infected women and men should be retested approximately 3 months after treatment, regardless of whether they believe that their sex partners were treated.

KEY POINTS

- Routine, periodic screening for *C. trachomatis* is recommended for all sexually active PWH at exposed anatomic sites, at initial evaluation and every 12 months thereafter, or more frequently as indicated by risk.

- Nucleic acid–based testing offers high sensitivity, ease of sample collection, and use of noninvasively acquired specimens (i.e., urine), though such tests are not FDA-cleared for use with all specimen types.

- Most *C. trachomatis* infections are asymptomatic and thus detected only by routine, periodic screening.

- Rectal *C. trachomatis* infection is especially common among MSM; in this population, the *C. trachomatis* subtypes that cause lymphogranuloma venereum (LGV) should be included in the differential diagnosis of those with severe symptoms of proctitis, especially when *C. trachomatis* is found to be the cause.

Chlamydia is the most commonly reported STD in the US in men and women. In 2018, a total of 1,758,668 chlamydial infections were reported to CDC from 50 states and the District of Columbia (CDC, Chlamydia—CDC Fact Sheet, 2018). However, underreporting might be substantial as the disease may be asymptomatic. Chlamydia infection is more frequent in younger age groups, racial/ethnic minorities, MSM, and incarcerated populations (Burstein et al., 1998;

Rietmeijer et al., 2008; Satterwhite et al., 2008). Genital and ocular chlamydial infections are caused by serotypes D to K, while LGV is caused by serotypes L1, L2, and L3.

CLINICAL PRESENTATION

Chlamydia genital infection secondary to serotypes D to K causes urethritis in men and cervicitis in women. Although most of the patients are asymptomatic, men may present with purulent urethral discharge (milder than gonorrhea) and women may complaint of vaginal discharge, intermenstrual bleeding, dyspareunia, and/or abdominal pain. Women may also present with symptoms exclusively of urethritis such as dysuria.

Serovars L1 to L3 cause LGV. LGV is not endemic in the US; prevalence is higher in Southeast Asia, the Caribbean, Latin America, and Africa. LGV presents as one or more genital ulcers or papules, followed by the development of unilateral or bilateral fluctuant inguinal lymphadenopathy called buboes. Since 2003, there have been reports of outbreaks in Western Europe and in the US of L2 serotype proctitis, particularly in MSM.

DIAGNOSIS

NAATs for chlamydia genital infections (by polymerase chain reaction assay or transcription-mediated amplification) have great sensitivity and specificity and can be performed on first-catch urine or vaginal swab without the need for a urethral swab. The diagnosis of LGV is challenging. Cell culture is the only diagnostic test approved by the FDA. Serology helps in the diagnosis as titers are typically elevated at the time of presentation.

Diagnosis of LGV proctitis is even more difficult. NAATs may be used if a local laboratory has validated them. The CDC recommends that when LGV is suspected, the provider should collect a specimen and send it to the state health department for referral to the CDC. If this is not possible, an antibiotic regimen effective against LGV should be included in empiric treatment for proctitis.

TREATMENT

Oral azithromycin (1 gram as a single dose) or doxycycline (100 mg twice a day for 7 days) are the treatments of choice. For proctitis, a 28-day treatment course with doxycycline (100 mg twice daily) is recommended.

HUMAN PAPILLOMAVIRUS

WHAT'S NEW?

There are three types of human papillomavirus (HPV) vaccines:

Cervarix™, a bivalent vaccine that targets HPV types 16 and 18

Gardasil™, a quadrivalent HPV vaccine that targets HPV types 6, 11, 16 and 18

Gardasil-9, a 9-valent vaccine that targets in addition HPV types 31, 33, 45, 52, and 58, which cause approximately 20% of cervical cancers and were not covered by Gardasil.

Only Gardasil-9 is available in the US.

KEY POINTS

- HPV is the most common STD in the US. There are more than 100 HPV types; however, certain strains are associated with genital warts and others with intraepithelial lesions and high-grade neoplasia.

- PWH have higher rates of HPV-related lesions; genital warts can be more aggressive and difficult to eradicate.

- A variety of patient- and provider-applied therapies are available.

- There are three types of human papillomavirus (HPV) vaccines:

  Cervarix™, a bivalent vaccine that targets HPV types 16 and 18

  Gardasil™, a quadrivalent HPV vaccine that targets HPV types 6, 11, 16 and 18

  Gardasil-9, a 9-valent vaccine that targets in addition HPV types 31, 33, 45, 52, and 58, which cause approximately 20% of cervical cancers and were not covered by Gardasil.

  Only Gardasil-9 is available in the US.

HPV is a double-stranded DNA virus that may infect the genital tract. There are more than 100 types of HPV; more than 40 may infect the genital area. HPV may cause two major clinical syndromes: genital warts (condylomata acuminata), associated mainly with types 6 and 11, and epithelial cervical or anal neoplasia, linked to serotypes 16 and 18. (For more information on cervical and anal neoplasia, refer to Chapter 29.)

HPV detection is significantly more common among HIV-infected women and men than among HIV-seronegative women and men (Mbulawa et al., 2009). Several studies have demonstrated that HPV increases the risk of HIV acquisition (Smith et al., 2010).

CLINICAL PRESENTATION

In most cases, HPV infection is transient, has no clinical manifestations or sequelae, and is self-limited. Genital warts typically present as single or multiple soft, fleshy, papillary or sessile, painless keratinized growths in the vulvovaginal area, penis, anus, urethra, or perineum. HIV-infected women have a higher prevalence of genital warts and they may progress more rapidly in the presence of a declining immune status. There are also higher rates of Pap smear–detected abnormalities, dysplasia, and progression to cervical cancer relative to uninfected women.

DIAGNOSIS

Diagnosis of warts is made clinically; laboratory confirmation is not needed. PWH, especially MSM, have a significantly increased risk of anal cancer due to oncogenic HPV types; therefore, routine anal Pap screening in HIV care settings is recommended.

TREATMENT

The main indications for treatment of vulvovaginal warts are bothersome symptoms and/or psychological distress. Vulvar biopsy to exclude precancerous or cancerous lesions is indicated when warts are identified in immunocompromised or postmenopausal women, when the lesions are visually atypical, or when warts fail to respond to standard therapy. The recommended treatment regimens for HPV in PWH are summarized in Table 37.3.

Table 37.3 RECOMMENDED TREATMENT REGIMENS FOR HPV/WARTS IN PWH

External genital warts, patient-applied	Podofilox 0.5% solution or gel *OR* Imiquimod 5% cream *OR* Sinecatechins 15% ointment
External genital warts. provider-administered	Cryotherapy with liquid nitrogen or cryoprobe. Repeat applications every 1–2 weeks. *OR* Trichloroacetic acid (TCA) or bichloroacetic acid (BCA) 80–90% *OR* Surgical removal either by tangential scissor excision, tangential shave excision, curettage, or electrosurgery
Vaginal warts	Cryotherapy with liquid nitrogen *OR* TCA or BCA 80–90% applied to warts *OR* Surgical removal
Urethral meatus warts	Cryotherapy with liquid nitrogen *OR* Surgical removal
Anal warts	Cryotherapy with liquid nitrogen *OR* TCA or BCA 80–90% applied to warts *OR* Surgical removal

PREVENTION

There are three types of HPV vaccines: a bivalent vaccine that targets HPV types 16 and 18 (Cervarix™); a quadrivalent HPV vaccine that targets HPV types 6, 11, 16, and 18 (Gardasil); and a 9-valent vaccine that prevents infection with HPV types 6, 11, 16, 18, 31, 33, 45, 52, and 58. Only Gardasil-9 is available in the US.

Routine vaccination is recommended for boys and girls at age 11 or 12 years. Gardasil-9 is approved until age 45. However, people older than 26 years may have prior exposure to different HPV types. The CDC emphasizes that immunocompromised or immunosuppressed patients, included PWH, MSM, and bisexual men, should also be vaccinated.

REFERENCES

Burstein GR, Waterfield G, Joffe A, et al. Screening for gonorrhea and chlamydia by DNA amplification in adolescents attending middle school health centers. Opportunity for early intervention. Sex Transm Dis 1998;25:395.

Centers for Disease Control and Prevention. Chlamydia Fact Sheet. 2021. https://www.cdc.gov/std/chlamydia/stdfact-chlamydia-detailed.htm

Centers for Disease Control and Prevention. Gonorrhea Fact Sheet. 2021. https://www.cdc.gov/std/gonorrhea/stdfact-gonorrhea-detailed.htm

Centers for Disease Control and Prevention. Sexually Transmitted Disease Surveillance 2018. Atlanta, GA: US Department of Health and Human Services, 2018.

Handsfield HH, Knapp JS, Diehr PK, et al. Correlation of auxotype and penicillin susceptibility of *Neisseria gonorrhoeae* with sexual preference and clinical manifestations of gonorrhea. Sex Transm Dis 1980;7:1–5.

Kent CK, Chaw JK, Wong W, et al. Prevalence of rectal, urethral, and pharyngeal chlamydia and gonorrhea detected in 2 clinical settings among men who have sex with men: San Francisco, California, 2003. Clin Infect Dis 2005;41:67–74.

Kirkcaldy RD, Weinstock HS, Moore PC, et al. The efficacy and safety of gentamicin plus azithromycin and gemifloxacin plus azithromycin as treatment of uncomplicated gonorrhea. Clin Infect Dis 2014;59:1083–1091

Lee M, Aynalem G, Kerndt P, et al. Symptomatic early neurosyphilis among HIV-positive men who have sex with men: four cities, United States, January 2002–June 2004. MMWR Morb Mortal Wkly Rep 2007;56:625–628.

Lewis DA, Sriruttan C, Muller EE, et al. Phenotypic and genetic characterization of the first two cases of extended-spectrum cephalosporin-resistant *Neisseria gonorrhoeae* infection in South Africa and association with cefixime treatment failure. J Antimicrob Chemother 2013;68:1267–1270.

Libois A, De Wit S, Poll B, et al. HIV and syphilis: when to perform a lumbar puncture. Sex Transm Dis 2007;34:141–144.

Maharajan M, Sampath Kumaar G. Cardiovascular syphilis in HIV infection: a case-control study at the Institute of Sexually Transmitted Diseases, Chennai, India. Sex Transm Infect 2005;81:361.

Marra CM, Maxwell CL, Smith SL, et al. Cerebrospinal fluid abnormalities in patients with syphilis: association with clinical and laboratory features. J Infect Dis 2004;189:369–376.

Mbulawa ZZ, Coetzee D, Marais DJ, et al. Genital human papillomavirus prevalence and human papillomavirus concordance in heterosexual couples are positively associated with human immunodeficiency virus coinfection. J Infect Dis 2009;199:1514.

Patton ME, Su JR, Weinstock H, et al. Primary and secondary syphilis—United States, 2005–2013. MMWR Morb Mortal Wkly Rep 2014;63(18):402–406.

Rietmeijer CA, Hopkins E, Geisler WM, et al. *Chlamydia trachomatis* positivity rates among men tested in selected venues in the United States: a review of the recent literature. Sex Transm Dis 2008;35:S8.

Rolfs RT, Joesoef MR, Hendershot EF, et al. A randomized trial of enhanced therapy for early syphilis in patients with and without human immunodeficiency virus infection. The Syphilis and HIV Study Group. N Engl J Med 1997;337:307–314.

Satterwhite CL, Joesoef MR, Datta SD, H W. Estimates of *Chlamydia trachomatis* infections among men: United States. Sex Transm Dis 2008;35:S3.

Smith JS, Moses S, Hudgens MG, et al. Increased risk of HIV acquisition among Kenyan men with human papillomavirus infection. J Infect Dis 2010;201:1677.

St Cyr S, Barbee L, Workowski KA, et al. Update to CDC's guidelines for gonococcal infection, 2020. *MMWR Reccom Rep.* 2020 Dec 18;69(50);1911–1916.

Su JR, Weinstock H. Epidemiology of co-infection with HIV and syphilis in 34 states, United States—2009. In: Proceedings of the 2011 National HIV Prevention Conference, August 13–17, 2011, Atlanta, GA.

Unemo M, Golparian D, Nicholas R, et al. High-level cefixime- and ceftriaxone-resistant *Neisseria gonorrhoeae* in France: novel penA mosaic allele in a successful international clone causes treatment failure. Antimicrob Agents Chemother 2012;56:1273–1280.

Weinert LS, Scheffel RS, Zoratto G, et al. Cerebral syphilitic gumma in HIV-infected patients: case report and review. Int J STD AIDS 2008;19:62.

Workowski KA, Berman S; Centers for Disease Control and Prevention. Sexually transmitted diseases treatment guidelines, 2015. *MMWR Recomm Rep.* 2015 Jun 5;64(RR-03):1–137.

38.

CARDIOVASCULAR DISEASE

Jeffrey T. Kirchner

LEARNING OBJECTIVES

- Discuss the pathophysiology of cardiovascular disease (CVD) and myocardial infarction (MI) in persons living with HIV (PWH).

- Describe the association between chronic HIV infection as it relates to an increased risk of CVD, MI, stroke, peripheral arterial disease, and sudden cardiac death.

- Explain the association between specific antiretroviral therapy (ART), CVD risk and MI.

- Assess CVD risk in PWH infection by application of the AHA/ACC ASCVD 10-year risk calculator.

- List medical therapies including statins and non-statins to lower the risk of CVD and MI in PWH.

- Discuss lifestyle interventions including diet, exercise, weight loss and smoking cessation to lower the risk of CVD and MI in PWH.

WHAT'S NEW?

- A meta-analysis completed in 2019 of 16 clinical studies found that PWH had higher acute MI incidence rates (absolute risk difference of 2.2/1,000 person-years [pys]) and twice the risk of acute MI (relative risk [RR] = 1.6).

- A modeling study suggests that by the year 2030 more than 70% of PWH will be over the age of 50 and 78% will have CVD.

- In past years, cardiomyopathy with systolic dysfunction related to advanced HIV infection was more common. In the post-ART era, asymptomatic systolic or diastolic heart failure (with reduced or preserved ejection fraction) is seen more frequently in PWH.

KEY POINTS

- Persons with HIV are at increased risk for CVD, including MI, stroke, heart failure, and sudden cardiac death.

- The excess risk of CVD has been linked to the double burden of high prevalent traditional risk factors (diabetes mellitus, hypertension, smoking) along with HIV-specific risk factors (inflammation, immune activation, immune suppression, viremia).

- Some ART regimens are thought to increase CVD risk by elevating lipid levels and other mechanisms, although this is less commonly seen in the modern treatment era.

- PWH should be screened regularly for established CVD risk factors, including hypertension, diabetes mellitus, dyslipidemia, and cigarette smoking.

- Changing ART to improve lipid profiles in PWH should considered but should not compromise virologic or immunologic control.

- PWH should be assessed for their 10-year CVD risk by using the ACC/AHA risk calculator.

- Statin therapies are recommended for primary and secondary prevention of CVD; additional medications may be indicated for select high-risk patients who need further lowering of LDL-cholesterol (LDL-C) levels.

- Proven interventions to lower the risk of CVD and MI include diet, exercise, smoking cessation, and the use of lipid-lowering agents and antihypertensive medications to treat modifiable risk factors.

- Gains in life expectancy for PWH due to successful ART will be lost if management of CVD is not optimized.

INTRODUCTION

There is considerable evidence that PWH are at increased risk for CVD, including MI and stroke. Epidemiologic studies published through the years have consistently found higher rates of CVD, especially MI and stroke, among PWH compared to HIV-negative persons (Freiberg et al., 2013; Rao et al., 2019). Premature atherosclerosis in PWH was noted almost 20 years ago in autopsy studies of PWH (Morgello et al., 2002). Many recent studies from the US and other parts of the world have found a greater frequency of coronary artery disease in PWH, including those treated with ART and having suppressed viremia, relative to uninfected controls (Hsue et al., 2019; Metkus et al., 2015; Post et al., 2014).

Most of these studies acknowledge a higher prevalence of known traditional risk factors for CVD among PWH and typically adjust for confounding variables. Cigarette smoking, in particular, is several-fold greater in PWH compared to the general population. After accounting for such traditional risks, significant differences between PWH and those without HIV generally persist—although the more factors added to these models, the greater the attenuation between HIV infection and CVD (Post et al., 2014; Rao et al., 2019).

Other factors, including poor diet, sedentary lifestyle, substance abuse, and even stress and mental illness, can increase the risk of CVD and could account for some of the excess CVD burden among PWH. However, data on these confounders are not typically collected (Khambaty et al., 2016; White et al., 2015).

There are now biologically plausible explanations for higher CVD risk accompanying HIV infection. Findings of higher levels of markers of immune activation and inflammation among infected patients with suppressed viremia compared to uninfected controls and a correlation between such markers and adverse events suggest infection-related pathogenic mechanisms for CVD in HIV (Deeks et al., 2013; Hunt, 2012; Scherzer et al., 2019). Moreover, although ART has been found to consistently reduce surrogate markers for inflammation, endothelial dysfunction, and immune activation, there has been evidence from observational studies that some ART regimens contribute to CVD. It remains unclear if such associations are affected by confounding variables and, if truly contributing, the mechanisms by which they act to cause CVD. The heightened risk for CVD in PWH, regardless of etiology, requires healthcare providers to be diligent in assessing for this risk and intervening when appropriate. Newer information has made it increasingly clear that the care for PWH requires not only chronic viral suppression but also early recognition and management of CVD risk factors (Rao et al., 2019). More research and subsequent data are greatly needed to elucidate the mechanisms of HIV-associated CVD and also therapeutic strategies to mitigate these risks.

EVIDENCE OF EXCESS RISK FOR CVD IN PWH

One of the largest epidemiologic studies examining differential rates of CVD among PWH and HIV-negative persons was conducted within a registry of patients receiving care in Boston that included 3,851 PWH and 1,044,589 HIV-negative patients (Triant et al., 2009). The difference in acute MI rates between HIV and non-HIV persons was significant, with an RR of 1.75 (95% confidence interval [CI], 1.51–2.02; $p < 0.0001$), adjusting for age, gender, race, hypertension, diabetes, and dyslipidemia.

Similar studies of the incidence of MI and stroke were conducted by the Kaiser Permanente system in California (Klein et al., 2014, 2015). Rates of both conditions were historically higher for PWH compared to HIV-negative members. However, a convergence over time was observed in the rates of MI and stroke experienced by PWH compared to HIV-negative patients. Improved detection and management of CVD risk factors plus better treatment of HIV infection is hypothesized to account for the decline in CVD rates in this cohort of patients. Similar declines in the rates of CVD over the past decade were reported from cohorts in Europe and British Columbia (Cheung et al., 2016; Hatleberg et al., 2016).

A paper from the Veterans Aging Cohort Study (VACS) that included 81,000 participants (33% HIV-positive) found that PWH veterans had twice the risk of acute MI compared to those who were HIV-negative (Paisible et al., 2015). However, it also found a low prevalence of optimization of cardiac health in this high-risk Veterans Administration population, including blood pressure (BP) control, treatment of hyperlipidemia, and smoking cessation. This alone may account for the increased risk of MI, and not HIV infection.

A 2018 systematic review by Shah et al. included data from 80 longitudinal studies of 793,635 PWH and a total follow-up of 3.5 million pys. The authors of this study reported an RR of 2.16 for MI and stroke in PWH compared to HIV-negative individuals (Shah et al., 2018). This is comparable to RRs of 2.48 with hypertension and 2.95 with smoking found in the multinational INTERHART study (Yusuf et al., 2004). Despite some variance in data from observational cohorts, the preponderance of these studies from the US, Europe, and sub-Saharan Africa support the fact that PWH indeed have an excess risk of CVD.

Beyond cohort studies, pathophysiologic evidence of excess CVD accompanying HIV infection has been found. Relatively high levels of inflammation within the aorta, possibly mediated by monocyte activation, were demonstrated by fluorodeoxyglucose positron emission tomography (FDG-PET) scanning in a small study of ART-receiving PWH without known CVD compared to uninfected controls with similar CVD risks. These data were later correlated with vulnerable coronary plaques (Subramanian et al., 2012; Tawakol et al., 2014). Similarly, a larger cross-sectional study from the Multicenter AIDS Cohort Study (MACS) examined coronary calcium scores and coronary plaque morphology in PWH and HIV-negative men who have sex with men (MSM) and found that plaque was highly prevalent in both groups (Post et al., 2014). After adjustment for major confounders, there remained a higher prevalence of plaque in male PWH (prevalence ratio [PR], 1.13; 95% CI, 1.04–1.23), who were also more likely to have noncalcified plaques (the most vulnerable to rupture) (PR, 1.25; 95% CI, 1.10–1.43). Older age was associated with noncalcified plaque in PWH but not HIV-negative men. This factor seemed to drive the overall differences between these groups. Adjustment for additional confounders reduced the association between HIV infection and noncalcified plaques.

The concept of HIV causing "accelerated" aging with CVD and other conditions (i.e., bone disease, frailty) possibly occurring earlier in PWH has been countered by data from the US Veterans Administration Aging Cohort and a large HIV case–control study from Denmark (Althoff et al., 2015;

Rasmussen et al., 2015). In both groups, excess risk of CVD with HIV infection was observed. However, this was detected at similar ages in HIV-positive and HIV-negative persons, and, over time, there was no observed increase in overall risk for those with HIV. In the North American NA-ACCORD cohort, the attributable risk of type 1 MI was much greater for PWH who smoked, had hypertension, and elevated lipid, levels as opposed to lower $CD4^+$ T-cell counts, elevated plasma HIV RNA level, or a diagnosis of AIDS (Althoff et al., 2017). Consequently, modeling studies have found that interventions that target the management of BP, glucose, and lipid levels, as well as smoking cessation, may have a much greater clinical impact than earlier initiation of HIV therapy or avoidance of ART regimens that have been associated with risk of CVD (Smit et al., 2018).

In recent years it is has become apparent that heart failure is more common in PWH. In the HIV-Heart Study being conducted within the Kaiser Permanente healthcare system, the rate of incident heart failure was compared between 39,000 PWH and more than 387,000 matched control (1:10) patients without HIV infection. Incident heart failure was higher among PWH (4% vs. 3%) with a hazard ratio indicating a 66% greater risk in the fully adjusted model that accounted for coronary syndrome events, suggesting an independent mechanism independent of atherosclerosis (Go et al., 2018). A recent study by Zanni et al. (2020) found that women with HIV had a higher incidence of myocardial fibrosis and subsequent reduced diastolic function, also referred to as heart failure with reduced ejection fraction.

PROPOSED MECHANISMS

While traditional and non-HIV-related factors appear to be driving much of the CVD events that PWH experience, factors related to HIV infection and treatment may play a role. Overall, the pathogenesis of atherosclerosis in the setting of HIV infection is likely more complex than the current level of understanding. Numerous mechanistic studies have examined the association between CVD (i.e., plaque, coronary calcium, arterial inflammation, and endothelial dysfunction) and markers of inflammation, immune activation, and microbial translocation across the gut (Deeks et al., 2013; Hunt, 2012). In the FDG-PET study, aortic wall inflammation was significantly correlated with markers of monocyte and macrophage activation, suggesting that these cell lines play a role in the observed changes. The monocyte activation marker soluble CD163 was also correlated with a noncalcified coronary plaque in men and women with HIV and well-controlled viral loads. In the MACS coronary imaging study, as in most other cohorts, smoking rates were higher among those who were HIV-positive. That smoking interacts with HIV and aging to accelerate CVD was observed by an examination of carotid intima-media thickness, suggesting HIV infection modifies the effect of smoking and age on cardiovascular health (Fitch et al., 2013). In a related report, smoking and obesity were each significantly associated with levels of inflammatory markers

including interleukin-6 (IL-6), sCD14, and sTNFR-I and -II (Krishnan et al., 2014). Similar findings linking smoking and inflammation were seen in the SUN cohort of PWH (Cioe et al., 2015). In that study, heavy alcohol intake was also associated with elevations of the coagulation marker D-dimer.

Data from Hsue et al. (2010) regarding T-cell activation and inflammation suggest that these certainly contribute to developing vascular disease. They have also suggested that HIV proteins such as transactivator of transcription (TaT) and negative factor (Nef) induce inflammation and endothelial dysfunction (Hsue et al., 2019). Residual immune activation secondary to incomplete control of HIV infection (despite undetectable viremia), coinfections (e.g., cytomegalovirus and hepatitis C virus), and irreversible translocation of microbial products across an altered gut lumen occur in PWH. They are thought to promote a pro-inflammatory milieu that is proatherogenic (Deeks et al., 2013; Hsue et al., 2019).

A number of studies have also shown that the risk of CVD among PWH is likely influenced by immunodeficiency—specifically, nadir $CD4^+$ T-cell count or low $CD4^+$ T-cell counts (Drozd et al., 2015). Nadir $CD4^+$ T-cell count has been linked to carotid intima-media thickness and arterial stiffness (Hsue et al., 2019). Two cohort studies found that low $CD4^+$ T-cell counts were associated with incident MI (Hsue et al., 2019). In the NA-ACCORD observational cohort, lower current $CD4^+$ T cell counts, as well as a history of AIDS and detectable plasma HIV RNA levels, were predictors of primary MI. Collectively, it appears that markers of immune damage and viremia are predictive of or related to CVD clinical events. However, the mechanisms linking damage to the immune system from HIV to atherosclerosis remain to be elucidated (Figure 38.1).

The pathogenesis of heart failure in the setting of HIV infection remains unclear. One hypothesis is that HIV acts directly on the myocardium, as well as indirectly via inflammation and autoimmunity (Remick et al., 2014). Some antiretroviral drugs (ARVs), including nucleoside reverse transcriptase inhibitors (NRTIs) in this theoretical model, could be contributing to the pathogenesis. Some preliminary data from the REPRIEVE study found that PWH who underwent cardiac magnetic resonance imaging (MRI) had increased prevalence of myocardial steatosis (increased myocardial triglyceride content), which predisposes to diastolic dysfunction and heart failure risk (Nelian et al., 2020). It was also found that for patients in this study, advanced age, low nadir $CD4^+$ T-cell count, and body mass index (BMI) 25 kg/m^2 or greater were all associated with heart failure.

EFFECT OF ART ON CVD

Multiple retrospective and some prospective studies have evaluated the impact of ART on CVD. As in the epidemiologic studies, these are often challenged by factors that confound analyses and/or lack an appropriate control group. The most obvious reason that ART increases CVD risk is due to effects on lipid levels, especially LDL-C and triglycerides. These

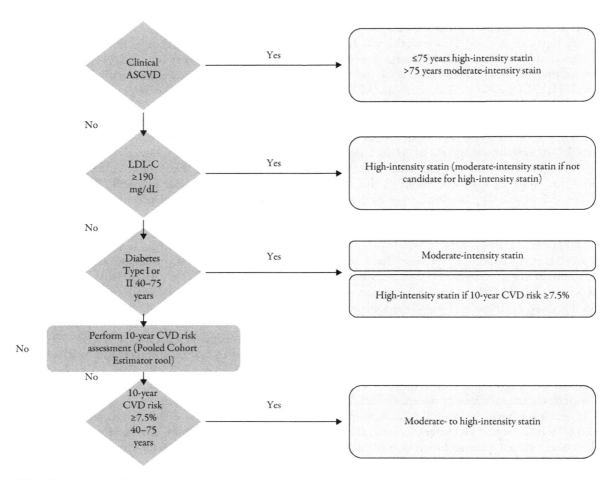

Figure 38.1 ACC/AHA statin benefit groups Adapted from Stone et al. (2014).

changes were more commonly seen with the older ritonavir-boosted protease inhibitors (PIs).

The most persuasive data on the issue of ART-related CVD risk comes from the Data Collection on Adverse Events of Anti-HIV Drugs (D:A:D) cohort. This is a large, ongoing, prospective, observational study of tens of thousands of PWH, the majority from Europe but also the US and Australia. In 2003, D:A:D investigators first reported the incidence of MI to be increased significantly with prolonged exposure to combination ART (Friis-Møller et al., 2003). The adjusted risk rate per year of exposure to ART ranged from 0.32 for no ART use to 2.93 for at least 6 years of ART use. Although there was a significant relative risk of MI with ART, the absolute risk of MI was low (over a period of 36,199 pys, only 126 patients had an MI). The initial association between ART and MI was mainly driven by PI therapy—specifically lopinavir-ritonavir and indinavir (D:A:D Study Group, 2007; Sabin et al., 2014). More recent data from D:A:D reported in 2018 found that ritonavir-boosted darunavir was associated with a 51% relative increased risk of MI and a 49% increased risk of stroke over a 5-year period (Ryom et al., 2018). However, a more recent study from the French Hospital Database found no significant association between MI and exposure to darunavir or atazanavir (Costagliola et al., 2020). Another study also found that the boosted PI atazanavir was not

associated with an increased MI risk. This may be due to the indirect hyperbilirubinemia that occurs with atazanavir, as other studies found a cardioprotective effect of higher bilirubin levels in the blood. This is further corroborated by a retrospective analysis from the VA cohort that found that veterans with and without HIV infection with elevated bilirubin levels had lower rates of CVD and heart failure after adjustment for traditional risk factors (Marconi et al., 2018).

An earlier link between the NRTI abacavir and MI from the D:A:D cohort ushered in a series of subsequent investigations that have reached mixed conclusions. Possible biomolecular mechanisms for this association have been sought and include increased platelet reactivity and/or endothelial cell and leukocyte interactions (induced by abacavir), but these remain to be proved (Baum et al., 2011; De Pablo et al., 2012). Another study of patients switching from abacavir to tenofovir alafenamide fumarate (TAF) found changes in platelet reactivity and collagen interaction, again suggesting that abacavir causes platelet dysfunction. The investigators believe this could explain the findings of an association between abacavir and CVD (Mallon et al., 2018). Per the latest US Department of Health and Human Services (USDHHS) and International Antiretroviral Association (IAS)-USA HIV treatment guidelines, abacavir should be avoided in patients with or at high risk for CVD (Saag et al., 2020; USDHHS,

Table 38.1 ACC/ AHA GUIDELINES FOR DIAGNOSIS AND MANAGEMENT OF HYPERTENSION.

BP CATEGORY	SYSTOLIC BP		DIASTOLIC BP	TREATMENT OR FOLLOW-UP
Normal	<120 mmHg	and	<80 mmHg	Evaluate yearly; encourage healthy lifestyle changes to maintain normal BP
Elevated	120–129 mmHg	and	<80 mmHg	Recommend healthy lifestyle changes and reassess in 3-6 months
Hypertension Stage 1	130–139 mmHg	or	80–89 mmHg	Assess the 10-year risk for heart disease and stroke using the atherosclerotic cardiovascular disease (AVSCD) risk calculator

				• If risk is <10%, start with healthy lifestyle recommendations and reassess 3-6 months
				• If risk is >10% or the patient has known clinical CVC, diabetes mellitus, chronic kidney disease, recommend lifestyle changes and BP-lowering medication (1 medication); reassess in 1 month for effectiveness of medication therapy
				  – If goals is met after 1 month, reassess in 3-6 months
				  – If goals is not met after 1 month, consider different medication or titration and continue monthly follow-up until control is achieved

Hypertension Stage 3	≥ 140 mmHg	or	≥90 mm Hg	• Recommend healthy lifestyle changes and BP-lowering medication (2 medications of different classes); reassess in 1 month for effectiveness • If goal is met after 1 month, reassess in 3-6 months • If goal is not met after 1 month, consider different medication or titration and continue follow-up until control is achieved

2020). The IAS guidelines also note that in PWH at moderate to high risk for a CVD-related event or those who have had an event (MI or stroke), switching from abacavir-based or PI-containing regimens (except atazanavir) is recommended (Saag et al., 2020). As HIV therapy evolves and exposure to new agents accumulates, the D:A:D investigators and other cohorts will regularly reexamine the risks associated with CVD events.

There are also other proposed mechanisms whereby ART increases cardiovascular risk in PWH. These included weight gain, insulin resistance, and lipodystrophy. Also worth noting is the risk of drug–drug interactions that could contribute to QT prolongation, which is associated with sudden cardiac death. At least one study found that PWH have a four times higher risk of sudden cardiac death compared to those without HIV (Tseng & Foisy, 2012) (Table 38.1).

SCREENING AND ASSESSING FOR CARDIOVASCULAR RISK

Given the higher risk of CVD among PWH, the standard of HIV care should include baseline screening for traditional risk factors and appropriate attention to management. This includes BP measurement and weight with calculation of BMI. Baseline laboratory parameters recommended are a lipid panel (total cholesterol, HDL-C, LDL-C, and triglycerides) and fasting blood glucose level or hemoglobin A1C. Baseline renal and hepatic function should be measured as well. After patients are started on ART, they should have a lipid profile repeated approximately 3 months after they stabilized on therapy. If the baseline and subsequent values are normal, then repeating a lipid panel yearly is recommended (Aberg et al., 2014). Risks for CVD and dyslipidemias should

generally be managed according to the most recent ACC/AHA guidelines (Grundy et al., 2019; Reiter-Brennan et al., 2020). An abundance of evidence suggests that the effects of cigarette smoking on CVD are magnified in those with HIV infection. Therefore, there is particular urgency for HIV care providers to ask patients about smoking and incorporate evidence-based interventions to facilitate cessation of smoking into their practice (see later discussion).

In the past, CVD risk for patients was usually assessed via the Framingham Heart Study risk calculator Older studies have used this in PWH and found it generally performed well in assessing the 10-year risk of CVD. However, in retrospect, Framingham likely underestimated the actual CVD risk compared to use in HIV-negative patients (Law et al., 2006). The newer 10-year CVD risk ACC/AHA risk calculator has become the standard of care in the US (Grundy et al., 2019) (Box 38.1). However, similar to the Framingham risk calculator, the ACC/AHA calculator appears to underestimate the risk of CVD in PWH (Regan et al., 2015; Thompson-Paul et al., 2015; Triant et al., 2018). More prospective data to validate these guidelines in PWH are needed to develop a risk calculator that includes HIV-specific factors, traditional CVD risk factors, and the ability to stratify patients based on sex.

Several inflammatory biomarkers of coagulation and inflammation have been studied for their potential role in predicting CVD events in PWH. Some of these are the highly sensitive C-reactive protein (hsCRP), D-dimer, IL-6, and fibrinogen. Combined data from three cohorts of PWH found that IL-6 and D-dimer were independently associated with the risk of serious non-AIDS events or death. Another study found that biomarkers in PWH can be clustered into a "cardiac phenotype" to risk-stratify these patients (Scherzer et al., 2018). Patients with high-levels of CRP, IL-6, and D-dimer had a higher prevalence of pulmonary hypertension and

- In all patients, regardless of age, emphasize a heart-healthy lifestyle to reduce ASCVD risk. In young adults 20–39 years of age, an assessment of lifetime risk facilitates the clinician–patient risk discussion.
- In patients with clinical ASCVD, the goal is to reduce low-density lipoprotein cholesterol (LDL-C) by >50% with high-intensity statin therapy or maximally tolerated statin therapy.
- In very-high-risk patients (history of multiple major ASCVD events or one event and multiple risk factors), with an LDL-C of >70 mg/dL on maximal statin therapy, consider adding ezetimibe. In patients whose LDL-C remains ≥70 mg/dL on maximally tolerated statin and ezetimibe therapy, adding a PCSK9 inhibitor is reasonable following a clinician–patient discussion about the net benefit, safety, and cost.
- In patients with severe primary hypercholesterolemia (LDL-C ≥ 190 mg/dL), begin high-intensity statin therapy without calculating 10-year ASCVD risk. If the LDL-C level remains ≥100 mg/dL, adding ezetimibe is reasonable. If the LDL-C on statin plus ezetimibe remains ≥100 mg/dL and the patient has multiple factors that increase the risk of ASCVD events, a PCSK9 inhibitor may be considered.
- In patients 40–75 years of age with diabetes mellitus and LDL-C ≥ 70 mg/dL, start moderate-intensity statin therapy without calculating 10-year ASCVD risk.
- In adults 40–75 years of age without diabetes mellitus with LDL-C ≥ 70 mg/dL and a 10-year ASCVD risk of ≥7.5%, start moderate-intensity statin if a discussion of treatment options favors statin therapy. If risk status is uncertain, consider using coronary artery calcium (CAC) to improve specificity. If CAC is zero, treatment with statin therapy may be withheld (except in cigarette smokers, those with diabetes mellitus, or a strong family history of premature ASCVD). A CAC score of 1 to 99 favors statin therapy, especially in those ≥55 years of age. If the CAC score is ≥100 Agatston units, statin therapy is indicated unless deferred by clinician–patient risk discussion.
- In adults 40–75 years of age without diabetes mellitus and 10-year risk of 7.5–19.9%, the presence of risk-enhancing factors (family history, LDL-C >160 mg/dL, metabolic syndrome, chronic kidney disease, premature menopause) favors statin therapy. The presence of inflammatory disorders, **including HIV**, with other risk-enhancing factors may favor statin therapy in patients at 10-year risk of only 5–7.5%.
- Assess adherence and response to lifestyle changes and cholesterol-lowering medications with repeat lipid measurement 4–12 weeks after statin initiation repeated every 3–12 months.

a threefold increase in mortality over approximately 7 years of follow-up. It is hoped that clustering of these biomarkers can help identify at-risk patients and target appropriate therapies to prevent or limit cardiovascular events.

INTERVENTIONS AND MANAGEMENT

There is currently no robust evidence base to determine if the management of CVD risks in PWH should differ from the general population. Modifiable risk factors, including diabetes mellitus, dyslipidemia, hypertension, obesity, and cigarette smoking, remain very important in PWH, and likely more so than for the general population. As noted previously, the ACC/AHA risk calculator may underestimate the risk of heart disease in PWH (Triant et al., 2018). Some experts believe the clinicians should adjust the calculated risk upward by 1.5 to 2 times on the basis of this underestimation (So-Armah et al., 2020). Regardless, risk-based assessment for CVD in PWH remains a rational starting point to guide lifestyle counseling, medical therapy (mainly statins), and other potential risk-reduction interventions (Grundy et al., 2019).

Aggressively treating HIV infection with ART to attain full viral suppression should remain the primary objective, even in the presence of CVD risk factors or established coronary artery disease. Data from the Strategies for Management of Antiretroviral Therapy (SMART) study as well as the ATHENA cohort (Van Lelyveld et al., 2012) found that ongoing viremia and incomplete immune recovery increase the risk

of cardiovascular events. In addition, a National Institutes of Health (NIH)-sponsored study of 6,517 patients, of whom 273 sustained an acute MI, found immunologic control was the most important HIV-related factor associated with acute MI (Triant et al., 2010).

Due to their potential effects on cholesterol (and thus CVD risk), the choice of ART should take into consideration a patient's individual CVD risk factors. Some combination ART regimens, such as ritonavir-boosted PIs, may increase lipid subsets, including LDL-C and triglycerides. The pharmacologic booster cobicistat appears to increase LDL-C, similar to ritonavir, but with a smaller impact on triglycerides. The NRTI abacavir increases LDL-C and triglycerides, whereas tenofovir disoproxil fumarate (TDF) has been observed to lower LDL-C (Tungsiripat et al., 2010). As noted earlier, in some studies, including D:A:D and SMART, abacavir has been associated with an increased risk of CVD and MI (Dorjee et al., 2018; SMART, 2008). In clinical trials, the NRTI TAF produced increases in fasting lipid parameters (total cholesterol, HDL, direct LDL, and triglycerides) compared to TDF and has been associated with weight gain (Sax et al., 2019). The more widely used integrase strand inhibitors (INSTIs) raltegravir, dolutegravir, elvitegravir, and bictegravir have not been found to significantly affect lipid levels when assessed in multiple clinical trials (Dorjee et al., 2018).

In patients with moderate to severe dyslipidemia and increased CVD risk, switching to an ART regimen with less effect on cholesterol and/or triglycerides is recommended by the USDHHS and IAS-USA treatment guidelines. However,

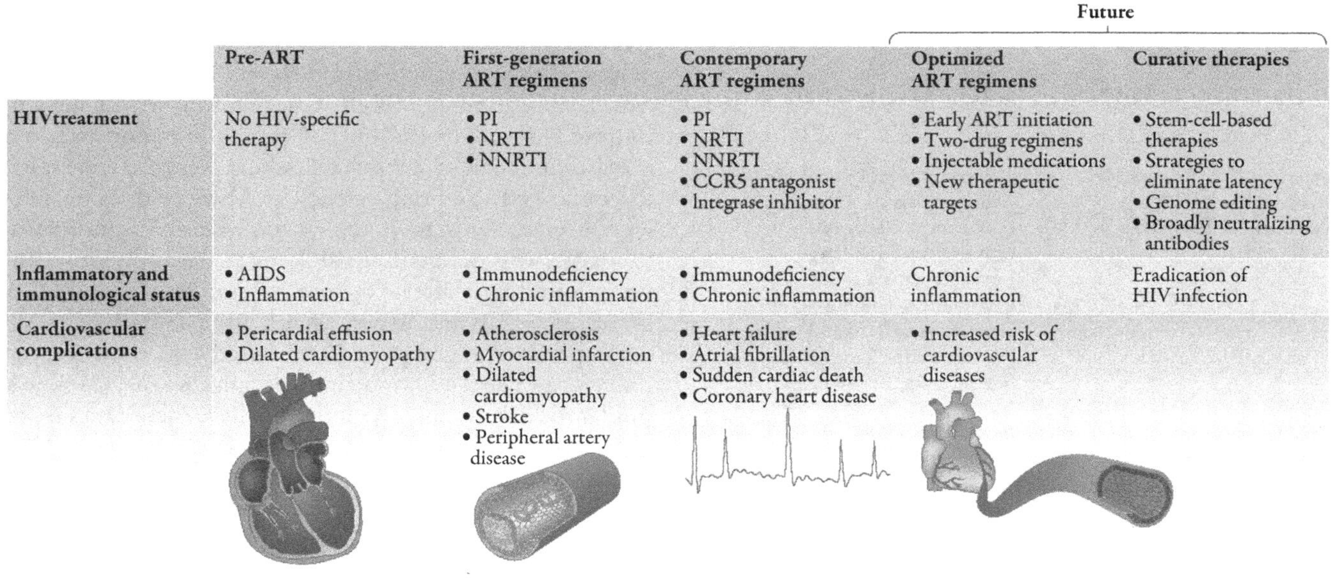

Figure 38.2 Overview of changes in HIV treatment and HIV-associated cardiovascular diseases.   SOURCE: Hsue P, et al. *Nat Rev Cardiol.* 2019. 16(12):745–759.

this should not be done at the expense of compromising virologic control. In the SPRIAL study, patients with stable HIV disease were switched from a ritonavir-boosted PI-based regimen to raltegravir, leading to significant improvement in lipid profiles (Martinez et al., 2010). In the SPIRIT study, changing from a ritonavir-boosted PI plus dual nucleoside regimen to rilpivirine plus TDF/emtricitabine led to significant reductions in LDL cholesterol (Palella et al., 2014). In the MARCH study, patients switched from a boosted-PI to maraviroc had significant reductions in mean total cholesterol over 96 weeks (Pett et al., 2018). Last, in the NEAT 022 study, all patients over the age of 50 and those over 18 with a 10-year CVD risk score of more than 10% were switched from a ritonavir-boosted PI to dolutegravir. At 48 weeks, the patients switched to dolutegravir had significant improvements in total cholesterol and other lipid fractions, and viral suppression was maintained by 93% in the dolutegravir group and 95% in the PI-ritonavir group (Gatell et al., 2017).

Management of lipid disorders in PWH should follow guidelines established for the general population. Attention should be paid to the potential for drug–drug interactions between lipid-lowering agents and ART. There are several published cholesterol guidelines, but most US practitioners follow those of the ACC/AHA (Figure 38.2 and Box 38.2). The most recent US recommendations for the management of cholesterol are based on several factors, including 10-year risk of ASCVD, presence of diabetes mellitus, baseline LDL-C levels, and chronic inflammatory conditions, including HIV infection (Grundy et al., 2019). The ACC/AHA guidelines note that if ASCVD risk is uncertain, coronary artery calcium may be used to determine indication for statin therapy (Grundy et al., 2019). The guidelines consider HIV to be a "risk-enhancing" factor that may influence starting medical therapy at a 10-year risk threshold below 7.5%. Depending on individual risk and the presence of risk-enhancing factors, this may include "high-intensity" or "moderate-intensity"

dosing with statins and the use of additional lipid-lowering agents (see later discussion).

STATIN THERAPY

The recommended therapy for CVD risk reduction in most patients is a 3-hydroxy-3-methylglutaryl coenzyme A reductase inhibitor ("statin"). These agents are very effective in lowering total cholesterol and LDL-C but vary in potency. There are a multitude of clinical trials supporting their role

---

Box 38.2 FACTORS INCLUDED IN THE ACC/AHA RISK CALCULATOR

10-Year ASCVD Risk: Pooled Cohort Equation

Demographics

- Age (40–79 years)
- Gender
- Race

History

- Hypertension
- Diabetes mellitus
- Tobacco use

Measurements

- Total cholesterol
- HDL
- Systolic blood pressure

Adapted from http://www.cvriskcalculator.com/

Table 38.2 HIGH- AND MODERATE-INTENSITY
STATIN THERAPY

HIGH-INTENSITY STATIN THERAPY	MODERATE-INTENSITY STATIN THERAPY
Lowers LDL-C by ~≥50%: Atorvastatin 40–80 mg Rosuvastatin 20–40 mg	Lowers LDL-C by ~30–49%: Atorvastatin 10–20 mg Fluvastatin 40 mg bid Fluvastatin XL 80 mg Lovastatin 40 mg [a] Pitavastatin 1–4 mg Pravastatin 40 mg (80 mg) Rosuvastatin (5 mg) 10 mg Simvastatin 20–40 mg [a]

[a] Should not be used with protease inhibitors.

Adapted from Grundy (2018).

for primary and secondary prevention of ASCVD (Grundy et al., 2019). Intensity of therapy should be determined by baseline risk and comorbidities (Table 38.2). Preferred statins for PWH include pravastatin, fluvastatin, atorvastatin, rosuvastatin, and pitavastatin. Of note, simvastatin and lovastatin should not be used in patients taking PIs. They are both metabolized by the cytochrome P3A4 isoenzyme, and inhibition of this enzyme system results in elevated statin levels, with an increased risk of rhabdomyolysis and hepatic toxicity. Conversely, the nonnucleoside reverse transcriptase inhibitor (NNRTI) efavirenz reduces the level of simvastatin and lovastatin and thus decreases efficacy of these drugs.

There are concerns regarding statin intolerance due to adverse effects of these drugs such as fatigue, myalgias, and myopathy—the latter is associated with creatinine kinase elevation. Myalgias are reported by about 15% of persons taking statins, but most do not have creatine kinase elevation (Guyton et al., 2014). It may be for this reason statins are less likely to be prescribed for PWH (Blackman et al., 2020). As statins remain the recommended drugs for CVD risk reduction, before considering a patient to be truly intolerant to statins it is prudent to rule out other causes of muscle-related symptoms, such as hypothyroidism, vitamin B12 or vitamin D deficiency, or other inflammatory musculoskeletal disorders. Rechallenging a statin-intolerant patient with a different agent or an alternative dosing strategy (e.g., once-a-week dosing) can also be done (Backes et al., 2017).

There was concern for hepatoxicity with statins, but in 2012 the US Food and Drug Administration (FDA) removed the recommendation for periodic monitoring of liver function tests in patients on statin therapy. Hepatic transaminase levels should be checked at baseline and only as clinically indicated thereafter. For PWH with hepatitis B or C infection it is prudent to monitor at least biannually for elevations in liver enzymes.

Regarding trials of statin efficacy, there are growing data supporting the use of statins in PWH (Eckard et al., 2016; Mosepele et al., 2018). An older retrospective cohort study of 700 PWHs taking atorvastatin, pravastatin, or rosuvastatin found that after a year of therapy on one of these agents,

decreases in total cholesterol and LDL-C were significantly greater with atorvastatin and rosuvastatin compared to pravastatin (Sing et al., 2011). The likelihood of achieving treatment goals for non-HDL-C at that time was higher with rosuvastatin (odds ratio [OR] of 2.3) but not atorvastatin or pravastatin. Toxicity rates were low and were the same for all three agents. In addition, a study by Aberg et al. compared 4 mg/day pitavastatin to 40 mg/day pravastatin in adult PWH ($n = 252$) who were taking ART for at least 6 months. This study found that after 12 weeks of statin therapy, LDL-C decreased by 31% in the pitavastatin group compared to 21% in the pravastatin group. At 52 weeks, adverse events, discontinuations (5% vs. 4%), and virologic failures (3% vs. 4%) were similar in both groups. The authors believe these data support pitavastatin as the "preferred drug" for dyslipidemia in PWH (Aberg et al., 2017).

The REPRIEVE trial was initiated by the NIH in 2015. This study is evaluating the use of pitavastatin versus placebo in 7,500 PWH aged 40 to 75 years at 100 clinical sites globally (https://clinicaltrials.gov/ct2/show/NCT02344290). Numerous primary outcomes will be measured, including time to the first event of a composite major cardiovascular event (including atherosclerotic or other CVD death, nonfatal MI, unstable angina hospitalization, coronary arterial revascularization, nonfatal stroke, or transient ischemic attack [TIA]). Secondary outcomes (change in lipid levels, inflammatory biomarkers, and all-cause mortality) are also being evaluated. Also embedded in REPRIEVE will be a sub-study of 800 patients who undergo coronary computed tomography to assess formation of coronary plaque. This study is now fully enrolled and there should be preliminary data forthcoming (Fitch et al., 2020; Grinspoon et al., 2020).

FIBRIC ACID DERIVATIVES

In PWH who have hypertriglyceridemia (defined as fasting serum level of >150 mg/dL), lifestyle management including weight loss and exercise is initially recommended. Historically, elevated triglyceride levels were seen in PWH taking boosted PIs, but the incidence has declined in recent years with diminished use of PIs. Fibric acid derivatives, including gemfibrozil or fenofibrate, remain a consideration for primary prevention of CVD in patients with high triglyceride levels (150–499 mg/dL) and borderline (5–7.4%) or intermediate (7.5–19.9%) risk. They are generally recommended in patients with severe triglyceride levels (≥500 mg/dL; Oh et al., 2020). These drugs effectively lower triglycerides but have little impact on other lipid parameters, including HDL-C, LDL-C, and apolipoprotein B (apo-B). Data from D:A:D suggested a very minor association between elevated triglycerides and MI after adjusting for other lipid and nonlipid risk factors. However, the D:A:D: Study Group (2011) also concluded that use of fibrates alone to lower triglycerides is unlikely to have a major impact on the incidence of MI. In the past, fibrates were also used to lower triglycerides in PWH due to the potential for acute pancreatitis with triglyceride levels greater than 1,000 mg/dL. The FDA-approved indications for fibrates include use as an adjunct to dietary modifications in adults with primary hypercholesterolemia or mixed dyslipidemia (Singh & Correa, 2020).

The current ACC/AHA treatment guidelines do not recommend this class of medications for dyslipidemia (Grundy et al., 2019). They cite a lack of data supporting an effect on CVD outcomes and note that their role in the primary prevention of CVD is less clear as it relates to a reduction in triglyceride levels. They note that in adults with fasting triglycerides of 500 mg/dL or higher, and especially fasting triglycerides of 1,000 mg/dL or more, it is important to identify and address causes of hypertriglyceridemia. If triglycerides are persistently elevated or increasing, they recommend a very-low-fat diet, avoidance of refined carbohydrates and alcohol, consumption of omega-3 fatty acids, and, if necessary to prevent acute pancreatitis, fibrate therapy (Grundy et al., 2019). A Cochrane review from 2016 concluded that there is "moderate-quality" evidence suggesting that fibrates lower the risk of CVD and coronary events in primary prevention, but the absolute risk reduction was less than 1% (Jakob et al., 2016). The ACC/AHA guidelines state that the combination of gemfibrozil and a statin should be avoided due to an increased risk for myopathy (Grundy et al., 2019).

EZETIMIBE

Ezetimibe is a drug that selectively inhibits gastrointestinal (GI) cholesterol absorption within the small intestine. Overall, this drug is safe, usually well tolerated, and effective in reducing LDL-C by an additional 12% to 19% when taken with statin therapy. Ezetimibe is neither a cytochrome P450 inhibitor nor a cytochrome P450 inducer, so metabolism with other drugs, including ARVs, is not a concern (Sizar et al., 2020). Studies with ezetimibe have been performed in PWH. They have examined ezetimibe as both monotherapy and adjunctive therapy for lipid management but did not specifically assess CVD outcomes (Grandi et al., 2014; Leyes et al., 2014; Saeedi et al., 2015, Wohl et al., 2008).

A study from Thailand that included PWH taking a PI plus a statin for at least 6 months found the addition of 10 mg/day ezetimibe produced a significant decline in mean serum total cholesterol, LDL, and triglycerides (Boonthos et al., 2018). Moreover, no adverse events or abnormal lab parameters were noted in study participants. The IMPROVE-IT trial demonstrated that ezetimibe significantly reduces the risk of major cardiovascular events in a group of high-risk patients with known CVD and already low LDL-C levels. In this trial, there was an absolute risk reduction of 2% in the cardiovascular event rate (32.7% vs. 34.7%) with the addition of ezetimibe in patients taking simvastatin compared to those taking simvastatin monotherapy (Cannon et al., 2015; Hammersley & Signy, 2017).

The ACC/AHA guidelines as well as the National Institute for Health and Care Excellence (NICE) guidelines from the United Kingdom recommend ezetimibe monotherapy for primary hyperlipidemia only in patients for whom a statin is contraindicated or who cannot tolerate statin therapy (Grundy et al., 2019; NICE, 2016). This is based on the lack of CVD outcome trials of ezetimibe monotherapy. A 2017 US update on non-statin therapies suggests the addition of 10 mg/day ezetimibe for patients in whom additional lowering of LDL-C is desired (Lloyd-Jones et al., 2017). The current US guidelines note that it is "reasonable" to add ezetimibe in very-high-risk patients with an LDL-C of greater than 70 mg/dL despite maximal statin therapy (Grundy et al., 2019). In a similar manner, the NICE guidelines and the European Society of Cardiology support ezetimibe as add-on therapy in "high or very high-risk patients" who fail to meet specific LDL targets.

OMEGA-3 FATTY ACIDS

A dosage of 3 to 5 g/day of omega-3 fatty acids (DHA/EPA or "fish oil") generally produces a 30% to 50% reduction in triglyceride levels. Their low cost, good tolerability, and lack of drug–drug interactions have made these agents historically attractive for use in the general population, including PWH. In December 2019, the FDA approved the omega-3 drug icosapent ethyl (Vascepa®) as adjunctive therapy to reduce the risk of CVD in adults with triglycerides above 150 mg/dL. Patients should have either established CVD disease or diabetes and two or more additional CVD risk factors. It is the first approved drug of this class to reduce CVD risk among patients with elevated triglycerides but as an add-on to maximally tolerated statin therapy (Oh et al., 2020). It is also considerably more expensive than over-the-counter generic formulations.

A recent meta-analysis was conducted of nine clinical trials ($n = 578$) evaluating the effect of omega-3 fatty acids on lipid patterns in PWH taking ART (Fogacci et al., 2020). The conclusion was that omega-3s significantly reduced triglycerides and increased HDL-C without affecting LDL-C or total cholesterol levels. They also noted the lack of adverse events with omega-3s. A systematic review with a meta-analysis of randomized clinical trials of patients with baseline triglyceride levels of greater than 200 mg/dL found the average combined reduction in triglycerides in patients taking omega-3 fatty acids was −114 mg/dL (Vieira et al., 2017). Several other studies have looked at the use of fish oil supplements in PWH to assess their effect on inflammatory biomarkers and oxidative stress (both with potential relationships to CVD) but found either no change or clinical benefit (Amador-Licona et al., 2016; Oliveira et al., 2015; Swanson et al., 2018).

The relationship between circulating triglyceride levels and atherosclerosis is still unclear. Current US cholesterol guidelines cite a lack of any randomized controlled trials evaluating this class of drugs and no proof of beneficial CVD outcomes. They may prevent pancreatitis in patients with severe triglyceride elevations (>1,000 mg/dL) but have been associated with some adverse events, including GI upset and infrequently skin conditions (rash and pruritus). Data from the British ASCEND trial found that 1 g omega-3 fatty acid daily did not reduce nonfatal MI or stroke, TIA, or CVD death compared to an olive oil placebo (8.9% vs. 9.2%) (Bowman et al., 2018). Two recent Cochrane reviews addressed the benefits of omega-3 fatty acids, including fish and plant-based sources (Abdelhamid et al., 2018, 2020). These extensive reviews note that increasing the intake of these compounds "probably slightly reduces the risk of coronary heart disease and CVD events but has little or no effect on all-cause CVD mortality". It is in this author's opinion that for select PWH with elevated triglycerides, it is reasonable to recommend or support generic fish oil supplementation.

PCSK9 INHIBITORS

There are currently two FDA-approved drugs in this class for use in select patient populations. The agents alirocumab and evolocumab are indicated for the treatment of high LDL-C. These medications are humanized monoclonal antibodies that inactivate proprotein convertase subtilisin-kexin type 9 (PCSK9) (Shahreyar et al., 2018). This inactivation results in decreased LDL-receptor degradation, increased recirculation of the receptor to the surface of hepatocytes, and consequent lowering of LDL-C levels in the bloodstream (Everett et al., 2015). These drugs can lower LDL-C by approximately 60% in patients on statin therapy and are generally safe and generally well tolerated. They are administered as a subcutaneous injection either every 2 weeks or once a month.

There are several studies providing evidence that PCKS9 inhibitors reduce CVD events when added to statin therapy (Giugliano et al., 2017; Sabatine et al., 2017). However, these agents, which originally came on the market at $14,000 per patient per year, have been reduced in price to about $6,000 per patient per year. The use of PCSK9 inhibitors remain limited to high-risk ASCVD patients—those with familial hypercholesterolemia or with known ASCVD who need further lowering of LDL-C levels despite maximal statin and ezetimibe therapy (Grundy et al., 2019; Lloyd Jones et al., 2017). Of note, PSCK9 levels are elevated in PWH and, in ART-naive patients, are positively associated with immunodeficiency and severity of HIV disease, but the role of treatment remains unknown (Boccara et al., 2017). There are currently no published studies of this drug class in PWH, although the BEIJERNICK study is enrolling patients to evaluate the use of monthly evolocumab in PWH who are on maximally tolerated statin therapy (Boccara et al., 2020). Results would be expected sometime in 2022.

BEMPEDOIC ACID

Bempedoic acid (Nexletol®) was approved by the FDA in 2020. This drug inhibits the cholesterol synthesis pathway several steps above where HMG CoA reductase inhibitors work. It has been shown to lower LDL-C levels by about 17% in clinical trials when combined with a moderate- or high-intensity statin (Ray et al., 2019). Pending further data, this drug is mainly recommended as add-on therapy for patients who need further LDL-C lowering despite optimal use of a statin and ezetimibe. An advantage over the PCSK9 inhibitors is that it can be given orally. There are currently no data on the use of bempedoic acid in PWH.

ASPIRIN

Aspirin (acetylsalicylic acid or ASA) has been recommended by healthcare providers for the prevention of CVD and associated clinical events, including MI and stroke. Recent surveillance data from the CDC found that 27% of US adults were taking aspirin for primary prevention and 74.9% for secondary CVD prevention (Wall, 2018). While the benefit of aspirin has been clearly demonstrated for people with established CVD, this risk/benefit equation is more complex in primary prevention of CVD and related clinical outcomes such as MI. Aspirin irreversibly inhibits cyclooxygenase-1 (COX-1) and blocks the formation and release of thromboxane A2, a strong platelet activator. The COX-1 enzyme is also responsible for producing prostaglandins that protect gastric mucosa; thus, patients who take aspirin may be susceptible to GI bleeding. Risk factors for GI bleeding with aspirin include higher dose and longer duration of use, history of GI ulcers, bleeding disorders, renal failure, advanced liver disease, and thrombocytopenia. Other factors that increase the risk for bleeding with low-dose aspirin use include concurrent anticoagulation with warfarin, direct-acting anticoagulants, or the use of nonsteroidal anti-inflammatory drugs.

The evidence for aspirin in the primary prevention of CVD, MI, or stroke remains limited, with very few published data in PWH (O'Brien et al., 2013; Suchindran et al., 2014). With the last update in 2016, the US Preventive Services Task Force (USPSTF) noted that, for primary prevention, "aspirin modestly reduces nonfatal MI/coronary events and major CVD events, but increases major GI bleeding risk" (Whitlock et al., 2016). The USPSTF gives a "B" recommendation for use of low-dose aspirin in person ages 50 to 59 years who have a 10% or greater 10-year CVD risk (http://tools.acc.org/ASCVD-Risk-Estimator), who are not at risk of bleeding, who have a life expectancy of at least 10 years, and who are willing to take low-dose aspirin for at least 10 years. For those 60 to 69 years old and with a 10% risk or greater, a "C" recommendation is given. The recommendation for aspirin as primary prevention of CVD in persons less than 50 years or greater than 70 years of age is given an "I" grade, meaning there is insufficient evidence to support this practice (Box 38.3).

There are several recently completed primary prevention trials with aspirin that provide updated guidance regarding use. The Aspirin in Reducing Events in the Elderly (ASPREE) trial included 19,000 patients 70 years and older from Australia and the US who took 100 mg aspirin daily or placebo (McNeil et al., 2018). During almost 5 years of follow-up, the use of low-dose aspirin resulted in a significantly higher risk of major hemorrhage and did not result in a significantly lower risk of CVD than placebo. In addition, all-cause mortality was higher in the ASA group. The

Box 38.3 USPSTF RECOMMENDATIONS FOR ASPIRIN THERAPY

ADULTS aged 50–59 years with a ≥10% 10-year CVD risk

The USPSTF recommends initiating low-dose aspirin for primary prevention of CVD in adults aged 50–59 years who have a 10% or greater 10-year CVD risk, are not at increased risk for bleeding, have a life expectancy of at least 10 years, and are willing to take low-dose aspirin daily for at least 10 years. [Level of evidence = B]

Adults aged 60–69 years with a ≥10% 10-YEAR CVD risk

The decision to initiate low-dose aspirin use for the primary prevention of CVD in adults aged 60–69 years who have a 10% or greater 10-year CVD risk should be an individual one. Persons who are not at increased risk for bleeding, who have a life expectancy of at least 10 years, and who are willing to take low-dose aspirin daily for at least 10 years are more likely to benefit. Persons who place a higher value on the potential benefits than the potential harms may choose to initiate low-dose aspirin. [Level of evidence = C]

Adults younger than 50 years

Current evidence is insufficient to assess the balance of benefits and harms of aspirin use for primary prevention of CVD. [Level of evidence = I]

Adults aged 70 years or older

Current evidence is insufficient to assess the balance of benefits and harms of aspirin use for primary prevention of CVD. [Level of evidence = I]

Adapted from Guirguis-Blake, 2016.

Aspirin to Reduce Risk of Initial Vascular Events (ARRIVE) trial from Europe randomized more than 12,500 adults with presumed moderate CVD risk to aspirin 100 mg/day or placebo. During 5 years of follow-up there was no reduction in CVD events by intent-to-treat analysis (Gaziano et al., 2018). There was a 19% relative reduction in the composite endpoint of CVD events in patients who took ASA but also a doubling in the rate of GI bleeding (0.5% in absolute terms). In the ASCEND trial, conducted in the United Kingdom, 15,480 patients older than 40 years with diabetes mellitus without CVD were randomized to aspirin 100 mg/day or placebo. After a mean follow-up of 7.4 years, the frequency of the primary endpoint (composite of nonfatal MI, nonfatal stroke, TIA, or death from any vascular cause) was 8.5% with aspirin and 9.6% with placebo. The minor benefit of aspirin came at the expense of more major bleeding events (Bowman et al., 2018).

The ACC/AHA guidelines note that low-dose aspirin may be considered among select adults 40 to 70 years of age who are at higher ASCVD risk but not at increased bleeding risk. They additionally note that aspirin should not be administered for the primary prevention of ASCVD among adults of any age who are at increased risk of bleeding (Marquis-Gravel et al., 2019).

Numerous studies have evaluated the role of aspirin in acute treatment of cardiac events and secondary prevention of CVD (Jones et al., 2018). There are strong data demonstrating that low-dose aspirin (75–100 mg/day) effectively reduces the risk of recurrence of vascular events in patients with a history of a previous MI, stroke, or TIA by approximately 20%. There has been FDA-approved labeling for this indication since the 1980s (Paikin & Eikelboom, 2012). Because of this consistently reported benefit, which has been found to outweigh the risk of major bleeding, aspirin therapy for secondary prevention is part of standard clinical practice.

BLOOD PRESSURE CONTROL

Hypertension has become more prevalent as the HIV population ages. It is one of the most important CVD risk factors and is strongly associated with CAD, stroke, heart failure, and renal disease. The prevalence varies with different HIV cohorts but is estimated to range from 10% to 50% (Boccara, 2017). Data from the CDC's Medical Monitoring Project found that 42% of PWH had hypertension (N = 8.631), but only 49% had their BP controlled (Olaiya et al., 2018). In a recent US study of Medicaid patients (n = 3,456), the prevalence of comorbidities increased from the fourth year to the first year prior to entry into care, including cardiovascular disease (28–40%), hypertension (24–37%), and hyperlipidemia (12–17%) (DerSarkissian et al., 2020). The global incidence of hypertension in adult PWH is estimated to be 35% compared to 30% in HIV-negative adults (Fahme et al., 2018).

Factors associated with elevated BP in PWH appear similar to those of the general population and include older age; male sex; African American, African, and Caribbean ethnicities; higher BMI; diabetes; and chronic kidney disease. Although less commonly seen than in the past, lipodystrophy and metabolic syndrome have also been associated with hypertension in PWH adults (Fahme et al., 2018). Older studies of BP changes in the D:A:D study and a US cohort found no evidence that ART increased the risk of hypertension (Medina-Torne et al., 2012; Thiébaut et al., 2005). Conversely, other studies have implicated both PIs and duration of ART as being associated with hypertension (Boccara et al., 2017). Some researchers also believe that immune activation and chronic inflammation contribute to the pathophysiology of hypertension in PWH (van Zoest et al., 2017).

It is appropriate to screen and manage hypertension in adult PWH per the current national guidelines (Whelton et al., 2018b) (Figure 38.3). It should be noted, however, that

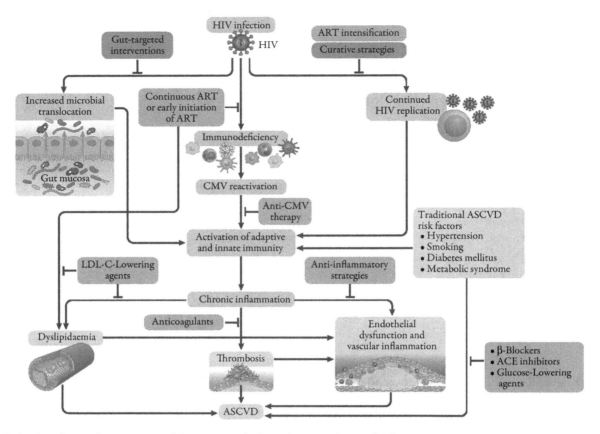

Figure 38.3 Pathophysiology and management of HIV-associated atherosclerotic cardiovascular disease. SOURCE: Hsue P, et al. *Nat Rev Cardiol.* 2019. 16(12):745–759.

current ACC/AHA US hypertension guidelines have been controversial and not collectively endorsed by all professional societies. The 2017 recommendation is for a diagnosis of "hypertension" rather than "pre-hypertension" for adults with a systolic BP of 130 mmHg or greater. They also recommend drug treatment for "high-risk" people with hypertension. These include those with existing CVD or a calculated 10-year CVD risk of 10% or greater, or another high-risk condition such as chronic kidney disease or diabetes (Whelton et al., 2018a). Some feel that by following the new ACC/AHA guidelines a large number of people will be subject to medical treatment with little or no benefit in terms of CVD risk reduction and mortality (Bell, 2018; Brunstrom & Carlberg, 2018). They believe the threshold for treating hypertension should remain at 140 mmHg. Regardless, for those for whom medical therapy is deemed necessary, it is important to be aware of potential drug–drug interactions with ART and antihypertensive agents. Moreover, management strategies should consider degree of frailty, comorbidities, and psychosocial factors and ideally should be individualized (Oliveros et al., 2020). Nonpharmacologic therapies, including the Dietary Approaches to Stop Hypertension (DASH) diet, restriction of sodium intake, and regular exercise, all play a role for some patients. Unfortunately, there have not been any large-scale studies of specific BP-lowering medications in PWH adults. However, there are small studies of renin-angiotensin antagonists showing very favorable results, and

many adult PWH will likely need two or more medications to reached recommended BP goals (Fahme et al., 2018).

Given that medication adherence is very important for PWH, it is worth noting that a recent study from Spain found that patients who took their BP medications at bedtime had a significant decrease in CVD events compared to morning dosing (Hermida et al., 2020). Better outcomes were seen for MI, coronary revascularization, and stroke over a 6-year follow-up of 1,752 subjects. In addition, there were no differences in adverse events, including hypotension and sleep disturbances, between the two groups.

SMOKING CESSATION

Smoking prevalence is remarkably high in many PWH cohorts, usually much higher than in the general population. Therefore, smoking cessation for PWH remains a very important part of CVD risk reduction. There is also an increased risk of lung cancer in PWH, which is directly influenced by smoking as well as immunosuppressive and inflammatory aspects of HIV (Sigel et al., 2017). The D:A:D study found that smoking cessation in PWH decreased the incident relative risk for MI from 3.73 in the first year of smoking cessation to 2.07 after 3 years of not smoking (Petoumenos et al., 2011). A study from 2017 estimated that smoking cessation in PWH could prevent 38% of acute MIs (Althoff et al., 2017).

Getting patients to stop smoking may significantly reduce their ACC/AHA risk scores by 50% or greater. Counseling, including the "5 A's" strategy (ask, advise, assess, assist, arrange follow-up), has proved successful (DeSocio et al., 2020). In addition, pharmacologic interventions including nicotine replacement, bupropion, and varenicline are all effective therapies to assist patients with smoking cessation (Box 38.4). The USPSTF recommends a combination of behavioral interventions and pharmacotherapy for all smokers. New guidelines now recommend varenicline over a nicotine patch or bupropion for most tobacco-dependent patients in whom treatment is initiated. They actually recommend dual therapy with varenicline plus a nicotine patch, although the evidence for combination treatment is limited (Leone et al., 2020). The new guidelines also recommend extended duration of these therapies (beyond the traditional 12 weeks) if clinically indicated.

A large multinational study of more than 8,000 adult smokers evaluated the safety of varenicline, bupropion, and 21-mg nicotine patches in regard to adverse cardiovascular effects. There was a very low incidence of cardiovascular events (<0.5%) during 12 weeks of treatment and after 12 additional weeks of follow-up (Benowitz et al., 2018). These data support these therapies by themselves or in combination to help patients stop smoking.

Regarding specifically PWH, a study from France found varenicline significantly more effective than placebo in helping maintain continuous abstinence at 48 weeks (Mercie et al., 2018). A Cochrane review of 12 studies assessing the effectiveness of interventions (behavioral and pharmacotherapy) to motivate and assist tobacco use cessation in PWH found moderate evidence that combined interventions were effective for long-term abstinence (Pool et al., 2016). The Cochrane authors concluded that tobacco cessation should be offered to all PWH as even nonsustained periods of abstinence are beneficial. In addition, office-based interventions that include focus groups, dedicated time to address smoking cessation as part of the clinic visit, and periodic phone follow-up have shown efficacy in helping PWH stop smoking (Cropsey et al., 2019; Pacek et al., 2020).

NONPHARMACOLOGIC INTERVENTIONS (DIET AND EXERCISE)

The process of atherosclerosis is thought to begin at a young age and progress over many decades before clinical CVD (e.g., acute coronary syndromes, stable or unstable angina, MI) becomes evident. As noted earlier, this progression appears to be accelerated in PWH due to chronic infection, inflammation, and some ART-related factors. Lifestyle modifications including a healthy diet, regular physical activity, maintaining a normal BMI, limited alcohol use, and not smoking have been associated with improvements in CVD risk (Ozemek et al., 2020).

Regarding physical activity, the ACC/AHA guidelines for both cholesterol and hypertension recommend that adults should be advised to engage in aerobic physical activity for three or four sessions per week, lasting on average 40 minutes per session and involving moderate- to vigorous-intensity physical activity (Grundy et al., 2019; Whelton et al., 2018a). These behaviors can lead to improvements in total cholesterol, LDL-C, HDL-C, blood glucose, and BP and ultimately lower 10-year and lifetime risk of CVD and subsequent clinical events.

Several published studies have found variable results in terms of exercise in PWH. One systematic review found that a low level of physical activity in PWH was consistently associated with older age, lower educational level, lower CD4 count, exposure to ART, and the presence of lipodystrophy. Other important barriers were the presence of bodily pain and depression (Vancampfort et al., 2018). A more recent and encouraging study found that 12 to 24 weeks of cardiovascular and resistance exercise significantly reduced total and visceral fat in PWH 50 to 75 years old (Jankowski et al., 2020). As PWH are living longer, it is important for providers to encourage engagement in multiple aspects of a healthy lifestyle, including regular physical activity.

ACKNOWLEDGMENT

The author would like to acknowledge the contributions of David Wohl, MD, to previous editions of this chapter.

Box 38.4 RECOMMENDATIONS FOR TREATING NICOTINE DEPENDENCE

- Tobacco dependence can be safely and effectively treated with counseling and pharmacotherapy.

- Varenicline is *strongly* recommended over nicotine patches and bupropion as first-line treatment due to higher abstinence rates and fewer adverse events.

- In patients with comorbid psychiatric conditions, varenicline is *strongly* recommended as first-line treatment as trials did not show an excess of neuropsychiatric events.

- Even in patients "not ready" to abstain, varenicline is still *strongly* recommended as it doubles the likelihood of abstinence.

- The combination of varenicline plus a nicotine patch is recommended over using varenicline alone for patients ready to quit, although there is only low-quality evidence to support this.

- When treatment is initiated, extended-duration therapy (>12 weeks) is *strongly* recommended over standard (6–12 week) regimens.

- Efficacy of electronic cigarettes has not been established and the FDA has not approved e-cigarettes as a smoking cessation aid. More research is needed on whether they are effective and to also better understand their health effects.

Leone FT, et al. *Am J Respir Crit Care Med* 2020;202(2):5–31.

REFERENCES

Abdelhamid AS, Brown TJ, Brainard JS, et al. Omega-3 fatty acids for the primary and secondary prevention of cardiovascular disease. *Cochrane Database Syst Rev.* 2018;11(11):CD003177.

Aberg JA, Gallant JE, Ghanem KG, et al. Primary care guidelines for the management of persons infected with HIV: 2013 update by the HIV Medicine Association of the Infectious Diseases Society of America. *Clin Infect Dis.* 2014;58(1):1–34.

Aberg JA, Sponseller CA, Ward DJ, et al. Pitavastatin versus pravastatin in adults with HIV-1 infection and dyslipidemia (INTREPID): 12 week and 52-week results of a phase 4, multicenter, randomized double-blind, superiority trial. *Lancet HIV.* 2017;4(7):e284–e294.

Althoff KN, McGinnis KA, Wyatt CM, et al. Comparison of risk and age at diagnosis of myocardial infarction, end-stage renal disease, and non-AIDS defining cancer in PWH versus uninfected adults. *Clin Infect Dis.* 2015;60:627–638.

Althoff KN, Palella FJ, Gebo K, et al. Impact of smoking, hypertension and cholesterol on myocardial infarction in HIV+ adults [Abstract 130]. CROI 2017, Boston.

Amador-Licona N, Díaz-Murillo TA, Gabriel-Ortiz G, et al. Omega 3 fatty acids supplementation and oxidative stress in HIV-seropositive patients: a clinical trial. *PLoS One.* 2016;11(3):e0151637.

Backes JM, Russinger JF, Gibson CA, et al. Statin-associated muscle symptoms—managing the highly intolerant. *J Clin Lipidol.* 2017;11(1):24–33.

Baum PD, Sullam PM, Stoddart CA, et al. Abacavir increases platelet reactivity via competitive inhibition of soluble guanylyl cyclase. *AIDS.* 2011;25(18):2243–2248.

Bell KJ. Incremental benefits and harms of the 2017 American College of Cardiology/American Heart Association high blood pressure guideline. *JAMA Intern Med.* 2018;178(6):755–757.

Benowitz NL, Pipe A, West R, et al. Cardiovascular safety of varenicline, bupropion, and nicotine patches in smokers: a randomized controlled trial. *JAMA Intern Med.* 2018;178(5):622–631.

Blackman AL, Pandit NS, Pincus KJ. Comparing rates of statin therapy in eligible patients living with HIV compared to uninfected patients. *HIV Med.* 2020;21(3):135–141.

Boccara F. Cardiovascular health in an aging HIV population. *AIDS.* 2017;31(suppl 2):S157–S163.

Boccara F, Ghislain M, Meyer L, et al. Impact of protease inhibitors on circulating PCSK9 levels in PWH antiretroviral-naïve patients from an ongoing prospective cohort. ANRS-COPANA Study Group. *AIDS.* 2017;31(17):2367–2376.

Boccara F, Kumar P, Caramelli B, et al. Evolocumab treatment in patients with HIV and hypercholesterolemia/mixed dyslipidemia: BEIJERNICK study design and baseline characteristics. *Am Heart J.* 2020;220:203–212.

Boonthos K, Puttilerpong C, Penssuparp T. Short-term efficacy and safety of adding ezetimibe to current regimen of lipid-lowering drugs in PWH Thai patients treated with protease inhibitors. *Japan J Infect Dis.* 2018;71:220–224.

Bowman L, Marion Mafham M, Wallendszus K, et al. Effects of aspirin for primary prevention in persons with diabetes mellitus: the ASCEND Study Collaborative Group. *N Engl J Med.* 2018;379:1529–1539.

Brunstrom M, Carlberg B. Association of blood pressure lowering with mortality and cardiovascular disease across blood pressure levels: a systematic review and meta-analysis. *JAMA Intern Med.* 2018;178(1):28–36.

Cannon C, Blazing M, Giugliano R, et al. Ezetimibe added to statin therapy after acute coronary syndromes. *N Engl J Med.* 2015;372:2387–2397.

Cheung CC, Ding E, Sereda P, et al. Reductions in all-cause and cause-specific mortality among PWH individuals receiving antiretroviral therapy in British Columbia, Canada: 2001-2012. *HIV Med.* 2016;17(9):694–701.

Cioe PA, Baker J, Kojic EM, et al. Elevated soluble CD14 and lower D-dimer are associated with cigarette smoking and heavy episodic alcohol use in persons living with PWH. *J AIDS.* 2015;70(4):400–405.

Costagliola D, Potard V, Lang S, et al. Is the risk of myocardial infarction in people with HIV associated with atazanavir or darunavir? A nested case-control study within the French hospital database on HIV. *J Infect Dis* 2020;221(4):516–522.

Cropsey KL, Bean MC, Haynes L, et al. Delivery and implementation of an algorithm for smoking cessation treatment for people with HIV and AIDS. *AIDS Care Psych Soc Aspect AIDS/HIV.* 2019;2:223–229.

Data Collection on Adverse Events of Anti-HIV Drugs (D:A:D) Study Group. Class of antiretroviral drugs and the risk of myocardial infarction. *N Engl J Med.* 2007;356:1723–1735.

Data Collection on Adverse Events of Anti-HIV Drugs (D:A:D) Study Group. The impact of fasting on the interpretation of triglyceride levels for predicting myocardial infarction risk in HIV-positive individuals: the D:A:D study. *J Infect Dis.* 2011;204(4):521–525.

Deeks S, Lewin SR, Havlir DA. The end of AIDS: HIV infection as a chronic disease. *Lancet.* 2013;283(9903):1525–1533.

De Pablo C, Orden S, Calatayud S, et al. Differential effects of tenofovir/emtricitabine and abacavir/lamivudine on human leukocyte recruitment. *Antivir Ther.* 2012;17(8):1615–1619.

DerSarkissian M, Bhak RH, Oglesby A, et al. Retrospective analysis of comorbidities and treatment burden among patients with HIV infection in a US Medicaid population. *Curr Med Res Opin.* 2020;36(5):781–788.

DeSocio GV, Ricci E, Maggi P, et al. Is it feasible to impact on smoking habits in PWH patients? *J AIDS.* 2020;83(5):496–503.

Dorjee K, Choden T, Baxi SM, et al. Risk of cardiovascular disease associated with exposure to abacavir among individuals with HIV: a systematic review and meta-analyses of results from seventeen epidemiologic studies. *Int J Antimicrob Agents.* 2018;52(5):541–553.

Drozd DR, Kitahata MM, Althoff KN, et al. Incidence and risk of myocardial infarction (MI) by type in the NA-ACCORD [Abstract 748]. CROI 2015, Seattle, WA.

Eckard AR, Meissner EG, Singh I, et al. Cardiovascular disease, statins, and HIV. *J Infect Dis.* 2016;214(suppl 2):S83–S92.

Everett BM, Smith RJ, Hiatt WR. Reducing LDL with PCSK9 inhibitors—the clinical benefit of lipid drugs. *N Engl J Med.* 2015;373:1588–1591.

Fahme SA, Bloomfield GS, Peck R. Hypertension and PWH adults: novel pathophysiologic mechanisms. *Hypertension.* 2018;72:44–55.

Fitch KV, Kileel EM, Looby SE, et al.; REPRIEVE Investigators. Successful recruitment of a multi-site international randomized placebo-controlled trial in people with HIV with attention to diversity of race and ethnicity: critical role of central coordination. *HIV Res Clin Pract.* 2020;21(1):11–23.

Fitch KV, Looby SE, Rope A, et al. Effects of aging and smoking on carotid intima-media thickness in HIV infection. *AIDS.* 2013;27(1):49–57.

Fogacci F, Strocchi E, Veronesi M, et al. Effect of omega-3 polyunsaturated fatty acids treatment on lipid pattern of HIV patients: a meta-analysis of randomized clinical trials. *Mar Drugs.* 2020;18(6):292.

Freiberg MS, Chang CC, Kuller LH, et al. HIV infection and the risk of acute myocardial infarction. *JAMA Intern Med.* 2013;173(8):614–622.

Friis-Møller N, Sabin CA, Weber R, et al.; the Data Collection on Adverse Events of Anti-HIV Drugs (D:A:D) Study Group. Combination antiretroviral therapy and the risk of myocardial infarction. *N Engl J Med.* 2003;349:1993–2003.

Friis-Møller N, Thiébaut R, Reiss P, et al. Predicting the risk of cardiovascular disease in PWH patients: the Data Collection on Adverse Effects of Anti-HIV Drugs Study. *Eur J Cardiovasc Prev Rehabil.* 2010;17(5):491–501.

Gatell JM, Assoumou L, Moyle G, et al. Switching from a ritonavir-boosted protease inhibitor to a dolutegravir-based regimen for maintenance of viral suppression in patients with high cardiovascular risk. *AIDS.* 2017;31:2503–2514.

Gaziano JM, Brotons C, Coppolecchia R. Use of aspirin to reduce the risk of initial vascular events in patients at moderate risk of cardiovascular disease (ARRIVE): a randomized double-blind placebo-controlled trial. *Lancet.* 2018;392:1035–1046.

Giugliano RP, Keech A, Murphy SA. Clinical efficacy and safety of evolocumab in high-risk patients receiving a statin: secondary analysis of patients with low LDL cholesterol levels and in those already receiving a maximal-potency statin in a randomized clinical trial. *JAMA*. 2017;2(12):1385–1391.

Go AS, Horberg M, Reynolds K, et al. HIV infection independently increases the risk of developing heart failure: The HIV HEART study [Abstract THAB0103]. AIDS 2018: 22nd International AIDS Conference, Amsterdam, Netherlands, July 23–27, 2018.

Grandi AM, Nicolini E, Rizzi L, et al. Dyslipidemia in HIV-positive patients: a randomized, controlled, prospective study on ezetimibe ± fenofibrate versus pravastatin monotherapy. *J Int AIDS Soc*. 2014;17:19004.

Grinspoon SK, Douglas PS, Hoffman U, et al. Leveraging a landmark trial of primary cardiovascular disease prevention in human immunodeficiency virus: introduction from the REPRIEVE coprincipal investigators. *J Infect Dis*. 2020;222:S1–S7.

Grundy SM, Stone NJ, Bailey AL, et al. 2018 ACC/AHA guideline on the management of blood cholesterol: a report of the American College of Cardiology/American Heart Association Task Force on Clinical Practice Guidelines. *Circulation*. 2019;139(25):e1046–e1081.

Guirguis-Blake JM, Evans CV, Senger CA, et al. Aspirin for the primary prevention of cardiovascular events: a systematic evidence review for the U.S. Preventive Services Task Force. *Ann Intern Med*. 2016;164(12):804–813.

Guyton JR, Bays HE, Grundy SM, et al. An assessment of the Statin Intolerance Panel: 2014 update. *J Clin Lipidol*. 2014;8(3 suppl):S72–S81.

Hatleberg CI, Ryom L, El-Sadr W, et al. Improvements over time in short-term mortality following myocardial infarction in HIV-positive individuals. *AIDS*. 2016;30(10):1583–1596.

Hammersley D, Signy M. Ezetimibe: an update on its clinical usefulness in specific patient groups. *Ther Adv Chronic Dis*. 2017;8(1):4–11.

Hermida RC, Crespo JJ, Domingues-Sardina M, et al. Bedtime hypertension treatment improves cardiovascular risk reduction. The Hygia Chronotherapy Trial. *Eur Heart J*. 2020;41(48):4565–4576.

Hsue P, Hunt P, Schnell A, et al. Inflammation is associated with endothelial dysfunction among individuals with treated and suppressed HIV infection [Abstract 708]. CROI 2010, San Francisco, CA.

Hsue PY, Waters DD. HIV infection and coronary heart disease: mechanisms and management. *Nat Rev Cardiol*. 2019;16(12):745–759.

Hunt PW. HIV and inflammation: mechanisms and consequences. *Curr HIV/AIDS Rep*. 2012;9(2):139–147.

Jakob T, Nordmann AJ, Schandelmaier S, et al. Fibrates for primary prevention of cardiovascular disease events. *Cochrane Database Syst Rev*. 2016 Nov 16;11(11):CD009753.

Jankowski CM, Mawhinney S, Wilson MP, et al. Body composition changes in response to moderate or high-intensity exercise among older adults with or without HIV infection. *JAIDS*. 2020;85(3):340–345.

Jones R, Arps K, Davis DM. Clinician guide to the ABCs of primary and secondary prevention of atherosclerotic cardiovascular disease. April 2018. https://www.acc.org/latest-in-cardiology/articles/2018/03/30/18/34/clinician-guide-to-the-abcs

Khambaty T, Stewart JC, Gupta SK, et al. Association between depressive disorders and incident acute myocardial infarction in human immunodeficiency virus-infected adults: Veterans Aging Cohort Study. *JAMA Cardiol*. 2016;1(8):929–937.

Klein DB, Leyden WA, Chao CR. No difference in the incidence of myocardial infarction for HIV+ and HIV− individuals in recent years. *Clin Infect Dis*. 2015;60(8):1278–1285.

Klein DB, Marcus JL, Leyden WA, et al. Infection and immunodeficiency as risk factors for ischemic stroke [Abstract 741]. CROI 2014, Boston, MA.

Krishnan S, Bosch RJ, Rodriguez B, et al. Correlates of inflammatory biomarkers one year after suppressive ART [Abstract 757]. CROI 2014, Boston, MA.

Law M, Friis-Møller N, El-Sadr WA, et al. The use of the Framingham equation to predict myocardial infarctions in PWH patients: comparison with observed events in the D:A:D study. *HIV Med*. 2006;7:218–230.

Leone FT, Zhang Y, Evers-Casey S, et al. Initiating pharmacologic treatment in tobacco-dependent adults—an official American Thoracic Society Clinical Practice guideline. *Am J Respir Crit Care Med*. 2020;202(2):5–31.

Leyes P, Martinez E, Larrousse M, et al. Effects of ezetimibe on cholesterol metabolism in PWH patients with protease inhibitor-associated dyslipidemia: a single-arm intervention trial. *BMC Infect Dis*. 2014;11(14):497.

Lloyd-Jones DM, Morris PB, Ballantyne CM, et al. 2017 Focused update of the 2016 ACC Expert Consensus Decision pathway on the role of non-statin therapies for LDL-cholesterol lowering in the management of atherosclerotic cardiovascular disease. *J Am Coll Cardiol*. 2017;70(14):1785–1822.

Mallon P, Winston A, Post F, et al. Platelet function upon switching to TAF vs. continuing ABC: a randomized sub-study [Abstract 80]. CROI 2018, Boston, MA.

Marconi VC, Duncan MS, So-Armah K, et al. Bilirubin is inversely associated with cardiovascular disease among HIV-positive and HIV-negative individuals in VACS (Veterans Aging Cohort Study). *J Am Heart Assoc*. 2018;7(10):e007792.

Marquis-Gravel G, Roe MT, Harrington RA. Revisiting the role of aspirin for the primary prevention of cardiovascular disease. *Circulation*. 2019;140:1115–1124.

Martinez E, Larrousse M, Llibre JM, et al. Substitution of raltegravir for ritonavir-boosted protease inhibitors in PWH patients: the SPIRAL study. *AIDS*. 2010;24(11):1697–1707.

McNeil JJ, Nelson MR, Woods RL, et al. Effect of aspirin on all-cause mortality in the healthy elderly. *N Engl J Med*. 2018;379(16):1519–1528.

Medical Letter on Drugs and Therapeutics. Drugs for tobacco dependence. *JAMA*. 2018;320(9):926–927.

Medina-Torne S, Ganesan A, Barahona I, et al. Hypertension is common among PWH persons, but not associated with HAART. *J Int Assoc Physicians AIDS Care*. 2012;11(1):20–25.

Mercie P, Arsandaux J, Katalama C, et al. Efficacy and safety of varenicline for smoking cessation in people living with HIV in France (ANRS 144 Inter-ACTIV): a randomized controlled phase 3 clinical trial. *Lancet HIV*. 2018;5(3):126–135.

Metkus TS, Brown T, Budoff M, et al. HIV infection is associated with an increased prevalence of coronary noncalcified plaque among participants with a coronary artery calcium score of zero: Multicenter AIDS Cohort Study (MACS). *HIV Med*. 2015;16(10):635–639.

Morgello S, Mahboob R, Yakoushina T, et al. Autopsy findings in human immunodeficiency virus-infected populations over 2 decades. *Arch Path Lab Med*. 2002;126:182–190.

Mosepele M, Molefe-Baikai OJ, Grinspoon SK, et al. Benefits and risks of statin therapy in the PWH population. *Curr Infect Dis Rep*. 2018;20:20. https://doi.org/10.1007/s11908-018-0628-7

National Institute for Health and Care Excellence. Ezetimibe for treating primary heterozygous familial and non-familial hypercholesterolemia. Guide TA385. 2016. http://nice.org.uk/guidance.

O'Brien S, Montenont E, Hu L, et al. Aspirin attenuates platelet activation and immune activation in HIV-1-infected subjects on antiretroviral therapy: a pilot study. *JAIDS*. 2013;63(3):280–288.

Oh RC, Trivette ET, Westerfield KL. Management of hypertriglyceridemia: common questions and answers. *Am Fam Phys*. 2020;102(6):347–354.

Olaiya O, Weiser J, Zhou W, et al. Hypertension among persons living with HIV in medical care in the United States—Medical Monitoring Project 2013–2014. *Open Forum Infect Dis*. 2018;5(3):ofy028.

Oliveira JM, Rondo PH, Lima LR, et al. Effects of low dose fish oil on inflammatory markers of Brazilian PWH adults on antiretroviral therapy: a randomized parallel placebo-controlled trial. *Nutrients*. 2015;7(8):6520–6528.

Oliveros E, Patel H, Kyung S, et al. Hypertension in older adults: assessment, management and challenges. *Clin Cardiol*. 2020;43(2):99–107.

Ozemek C, Erlandson KM, Jankowski CM. Physical activity and exercise to improve cardiovascular health for adults living with HIV. *Prog Cardiovasc Dis*. 2020;63(2):178–183.

Pacek LR, Holloway AD, Cropsey KL, et al. Cigarette smoking and cessation-related interactions with health care providers in the context of living with HIV: focus group study findings. *J Assoc Nurses AIDS Care*. 2020 [E-pub before print].

Paikin JS, Eikelboom JW. Cardiology patient page: aspirin. *Circulation*. 2012;125(10):e439–e442.

Paisible AL, Chang CH, So-Armah KA, et al. HIV infection, cardiovascular disease risk factor profile, and risk for acute myocardial infarction. *J AIDS*. 2015;68:209–216.

Palella FJ Jr, Fisher M, Tebas P, et al. Simplification to rilpivirine/emtricitabine/tenofovir disoproxil fumarate from ritonavir-boosted protease inhibitor antiretroviral therapy in a randomized trial of HIV-1 RNA-suppressed participants. *AIDS*. 2014;28(3):335–344

Petoumenos K, Worm S, Reiss P, et al.; D:A:D Study Group. Rates of cardiovascular disease following smoking cessation in patients with HIV infection: results from the D:A:D study. *HIV Med*. 2011;12(7):412–421.

Pett SL, Amin J, Horban A, et al. Week 96 results of the randomized, multicenter Maraviroc Switch (MARCH) Study. *HIV Med*. 2018;19:65–71.

Pool ER, Dogar O, Lindsay RP, et al. Interventions for tobacco use cessation in people living with HIV and AIDS. *Cochrane Database Syst Rev*. 2016;13(6):CD011120.

Post WS, Budoff M, Kingsley L, et al. Associations between HIV infection and subclinical coronary atherosclerosis. *Ann Intern Med*. 2014;160:458–467.

Rao SG, Galaviz KI, Hawkins GC, et al. Factors associated with excess myocardial infarction risk in PWH adults: a systemic review and meta-analysis. *J AIDS*. 2019;81(2):224–230.

Rasmussen LD, May MT, Kronborg G, et al. Time trends for risk of severe age-related diseases in individuals with and without HIV infection in Denmark: a nationwide population-based cohort study. *Lancet HIV*. 2015;2(7):e288–e298.

Ray KK, Bays HE, Catapano AL, et al.; CLEAR Harmony Trial. Safety and efficacy of bempedoic acid to reduce LDL cholesterol. *N Engl J Med*. 2019;380(11):1022–1032.

Regan S, Meigs JB, Massaro J, et al. Evaluation of the ACC/AHA CVD risk prediction algorithm among PWH patients [Abstract 751]. CROI 2015, Seattle, WA.

Reiter-Brennan C, Osei AD, Iftekhar Uddin SM, et al. ACC/AHA lipid guidelines: personalized care to prevent cardiovascular disease. *Cleve Clin J Med*. 2020;87(4):231–239.

Remick J, Georgiopoulou V, Marti C, et al. Heart failure in patients with human immunodeficiency virus infection: epidemiology, pathophysiology, treatment, and future research. *Circulation*. 2014;129(17):1781–1789.

Ryom L, Lundgren JD, El-Sadr W, et al. Cardiovascular disease and use of contemporary protease inhibitors: the D:A:D international prospective multicohort study. *Lancet HIV*, 2018;6:e291–e300.

Saag MS, Gandhi RT, Hoy JF, et al. Antiretroviral drugs for treatment and prevention of HIV infection in adults: 2020 recommendations of the International Antiviral Society–USA Panel. *JAMA*. 2020;324(16):1651–1669.

Sabatine MS, Giugliano RP, Keech AC, et al. Evolocumab and clinical outcomes in patients with cardiovascular disease. *N Engl J Med*. 2017;376:1713–1722.

Sabin C, Reiss P, Ryom L, et al. Is there continued evidence for an association between abacavir and myocardial infarction risk? [Abstract 747]. CROI 2014, Boston, MA.

Saeedi R, Johns K, Frohlich J, et al. Lipid-lowering efficacy and safety of ezetimibe combined with rosuvastatin compared with titrating rosuvastatin monotherapy in HIV-positive patients. *Lipids Health Dis*. 2015;14:57.

Sax PC, Zolopa A, Eleon R. Tenofovir alafenamide vs. tenofovir disoproxil fumarate in single tablet regimens for initial HIV-1 therapy: a randomized phase 2 study. *J AIDS*. 2014;67(1):52–58.

Shah ASV, Stelze D, Lee KK, et al. Global burden of atherosclerotic vascular disease in people living with HIV: systematic review and meta-analysis. *Circulation*. 2018;138:1100–1112.

Shahreyar M, Salem SA, Nayyar M. Hyperlipidemia: management with proprotein convertase subtilisin/kexin type 9 (PCSK9) inhibitors. *J Am Board Fam Med*. 2018;31(4):628–634.

Scherzer R, Shah SJ, Secemsky E, et al. Association of biomarker clusters with cardiac phenotypes and mortality in patients with HIV infection. *Circ Heart Fail*. 2018;11(4):e004312.

Sigel K, Makinson A, Thaler J. Lung cancer in persons with HIV. *Curr Opin HIV AIDS*. 2017;12(1):31–38.

Sing S, Willig JH, Mugavero MJ, et al. Comparative efficacy and toxicity among statins in PWH patients. *Clin Infect Dis*. 2011;52(3):387–395.

Singh G, Correa R. Fibrate medications. StatPearls, 2020.

Sizar O, Nassereddin A, Talati R. Ezetimibe. StatPearls, 2020.

Smit M, van Zoest RA, Nichols BE, et al. Cardiovascular disease prevention policy in human immunodeficiency virus: recommendations from a modeling study. *Clin Infect Dis*. 2018;66(5):743–750.

So-Armah K, Benjamin LA, Bloomfield GS, et al. HIV and cardiovascular disease. *Lancet HIV*. 2020;7:e279–e293.

Strategies for Management of Antiretroviral Therapy (SMART)/INSIGHT/D:A:D Study Groups. Use of nucleoside reverse transcriptase inhibitors and risk of myocardial infarction in PWH patients. *AIDS*. 2008;22:F17–F24.

Stone NJ, Robinson JG, Lichtenstein AH, et al. 2013 ACC/AHA guideline on the treatment of blood cholesterol to reduce atherosclerotic cardiovascular risk in adults: a report of the American College of Cardiology/American Heart Association Task Force on Practice Guidelines. *Circulation*. 2014;129(25 Suppl 2):S1–45.

Subramanian S, Tawakol A, Burdo TH, et al. Arterial inflammation in patients with HIV. *JAMA*. 2012;308:379–386.

Suchindran S, Regan S, Meigs JB, et al. Aspirin use for primary and secondary prevention in human immunodeficiency virus (HIV)-infected and HIV-uninfected patients. *Open Forum Infect Dis*. 2014;1(3):ofu076.

Swanson B, Keithley J, Baum L, et al. Effects of fish oil on HIV-related inflammation and markers of immunosenescence: a randomized clinical trial. *J Altern Complement Med*. 2018;24(7):709–716.

Tawakol A, Lo J, Zanni MV, et al. Increased arterial inflammation relates to high-risk coronary plaque morphology in PWH patients. *J AIDS*. 2014;66(2):164–171.

Thiébaut R, El-Sadr W, Friis-Møller N, et al.; the D:A:D Study Group. Predictors of hypertension and changes in blood pressure in PWH patients. *Antiviral Ther*. 2005;10:811–823.

Thompson-Paul A, Buchacz K, Wei S, et al. Evaluation of the ACC/AHA CVD risk prediction algorithm among PWH patients [Abstract 747]. CROI 2015, Seattle, WA.

Triant V, Perez J, Regan S et al. Cardiovascular risk prediction functions underestimate risk in HIV infection. *Circulation*. 2018;137(21):2203–2214.

Triant V, Regan S, Lee H, et al. Association of immunologic and virologic factors with myocardial infarction rates in the U.S. health care system. *J AIDS*. 2010;55(5):615–619.

Tseng A, Foisy M. Important drug–drug interactions in PWH persons on antiretroviral therapy: an update on new interactions between HIV and non-HIV drugs. *Curr Infect Dis Rep*. 2012;14(1):67–82.

Tungsiripat M, Kitch D, Glesby MJ, et al. A pilot study to determine the impact on dyslipidemia of adding tenofovir to stable background antiretroviral therapy: ACTG 5206. *AIDS*. 2010;24(11):1781–1784.

US Department of Health and Human Services, Panel on Antiretroviral Guidelines for Adults and Adolescents. Guidelines for the use of antiretroviral agents in adults and adolescents living with HIV. 2020. https://clinicalinfo.hiv.gov/sites/default/files/inline-files/AdultandAdolescentGL.pdf

Vancampfort D, Mugisha J, Richards J, et al. Physical activity correlates in people living with HIV/AIDS: systematic review of 45 studies. *Disabil Rehabil*. 2018;40(14):1618–1629.

Van Lelyveld SF, Gras L, Kesselring A, et al. ATHENA national observational cohort study: long-term complications in patients with poor immunological recovery despite virological successful HAART in Dutch ATHENA cohort. *AIDS*. 2012;26(4):465–474.

van Zoest RA, van den Born BH, Reiss P. Hypertension in people living with HIV. *Curr Opin HIV AIDS*. 2017;12(6):513–522.

Vieira AD, Silveira GR. Effectiveness of omega-3 fatty acids in the treatment of hypertriglyceridemia in HIV/AIDS patients: a meta-analysis. *Cien Saude Colet*. 2017;22(8):2659–2669.

Wall HK, Ritchey MD, Gillespie C, et al. Vital signs: prevalence of key cardiovascular disease risk factors for Million Hearts 2022—United States, 2011–2016. *MMWR Morb Mortal Wkly Rep*. 2018;67:983–991.

Whelton PK, Carey RM, Aronow WS, et al. 2017 ACC/AHA/AAPA/ABC/ACPM/AGS/APhA/ASH/ASPC/NMA/PCNA guideline for the prevention, detection, evaluation, and management of high blood pressure in adults: executive summary: a report of the American College of Cardiology/American Heart Association Task Force on Clinical Practice Guidelines. *Circulation*. 2018a;138(17):e426–e483.

Whelton PK, Carey RM, Aronow WS, et al. ACC/AHA/AAAP/ABC/ACPM/AGS/ASH/ASPC/NMA/PCNA guideline for the prevention, detection, and management of high blood pressure in adults. *Hypertension*. 2018b;71:e13–e115.

White JR, Chang CC, So-Armah KA, et al. Depression and HIV infection are risk factors for incident heart failure among veterans: VACS. *Circulation*. 2015;132(17):1630–1638.

Whitlock EP, Burda BU, Williams SB, et al. Bleeding risks with aspirin use for primary prevention in adults: a systematic review for the U.S. Preventive Services Task Force. *Ann Intern Med*. 2016;164(12):826–835.

Wohl D, Waters D, Simpson R, et al. Ezetimibe alone reduces low-density lipoprotein cholesterol in PWH patients receiving combination antiretroviral therapy. *Clin Infect Dis*. 2008;47:1105–1108.

Yusuf S, Hawken S, Ounpuu S, et al. Effect of potentially modifiable risk factors associated with myocardial infarction in 52 countries (the INTERHEART Study): case-control study. *Lancet*. 2004;364:937–952.

Zanni MV, Awadalla M, Toibio M, et al. Immune correlates of diffuse myocardial fibrosis and diastolic dysfunction among aging women with human immunodeficiency virus. *J Infect Dis*. 2020;221:1315–1320.

39.

RENAL COMPLICATIONS

Jonathan Lim, Steven Menez, and Derek M. Fine

LEARNING OBJECTIVES

Upon completion of this chapter, the reader should be able to:

- Discuss the broad pathologic spectrum of renal disease in PWH including medication-induced renal injury HIV

- Explain the importance of screening and monitoring PWH for chronic kidney disease along with the indications for nephrology referral and renal biopsy

WHAT'S NEW?

- The spectrum of kidney disease in patients with HIV is changing in the current era of combined ART.

- There are updates from the 2017 Kidney Disease: Improving Global Outcomes (KDIGO) conference regarding the diagnosis and management of kidney disease in the setting of HIV infection.

EPIDEMIOLOGY OF RENAL DISEASE IN PWH

Although the incidence of HIV-associated nephropathy (HIVAN) has greatly declined, the overall prevalence of kidney disease in PWH has increased as a result of improved survival. With improved life expectancy and ART-related metabolic abnormalities, chronic kidney disease (CKD) is a significant comorbidity in PWH. Risk factors for kidney disease include Black race, CD4+ T-cell counts of less than 200 cells/mm³, HIV RNA levels of greater than 10,000 copies/mL, family history of CKD, diabetes mellitus, hypertension, and hepatitis coinfection. The spectrum of kidney disease is being driven by traditional risk factors such as obesity, diabetes, hypertension, the use of nephrotoxic medications, and aging of the HIV population (Heron et al., 2020; Waheed & Atta, 2014).

Despite widespread use of ART, PWH remain at a higher risk of renal insufficiency, cardiovascular disease, and overall mortality than matched cohorts of HIV-negative people

(Kalayjian, 2011). Up to 30% of PWH are at risk of developing proteinuria, a key marker of kidney disease. Moreover, cross-sectional cohorts from Europe, Asia, and North America have demonstrated high CKD rates in PWH, with about 6% of PWH having stages 3 to 5 CKD (Post & Holt, 2009). Based on another large sample of US veterans, the incidence rate of ESRD in Black PWH is even higher than that of patients with diabetes (incidence rates per 1,000 person-years [pys]: 71.1 for HIV, 59.9 for diabetes mellitus, and 27.9 for individuals with neither HIV nor diabetes; Choi et al., 2007). Compared to the general population, PWH have a 16-fold higher risk of requiring renal replacement therapy.

PATHOGENESIS

The apolipoprotein 1 (*ApoL1*) gene, which encodes a factor to lyse the parasite *Trypanosoma brucei*, is the key susceptibility allele in HIVAN and other kidney diseases in the APOL1 nephropathy spectrum. HIV RNA localizes to podocytes and tubular epithelial cells in the kidney, suggesting a direct role of the virus in kidney disease. Furthermore, the role of viral proteins is supported by animal studies. The HIV regulatory protein *nef* and HIV accessory protein *vpr* are overexpressed in mice reproducing the HIV-associated nephropathy phenotype.

Kidney disease is a major cause of mortality from non–AIDS-related conditions in PWH, along with malignancies, cardiovascular disease, and liver disease (Ryom et al., 2019). Renal pathology in PWH was originally reported in 1984 and was called "acquired immune deficiency syndrome (AIDS) nephropathy" (Rao et al., 1984). The histopathology on kidney biopsy of these persons showed a collapsing type of focal and segmental glomerulosclerosis, and the clinical presentation was that of proteinuria, usually nephrotic, and rapid progression to ESRD. Subsequently, HIVAN became more commonly recognized as a major cause of kidney disease in PWH. In the US, the incidence of HIVAN peaked in the mid-1990s and dropped significantly after the introduction of highly active ART by the late 1990s (Ross & Klotman, 2002). More recent data show the annual incidence of ESRD in PWH in the US is now about 800 to 900 cases per year (Cohen et al., 2017).

RISK FACTORS FOR NEPHROPATHY

Risk factors for the development of kidney disease in PWH include Black race, diabetes mellitus, hypertension, hepatitis C coinfection, cardiovascular disease, and family history of CKD (Mocroft et al., 2015; Naicker & Fabian, 2010). In addition, individuals with advanced undiagnosed and/or untreated HIV infection with CD4$^+$ T-cell counts of less than 200 cells/mm^3 and active viral replication are at high risk for developing HIVAN (Bige et al., 2012; Lescure et al., 2012).

GENETIC PREDISPOSITION

The major genetic risk factor for developing HIVAN and non-HIVAN focal segmental glomerulosclerosis (FSGS) in persons of African descent is the presence of polymorphisms in the *APOL1* gene, which is also located on chromosome 22 (Genovese et al., 2010; Lescure et al., 2012; Tzur et al., 2010). *APOL1* encodes a serum factor that lyses *T. brucei*. Thus, selective mutations in Africans to counter an endemic parasite may have contributed to the current rates of HIVAN and FSGS in Black populations. Two *APOL1* risk alleles, G1 and G2, are associated with the increased susceptibility for the development of HIVAN and other types of kidney disease collectively termed *APOL1* nephropathy (Friedman & Pollak, 2021; Genovese et al., 2010; Papeta et al., 2011). It is hypothesized that *APOL1* risk variants create pores in cell membranes within the kidney much like they do in trypanosomal organelles, but other studies suggest overexpression of risk variants leads to mitochondrial dysfunction and injury. There is still no consensus on the molecular mechanism of *APOL1* nephropathy (Friedman & Pollak, 2021). In PWH who carry the two *APOL1* risk alleles, this alone can explain 35% of cases of HIVAN and 18% of FSGS cases (Kopp et al., 2011). Two risk variants confer an odds ratio of approximately 7 to 10 for hypertension-associated ESRD, 17 for FSGS, 29 for HIVAN in the US, and 89 for HIVAN in Africa. These data suggest that these diseases have some overlapping mechanism of pathogenesis (Friedman & Pollak, 2021). *APOL1* homozygosity, present in 13% of the general Black American population, was noted in more than 60% of Black Americans with HIVAN and non-HIVAN FSGS (Kopp et al., 2011).

In animal models, HIV gene expression within kidney cells is required for the development of HIVAN (Bruggeman et al., 1997). Even in HIVAN persons with undetectable plasma HIV-RNA levels, proviral DNA can be found in the renal tissue of all PWH (Izzedine et al., 2011). This implies that the kidney acts as a separate compartment from blood, allowing HIV to replicate in the kidney even in PWH who achieve viral suppression in their plasma with treatment (Medapalli et al., 2011). HIV-RNA localizes to podocytes and tubular epithelial cells in the kidney. HIV regulatory protein *nef* and HIV accessory protein *vpr* are overexpressed

---

in mice reproducing the HIV-associated nephropathy phenotype (Cohen et al., 2017). HIV induces apoptosis of cells in addition to causing cytopathic effects. These effects, in combination with cytokine release, are thought to play a role in the development of HIVAN (Box 39.1).

MARKERS OF KIDNEY INJURY

Markers of kidney injury include an elevated serum creatinine, proteinuria, glycosuria, and an increased fractional excretion of uric acid (Makris & Spanou, 2016). Risk factors for proteinuria include older age, Black race, insulin resistance, hypertension, and a low CD4$^+$ T-cell count (Heron et al., 2020). The presence of albuminuria and overt proteinuria is also associated with increased cardiovascular morbidity and mortality in this population (Wyatt et al., 2011). In a study of PWH and albuminuria, the 5-year mortality rate was 20%

in persons with albuminuria and 48% in individuals with a glomerular filtration rate (GFR) of less than 60 mL/min and albuminuria (Choi et al., 2010).

ASSESSMENT OF KIDNEY FUNCTION

Like the general population, kidney damage in PWH is assessed by using creatinine-based estimates of glomerular filtration rate (eGFR) with the Cockcroft–Gault equation, Modification of Diet in Renal Disease (MDRD), and CKD Epidemiology Collaboration (CKD-EPI) equation, but none of these estimates has been systematically validated in PWH.

Cystatin C is an alternative marker of eGFR that does not depend on muscle mass and is more sensitive for kidney damage than creatinine-based formulas. Its role in diagnosis and as a prognostic marker in PWH remains to be defined. Dragović et al. (2018) found that cystatin C may be elevated in PWH with metabolic syndrome. Out of 89 PWH, the 33 individuals with metabolic syndrome had a statistically significantly higher cystatin C level compared to those without. Notably, there were no significant differences with respect to CD4 level, time on ART, smoking status, or hepatitis B or C status. Another study found that cystatin C may assist in plasma creatinine fluctuations after dolutegravir initiation, particularly in high-risk renal PWH (Palich et al., 2018). Pending data from clinical studies, cystatin C is not recommended as a screening or diagnostic tool in clinical practice to assess renal function in PWH.

PATHOLOGIC SPECTRUM OF KIDNEY DISEASE

PWH can develop multiple forms of renal disease, including acute kidney injury (AKI), HIVAN, HIV immune complex kidney disease (HIVICK), thrombotic microangiopathy (TMA), and medication-induced nephrotoxicity. However, kidney disease in PWH has been evolving over time with the high rates of ART usage and longer life expectancy in PWH. This has increased the accumulation of traditional CKD risk factors in the HIV population, broadening the spectrum of etiologies of renal disease seen (Box 39.2) (Swanepoel et al., 2018). In a large academic center, renal biopsies from 437 PWH (80% on ART) were reevaluated to reassess spectrum of disease. This cohort of biopsies from 2010 to 2018 showed the most common pathology to be immune complex glomerulonephritis (ICGN; 17%), follow by diabetic nephropathy (16%), HIVAN (14%), tenofovir (TFV) nephrotoxicity (13%), FSGS–not otherwise specified (NOS; 12%), and global glomerulosclerosis-NOS (9%). In regard to the trend during this 9-year timeframe, TFV nephrotoxicity decreased while FSGS-NOS and diabetic nephropathy increased. In contrast, the same institution in 1987 reported that HIVAN made up 76% of kidney biopsies done on PWH, followed by ICGN (9%) and interstitial nephritis (6%). These researchers also showed that serologies and clinical syndromes, besides

---

Box 39.2 HIV-RELATED KIDNEY DISEASES

I. Glomerular-dominant
   a. Immune complex–mediated glomerular disease (ICGN)
      i. IgA nephropathy
      ii. Lupus nephritis
      iii. Membranous nephropathy
      iv. Membranoproliferative pattern glomerulonephritis
      v. Bacterial infection–related glomerulonephritis
      vi. ICGN with no etiology other than HIV
      vii. Other immune complex diseases in the setting of HIV
   b. Podocytopathies
      i. Classic HIVAN
      ii. FSGS-NOS in the setting of HIV
      iii. Minimal-change disease in the setting of HIV
      iv. Other podocytopathy in the setting of HIV
   c. Other glomerular diseases
      i. Diabetic nephropathy
      ii. AA amyloidosis
      iii. Pauci-immune glomerulonephritis

II. Tubulointerstitial-dominant
   a. Tenofovir toxicity
   b. Tubulointerstitial injury in the setting of classic HIVAN
   c. Acute tubular injury or acute tubular necrosis (associated with ART vs. other drugs)
   d. Tubulointerstitial nephritis (associated with ART vs. other drugs)
   e. Renal parenchymal infection by bacterial, viral, or fungal pathogens
   f. Immunologic dysfunction–related tubulointerstitial inflammation
      i. Diffuse infiltrative lymphocytosis syndrome (DILS)
      ii. Immune reconstitution inflammatory syndrome (IRIS)
   g. Other tubulointerstitial inflammation in the setting of HIV

III. Vascular-dominant
   a. Thrombotic microangiopathy in the setting of HIV
   b. Arteriosclerosis and/or cholesterol emboli
   c. Infarction

IV. Other, in the setting of HIV infection
   a. Diabetic nephropathy
   b. Age-related nephrosclerosis

Adapted from Swanepoel CR et al. Kidney Disease in The Setting of HIV Infection: Conclusions from A Kidney Disease: Improving Global Outcomes (KDIGO) Controversies Conference. *Kidney International*. 2018; 22(6), 84–100.

Fanconi syndrome concerning for TFV toxicity, were not predictive of biopsy findings (Kudose et al., 2020). Therefore, renal biopsy remains an important diagnostic strategy in most PWH with kidney disease to determine the underlying renal pathology, as treatment strategies often differ based on histopathologic findings Cohen & Kimmel, 2009).

ACUTE KIDNEY INJURY

Poor nutritional state of patients, dehydration, polypharmacy, and less commonly opportunistic infections in PWH predispose to development of AKI, with incidence rates of 2.7 to 6.9 per 100 pys (Campos et al., 2016). Higher incidence of AKI is also associated with advanced age, diabetes mellitus, CKD, acute or chronic liver failure, CD4+ T-cell counts of less than 200 cells/mm³, HIV-1 RNA levels of more than 10,000 copies/mL, and hepatitis coinfection (Wyatt et al., 2006). Common causes of AKI in PWH are similar to those in HIV-negative individuals, with prerenal states and acute tubular necrosis accounting for about one-third of cases. Less common causes of AKI in PWH include obstruction from lymphadenopathy related to malignancy, tumor lysis syndrome, and polyoma virus–induced renal dysfunction. Regardless of the etiology, short- and long-term mortality is increased in PWH with AKI by as much as fivefold. In one study from Portugal of 489 hospitalized PWH, mortality was 27.3% for those with AKI versus 8% for those without AKI (Campos et al., 2016). Other studies have shown that long-term mortality is higher in PWH with AKI. In a study of 433 PWH who were hospitalized, at 1, 2, and 5 years of follow-up, the cumulative probability of death in those with AKI was 21%, 25%, and 31%, respectively, compared to 10%, 13%, and 16.5% in patients without AKI (Lopes et al., 2016).

HIV-ASSOCIATED NEPHROPATHY

HIVAN is the most aggressive form of kidney disease associated with HIV infection and generally presents in patients with advanced HIV infection who exhibit a rapidly declining GFR and significant proteinuria. The incidence of HIVAN significantly declined after the widespread use of ART, but it remains a cause of ESRD in young Black patients. HIVAN is pathologically characterized by a collapsing form of focal and segmental sclerosis, prominent tubular microcysts, and tubulointerstitial inflammation (D'Agati et al., 1989).

FSGS-NOS has become a more common finding in renal biopsies in the ART era (Kudose et al., 2020). A subset of these patients with FSGS-NOS are believed to have an attenuated form of HIVAN given similar median severity of tubular atrophy, interstitial fibrosis, and inflammation to HIVAN cases. Additionally, many of these samples had presence of tubuloreticular inclusions (TRIs), tubular microcysts, and moderate foot-process effacement seen in HIVAN. Differentiating between FSGS-NOS and attenuated HIVAN is difficult without molecular studies addressing viral infection of renal epithelia, infiltrating leukocytes phenotype, and dysregulation of host-signaling pathways. However, patients with FSGS-NOS tend to be older and hypertensive with cardiovascular disease and are usually on ART (Kudose et al., 2020).

IMMUNE COMPLEX GLOMERULONEPHRITIS AND HIVICK

Various immune complex kidney diseases have been reported in PWH, such as postinfectious glomerulonephritis, membranoproliferative glomerulonephritis, membranous nephropathy, immunoglobulin A nephropathy, and lupus-like glomerulonephritis, and they were previously referred to collectively as HIVICK (Balow et al., 2005; Kalayjian, 2011). However, in 2017, KDIGO replaced HIVICK in favor of a more descriptive pattern of immune complex disease due to lack of certainty of HIV causality in most cases. The previously eluted glomerular immune deposits with specific anti-HIV antibodies in previous HIVICK cases were done in the research setting and not replicable in routine pathology laboratories. The transition away from collectively naming all immune complex disease as HIVICK was to encourage workup of secondary and possibly treatable causes of immune complex deposition (Swanepoel et al., 2018). In a review of renal biopsies in patient with HIV, immune complex glomerulonephritis was the most prevalent finding. Furthermore, in those 75 cases of immune complex glomerulonephritis, 79% had an identifiable etiology other than HIV infection. Of the remaining 21%, two-thirds of them were not on ART, raising suspicion for true HIVICK in those cases (Kudose et al., 2020).

TUBULOINTERSTITIAL DISEASE

This can include HIVAN, which has a tubulointerstitial component in addition to a glomerular component. TFV and protease inhibitor (PI) toxicity can play a role and will be discussed later in the chapter. PWH are also at risk for tubular injury by the same etiologies seen in the general population, such as toxic, ischemic, septic, and hypovolemic insults. Antibiotics, proton pump inhibitors, and other medications can cause tubulointerstitial nephritis in the general and HIV population as well. However, two rare but notable causes of tubulointerstitial injury involve immune dysfunction from HIV and are characterized by prominent CD8 T-cell infiltrates. Diffuse infiltrative lymphocytosis syndrome (DILS) affects the kidneys 10% of the time as a result of a hyperimmune reaction against HIV. Immune reconstitution inflammatory syndrome (IRIS) rarely involves the kidney but may occur in patients with advanced HIV infection after ART initiation unmasks a subclinical infectious process (Swanepoel et al., 2018).

VASCULAR CONDITIONS

Progressive vascular disease may occur in PWH from a direct effect of HIV on renal vasculature but is also associated with dyslipidemia and chronic inflammation (Heron et al., 2020). TMA is a rare complication of HIV-1 infection, with an incidence of isolated renal TMA of 0.3% (Becker et al., 2004). It manifests as thrombocytopenia, microangiopathic hemolytic anemia, with or without fever, and neurologic deficits. Opportunistic infections, high plasma HIV viral load, low

CD4 counts, and various drugs used in advanced HIV disease can all contribute to development of TMA. In the post–combination ART era, atherosclerotic disease has become the dominant vascular cause of kidney disease in PWH, with management focused on modifiable risk factors such as lipid-lowering agents and ART (Swanepoel et al., 2018).

TREATMENTS

Specific recommendations regarding therapy of the preceding conditions are limited due to the lack of randomized prospective controlled trials. Most of the treatment options, including supportive care, ART, inhibition of the renin–angiotensin-aldosterone system, and corticosteroids, are based on retrospective studies and nonrandomized trials.

ANTIRETROVIRAL THERAPY

Multiple observational studies have supported the benefit of ART in slowing the progression or reversing renal disease in persons with HIVAN. In an older Johns Hopkins Clinic cohort of 4,000 PWH, ART was associated with a 60% risk reduction for HIVAN, with 6.8 and 26.4 episodes per 1,000 pys in PWH who did or did not receive ART, respectively. In addition, no persons in the Hopkins cohort developed HIVAN when ART was initiated before the development of AIDS (Lucas et al., 2004).

Consistent evidence demonstrates preservation of renal function with ART in HIV populations. In the Strategies for Management of Antiretroviral Therapy (SMART) study, continuous therapy versus episodic use of ART was evaluated in 5,472 PWH with CD4$^+$ T-cell counts of more than 350 cells/μL. In the continuous-use group, fewer persons developed renal disease compared to the episodic-use group (0.2 vs. 0.1 events/100 pys) (SMART Study Group, 2006). In addition, in a prospective, multicenter cohort involving 1,776 PWH, ART intervention in persons with CKD stage 2 or greater and low CD4$^+$ T-cell counts led to an average increase of 9.2 mL/min in GFR at a median follow-up of 160 weeks. These results were magnified in those with a lower baseline GFR and greater decreases in viral load (Longenecker et al., 2009).

ANGIOTENSIN-CONVERTING ENZYME INHIBITOR AND ANGIOTENSIN II BLOCKADE

Multiple randomized controlled trials in CKD patients from the general population have demonstrated the efficacy of angiotensin-converting enzyme (ACE) inhibitors and angiotensin receptor blockers (ARBs) in decreasing proteinuria, slowing the progression of kidney disease, and also reducing the incidence of cardiovascular disease and death. However, data regarding their use in PWH are limited. In an older study of 18 PWH with biopsy-proven HIVAN, the 9 who were treated with captopril had an enhanced renal survival compared to controls (mean renal survival, 156 ± 71 vs. 37 ± 5 days) (Kimmel et al., 1996). In another study of 44 patients with biopsy-proven HIVAN, patients treated with

ACE inhibition had significantly less progression to ESRD compared to those without therapy (14% vs. 100% at 5 years) (Wei et al., 2003). Based on these results and data from non-HIV populations, ACE inhibitors or ARBs are recommended for most PWH with CKD and glomerular diseases in the absence of contraindications to these medications.

CORTICOSTEROIDS

In patients with HIVAN, older studies found that tubulointerstitial inflammation improves after treatment with steroids (Briggs et al., 1996). However, there are no randomized trials to support steroid use in this population. In a retrospective cohort study of 21 patients, 13 of whom received corticosteroids, the relative risk for progressive renal failure with corticosteroid treatment at 3 months was 0.20 ($p < 0.05$) (Eustace et al., 2000). This association remained significant despite adjustment in logistical regression analyses for baseline creatinine, 24-hour proteinuria, CD4$^+$ count, and history of intravenous drug use and hepatitis B or hepatitis C coinfection (Eustace et al., 2000). However, there were 18 infections in corticosteroid-treated patients compared to 8 in the non–corticosteroid-treated group. Larger studies are needed to further clarify the value of steroids in patients with HIV-related kidney disease, but in the post-ART era these are unlikely to be performed. On the basis of older data noted above, some experts would still recommend a short course of corticosteroid therapy in those with a new diagnosis of HIVAN (Atta et al., 2008; Fine et al., 2008). Risks of adverse effects, such as glucose intolerance, bone disease, and further immunosuppression, must always be weighed against the benefits when steroids are used in PWH.

NOVEL MEDICAL THERAPIES

In animal models, all-*trans*-retinoic acid has been shown to reverse the *nef*-induced signaling pathway with improvement in proteinuria and glomerulosclerosis (Ratnam et al., 2011). Moreover, when phosphodiesterase inhibitors are used in combination, they increase the renal protective effect of retinoids in animal models (Zhong et al., 2012). However, further studies are needed before their use can be recommended. There are some data to support the use of plasma exchange or eculizumab in patients with TMA (Cohen et al., 2017). Sodium-glucose cotransporter 2 (SGLT2) inhibitors have been shown to reduce the risk of adverse renal outcomes, including dialysis, transplantation, and death, through multiple studies. This class of drugs has also been shown to have an additive effect to RAS blockade in patients with diabetes and albuminuric kidney disease (Neuen et al., 2019). They may confer similar benefits if clinically indicated in PWH.

RENAL REPLACEMENT THERAPY (DIALYSIS)

Compared to the general population, PWH have a 2- to 20-fold higher incidence of requiring renal replacement therapy (Campos et al., 2016). This number varies depending on patient populations and geographic location. Overall survival of HIV patients on dialysis historically was worse compared to that of the general ESRD population, mainly due to increased risk of infections (Atta et al., 2007). Older age, lower serum albumin level, lower CD4[+] T-cell count, and lack of ART have all been associated with poor survival in PWH undergoing hemodialysis or peritoneal dialysis. It appears that the incidence of ESRD has plateaued, but the prevalence of PWH undergoing dialysis in the US has increased, likely due to the aging of the HIV population (Cohen et al., 2017). Survival among these patients receiving dialysis is now similar to persons without HIV disease (Campos et al., 2016; Razzak et al., 2015). Peritoneal dialysis is also an option for some PWH, with data supporting its use. In one study of 70 PWH on continuous peritoneal dialysis, there was no increase in technique failure rates or catheter patency compared to non-HIV patients at 1 year, although the rate of hospital admission and all-cause mortality was higher in the HIV-infected group (Ndlovu & Assounga, 2017).

RENAL TRANSPLANTATION

Renal transplantation was previously contraindicated in PWH due to the concern of using immunosuppressive agents in persons with an impaired immune system. However, increasing data show that renal transplantation is both safe and effective in PWH (Locke et al., 2015; Zheng et al., 2019). A single-center study examined the transplant outcomes of 16 PWH undergoing renal transplant. Despite higher rates of acute rejection at 1 and 3 years (18% and 27%, respectively), 1- and 3-year graft survival rates were 100% and 81%, respectively (Waheed et al., 2015). Initially, renal transplantation in HIV patients was performed without induction therapy. However, the use of antithymocyte globulin as induction therapy is associated with a 2.6-fold lower risk of rejection, as shown in a study of 516 PWH (Locke et al., 2014). Many of the agents used in post-transplantation immunosuppression have antiretroviral properties. Mycophenolate mofetil has virostatic properties by depleting the guanosine nucleosides necessary for the viral life cycle. Calcineurin inhibitors (tacrolimus and cyclosporine) selectively inhibit infected cell growth, and sirolimus disrupts infective viral replication by suppressing antigen-presenting cell function.

Currently undergoing investigation is the *APOL1* status of the donor and reports suggesting increased rates of kidney failure after donation from persons with high-risk *APOL1* genotypes. Recipient *APOL1* status does not appear to affect graft survival, which suggests that renal *APOL1* and not circulating *APOL1*, derived from the liver, is the main driver of *APOL1* kidney disease (Freedman & Julian, 2015). There are limited data from large prospectively designed trials, but the *APOL1* Long-Term Kidney Transplantation Outcomes Network (APOLLO) study is currently under way. Additional evaluation of these patients is needed to determine causality to the *APOL1* donor kidney. This would help donor and recipient education as they weigh the risks and benefits of *APOL1* high-risk kidney donation against remaining on dialysis. A more comprehensive analysis is needed as it has the potential to change the allocation and outcomes of kidney transplantation (Friedman & Pollak, 2021).

PWH considered eligible for renal transplant should have a CD4[+] T-cell count greater than 200/mm^3 and an undetectable viral load while on a stable ART regimen. There is concern for drug–drug interactions between some antiretroviral drugs (ARVs) and immunosuppressive agents. This is especially true for ritonavir or cobicistat-boosted PIs that are metabolized through the cytochrome P450 system. Thus, although kidney transplantation is effective in PWH, it requires close monitoring of drug levels and rejection risk. The HIV Organ Policy Equity (HOPE) was signed into law in November 2013 and implemented in 2015. This legislation allows for the transplantation of kidneys and other organs from HIV-infected donors to HIV-positive recipients. It should increase the donor pool and shorten wait time and may make transplant a viable option for a greater number of patients with ESRD (Cohen et al., 2017).

RECOMMENDED READING

Naicker S. HIV/AIDS and chronic kidney disease. *Clin Nephrol.* 2020;93(1):87–93.
Wojciechowski D, Ghandi RT, Rosales IA. Case 11-2019: a 49-year-old man with HIV infection and chronic kidney disease. *N Engl J Med.* 2019;380:1464–1472.

ART-RELATED KIDNEY COMPLICATIONS

ART has been known for many years to cause both acute and chronic injury. This was seen early in the epidemic with several of the PIs, including indinavir sulfate. Later it was found that tenofovir disoproxil fumarate (TDF) could cause AKI and proximal, sometimes irreversible tubular dysfunction. Other agents, as will be discussed in this section, are not inherently nephrotoxic but can increase serum creatinine levels by blocking tubular secretion. Lastly, with the aging of the HIV population and associated comorbidities, polypharmacy related to ART and medications for other comorbid conditions can increase the risk of acute and chronic kidney disease in PWH.

NUCLEOS(T)IDE REVERSE TRANSCRIPTASE INHIBITORS

TDF is a nucleotide reverse transcriptase inhibitor (NRTI) that is used in HIV patients and has been associated with chronic kidney disease. It is cleared by the kidneys via active proximal tubular secretion and glomerular filtration. Due to high renal toxicity rates of its acyclic nucleotide predecessors adefovir and cidofovir, both of which cause AKI and proximal tubular toxicity, there was initial concern regarding the potential renal toxicity of TDF. Early studies did not reveal significant toxicity related to TDF, but after approval by the US Food and Drug Administration (FDA), case reports emerged of Fanconi syndrome, kidney injury, and diabetes insipidus (Gaspar et al., 2004; Karras et al., 2003). The active ingredient of TDF is TFV, and nephrotoxicity is proportional to plasma TFV concentrations. TFV undergoes glomerular filtration and active secretion by the renal proximal tubule cells (PTC) via the organic anion transporter pathway. As it accumulates in the renal PTC, TFV alters DNA expression of endothelial nitric oxide synthase, the sodium-phosphorus cotransporter, sodium/hydrogen exchanger 3, and aquaporin 2. It is manifested as intense renal vasoconstriction, phosphaturia, proximal tubular acidosis, polyuria, and impaired urine-concentrating ability (Novick et al., 2017). Proximal tubular dysfunction, which may manifest as a Fanconi syndrome or a limited defect, is the most common manifestation of mitochondrial disease and supports the hypothesis that TFV exposure causes mitochondrial dysfunction (Kalyesubula & Perazella, 2011). Fanconi syndrome is characterized by proximal tubular kidney dysfunction, with decreased tubular reabsorption and urinary wasting of phosphate, glucose, amino acids, bicarbonate, and sodium. This solute loss leads to acidosis, bone disease, and electrolyte abnormalities. Most patients do not develop full Fanconi syndrome but instead manifest primarily with urinary phosphate wasting and, hence, hypophosphatemia in most cases (Waheed et al., 2015). This may occur in isolation or in conjunction with AKI. Urinary phosphate wasting is a more sensitive marker of TDF-induced nephrotoxicity because hypophosphatemia is not present in all cases. Patients with low $CD4^+$ T-cell counts, advanced age, lower body weight, and higher baseline serum creatinine are most at risk for developing TDF-induced nephrotoxicity.

A long-term follow-up of 23,905 PWH in the Data Collection on Adverse Events of Anti-HIV Drugs (D:A:D) study cohort who initiated ARVs with normal eGFR (>90 mL/min/1.73 m²) showed a significant increase in the development of CKD with exposure to TFV, ritonavir-boosted atazanavir, and ritonavir-boosted lopinavir but not other ritonavir-boosted PIs or abacavir (Mocroft et al., 2015). These findings are similar to those of previous studies in the cohort and added to the expanding literature on the long-term effects of ARVs on the kidney.

Tenofovir alafenamide (TAF) is a prodrug of TDF that has potent anti-HIV-1 activity and a higher intracellular concentration in peripheral blood mononuclear cells compared to TDF while maintaining a lower plasma concentration (Markowitz et al., 2014). With TAF's increased stability and lower plasma concentrations of TFV compared to TDF, it has a much better renal side-effect profile. Additionally, TFV released from TDF undergoes active renal secretion via organic anion transporters (OAT1 and OAT3), leading to higher exposure of renal proximal tubules to TFV and a potential for toxicity. Unlike TDF, TAF does not interact with renal transporters OAT1 and OAT3 and therefore is considered safer (Bam et al., 2014). In a randomized controlled trial of PWH who had achieved virologic suppression (viral load <50 mL/min) on a TDF-based regimen with a GFR of 50 mL/min or higher, patients were randomly assigned to continue the same ART or were switched to a TAF-based regimen (in combination with elvitegravir, cobicistat, and emtricitabine). The TAF-containing regimen led to continued viral suppression with improvement in bone mineral density and renal function (Mills et al., 2016). Other "switch" studies have also found that laboratory markers of moderately/severely increased proteinuria improved after patients were changed from TDF-based to TAF-based ART (Schwarze-Zande et al., 2020).

Although uncommon, at least one case report showed that accumulation of TFV from TAF could still be sufficient to cause mitochondrial dysfunction. Confounding variables in this case included previous TDF exposure, supratherapeutic TAF levels from preexisting kidney disease, and diabetic kidney disease altering proximal tubule mitochondria as possible etiologies for the enlarged dysmorphic mitochondria seen on biopsy. However, the most compelling evidence that TAF was the offending agent was that withdrawing the drug from the patient's ART resulted in recovery off dialysis. In addition, the patient's renal biopsy showed no evidence of other acute insults (Novick et al., 2017). Based on current knowledge of TDF toxicities, there is no absolute consensus regarding the monitoring of kidney function in patients on TFV-based ART regimens. Some experts recommend a GFR-based approach while others advocate periodic monitoring of additional markers of renal function in all patients on TFV regardless of GFR (Fine & Gallant, 2013; Holt et al., 2014). Although the renal toxicity of TDF is mostly reversible with the cessation of this drug, patients often do not achieve their pre-TDF creatinine clearance levels (Waheed et al., 2015). With the increased availability of single-table ART regimens that contain TAF, the use of TDF in the US has significantly declined. Clinicians should be vigilant regarding monitoring patients for renal toxicity, with early change in the regimen when toxicity is identified.

PROTEASE INHIBITORS

PIs are used less frequently with the availability of newer and safer ARVs but still have a role for some patients, especially those with high-level drug resistance. Two of these agents, indinavir and atazanavir, can cause urolithiasis. This was most frequently seen with indinavir, one of the first PIs first approved by the FDA in 1996, but has also been observed with other PIs (Huynh et al., 2011; Rockwood et al., 2011). With expanded use, indinavir was also associated with progression of CKD. As noted earlier, this drug is rarely used in the US, so its toxicity has become more of historical importance (McLaughlin et al., 2018).

Several studies found nephrotoxicity associated with atazanavir use after its approval in 2003. The largest included 22,603 D:A:D cohort participants with normal baseline kidney function (eGFR >90 mL/min). The decline in eGFR by more than 20 mL/min to less than 70 mL/min was associated with the use of TFV with ritonavir-boosted atazanavir. An earlier study of the EuroSIDA cohort (a subset of the D:A:D cohort) found similar results in a smaller study of PWH (Mocroft et al., 2010). In a study of a large Veterans Health Administration population, Scherzer et al. (2012) showed an association between atazanavir use and rapid GFR decline. The formation of kidney stones with atazanavir use has been well described in the literature (Chan-Tack et al., 2007).

Therefore, a plausible mechanism for the potential toxicity may be related to the predilection for atazanavir to crystallize in renal interstitial tissues and urine. With many studies confirming an association of nephrotoxicity with atazanavir, close monitoring of renal function in patients taking this PI is recommended. If a decline in GFR or other evidence of nephrotoxicity is noted, it should be discontinued. If a PI is needed to maintain viral suppression, switching to an alternative agent such as darunavir, which has not been associated with kidney stones or nephrotoxicity, is recommended (McLaughlin et al., 2018).

INTEGRASE STRAND TRANSFER INHIBITORS

Integrase strand transfer inhibitors (INSTIs) have become the most commonly used class of drugs to treat HIV disease due to their efficacy, safety, and tolerability. Raltegravir was the first FDA-approved INSTI, and several published studies assessed its effect on renal function. A retrospective study of 29 PWH started on raltegravir noted a small but nonsignificant increase in serum creatinine. The authors concluded there was no evidence of direct nephrotoxicity but the increases were likely due to inhibition of renal organic cation transporter 2 (OCT2) (Lindeman et al., 2016).

In a similar fashion, it was subsequently found that another INSTI, dolutegravir, inhibits the tubular secretion of creatinine through OCT2 at the basolateral membrane of the proximal tubular cells. This raises the serum creatinine concentration without affecting the actual GFR (Rathbun et al., 2014). A phase 1 study by Koteff et al. (2013) included 34 healthy individuals who received 50 mg dolutegravir twice daily or placebo for 14 days. Participants received iohexol, which is freely filtered, and para-aminohippurate (PAH) on days 1, 7, and 14 to see if dolutegravir impacted GFR or renal blood flow. Additional tubular function biomarkers, including albumin, cystatin C, and total protein, were also measured. The authors determined that dolutegravir increased serum creatinine levels by 10% to 14% but did not impact renal blood flow or glomerular filtration (Koteff et al., 2013).

In the SPRING-1 and SPRING-2 HIV clinical trials that enrolled treatment-naive patients, a noticeable rise in serum creatinine was noted in patients who received dolutegravir, without any significant clinical adverse effects (Raffi et al., 2013; Stellbrink et al., 2013). The rise in creatinine was typically seen in the first week of therapy, then stabilized. In the VIKING trial, a similar pattern was noted for PWH who had developed resistance to raltegravir and switched to dolutegravir (Eron et al., 2013).

Elvitegravir, another INSTI, is primarily metabolized by the liver into two metabolites. A very small amount is excreted unchanged in the urine (McLaughlin et al., 2018). It is therefore not felt to present any risks of nephrotoxicity. However, it is coadministered with cobicistat (COBI), so small increases in serum creatinine in patients taking this drug have also been reported (Imaz et al., 2017).

Bictegravir is a second-generation INSTI that is currently widely used in the US and developing countries in both treatment-naive and -experienced patients. This drug has

been evaluated in several large phase 3 clinical trials, with in vitro studies showing a relatively higher barrier to resistance compared to other ARVs. Coformulated bictegravir, emtricitabine, and TAF was compared to dolutegravir-based combination ART in two noninferiority trials (Gallant et al., 2017; Sax et al., 2017). In these studies, the estimated GFR declined by −7.0 mL/min in the bictegravir arm and −11.3 mL/min in the dolutegravir arm at week 48, but there were no patient discontinuations due to kidney-related adverse events and no cases of tubulopathy.

Several subsequent studies evaluated the efficacy and safety of switching to a bictegravir-based regimen from either a dolutegravir-based or PI-based regimen (Daar et al., 2018; Molina et al., 2018). There were no discontinuations of therapy due to renal adverse effects. Changes in serum creatinine, serum eGFR, and urinary markers such as albumin-to-creatinine ratio were also not significant.

PHARMACOKINETIC ENHANCER

Several ARVs are coformulated with COBI, a cytochrome P450 inhibitor. COBI increases serum levels of specific ARVs and allows once-daily dosing of these drugs (Johnson & Saravolatz, 2014). Although COBI has no inherent nephrotoxicity, it inhibits the cationic renal transporter MATE1 (multidrug and toxin extrusion protein-efflux) at the apical membrane of the proximal tubular cells, which blocks tubular secretion of creatinine (Figure 39.1) (Lepist et al., 2011). This leads to an increase in the plasma creatinine concentration without any effect on the actual GFR. This finding was evaluated in a study of 36 patients in which COBI use was associated with an increase in serum creatinine and an approximately 10-mL/min decrease in eGFR. The decrease in

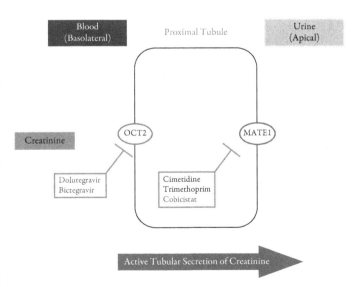

Figure 39.1: Effect of drugs on creatinine secretion. Inhibition of creatinine transporter by drugs shown will result in increase in serum creatinine without GFR effects.

Model for effect of tested drugs on creatinine secretion. BCRP, breast cancer resistance protein; MATE, multidrug and toxin extrusion protein; MRP, multidrug resistance protein; OCT, organic cation transporter; OCTN, organic cation/ergothioneine transporter; Pgp, P-glycoprotein.
SOURCE: From Lepist I, et al., ICAAC 2011, Chicago. Poster A1-1724.

eGFR was reversible upon discontinuation of the medication, thus highlighting that this drug has no adverse effect on the actual GFR (German et al., 2010). The timing of the increase in creatinine and subsequent resolution after COBI discontinuation was consistent with altered proximal tubular creatinine secretion.

DOSE ADJUSTMENT OF ART IN RENAL INSUFFICIENCY

Most nonnucleoside reverse transcriptase inhibitors (NNRTIs), integrase inhibitors, and PIs do not require dose modification in CKD or ESRD and can therefore can be safely used. TDF alone or coformulated with other ARVs should be avoided in PWH with a creatinine clearance of less than 50 mL/min and stopped in those with declining eGFR. There may be instances in which other options are not available, and dose adjustments with TDF, including giving this drug three times weekly, can be made. In general, the availability of TAF makes this less of a clinical issue for most patients taking TFV as part of their ART regimen.

Patient who are taking combination single-tablet regimens often will require separation of the component drugs for individual dosing if they have a decline in renal function. However, a small study ($n = 55$) found that a once-daily single tablet comprising elvitegravir, COBI, emtricitabine, and TAF was effective in maintaining virologic suppression in PWH on chronic hemodialysis over 96 weeks of follow-up. It was well tolerated and associated with improved patient satisfaction (Eron et al., 2019).

CKD SCREENING AND MONITORING IN PWH

CKD may have a prolonged asymptomatic period; therefore, all PWH should be monitored on a regular basis for CKD. Appropriate diagnosis and management of other risk factors for CKD, including diabetes and hypertension, should also be part of routine care of PWH. In 2017, KDIGO made specific recommendations regarding screening and monitoring for renal dysfunction in persons with HIV (Swanepoel et al., 2018). They noted that kidney disease risk stratification should be considered when choosing an ART regimen for PWH. This document states that "standard ART" as recommended by treatment guidelines may be used in those with "low risk" for CKD (eGFR >90 mL/min, urine protein/creatinine ratio [uPCR] <200 mg/g, <50 years of age). Avoidance of potentially nephrotoxic ART agents (e.g., TDF, indinavir, atazanavir, and lopinavir) is recommended in those with "high risk" for CKD (eGFR <70 mL/min, uPCR >500 mg/g, >60 years of age, hepatitis C coinfection, diabetes mellitus, uncontrolled hypertension, or cardiovascular disease). Yearly screening of PWH for proteinuria and eGFR is recommended for those who are clinically stable and virologically suppressed on ART. Proteinuria can be quantified by a urine albumin/creatinine ratio or uPCR. Those at higher risk should have

assessment of eGFR screening for proteinuria at least twice per year. All PWH should have renal function reassessed at baseline and then at 1 month after ART modification. Those on TDF with a ritonavir- or COBI-boosted PI should be assessed two to four times per year with eGFR, proteinuria, serum phosphorus, urinalysis, and fractional excretion of phosphate (Swanepoel et al., 2018).

RECOMMENDED READING

Wearne N, Davidson B, Blockman M, et al. HIV, drugs and the kidney. *Drugs in Context*. 2020;9:2019-11-1.

REFERENCES

Atta MG, Fine DM, Kirk GD, et al. Survival during renal replacement therapy among African Americans infected with HIV type 1 in urban Baltimore, Maryland. *Clin Infect Dis.* 2007;45(12):1625–1632.

Atta MG, Lucas GM, Fine DM. HIV-associated nephropathy: epidemiology, pathogenesis, diagnosis and management. *Expert Rev Anti Infect Ther.* 2008;6(3):365–371.

Balow JE. Nephropathy in the context of HIV infection. *Kidney Int.* 2005;67(4):1632–1633.

Bam RA, Birkus G, Babusis D, et al. Metabolism and antiretroviral activity of tenofovir alafenamide in CD4+ T-cells and macrophages from demographically diverse donors. *Antivir Ther.* 2014;19(7):669–677.

Becker S, Fusco G, Fusco J, et al. HIV-associated thrombotic microangiopathy in the era of highly active antiretroviral therapy: an observational study. *Clin Infect Dis.* 2004;39(Suppl 5):S267–S275.

Bige N, Lanternier F, Viard JP, et al. Presentation of HIV-associated nephropathy and outcome in HAART-treated patients. *Nephrol Dial Transplant.* 2012;27(3):1114–1121.

Briggs WA, Tanawattanacharoen S, Choi MJ, et al. Clinicopathologic correlates of prednisone treatment of human immunodeficiency virus-associated nephropathy. *Am J Kidney Dis.* 1996;28(4):618–621.

Bruggeman LA, Dikman S, Meng C, et al. Nephropathy in human immunodeficiency virus-1 transgenic mice is due to renal transgene expression. *J Clin Invest.* 1997;100(1):84–92.

Campos P, Ortiz A, Soto K. HIV and kidney diseases: 35 years of history and consequences. *Clin Kidney J.* 2016;9(6):772–781.

Chan-Tack KM, Truffa MM, Struble KA, et al. Atazanavir-associated nephrolithiasis: cases from the US Food and Drug Administration's Adverse Event Reporting System. *AIDS.* 2007;21(9):1215–1218.

Choi A, Rodriguez RA, Bacchetti P, et al. The impact of HIV on chronic kidney disease outcomes. *Kidney Int.* 2007;72(11):1380–1387.

Choi A, Scherzer R, Bacchetti P, et al. Cystatin C, albuminuria, and 5-year all-cause mortality in HIV-infected persons. *Am J Kidney Dis.* 2010;56(5):872–882.

Cohen SD, Kimmel PL. Renal biopsy is necessary for the diagnosis of HIV-associated renal diseases. *Nat Clin Pract Nephrol.* 2009;5(1):22–23.

Cohen SD, Kopp JB, Kimmel PL. Kidney diseases associated with human immunodeficiency virus infection. *N Engl J Med.* 2017;377(24):2363–2375.

Daar ES, DeJesus E, Ruane P, et al. Efficacy and safety of switching to fixed-dose bictegravir, emtricitabine, and tenofovir alafenamide from boosted protease inhibitor-based regimens in virologically suppressed adults with HIV-1: 48-week results of a randomised, open-label, multicenter, phase 3, non-inferiority trial. *Lancet HIV.* 2018;5(7):347–356.

D'Agati V, Suh J, Carbone L, et al. Pathology of HIV-associated nephropathy: a detailed morphologic and comparative study. *Kidney Int.* 1989;35(6):1358–1370.

Dragović G, Srdić D, Al Musalhi K, et al. Higher levels of cystatin C in HIV/AIDS patients with metabolic syndrome. *Basic Clin Pharmacol Toxicol*. 2018;122:396–401.

Eron J, Clotet B, Katlama C, et al. Safety and efficacy of dolutegravir in treatment-experienced subjects with ratlegravir-resistant HIV type 1 infection: 24-week results of the VIKING Study. *J Infect Dis*. 2013;207(5):740–748.

Eron J, Lelievre JD, Kalayjian R. Longer-term safety and efficacy of elvitegravir/cobicistat/emtricitabine/tenofovir alafenamide in virologically suppressed adults living with HIV and ESRD on chronic hemodialysis. *Open Forum Infect Dis*. 2019;6(S-2):864.

Eustace JA, Nuermberger E, Choi M, et al. Cohort study of the treatment of severe HIV-associated nephropathy with corticosteroids. *Kidney Int*. 2000;58(3):1253–1260.

Fine DM, Gallant JE. Nephrotoxicity of antiretroviral agents: is the list getting longer? *J Infect Dis*. 2013;207(9):1349–1351.

Fine DM, Perazella MA, Lucas GM, et al. Kidney biopsy in HIV: beyond HIV-associated nephropathy. *Am J Kidney Dis*. 2008;51(3):504–514.

Freedman BI, Julian BA, Pastan SO, et al. Apolipoprotein L1 gene variants in deceased organ donors are associated with renal allograft failure. *Am J Transplant*. 2015;15(6):1615–1622.

Friedman DJ, Pollak MR. *APOL1* nephropathy: from genetics to clinical applications. *Clin J Am Soc Nephrol*. 2021;16(2):294–303.

Gallant JE, Lazzarin A, Mills A, et al. Bictegravir, emtricitabine, and tenofovir alafenamide versus dolutegravir, abacavir, and lamivudine for initial treatment of HIV-1 infection (GS-US-380-1489): a double-blind, multicentre, phase 3, randomised controlled non-inferiority trial. *Lancet*. 2017;390(10107):2063–2072.

Gaspar G, Monereo A, Garcia-Reyne A, et al. Fanconi syndrome and acute renal failure in a patient treated with tenofovir: a call for caution. *AIDS*. 2004;18:351–352.

Genovese G, Friedman DJ, Ross MD, et al. Association of trypanolytic ApoL1 variants with kidney disease in African Americans. *Science*. 2010;329(5993):841–845.

German P, Warren D, West S, et al. Pharmacokinetics and bioavailability of an integrase and novel pharmacoenhancer-containing single-tablet fixed-dose combination regimen for the treatment of HIV. *J AIDS*. 2010;55(3):323–329.

Heron JE, Bagnis CI, Gracey DM. Contemporary issues and new challenges in chronic kidney disease amongst people living with HIV. *AIDS Res Ther*. 2020;17(1):11. doi:10.1186/s12981-020-00266-3

Holt SG, Gracey DM, Levy MT, et al. A consensus statement on the renal monitoring of Australian patients receiving tenofovir based antiviral therapy for HIV/HBV infection. *AIDS Res Ther*. 2014;11:35.

Huynh J, Hever A, Tom T, et al. Indinavir-induced nephrolithiasis three and one-half years after cessation of indinavir therapy. *Int Urol Nephrol*. 2011;43(2):571–573.

Izzedine H, Acharya V, Wirden M, et al. Role of HIV-1 DNA levels as clinical marker of HIV-1-associated nephropathies. *Nephrol Dial Transplant*. 2011;26(2):580–583.

Johnson LB, Saravolatz LD. The quad pill, a once-daily combination therapy for HIV infection. *Clin Infect Dis*. 2014;58(1):93–98.

Kalayjian RC. Renal issues in HIV infection. *Curr HIV AIDS Rep*. 2011;8(3):164–171.

Kalyesubula R, Perazella MA. Nephrotoxicity of HAART. *AIDS Res Treat*. 2011;2011:562790.

Karras A, Lafaurie M, Furco A, et al. Tenofovir-related nephrotoxicity in human immunodeficiency virus-infected patients: three cases of renal failure, Fanconi syndrome, and nephrogenic diabetes insipidus. *Clin Infect Dis*. 2003;36:1070–1073.

Kimmel PL, Mishkin GJ, Umana WO. Captopril and renal survival in patients with human immunodeficiency virus nephropathy. *Am J Kidney Dis*. 1996;28(2):202–208.

Kopp JB, Nelson GW, Sampath K, et al. Genetic variants in focal segmental glomerulosclerosis and HIV-associated nephropathy. *J Am Soc Nephrol*. 2011;22(11):2129–2137.

Koteff J, Borland J, Chen S, et al. A phase 1 study to evaluate the effect of dolutegravir on renal function via measured iohexol and PAH clearance in healthy subjects. *Br J Clin Pharmacol*. 2013;75:990–996.

Kudose S, Santoriello D, Bomback AS, et al. The spectrum of kidney biopsy findings in HIV-infected patients in the modern era. *Kidney Int*. 2020;97(5):1006–1016.

Lepist EI, Murray BP, Tong L, et al. Effect of cobicistat and ritonavir on proximal renal tubular cell uptake and efflux transporters [Abstract A1-1724]. Presented at the 51st Interscience Conference on Antimicrobial Agents and Chemotherapy (ICAAC), Chicago, September 17–20, 2011.

Lescure FX, Flateau C, Pacanowski J, et al. HIV-associated kidney glomerular diseases: changes with time and HAART. *Nephrol Dial Transplant*. 2012;27:2349–2355.

Lindeman TA, Dugan JM, Sahloff EG. Evaluation of serum creatinine changes with integrase inhibitor use in HIV-1 infected adults. *Open Forum Infect Dis*. 2016;3(2):1–3.

Locke JE, James NT, Mannon RB, et al. Immunosuppression regimen and the risk of acute rejection in HIV-infected kidney transplant recipients. *Transplantation*. 2014;97(4):446–450.

Locke JE, Mehta S, Reed RD, et al. A national study of outcomes among HIV-infected kidney transplant recipients. *J Am Soc Nephrol*. 2015;26(9):2222–2229.

Longenecker CT, Scherzer R, Bacchetti P, et al. HIV viremia and changes in kidney function. *AIDS*. 2009;23(9):1089–1096.

Lopes JA, Melo MJ, Raimundo M, et al. Long-term risk of mortality for acute kidney injury in HIV-infected patients: a cohort analysis. *BMC Nephrol*. 2013;14:32.

Lucas GM, Eustace JA, Sozio S, et al. Highly active antiretroviral therapy and the incidence of HIV-1-associated nephropathy: a 12-year cohort study. *AIDS*. 2004;18(3):541–546.

Makris K, Spanou L. Acute kidney injury: definition, pathophysiology, and clinical phenotypes. *Clin Biochem Review*. 2016;37(2):85–98.

Markowitz M, Zolopa A, Squires K, et al. Phase I/II study of the pharmacokinetics, safety and antiretroviral activity of tenofovir alafenamide, a new prodrug of the HIV reverse transcriptase inhibitor tenofovir, in HIV-infected adults. *J Antimicrob Chemother*. 2014;69(5):1362–1369.

McLaughlin MM, Guerrero AJ, Merker A. Renal effects of non-tenofovir antiretroviral therapy in patients living with HIV. *Drugs in Context*. 2018;7:1–15.

Medapalli RK, He JC, Klotman JP. HIV-associated nephropathy: pathogenesis. *Curr Opin Nephrol Hypertens*. 2011;20(3):306–311.

Mills A, Arribas JR, Andrade-Villanueva J, et al. Switching from tenofovir disoproxil fumarate to tenofovir alafenamide in antiretroviral regimens for virologically suppressed adults with HIV-1 infection: a randomised, active-controlled, multicentre, open-label, phase 3, non-inferiority study. *Lancet Infect Dis*. 2016;16(1):43–52.

Mocroft A, Kirk O, Reiss P, et al. Estimated glomerular filtration rate, chronic kidney disease and antiretroviral drug use in HIV-positive patients. *AIDS*. 2010;24(11):1667–1678.

Mocroft A, Lundgren JD, Ross M, et al.; D:A:D Study Group Royal Free Hospital Clinic Cohort, Insight Study Group, Smart Study Group and Esprirt Study Group. Development and validation of a risk score for chronic kidney disease in HIV infection using protective cohort data from the D:A:D study. *PLoS Med*. 2015;12(3):e1001809.

Molina JM, Ward D, Brar I, et al. Switching to fixed-dose bictegravir, emtricitabine, and tenofovir alafenamide from dolutegravir plus abacavir and lamivudine in virologically suppressed adults with HIV-1: 48-week results of a randomised, double-blind, multicentre, active-controlled, phase 3, non-inferiority trial. *Lancet HIV*. 2018;5(7):357–365.

Naicker S, Fabian J. Risk factors for the development of chronic kidney disease with HIV/AIDS. *Clin Nephrol*. 2010;74(Suppl 1):S51–S56.

Neuen BL, Young T, Heerspink HJL, et al. SGLT2 inhibitors for the prevention of kidney failure in patients with type 2 diabetes: A systematic review and meta-analysis. *Lancet Diabetes Endocrinol*. 2019;7(11):845–854.

Novick TK, Choi MJ, Rosenberg AZ, et al. Tenofovir alafenamide nephrotoxicity in an HIV-positive patient. *Medicine*. 2017;96(36):e8046.

Ndlovu KCZ, Assounga A. Continuous ambulatory peritoneal dialysis in patients with HIV and end-stage renal failure. *Perit Dial Int*. 2017;37(3):321–330.

Palich R, Tubiana R, Abdi B, et al. Plasma cystatin C as a marker for estimated glomerular filtration rate assessment in HIV-1-infected patients treated with dolutegravir-based ART. *J Antimicrob Chemother.* 2018;73(7):1935–1939.

Papeta N, Kiryluk K, Patel A, et al. APOL1 variants increase risk for FSGS and HIVAN but not IgA nephropathy. *J Am Soc Nephrol.* 2011;22(11):1991–1996.

Post FA, Holt SG. Recent developments in HIV and the kidney. *Curr Opin Infect Dis.* 2009;22(1):43–48.

Raffi F, Rachlis A, Stellbrink HJ, et al. Once-daily dolutegravir versus raltegravir in antiretroviral-naïve adults with HIV-1 infection: 48-week results from the randomized, double-blind, non-inferiority SPRING-2 Study. *Lancet.* 2013;381(9868):735–743.

Rao TK, Filippone EJ, Nicastri AD, et al. Associated focal and segmental glomerulosclerosis in the acquired immunodeficiency syndrome. *N Engl J Med.* 1984;310(11):669–673.

Rathbun RC, Lockhart SM, Miller MM, et al. Dolutegravir, a second-generation integrase inhibitor for the treatment of HIV-1 infection. *Ann Pharmacother.* 2014;48(3):395–403.

Ratnam KK, Feng W, Chuang PY, et al. Role of the retinoic acid receptor-alpha in HIV-associated nephropathy. *Kidney Int.* 2011;79(6):624–634.

Razzak CS, Workeneh BT, Montez-Rath ME, et al. Trends in the out-comes of end-stage renal disease secondary to HIV-associated nephropathy. *Nephrol Dial Transplant.* 2015;30:1734–1740.

Rockwood N, Mandalia S, Bower M, et al. Ritonavir-boosted atazanavir exposure is associated with an increased rate of renal stones compared with efavirenz, ritonavir-boosted lopinavir and ritonavir-boosted darunavir. *AIDS.* 2011;25(13):1671–1673.

Ross MJ, Klotman PE. Recent progress in HIV-associated nephropathy. *J Am Soc Nephrol.* 2002;13(12):2997–3004.

Ryom L, Lundgren JD, Law M, et al. Serious clinical events in HIV-positive persons with chronic kidney disease. *AIDS.* 2019;33(14):2173–2188.

Sax PE, Pozniak A, Montes ML, et al. Co-formulated bictegravir, emtricitabine, and tenofovir alafenamide versus dolutegravir with emtricitabine and tenofovir alafenamide, for initial treatment of HIV-1 infection (GS-US-380-1490): a randomised, double-blind, multicentre, phase 3, non-inferiority trial. *Lancet.* 2017;390(10107):2073–2082.

Scherzer R, Estrella M, Li Y, et al. Association of tenofovir exposure with kidney disease risk in HIV infection. *AIDS.* 2012;26(7):867–875.

Schwarze-Zander C, Piduhn H, Boesecke C, et al. Switching tenofovir disoproxil fumarate to tenofovir alafenamide in a real-life setting: what are the implications? *HIV Med.* 2020;21(6):378–385.

Stellbrink HJ, Reynes J, Lazzarin A, et al. Dolutegravir in antiretroviral-naive adults with HIV-1: 96-week results from a randomized dose-ranging study. *AIDS.* 2013;27(11):1771–1778.

Strategies for Management of Antiretroviral Therapy (SMART) Study Group. CD4+ count-guided interruption of antiretroviral treatment. *N Engl J Med.* 2006;355(22):2283–2296.

Swanepoel CR, Atta MG, D'Agati VD, et al. Kidney disease in the setting of HIV infection: conclusions from a Kidney Disease: Improving Global Outcomes (KDIGO) Patient Controversies Conference. *Kidney Int.* 2018;22(6):84–100.

Tzur S, Rosset S, Shemer R, et al. Missense mutations in the APOL1 gene are highly associated with end-stage kidney disease risk previously attributed to the MYH9 gene. *Hum Genet.* 2010;128(3):345–350.

Waheed S, Atta MG. Predictors of HIV-associated nephropathy. *Expert Rev Anti Infect Ther.* 2014;12(5):555–563.

Waheed S, Sakr A, Chheda N, et al. Outcomes of renal transplantation in HIV-1 associated nephropathy. *PLoS One.* 2015;10(6):e0129702.

Wei A, Burns G, Williams CM, et al. Long-term renal survival in HIV-associated nephropathy with angiotensin-converting enzyme inhibition. *Kidney Int.* 2003;64(4):1462–1471.

Wyatt CM, Hoover DR, Shi Q, et al. Pre-existing albuminuria predicts AIDS and non-AIDS mortality in women initiating antiretroviral therapy. *Antiviral Ther.* 2011;16(4):591–596.

Zheng X, Gong L, Xue W, et al. Kidney transplant outcomes in HIV-positive patients: a systematic review and meta-analysis. *AIDS Res Ther.* 2019;16(1):37.

Zhong Y, Wu Y, Liu R, et al. Roflumilast enhances the renal protective effects of retinoids in an HIV-1 transgenic mouse model of rapidly progressive renal failure. *Kidney Int.* 2012;81(9): 856–864.

40.

HIV AND BONE HEALTH

Edgar T. Overton

LEARNING OBJECTIVES

- Discuss the concept that metabolic bone disease is a common manifestation of HIV infection leading to an increased risk of fracture

- List the screening indications and diagnostic tests used to identify bone disease in PWH

WHAT'S NEW?

- Beyond the detrimental effects of active HIV replication, viral proteins that are released into the circulation likely alter normal bone metabolism through numerous detrimental bystander effects, including apoptosis, oxidative stress, and mitochondrial toxicity. These effects persist even after viral suppression with antiretroviral therapy (ART) and can exacerbate bone loss (Agidigi & Kim, 2019; Liu et al., 2017).

- Frailty, a phenotype usually described among geriatric populations, has been identified as occurring at higher rates in PWH and is associated with both osteoporosis and increased risk of fragility fractures (Pramukti et al., 2020).

- Women with HIV experience a twofold higher rate of bone loss than men with HIV (Erlandson et al., 2018).

- In the Women's Interagency HIV Study (WIHS) Study, women with HIV had similar BMD as an HIV-negative cohort matched for socioeconomic status; however, the microarchitecture or quality of bone in women with HIV was significantly worse than in HIV-negative women (Sharma et al., 2018).

- A recent study of women with HIV highlighted that HIV is associated with increased rates of prolonged secondary amenorrhea that placed these women at greater risk for declines in BMD compared to women without HIV (King et al., 2020).

- A recent meta-analysis confirmed that HIV increases the risk of fragility fracture (by 1.51 times) and of hip fracture (by 4.05 times). The increased risk is not completely explained by differences in BMD alone, indicating that differences due to quality of bone or other HIV-related factors may be contributing to the marked fracture risk (Starup-Linde et al., 2020).

- Two recent studies demonstrated that zoledronate, an intravenous bisphosphonate, is safe and durable for preserving BMD in HIV. One study demonstrated beneficial bone effects through 11 years (Bolland et al., 2019; Ofokotun et al., 2019).

- Another study highlighted that perinatally infected youth (aged 11–24) have reduced BMD and that oral alendronate is safe and effective at preserving BMD in this young population (Jacobson et al., 2020).

KEY POINTS

- Multiple cohort studies have found a higher-than-expected prevalence of low BMD in populations of adults living with HIV.

- Fracture prevalence is greater in PWH compared to the general population. Incident fracture rates among PWH in the HIV Outpatient Study (HOPS) were increased nearly threefold compared to those for the general US population. These data have been corroborated in two other recent meta-analyses.

- Asymptomatic vertebral fractures are highly prevalent among PWH over the age of 50.

- Cohort studies suggest that, in addition to traditional factors such as age, smoking, hepatitis C virus (HCV) coinfection, frailty, prolonged amenorrhea, and proteinuria. HIV disease-associated factors and ART factors are predictive indicators of fracture risk in PWH.

- ART initiation is associated with a BMD decrease of 2% to 6%, with the largest decrease occurring in the first 6 to 12 months of treatment and then stabilizing.

- Greater BMD losses occur with initiation of zidovudine (AZT), tenofovir disoproxil fumarate (TDF), and protease inhibitors (PIs).

- Bisphosphonates can safely be administered to PWH with evidence supporting durable gains in BMD, including among youth with HIV.
- There are limited HIV-specific evidence-based recommendations regarding screening for bone disease, although extrapolation of screening recommendations from the general population is reasonable. Several organizations recommend using dual-energy X-ray absorptiometry (DXA) and/or the Fracture Risk Assessment Tool (FRAX) for screening PWH at risk of fractures.

INTRODUCTION

With improved long-term survival among PWH, age-related comorbidities, including osteoporosis and fragility fractures, have become more prevalent (Justice & Falutz, 2014; Pramukti et al., 2020; Premaor & Compston, 2018). There is increasing evidence that cardiovascular, renal, and bone disease and neurocognitive deficits are more common among long-term PWH, with negative interactions between these comorbidities. Data from cohort and prospective randomized studies suggest that for a multitude of reasons, PWH are at increased risk of metabolic bone disease and related fractures (Battalora et al., 2016; Womack et al., 2011).

BONE MINERALIZATION ABNORMALITIES

The World Health Organization (WHO) defines two categories of bone abnormalities based on comparison with the mean BMD of young healthy women (T-score): (1) osteoporosis—low bone mass and microarchitectural deterioration of bone tissue, BMD value more than 2.5 standard deviations (SD) below the mean BMD of young adult women (BMD T-score < −2.5) and (2) osteopenia—low bone mass, BMD value between 1 and 2.5 SD below the mean BMD of young adult women (−2.5 < bone mineral density T-score < −1) (WHO, 1994; Woolf & Pfleger, 2003). Osteomalacia is a third type of bone mineralization abnormality and refers to softening of bones due to impaired bone mineralization typically resulting from severe vitamin D deficiency (McComsey et al., 2010; WHO, 2002). Osteonecrosis or avascular necrosis, another bone abnormality, results from interrupted blood supply to a bone or part of a bone, commonly occurring as a complication of trauma or fracture and typically located at the articular end of a bone (WHO, 2002).

In the general population, BMD peaks at approximately 22 to 35 years of age (Orwoll & Klein, 1995). Bone mineral density appears to decrease by 2% to 6% during the first 1 to 2 years of ART (Brown et al., 2009). Until recently, it was believed that PWH subsequently experienced relative stability regarding BMD, but a recent longitudinal study contradicts this belief. Grant et al. (2016) followed 97 PWH for a median of 7.5 years after ART initiation and compared their BMD data to data from 614 HIV-negative controls. While the rate of BMD loss after week 96 slowed in the cohort of PWH, the decline in lumbar spine BMD remained significantly greater than that seen in the HIV-negative cohort. These data suggest ongoing metabolic bone disease despite HIV suppression with ART. The long-term metabolic consequences of HIV and ART need further evaluation. Additional data highlight significant differences between men and women living with HIV.

A recent study included 839 female and 1,759 male PWH with two or more DXA scans. The group reflected the aging HIV epidemic, with 82% older than 50 years of age and 76% with virologic suppression (<50 copies/mL). BMD loss was associated with ART exposure, HCV coinfection, lower physical activity, and vitamin D insufficiency. Among the women, BMD at the femoral neck declined twice as fast as among men after adjusting for traditional risk factors. More attention needs to be paid to aging-associated diseases among women with HIV (Erlandson et al., 2018).

Bone strength is a function of bone density and bone quality. Bone quality refers to rate of remodeling, microarchitecture, size, shape, amount of mineralization in the bone, and matrix quality (Yin, 2012). Rate of remodeling is measured from serum levels of the bone turnover markers osteocalcin (OCN, a formation marker) and N-terminal telopeptide (NTX, a resorption marker). Microarchitecture is observed with computed tomography (CT) imaging. Mineralization quantity and matrix quality can be determined by biopsy, but this is rarely indicated. The importance of considering the microarchitecture or quality of bone was highlighted in a recent study from the WIHS (Sharma et al., 2018). In this analysis including 319 women with HIV and 118 without HIV, loss of BMD by DXA was similar between the two groups. However, the bone microarchitecture or quality of bone was significantly worse in the women with HIV. The effects of HIV on bone health are more complex than mere quantification by DXA alone.

PREVALENCE OF LOW BMD IN THE HIV POPULATION

Multiple cohort studies have found a higher-than-expected prevalence of low BMD in populations of adults living with HIV (Brown & Qaqish, 2006). Notably, these studies represent diverse populations of PWH, including ART-naive and ART-experienced patients (Bedimo et al., 2012; Escota et al., 2016; McComsey et al., 2011). A meta-analysis of 29 studies of BMD in PWH confirmed the preceding information (Goh et al., 2018). The prevalence of osteopenia and osteoporosis was 2.4 to 3.4 times higher in PWH compared to HIV-uninfected adults depending on site (lumbar spine and hip). Traditional risk factors (low body mass index [BMI], history of fracture, older age, being Hispanic or Caucasian, low testosterone levels, smoking, low CD4$^+$ T-cell counts, low lean and fat mass, and lipodystrophy) were associated with low BMD. Persons treated with TDF as part of their ART regimen were also more likely to have low BMD compared to nonusers (53% vs. 43%), but the difference was not statistically significant.

Using data from the Study to Understand the Natural History of HIV and AIDS in the Era of Effective Therapy

(SUN Study)—a prospective, observational cohort study funded by the US Centers for Disease Control and Prevention (CDC)—Escota et al. (2016) determined that low BMD at the hip and femoral neck was significantly more prevalent in PWH than in matched controls from the National Health and Nutrition Examination Survey (NHANES) (47% vs. 29%; $p < 0.001$). In this cohort of 653 participants (77% male, median age 41 years, median CD4+ T-cell count 464; 89% with HIV RNA levels <400 copies/mL), 51% of participants had osteopenia and 10% had osteoporosis at baseline.

Postmenopausal women with HIV demonstrate a greater decline in BMD. In a longitudinal study of bone loss in this specific population, higher rates of bone decline at the spine and forearm were observed compared to HIV-negative women (Yin & Overton, 2011). Thus, higher rates of bone loss at the spine and forearm of women described in this study coupled with increased fracture prevalence among PWH suggest that an increased rate of fractures in postmenopausal women with HIV is concerning (Triant et al., 2008). Similarly, an older study found higher rates of bone loss in men with HIV older than 50 years (Orwoll & Klein, 1995). However, there is still little information on bone loss for PWH over the age of 65 years, the period in which fractures are most prevalent in the general population.

There are some data from resource-limited settings regarding low BMD in HIV-infected populations. In one South African cohort of 444 HIV-infected individuals (median age 35 years; 77% women), low BMD (Z-score < −2 SD) was found in 17% of participants at the lumbar spine and 5% at the hip (Dave et al., 2015). This study found that median total hip and femoral neck BMDs were lower among those receiving ART than in ART-naive participants. Similarly, femoral neck BMD was lower among ART-receiving participants compared to ART-naive participants. In addition, vitamin D deficiency was found in 15% of cohort participants and was associated with efavirenz use. In multivariate analysis, exposure to efavirenz- or lopinavir/ritonavir-based ART was associated with lower total hip BMD. Having a higher weight, being male, and having increased vitamin D levels were associated with higher total hip BMD. Additional factors independently associated with lower lumbar spine BMD included advanced age, weight, sex, and efavirenz use (Dave et al., 2015).

Hoy et al. (2015) reported results from the Strategic Timing of Antiretroviral Treatment (START) BMD sub-study (INSIGHT START Study Group, 2015). The primary START study enrollment consisted of 4,685 adult PWH from 35 countries with CD4+ T-cell counts of greater than 500 cells/mm³; the median age was 36 years, and 27% were female. Participants were randomized to start ART at study entry or delay therapy until their CD4+ T-cell count fell below 350 cells/mm³ or they developed AIDS or another condition that dictated the use of ART (deferred-initiation group). In the BMD sub-study of this trial, 193 participants were randomized to the early ART group and 204 to the deferred ART group (Hoy et al., 2015). Sub-study participants underwent DXA scans of the lumbar spine, total hip, and femoral

neck at baseline and annually thereafter. Mean follow-up was 2.2 years. Hoy et al. reported significantly greater loss of BMD at both the hip and the spine in participants randomized to early ART. There was no difference in the development of osteoporosis between groups or incident fractures in the main START study (Hoy et al., 2015). More data are needed on the change in BMD among persons who initiate ART with a high/normal CD4+ T-cell count, as in the START trial.

HIGHER PREVALENCE AND INCIDENCE OF FRACTURES IN THE HIV POPULATION

Numerous studies have concluded that PWH are at greater risk of bone fractures. Triant et al. (2008) presented findings in 2008 that fracture prevalence was greater in HIV-infected women and men compared to the general population. Based on an analysis of more than 11 years of data from a large US single healthcare database, they determined that PWH had a higher number of vertebral, hip, wrist, and combined fractures compared with non–HIV-infected participants. These findings were consistent across age, race, and sex categories, but no correlations were made as to specific risk factors due to lack of data. A recent review article highlighted that the heterogeneity and small sample size of studies of fractures among PWH make this a challenging topic to study (Premaor & Compston, 2018). However, despite a wide range of incident fractures among PWH, ranging from 0.1 to 11.3 fractures/1,000 person-years (pys), HIV is consistently associated with an approximately twofold increased risk of fracture (Pramukti et al., 2020).

Several large observational studies published findings correlating fracture incidence in PWH compared to control groups. Differences in population, controls, and fracture definitions (i.e., fracture and fragility fracture definitions) were unique to each study. The WIHS reported fracture incidence in 1,728 HIV-infected and 663 HIV-negative premenopausal women (Yin et al., 2010). Rates of fracture were not increased in women with HIV compared to HIV-negative women. However, in the women with HIV, having a history of an AIDS-defining illness was a more predictive indicator of fracture than being on ART.

Incident fracture rates among PWH in the HOPS study were increased nearly threefold compared to rates in the general US population between 2000 and 2006 (Young et al., 2011). Rates of first fractures at any anatomic site were analyzed in 5,826 participants (median baseline age 40 years, 79% male, and 73% on ART).

Rates of fracture were indirectly standardized to the general population by age and sex using data from patients in the National Hospital Ambulatory Medical Care Survey (NHAMCS-OPD). Greater proportions of fractures were located at the hip, wrist, or spine in PWH. In this cohort, fractures were associated with lower nadir CD4+ T-cell count, longer duration of HIV diagnosis, and HIV/HCV coinfection. The study suggested that younger PWH, particularly those aged 25 to 54 years, are at an increased risk of bone fracture compared to the general population. On the basis of these data, the authors recommended regular assessment of PWH for fracture risk, particularly those with low nadir CD4[+] T-cell counts and other recognized fracture risk factors.

In the all-male Veterans Aging Cohort Study Virtual Cohort (VACS-VC) study, Womack et al. (2011) reported that men with HIV were at greater risk for fragility fracture compared to HIV-negative counterparts. In this study of 119,318 men, 33% were HIV-positive, 34% were 50 years or older at baseline, and 55% were Black or Hispanic. Fracture risk factors included age, race, alcohol dependency, liver disease, tobacco smoking, or current use of corticosteroids or proton pump inhibitors.

Hansen et al. (2012) studied the incidence of fragility fractures in PWH not receiving ART and PWH on ART in the Danish HIV Cohort. This was a comparative, sex- and age-matched study involving 5,306 PWH and a general population cohort of 26,530 HIV-negative participants. The PWH had an increased overall rate of fractures and an increased risk of low-energy fractures but not high-energy fractures. There was a moderate increased risk of low-energy fracture in PWH receiving ART when controlled for traditional osteoporosis risk factors of age and cigarette smoking.

In the AIDS Clinical Trials Group A5224s, a sub-study of ACTG A5202, McComsey et al. concluded that fracture rates increased in 269 subjects during the first 2 years of ART initiated during the clinical trial compared to additional years of therapy. Although differences in BMD change were observed between patients who initiated different ART regimens, no significant differences in fracture rate were reported, although the cohort was young and follow-up was limited (McComsey et al., 2011; Yin & Overton, 2011).

Osteoporotic fractures were associated with cumulative exposure to TDF and other ART in a large retrospective cohort study (56,600 patients) with a mean age of 45 years (Bedimo et al., 2012). However, 95% of this cohort was male, limiting the ability to generalize the conclusion to females.

Another recent publication highlighted an underappreciated fracture: asymptomatic vertebral fractures (Llop et al., 2018). In this cohort of 93 males and 35 females (mean age 57 years), with more than 70% having low BMD at both hip and spine by DXA, 20% were found to have an asymptomatic vertebral fracture. Factors associated with these fractures included older age, longer time since HIV diagnosis, and renal insufficiency. The authors concluded that routine spinal imaging with plain x-rays should be considered in the aging HIV population.

Starup-Linde et al. (2020) performed a meta-analysis that included 84 papers focused on bone health and fracture risk in the setting of HIV. They concluded that HIV infection is associated with a significant increase in incident fragility fracture (hazard ratio [HR] 1.51) and a marked increased risk of hip fracture (HR 4.05) The increased risk was not explained by the differences in BMD alone, indicating a difference in quality of bone or other factors related to HIV disease.

Findings from several cohort studies have contributed to the developing field of fracture incidence in PWH. Among 1,006 participants from two CDC-funded cohorts (median age 43 years; 83% male; median CD4[+] T-cell count 461 cells/

mm³), osteopenia was found in 36% of participants and osteoporosis in 4%. A prior fracture was documented in 67 participants. During 4,068 pys of observation after DXA scanning, 85 incident fractures occurred. These were predominantly rib/sternum (n = 18), hand (n = 14), foot (n = 13), and wrist (n = 11). Low BMD (osteopenia and/or osteoporosis) was diagnosed in nearly 40% of the participants. Associated risk factors for fractures included older age, lower nadir CD4[+] T-cell count, male–male sex HIV transmission risk, and prior history of fracture. Fourfold higher fracture rates were observed in HIV-positive participants with osteoporosis compared to PWH with normal BMD. In multivariable analyses, osteoporosis and current/prior tobacco use were associated with incident fracture (Battalora et al., 2016).

In addition to traditional risk factors such as older age and smoking, HIV-associated factors (nadir CD4[+] T-cell count) and ART factors are important predictive indicators of fracture risk in PWH (Yin, 2012). In the *Clinician's Guide to Prevention and Treatment of Osteoporosis*, the National Osteoporosis Foundation (2014) included AIDS/HIV as disease risk factors for osteoporosis and fragility fractures (Battalora et al., 2014).

Recent research has identified additional mediators of fracture risk in the setting of HIV. Frailty, a phenotype generally seen in geriatric populations, has been recognized to occur at an earlier age among PWH. Sharma et al. (2019) from the WIHS Cohort reported that frailty was not only more common among women with HIV than their HIV-negative counterparts, but it was also independently associated to time to first fracture as well as second fracture. Sarcopenia, or the gradual loss of muscle mass, is a key component of frailty and has long been recognized as a complication of HIV infection. It is not surprising that frailty is linked to fracture risk.

From the MACS cohort, Gonciulea et al. (2019) have also linked proteinuria to fragility fractures. In this cohort of both HIV-negative men and men with HIV, the presence of proteinuria, which was more common among men with HIV, conferred a 230% increased risk of fragility fracture (Gonciulea et al., 2019). These data highlight how chronic comorbidities often cluster in PWH and can significantly complicate long-term management beyond the use of ART.

PATHOPHYSIOLOGY AND RISK FACTORS

Bone loss in PWH is likely multifactorial, involving three common elements: the host, the virus, and ART. Lower bone density in PWH is attributable to host risks, including smoking, alcohol consumption, exposure to glucocorticoids, decreased activity, lipodystrophy, HCV coinfection, vitamin D deficiency, weight loss, hypogonadism, and chronic kidney disease.

At least one genetic marker or HLA supertype, specifically HLA-DQ3, has been associated with bone density status in one cohort study of HIV-positive adults (Haskelberg et al., 2014). HIV may directly affect bone cells by viral protein induction of osteoclastogenesis or by causing osteoblast apoptosis (Raynaud-Messina et al., 2018). Recent data highlight that the effects of HIV proteins on bone loss may not be a direct effect but rather an indirect or bystander effect through mitochondrial toxicity, oxidative stress, or effects on other cell processes (Agidigi & Kim, 2019; Liu et al., 2017). Moreover, T-cell and B-cell activation during HIV infection results in increased circulating cytokines, including tumor necrosis factor-α, interleukin-6 (IL-6), and RANKL, which appear to induce osteoclast bone resorption (Titanji, 2017). In a study by Hileman et al. (2014), elevated levels of IL-6 were associated with risk of progression to osteoporosis among PWH. Similar increases in cytokine levels have been reported in other chronic inflammatory diseases (e.g., rheumatoid arthritis).

It is worth noting that ART initiation has been associated with a BMD decrease of 2% to 6%, with the largest decrease occurring in the first 6 to 12 months of treatment and then stabilizing (Brown et al., 2009). Greater BMD loss was also seen with the older nucleoside agent AZT (van Vonderen et al., 2009) and was well documented with the use of TDF (McComsey et al., 2011; Yin & Overton, 2011). In addition, PIs contribute to bone loss in the setting of HIV infection, which appears to be a class effect observed with all PIs that have been studied (McComsey et al., 2011; Moran et al., 2016). Fracture rates, both fragility and nonfragility, as noted previously, are higher in PWH and associated with HCV coinfection and possibly ART (Bedimo et al., 2012; Maalouf et al., 2013). Currently, the pooled estimate of fracture incidence is noted to be 11.3/1,000 pys, a figure that will likely increase as the population of PWH ages (Pramukti et al., 2020).

CLINICAL MANAGEMENT

SCREENING FOR BONE DISEASE

There are limited evidence-based recommendations for PWH regarding screening for bone disease, although extrapolation of recommendations from the general population is, at a minimum, reasonable.

The National Osteoporosis Foundation (2014) published recommendations to clinicians for postmenopausal women and men aged 50 years or older. The reader is advised to consult the complete list of recommendations in the foundation's *Clinician's Guide to Prevention and Treatment of Osteoporosis*. A brief listing of the major recommendations is provided here:

- Counsel patient on risk of osteoporosis and related fractures.

- Assess for secondary causes of osteoporosis.

- Advise patient on adequate intake of calcium (at least 1,200 mg/day) and vitamin D (800–1,000 IU/day), including supplements if necessary, for individuals aged 50 years or older.

- Recommend regular weight-bearing and muscle-strengthening exercise to reduce risk of falls and fractures.

- Advise against tobacco smoking and excessive alcohol consumption.

- Recommend BMD testing in women aged 65 years or older and men aged 70 years or older.

- In postmenopausal women and men aged 50 to 69 years, recommend BMD testing based on risk factor profile.

- In postmenopausal women and men older than age 50 years who have had an adult-age fracture, diagnose and determine degree of osteoporosis.

- Initiate medical therapies for patients with hip or vertebral (clinical or morphometric) fractures.

- Initiate therapy in patients with BMD T-scores of −2.5 or less at the femoral neck or spine by DXA, after appropriate evaluation.

- Initiate treatment in postmenopausal women and men aged 50 years or older with low bone mass (T-score between −1.0 and −2.5, osteopenia) at the femoral neck or spine and a 10-year hip fracture probability 3% or greater or a 10-year major osteoporosis-related fracture probability of 20% or greater based on the US-adapted WHO absolute fracture risk model FRAX.

- Current US Food and Drug Administration (FDA)-approved pharmacologic options for osteoporosis are bisphosphonates (alendronate, alendronate, ibandronate, risedronate, and zoledronic acid), calcitonin, estrogen agonist/antagonist (raloxifene), estrogens and/or hormone therapy, tissue-selective estrogen complex (conjugated estrogens/bazedoxifene; parathyroid hormone [PTH] amino acid sequence 1–34 [teriparatide]), and the RANKL inhibitor denosumab.

- BMD testing performed in DXA centers using accepted quality assurance measures is appropriate for monitoring bone loss (FDA, 2013).

- Patients taking FDA-approved medications for low BMD should have laboratory and bone density reevaluation after 2 years or more frequently when medically appropriate (National Osteoporosis Foundation, 2014).

Brown et al. (2015) published recommendations for evaluation and management of bone disease in PWH. Input on these recommendations was provided by 34 HIV specialists from 16 countries. Noting global variation in practice and thus difficulty in determining one set of recommendations for evaluation and management of bone disease, use of the FRAX risk calculator (see later in the chapter) without BMD assessment is recommended for patient assessment in resource-limited settings without access to DEXA scanning. The reader is referred to this publication for a complete listing of their recommendations and clinical rationale. With future observational data from HIV cohorts, updates to these recommendations can be anticipated.

SCREENING FOR VITAMIN D INSUFFICIENCY

Vitamin D testing and supplementation remains an area of debate among clinicians. Various groups and institutions have published guidance regarding vitamin D deficiency, although none are specific for PWH. The Institute of Medicine (2010) published dietary reference intakes for calcium and vitamin D but did not provide screening recommendations or specific reference intakes for PWH. The Endocrine Society (2011) and the European AIDS Clinical Society (2020) recommended screening at-risk patients and those on ART and having risk factors for low vitamin D or fracture risks. The US Preventive Service Task Force and the American Academy of Family Physicians have concluded that the current evidence is insufficient to assess the balance of benefits and harms of screening for vitamin D deficiency in asymptomatic adults (LeFevre & LeFevre, 2018). There are limited data on vitamin D supplementation in PWH, although several studies have demonstrated benefit for BMD and reduction in PTH and bone turnover markers (Havens et al., 2018b; Overton et al., 2015).

SCREENING FOR FALL RISK

Fall risk assessment tools are used to determine the probability of future falls. Typical categories of the assessment tools include fall risk factors (e.g., recent falls, medications, psychological, cognitive status, vision, mobility, transfer, behaviors, activities of daily living, environment, nutrition, continence, and other risk factors). Screening for frailty in the office setting is reasonable and may help identify PWH at heightened risk for falls and fragility fractures.

SCREENING FOR FRACTURE RISK

FRAX

FRAX was developed by the WHO Metabolic Bone Disease Group (2008) to assess fractures with improved predictors of fracture risk compared to *T*-scores (van den Bergh et al., 2010). This assessment tool is not specific for PWH. FRAX provides the 10-year probability of hip fracture and the 10-year probability of a major osteoporotic fracture (hip, spine, shoulder, or forearm). Probability is estimated based on clinical risk factors and BMD values from the femoral neck (WHO Metabolic Bone Disease Group, 2008). Models have been developed based on location (i.e., Asia, Europe, Middle East and Africa, North America, Latin America, and Oceania) and ethnicity. Risk factors included in the calculation tool are age, sex, weight (kilograms), height (centimeters), previous fracture, parent fractured hip, current tobacco smoking, exposure to glucocorticoids, rheumatoid arthritis, secondary osteoporosis, alcohol intake of three or more units per day, and BMD (g/cm²) or, alternatively, *T*-score based on the NHANES III female reference data (Kanis, 2007).

The International Osteoporosis Foundation, the National Osteoporosis Foundation, the American Society for Bone and Mineral Research, and the International Society for Clinical Densitometry all endorse the use of FRAX (van den Bergh et

al., 2010). The National Osteoporosis Foundation (2014) recommends using FRAX for postmenopausal women and men aged 50 years or older who are not on treatment, who have not had spine or hip fractures, and who have *T*-scores between −1.0 and −2.5 SD (van den Bergh et al., 2010). If the FRAX 10-year probability exceeds 20% for major osteoporotic fractures or 3% risk for hip fracture, the National Osteoporosis Foundation's 2014 guidelines recommend initiating drug treatment.

Increasing baseline FRAX 10-year probability was consistently associated with increased rates of incident fractures in a large cohort of adults with HIV (Battalora et al., 2014). Although FRAX may underestimate fracture risk in PWH, the European AIDS Clinical Society (2020) recommends FRAX screening in all persons older than 40 years.

DXA

BMD measurements are widely obtained using DXA scan. Relevant measurement locations include the hip, spine, and forearm. DXA is a two-dimensional system in which the size of the specimen is directly proportional to the estimate of area density. Overestimation of BMD values obtained from larger patients is a concern (Amorosa & Tebas, 2006a). Of greater concern is that DXA has not been validated for fractures among PWH. Furthermore, fewer data exist on younger adults except in those taking TDF for preexposure prophylaxis. Additional concerns are the application of WHO definitions for osteoporosis and osteopenia to populations and skeletal sites other than those serving as the basis for the DXA correlations on which these bone abnormality definitions are described (Amorosa & Tebas, 2006b).

DXA is noninvasive and convenient, but it does not assess bone condition, bone structure, or bone quality, a factor directly linked to load-bearing strength (Ofotokun & Weitzmann, 2011). It has been suggested that DXA may underestimate fracture risk in PWH (Ofotokun & Weitzmann, 2011). In 2007, Nguyen et al. demonstrated that approximately 50% of postmenopausal women experiencing a fracture did not meet the clinical definition of osteoporosis based on DXA values (Ofotokun & Weitzmann, 2011).

Other BMD measurement tools exist and assist in the prediction of fragility fracture risk but have inherent limitations. Quantitative CT scanning (QCT) detects volumetric density and in some studies has been shown to detect a higher occurrence of osteoporosis and osteopenia (Pitukcheewanont et al., 2005). However, QCT is more expensive than DXA, requires a higher radiation dose, and is mainly used in research settings (Amorosa & Tebas, 2006a). Other tools, including quantitative ultrasound and analysis of biochemical and hormonal markers, may prove increasingly useful in the future.

The National Osteoporosis Foundation (2014) recommends DXA screening for osteoporosis in the general population for women aged 65 years or older and men aged 70 years or older, regardless of clinical risk factors. They also recommend that women in menopausal transition and men aged 50 to 69 years with clinical risk factors for fracture should be screened. Men and women aged 50 years or older who have had a fracture and persons with other established risk factors, including rheumatoid arthritis or glucocorticoid use, should be screened (National Osteoporosis Foundation, 2014). The foundation does not provide HIV-specific guidelines for DXA screening.

In 2014, the Infectious Diseases Society of America and the HIV Medicine Association issued guidance that recommended baseline DXA screening in HIV-positive postmenopausal women and men aged 50 years or older (Aberg et al., 2014). This recommendation was based on expert opinion and not evidence from randomized controlled trials. Following baseline DXA, the Infectious Diseases Society of America's guidelines recommend periodic monitoring of risk factors for premature bone loss. Risk factors to consider include White race, small body habitus, sedentary lifestyle, cigarette smoking, alcoholism, phenytoin therapy, corticosteroid therapy, hyperparathyroidism, vitamin D deficiency, thyroid disease, and hypogonadism.

The European HIV guidelines (European AIDS Clinical Society, 2020) recommend DXA screening for any of the following patients, preferably prior to initiation of ART:

- Postmenopausal women

- Men aged 50 years or older

- History of low-impact fracture or high risk for falls

- Clinical hypogonadism

- Oral glucocorticoid use

- Those between 40 and 50 years with high fracture risk

TREATMENT

Treatment of PWH with low BMD and associated complications should consider multiple factors. These include patient profile, patient age, risk factor reduction, potential for drug–drug interactions, underlying hepatic or renal disease, and likelihood of medication adherence.

IDENTIFY AND TREAT SECONDARY CAUSES OF LOW BMD

For persons with abnormal DXA scans (T-scores of 1 or less) or with a history of a fragility fracture, clinicians should evaluate and address secondary causes of osteoporosis, particularly in cases in which vitamin D deficiency or phosphate wasting is observed. These conditions can cause osteomalacia or bone mineralization deficiency and may be difficult to differentiate from osteoporosis based on DXA scans (Yin, 2012).

BEHAVIORAL AND LIFESTYLE ADVICE

Several lifestyle factors. including being sedentary and cigarette smoking. are associated with low BMD and/or fractures in the general population. Dietary modification to optimize calcium and vitamin D intake, increasing weight-bearing exercise, and smoking cessation are prudent in general but especially among persons at increased risk of low BMD or fractures. In addition, because excess alcohol consumption (>3 units/day) and substance dependency are associated with fracture risk, strategies to limit or abstain from alcohol consumption should be discussed with patients.

VITAMIN D AND CALCIUM REPLACEMENT

Vitamin D deficiency is common among PWH and may contribute to low BMD and fractures. Although there are no standardized guidelines for vitamin D and calcium repletion or supplementation, the Institute of Medicine (2011) published a report providing dietary recommendations for calcium and vitamin D. It suggests 1,000 mg/day of calcium for most adults aged 19 to 50 years and for men up to age 71 years. No more than 1,200 mg/day of calcium is suggested for women over aged 50 years and for men and women aged 71 years or older (Institute of Medicine, 2011).

Specific to PWH, a 2014 study (ACTG A5280) evaluated the effect of high-dose vitamin D3 (4,000 IU/day) plus calcium supplementation (1,000 mg/day calcium carbonate) on BMD in 142 PWH (90% male; median 33 years; BMI 24.4 kg/m^2; CD4$^+$ cell count, 341 cells/mm^3; HIV-1 RNA level, 4.5 log$_{10}$ copies/mL; mean 25(OH) vitamin D, 23 ng/mL) with DXA scanning done at baseline and then at week 48 after initiating ART with efavirenz/emtricitabine/tenofovir disoproxil (EFV/FTC/TDF). Supplementation with vitamin D/calcium mitigated loss of BMD, particularly at the total hip (Overton et al., 2014). The effect of vitamin D supplementation has subsequently been corroborated by others. Most notably, Havens et al. (2018a) reported on a randomized controlled trial of high-dose vitamin D. In this study of 214 young PWH (median age 22 years), 50,000 units of vitamin D monthly was associated with a significant increase in lumbar spine BMD (1.2% increase vs. no change in the placebo arm). No effect was seen on hip BMD. The group receiving vitamin D also experienced a significant decline in PTH and bone turnover markers and an increase in serum vitamin D levels.

Assuming minimal sun exposure in geographic regions of the US and Canada, the Institute of Medicine (2011) suggests 600 IU/day of vitamin D for most persons aged 1 to 70 years and 800 IU/day for persons aged 71 years or older. These recommendations are not specific for PWH. However, it may be reasonable to monitor 25-hydroxy vitamin D levels in this population and to recommend supplementation in situations of ART initiation and continued therapy if vitamin D levels are low (Overton et al., 2014; Yin, 2012).

TESTOSTERONE REPLACEMENT

Testosterone deficiency is relatively common in men with HIV, especially in the aging population, and is associated with a decrease in BMD. A recent publication identified the BMD benefits of testosterone supplementation in a cohort of men with and without HIV (Grant et al., 2019). Testosterone use was more frequently reported in HIV-positive men compared to HIV-negative men (4% vs. 2%, $p < 0.001$). In the overall study population, testosterone use was associated with significantly higher BMD at both the lumbar spine and hip when compared to men not receiving testosterone. Clinicians should assess the risks and benefits of testosterone replacement in PWH with low BMD and low serum testosterone levels.

BISPHOSPHONATES

Currently, there are no specific guidelines for the treatment of BMD disorders among PWH. As noted earlier, diagnosis and management of bone disease among PWH generally follows guidance from the non-HIV population. The National Osteoporosis Foundation (2014) currently recommends pharmacologic treatment of postmenopausal women and men aged 50 or older with hip or vertebral fractures or a T-score of −2.5 or less at the femoral neck or spine after evaluation to exclude secondary causes. In addition, patients with a T-score between −1.0 and −2.5 at the femoral neck or spine and 10-year probability fracture by FRAX of 3% or greater at the hip and of 20% or greater for any osteoporosis-related fracture should be considered for treatment (National Osteoporosis Foundation, 2014).

The class of drugs referred to as bisphosphonates inhibit osteoclast resorption and can reduce vertebral and nonvertebral fractures by 25% to 50% in HIV-negative individuals. The agents are indicated for prevention and treatment of osteoporosis and other bone diseases, including Paget's disease (Barbosa, 2021).

The effectiveness of these antiresorptive therapies in PWH has been evaluated in numerous placebo-controlled randomized trials. Five older studies evaluated patients with T-scores not within the osteoporotic range (Bolland et al., 2007; Guaraldi et al., 2004; Huang et al., 2009; McComsey et al., 2007; Mondy et al., 2005). Another trial included patients with T-scores of less than −2.5 (Rozenberg et al., 2012). Resulting data showed significant increases in BMD at the lumbar spine in all six studies and a large increase at the hip in three (Bolland et al., 2007; Huang et al., 2009; McComsey et al., 2007). The 2-year treatment trials (Bolland et al., 2007; Rozenberg et al., 2012) demonstrated the greatest change in BMD. Notably, an increase in BMD was detected in the placebo groups that were also given calcium and vitamin D.

A publication by Hoy et al. (2018) evaluated the use of the intravenous bisphosphonate zoledronic acid to mitigate bone loss associated with ART. This study included subjects on TDF and with low BMD and randomized them to a switch from TDF or administration of a single dose of zoledronic acid or placebo. This drug was found to be safe and well tolerated and was associated with a greater increase in BMD at the hip and lumbar spine (4.6% vs. 2.6% and 7.4% vs. 2.9%, respectively).

Long-term data have been published confirming the beneficial effect of bisphosphonates among PWH. Bolland et al. (2019) reported data on BMD on 25 men with HIV 11 years after receiving two doses of intravenous zoledronate. Their BMD remained significantly higher at the lumbar spine (3.7% higher), total hip (3.7% higher), and femoral neck (5.0% higher) compared to those given placebo. Bone turnover markers remained lower in the treatment arm as well, suggesting that the effect of the bisphosphonate was mediated through reduced bone turnover (Bolland et al., 2019).

These data were corroborated by another randomized controlled trial of zoledronate versus placebo that followed 63 PWH with bone loss for 3 years after treatment. The participants who received a single dose of zoledronate had an 11% increase in BMD at the lumbar spine at 3 years compared to a 4.3% loss in the placebo arm. More modest differences were seen in the femoral neck and total hip, but these changes did not reach statistical significance (Ofotokun et al., 2020).

A pediatric study evaluated the use of alendronate in perinatally infected children and adolescents with low BMD for age. Fifty-two youths (aged 11–24 years) were randomized to weekly alendronate or placebo for 2 years. The therapy was well tolerated, with similar adverse effects in both groups and no cases of osteonecrosis or nonhealing fractures. The group who received alendronate experienced 20% BMD gains in the lumbar spine at 1 year versus 7% in the placebo arm. with similar differences in the whole-body BMD (Jacobson et al., 2020).

Taken as a whole, these data suggest that bisphosphonates are safe and effective for use in PWH. It is this author's opinion that HIV providers should be more aggressive with the use of bisphosphonates in this high-risk population.

Adverse effects of bisphosphonates include osteonecrosis of the jaw (<1 case per 100,000 pys of exposure) and subtrochanteric fractures or atypical femoral shaft fractures (uncommon in patients with <5 years of treatment) (Yin, 2012). Thus, only patients with appropriate indications for treatment should be administered bisphosphonates, and the FDA recommends stopping treatment after 5 years (Yin, 2012).

Other treatments for osteoporosis include teriparatide, a recombinant form of PTH that stimulates osteoblasts and is used in patients who do not respond to bisphosphonates. However, no data exist on teriparatide's efficacy in PWH (Yin, 2012). Denosumab, a monoclonal RANKL antibody, blocks the RANKL/RANKL interaction but may increase the likelihood of infection (Yin, 2012). For this reason, more data are needed to determine the safety of denosumab in PWH (National Osteoporosis Foundation, 2014; Yin, 2012). Hormone replacement therapy including estrogen and raloxifene may be appropriate in some women with HIV. but the benefits may be countered by increased risk of malignancy, thrombotic events, and cardiovascular disease.

ROLE OF ART SELECTION AND SWITCHING

Because TDF is associated with greater initial loss of BMD compared to other antiretrovirals, the US Department of Health and Human Services HIV adult treatment guidelines (2020) recommend the avoidance of TDF in patients with osteoporosis. Tenofovir alafenamide (TAF), a prodrug of tenofovir, is associated with less BMD loss compared to

TDF in both initial and ART switch settings, and it may mitigate the BMD effect of TDF (Mills et al., 2016; Sax et al., 2014). There are limited data on the efficacy of ART switch strategies. HIV clinicians should generally consider avoiding TDF or ritonavir-boosted PIs in patients at risk for bone loss. Some older short-term studies found that switching virologically suppressed patients to abacavir or raltegravir resulted in improvement in BMD compared to TDF (Haskelberg et al., 2012; Yin et al., 2012). For many PWH, TAF would be the preferred nucleoside analog to use instead of TDF.

CONCLUSION

The field of metabolic bone disease in PWH remains a critical area of research—especially as this population of patients successfully ages into the seventh and eighth decades of life and beyond. Additional data from clinical trials and observational cohorts are needed to identify the best preventive, screening, and treatment strategies for osteoporosis and fragility fractures for PWH.

REFERENCES

Aberg JA, Gallant JE, Ghanem KG, et al. Primary care guidelines for the management of persons infected with HIV: 2013 update by the HIV Medicine Association of the Infectious Diseases Society of America. *Clin Infect Dis.* 2014;58(1):e1–e34.

Agidigbi TS, Kim C. Reactive oxygen species in osteoclast differentiation and possible pharmaceutical targets of ROS-mediated osteoclast diseases. *Int J Mol Sci.* 2019;20:3576. doi:10.3390/ijms2014357

Amorosa V, Tebas P. Bone disease and HIV infection. *Clin Infect Dis.* 2006a;42(1):108–114.

Amorosa V, Tebas P. Reply to Rojo and Ramos and to Vignolo et al. *Clin Infect Dis.* 2006b;43(1):113–114.

Barbosa JS, Almeida Paz FA, Santos Braga S, et al. Bisphosphonates, Old Friends of Bones and New Trends in Clinics. *J Med Chem.* 2021;64(3):1260–1282.

Battalora L, Buchacz K, Armon C, et al. Low bone mineral density is associated with increased risk of incident fracture in HIV-infected adults. *Antivir Ther.* 2016;21(1):45–54.

Battalora LA, Young B, Overton ET. Bones, fractures, antiretroviral therapy and HIV. *Curr Infect Dis Rep.* February 2014;16(2):393.

Bedimo R, Maalouf NM, Zhang S, et al. Osteoporotic fracture risk associated with cumulative exposure to tenofovir and other antiretroviral agents. *AIDS.* 2012;26(7):825–831.

Bolland MJ, Grey AB, Horne AM, et al. Annual zoledronate increases bone density in highly active antiretroviral therapy-treated human immunodeficiency virus-infected men: a randomized controlled trial. *J Clin Endocrinol Metab.* 2007;92(4):1283–1288.

Bolland MJ, Horne AM, Briggs SE, et al. Effects of intravenous zoledronate on bone turnover and bone density persist for at least 11 years in HIV-infected men. *J Bone Miner Res.* 2019;34:1248–1253.

Brown TT, Hoy J, Borderi M, et al. Recommendations for evaluation and management of bone disease in HIV. *Clin Infect Dis.* 2015;60:1242–1251.

Brown TT, McComsey GA, King MS, et al. Loss of bone mineral density after antiretroviral therapy initiation, independent of antiretroviral regimen. *J AIDS.* 2009;51:554–561.

Brown TT, Qaqish RB. Antiretroviral therapy and the prevalence of osteopenia and osteoporosis: a meta-analytic review. *AIDS.* 2006;20(17):2165–2174.

Dave JA, Cohen K, Micklesfield LK, et al. Antiretroviral therapy, especially efavirenz, is associated with low bone mineral density in HIV-infected South Africans. *PLoS One.* 2015;10(12):e0144286.

Endocrine Society. Clinical guidelines: evaluation, treatment and prevention of vitamin D deficiency: an Endocrine Society clinical practice guideline. 2011. https://academic.oup.com/jcem/article/96/7/1911/2833671

Erlandson KM, Lake JE, Sim M, et al. Bone mineral density declines twice as quickly among HIV-infected women compared with men. *J AIDS.* 2018;77(3):288–294.

Escota GV, Mondy K, Bush T, et al. High prevalence of low bone mineral density and substantial bone loss over 4 years among HIV-infected persons in the era of modern antiretroviral therapy. *AIDS Res Human Retroviruses.* 2016;32(1):59–67.

European AIDS Clinical Society. Guidelines Version 10.1. October 2020. https://eacs.sanfordguide.com/

Goh SSL, Lai PSM, Tan ATB, et al. Reduced bone mineral density in human immunodeficiency virus-infected individuals: a meta-analysis of its prevalence and risk factors. *Osteoporos Int.* 2018;29(3):595–613.

Gonciulea A, Wang R, Althoff KN, et al. Proteinuria is associated with increased risk of fragility fracture in men with or at risk of HIV infection. *J AIDS.* 2019;81(3):e85–e91.

Grant PM, Kitch D, McComsey GA, et al. Long-term bone mineral density changes in antiretroviral-treated HIV-infected individuals. *J Infect Dis.* 2016;214(4):607–611.

Grant PM, Li X, Jacobson LP, et al. Effect of testosterone use on bone mineral density in HIV-infected men. *AIDS Res Hum Retroviruses.* 2019;35(1):75–80.

Guaraldi G, Orlando G, Madeddu G, et al. Alendronate reduces bone resorption in HIV-associated osteopenia/osteoporosis. *HIV Clin Trials.* 2004;5(5):269–277.

Hansen AB, Gerstoft J, Kronborg G, et al. Incidence of low and high-energy fractures in persons with and without HIV infection: a Danish population-based cohort study. *AIDS.* 2012;26(3):285–293.

Haskelberg H, Cordery DV, Amin J, et al. HLA alleles association with changes in bone mineral density in HIV-1-infected adults changing treatment to tenofovir–emtricitabine or abacavir–lamivudine. *PLoS One.* 2014;9(3):e93333.

Haskelberg H, Hoy JF, Amin J, et al. Changes in bone turnover and bone loss in HIV-infected patients changing treatment to tenofovir–emtricitabine or abacavir–lamivudine. *PLoS One.* 2012;7(6):e38377.

Havens PL, Long D, Schuster GU; Adolescent Medicine Trials Network for HIV/AIDS Interventions (ATN) 117 and 109 study teams. Tenofovir disoproxil fumarate appears to disrupt the relationship of vitamin D and parathyroid hormone. *Antivir Ther.* 2018a;23(7):623–628. doi:10.3851/IMP3269

Havens PL, Stephensen CB, Van Loan MD; Adolescent Medicine Trials Network for HIV/AIDS Interventions (ATN) 109 Study Team. Vitamin D3 supplementation increases spine bone mineral density in adolescents and young adults with human immunodeficiency virus infection being treated with tenofovir disoproxil fumarate: a randomized, placebo-controlled trial. *Clin Infect Dis.* 2018b;66(2):220–228.

Hileman CO, Labbato DE, Storer NJ, et al. Is bone loss linked to chronic inflammation in antiretroviral-naïve HIV-infected adults? A 48-week matched cohort study. *AIDS.* 2014;28(12):1759–1767.

Hoy J, Grund B, Roediger M, et al.; INSIGHT START Bone Mineral Density Substudy Group. Effects of immediate versus deferred initiation of antiretroviral therapy on bone mineral density: a substudy of the INSIGHT Strategic Timing of Antiretroviral Therapy (START) Study [Abstract ADRLH-62]. Paper presented at the 15th European AIDS Conference and 17th International Workshop on Comorbidities and Adverse Drug Reactions in HIV, Barcelona, Spain, October 21–24, 2015.

Hoy JF, Richardson R, Ebeling PR; ZEST Study Investigators. Zoledronic acid is superior to tenofovir disoproxil fumarate-switching for low bone mineral density in adults with HIV. *AIDS.* 2018;32(14):1967–1975.

Huang J, Meixner L, Fernandez S, et al. A double-blinded, randomized controlled trial of zoledrone therapy for HIV-associated osteopenia and osteoporosis. *AIDS*. 2009;23(1):51–57.

INSIGHT START Study Group. Initiation of antiretroviral therapy in early asymptomatic HIV infection. *N Engl J Med*. 2015;373:795–807.

Institute of Medicine. *Dietary reference intakes for calcium and vitamin D*. Washington, DC: National Academies Press. 2010. http://iom.nationalacademies.org/~/media/Files/Report%20Files/2010/Dietary-Reference-Intakes-for-Calcium-and-Vitamin-D/Vitamin%20D%20and%20Calcium%202010%20Report%20Brief.pdf

Jacobson DL, Lindsey JC, Gordon C, et al. Alendronate improves bone mineral density in children and adolescents perinatally infected with human immunodeficiency virus with low bone mineral density for age. *Clin Infect Dis*. 2020;71:1281–1288.

Justice A, Falutz J. Aging and HIV: an evolving understanding. *Curr Opin HIV AIDS*. 2014;9(4):291–293.

LeFevre ML, LeFevre NM. Vitamin D screening and supplementation in community-dwelling adults: common questions and answers. *Am Fam Physician*. 2018;97(4):254–260.

Kanis JA, on behalf of the World Health Organization Scientific Group. *Assessment of Osteoporosis at the Primary Health-Care Level. Technical Report*. World Health Organization Collaborating Centre for Metabolic Bone Diseases, University of Sheffield, UK. 2007. https://www.shef.ac.uk/FRAX/pdfs/WHO_Technical_Report.pdf

King EM, Nesbitt A, Albert AY, et al. Prolonged amenorrhea and low hip bone mineral density in women living with HIV: a controlled cross-sectional study. *J AIDS*. 2020;83:486–495.

Liu Z, Xiao Y, Torresilla C, et al. Implication of different HIV-1 genes in the modulation of autophagy. *Viruses*. 2017;9:389. doi:10.3390/v9120389

Llop M, Sifuentes WA, Bañón S, et al. Increased prevalence of asymptomatic vertebral fractures in HIV-infected patients over 50 years of age. *Arch Osteoporos*. 2018;13(1):56.

Maalouf NM, Zhang S, Drechsler H, et al. Hepatitis C co-infection and severity of liver disease as risk factor for osteoporotic fractures among HIV-infected patients. *J Bone Miner Res*. 2013;28(12):2577–2583.

McComsey GA, Kendall MA, Tebas P, et al. Alendronate with calcium and vitamin D supplementation is safe and effective for the treatment of decreased bone mineral density in HIV. *AIDS*. 2007;21(18):2473–2482.

McComsey GA, Kitch D, Daar ES, et al. Bone mineral density and fractures in antiretroviral-naive persons randomized to receive abacavir–lamivudine or tenofovir disoproxil fumarate–emtricitabine along with efavirenz or atazanavir–ritonavir: AIDS Clinical Trials Group A5224s, a substudy of ACTG A5202. *J Infect Dis*. 2011;203(12):1791–1801.

McComsey GA, Tebas P, Shane E, et al. Bone disease in HIV infection: a practical review and recommendations for HIV care providers. *Clin Infect Dis*. 2010;51(8):937–946.

Mills A, Arribas JR, Andrade-Villanueva J, et al. Switching from tenofovir disoproxil fumarate to tenofovir alafenamide in antiretroviral regimens for virologically suppressed adults with HIV-1 infection: a randomised, active-controlled, multicentre, open-label, phase 3, non-inferiority study. *Lancet Infect Dis*. 2016;16(1):43–52.

Mondy K, Powderly WG, Claxton SA, et al. Alendronate, vitamin D, and calcium for the treatment of osteopenia/osteoporosis associated with HIV infection. *J AIDS*. 2005;38(4):426–431.

Moran CA, Weitzmann MN, Ofotokun I. The protease inhibitors and HIV-associated bone loss. *Curr Opin HIV AIDS*. 2016;11(3):333–342.

National Osteoporosis Foundation. *Clinician's Guide to Prevention and Treatment of Osteoporosis*. Washington, DC: National Osteoporosis Foundation; 2014.

Nguyen ND, Eisman JA, Center JR, et al. Risk factors for fracture in nonosteoporotic men and women. *J Clin Endocrinol Metab*. 2007 Mar;92(3):955–962.

Ofotokun I, Weitzmann MN. HIV and bone metabolism. *Discov Med*. 2011;11(60):385–393.

Ofotokun I, Collins LF, Titanji K, et al. Antiretroviral therapy-induced bone loss is durably suppressed by a single dose of zoledronic acid in treatment-naïve persons with HIV infection: a phase IIB trial. *Clin Infect Dis*. 2020;71(7):1655–1663. doi:10.1093/cid/ciz1027

Orwoll ES, Klein RF. Osteoporosis in men. *Endocr Rev*. 1995;16(1):87–116.

Overton ET, Chan ES, Brown TT, et al. Vitamin D and calcium attenuate bone loss with antiretroviral therapy initiation: a randomized trial. *Ann Intern Med*. 2015;162(12):815–824.

Pitukcheewanont P, Safani D, Church J, et al. Bone measures in HIV-1 infected children and adolescents: disparity between quantitative computed tomography and dual-energy X-ray absorptiometry measurements. *Osteoporosis Int*. 2005;16(11):1393–1396.

Pramukti I, Lindayani L, Chen YC, et al. Bone fracture among people living with HIV: a systematic review and meta-regression of prevalence, incidence, and risk factors. *PloS One*. 2020;15(6):e0233501.

Premaor MO, Compston JE. The hidden burden of fractures in people living with HIV. *JBMR Plus*. 2018;2(5):247–256.

Raynaud-Messina B, Bracq L, Dupont M, et al. Bone degradation machinery of osteoclasts: an HIV-1 target that contributes to bone loss. *Proc Natl Acad Sci USA*. 2018;115(11):E2556–E2565.

Rozenberg S, Lanoy E, Bentata M, et al. Effect of alendronate on HIV-associated osteoporosis: a randomized, double-blind, placebo-controlled, 96-week trial (ANRS 120). *AIDS Res Hum Retroviruses*. 2012;28(9):972–980.

Sax PE, Zolopa A, Brar I, et al. Tenofovir alafenamide vs. tenofovir disoproxil fumarate in single tablet regimens for initial HIV-1 therapy: a randomized phase 2 study. *J AIDS*. 2014;67(1):52–58.

Sharma A, Ma Y, Tien PC, et al. HIV infection is associated with abnormal bone microarchitecture: measurement of trabecular bone score in the Women's Interagency HIV Study. *J AIDS*. 2018;78(4):441–449.

Sharma A, Shi Q, Hoover DR, et al. Frailty predicts fractures among women with and at risk for HIV: results from the Women's Interagency HIV Study. *AIDS*. 2019;33:455–463.

Starup-Linde J, Rosendahl SB, Storgaard M, et al. Management of osteoporosis in patients living with HIV: a systematic review and meta-analysis. *J AIDS*. 2020;83(1):1–8.

Titanji K. Beyond antibodies: B cells and the OPG/RANK-RANKL pathway in health, non-HIV disease and HIV-induced bone loss. *Front Immunol*. 2017;8:1851.

Triant VA, Brown TT, Lee H, et al. Fracture prevalence among human immunodeficiency virus (HIV)-infected versus non-HIV-infected patients in a large US healthcare system. *J Clin Endocrinol Metab*. 2008;93(9):3499–3504.

US Department of Health and Human Services, Panel on Antiretroviral Guidelines for Adults and Adolescents. Guidelines for the use of antiretroviral agents in HIV-1-infected adults and adolescents. 2020; https://clinicalinfo.hiv.gov/sites/default/files/inline-files/AdultandAdolescentGL.pdf

van den Bergh JP, van Geel TA, Lems WF, et al. Assessment of individual fracture risk: FRAX and beyond. *Curr Osteoporosis Rep*. 2010;8(3):131–137.

van Vonderen MG, Lips P, van Agtmael MA, et al. First line zidovudine/lamivudine/lopinavir/ritonavir leads to greater bone loss compared to nevirapine/lopinavir/ritonavir. *AIDS*. 2009;23(11):1367–1376.

Womack JA, Goulet JL, Gibert C, et al. Increased risk of fragility fractures among HIV infected compared to uninfected male veterans. *PloS One*. 2011;6(2):e17217.

Woolf AD, Pfleger B. Burden of major musculoskeletal conditions. *Bull World Health Organ*. 2003;81(9):646–656.

World Health Organization. WHO Technical Report Series 843: assessment of fracture risk and its application to screening for postmenopausal osteoporosis. Report of a WHO Study Group. *World Health Organ Tech Rep Ser*. 1994;843:1–129.

World Health Organization. WHO manual of diagnostic imaging. 2002. http://apps.who.int/iris/bitstream/10665/42457/1/9241545550_eng.pdf

World Health Organization. Metabolic Bone Disease Group. FRAX tool. 2008. http://www.shef.ac.uk/FRAX.

Yin M. Bone loss in HIV: virus, host or ART. Paper presented at the Conference on Retroviruses and Opportunistic Infections (CROI), Seattle, WA, March 5–8, 2012.

Yin MT, Overton ET. Increasing clarity on bone loss associated with antiretroviral initiation. *J Infect Dis*. 2011;203(12):1705–1707.

Yin MT, Shi Q, Hoover DR, et al. Fracture incidence in HIV-infected women: results from the Women's Interagency HIV Study. *AIDS*. 2010;24(17):2679–2686.

Young B, Dao CN, Buchacz K, et al. Increased rates of bone fracture among HIV-infected persons in the HIV Outpatient Study (HOPS) compared with the US general population, 2000–2006. *Clin Infect Dis*. 2011;52(8):1061–1068.

41.

HIV-ASSOCIATED LIPODYSTROPHY AND LIPOATROPHY

Rajagopal V. Sekhar

LEARNING OBJECTIVES

Upon completion of this chapter, the reader should be able to:

- Understand what is known about HIV-associated lipodystrophy (HAL)

- Understand the clinical implications of lipodystrophy in persons with HIV (PWH)

- Be aware of therapeutic interventions to treat and improve the health status of PWH with lipodystrophy

WHAT'S NEW?

- The incidence of new-onset lipoatrophy has declined in recent years.

- There is a greater risk and prevalence of abdominal obesity, especially with integrase strand transfer inhibitor (INSTI) drugs.

KEY POINTS

- HIV is associated with abnormal fat distribution, which is termed *lipodystrophy*.

- HIV lipodystrophy can manifest as fat loss (lipoatrophy), fat gain (lipohypertrophy), or a mixed pattern.

- Therapeutic options are limited and treatment is challenging.

- HIV lipodystrophy is associated with increased risk of developing cardiovascular disease (CVD), fatty liver disease, and renal disease.

INTRODUCTION

The advent of combination antiretroviral therapy (ART) in the mid- to late 1990s resulted in significant health benefits for PWH by reducing AIDS-related mortality and increasing life expectancy. Additional collateral benefits were an improvement in nutritional status and a reduction in HIV-associated opportunistic infections. In parallel with these benefits, PWH began to develop unusual changes in body habitus with variable combinations of loss of peripheral fat in the limbs, buttocks, and face (termed *lipoatrophy*) and central fat accumulation in the abdomen (termed *lipohypertrophy*). These changes were described as a lipodystrophic syndrome afflicting these individuals (Carr et al., 1998), and the condition was referred to as *HIV-associated lipodystrophy* (HAL).

Although the origins of HAL are unclear, its onset has been associated with several factors. Since improvements in ART regimens have increased the lifespan of PWH, it is possible that the HAL phenotype is simply a representation of HIV as a chronic disease. The specific effects of antiretroviral medications (ARVs) have also been implicated. The initial usage of combination ART in the 1990s was accompanied by multiple reports of abnormalities in body fat distribution linked to the protease inhibitor (PI) and nucleoside reverse transcriptase inhibitor (NRTI) classes of drugs, with terminologies ranging from "protease paunch," "Crixivan belly," and "buffalo hump" to reporting breast enlargement in women and men (Carr et al., 1998; Herry et al., 1997; Lo et al., 1998; Massip et al., 1997; Miller et al., 2003; Vazquez, 1999). Factors other than ART implicated in the pathogenesis of HAL included immune phenomenon and effects mediated directly by HIV itself. However, despite more than two decades of intensive research to understand the mechanistic underpinnings of HIV lipodystrophy and lipoatrophy, the answers remain elusive (Bacchetti et al., 2005; Sattler, 2003; Tien & Grunfeld, 2004).

LIPODYSTROPHY, LIPOHYPERTROPHY, AND LIPOATROPHY

"Lipodystrophy" is a broad term that collectively describes a variable combination of accumulation of fat in several regions, including the abdomen (Engelson et al., 1999; Miller et al., 2003; Vigano et al., 2005; Yin & Glesby, 2005); interscapular dorsocervical region, termed the "buffalo hump" (Lo et al., 1998; Roth et al., 1998; Torres et al., 1999); and the submental region, where it was termed the "bull neck" (Meinrenken et al., 1998), together with a simultaneous loss of fat from the limbs, face, and buttocks (Bacchetti et al., 2005; Lichtenstein et al., 2003; Martin & Mallon, 2005; Parruti & Toro, 2005). This "mixed" pattern of lipodystrophy includes a variable and simultaneous expression of both lipoatrophy (fat loss) and lipohypertrophy (fat gain) occurring concomitantly in the same person. These abnormalities in body habitus are often accompanied by distinct biochemical abnormalities, including dyslipidemia (mainly hypertriglyceridemia) and insulin resistance. In 2001, the US Cholesterol Education Program Adult Treatment Panel III (ATP III) defined metabolic syndrome to include three of the following five criteria: increased waist circumference (>102 cm men, >88 cm women), increased triglycerides (>150 ng/dL), reduced high-density lipoprotein cholesterol (HDL-C; <40 mg/dL men, <50 mg/dL women), high blood pressure (>130/>85 mmHg), and elevated fasting glucose (>110 mg/dL) (National Cholesterol Education Program, 2001). This remains the standard definition used by most epidemiologic studies of populations with this condition. A study that evaluated PWH reported a 14% prevalence of metabolic syndrome by the International Diabetes Federation criteria and 18% by ATP III criteria (Samaras et al., 2007). In effect, the changes associated with HAL, especially with the mixed pattern, resemble an accelerated form of metabolic syndrome.

DEFINITION AND PREVALENCE OF HAL

The initial description of HAL by Carr et al. in 1998 was followed by numerous reports of this condition by the HIV medical and scientific community. However, the prevalence varied widely due to the absence of a consensus case definition, leading to wide fluctuations in the clinical diagnosis of HAL (Carter et al., 2001). Since it became necessary to have a standard and uniformly accepted case definition for HAL, the HIV Lipodystrophy Case Definition Study Group developed a statistical model for the diagnosis of lipodystrophy (including age, sex, duration of HIV infection, HIV disease stage, waist-to-hip ratio [WHR], anion gap, serum HDL-C concentration, trunk-to-peripheral fat ratio, percentage leg fat, and intra- and extra-abdominal fat ratio as variables), with a quantitative scale for identification (Carr et al., 2003; Carr & Law, 2003). This model identified HIV lipodystrophy with a fair degree of accuracy, but it required multiple parameters whose measurement was not feasible or practical in a clinical outpatient setting. Thus, the field is still challenged by the lack of a simple, effective, practical, clinically applicable, and relevant case definition for HAL. The current practical approach to the PWH with mixed lipodystrophy is for the treating clinician to document objective evidence of central obesity and peripheral lipoatrophy, with evidence of dyslipidemia, insulin resistance, or both.

Despite these uncertainties, HIV infection was associated with an increased prevalence of lipodystrophy at the turn of the century, with multiple studies reporting peripheral fat wasting, increased central fat accumulation, or both in PWH (Bergersen et al., 2004; Bernasconi et al., 2002; Miller et al., 2003; Worm et al., 2002), with a higher association of lipoatrophy with the use of nucleoside analog therapy,

especially stavudine (Bernasconi et al., 2002; Chêne et al., 2002). When fat accumulation and fat loss were analyzed, it was found that the prevalence of fat accumulation was 56%, that of fat loss was 24%, and the mixed form occurred in 83% of PWH (Safrin & Grunfeld, 1999). More stringent analyses of the relative prevalence of the individual components of lipodystrophy have reported on average 45% central obesity, up to 62% for any lipodystrophy, and 38% for peripheral lipoatrophy (Lichtenstein et al., 2004; Paparizos et al., 2000; Saves et al., 2002; Tien & Grunfeld, 2004). HAL has also been described to affect children. A study from India found that lipodystrophy was observed in 34% of children, with lipoatrophy being the most common subtype, followed by lipohypertrophy (Bhutia et al., 2014). These data confirm a significant presence of the lipodystrophic phenotype in the HIV-infected population. However, since the use of stavudine appeared to be closely linked to lipoatrophy, phasing out the use of this drug has lowered the incidence of new-onset lipoatrophy (Innes et al., 2018; Ribera et al., 2008). Alongside these changes, the risk of abdominal obesity in PWH appears to be rising for any given body mass index (BMI), and the excess odds of abdominal obesity is stronger with older age, hypertension, and hypertriglyceridemia (Gelpi et al., 2018). This is also the clinical experience of this author, where the incidence of de novo HAL with a mixed pattern of lipodystrophy has declined significantly over the past decade, with almost no persons presenting with lipoatrophy, although the proportion of PWH with abdominal obesity has substantially increased. These observed changes are likely due to the advent of improved and newer classes of ARVs, suggesting that older ARVs may have played even a greater contributory role in the pathogenesis of HAL than originally suspected. An alternative possibility is that when lipodystrophy was described in the 1990s, it could simply have been a coincidental juxtaposition of nucleoside analog–induced lipoatrophy, abdominal obesity due to other causes, and a coincidental occurrence of both phenotypes in some PWH. This hypothesis provides the most parsimonious explanation to link the HAL phenotype from the 1990s to the current phenotype of abdominal obesity with its associated metabolic and cardiovascular risk profile. The lipoatrophic phenotype is rapidly disappearing, whereas the central obesity phenotype persists and is increasing in prevalence. Additional studies are needed to understand the dynamic evolution of the HIV body phenotype. Despite these observations, since HAL is linked to an increased risk of metabolic complications, including CVD, diabetes, and liver fat accumulation, it is still important to understand the underlying contributory mechanisms.

DIAGNOSING HAL

The clinical diagnosis of HAL is based on multiple approaches, including self-reporting, use of questionnaires, clinical scales with scores, anthropometric formulas, and radiographic techniques. Standard anthropometric tests have the advantage of being readily available to clinicians (Schwenk, 2002; Schwenk et al., 2001). Computed tomography, magnetic resonance imaging, and dual-energy X-ray absorptiometry (DXA) scans provide quantifiable data on the location and mass of visceral fat, subcutaneous adipose tissue, and subcutaneous limb fat (Cavalcanti et al., 2005; Schambelan et al., 2002). However, the usefulness of these imaging modalities in the outpatient clinical setting is limited due to availability, expense, radiation exposure, and dependence on single-slice data instead of whole-body studies. Therefore, they are impractical for use in routine clinical practice. A study of 100 PWH on ART used DXA scan for anthropometric measures and proposed a fat mass ratio of 1.26, waist:thigh ratio of 1.74, and arm:trunk ratio of 2.08 to diagnose lipodystrophy (Beraldo et al., 2015). Routine measurement of body weight, waist circumference, and/or waist-to-hip ratio may be helpful and is recommended for all PWH, especially since the phenotype of central fat accumulation is more prevalent in this population.

MECHANISMS UNDERLYING THE DEVELOPMENT OF HAL

The notion of fat loss in some regions of the body concomitant with fat accumulation in other regions has led to questions of whether fat is reciprocally "redistributed" from one site to another. However, evidence to support this hypothesis is lacking. A large cross-sectional study of PWH and HIV-negative persons did not find any correlation between changes in central and peripheral fat in men with HIV (Bacchetti et al., 2005). These data suggest that, in HIV, central fat accumulation and peripheral fat loss are independent of each other, which means that two distinctly separate phenomena are operating in these individuals—one to cause lipoatrophy and the other to cause abdominal obesity.

Several mechanistic studies using stable isotope tracer methodologies shed light on some of the fundamental biochemical defects underlying HIV (Reeds et al., 2003; Sekhar et al., 2002). It has been shown that HAL is associated with accelerated rates of adipocyte lipolysis. Although there is a significant increase in adipocyte re-esterification, most of the fatty acids released by adipocyte lipolysis are released into the plasma. Since oxidation of plasma fatty acids is blunted, they are available for increased re-esterification and accumulation in the liver and the central compartment, including the abdomen. These fundamental defects may account for the phenotypic appearance of lipodystrophy, where lipoatrophy may be accounted for by the increased lipolysis, and lipohypertrophy in selected sites may be the result of increased adipocyte re-esterification. In addition, the increased delivery of fatty acids to the liver raises the possibility of an increased risk of fatty liver disease, which is increasingly being described in PWH (Morrison et al., 2019). The factors contributing to these metabolic defects are unclear, but ARVs, immune phenomena, adipokines, and HIV itself are involved.

ARVs have been implicated in the mechanistic origins of HAL. As noted earlier, one of the older drugs, stavudine, approved by the US Food and Drug Administration (FDA) in 1994, has been strongly linked to the development of lipoatrophy (Bernasconi et al., 2002; Chêne et al., 2002). The incidence of lipoatrophy receded significantly after discontinuing this NRTI as part of standard ART regimens, replacing it with abacavir or tenofovir (Innes et al., 2018; Ribera et al., 2008). PIs have also been linked to the development of lipohypertrophy. A study using a human preadipocyte cell line found that the PI ritonavir caused massive apoptosis, whereas atazanavir triggered both autophagy and mitophagy (Gibellini et al., 2012). The progression of HAL has been a dynamic process with a high incidence and prevalence in the late 1990s and early 2000s, but decreasing lipoatrophy and increasing central obesity since that time. As PWH with HAL are living longer and there are improvements and changes in the use of ART, it is important to follow and monitor the natural progression of this condition in these individuals.

INCIDENCE OF NEW-ONSET HAL

The incidence of the mixed phenotype of HAL (especially new-onset lipoatrophy) has been declining over the past decade. Most of the descriptions of HAL span the 1995–2010 timeframe, but there are limited data regarding new-onset HAL in the 2010–2020 timeframe. The experience of this author in a busy HIV clinic is a sharply declined incidence of mixed and lipoatrophic phenotypes of HAL over the past decade, but the phenotypic features of those PWH who already had HAL have not resolved. Reasons for this decline in new-onset HAL are not well understood but could be related to the introduction and use of newer ART medications, while omitting PIs and the older nucleoside analogs such as stavudine and didanosine. In support of these observations, a recent study in children and adolescents reported a low prevalence of HAL in Senegalese children on a long-term stavudine-sparing ART regimen (Cames et al., 2018).

CLINICAL IMPLICATIONS OF HAL

PWH with HAL may develop several clinical complications as a result of lipodystrophy. Abdominal obesity and peripheral lipoatrophy lead to the psychological discomfort of a potentially disfiguring condition (Persson, 2005; Peterson et al., 2008; Turner et al., 2006). Abdominal obesity may also produce physical discomfort from abdominal distension, along with the potential for umbilical herniation and gastroesophageal reflux disease (Miller et al., 2003). Visceral fat accumulation has also been linked to an elevated risk of developing insulin resistance, CVD, and fatty liver disease. In addition, visceral fat accumulation is a known predictor of all-cause mortality in non–HIV-infected people (Kuk et al., 2006).

DYSLIPIDEMIA

The increased association of HAL with dyslipidemia and its management represent an important clinical consideration, especially in the context of an increasing incidence of HIV-associated CVD. See Chapter 38, "Cardiovascular Disease," for a discussion regarding the management of hyperlipidemia in PWH.

INSULIN RESISTANCE

PWH with HAL have an increased predisposition to insulin resistance and diabetes mellitus. Factors contributing to this include ARVs, lipotoxicity, immunocytokine factors, and hepatic steatosis. An estimated 30% to 90% of persons receiving PIs may develop insulin resistance, although the incidence of diabetes mellitus is less than 10% (van der Valk et al., 2001). Lipodystrophy (peripheral lipoatrophy and/or lipohypertrophy) and the presence of the dorsocervical fat pad or "buffalo hump" have also been linked to hyperinsulinemia and insulin resistance (Balasubramanyam et al., 2004; Calza et al., 2004; Hadigan et al., 2006).

ARVs may also play a role in the development of insulin resistance in HIV. PIs predispose to insulin resistance by inhibiting the insulin-sensitive glucose transporter Glut4 (Mallon et al., 2005). Thirty-five percent of PWH in one study was reported to have developed insulin resistance on PI therapy (Murata et al., 2002). PIs also predispose to impaired glucose tolerance and fasting hyperinsulinemia (Hadigan et al., 2001). NRTIs, especially the thymidine analogs, also promote insulin resistance in HIV, induce lipotoxicity by disrupting mitochondrial oxidative phosphorylation, and cause defective mitochondrial fatty acid oxidation.

Defective lipid kinetics together with impaired fat oxidation (Reeds et al., 2003; Sekhar et al., 2002, 2005) promote accumulation of ectopic fat in critical metabolic sites of insulin action (e.g., liver and skeletal muscle), resulting in insulin resistance (Gan et al., 2002; Sutinen et al., 2002). Studies in rodents and humans have reported that correcting the deficiency of the endogenous antioxidant glutathione (GSH) significantly improves insulin sensitivity. A pilot study using the gold standard "hyperinsulinemic–euglycemic clamp" to measure insulin sensitivity found that improving levels of GSH using oral supplementation with N-acetylcysteine and glycine in PWH increased insulin sensitivity by 32% within 2 weeks (Nguyen et al., 2014). HAL is associated with defects in adipocyte function that result in altered secretion of critical adipokines such as adiponectin. Deficiency of adiponectin is strongly linked to insulin resistance, and it also occurs in PWH with HAL (Addy et al., 2003; Kim et al., 2007; Samaras et al., 2007).

CARDIOVASCULAR RISKS

It has been known for many years that PWH are at increased risk for CVD (d'Arminio et al., 2004; Friis-Moller et al., 2003) and myocardial infarction (Beires et al., 2018; Friis-Moller et al., 2007; Glesby et al., 2018; Triant et al., 2007; Varriale et al., 2004). The mechanistic underpinnings of this increased risk are complex and likely include a combination of factors, including chronic inflammation, adipocyte dysfunction, excessive lipolysis, elevated low-density lipoprotein cholesterol (LDL-C) and decreased HDL-C, proatherogenic lipoprotein particle sizes with small dense LDL-C, along with adipokine, and immunokine factors. Further impacting the prevalence of CVD in PWH are traditional Framingham risk factors such as diabetes, hypertension, smoking, and family history.

RENAL COMPLICATIONS

HIV lipodystrophy may adversely affect renal function. Data from the LIPOKID study, a prospective cohort study of HIV patients in Switzerland published in 2018, suggest that HAL is independently associated with chronic kidney disease (Bouatou et al., 2018). It is not clear whether this is unique to HAL since renal complications have also been described in patients with generalized lipodystrophy (Akinci et al., 2018). Nonetheless, it is important to regularly monitor renal function in the clinical care of all PWH and perhaps more closely in those with features of lipodystrophy (see Chapter 39, "Renal Complications").

SYSTEMIC STEATOSIS

There are reports of hepatic and intramyocellular fat accumulation in HAL. In HIV, fatty liver disease may be induced by a combination of factors, including coinfection with hepatitis B or C, chronic inflammation, and metabolic defects in lipid cycling, as described previously (Ristig et al., 2005). Interestingly, in PWH with HAL, insulin resistance appears to be related to hepatic fat accumulation more than intra-abdominal fat accumulation (Sutinen et al., 2002). Excess circulating free fatty acids due to excessive lipolysis can be stored in other ectopic sites and contribute to systemic steatosis. An important site for fat deposition is skeletal muscle, and elevated levels of intramyocellular triglycerides have been reported in the soleus and tibialis anterior muscles (Luzi et al., 2003). An important consequence of increased myocellular fat is the development of insulin resistance in these persons. More recently the ART class of INSTIs have been associated with significant weight gain in PWH. The NA-ACCORD, a large observational cohort study in the US and Canada, compared 22,972 adult, treatment-naive PWH who were initiated with INSTI, PI, or NNRTI-based ART. The study found that compared to PIs and NNRTIs, the INSTIs were most associated with weight gain, with the highest weight gain being with dolutegravir (+7.2 kg), followed by raltegravir (+5.8 kg) and elvitegravir (+4.1 kg) (Bourgi et al., 2020a). Similar findings have been reported in other studies in patients on dolutegravir-based regimens (Bourgi et al., 2020b). Although the mechanisms have not been determined, weight gain with INSTIs has become a growing concern, especially in women with HIV (Kerchberger et al., 2020). A recent pooled analysis of eight randomized controlled clinical trials involving over 5,000 treatment-naive PWH who initiated ART between 2003 and 2015 found evidence of higher weight gain in those taking newer ARVs, especially INSTIs (Sax et al., 2020). Again, INSTIs were associated with higher weight gain than PIs and NNRTIs. The study also found that demographic factors such as lower CD4[+] T-cell count, higher HIV viral load, female gender, and Black race were associated with weight gain (Sax et al., 2020).

ECTOPIC FAT ACCUMULATION

In patients with HAL, ectopic fat accumulation occurs in the interscapular dorsocervical "buffalo hump" area and the submental "bull neck" area (Lo et al., 1998). Such patterns of ectopic fat accumulation predispose to other comorbidities, such as obstructive sleep apnea, limited neck motion, and neck and back discomfort (Gold & Annino, 2005; Reynolds et al., 2006).

METABOLIC SYNDROME

The combination of the previously discussed defects has led to an increase in metabolic syndrome in many PWH. A study of Hispanic PWH found that the presence of lipodystrophy was associated with a higher prevalence of metabolic syndrome (69%) compared to nonlipodystrophic patients (39%) (Ramírez-Marrero et al., 2014). A more recent study of 1,861 PWH in four southern states (Texas, Mississippi, Florida, and Georgia) found a prevalence of metabolic syndrome of 34%. The participants were 55% Black and 72% male, 46% were at least 50 years old, 69% had undetectable viral loads, and 98% were on ART (Sears et al., 2019).

TREATMENT OF HAL AND RELATED COMPLICATIONS

There is no single therapy for all the clinical manifestations of HAL as described here. Treatments are generally directed to the individual components and complications of HAL. Medical management has included trials of underlying pathophysiologic defects, including the use of thiazolidinedione drugs to increase fat deposition in lipodystrophic sites. Although data from clinical studies are conflicting (Carr et al., 2004; Hadigan et al., 2004; Sutinen et al., 2003), a small stable isotope-based study examining the interplay of kinetic factors of fat metabolism in the adipocytes suggested that rosiglitazone increased fat deposition in adipocytes. However, this benefit was offset by elevated rates of lipolysis, which results in the inability of adipocytes to retain triglycerides (Sekhar et al., 2011).

Growth hormone (GH) has been used in an attempt to lower abdominal fat, but doses used in several clinical trials were supraphysiologic. Using GH at a physiologic dose resulted in some decrease in lipolysis (D'Amico et al., 2006). A more recent study evaluated the combination of rosiglitazone and human GH in 72 patients with HIV-associated abdominal obesity and insulin resistance (Leung et al., 2016). This study found beneficial effects on adiponectin concentrations with a combination of rosiglitazone and GH, but GH alone did not demonstrate any significant impact on adiponectin levels despite reductions in visceral adipose tissue. More studies are needed to determine a role for GH in treatment of select PWH.

The GH analog tesamorelin (Egrifta™) was approved by the FDA in 2010 and has been shown to have benefits in lowering central fat and improving dyslipidemia (Falutz et al., 2007; Stanley et al., 2014). Use of this product has been limited by the need for daily subcutaneous injections and uncertainty regarding long-term benefits. It also is expensive, with a monthly cost of about $3,000 (Pharmacoeconomic Review, 2016).

A recent study that used the farnesyltransferase inhibitors (FTIs) tipifarnib and lonafarnib was successful in preventing lipodystrophy and metabolic syndrome induced by lopinavir/ritonavir in mice (Tanaka et al., 2018). The authors believe these data support FTIs as a possible strategy to prevent or treat PI-associated lipodystrophy and metabolic syndrome in PWH. Further human studies are needed to understand and clarify a therapeutic for role of FTIs.

Surgical treatment of excess fat accumulation has been done with liposuction, but long-term success is limited by the tendency of fat to reaccumulate (Hultman et al., 2007). Facial lipoatrophy has been treated with lipofilling with autologous fat transfer (Uzzan et al., 2012) or polyalkylimide gel (De Santis et al., 2012). Other artificial fillers, including silicone, have been used with psychological improvement in body image perception (Mori et al., 2006).

CONCLUSION

HIV infection and ART continue to be associated with HAL. Although these complications affected many patients in the mid- to late 1990s and early 2000s, the relative incidences of lipoatrophy and lipohypertrophy are changing over time, with a decrease in the former and an increase in the latter, especially in the aging HIV population. Nevertheless, these changes in body morphology are complicated by physical symptoms due to the nature of fat accumulation, psychological discomfort due to abnormal body image perception, and metabolic complications such as dyslipidemia and insulin resistance with an increased risk of CVD and fatty liver disease. Effective preventive therapies are needed for these complications as current treatment options are limited and often are just focused on symptoms or complications. In addition, there is an vital need for further research to understand the pathophysiologic mechanisms of HAL in PWH.

REFERENCES

Addy CL, Gavrila A, Tsiodras S, et al. Hypoadiponectinemia is associated with insulin resistance, hypertriglyceridemia, and fat redistribution in human immunodeficiency virus-infected patients treated with highly active antiretroviral therapy. *J Clin Endocrinol Metab.* 2003;88:627–636.

Akinci B, Unlu SM, Simsir IY, et al. Renal complications of lipodystrophy: a closer look at the natural history of kidney disease. *Clin Endocrinol.* 2018;89(1):65–75. doi:10.1111/cen.13732

Bacchetti P, Gripshover B, Grunfeld C, et al.; Study of Fat Redistribution and Metabolic Change in HIV Infection (FRAM). Fat distribution in men with HIV infection. *J AIDS.* 2005;40(2):121–131.

Balasubramanyam A, Sekhar RV, Jahoor F, et al. Pathophysiology of dyslipidemia and increased cardiovascular risk in HIV lipodystrophy: a model of "systemic steatosis." *Curr Opin Lipidol.* 2004;15:59–67.

Beires MT, Silva-Pinto A, Santos AC, et al. Visceral adipose tissue and carotid intima-media thickness in HIV-infected patients undergoing cART: a prospective cohort study. *BMC Infect Dis.* 2018;18(1):32.

Beraldo RA, Vassimon HS, Aragon DC, et al. Proposed ratios and cut-offs for the assessment of lipodystrophy in HIV-seropositive individuals. *Eur J Clin Nutr.* 2015;69(2):274–278.

Bergersen BM, Sandvik L, Bruun JN. Body composition changes in 308 Norwegian HIV-positive patients. *Scand J Infect Dis.* 2004;36:186–191.

Bernasconi E, Boubaker K, Junghans C, et al. Abnormalities of body fat distribution in HIV-infected persons treated with antiretroviral drugs: the Swiss HIV Cohort Study. *JAIDS.* 2002;31:50–55.

Bhutia E, Hemal A, Yadav TP, et al. Lipodystrophy syndrome among HIV infected children on highly active antiretroviral therapy in northern India. *Afr Health Sci.* 2014;14(2):408–413.

Bouatou Y, Gayet Ageron A, Bernasconi E, et al. Lipodystrophy increases the risk of CKD development in HIV positive patients in Switzerland: the LIPOKID study. *Kidney Int Rep.* 2018;3(5):1089–1099.

Bourgi K, Jenkins CA, Rebeiro PF, et al. Weight gain among treatment-naïve persons with HIV starting integrase inhibitors compared to non-nucleoside reverse transcriptase inhibitors or protease inhibitors in a large observational cohort in the United States and Canada. *J Int AIDS Soc.* 2020a;23(4):325484.

Bourgi K, Rebeiro PF, Turner M, et al. Greater weight gain in treatment-naive persons starting dolutegravir-based antiretroviral therapy. *Clin Infect Dis.* 2020b;70(7):1267–1274.

Calza L, Manfredi R, Chiodo F. Insulin resistance and diabetes mellitus in HIV infected patients receiving antiretroviral therapy. *Metab Syndr Relat Disord.* 2004;2:241–250.

Cames C, Pascal L, Ba A, et al. Low prevalence of lipodystrophy in HIV-infected Senegalese children on long-term antiretroviral treatment: the ANRS 12279 MAGGSEN Pediatric Cohort Study. *BMC Infect Dis.* 2018;18:374.

Carr A, Emery S, Law M, et al. An objective case definition of lipodystrophy in HIV-infected adults: a case–control study. *Lancet.* 2003;361:726–735.

Carr A, Law M. An objective lipodystrophy severity grading scale derived from the lipodystrophy case definition score. *J AIDS.* 2003;33:571–576.

Carr A, Samaras K, Burton S, et al. A syndrome of peripheral lipodystrophy, hyperlipidemia and insulin resistance in patients receiving HIV protease inhibitors. *AIDS.* 1998;12:F51–F58.

Carr A, Workman C, Carey D, et al. No effect of rosiglitazone for treatment of HIV-1: randomized, double-blind, placebo-controlled trial. *Lancet.* 2004;363(9407):429–438.

Carter VM, Hoy JF, Bailey M, et al. The prevalence of lipodystrophy in an ambulant HIV-infected population: it all depends on the definition. *HIV Med.* 2001;2(3):174–180.

Cavalcanti RB, Cheung AM, Raboud J, et al. Reproducibility of DXA estimations of body fat in HIV lipodystrophy: implications for clinical research. *J Clin Densitom.* 2005;8:293–297.

Chêne G, Angelini E, Cotte L, et al. Role of long-term nucleoside-analogue therapy in lipodystrophy and metabolic disorders in human immunodeficiency virus-infected patients. *Clin Infect Dis.* 2002;34(5):649–657.

D'Amico S, Shi J, Sekhar RV, et al. Physiologic growth hormone replacement improves fasting lipid kinetics in patients with HIV lipodystrophy syndrome. *Am J Clin Nutr.* 2006;84(1):204–211.

d'Arminio A, Sabin CA, Phillips AN, et al. Cardio- and cerebrovascular events in HIV-infected persons. *AIDS.* 2004;18(13):1811–1817.

De Santis G, Pignatti M, Baccarani A, et al. Long-term efficacy and safety of polyacrylamide hydrogel injection in the treatment of human immunodeficiency virus-related facial lipoatrophy: a 5-year follow-up. *Plastic Reconstruct Surg.* 2012;129(1):101–109.

Engelson ES, Kotler DP, Tan Y, et al. Fat distribution in HIV-infected patients reporting truncal enlargement quantified by whole-body magnetic resonance imaging. *Am J Clin Nutr.* 1999;69:1162–1169.

Falutz J, Allas S, Blot K, et al. Metabolic effects of a growth hormone-releasing factor in patients with HIV. *N Engl J Med.* 2007;357(23):2359–2370.

Friis-Moller N, Reiss P, Sabin CA, et al. Class of antiretroviral drugs and the risk of myocardial infarction. *N Engl J Med.* 2007;356:1723–1735.

Friis-Moller N, Weber R, Reiss P, et al. Cardiovascular disease risk factors in HIV patients—association with antiretroviral therapy. Results from the D:A:D study. *AIDS.* 2003;17(8):1179–1193.

Gan SK, Samaras K, Thompson CH, et al. Altered myocellular and abdominal fat partitioning predict disturbance in insulin action in HIV protease inhibitor-related lipodystrophy. *Diabetes.* 2002;51:3163–3169.

Gelpi M, Afzal S, Lundgren J, et al. Higher risk of abdominal obesity, elevated LDL cholesterol, hypertriglyceridemia, but not of hypertension in PLWH: results from the Copenhagen Comorbidity in HIV Infection (COCOMO) Study. *Clin Infect Dis.* 2018;67(4):579–586. doi:10.1093/cid/ciy146

Gibellini L, De Biasi S, Pinto M, et al. The protease inhibitor atazanavir triggers autophagy and mitochoagy in human preadipocytes. *AIDS.* 2012;26(16):2017–2026.

Glesby MJ, Hanna DB, Hoover DR, et al. Abdominal fat depots and subclinical carotid artery atherosclerosis in women with and without HIV Infection. *JAIDS.* 2018;77(3):308–316.

Gold DR, Annino DJ, Jr. HIV-associated cervicodorsal lipodystrophy: etiology and management. *Laryngoscope.* 2005;115:791–795.

Hadigan C, Kamin D, Liebau J, et al. Depot-specific regulation of glucose uptake and insulin sensitivity in HIV-lipodystrophy. *Am J Physiol Endocrinol Metab.* 2006;290:E289–E298.

Hadigan C, Meigs JB, Corcoran C, et al. Metabolic abnormalities and cardiovascular disease risk factors in adults with human immunodeficiency virus infection and lipodystrophy. *Clin Infect Dis.* 2001;32:130–139.

Hadigan C, Yawetz S, Thomas A, et al. Metabolic effects of rosiglitazone in HIV lipodystrophy: a randomized, controlled trial. *Ann Intern Med.* 2004;140(10):786–794.

Herry I, Bernand L, de Truchis P, et al. Hypertrophy of the breasts in a patient treated with indinavir. *Clin Infect Dis.* 1997;25:937–938.

Hultman CS, McPhail LE, Donaldson JH, et al. Surgical management of HIV-associated lipodystrophy: role of ultrasonic-assisted liposuction and suction-assisted lipectomy in the treatment of lipohypertrophy. *Ann Plast Surg.* 2007;58(3):255–263.

Innes S, Harvery J, Collins IJ, et al. Lipoatrophy/lipohypertrophy outcomes after antiretroviral therapy switch in children in the UK/Ireland. *PLoS One.* 2018;13(4):e0194132.

Kerchberger AM, Sheth AN, Angert CD, et al. Weight gain associated with integrase stand transfer inhibitor use in women. *Clin Infect Dis.* 2020;71(3):593–600.

Kim RJ, Carlow DC, Rutstein JH, et al. Hypoadiponectinemia, dyslipidemia, and impaired growth in children with HIV-associated facial lipoatrophy. *J Pediatr Endocrinol Metab.* 2007;20:65–74.

Kuk JL, Katzmarzyk PT, Nichaman MZ, et al. Visceral fat is an independent predictor of all-cause mortality in men. *Obesity.* 2006;14:336–341.

Leung V, Chiu YL, Kotler DP, et al. Effect of recombinant human growth hormone and rosiglitazone for HIV-associated abdominal fat accumulation on adiponectin and other markers of inflammation. *HIV Clin Trials.* 2016;17(2):55–62

Lichtenstein K, Delaney KM, Armon C, et al. Incidence of and risk factors for lipoatrophy (abnormal fat loss) in ambulatory HIV-1-infected patients. *J AIDS.* 2003; 32:48–56.

Lichtenstein K, Wanke C, Henry K, et al. Estimated prevalence of HIV-associated adipose redistribution syndrome (HARS): abnormal abdominal fat accumulation in HIV-infected patients. *Antiviral Ther.* 2004;9:L33.

Lo JC, Mulligan K, Tai VW, et al. "Buffalo hump" in men with HIV-1 infection. *Lancet.* 1998;351:867–870.

Luzi L, Perseghin G, Tambussi G, et al. Intramyocellular lipid accumulation and reduced whole body lipid oxidation in HIV lipodystrophy. *Am J Physiol Endocrinol Metab*. 2003;284:E274–E280.

Mallon PW, Wand H, Law M, et al.; HIV Lipodystrophy Case Definition Study; Australian Lipodystrophy Prevalence Survey Investigators. Buffalo hump seen in HIV-associated lipodystrophy is associated with hyperinsulinemia but not dyslipidemia. *J AIDS*. 2005;38:156–162.

Martin A, Mallon PW. Therapeutic approaches to combating lipoatrophy: do they work? *J Antimicrob Chemother*. 2005;55:612–615.

Massip P, Marchou B, Bonnet E, et al. Lipodystrophy with protease inhibitors in HIV patients. *Thérapie*. 1997;52:615.

Meinrenken S. "Bull-neck" in HIV-positive patients: result of therapy? *Dtsch Med Wochenschr*. 1998;22:123(21):A9.

Miller J, Carr A, Emery S, et al. HIV lipodystrophy: prevalence, severity and correlates of risk in Australia. *HIV Med*. 2003;4:293–301.

Mori A, Lo Russo G, Agostini T, et al. Treatment of human immunodeficiency virus-associated facial lipoatrophy with lipofilling and submalar silicone implants. *J Plastic Reconstruct Aesthetic Surg*. 2006;59(11):1209–1216.

Morrison M, Hughes HY, Naggie S, et al. Nonalcoholic fatty liver disease among individuals with HIV infection: a growing concern? *Dig Dis Sci*. 2019;64(12):3394–3401.

Murata H, Hruz PW, Mueckler M. Indinavir inhibits the glucose transporter isoform Glut4 at physiologic concentrations. *AIDS*. 2002;16:859–863.

National Cholesterol Education Program. Executive summary of the third report of the National Cholesterol Education Program (NCEP) Expert Panel on Detection, Evaluation, and Treatment of High Blood Cholesterol in Adults (Adult Treatment Panel III). *JAMA*. 2001;285:2486–2497.

Nguyen D, Hsu JW, Jahoor F, et al. Effect of increasing glutathione with cysteine and glycine supplementation on mitochondrial fuel oxidation, insulin sensitivity, and body composition in older HIV-infected patients. *J Clin Endocrinol Metab*. 2014;99(1):169–177.

Paparizos VA, Kyriakis KP, Polydorou-Pfandl D, et al. Epidemiologic characteristics of Koebner's phenomenon in AIDS-related Kaposi's sarcoma. *J AIDS*. 2000;25:283–284.

Parruti G, Toro GM. Persistence of lipoatrophy after a four-year long interruption of antiretroviral therapy for HIV1 infection: case report. *BMC Infect Dis*. 2005;5:80.

Persson A. Facing HIV: body shape change and the (in) visibility of illness. *Med Anthropol*. 2005;24:237–264.

Peterson S, Martins CR, Cofranscesci J Jr. Lipodystrophy in the patient with HIV: social, psychological and treatment considerations. *Anesthet Surg J*. 2008;28(4):443–451.

Pharmacoeconomic Review Report: Tesamorelin (Egrifta). Ottawa (ON): Canadian Agency for Drugs and Technologies in Health; 2016 Aug. Executive Summary.

Ramírez-Marrero FA, Santana-Bagur JL, Joyner MJ, et al. Metabolic syndrome in relation to cardiorespiratory fitness, active and sedentary behavior in HIV+ Hispanics with and without lipodystrophy. *P R Health Sci J*. 2014;33(4):163–169

Reeds DN, Middendorf B, Patterson BW, et al. Alterations in lipid kinetics in men with HIV-dyslipidemia. *Am J Physiol Endocrinol Metab*. 2003;285:E490–E497.

Reynolds NR, Neidig JL, Wu AW, et al. Balancing disfigurement and fear of disease progression: patient perceptions of HIV body fat redistribution. *AIDS Care*. 2006;18:663–673.

Ribera E, Paradineiro JC, Curran A, et al. Improvements in subcutaneous fat, lipid profile, and parameters of mitochondrial toxicity in patients with peripheral lipoatrophy when stavudine is switcher to tenofovir (LIPOTEST study). *HIV Clin Trials*. 2008;9(6):407–417.

Ristig M, Drechsler H, Powderly WG. Hepatic steatosis and HIV infection. *AIDS Patient Care STDs*. 2005;19:356–365.

Roth VR, Kravcik S, Angel JB. Development of cervical fat pads following therapy with human immunodeficiency virus type 1 protease inhibitors. *Clin Infect Dis*. 1998;27:65–67.

Safrin S, Grunfeld C. Fat distribution and metabolic changes in patients with HIV infection. *AIDS*. 1999;13(18):2493–505.

Samaras K, Wand H, Law M, et al. Prevalence of metabolic syndrome in HIV-infected patients receiving highly active antiretroviral therapy using International Diabetes Foundation and Adult Treatment Panel III Criteria: associations with insulin resistance, disturbed body fat compartmentalization, elevated C-reactive peptide, and hypoadiponectinemia. *Diabetes Care*. 2007;30:113–119.

Sattler F. Body habitus changes related to lipodystrophy. *Clin Infect Dis*. 2003;36:S84–S90.

Saves M, Raffi F, Capeau J, et al. Factors related to lipodystrophy and metabolic alterations in patients with human immunodeficiency virus infection receiving highly active antiretroviral therapy. *Clin Infect Dis*. 2002;34:1396–1405.

Sax PE, Erlandson KM, Lake JE, et al. Weight gain following initiation of antiretroviral therapy: risk factors in randomized clinical trials. *Clin Infect Dis*. 2020;71:1380–1389.

Schambelan M, Benson CA, Carr A, et al. Management of metabolic complications associated with antiretroviral therapy for HIV-1 infection: recommendations of an International AIDS Society–USA panel. *J AIDS*. 2002;31:257–275.

Schwenk A. Methods of assessing body shape and composition in HIV-associated lipodystrophy. *Curr Opin Infect Dis*. 2002;15:9–16.

Schwenk A, Breuer P, Kremer G, et al. Clinical assessment of HIV-associated lipodystrophy syndrome: bioelectrical impedance analysis, anthropometry and clinical scores. *Clin Nutr*. 2001;20:243–249.

Sears S, Buendia JR, Odem S, et al. Metabolic syndrome among people living with HIV receiving medical care in southern United States: prevalence and risk factors. *AIDS Behav*. 2019;23(11):2916–2925.

Sekhar RV, Jahoor F, Pownall HJ, et al. Severely dysregulated disposal of postprandial triacylglycerols exacerbates hypertriacylglycerolemia in HIV lipodystrophy syndrome. *Am J Clin Nutr*. 2005;81:1405–1410.

Sekhar RV, Jahoor F, White AC, et al. Metabolic basis of HIV lipodystrophy syndrome. *Am J Physiol Endocrinol Metab*. 2002;283:E332–E337.

Sekhar RV, Patel SG, D'Amico S, et al. Effects of rosiglitazone on abnormal lipid kinetics in HIV-associated dyslipidemic lipodystrophy: a stable isotope study. *Metabolism*. 2011;60(6):754–760.

Stanley TL, Feldpausch MN, Oh J, et al. Effect of tesamorelin on visceral fat and liver fat in HIV-infected patients with abdominal fat accumulation: a randomized clinical trial. *JAMA*. 2014;312(4):380–389

Sutinen J, Hakkinen AM, Westerbacka J, et al. Increased fat accumulation in the liver in HIV-infected patients with antiretroviral therapy-associated lipodystrophy. *AIDS*. 2002;16:2183–2193.

Sutinen J, Hakkinen AM, Westerbacka J, et al. Rosiglitazone in the treatment of HAART-associated lipodystrophy: a randomized double-blind placebo-controlled study. *Antiviral Ther*. 2003;8(3):199–207.

Tanaka T, Nakazawa H, Kuriyama N, et al. Farnesyltransferase inhibitors prevent HIV protease inhibitor (lopinavir/ritonavir) induced lipodystrophy and metabolic syndrome in mice. *Exp Ther Med*. 2018;15(2):1314–1320.

Tien PC, Grunfeld C. What is HIV-associated lipodystrophy? Defining fat distribution changes in HIV infection. *Curr Opin Infect Dis*. 2004;17:27–32.

Torres RA, Unger KW, Cadman JA, et al. Recombinant human growth hormone improves truncal adiposity and "buffalo humps" in HIV-positive patients on HAART. *AIDS*. 1999;13:2479–2481.

Triant VA, Lee H, Hadigan C, et al. Increased acute myocardial infarction rates and cardiovascular risk factors among patients with HIV disease. *J Clin Endocrinol Metab*. 2007;92:2506–2512.

Turner R, Testa MA, Su M, et al. The impact of HIV-associated adipose redistribution syndrome (HARS) on health-related quality of life. *Antiviral Ther*. 2006;11:L25.

Uzzan C, Boccara D, Lacheré A, et al. Treatment of facial lipoatrophy by lipofilling in HIV infected patients: retrospective study on 317 patients on 9 years. *Ann Chir Plast Esthet*. 2012;57(3):210–216.

van der Valk M, Bisschop PH, Romijn JA. Lipodystrophy in HIV-1-positive patients is associated with insulin resistance in multiple metabolic pathways. *AIDS*. 2001;15:2093–2100.

Varriale P, Saravi G, Hernandez E, et al. Acute myocardial infarction in patients infected with human immunodeficiency virus. *Am Heart J*. 2004;147(1):55–59.

Vazquez E. Understanding and treating protease paunch. *Posit Aware*. 1999;10(4):59–63.

Vigano A, Mora S, Manzoni P, et al. Effects of recombinant growth hormone on visceral fat accumulation: pilot study in human immunodeficiency virus-infected adolescents. *J Clin Endocrinol Metab*. 2005;90:4075–4080.

Worm D, Kirk O, Anderson O, et al. Clinical lipoatrophy in HIV-1 patients on HAART is not associated with increased abdominal girth, hyperlipidemia or glucose intolerance. *HIV Med*. 2002;3(4): 239–246.

Yin MT, Glesby MJ. Recombinant human growth hormone therapy in HIV-associated wasting and visceral adiposity. *Expert Rev Anti Infect Ther*. 2005;3:727–738.

42.

IMMUNE RECONSTITUTION INFLAMMATORY SYNDROME (IRIS)

Dagan Coppock

CHAPTER GOALS

Upon completion of this chapter, the reader should be able to:

- Understand the epidemiology of IRIS and its associated opportunistic infections (OIs)

- Recognize the timing considerations regarding opportunistic infection treatment and antiretroviral therapy (ART) initiation as related to the risk for IRIS

- Understand the management approaches to IRIS, based upon its presentation and the underlying OI

LEARNING OBJECTIVE

- Review the current status of research and clinical recommendations regarding IRIS

WHAT'S NEW?

- Clinical trial data suggest that the use of integrase strand transfer inhibitor (INSTI)-based ART regimens do not increase the risk for IRIS.

- For people with HIV (PWH) who are coinfected with hepatitis C virus (HCV) and active hepatitis B virus (HBV), ART that is active against HBV should be initiated before starting HCV treatment.

KEY POINTS

- IRIS is associated with either worsening of a recognized infection (paradoxical IRIS) or an unrecognized infection (unmasking IRIS), which occurs in the setting of improved immunologic function.

- Most people presenting with IRIS should be maintained on ART along with treatment for the associated infection.

INTRODUCTION

The hallmark of HIV pathogenesis is the gradual destruction of the cell-mediated immune system over a period of many years, as evidenced by a progressive and profound decline in CD4[+] T-helper lymphocytes. This decline leads to increased susceptibility to OIs, malignancies, and the development of AIDS. ART can suppress HIV replication, preventing further deterioration, and it allows for the regeneration of the immune system. Even people with advanced AIDS have a marked improvement in both quantity and quality of their immune system after starting ART. However, in a subset of those initiating ART, the harmonious, gradual reconstitution of the immune system does not occur; rather, there is a rapid immunologic recovery with an abrupt transition to a pathologic inflammatory state often causing clinical deterioration. Opportunistic and other infections, previously unrecognized or tolerated by the failing immune system, suddenly become the targets of this overzealous immunologic recovery. In this inflammatory state, people can clinically worsen despite an otherwise excellent response to ART, as evidenced by a decreased viral load and increased CD4[+] T-cell counts. This paradoxical inflammatory response has been termed *immune reconstitution inflammatory syndrome* or IRIS (French et al., 2004), which is used an umbrella term encompassing two clinical entities: (1) paradoxical IRIS, an exacerbation of a known OI, and (2) unmasking IRIS, a flare of an undiagnosed (subclinical) OI.

INCIDENCE AND ASSOCIATED OIS

The incidence of IRIS depends on the population being studied. It occurs more frequently in persons with specific OIs, a higher viral load, and more significant immunosuppression (Müller et al., 2010). The HIV Outpatient Study—an eight-city, US-wide, prospective cohort study—evaluated 2,610 persons with 370 cases of IRIS (occurring in 276 people) who initiated or resumed ART and, during the next 6 months, demonstrated a decline in plasma HIV RNA viral load of at least 0.5 $\log_{10}$ copies/mL or an increase of at least 50% in CD4[+] T-cell count per microliter. It reported that the incidence of IRIS was 10.6%. The most common IRIS-defining diagnoses were candidiasis (23%), cytomegalovirus (CMV) infection (3.5%), disseminated *Mycobacterium avium intracellulare* (3.2%), *Pneumocystis* pneumonia (2.7%), *Varicella zoster* (2.4%), Kaposi's sarcoma (KS) (2.4%), non-Hodgkin's lymphoma (2.2%), and *Mycobacterium tuberculosis* (0.3%). IRIS was independently associated with CD4+ T-cell counts of less than 50 cells/mL versus at least 200 cells/mL (odds ratio [OR], 5.0) and a viral load of at least 5.0 $\log_{10}$ copies/mL versus less than 4.0 $\log_{10}$ copies/mL (OR, 2.3) (Novak et al., 2012). In contrast, a study from the University of Washington HIV Cohort demonstrated a higher rate of IRIS in people with KS (29%), with no evident cases in people with CMV disease or *Candida* esophagitis. In this study, the highest IRIS-associated morbidity was in cases of visceral KS. The differences in clinical characteristics between these two studies may reflect population and geographic variability.

IRIS AND ART

In addition to the potential demographic factors that might affect the presentation of IRIS, the choice of ART regimen may also play a role. The AIDS Clinical Trial Group (ACTG) reported the incidence and associations with IRIS in ACTG 5202, a phase 3b, randomized clinical trial conducted in the US that compared the safety, tolerability, and efficacy of four commonly used, once-daily, initial ART regimens. Two dual nucleoside/nucleotide reverse transcriptase inhibitor (NRTI) fixed-dose combinations (tenofovir disoproxil fumarate/emtricitabine or abacavir/lamivudine) were compared when used in combination with either the nonnucleoside reverse transcriptase inhibitor (NNRTI) efavirenz or a ritonavir-boosted protease inhibitor, atazanavir/ritonavir. Among 1,848 eligible participants who initiated in this study, IRIS events occurred in 52 participants by week 48, with 4 participants having two events. Incidence rates were 6.05 (95% confidence interval [CI], 4.57–8.00) and 3.30 (95% CI, 2.51–4.33) cases/100 person-years (pys) through 24 and 48 weeks, respectively. IRIS occurred 1 to 298 days after the initiation of ART, with 75% of cases occurring within 67 days and 3 cases after 24 weeks. IRIS events included the following associated OIs or other clinical diagnoses: *Mycobacterium avium* complex (MAC) ($n = 11$); *Varicella zoster* virus ($n = 11$); herpes simplex virus ($n = 8$); KS ($n = 5$); HCV, tuberculosis (TB), and *Pneumocystis jirovecii* pneumonia (PCP) ($n = 4$ each); toxoplasmosis and cryptococcosis ($n = 2$ each); and CMV-associated colitis, progressive multifocal leukoencephalopathy (PML), *Mycobacterium kansasii*, eosinophilic folliculitis, and swollen lymph node ($n = 1$ each). The most commonly reported symptoms were fever and pain. There were no deaths from IRIS in this cohort. Among participants with IRIS, median baseline HIV RNA was 4.9 $\log_{10}$ copies/mL, median CD4+ T-cell count was 49 cells/mL, and 50% had prior AIDS illness. In univariate Cox proportional hazards models, an increased risk of IRIS was associated with baseline prior AIDS illness, higher HIV RNA level, lower CD4+ T-cell

count and percentage, lower CD8+ T-cell count and higher percentage, and lower CD4+:CD8+ T-cell ratio (all $p \leq 0.01$). No significant association was observed with sex, age, or race/ethnicity ($p > 0.19$). Of note, IRIS events were more common with abacavir/lamivudine relative to tenofovir/emtricitabine for participants with low CD4+ T-cell counts. This finding may reflect the more rapid CD4+ T-cell increases observed with abacavir/lamivudine regimens (Fischl et al., 2010).

Recently, observational data have raised concerns regarding INSTI-based regimens and their associations with IRIS, although subsequent clinical trial data do not bear out these findings. In a retrospective cohort trial, 2,287 persons with CD4+ T-cell counts below 200/mL were evaluated by ART regimen. Cohorts consisted of participants receiving either INSTI-based or non-INSTI-based ART regimens. The OR for developing IRIS was 1.99 (1.09–3.47) ($p = 0.04$) for the INSTI-based group (Dutertre et al., 2017). Similarly, the ATHENA observational study evaluated the association of INSTI initiation with the development of IRIS, as defined by either previously established criteria (French et al., 2004) or the French criteria plus clinical diagnosis. The study found that the use of INSTI-based treatment was independently associated with IRIS based on the French criteria (HR 2.6; 95% CI, 1.3–5.1; $p = 0.004$) as well as IRIS based on the French criteria plus clinical diagnosis (HR 2.6; 95% CI, 1.6–4.4; $p = 0.0001$) (Wijting et al., 2017). However, a subsequent clinical trial demonstrated no significant risk of IRIS despite the use of INSTI-based therapy. In this trial, 1,805 participants were randomized to receive either standard therapy (2NRTI + NNRTI) or standard therapy plus raltegravir. Looking at an outcome of fatal/nonfatal IRIS-compatible events, there was no significant difference between the standard arm compared with the standard-plus-raltegravir arm (9.5% vs. 9.9%, $p = 0.79$) (Gibb et al., 2018). Subsequent publication of the ATHENA data suggested that channeling bias may partially account for the study's findings (Wijting et al., 2019).

ETIOLOGY AND PATHOGENESIS

Recovery of pathogen-specific T-cell responses and an increased production of pro-inflammatory chemokines and cytokines produced by the innate immune response after commencing ART may contribute to the immunopathogenesis of IRIS. Higher T-cell responses to nonstructural antigens of HCV in enzyme-linked immunosorbent spot assays and higher serum levels of antibodies to a mixture of virus proteins were demonstrated in PWH and HCV coinfection who experienced an increase in serum liver enzyme levels after commencing ART (Cameron et al., 2011). People who develop TB IRIS have lower plasma levels of the chemokine CCL2 before commencing ART (Oliver et al., 2010).

The identification of biomarkers could be used to diagnose IRIS in the future and predict which persons might be at risk. A cohort of 45 HIV-1–infected, treatment-naive persons with baseline CD4+ T-cell counts of 100 cells/μL or less who were started on ART, who suppressed HIV RNA to less than 50 copies/mL, and who were seen every 1 to 3 months for 1 year were retrospectively evaluated for suspected or confirmed IRIS. Pre-ART levels of both D-dimer and the inflammatory biomarker C-reactive protein (CRP) were higher in IRIS cases versus controls (Porter et al., 2010). In another study, individuals with elevated baseline levels of CRP and the fibrosis biomarker hyaluronic acid were more likely to progress to AIDS, develop IRIS, or die within the first month after starting ART (Boulware et al., 2011). Large prospective studies to elucidate the predictive and diagnostic values of IRIS biomarkers are needed.

GUIDELINES FOR ART INITIATION

Current guidelines recommend the early initiation of ART except in select clinical scenarios. US Department of Health and Human Services (USDHHS, 2018) guidelines recommend early initiation of ART despite the presence of OIs, with the exception of cryptococcal and tuberculous meningitis, for which a "short delay" may be warranted. Recommendations of the International Antiviral Society (IAS)-USA Panel agree that, in the setting of most OIs, ART should be initiated within 2 weeks (Saag et al., 2020). However, the guidelines go on to elaborate that for pulmonary TB, ART can be initiated within 2 weeks of starting TB treatment for persons with a CD4+ T-cell count less than 50 cells/mL and between 2 to 8 weeks for persons with a CD4+ T-cell count greater than 50 cells/mL The IAS-USA guidelines go on to state that, in cases of cryptococcal meningitis in resource-rich areas, ART can be initiated within 2 weeks, albeit with careful monitoring and aggressive management of intracranial pressure.

ART INITIATION AND THE RISK OF NON–TB-ASSOCIATED IRIS

The timing of ART initiation and its association with OI-specific IRIS remains a concern for clinicians. In the ACTG 5164 study, 282 participants with an acute OI and a baseline median CD4+ T-cell count of 29 cells/mL were prospectively randomized to immediate (<14 days) versus delayed (>28 days) initiation of ART. In this study, which included participants diagnosed with PCP (63%), cryptococcal meningitis (12%), and bacterial infections (12%), earlier initiation of ART resulted in less progression to AIDS and/or death and no increase in adverse events or loss of virologic response compared to deferred ART. Participants with or on treatment for TB were excluded. Rates of IRIS in this study were low (7%) and did not differ by timing of ART (Zolopa et al., 2009). IRIS was reported in 23 cases and confirmed in 20, 8 participants in the immediate arm and 12 in the deferred arm. There was no evidence of an association of IRIS with the entry OI/bacterial infection: 13 (65%) IRIS cases were in participants with PCP, who made up 63% of the study population. IRIS developed a median of 33 days (interquartile range, 26–72 days) after initiation of ART. There was no significant difference in the frequency of IRIS between participants who received corticosteroids during the treatment of their OI and those who did not receive corticosteroids: 9/150 (6%) versus 11/112 (9.8%), respectively ($p = 0.35$).

The optimal timing of ART initiation in cryptococcal meningitis is controversial. Approximately 25% of PWH and treated cryptococcal meningitis will experience IRIS after commencing ART (Haddow et al., 2010). It is associated with mortality in more than 25% of persons from resource-poor countries, and it is an important cause of early mortality after starting ART in PWH from these countries. Early initiation of ART (within 72 hours) in people with treated cryptococcal meningitis was associated with a higher rate of mortality compared to those who waited for at least 10 weeks in one study (Makadzange et al., 2010). However, a more recent study suggested that, in high-resource areas, there is no significant difference in mortality for people who initiate ART within 2 weeks of beginning antifungal treatment (Ingle et al., 2015). Based on the studies completed and expert opinion, it is prudent to delay initiation of ART until after the completion of induction therapy (the first 2 weeks) and possibly until the total induction/consolidation (10 weeks) phase has been completed. There are certain scenarios where a delay in ART may be important, such as when there is evidence of increased intracranial pressure or in those with low cerebrospinal fluid (CSF) white cell counts.

IRIS related to JC polyoma virus infection remains a clinical challenge as ART initiation and immune reconstitution is the only available treatment. Prior to ART, JC virus infection can lead to PML in people with advanced HIV infection. However, approximately 15% of individuals experience an exacerbation of PML after ART is commenced (Martin-Blondel et al., 2011). A review of 54 cases of PML IRIS evaluated the mortality of persons as stratified by steroid use. Five of the 12 persons receiving steroids and 14 of the 42 persons not receiving steroids died, suggesting a high mortality of PML IRIS, regardless of steroid use (Tan et al., 2009).

In people coinfected with HIV and viral hepatitides, IRIS is a frequent concern. Up to 25% of PWH with HBV or HCV coinfection experience a flare of hepatitis and/or elevation of serum liver enzyme levels after commencing ART (Cameron et al., 2011; Crane et al., 2009). Hepatitis flares in PWH and HBV coinfection are associated with a higher plasma HBV DNA level before ART (Crane et al., 2009), suggesting that pathogen load is an important determinant of disease. Even when ART with activity against HBV is selected for treatment, HBV IRIS can still occur, complicating the differential of a hepatitis flare (Crane et al., 2008). In recent years, the use of direct-acting antivirals for treating HCV has further complicated the differential. The use of direct-acting antivirals has been associated with HBV reactivation (Bersoff-Matcha et al., 2017). This has led to changes in guidelines regarding the timing of ART initiation in people with viral hepatitis. For people who are both coinfected with HIV/HCV and who have active HBV infection, USDHHS guidelines now recommend first initiating ART with activity against HBV before starting direct-acting antivirals.

TB IRIS AND ART INITIATION

For PWH and TB coinfection, unmasking and paradoxical IRIS can lead to two distinct clinical scenarios. In the context of TB, unmasking IRIS is the development of overt TB in people who initially screened negative for this infection, typically seen within the first 60 days following ART initiation (Dheda et al., 2004; Shelburne et al., 2006). It is thought to be due to an increase in circulating memory T cells that were sequestered in lymphatic tissue prior to therapy. Alternatively, paradoxical IRIS involves worsening of signs and symptoms of TB in individuals with a known history of TB after they have been started on ART.

The HIV-CAUSAL Collaboration demonstrated that the incidence of TB decreased after ART initiation but not among persons older than age 50 years or those with a CD4+ T-cell count of less than 50 cells/mL. Despite an overall decrease in TB incidence, the increased rate during 3 months of ART suggests unmasking IRIS. This is a multinational cohort study among PWH from high-income countries. Among 65,121 individuals, 712 developed TB during 28 months of median follow-up (incidence, 3.0 cases per 1,000 pys). The hazard ratio (HR) for TB for ART versus no ART was 0.56 (95% CI, 0.44–0.72) overall, 1.04 (95% CI, 0.64–1.68) for individuals aged older than 50 years, and 1.46 (95% CI, 0.70–3.04) for people with a CD4+ T-cell count of less than 50 cells/mL. Compared with people who had not started ART, HRs differed by time since ART initiation: 1.36 (95% CI, 0.98–1.89) for initiation less than 3 months previously and 0.44 (95% CI, 0.34–0.58) for initiation 3 months or more previously. Compared with people who had not initiated ART, HRs less than 3 months after ART initiation were 0.67 (95% CI, 0.38–1.18), 1.51 (95% CI, 0.98–2.31), and 3.20 (95% CI, 1.34–7.60) for people younger than age 35, aged 35 to 50, and older than age 50 years, respectively, and 2.30 (95% CI, 1.03–5.14) for people with a CD4+ T-cell count of less than 50 cells/mL (HIV-CAUSAL Collaboration, 2012).

In a South African cohort of 498 persons with advanced HIV, symptomatic individuals were screened for TB by chest x-ray and/or sputum examination. People who screened positive were initiated on anti-TB therapy prior to starting ART. Individuals who screened negative and went on to develop unmasking IRIS were found to have significantly elevated levels of interferon-γ (IFN-γ) and CRP at baseline prior to ART compared to non-IRIS, non-TB controls. These results suggest the presence of subclinical TB infection despite negative screening that was done prior to the initiation of ART (Haddow et al., 2009). Persons who exhibit paradoxical IRIS have been reported to have elevated tuberculin-specific effector memory CD4+ T cells prior to initiation of ART. Following the commencement of ART, increased levels of Th1-associated cytokines, IFN-γ, and tumor necrosis factor-α most likely contribute to the overwhelming inflammatory reaction to the TB antigen present (Bourgarit et al., 2009). Persons with HIV and latent TB (defined as >5 mm of skin test induration or positive IFN-γ release assay) are at increased risk for progression to active TB compared to the HIV-negative population, which underscores the need to identify and treat people with latent disease. Active TB in PWH requires immediate treatment. However, optimal timing of ART has yet to be established. The potential for multiple adverse drug reactions, drug–drug interactions, and IRIS reactions has led to increased difficulty in defining the proper timing of ART.

TIMING OF ART WITH TB IRIS

In recent years, there has been debate on the timing of ART initiation relative to the initiation of TB treatment in known coinfected people. However, based on a number of trials, as discussed here, current USDHHS guidelines recommend an early, integrative approach to ART and TB treatment initiation.

In the SAPiT trial, there were no differences in rates of AIDS or death between people who started ART within 4 weeks after initiating TB treatment and those who started ART at 8 to 12 weeks (i.e., within 4 weeks after completing the intensive phase of TB treatment) (Abdool Karim, 2010). However, in people with baseline CD4+ T-cell counts of less than 50 cells/mL, the rate of AIDS or death was lower in the earlier therapy group than in the later therapy group (8.5 vs. 26.3 cases per 100 pys, a strong trend favoring the earlier treatment arm [p = 0.06]). For all people, regardless of CD4+ T-cell count, earlier therapy was associated with a higher incidence of IRIS and of adverse events that required a switch in antiretroviral drugs compared to those who started therapy later. In this study, two deaths were attributed to IRIS.

In the CAMELIA study, people who had CD4+ T-cell counts of less than 200 cells/mL were randomized to initiate ART at 2 or 8 weeks after initiation of TB treatment (Blanc et al., 2011). Study participants had a median CD4+ T-cell count of 25 cells/mL and high rates of disseminated TB disease. ART initiated at 2 weeks resulted in a 38% reduction in mortality (p = 0.006) compared with that of therapy initiated at 8 weeks. A significant reduction in mortality was seen in people with CD4+ T-cell counts of 50 cells/mL or less and in people with CD4+ T-cell counts of 51 to 200 cells/mL. Overall, six deaths were associated with TB IRIS.

The ACTG 5221 (STRIDE) trial, a multinational study, randomized ART-naive individuals with confirmed or probable TB and CD4+ T-cell counts of less than 250 cells/mL to earlier (<2 weeks) or later (8–12 weeks) ART (Havlir et al., 2011). At study entry, the participants' median CD4+ T-cell count was 77 cells/mL. The rates of mortality and AIDS diagnoses were not different between the earlier and later arms, although higher rates of IRIS were seen in the earlier arm. However, a significant reduction in AIDS or death was seen in the subset of people with CD4+ T-cell counts of less than 50 cells/mL who were randomized to the earlier ART arm (p = 0.02).

Given the previously discussed data, USDHHS guidelines recommend the initiation of HAART within 2 weeks when an individual's CD4+ T-cell count is less than 50 cells/mL and by 8 to 12 weeks for all others. This reflects the observation that earlier ART initiation in TB-infected people improves mortality.

TREATMENT OF IRIS

Although the nonsteroidal anti-inflammatory agents or steroids are commonly used in clinical practice, the dosage and timing have not been well established in the medical literature. A double-blind, placebo-controlled, randomized clinical trial, including those receiving both ART and anti-TB therapy and experiencing paradoxical IRIS, evaluated a tapering course of prednisone over 4 weeks. Individuals on steroid therapy had a significantly decreased length of hospitalization and marked improvement of symptoms related to IRIS, suggesting a potential role for steroids in the management of paradoxical IRIS (Meintjes et al., 2010). In the previously described ACTG 5164 study, 63% of participants reported having *Pneumocystis* pneumonia as an OI. There was no significant difference in the frequency of IRIS between participants who received corticosteroids during the treatment and those who did not receive corticosteroids: 9/150 (6%) versus 11/112 (9.8%), respectively ($p = 0.35$).

In other forms of IRIS, such as MAC, surgical drainage of necrotic lymphadenitis may be of benefit. In people with cryptococcal meningitis IRIS, CSF drainage may provide relief of increased intracranial pressure. While the data to support the use of corticosteroids in cryptococcal meningitis IRIS are sparse, Infectious Disease Society of America guidelines recommend considering their use in the setting of central nervous system inflammation and increased intracranial pressure (Perfect, 2010). Corticosteroid or other anti-inflammatory therapies may also be effective for treating some forms of IRIS, such as PML-associated IRIS (Martin-Blondel et al., 2011).

As a general approach, in unmasking IRIS, management should focus on diagnosing the OI and instituting appropriate treatment. Screening for latent TB infection should be undertaken in all PWH. In paradoxical IRIS, it is crucial to exclude alternative diagnoses and ensure the individual is receiving appropriate treatment for the condition. In the majority of cases, ART is continued, but on rare occasions, cessation of ART is warranted in severe IRIS, particularly when it is life-threatening.

REFERENCES

Abdool Karim SS. Timing of initiation of antiretroviral drugs during tuberculosis therapy. *N Engl J Med.* 2010;362(8):697–706.

Bersoff-Matcha SJ, Cao K, et al. Hepatitis B virus reactivation associated with direct-acting antiviral therapy for chronic hepatitis C virus: a review of cases reported to the US Food and Drug Administration adverse event reporting system. *Ann Intern Med.* 2017;166(11):792–798.

Blanc FX, Sok T, Laureillard D, et al. Earlier versus later start of antiretroviral therapy in HIV-infected adults with tuberculosis. *N Engl J Med.* 2011;365(16):1471–1481.

Boulware DR, Hullsiek KH, Puronen CE, et al.; INSIGHT Study Group. Higher levels of CRP, D-dimer, IL-6, and hyaluronic acid

before initiation of antiretroviral therapy (ART) are associated with increased risk of AIDS or death. *J Infect Dis.* 2011;203(11):1637–1646.

Bourgarit A, Carcelain G, Samri A, et al. TB-associated immune restoration syndrome in HIV-1-infected patients involves tuberculin-specific CD4 Th1 cells and can be predicted by KIR-negative gammadelta T cells [Abstract 772]. Paper presented at the 16th Conference on Retroviruses and Opportunistic Infections, February 8–11, 2009, Montréal, Canada.

Cameron BA, Emerson CR, Workman C, et al. Alterations in immune function are associated with liver enzyme elevation in HIV and HCV co-infection after commencement of combination antiretroviral therapy. *J Clin Immunol.* 2011;31:1079–1083.

Crane M, Matthews G, Lewin SR. Hepatitis virus immune restoration disease of the liver. *Curr Opin HIV AIDS.* 2008;3(4):446–452.

Crane M, Oliver B, Matthews G, et al. Immunopathogenesis of hepatic flare in HIV/hepatitis B virus (HBV)-coinfected individuals after the initiation of HBV-active antiretroviral therapy. *J Infect Dis.* 2009;199:974–981.

Dheda K, Lampe FC, Johnson MA, et al. Outcome of HIV-associated tuberculosis in the era of highly active antiretroviral therapy. *J Infect Dis.* 2004;190(9):1670.

Dutertre M, Cuzin L, Demonchy E, et al. Initiation of antiretroviral therapy containing integrase inhibitors increases the risk of IRIS requiring hospitalization. *J AIDS.* 2017;76(1):e23–e26.

Fischl M, Mollan K, Pahwa S, et al. IRIS among US subjects starting ART in AIDS Clinical Trials Group Study A5202 [Abstract 791]. Paper presented at the 15th Conference on Retroviruses and Opportunistic infections, February 16–19, 2010, San Francisco, CA.

French MA, Price P, Stone SF. Immune restoration disease after antiretroviral therapy. *AIDS.* 2004;18:1615–1627.

Gibb D, Szubert AJ, Chidziva E, et al. Impact of raltegravir intensification of first-line ART on IRIS in the REALITY trial [Abstract 23]. Paper presented at the 25th Conference on Retroviruses and Opportunistic Infections, March 4–7, 2018.

Haddow L, Borrow P, Dibben O, et al. Cytokine profiles predict unmasking TB immune reconstitution inflammatory syndrome and are associated with unmasking and paradoxical presentations of TB immune reconstitution inflammatory syndrome [Abstract 773]. Paper presented at the 16th Conference on Retroviruses and Opportunistic Infections, February 8–11, 2009, Montréal, Canada.

Haddow LJ, Colebunders R, Meintjes G, et al. Cryptococcal immune reconstitution inflammatory syndrome in HIV-1-infected individuals: proposed clinical case definitions. *Lancet Infect Dis.* 2010;10:791–802.

Havlir DV, Kendall MA, Ive P, et al. Timing of antiretroviral therapy for HIV-1 infection and tuberculosis. *N Engl J Med.* 2011;365(16):1482–1491.

HIV-CAUSAL Collaboration. Impact of antiretroviral therapy on tuberculosis incidence among HIV-positive patients in high-income countries. *Clin Infect Dis.* 2012;54(9):1364–1372.

Ingle SM, Miro JM, Furrer H, et al. Impact of ART on mortality in cryptococcal meningitis patients: high-income settings [Abstract 837]. Paper presented at 22nd Conference on Retroviruses and Opportunistic Infections. February 23–26, 2015, Seattle, WA.

Makadzange AT, Ndhlovu CE, Takarinda K, et al. Early versus delayed initiation of antiretroviral therapy for concurrent HIV infection and cryptococcal meningitis in sub-Saharan Africa. *Clin Infect Dis.* 2010;50:1532–1538.

Martin-Blondel G, Delobel P, Blancher A, et al. Pathogenesis of the immune reconstitution inflammatory syndrome affecting the central nervous system in patients infected with HIV. *Brain.* 2011;134:928–946.

Meintjes G, Wilkinson RJ, Morroni C, et al. Randomized placebo-controlled trial of prednisone for paradoxical tuberculosis-associated immune reconstitution inflammatory syndrome. *AIDS.* 2010;24(15):2381–2390.

Müller M, Wandel S, Colebunders R, et al. Immune reconstitution inflammatory syndrome in patients starting antiretroviral therapy for HIV infection: a systematic review and meta-analysis. *Lancet Infect Dis.* 2010;10:251–261.

Novak RM, Richardson JT, Buchacz K, et al.; HIV Outpatient Study (HOPS) Investigators. Immune reconstitution inflammatory syndrome: incidence and implications for mortality. *AIDS.* 2012;26(6):721–730.

Oliver BG, Elliott JH, Price P, et al. Mediators of innate and adaptive immune responses differentially affect immune restoration disease associated with *Mycobacterium tuberculosis* in HIV patients beginning antiretroviral therapy. *J Infect Dis.* 2010;202:1728–1737.

Porter BO, Ouedraogo GL, Hodge JN, et al. d-Dimer and CRP levels are elevated prior to antiretroviral treatment in patients who develop IRIS. *Clin Immunol.* 2010;136(1):42–50.

Perfect JR. Clinical practice guidelines for the management of cryptococcal disease: 2010 update by the Infectious Diseases Society of America. *Clin Infect Dis.* 2010;50(3):291–322.

Saag M, Benson CA, Gandhi RT, et al. Antiretroviral drugs for treatment and prevention of HIV infection in adults: 2018 recommendations of the International Antiviral Society–USA Panel. *JAMA.* 2018;320(4):379–396.

Shelburne SA, Montes M, Hamill RJ. Immune reconstitution inflammatory syndrome: more answers, more questions. *J Antimicrob Chemother.* 2006;57(2):167.

Tan K, Roda R, Ostrow L, et al. PML-IRIS in patients with HIV infection: clinical manifestations and treatment with steroids. *Neurology.* 2009;72(17):1458–1464.

US Department of Health and Human Services. Guidelines for the use of antiretroviral agents in adults and adolescents living with HIV. 2018. https://aidsinfo.nih.gov/guidelines

Wijting I, Rokx C, Wit F, et al. Integrase inhibitors are an independent risk factor for IRIS: an ATHENA-Cohort study [Abstract 731]. Paper presented at the 24th Conference on Retroviruses and Opportunistic Infections, February 13–16, 2017.

Wijting I, Wit F, Rokx C, et al. Immune reconstitution inflammatory syndrome in HIV infected late presenters starting integrase inhibitor containing antiretroviral therapy. *EClinicalMedicine.* 2019;17.

Zolopa AR, Anderson J, Komarow L, et al. Early antiretroviral therapy reduces AIDS progression/death in individuals with acute opportunistic infections: a multicenter randomized strategy trial. *PLoS One.* 2009;4(5):e5575.

43.

US HEALTHCARE SYSTEMS, HIV PROGRAMS, AND COVERAGE POLICY ISSUES

Bruce J. Packett, II

LEARNING OBJECTIVE

Upon completion of this chapter, the reader should be able to:

- Broadly understand the landscape of US healthcare systems and payers as they relate to the provision of HIV care (treatment and prevention) and medical coding/billing for reimbursement

WHAT'S NEW?

Implementation of the Affordable Care Act (ACA), primarily in 2014, greatly expanded the availability of health coverage for persons with HIV (PWH) in the US. However, serious challenges such as affordability and access to treatment remain and are especially evident in states that have chosen not to expand their Medicaid coverage or have instituted other waivers and entitlement restrictions. The 30th anniversary of the Ryan White Comprehensive AIDS Resources Emergency (CARE) Act was commemorated on August 18, 2020. The CARE Act has been reauthorized four times since it was initially signed into law and aims to accommodate new and emerging needs of PWH as well as address ongoing disparities in access to care to improve HIV-related health outcomes.

KEY POINTS

- The ACA's 2014 implementation required all US citizens by law to have some form of health coverage, although the nature of that coverage varied widely. Subsequently, the passage of the Tax Cuts and Jobs Act of 2017 repealed the ACA's "individual mandate" to purchase insurance. As a result, individuals who are unable to afford insurance have been heavily impacted by chronic lack of access to health coverage. The COVID-19 pandemic has significantly undermined health insurance coverage, as broad surges in unemployment have caused many to lose employer-sponsored insurance and disrupted access to care.

- Many states have implemented Medicaid expansion, making Medicaid coverage available to all citizens at or under

138% of the federal poverty level. However, several states still have not, and some states are considering Medicaid expansion but have not yet implemented it. Health coverage systems across states are evolving rapidly based largely on state politics.

- Access to (and affordability of) HIV treatment varies greatly across payers and geography; further, coverage and reimbursement for HIV services varies widely by payer, coverage source, and state of residence.

- The Ryan White HIV/AIDS Program is a federal "wraparound" or "payer of last resort" program designed to provide services to PWH with insufficient coverage and benefits.

INTRODUCTION

HIV healthcare services in the US have historically been covered or provided by an assortment of federal, state, and local programs, such as Medicare, Medicaid, the US Department of Health and Human Services Health Resources and Services Administration (HRSA)'s Ryan White HIV/AIDS Program, and state and local health programs. HIV/AIDS service organizations and private and charitable health organizations have also provided services for PWH who do not carry health coverage. These programs collectively constitute the longstanding pathways to insurance coverage, care provision, and access to HIV-related treatment and prevention for PWH and those at risk for contracting HIV. Some of these programs also supply coverage for, or access to, medications that treat co-occurring conditions common among PWH.

AFFORDABLE CARE ACT

The Patient Protection and Affordable Care Act (also called the "Affordable Care Act" or "ACA") was signed into law by President Obama and was designed to reform healthcare coverage in the US (Levy, 2015). It represents the broadest reform to US healthcare systems since the 1960s. When the ACA was enacted in 2010, approximately 46.5 million non-elderly Americans had no health insurance. The number dropped rapidly and reached a historic low of 27 million in 2016. Under the Trump administration starting in 2017, however, the trend has reversed. According to 2019 estimates, approximately 500,000 people became uninsured annually in 2017 and 2018 (Henry J. Kaiser Family Foundation, "Key Facts About the Uninsured Population"). The rate of uninsured Americans rose to 8.5% between 2017 and 2018, an increase that deprived 1.9 million people of their insurance. The landscape of coverage options, including Medicaid, now varies widely among states (Berchick et al., 2019).

Passage of the ACA also directly affected provision of HIV care. Reforms that had a significant impact on PWH include:

1. Prohibiting discrimination by insurers against individuals with preexisting conditions

2. Requiring that all US citizens obtain health insurance coverage (this was subsequently effectively repealed, as noted earlier)

3. Expanding the Medicaid program to cover all individuals under 138% of the federal poverty level (this was made optional for states by a 2012 Supreme Court ruling; see the next paragraph)

4. Creating individual and small-group insurance markets ("exchanges") in each state. Along with the addition of federal tax credits for qualified individuals, these mechanisms have enabled low-income individuals to purchase more affordable insurance.

Ongoing public policy maneuvers, however, have brought about diverse changes in availability and affordability of private insurance coverage for PWH in many cases, depending in part on state of residence.

The constitutionality of various aspects of the ACA has been repeatedly challenged, even up to the US Supreme Court. The most momentous of these was a 2012 decision effectively making Medicaid expansion an optional, state-by-state decision. As of July 2020, 38 states and the District of Columbia have chosen to adopt Medicaid expansion. The remaining 13, to date, have declined. Four of these states are located outside of the US South and the remaining nine are southern. As of June 2020, Texas had 5 million uninsured citizens who would qualify for coverage if the state had Medicaid expansion. Florida has the second largest uninsured population, with 2.72 million. In its annual HIV Prevention Progress Report, the Centers for Disease Control and Prevention (CDC, 2019) for the first time listed "persons residing in the southern United States" as a specific population at increased risk of acquiring HIV, along with people of color, men who have sex with men, and various other groups.

Importantly, Medicaid remains the largest source of coverage for PWH in the US, covering 42% of the population with HIV (Henry J. Kaiser Family Foundation, "Medicaid and HIV"). In states that reject Medicaid expansion, individuals who are not below the poverty line but cannot afford commercial insurance remain uninsured. Low-income adults who do not qualify for Medicaid through other qualifying categories (e.g., are not disabled, elderly, caring for children, or pregnant) are left without access to any affordable health coverage options whatsoever. The lack of universal Medicaid expansion at present, coupled with significant flexibility provided to state lawmakers and insurers in the state insurance markets, has left PWH in each state with insurance coverage options of widely varying value. Although the Ryan White HIV/AIDS Program (see later in this chapter) is a safety net program designed to "wrap around" other forms of health coverage, it is also affected by what each state can offer to its residents with HIV. With the COVID-19 pandemic, states declining Medicaid expansion are experiencing a "skyrocketing number of uninsured, and a fragility of our health care system [that offers] compelling reasons for non-expansion states to take another look" (Mann, 2020).

Since the 2016 presidential election, opponents of the ACA have expended considerable political and financial efforts in hopes of overturning it and repudiating a hallmark of the Obama administration. In 2018, an ACA repeal by Congress was narrowly avoided, and whether the next administration will support or further attempt to undermine the ACA remains to be seen. The Centers for Medicare and Medicaid Services (CMS) also issued a final rule in 2018 to increase the maximum use of ACA-noncompliant "short-term" insurance policies from 3 months to 364 days, thus facilitating uptake of these policies by people who want or need to buy their insurance as inexpensively as possible. Often referred to as "junk insurance," these policies usually do not cover prescription drugs, maternity care, or care for people with preexisting medical conditions. Purchasers are often not fully aware of their very limited utility at the time of purchase.

PRIVATE INSURANCE

Private health insurance in the US is typically offered by private, for-profit, or nonprofit companies to various markets. In 2008, employment-based health insurance was the primary source of coverage for US workers (Rho & Schmitt, 2010), offered as benefits or in the form of other compensation to employees by their employer. Individual insurance plans were less common before the 2014 ACA implementation.

Some common forms of private insurance are indemnity plans, preferred provider plans, and health maintenance organizations. With indemnity plans, individuals can generally choose any healthcare provider and have a portion of the fees paid by the insurance. With preferred provider plans, individuals must choose from a defined network of clinicians, but the clinicians are generally employed by different groups. With health maintenance plans, individuals receive care from one or a small number of clinician groups hired by the insurer.

Reimbursement to clinicians varies widely with private insurance policies, with lower rates generally paid by managed care organizations. The provider networks within insurance plans can also affect reimbursement levels, as can plan benefits, co-pays, and cost-sharing mechanisms. Coverage of particular medications and treatments varies widely under private insurance plans.

Importantly, the ACA prohibits health insurance discrimination based on health status or gender, as well as lifetime limits on coverage, preexisting condition exclusions, and charging higher premiums based on gender or health status (Obamacare Facts, "Pre-Existing Conditions"; Obamacare Facts, "No Discrimination"). As noted previously, the ACA also created an "individual mandate" requiring all US citizens, beginning in 2014, to obtain health coverage or face federal tax penalties (Obamacare Facts, "Obamacare Individual Mandate"; HealthCare.gov, "If You Don't Have Health Insurance: How Much You'll Pay"). However, this individual mandate (in the form of tax penalties) effectively disappeared beginning in 2019. Individuals who do not have access to employer-based insurance or other insurance coverage and do not qualify for public health coverage programs such as Medicaid can purchase individual insurance through the state insurance exchanges ("marketplaces," discussed in the next section), assuming they can afford to do so.

STATE INSURANCE EXCHANGES

One of the most significant accomplishments of the ACA was the creation of marketplaces for individual and small-group insurance plans in each state (Center for Consumer Information & Oversight, "State Health Insurance Marketplaces"). Each state insurance exchange is simply a market forum where private insurance companies offer various qualified health plans to residents of that state. Individuals can access the marketplace online, by phone, or in person through assistants. Potential customers also use the marketplace to determine their eligibility for Medicaid or Children's Health Insurance Program (CHIP) benefits (HealthCare.gov, "Medicaid and CHIP Coverage Health Insurance Marketplace").

The ACA also makes tax credit subsidies available to some low- and middle-income individuals in order to purchase insurance through the state exchanges. Tax credits of gradated amounts are available to those with income levels between 138% and 400% of the federal poverty level, and they are taken as upfront subsidies to the plan premium (HealthCare.gov, "Premium Tax Credit").

Plans offered within the markets vary widely in cost as well as coverage and benefit design. However, all are required to provide essential health benefits as a part of the insurance package, including services within the following 10 categories: ambulatory patient services; emergency services; hospitalizations; maternity and newborn care; mental health and substance use disorder services (including behavioral health treatment); prescription drugs; rehabilitative and habilitative services and devices; laboratory services; preventive and wellness services and chronic disease management; and pediatric services (including oral and vision care) (HealthCare.gov, "Essential Health Benefits"; HealthCare.gov, "What marketplace health insurance plans cover"). In addition, all state exchange plans are required to include a minimum percentage of all the essential community providers in a geographic area in their provider networks. Essential community providers are those who serve predominately low-income, medically underserved individuals. This includes Ryan White HIV/AIDS Program providers.

MEDICAID

Medicaid has long been the nation's public health insurance program for people with low-income status, limited resources, and disability. Originally, the program covered only certain populations, such as the medically disabled and pregnant persons, infants, and children living in poverty.

The ACA sought to expand the program's coverage to include all citizens below 138% of the federal poverty level regardless of other categorizations. However, as discussed earlier, this was not accepted by all states. Some states have partially expanded their Medicaid program in a variety of ways, and others have declined expansion altogether, largely for political reasons. Individuals in those states are exempt from the tax penalties under the individual mandate (Obamacare Facts, "Obamacare Mandate: Exemption and Tax Penalty"), but many are also left with little or no access to healthcare except through free clinics or local health department services when and where they are available.

Medicaid covers inpatient, ambulatory care, and skilled nursing care. Medicaid also covers prescription medications except for persons who also have Medicare coverage (Medicaid.gov, "Dual Eligibles"). Coverage levels, eligibility criteria, and program benefits vary widely from state to state (Medicaid.gov, "Benefits").

Medicaid is financed jointly by the federal government and states. It is administered by state governments in accordance with certain basic federal eligibility and benefit standards (Medicaid.gov, "Financing & Reimbursement"). At the federal level, the Medicaid program is run by CMS under the US Department of Health and Human Services. Medicaid is the third largest domestic program in the federal budget, after Social Security and Medicare (Rudowitz & Musumeci, 2015; Rudowitz & Snyder, 2015). It is also the second largest program in most state budgets. The federal government matches state spending in Medicaid, paying for 56% of the program's spending overall (Rudowitz & Musumeci, 2015; Rudowitz & Snyder, 2015).

In 2019, 40 states reported that they used capitated managed care models to deliver Medicaid services to mitigate Medicaid budgetary costs through reductions of benefits, limitations to drug formularies, and other efforts (Henry J. Kaiser Family Foundation, "10 Things to Know About Managed Care"). Some others also offer managed care–type programs to particular populations in efforts to reduce costs.

Managed care organizations contract directly with the state to provide services and benefits in a variety of capacities (Henry J. Kaiser Family Foundation, "Medicaid Managed Care Market Tracker"). Some managed care organizations are operated by a parent firm that also participates in the private insurance market.

Traditional Medicaid programs offer provider reimbursement through fee-for-service rates that are determined by the state. Managed care organizations make agreements for provider reimbursement based on monthly capitation rates.

MEDICARE

Medicare is the federal health insurance program for people older than 65 years and also for those younger than 65 who have permanent disabilities. The Medicare program is also administered by CMS. About one-quarter of PWH receive medical care through Medicare (Henry J. Kaiser Family Foundation, "Medicare and HIV").

Medicare eligibility is tied to work history and contributions to Medicare through employment-based withholding. Some individuals are eligible for both Medicare and Medicaid ("dual eligible") based on their income and disability status. The number of PWH who use Medicare has increased due to both the increased survival rates and aging attributable to effective ART and development of multiple chronic health conditions. Medicare covers inpatient and outpatient care, some skilled nursing and home care, and medications. It also covers HIV testing for beneficiaries.

Since Medicare Part D was launched in 2006, Medicare has provided prescription drug coverage under the Medicare Part D drug benefit. Most Medicare-eligible individuals can decide whether to participate through enrollment in one of several prescription drug plans that are marketed as stand-alone coverage or to rely on managed care plans ("Medicare Advantage"). When Medicare Part D was launched, Congress identified six types of prescription drugs as "protected classes" and required that they be covered by Part D plans. Antiretroviral drugs were one of the protected classes, as well as cancer drugs, mental health treatments, and other medications that also require uninterrupted use. These protected classes were exempted from any prior authorization, step therapy, or other "utilization management" techniques that would interrupt or delay patients' access to these drugs.

In 2018, CMS proposed a new rule to discard the "protected classes" designation, despite the fact that doing so would subject patients to treatment interruptions due to utilization review and step therapy practices (these involve requirements to start patients on a less expensive treatment regimen; the patient then needs to "fail" one or more plan drugs prior to moving to the prescriber's chosen regimen) in order to reduce Medicare costs. Through strong public opposition mobilized by American Academy of HIV Medicine members and staff, the HIV Medicine Association, and other advocacy organizations, the proposal to remove ART from the protected classes was halted.

Medicare Part D also includes an "exceptions and appeals" process that can be used to request coverage of drugs not covered by the plan. Individual Part D plans differ widely in terms of premiums and other cost-sharing requirements. Specifically, Medicare Part D includes a sequence of cost-sharing requirements, including an initial deductible and subsequent "out-of-pocket" costs. Most Part D plans also have a coverage gap (also referred to as the Part D "donut hole") in which, after a certain amount of the cost have been paid through the coverage plan, any additional costs become the responsibility of the individual (Medicare.gov, "Costs in the Coverage Gap") until the costs reach the catastrophic coverage threshold (Medicare.gov, "Catastrophic Coverage"). At that point, nearly all costs are then covered by Medicare. The ACA plans to close this gap in coverage gradually in 2020, and it provides some rebates for those who encounter the coverage gap in the interim (Medicare.gov, "Costs in the Coverage Gap").

Medicare reimbursement rates are similar to those of private insurance. Clinicians who accept Medicare reimbursement are subject to federal audits of their charts to check billed amounts against services documented.

RYAN WHITE HIV/AIDS PROGRAM

The Ryan White HIV/AIDS Program is a federal program designed specifically to ensure provision of care, treatment, and supportive services for PWH in the US. First enacted in 1990, it is administered by the HRSA under the US Department of Health and Human Services (HRSA HIV AIDS Programs, "About the Ryan White HIV/AIDS Program").

Fundamentally, the Ryan White Program provides a "safety net" for healthcare services to PWH who have no other source of health coverage or are confronted with coverage limits (HRSA HIV AIDS Programs, "About the Ryan White HIV/AIDS Program"). The program is designed to "wrap around" other forms of coverage and is—from a legal perspective—the "payer of last resort." This designation means that individuals who are eligible for any other program must access that coverage and benefits before accessing the Ryan White Program (HRSA.gov, "Eligible Individuals & Allowable Uses of Funds for Discretely Defined Categories of Services").

As the third largest source of federal funding for HIV care in the US after Medicare and Medicaid, the Ryan White Program is estimated to reach over half a million PWH each year (HRSA, 2018). Funding for the Ryan White Program is subject to congressional appropriations each year. In addition to federal funding, some states and localities also provide funding to their Ryan White services through state matching funds requirements.

Part A of the Ryan White Program provides funding to "Eligible Metropolitan Areas and Transitional Grant Areas" hardest hit by the HIV/AIDS epidemic for a wide range of services and efforts.

Part B provides funding to states and territories (HRSA HIV AIDS Programs, "About the Ryan White HIV/AIDS Program"). A vitally important component is the AIDS Drug Assistance Program, which is specifically funded through allocations to the states under Part B along with state funding contributions. Each state's AIDS Drug Assistance Program provides HIV-related prescription drugs to low-income individuals with limited or no prescription drug coverage (Henry J. Kaiser Foundation, "AIDS Drug Assistance Programs"). Many states also use AIDS Drug Assistance Program funding to purchase health insurance and/or pay insurance premiums, co-payments, or deductibles for PWH. All AIDS Drug Assistance Programs participate in the federal 340B Program, enabling them to purchase drugs at or below the statutorily defined 340B ceiling price. Because of "shelter in place" mandates issued during the COVID-19 pandemic, many AIDS Drug Assistance Programs around the country have adjusted some policies and processes to ensure PWH uninterrupted access to needed medications without introducing unnecessary health risks (HRSA.gov, "Ryan White HIV/AIDS Program: COVID-19 Frequently Asked Questions," 2020).

Part C of the Ryan White Program funds providers and medical clinics to deliver comprehensive medical care and treatment to PWH who have no other source for care (HRSA HIV AIDS Programs, "About the Ryan White HIV/AIDS Program"). Part C also funds early intervention services, ambulatory care, and primary health care services for PWH in underserved or rural communities and communities of color. Finally, Part C also provides planning grants and capacity grants to support organizations in the delivery of high-quality, effective HIV care.

Part D of the Ryan White Program grants for support services for women, infants, children, and youth (HRSA HIV AIDS Programs, "About the Ryan White HIV/AIDS Program").

Part F provides funding for a variety of initiatives, including the Special Projects of National Significance, AIDS Education & Training Centers, dental programs, and the Minority AIDS Initiative (HRSA HIV AIDS Programs, "About the Ryan White HIV/AIDS Program").

The benefits available through the ACA (even despite its recent rollbacks), together with supports provided by Medicaid expansion in the majority of states, are now in place to provide some supports to PWH that were not available when the CARE Act was created in 1990. Simultaneously, however, the number of PWH has increased over those decades and the proportion of PWH needing services provided by these programs is climbing.

In the 30 years since the Ryan White Program was founded, organizations have learned how to try and make these programs dovetail to best meet the needs of PWH in a country without a national healthcare system or the other safety net/public health systems that most countries have in place. The early passage and development of the CARE Act set a critical precedent for the delivery of functional, HIV-focused services. This prototype, designed in close collaboration with the people it serves, subsequently influenced the ACA and Medicare expansion as these programs were similarly designed in consultation with program users. The Kaiser Family Foundation has asserted that "the Ryan White Program remains a critical component of the nation's response to HIV in the ACA era" (Ryan White HIV/AIDS Program, "The Basics").

NETWORKS OF CARE

For HIV providers, inclusion in networks of care for health programs is of great importance. Most patients' health coverage limits them to (1) seeing only certain providers who are "in network"; (2) being charged substantially higher fees for seeing "out of network" providers; or (3) being declined services by providers not included in the network.

The ACA requires that all plans in the state exchanges include a minimum percentage of all the essential community providers in a geographic area in their provider network. As indicated previously, essential community providers serve predominately low-income, medically underserved individuals (Henry J. Kaiser Family Foundation, "Definition of Essential Community Providers in Marketplaces"). This includes Ryan White HIV/AIDS Program providers.

Reimbursement rates and schedules for providers who are part of the network are set by or negotiated with health coverage issuers and entities.

PROVIDER REIMBURSEMENT

Reimbursement for medical encounters and procedures depends heavily on thorough and accurate documentation of the medical visit, diagnosis, treatment, and services as recorded and submitted through coding claims. The level of complexity and severity of the medical encounter—and thus the level of reimbursement owed—is defined by the nature of the problem(s), the number of problems at issue, the amount of time spent with the patient, and other factors. Careful documentation of these factors is required to ensure adequate and appropriate reimbursement and is also generally considered a best practice to accurately communicate a provider's clinical decision-making. Other factors that are essential to document are the specific elements of the medical history, the physical examination, and medical decision-making. Documenting time spent on prevention services (e.g., counseling the patient about consistent condom use and disclosure to partners) and on promoting other behavioral changes (e.g., tobacco cessation, weight loss) is also essential for accurate reimbursement of these services.

Standardized coding systems are used in the US to process billing claims to private and public insurers. The two principal systems used for coding medical information in the US are the World Health Organization (WHO)'s International Classification of Diseases (ICD) and the Current Procedural Terminology (CPT) codes that make up the Healthcare Common Procedure Coding System (HCPCS). In general, CPT/HCPCS codes identify the services rendered, whereas ICD codes focus more on the diagnosis. CPT codes are created, maintained, and trademarked by the American Medical Association (AMA, " CPT overview and code approval").

The HCPCS was created by the federal CMS. It is based on CPT codes but provides for two levels of coding. Level I consists of AMA's CPT codes and provides for medical services and procedures furnished by clinicians. Level I codes are numeric. Level II codes are alphanumeric and apply primarily to medical devices and non-clinician services, such as ambulatory care, immunizations, diagnostic procedures, family counseling, and services provided by other health professionals (e.g., clinical nurses, psychologists, and pharmacists) (CMS, "HCPCS—General Information"). Medicaid and

Medicare services are reimbursed by CMS on the basis of the HCPCS codes for clinician activities.

The ICD is the international standard diagnostic classification for all epidemiologic, health, and clinical usage. It is a coding and classification system of diseases, symptoms, injuries, and abnormal findings. It also documents the social circumstances and external causes of injury or diseases, as classified by the WHO. The most recent iteration of these codes, ICD-11, was unanimously endorsed by members of the World Health Assembly in 2019. With its 11th update, many technological and infrastructural improvements are expected to enhance transition and usability. The ICD-11 is scheduled to be implemented beginning in January 2022.

Though it was first used by World Health Assembly member states as early as 1994, US providers did not fully transition to the ICD-10 system until October 2015 (CDC, "International Classification of Diseases"; CMS, "ICD-10").

In the context of reimbursement, ICD codes are used in conjunction with CPT codes to classify vital records and health condition codes associated with outpatient, inpatient, medical office utilization, and hospital charges.

REFERENCES

American Medical Association. https://www.ama-assn.org/practice-management/cpt/cpt-overview-and-code-approval

Berchick ER, Barnett JC, Upton RD. Health insurance coverage in the United States: 2018. November 2019. https://www.census.gov/content/dam/Census/library/publications/2019/demo/p60-267.pdf

Center for Consumer Information & Oversight. State health insurance marketplaces. https://www.cms.gov/cciio/resources/fact-sheets-and-faqs/state-marketplaces.html

Centers for Disease Control and Prevention. HIV prevention progress report, 2019. https://www.cdc.gov/hiv/pdf/policies/progressreports/cdc-hiv-preventionprogressreport.pdf

Centers for Disease Control and Prevention. International Classification of Diseases, Tenth Revision, Clinical Modification (ICD-10-CM). National Coding with CPT for proper reimbursement Center for Health Statistics. https://www.cdc.gov/nchs/icd/icd10cm.htm

Centers for Medicare and Medicaid Services. HCPCS—general information. https://www.cms.gov/medicare/coding/medhcpcsgeninfo/index.html

Centers for Medicare and Medicaid Services. ICD-10. https://www.cms.gov/medicare/Coding/ICD10/index.html

HealthCare.gov. Essential health benefits. https://www.healthcare.gov/glossary/essential-health-benefits

HealthCare.gov. Health insurance marketplace. https://www.healthcare.gov/glossary/health-insurance-marketplace-glossary

HealthCare.gov. If you don't have health insurance: how much you'll pay. https://www.healthcare.gov/fees

HealthCare.gov. Medicaid and CHIP coverage health insurance overview. https://marketplace.cms.gov/technical-assistance-resources/medicaid-chip-overview.pdf

HealthCare.gov. Premium tax credit. https://www.healthcare.gov/glossary/premium-tax-credit

HealthCare.gov. What Marketplace health insurance plans cover. https://www.healthcare.gov/coverage/what-marketplace-plans-cover/

Henry J. Kaiser Family Foundation. 10 things to know about managed care. December 16, 2019. https://www.kff.org/medicaid/issue-brief/10-things-to-know-about-medicaid-managed-care/

Henry J. Kaiser Family Foundation. AIDS drug assistance programs. April 8, 2014. http://kff.org/hivaids/fact-sheet/aids-drug-assistance-programs/

Henry J. Kaiser Family Foundation. Definition of essential community providers (ECPs) in marketplaces. http://kff.org/other/state-indicator/definition-of-essential-community-providers-ecps-in-marketplaces

Henry J. Kaiser Family Foundation. Key facts about the uninsured population. December 13, 2019. https://www.kff.org/uninsured/issue-brief/key-facts-about-the-uninsured-population/

Henry J. Kaiser Family Foundation. Medicaid managed care market tracker. http://kff.org/data-collection/medicaid-managed-care-market-tracker

Henry J. Kaiser Family Foundation. Medicaid and HIV. October 1, 2019. https://www.kff.org/hivaids/fact-sheet/medicaid-and-hiv/

Henry J. Kaiser Family Foundation. Medicare and HIV. October 14, 2016. https://www.kff.org/hivaids/fact-sheet/medicare-and-hiv/

HRSA HIV AIDS Programs. About the Ryan White HIV/AIDS Program. http://hab.hrsa.gov/abouthab/aboutprogram.html

HRSA.gov. Eligible individuals & allowable uses of funds for discretely defined categories of services. http://hab.hrsa.gov/manageyourgrant/pinspals/eligible1002.html

HRSA.gov. Ryan White HIV/AIDS Program. COVID-19 frequently asked questions. https://hab.hrsa.gov/coronavirus/frequently-asked-questions

Levy M. Patient Protection and Affordable Care Act (PPACA). *Encyclopedia Britannica*, June 26, 2015. https://www.britannica.com/topic/Patient-Protection-and-Affordable-Care-Act

Mann C. The Commonwealth Fund. The COVID-19 Crisis Is Giving States That Haven't Expanded Medicaid New Reasons to Reconsider. 2020. https://www.commonwealthfund.org/blog/2020/covid-19-crisis-giving-states-havent-expanded-medicaid-new-reconsideration

Medicaid.gov. Benefits. https://www.medicaid.gov/medicaid-chip-program-information/by-topics/benefits/medicaid-benefits.html

Medicaid.gov. Dual eligibles. https://www.medicaid.gov/affordablecare-act/provisions/dual-eligibles.html

Medicaid.gov. Financing & reimbursement. https://www.medicaid.gov/medicaid-chip-program-information/by-topics/financing-and-reimbursement/financing-and-reimbursement.html

Medicare.gov. Catastrophic coverage. https://www.medicare.gov/part-d/costs/catastrophic-coverage/drug-plan-catastrophic-coverage.html

Medicare.gov. Costs in the coverage gap. https://www.medicare.gov/part-d/costs/coverage-gap/part-d-coverage-gap.html

Obamacare Facts. No discrimination. http://obamacarefacts.com/no-discrimination

Obamacare Facts. Obamacare individual mandate. http://obamacarefacts.com/obamacare-individual-mandate

Obamacare Facts. Obamacare mandate: exemption and tax penalty. http://obamacarefacts.com/obamacare-mandate-exemption-penalty

Obamacare Facts. Pre-existing conditions. http://obamacarefacts.com/pre-existing-conditions

Rho HJ, Schmitt J. Health-insurance coverage rates for US workers, 1979–2008. March 2010. http://cepr.net/documents/publications/hc-coverage-2010-03.pdf

Rudowitz R, Musumeci M. The ACA and medicaid expansion waivers. Henry J. Kaiser Family Foundation. November 20, 2015. http://kff.org/medicaid/issue-brief/the-aca-and-medicaid-expansion-waivers

Rudowitz R, Snyder L. The ACA and medicaid expansion waivers. Henry J. Kaiser Family Foundation, May 20, 2015. http://kff.org/medicaid/issue-brief/medicaid-financing-how-does-it-work-and-what-are-the-implications/

Ryan White HIV/AIDS Program. The basics. Kaiser Family Foundation. February 2017. http://files.kff.org/attachment/fact-sheet-pdf-the-ryan-white-program

World Health Organization. International Classification of Diseases (ICD). http://www.who.int/classifications/icd/en

44.

LEGAL ISSUES

Jeffrey T. Schouten

ROUTINE HIV TESTING (WITH CONSENT)

LEARNING OBJECTIVE

- Discuss the Centers for Disease Control and Prevention's (CDC) recommendations for routine HIV testing in various healthcare settings

WHAT'S NEW?

- The US Preventive Services Task Force (USPSTF) recommended that clinicians screen for HIV infection in all pregnant persons, including those who present in labor or at delivery whose HIV status is unknown.

- The USPSTF recommended that clinicians screen for HIV infection in adolescents and adults aged 15 to 65 years. Younger adolescents and older adults who are at increased risk of infection should also be screened.

KEY POINTS

- It is estimated that the 15% of people who do not know they are HIV-infected account for 40% of new cases of HIV infection.

- The CDC recommends that all people aged 13 to 65 years receive an HIV test at least once as part of routine healthcare. Persons identified as high risk for HIV infection should be retested at least annually.

- Routine testing delinks pre- and posttest counseling from testing.

- Both in routine and emergency care settings, many opportunities for routine HIV testing are missed.

An estimated 1.2 million people in the US have HIV, including about 161,800 people who are unaware of their status. Nearly 40% of new HIV infections are transmitted by people who don't know they have the virus (CDC, 2006). Approximately half of unaware men who have sex with men (MSM) and people who inject drugs (PWID) who reported not having been tested in the past year reported not being offered HIV testing by any clinician despite having seen one.

A Morbidity and Mortality Weekly Report (MMWR) from the CDC in June 2018 evaluated a sample of 333 healthcare-seeking, heterosexual adults at increased risk for acquiring HIV infection: 194 (58%) reported not receiving an HIV test offer at a recent medical visit(s), and men (vs. women) had a significantly lower prevalence of provider-initiated HIV test offers (32% vs. 48%). Recent HIV testing was higher among recipients of provider-initiated offers compared with nonrecipients (71% vs. 16%). Provider-initiated HIV test offers are an important strategy for increasing HIV testing among heterosexual populations. More provider-initiated HIV screening among heterosexual adults at increased risk for acquiring HIV infection, especially men, is needed.

A meta-analysis of 11 independent studies showed that the prevalence of high-risk sexual behavior is reduced substantially after people become aware that they are HIV-infected (Marks et al., 2006). Estimated transmission is 3.5 times higher among persons who are unaware of their infection than among persons who are aware of their infection, which contributes disproportionately to the number of new HIV infections each year in the US (Marks et al., 2006). Modeling data showed that an estimated 49% of transmissions were from the 20% of persons unaware of their HIV infection (Hall et al., 2012).

A study in South Carolina found that among the persons identified as late testers (persons who received an AIDS diagnosis within 1 year of HIV diagnosis), approximately three-fourths had visited a South Carolina healthcare facility prior to their HIV diagnosis. In addition, most of the late testers had made multiple visits, and most of their visits occurred 1 year or more before diagnosis of HIV infection. According to the report, the majority of diagnoses for these previous visits probably would not have prompted HIV testing under a risk-based testing strategy (CDC, 2006). The CDC published revised recommendations concerning routine HIV testing in healthcare settings in September 2006. The major recommendations are as follows:

- For patients in all healthcare settings
  - HIV screening is recommended for patients in all healthcare settings after patients are notified that testing will be performed, unless patients decline (opt-out screening).
  - Persons at high risk for HIV infection should be screened for HIV at least annually.
  - Separate written consent for HIV testing should not be required; general consent for medical care should be considered sufficient to encompass consent for HIV testing.
  - Prevention counseling should *not* be required as part of HIV diagnostic testing or HIV screening programs in healthcare settings.

- For pregnant women
  - HIV screening should be included in the routine panel of prenatal screening tests for all pregnant women.
  - HIV screening is recommended after the patient is notified that testing will be performed unless the patient declines (opt-out screening).
  - Separate written consent for HIV testing should not be required; general consent for medical care should be considered sufficient to encompass consent for HIV testing.
  - Repeat screening in the third trimester is recommended in certain jurisdictions with elevated rates of HIV infection among pregnant women.

Although the CDC recommends that prevention counseling should not be required with HIV diagnostic testing in healthcare settings, the elements of informed consent include some of the information communicated during pretest counseling. Also, risk assessment is needed to identify patients at high risk for HIV infection who should be screened at least annually. The CDC recommendations define informed consent as follows (CDC, 2006):

A process of communication between patient and provider, through which an informed patient can choose whether to undergo HIV testing or decline to do so. Elements of informed consent typically include providing oral or written information regarding HIV, the risks and benefits of testing, the implications of HIV test results, how test results will be communicated, and the opportunity to ask questions.

Routine testing means that HIV testing is offered to all patients. Testing requires informed consent, but that consent can be included in the general consent-to-care agreements. Patients can choose to opt out of routine testing if they do not want to be tested.

The CDC recommends providers in clinical settings should offer HIV screening at least annually to all sexually active MSM. "Clinicians can also consider the potential benefits of more frequent HIV screening (e.g., every 3 or 6 months) for some asymptomatic sexually active MSM based on their individual risk factors, local HIV epidemiology, and local policies" (DiNenno et al., 2017). The CDC also noted that "additional research is needed to establish the individual- or community-level factors that might increase the risk for HIV acquisition for MSM and merit more frequent HIV screening. For MSM who are prescribed preexposure prophylaxis, HIV testing every 3 months and immediate testing whenever signs and symptoms of acute HIV infection are reported is indicated" (DiNenno et al., 2017).

The USPSTF Recommendation Summary found convincing evidence that identification and early treatment of HIV infection is of substantial benefit in reducing the risk of AIDS-related events or death. The USPSTF found convincing evidence that the use of antiretroviral therapy (ART) is of substantial benefit in decreasing the risk of HIV transmission to uninfected sex partners. The USPSTF also found convincing evidence that identification and treatment of pregnant women living with HIV infection is of substantial benefit in reducing the rate of mother-to-child transmission. The overall magnitude of the benefit of screening for HIV infection in adolescents, adults, and pregnant women is substantial (USPSTF, 2019) (Table 44.1).

Laws governing consent for HIV testing are state specific. Although all states require consent for an HIV test, most states that had required explicit written consent prior to the 2006 CDC revised HIV testing recommendations have changed their laws (Neff & Goldschmidt, 2011). This remains a dynamic area of law and regulation. A good resource is the Compendium of State HIV Testing Laws maintained by the National Clinician Consultation Center, although it is no longer updated.

Challenges in implementing routine HIV testing include cost of testing, follow-up notification of positive results in

Table 44.1 US PREVENTIVE SERVICES TASK FORCE HIV SCREENING RECOMMENDATIONS

POPULATION	RECOMMENDATION	GRADE
Pregnant persons	The USPSTF recommends that clinicians screen for HIV infection in all pregnant persons, including those who present in labor or at delivery whose HIV status is unknown.	A
Adolescents and adults aged 15–65 years	The USPSTF recommends that clinicians screen for HIV infection in adolescents and adults aged 15–65 years. Younger adolescents and older adults who are at increased risk of infection should also be screened. See the Clinical Considerations section of the recommendations for more information about assessment of risk, screening intervals, and rescreening in pregnancy.	A

SOURCE: The US Preventative Services Task Force. Available at: https://uspreventiveservicestaskforce.org/uspstf/recommendation/human-immunodeficiency-virus-hiv-infection-screening. Accessed September 14, 2020.

emergency departments and inpatient settings, and adoption of rapid testing. The USPSTF recommends that clinicians screen for HIV infection in adolescents and adults aged 15 to 65 years. Younger adolescents and older adults who are at increased risk should also be screened.

REFERENCES/RECOMMENDED READING

American Medical Association. AMA Code of Medical Ethics Opinion 8.1—Routine universal screening for HIV. https://www.ama-assn.org/delivering-care/ethics/routine-universal-screening-hiv

Centers for Disease Control and Prevention. Revised recommendations for HIV testing of adults, adolescents, and pregnant women in healthcare settings. *MMWR Morbid Mortal Wkly Rep.* 2006;55(RR14):1–17. www.cdc.gov/mmwr/preview/mmwrhtml/rr5514a1.htm

Cossarini F, Hanna DB, Ginsberg MS, et al. Missed opportunities for HIV prevention: individuals who HIV seroconverted despite accessing healthcare. *AIDS Behav.* 2018;22(11):3519–3524. https://www.ncbi.nlm.nih.gov/pmc/articles/PMC6204105/pdf/nihms971562.pdf

Dailey AF, Hoots BE, Hall HI, et al. Vital signs: human immunodeficiency virus testing and diagnosis delays—United States. *MMWR Morb Mortal Rep.* 2017;66(47):1300–1306. https://www.cdc.gov/mmwr/volumes/66/wr/mm6647e1.htm

Diepstra KL, Cunningham T, Rhodes AG, et al. Prevalence and predictors of provider-initiated HIV test offers among heterosexual persons at increased risk for acquiring HIV infection—Virginia, 2016. *MMWR Morb Mortal Wkly Rep.* 2018;67(25):714–717. https://www.ncbi.nlm.nih.gov/pmc/articles/PMC6023187/pdf/mm6725a3.pdf

DiNenno EA, Prejean J, Irwin K, et al. Recommendations for HIV screening of gay, bisexual, and other men who have sex with men—United States, 2017. *MMWR Morb Mortal Wkly Rep.* 2017;66(31):830–832. https://www.ncbi.nlm.nih.gov/pmc/articles/PMC5687782/pdf/mm6631a3.pdf

Hall HI, Holtgrave D, Maulsby C. HIV transmission rates from persons living with HIV who are aware and unaware of their infection. *AIDS.* 2012;26:893–896.

Hughes C. ICD-10 simplifies preventive care coding, sort of. *Fam Pract Manag.* 2014;21(4):OA1–OA4. http://www.aafp.org/fpm/2014/0700/oa1.html

Marks G, Crepaz N, Janssen RS. Estimating sexual transmission of HIV from persons aware and unaware that they are infected with the virus in the USA. *AIDS.* 2006;20:1447–1450.

Neff S, Goldschmidt, R. Centers for Disease Control and Prevention 2006 human immunodeficiency virus testing recommendations and state testing laws. *JAMA.* 2011;305(17):1767–1768.

US Preventive Services Task Force. Screening for HIV infection: US Preventive Services Task Force recommendation statement. *JAMA.* 2019;321(23):2326–2336. https://jamanetwork.com/journals/jama/fullarticle/2735345

Wejnert C, Prejean J, Hoots B, et al. Prevalence of missed opportunities for HIV testing among persons unaware of their infection. *JAMA.* 2018;319(24):2555–2557. https://jamanetwork.com/journals/jama/fullarticle/2685972

HIV TESTING WITHOUT CONSENT

LEARNING OBJECTIVE

- Discuss the circumstances under which it is allowable to test a patient for HIV without consent, including reference to applicable legal regulations

WHAT'S NEW?

The information on HIV testing without consent has remained consistent during the past few years.

KEY POINTS

- Many states allow HIV testing without consent in limited situations, such as emergency situations or when a healthcare worker or public safety officer has had a potential exposure to HIV.

- Some states require HIV testing of convicted sex offenders, and some states allow testing of persons charged with a crime capable of transmitting HIV, such as rape.

Although all states require consent for HIV testing (Halpern, 2005), there are situations in which it is possible to obtain an HIV test without the consent of the person to be tested. In some cases, HIV testing without consent may be standard practice. For example, in New York, newborn infants are tested without parental consent if their mother did not consent to HIV testing during pregnancy. Some states require HIV testing of convicted sex offenders (e.g., Revised Code of Washington RCW 70.24.340).

A minority of states provide explicit exceptions for consent for HIV testing in emergency medical situations (Halpern, 2005). Some states allow for testing of source patients when there has been a potential exposure to HIV in a healthcare setting or when a public safety officer has had potential exposure. California and several other states allow for HIV testing of persons accused of a criminal act capable of transmitting HIV. California requires a court hearing showing there is probable cause to believe that the accused committed the offense and that blood, semen, or another bodily fluid capable of transmitting HIV (as identified in State Department of Health Services regulations) has been transferred from the accused to the victim (California Penal Code 1524.1(b)(3)(A)). A major challenge with testing without consent is getting the court order (if required) from the appropriate authority so that testing and initiation of postexposure prophylaxis can take place in a timely manner (see Chapter 4). A survey showed that intensivists' decisions to pursue testing without consent, a not uncommon situation, are associated with their personal ethics and often erroneous perceptions of state laws but not with the laws themselves (Halpern et al., 2007). Because laws and regulations vary by state, clinicians are responsible for knowing the appropriate rules in the state in which they practice. Consultation with the local public health officer is advised whenever HIV testing without consent is believed to be necessary.

REFERENCES/RECOMMENDED READING

Halpern SD. HIV testing without consent in critically ill patients. *JAMA.* 2005;294(6):734–737.

Halpern SD, Metkus TS, Fuchs BD, et al. Nonconsented human immunodeficiency virus testing among critically ill patients: intensivists' practices and the influence of state laws. *Arch Intern Med.* 2007;167(21):2323–2328.

DISEASE REPORTING SYSTEM

LEARNING OBJECTIVE

- Discuss the system of disease reporting in the US and identify reportable conditions related to HIV care

WHAT'S NEW?

- The CDC and many states have implemented molecular surveillance, based on resistance testing data, to rapidly identify cluster outbreaks of community HIV transmission.

KEY POINTS

- All state and local departments of health use name-based HIV diagnosis and AIDS reporting to track HIV infection.

HIV/AIDS SURVEILLANCE

Since HIV/AIDS was first recognized as a disease, most state and city departments of health have used the reporting of AIDS cases to track the incidence and prevalence of HIV infections and HIV-related complications. Data on AIDS cases are reported in a standardized format to the CDC by all 50 states, the District of Columbia, and US dependencies and possessions.

The rationale frequently cited for using HIV rather than AIDS case surveillance is that it allows for a more thorough and accurate characterization of the populations in which HIV infection has been newly diagnosed and helps in the prioritization of prevention services (CDC, 2005; Holtgrave, 2004). Significant changes in HIV transmission and behavior can be achieved by appropriate programs. For example, aggressive efforts to prevent maternal–fetal transmission have been credited with the steep decline in mother-to-child HIV transmission, the increase in the proportion of HIV-infected pregnant women who have been tested prior to delivery, and the high proportion of HIV-infected pregnant women who accept antiretroviral prophylaxis (Wortley et al., 2001). Lab-based reporting of CD4 counts and HIV RNA for surveillance has become a helpful tool to assess engagement, linkage, and retention in care (Lubelchek et al., 2015; Wiewel et al., 2015).

In 2005, the CDC recommended that name-based HIV reporting be implemented using the same approach that is used for nationwide AIDS surveillance. All states successfully implemented confidential name-based HIV infection reporting by April 2008.

HIV MOLECULAR SURVEILLANCE

Name-based HIV case surveillance data can identify patterns in diagnosis rates, but in high-incidence areas, recent, rapid transmission may not be identifiable amid large numbers of cases. Partner notification services staff interview persons with HIV to collect information about their partners; however, not all index cases are interviewed and partners may not be known or located. However, analysis of HIV-1 genetic sequence data (molecular surveillance) can identify transmission clusters, enabling high-impact prevention efforts for social networks at high risk of HIV infection (Oster et al., 2018). Molecular clusters are identified through analysis of HIV molecular sequence data that are generated from HIV drug resistance testing. This is also referred to as cluster response. Cluster response uses data routinely reported to health departments to identify communities where HIV may be spreading quickly. This information can then be used to identify gaps in prevention and care services and ensure that services reach the populations that need them the most (CDC, "HIV Cluster Response" and "HIV Cluster and Outbreak Detection and Response"). The technology in use by the CDC and provided to local health departments is HIV-TRACE (TRAnsmission Cluster Engine), which is a platform that has been used extensively for rapid inference of transmission networks from large sets of pathogen genetic sequences to identify potential transmission links and to describe putative transmission clusters. HIV-TRACE identifies groups of putative transmission partners and assembles these partners in transmission clusters but cannot determine transmission directionality (Kosakovsky Pond et al., 2018).

As emphasized in the CDC draft document:

Although some tools, such as Secure HIV-TRACE and MicrobeTrace, generate network diagrams of clusters based on genetic distance data, there are important limitations to drawing inferences from these data at an individual level. Although two persons infected with highly similar HIV strains could be directly linked through transmission, other transmission relationships could be consistent with this sequence similarity: both could have been infected from a third source, or they could be connected indirectly through a transmission chain including one or more intermediaries. Because of this scientific uncertainty, the potential for the misuse and misinterpretation of these data presents a concern. Moreover, presence of or patterns of linkages can be affected by timing of diagnoses and drug resistance testing. Although analysis of molecular data to identify growing transmission clusters can identify important opportunities for individual- and cluster-level public health interventions, inferences about specific transmission linkages or indirect inferences about sexual or other risk behaviors should not be used to guide services or follow-up at the individual level. Because of the potential for misinterpretation of these diagrams, it is not recommended to disseminate genetic network diagrams beyond the group of staff involved in the analysis of sequence data. (HIV Cluster Guidance Working Group, 2020)

The National Alliance of State and Territorial AIDS Directors (NASTAD, 2018) notes that:

Emerging data-use and data-sharing activities raise questions about data privacy and confidentiality protections and the ethical uses and sharing of personally identifiable data. The fact that HIV surveillance data is, by and large, collected without explicit patient consent for enumerated data uses triggers additional ethical considerations for how health departments use and share this data. Data-sharing protections and limitations are important not only to inform emerging public health data-sharing activities, but also to restrict data sharing for non-public health purposes, such as criminal HIV exposure and transmission prosecutions.

NASTAD focused this analysis on 10 states (Illinois, Iowa, Louisiana, Massachusetts, Michigan, North Carolina, Tennessee, Virginia, Wisconsin and Utah). Community engagement is an important component of this rapidly evolving surveillance methodology (NASTAD, 2018).

ANONYMOUS AND CONFIDENTIAL HIV TESTING

Although most studies have not shown a decrease in HIV testing in states that have adopted name-based reporting, data indicate that some people prefer anonymous HIV testing to name-based confidential testing (Charlebois et al., 2005). Many people are understandably reluctant to have their name entered in a database of persons with HIV infection. Although the states have established elaborate precautions to prevent breaches of security, the risk of revelation of HIV status can be intimidating. Therefore, in many areas, individuals can choose to be tested for HIV either anonymously (without giving any identifying information) or confidentially (with the HIV test result linked to identifying information, such as patient name).

In states that require HIV case reporting, only confidential testing results must be reported to public health authorities. Test results from anonymous testing are not reportable. However, they do provide the clinician with an important opportunity for educating and counseling patients about reducing high-risk behaviors and seeking HIV treatments, at which point they would be captured in systems linking HIV viral load and CD4 testing to the reporting database.

REPORTABLE HIV-RELATED DISEASES

Most states require reporting of conditions that commonly occur or are associated with HIV infection, including syphilis and other sexually transmitted diseases (STDs), tuberculosis, acute hepatitis (A, B, or C), histoplasmosis, and HIV-related opportunistic infections. Certain microbiologic diagnoses that are made by culture or serology are reported directly by the laboratory to the appropriate state or local health authority.

THE CLINICIAN'S ROLE

Healthcare providers should know which illnesses and complications must be reported to their state health departments and the timeframe within which reporting is required. They should understand that reporting of notifiable conditions depends on the jurisdiction, that a legal obligation is imposed upon practitioners by those states, and that sanctions (e.g., fines) can be imposed upon practitioners for failure to report (CDC, 2020).

REFERENCES/RECOMMENDED READING

Boyle BA, Bradley T, Bradley H, et al. Health Insurance Portability and Accountability Act of 1996: new national medical privacy standards. *AIDS Read.* 2003;13:261–262, 265–266.

Centers for Disease Control and Prevention. HIV cluster and outbreak detection and response. https://www.cdc.gov/hiv/programresources/guidance/cluster-outbreak/index.html

Centers for Disease Control and Prevention. HIV cluster response. https://www.cdc.gov/hiv/effective-interventions/respond/hiv-cluster-response/index.html

Centers for Disease Control and Prevention. State Laboratory Reporting Laws: Viral Load and CD4 Requirements. 2020. https://www.cdc.gov/hiv/policies/law/states/reporting.html

Centers for Disease Control and Prevention. Trends in HIV/AIDS diagnosis—33 states, 2001–2004. *MMWR Morb Mortal Wkly Rep.* 2005;54(45):1149–1153.

Charlebois ED, Maiorana A, McLaughlin M, et al. Potential deterrent effect of name-based HIV infection surveillance. *J AIDS.* 2005;39(2):219–227.

HIPAA Privacy Rule and Public Health: Guidance from CDC and the U.S. Department of Health and Human Services. *MMWR Morb Mortal Wkly Rep.* 2003;52(S-1):1–12. https://www.cdc.gov/mmwr/preview/mmwrhtml/su5201a1.htm

HIV Cluster Guidance Working Group. Detecting and responding to HIV transmission clusters: a guide for health departments (draft). 2020. https://www.cdc.gov/hiv/pdf/funding/announcements/ps18-1802/CDC-HIV-PS18-1802-AttachmentE-Detecting-Investigating-and-Responding-to-HIV-Transmission-Clusters.pdf

Holtgrave DR. Estimation of annual HIV transmission rates in the United States, 1978–2000. *J AIDS.* 2004;35(1):89–92.

Kosakovsky Pond SL, Weaver S, Leigh Brown AJ, et al. BHIV-TRACE (TRAnsmission Cluster Engine). *Mol Biol Evol.* 2018;35(7):1812–1819.

Lubelchek RJ, Finnegan KJ, Hotton AL, et al. Assessing the use of HIV surveillance data to help gauge patient retention-in-care. *J AIDS.* 2015;69:S25–S30.

National Alliance of State and Territorial AIDS Directors. HIV data privacy and confidentiality legal & ethical considerations for health department data sharing. June 2018. https://www.nastad.org/sites/default/files/Uploads/2018/nastad-hiv-data-privacy-06062018.pdf

Oster AM, France AM, Panneer N, et al. Identifying clusters of recent and rapid HIV transmission through analysis of molecular surveillance data. *J AIDS.* 2018;79(5):543–550. https://www.ncbi.nlm.nih.gov/pmc/articles/PMC6231979/

US Department of Health and Human Services, Office for Civil Rights. HIPAA. Summary of the HIPAA Privacy Rule. https://www.

hhs.gov/hipaa/for-professionals/privacy/laws-regulations/index.html?language=en

Wiewel E, Braunstein SL, Xiaet Q, et al. Monitoring outcomes for newly diagnosed and prevalent HIV cases using a care continuum created with New York City surveillance data. *J AIDS*. 2015;68:217–226.

Wortley PM, Lindegren ML, Fleming PL. Successful implementation of perinatal HIV prevention guidelines: a multistate surveillance evaluation. *MMWR Morbid Mortal Wkly Rep*. 2001;50(RR-6):17–28. https://www.cdc.gov/mmwr/preview/mmwrhtml/rr5006a2.htm

PARTNER NOTIFICATION AND PREVENTION FOR HIV-POSITIVE PATIENTS

LEARNING OBJECTIVE

- Describe the requirements for partner notification practices in HIV disease

WHAT'S NEW?

Information regarding partner notification and prevention for HIV-positive people has remained consistent during the past several years.

KEY POINTS

- Many states require healthcare providers to discuss partner notification options with their HIV-infected patients. The federal 1996 Ryan White CARE Act requires all states to adopt laws requiring notification of spouses of HIV-infected patients.

- Many HIV-infected individuals do not disclose their HIV status to their partners out of fear of rejection, loss of financial support, and/or abuse. Their partners then remain unaware of their own potential HIV exposure.

- Partner notification programs typically allow HIV-infected persons to anonymously inform their sexual and needle-sharing partners that they may have been exposed to HIV.

PARTNER NOTIFICATION LEGAL REQUIREMENTS

In many states, healthcare providers are required to discuss partner notification options with HIV-infected patients. This is not only a legal requirement, carrying the possibility of civil and/or legal sanctions for violation of partner notification laws, but also an ethical issue. Amendments to the federal Ryan White CARE Act in 1996 require states to take "administrative or legislative action to require that a good faith effort" is made to notify the spouse of a known HIV-infected patient of the spouse's potential exposure to HIV. This action must be taken by states in order to be eligible for CARE Act funds (Webber, 2004).

States can be categorized into three groups based on their rules and regulations for partner notification programs: (1)

states that require healthcare providers to give the contact's name to the local health officer, and the public health official then notifies the contact; (2) states that give the healthcare provider the choice of notifying either the local health officer or the contacts named by the source patient directly; and (3) states that make such disclosures to a state agency discretionary or optional (Lin & Liang, 2005). Healthcare providers should seek advice from local public health departments and their own attorneys to specifically understand their legal responsibilities.

THE CLINICIAN'S ROLE

Preventing harm not only to the patient but also to others should be the goal of every clinician. The CDC has recommended an increased emphasis on prevention efforts in the primary care of HIV-infected people (Box 44.1).

In general, HIV-infected persons should be given the option of directly informing their sexual or needle-sharing contacts. A study of MSM found that knowledge of HIV status resulted in a significant decrease in behaviors capable of transmitting HIV; however, the behavioral changes were not permanent (Colfax et al., 2002).

Many HIV-infected individuals do not disclose their HIV status to their partners, fearing that they would be threatened, harmed, or abandoned. Nondisclosers, however, are not more likely than disclosers to use condoms or other disease prevention measures (Stein et al., 1998; Wolitski et al., 1998). When individuals are reluctant to disclose their HIV status to their partners themselves, partner notification programs can assist (CDC, 2008).

PARTNER NOTIFICATION PROGRAMS

Partner notification programs are designed to allow HIV-infected individuals to inform their sexual and needle-sharing partners that they may have been exposed to HIV. For HIV-infected persons who opt not to inform their partners themselves, these programs typically provide counselors who will

---

Box 44.1 METHODS FOR HEALTHCARE PROVIDERS TO HELP REDUCE HIV INFECTION

- HIV testing and linkage to care
- HIV medications
- Access to condoms
- Prevention programs for people with HIV and their partners
- Prevention programs for people at high risk for HIV infection
- Substance abuse treatment and access to sterile needles and syringes
- Screening and treatment for sexually transmitted infections

SOURCE: CDC (2016).

---

inform the at-risk persons of possible HIV exposure without revealing the identity of the HIV-infected person who may have exposed them.

Partner notification programs maximize the opportunity for persons to become aware of their HIV exposure and to access HIV testing and counseling. Partner notification may prevent an at-risk individual from acquiring HIV or, if he or she already has HIV, allow him or her to receive appropriate treatment and learn how to prevent the transmission of HIV infection to others.

REFERENCES/RECOMMENDED READING

Centers for Disease Control and Prevention. Incorporating HIV prevention into the medical care of persons living with HIV. Recommendations of CDC, the Health Resources and Services Administration, the National Institutes of Health, and HIV Medicine Association of the IDSA. *MMWR Morbid Mortal Wkly Rep.* 2003;52:1–24. http://www.cdc.gov/mmwr/preview/mmwrhtml/rr5212a1.htm

Centers for Disease Control and Prevention. Recommendations for partner services programs for HIV infection, syphilis, gonorrhea, and chlamydial infection. *MMWR Recomm Rep.* 2008;57(RR-9):1–84. https://www.cdc.gov/mmwr/preview/mmwrhtml/rr5709a1.htm

Colfax GN, Buchbinder SP, Cornelisse PGA, et al. Sexual risk behaviors and implications for secondary HIV transmission during and after HIV seroconversion. *AIDS.* 2002;16:1529–1535.

Laar AK, DeBruin DA, Craddock S. Partner notification in the context of HIV: an interest-analysis. *AIDS Res Ther.* 2015;12:15. http://www.biomedcentral.com/content/pdf/s12981-015-0057-8.pdf

Lin L, Liang BA. HIV and health law: striking the balance between legal mandates and medical ethics. *Virtual Mentor AMA J Ethics.* 2005;7(10). http://journalofethics.ama-assn.org/2005/10/hlaw1-0510.html

Stein MD, Freedberg KA, Sullivan LM, et al. Sexual ethics: disclosure of HIV-positive status to partners. *Arch Intern Med.* 1998;158:253–257.

Webber DW. Self-incrimination, partner notification, and the criminal law: negatives for the CDC's "prevention for positives" initiative. *AIDS Public Policy J.* 2004;19:54–66. https://www.hivlawandpolicy.org/sites/default/files/APPJ%202004%20Webber.pdf

Wejnert C, Prejean J, Hoots B, et al. Prevalence of missed opportunities for HIV testing among persons unaware of their infection. *JAMA.* 2018;319(24):2555–2557.

ISSUES IN DISCLOSURE

LEARNING OBJECTIVE

- Discuss the healthcare provider's legal responsibilities to HIV-infected patients who do not disclose their HIV status to sexual and needle-sharing partners

WHAT'S NEW?

Information regarding disclosure issues has remained consistent during the past several years.

KEY POINTS

- The obligation of healthcare providers to maintain patient confidentiality may be overridden to protect the public health or individuals who are endangered by HIV-infected persons.

- Healthcare providers should consult an attorney or their state laws and regulations before making any such disclosures.

- Healthcare providers may have a "duty to warn" if there is an ongoing exposure to potential HIV infection. Conversely, there may be criminal actions brought against patients based on information provided to local health departments about ongoing behaviors endangering the public health.

Information disclosed by a patient to a healthcare provider during the course of the provider–patient relationship is considered confidential. This confidentiality is essential for a full and free disclosure of information so that effective counseling and therapy can be provided. In general, unless required by the law to do so, a healthcare provider is ethically barred from revealing confidential communications or information without the patient's consent.

The obligation to maintain patient confidence is not without limits, however, and it may be overridden by exceptions that are ethically and legally justified. Such justification may occur when patients threaten to inflict bodily harm to another person or to themselves and there is a reasonable probability that they may carry out the threat, and also when reports are required by law, such as with communicable diseases and gunshot and knife wounds. California established a physician's duty to warn third parties if there is an imminent threat of serious harm to a known third party (*Tarasoff*, 1976). Subsequent to the *Tarasoff* case, many other states have adopted this duty-to-warn requirement and even expanded it to the unknown third parties. However, it is still not clear whether the duty to warn as identified in the *Tarasoff* case would apply to a sexual or needle-sharing partner of an HIV-infected patient who had not disclosed his or her HIV status.

It is important to differentiate "permissive" disclosures allowed under state laws, usually to local public health officers, from "mandatory" disclosures as required by law. A mandatory disclosure is one that a healthcare provider must make, such as disclosure of reportable diseases or suspected child abuse. In a permissive disclosure, local regulations allow a healthcare provider to discuss a specific patient with local public health officials (e.g., to seek their assistance in modifying a patient's behavior).

It is within this legal and ethical framework that providers should consider their obligations when they are aware that an HIV-infected patient is endangering others by engaging in acts that may lead to transmission of HIV. American Medical Association (AMA) guidelines issued in 1992 and updated in 1994, while recognizing a physician's obligation to protect the patient's confidentiality whenever possible, acknowledge that there are exceptions to this confidentiality:

When necessary to protect the public health or when necessary to protect individuals, including healthcare workers, who are endangered by persons infected with HIV. If a physician knows that a seropositive individual is endangering a third party, the physician should, within the constraints of the law: (1) attempt to persuade the infected patient to cease endangering the third party; (2) if persuasion fails, notify authorities; and (3) if the authorities take no action, notify the endangered third party.

Given the legal implications of divulging a person's HIV status, healthcare providers should consult an attorney or become familiar with state laws and regulations before making any such disclosures.

PERINATAL/ADOLESCENT HIV DISCLOSURE

Complex disclosure challenges may arise during the peri/neonatal period. Local, regional and national laws should be consulted in determining disclosure and privacy laws as they apply to the peri/neonatal period. Likewise, disclosure of HIV infection to young children or adolescents is a difficult challenge. HIV status disclosure to children is quite low in sub-Saharan Africa. This may be due to several factors, including parents'/caregivers' fear of the child disclosing status to others, a lack of knowledge on how to make the disclosure, and the assessment of whether the child can cope with the psychological impact of the diagnosis (Doat et al., 2019).

The World Health Organization (WHO) recommends disclosing HIV status between 6 and 12 years, and the American Academy of Pediatrics recommends that children are informed at "school age." The WHO guidance notes that healthcare workers are often without the support of definitive, evidence-based policies and guidelines on when, how, and under what conditions children should be informed about their own or their caregivers' HIV status (Krauss et al., 2011).

Key conclusions of the WHO guideline on HIV disclosure counseling for children up to 12 years of age are as follows (Krauss et al., 2011):

Disclosure to children of their own HIV status

- There is evidence of health benefit (e.g. reduced risk of death) and little evidence of psychological or emotional harm from disclosure of HIV status to HIV-positive children. Immediate emotional reactions dissipate with time and respond to programme interventions.

- Disclosure of diagnosis, as described by published researchers and by practitioners, is not an isolated event but rather a step in the process of adjustment by the child, caregivers, and the community to an illness and the life challenges that it poses.

Disclosure to children of their parent's or caregivers' HIV status

- There is evidence of benefit to health for HIV-positive and HIV-negative children of HIV-positive caregivers if the caregiver discloses to them.

- The concerns of some caregivers that disclosure leads to increased behavioural problems in children and decreases the quality of the relationship are not supported by children's reports about their reactions to disclosure of their caregivers' HIV status. Even by parents' reports, anticipating and preparing for the understandable initial emotional reactions can improve the child's responses, and responses improve with time.

- There appears to be no harm to caregivers when they disclose their status to their children or wards.

Given that virally suppressed people do not transmit HIV and that interrupting the transmission cycle is critical to ending the HIV epidemic, Budhwani et al. (2020) examined the relationship between age of disclosure and viral load suppression by evaluating data from a pediatric HIV clinic in the southern US. Records from 61 perinatally infected patients seen between 2008 and 2018 were analyzed. The preliminary findings suggest that disclosing HIV status between age 10 and 12 years may promote viral suppression through medication adherence.

REFERENCES/RECOMMENDED READING

Budhwani H, Mills L, Marefka LEB, et al. Preliminary study on HIV status disclosure to perinatal infected children: retrospective analysis of administrative records from a pediatric HIV clinic in the southern United States. *BMC Res Notes* 2020;13:253.

Doat AR, Negarandeh R, Hasanpour M. Disclosure of HIV status to children in sub-Saharan Africa: a systematic review. *Medicina*. 2019;55(8):433.

Downs L. The duty to protect a patient's right to confidentiality: Tarasoff, HIV, and confusion. *J Forensic Psychol Pract*. 2015;15(2):160–170. http://dx.doi.org/10.1080/15228932.2015.1007776

HIV.gov. HIV disclosure policies and procedures. https://www.hiv.gov/hiv-basics/living-well-with-hiv/your-legal-rights/limits-on-confidentiality

Krauss B, Letteney S, de Baets A, et al. Guideline on HIV disclosure counselling for children up to 12 years of age. Geneva: World Health Organization; 2011. https://apps.who.int/iris/bitstream/handle/10665/44777/9789241502863_eng.pdf;jsessionid=27A6CA8DA056F1823129425B95692717?sequence=1

Lin L, Liang BA. HIV and health law: striking the balance between legal mandates and medical ethics. *Virtual Mentor Am Med Assoc J Ethics*. 2005;7(10). http://journalofethics.ama-assn.org/2005/10/hlaw1-0510.html

Obermeyer CM, Baijal P, Pegurri E. Facilitating HIV disclosure across diverse settings: a review. *Am J Pub Health*. 2011;101(6):1011–1023.

Richardson R, Golden S, Hanssens C. *Ending and defending against HIV criminalization—A manual for advocates: Vol. 1. State and federal laws and prosecutions*. 2nd ed., Winter 2015. http://www.hivlawandpolicy.org/sites/www.hivlawandpolicy.org/files/HIV%20Crim%20Manual%20%28updated%205.4.15%29.pdf

Simoni JM, Davis ML, Drossman JA, et al. Mothers with HIV/AIDS and their children: disclosure and guardianship issues. *Womens Health*. 2000;31:39–54.

Tarasoff v. Regents of U. of California, 131 Cal. Rptr. 14, 551 P.2d 334 (1976).

Webber DW. Self-incrimination, partner notification, and the criminal law: negatives for the CDC's "prevention for positives" initiative. *AIDS Public Policy J*. 2004; 9:54–66.

HIV CRIMINALIZATION

LEARNING OBJECTIVE

- Describe the scientific rationale of the International AIDS Society's expert consensus statement on the science of HIV in the context of criminal law and the recommendations from the National HIV/AIDS Strategy (NHAS) concerning criminal laws regarding HIV transmission and prevention

WHAT'S NEW?

Some states have modified their HIV criminalization statutes in keeping with the data about U=U ("Undetectable = Untransmittable") in the past few years.

KEY POINTS

- Stigma and discrimination continue to be major challenges to the comprehensive response necessary to address the HIV public health crisis.

- The NHAS recommends that evidence-based public health approaches to HIV prevention and care be implemented and that state legislatures should review HIV-specific criminal statutes to ensure that they are consistent with current scientific knowledge of HIV transmission and support public health approaches to preventing and treating HIV.

- The International AIDS Society recommends that those working in legal and judicial systems pay close attention to the significant advances in HIV science that have occurred over the past three decades to ensure that current scientific knowledge informs application of the law in cases related to HIV.

In an attempt to limit the spread of HIV, many states have enacted laws that criminalize willful or knowing exposure of another person to HIV infection (Gostin, 1989). During the early years of the HIV epidemic, many states implemented HIV-specific criminal exposure laws (statutes and regulations). Some of these state laws criminalize behaviors that cannot transmit HIV and apply regardless of actual transmission. As of 2020, 37 states have laws that criminalize HIV exposure.

The laws for the 50 states and the District of Columbia were assessed and categorized into five categories:

1. HIV-specific laws that criminalize or control behaviors that can potentially expose another person to HIV

2. Laws specific to an STD, communicable disease, contagious disease, or infectious disease that criminalize or control behaviors that can potentially expose another person to such a disease. This might include HIV.

3. Sentence enhancement laws specific to HIV that do not criminalize a behavior but increase the sentence length when a person with HIV commits certain crimes

4. Sentence enhancement laws specific to STDs that do not criminalize a behavior but increase the sentence length when a person with an STD commits certain crimes. This might include HIV.

5. No specific criminalization laws

Some statutes do not require proof of intent to harm, only proof that the person knew that he or she was HIV-infected and, despite that knowledge, failed to inform at-risk contacts or use appropriate precautions (e.g., safer sex or clean needles) to prevent contacts from becoming infected. These laws have also been applied to HIV-positive people who solicited sex for money, a prisoner who bit a prison guard, and individuals who spat on another person. Although these statutes have been challenged on the alleged grounds of unconstitutional vagueness or violations of free speech or free association, most have been upheld. In addition to these laws, prosecutors have brought other criminal charges against HIV-infected individuals who unreasonably risk transmission of HIV through such acts as attempted murder, assault or assault with a dangerous or deadly weapon, and reckless endangerment (Gostin, 1989; Webber, 2004). The tension between the public health approach and a criminal justice approach and the effect on disclosure continues as applied to HIV transmission (Csete, 2011; Obermeyer et al., 2011).

An analysis by CDC and US Department of Justice researchers found that, through 2011, a total of 67 laws explicitly focused on persons with HIV had been enacted in 33 states. These laws vary as to what behaviors are criminalized or result in additional penalties. In 24 states, laws require persons who are aware that they have HIV to disclose their status to sexual partners, and 14 states require disclosure to needle-sharing partners. Twenty-five states have laws that criminalize one or more behaviors that, as noted by Lehman et al. (2014), pose low or negligible risk for HIV transmission. The majority of laws were passed before studies showed that ART reduces HIV transmission risk, and most laws do not account for HIV prevention measures that reduce transmission risk, such as condom use, ART, or preexposure prophylaxis (PrEP). Punishing people for behavior that is either consensual or poses no risk of HIV transmission only serves to further stigmatize already marginalized communities while missing opportunities for prevention education.

The American Academy of HIV Medicine (AAHIVM) and its members are opposed to laws that distinguish HIV disease from other comparable diseases or that create disproportionate penalties for disclosure, exposure, or transmission of HIV disease beyond normal public health ordinances. The AAHIVM supports nonpunitive prevention approaches to HIV centered on current scientific understanding and evidence-based research. The HIV Medicine Association (HIVMA) urged repeal of HIV-specific criminal statutes and noted that stigma and discrimination continue to be major impediments to the comprehensive response necessary to address the HIV public health crisis. HIVMA noted that policies and laws that create HIV-specific crimes or that impose penalties for persons who are HIV-infected are unjust and harmful to public health throughout the world.

The NHAS, released by the White House in July 2010 and updated in 2015 with goals through 2020, recommends that federal and state governments should ensure that federal and state criminal laws reflect current scientific information regarding HIV transmission and prevention. The NHAS document also recommends evidence-based public health approaches to HIV prevention and care. The document notes that state legislatures should review HIV-specific criminal statutes to ensure that they are consistent with current scientific knowledge of HIV transmission and support public health approaches to preventing and treating HIV.

An expert consensus statement on the science of HIV in the context of criminal law was published in July 2018. The statement concluded that:

> We strongly recommend that more caution be exercised when considering criminal prosecution, including careful appraisal of current scientific evidence on HIV-related risks and harms. This is instrumental to reduce stigma and discrimination and to avoid miscarriages of justice. In this context, we hope this Consensus Statement will encourage governments and those working in the legal and judicial system to pay close attention to the significant advances in HIV science that have occurred over the last three decades, and make all efforts to ensure that a correct and complete understanding of current scientific knowledge informs any application of the criminal law in cases related to HIV. (Barre-Sinoussi et al., 2018)

The Sero Project is a network of persons with HIV and their allies fighting for freedom from stigma and injustice. Sero is particularly focused on ending inappropriate criminal prosecutions of people with HIV, including for nondisclosure of their HIV status and potential or perceived HIV exposure or HIV transmission. Iowa and California have both revised their HIV criminalization laws to better reflect the current scientific information about HIV transmission.

The CDC notes that since 2014, at least five states have modernized their HIV criminal laws. Changes include removing HIV prevention issues from the criminal code and including them under disease control regulations, requiring intent to transmit and actual HIV transmission, or providing defenses for taking measures to prevent transmission such as viral suppression or being noninfectious, condom use, and partner PrEP use. The states are California, Colorado, Iowa, Michigan, and North Carolina. (CDC). Additionally, Washington state changed its HIV criminalization laws in 2020: the change reduced penalties for HIV exposure from a felony to a misdemeanor, requires specific intent to transmit HIV and for transmission to occur, and removes the requirement for sex offender registration (Center for HIV Law and Policy, 2020a, 2020b).

REFERENCES/RECOMMENDED READING

Adam BD, Corriveau P, Elliott R, et al. HIV disclosure as practice and public policy. *Crit Public Health*. 2015;25(4):386–397. http://dx.doi.org/10.1080/09581596.2014.980395

American Academy for HIV Medicine. Confidentiality. https://www.ama-assn.org/delivering-care/ethics/confidentiality

American Academy for HIV Medicine. HIV criminalization. https://aahivm.org/hiv-criminalization/

Barre-Sinoussi F, Abdool Karim SS, Albert J, et al. Expert consensus statement on the science of HIV in the context of criminal law. *J Int AIDS Soc*. 2018;21(7):e25161.

Center for HIV Law and Policy. HIV criminalization in the United States (updated July 2020a). http://www.hivlawandpolicy.org/sites/default/files/HIV%20Criminalization%20in%20the%20US%20%282020%29.pdf

Center for HIV Law and Policy. Washington state advocates succeed in reforming state's HIV criminal law. 2020b. https://www.hivlawandpolicy.org/news/washington-state-advocates-succeed-reforming-state%E2%80%99s-hiv-criminal-law

Francis LP, Francis JG. Criminalizing health-related behaviors dangerous to others? Disease transmission, transmission-facilitation, and the importance of trust. *Criminal Law Philosophy*. 2012;6:47–63.

Gostin LO. Public health strategies for confronting AIDS. Legislative and regulatory policy in the United States. *JAMA*. 1989;261(11):1621–1630.

Haire B, Kaldor J. HIV transmission law in the age of treatment-as-prevention. *J Med Ethics*. 2015;41:982–986.

HIV Criminalization Resources. http://www.seroproject.com/resources

HIV.gov. National HIV/AIDS Strategy for the United States. Updated to 2020. https://files.hiv.gov/s3fs-public/nhas-update.pdf

HIV Medicine Association. HIV criminalization reform and advocacy. https://www.hivma.org/policy--advocacy/hiv-criminalization-reform-and-advocacy/

Lehman JS, Carr MH, Nichol AJ, et al. Prevalence and public health implications of state laws that criminalize potential HIV exposure in the United States. *AIDS Behav*. 2014;18(6):997–1006. http://rd.springer.com/article/10.1007/s10461-014-0724-0/fulltext.html

Mykhalovskiy E. The public health implications of HIV criminalization: past, current, and future research directions. *Crit Public Health*. 2015;25(4):373–385. http://dx.doi.org/10.1080/09581596.2015.1052731

Obermeyer CM, Baijal P, Pegurri E. Facilitating HIV disclosure across diverse settings: a review. *Am J Pub Health*. 2011;101(6):1011–1023.

Webber DW. Self-incrimination, partner notification, and the criminal law: negatives for the CDC's "prevention for positives" initiative. *AIDS Public Policy J*. 2004;19:54–66. https://www.hivlawandpolicy.org/sites/default/files/APPJ%202004%20Webber.pdf

TREATING MINORS

LEARNING OBJECTIVE

- Describe legal issues related to treatment of minors with HIV infection

WHAT'S NEW?

Information regarding treatment of minors has remained consistent during the past several years.

- Medical treatment of minors (persons younger than 18 years) must generally be authorized by a parent or legal guardian, with specific exceptions that vary across states.

- This area of law is often complex and variable. Healthcare providers unsure of their state laws and regulations should seek legal advice before treating minors for HIV.

The medical care of minors—defined in most states as persons younger than 18 years—must generally be authorized by their parent or legal guardian. This usually means that a parent or guardian of a minor is required to give informed consent on behalf of the minor for most medical decisions. However, there are exceptions to this rule, and certain minors can consent to certain types of medical care without the authority of a parent or legal guardian.

CONSENT FOR STD SERVICES AND MEDICAL TREATMENT

All 50 states and the District of Columbia explicitly allow minors to consent to STD services, although 11 states require that a minor be of a certain age (generally 12–14 years) before being allowed to consent. Thirty-two states explicitly include HIV testing and treatment in the package of STD services to which minors may consent.

Most states have laws that authorize minors to consent to certain types of medical treatment, such as care for pregnancy; contraception and abortion care; treatment for contagious diseases, STDs, rape, sexual assault, mental health, and drug or alcohol abuse; and HIV testing. In many states, absent exceptional circumstances, a minor is not able to consent to HIV treatment, and consent must be obtained from the parent or legal guardian (e.g., see New York State Public Health Law 2504).

Almost all states have laws that authorize minors who have attained a certain status to make the majority of their own healthcare decisions. These may include minors who are married (or divorced), on active duty with the US Armed Forces, emancipated by a court order, or self-sufficient such that they have attained a designated age and live away from home and manage their own financial affairs.

LAWS RELATED TO INFORMING PARENTS

Eighteen states allow healthcare providers to inform a minor's parents that he or she is seeking or receiving STD services. With the exception of one state (Iowa requires parental notification in the case of a positive HIV test), no state requires that providers notify parents (Guttmacher Institute, 2020; Ho et al., 2005). In some states, healthcare providers are prohibited from telling the minor's parent(s) or legal guardian about any test-related medical care unless the minor authorizes it (e.g., see New York State Public Health Law 2780.5).

SEEKING LEGAL ADVICE

Healthcare providers should be aware that this area of the law is very complex, highly variable by state, and rife with legal risks and exposure if an incorrect decision regarding treatment is made. Therefore, it is highly advisable that healthcare providers who are unsure of the law in their state consult a lawyer before providing HIV testing or treatment to a minor. Healthcare providers must be acutely aware of the importance of consulting and obtaining the informed consent of a parent or legal guardian of the minor when required by law.

REFERENCES/RECOMMENDED READING

Center for HIV Law and Policy. Minors' consent laws for HIV and STD services. https://www.cdc.gov/hiv/policies/law/states/minors.html

Center for HIV Law and Policy. State HIV laws HIV-specific criminal laws, state guidelines for health care workers with HIV, youth access to STI and HIV testing and treatment, HIV testing. http://www.hivlawandpolicy.org/state-hiv-laws

Guttmacher Institute. Minors' access to STD services: state laws and policies. September 1, 2020. http://www.guttmacher.org/statecenter/spibs/spib_MASS.pdf

Ho WW, Brandfield J, Retkin R, et al. Complexities in HIV consent in adolescents. *Clin Pediatr.* 2005;44:473–478.

Kaiser Foundation. Minors' authority to consent to STI services. http://kff.org/hivaids/state-indicator/minors-right-to-consent

CONFIDENTIALITY

LEARNING OBJECTIVE

- Discuss legal issues related to confidentiality and HIV, including health information protected under the Health Insurance Portability and Accountability Act of 1996 (HIPAA) along with HIPAA's Privacy Rule and its impact on communicating a patient's personal health information.

WHAT'S NEW?

Information regarding confidentiality has remained consistent during the past several years.

KEY POINTS

- There are many reasons for maintaining strict confidentiality in the medical setting, including the need to maintain effective clinician–patient relationships.

- Various state and federal regulations govern confidentiality of medical information. Noncompliance carries the risk of civil and/or criminal penalties.

- Federal provisions governing confidentiality were established in HIPAA. The act defines which health entities are covered, the types of medical information covered, how information can be used, and requirements for notifying patients. The deadline for compliance with the HIPAA Privacy Rule was April 14, 2003.

- The HIPAA Security Standards dictate that "administrative, physical, and technical" safeguards must be in place to protect confidential information and its transmission and storage. Healthcare providers had to comply with the HIPAA Security Standards by April 21, 2005, with a 1-year extension permitted for small health plans.

- Available resources may assist clinicians in complying with HIPAA and other confidentiality provisions.

The rationale for confidentiality in the medical setting is that an effective clinician–patient relationship is based on trust and strict confidentiality regarding the patient's medical information. Maintaining patient confidentiality has particular importance when the patient is infected with HIV. Patients may choose to keep their status private in order to avoid the significant emotional, social, and financial stigmatization, isolation, and loss that many HIV-infected persons encounter when their status becomes known. Therefore, all clinicians should seek to respect the privacy of their patients, including persons with HIV, and their wishes not to have personal information about themselves made available to others.

The Hippocratic Oath and other ethical guidelines instruct providers that information gained through the provider–patient relationship is confidential. Confidentiality requirements are also underscored by various state laws and federal provisions. HIPAA has implications for nearly all healthcare providers and facilities, including federally funded facilities that provide substance abuse treatment services.

In general, both state and federal confidentiality requirements address the areas discussed in the following sections.

HANDLING OF MEDICAL INFORMATION

State laws require patient consent for releasing information to all or only certain requestors. HIPAA provides criteria to oversee transmission of information within the current interrelated healthcare system for purposes of treatment, payment, or other healthcare functions. HIPAA regulates the sharing of information among multiple providers and payers.

PROCEDURES FOR HANDLING EXCEPTIONAL SITUATIONS

State laws typically provide for disclosure of information for public health purposes, such as the "duty to warn" an individual facing imminent harm from a patient. Assaults and communicable diseases are reportable, and their reporting may be legally mandated (American Medical Association, 2005). Physician–patient confidentiality is not absolute under the law of most states. The courts and legislators in many states have attempted to strike a balance between competing rights: those of patients to confidentiality and those of others to information about the significant dangers they may face. It seems reasonable that the patient's right to privacy should be breached only when it is necessary to avoid imminent and serious harm. If the chance of contracting HIV from contact with the patient is remote (i.e., a household contact), then the right to confidentiality should be considered paramount. However, if the chance of contracting HIV is high (i.e., through sexual contact), then the duty to warn may take precedence (see Objective 60.5, Issues in Disclosure).

PENALTIES

Providers treating HIV-infected patients must seek to balance these legal and ethical obligations. There is no guarantee that the balance struck by the clinician will be the same struck by a court should the matter end up in litigation. Almost half of the states have provisions for revoking a healthcare provider's medical license or exercising other disciplinary action when confidential patient information is inappropriately or unlawfully disclosed. HIPAA also contains penalty provisions. When in doubt, clinicians should consult an attorney before taking any action or making any disclosure without consent.

HIPAA

In 2003, Boyle et al. described the HIPAA regulations on privacy and disclosure of medical information (i.e., the "Privacy Rule"). HIPAA places the burden on healthcare providers and others who have access to confidential medical information to keep that information private and protected. HIPAA outlines who must comply, what information is protected, and what providers must do to comply. Similar state laws take precedence if they are more stringent than HIPAA.

The Privacy Rule definition of who must comply ("covered entities") covers most clinicians and health plans because it essentially applies to anyone who bills for services electronically. "Protected health information" (PHI) also is broadly defined (i.e., medical records and other identifying information). Covered entities were required to comply with the Privacy Rule by April 14, 2003.

The Privacy Rule stipulates in great detail how information may be used and disclosed. A key example of allowed uses is the release of information to the patient in question. Patients must have access to their medical records along with information about who has been granted access to them. Information also can be used in treatment and payment processes. HIPAA contains provisions for special circumstances in which medical information can be released, such as the "duty to warn" provisions cited previously.

Patient consent must be obtained for most disclosures of medical information. Covered entities are also required to provide patients with a written "Notice of Privacy Practices" that clearly explains the provider's privacy policy, and providers must document that their patients received it (Boyle et al., 2003). In general, healthcare providers must institute reasonable measures to prevent incidental disclosure of patient information. Such measures include ensuring that unauthorized persons cannot wander into record rooms, access computer databases, or overhear names during in-person or telephone communications. However, HIPAA is not intended to impede customary communications, nor does it require protection against any conceivable incidental disclosure, such as when a visitor glimpses patient names on a sign-in sheet.

In addition to the Privacy Rule, HIPAA also requires clinicians and health plans to protect the security of patients' medical information that is stored or transmitted electronically (the "Security Standards"). The Security Standards call for all covered entities to enact administrative, physical, and technical safeguards for electronic data. Examples of such safeguards in an office setting are policies that limit access to database software to those who require it (physical safeguard), sanctions for employees who violate the standards (administrative safeguard), and the maintenance of electronic "audit logs" on computer systems that are equipped to access PHI (technical safeguard).

IDEAS FOR COMPLIANCE

Clinicians should establish compliance provisions not only to fulfill HIPAA requirements but also to be prepared to handle confidentiality in a responsible manner. Among the methods used is the securing of written informed consent from patients (required by HIPAA for certain situations) and formulation of clear procedures for handling patient information (e.g., secure storage, definitions of what information is to be protected and with whom it can be shared, and strategies for handling special circumstances). Other options include designating a privacy officer who is knowledgeable about the details of HIPAA and providing staff training on confidentiality.

For handling situations in which a "duty to warn" another individual arises, such as a sex partner or injection drug-using partner, clinicians can seek assistance. Most local or state health departments have partner notification programs that do this work. A number of internet resources can assist clinicians in complying with HIPAA and other confidentiality provisions (Table 44.2).

The Patient Safety and Quality Improvement Act of 2005 (PSQIA) establishes a voluntary reporting system to enhance the data available to assess and resolve patient safety and healthcare quality issues. To encourage the reporting and analysis of medical errors, PSQIA provides federal privilege and confidentiality protections for patient safety information called *patient safety work product*. The patient safety work product includes information collected and created during the reporting and analysis of patient safety events. The regulation implementing the PSQIA became effective on January 19, 2009 (42 C.F.R. Part 3).

PSQIA authorizes the US Department of Health and Human Services (USDHHS) to impose civil monetary penalties for violations of patient safety confidentiality. PSQIA also authorizes the Agency for Healthcare Research and Quality (AHRQ) to list patient safety organizations. Patient safety organizations are the external experts that collect and review patient safety information.

The Administrative Simplification provisions of HIPAA (Title II) require the USDHHS to adopt national standards for electronic healthcare transactions and national identifiers from providers, health plans, and employers. To date, the implementation of HIPAA standards has increased the use of electronic data interchange. Provisions under the Affordable Care Act of 2010 include requirements to adopt the following:

- Operating rules for each of the HIPAA-covered transactions

- A unique, standard Health Plan Identifier (HPID)

- Standard and operating rules for electronic funds transfer and electronic remittance advice and claims attachments

In addition, health plans will be required to certify their compliance. The Affordable Care Act provides for substantial penalties for failures to comply with the new standards and operation rules.

Table 44.2 WEB-BASED HIPAA AND PRIVACY COMPLIANCE RESOURCES FOR HEALTHCARE PROVIDERS

ORGANIZATION	URL	CONTENTS
American Medical Association	http://www.ama-assn.org/ama/pub/physician-resources/solutions-managing-your-practice/coding-billing-insurance/hipaahealth-insurance-portability-accountability-act.page?	- HIPAA information - FAQ page - Sample documents - Links to other resources - Complaint form for out-of-compliance health plans and other payers
US Department of Health and Human Services Office of Civil Rights	www.hhs.gov/ocr/hipaa	- HIPAA information for clinicians and patients - Fact sheets - Sample documents - Educational materials
Centers for Medicare and Medicaid Services	https://www.cms.gov/Regulations-and-Guidance/Administrative-Simplification/HIPAA-ACA/index.html	- Standards - Educational materials

REFERENCES/RECOMMENDED READING

American Medical Association. The AMA Code of Medical Ethics' opinions on confidentiality of patient information. Opinion 505—Confidentiality. http://journalofethics.ama-assn.org/2012/09/coet1-1209.html

American Medical Association. The AMA Code of Medical Ethics' opinions on confidentiality of patient information. Opinion 9.124—Professionalism in the use of social media. http://journalofethics.ama-assn.org/2011/07/coet1-1107.html

Boyle BA, Bradley T, Bradley H, et al. Health Insurance Portability and Accountability Act of 1996: new national medical privacy standards. *AIDS Read*. 2003;13:261–262, 265–266.

ADVANCE PLANNING

LEARNING OBJECTIVE

• Discuss the use of advance directives, durable power of attorney, health proxy, and arranging for custody of minors for HIV-infected patients

WHAT'S NEW?

Information regarding advance planning has remained consistent during the past few years.

People newly diagnosed with HIV infection (or any potentially life-threatening illness) face a myriad of legal concerns that affect almost every facet of their lives. At times, this may seem overwhelming to patient and provider alike. However, legal planning can greatly benefit HIV-infected patients and their families. Providers can play an important role in informing patients of the benefits of planning ahead.

All providers should advise their patients to investigate and prepare three essential tools of effective legal planning:

1. A durable power of attorney for medical decision-making

2. An advance directive ("living will")

3. A will

DURABLE POWER OF ATTORNEY

A durable power of attorney makes legal provision for someone to make decisions in a patient's stead if he or she is no longer able to do so. Patients should consider two such documents to best protect their legal interests: one for healthcare decisions and one for legal and financial decisions. A patient may choose a single person to fill both roles, but the responsibilities are different. A durable power of attorney for financial issues may cover any and all financial concerns or may stipulate only specific tasks, such as paying standard household expenses or filing tax returns (NOLO, "Estate Planning"). A durable power of attorney for healthcare may cover any and all medical decisions or may stipulate only specific decisions can be made, such as consenting to or refusing any medical treatment. These documents are particularly important for couples who are not legally married, including gay and lesbian couples, because without a durable power of attorney, hospitals and courts usually defer to the closest biological relative to make medical decisions.

A power of attorney may take effect immediately when a patient signs it, or it may become effective only at a time or circumstance that the patient designates—for example, upon the patient's incapacity or other disability that hinders medical or financial decision-making (NOLO, "Estate Planning"). Patients must state in the document that a power of attorney is durable, or it will automatically end if the patient becomes incapacitated. In all cases, a power of attorney ends when the patient dies. Patients may choose to revoke the power of attorney at any time. If married patients grant power of attorney to a spouse, in some states (e.g., California, Illinois, and Texas) the power terminates if the couple divorces (NOLO, "Estate Planning"). Patients should consult an attorney in drafting a durable power of attorney to ensure that it is drawn up correctly.

ADVANCE DIRECTIVES

An advance directive is a document in which patients provide specific instructions about the kind of healthcare they do or do not want in the event that they have an incapacity that makes them unable to make or communicate medical decisions. These instructions are commonly referred to as a "living will." However, there is an important distinction: living wills generally are limited to cases of terminal illness, whereas advance directives may apply to any situation in which a patient is incapacitated, even temporarily. This distinction is especially compelling regarding HIV-infected patients, who may experience AIDS-related dementia or other complications that may impair rational decision-making, but they may subsequently have improved executive function as a result of ART. Patients should know that an advance directive "may be the most convincing evidence of your wishes you can create" (AARP, "Advance Directive Forms"). However, in a large national study of HIV-infected patients, fewer than half reported having advance directives. The most important factor associated with having an advance directive was whether their practitioner had discussed end-of-life issues (Wenger et al., 2001). As the HIV population ages, these discussions should routinely be part of intake medical visits and should be reviewed periodically.

Advance directives are valid in every US state and the District of Columbia, but the specifics of the law vary from state to state. Therefore, patients who spend significant time in more than one state or who move to another state should have directives adjusted to follow each state's guidelines (Caring Connections, "Advance Care Planning"). In creating an advance directive, the patient should consult an expert and should attempt to answer three important questions:

• What are my goals for treatment? Among other things, patients should consider their values relative to independence and their environment and their religious beliefs.

- How specific should I be? No directive can cover all eventualities, but it is suggested that patients address anything that is especially important to them.

- How can I make sure that healthcare providers will follow my advance directive?

Most states give healthcare providers the right to refuse to honor directives on grounds of conscience. In such cases, healthcare providers generally are obligated to refer patients to other healthcare providers who will honor the directive. It is important to ask patients about their wishes. Generally, patients need both a durable power of attorney and an advance directive. In essence, the advance directive expresses a patient's specific wishes, and the durable power of attorney grants someone the authority to execute those wishes or to make healthcare decisions that could not be anticipated by the advance directive.

A study by Stein and Bonuck (2001) found that gay men and lesbians were more likely than the general population to have executed advance directives. However, given the importance of these documents to HIV-infected patients, and because fewer than half of those studied had executed formal directives, healthcare providers are urged to assume a larger role in educating patients about advance care planning. Another study (Ho et al., 2000) affirmed previous results that intervention in an outpatient setting significantly increased the likelihood that HIV-infected patients would execute advance care planning.

Although the focus of advance care planning is usually on the healthcare and legal value of the process, another study showed that advance care planning also increased patients' sense of control and strengthened their relationships with their loved ones (Martin, 1999). However, more than 75% of all respondents in the Stein and Bonuck (2001) study said that their healthcare provider had never asked who should make medical decisions if patients were unable to do so themselves. Healthcare providers are encouraged to discuss these issues with patients.

PHYSICIAN ORDER FOR LIFE-SUSTAINING TREATMENT

A physician order for life-sustaining treatment (POLST) form is becoming more commonly implemented as a part of advance care planning in many states. This form should be done with the healthcare provider, and it specifies medical treatments that a patient may or may not want in the event of a medical emergency or life-threatening event. In many cases it can complement the advance directive and may be more appropriate for persons with a serious illness or advanced frailty near the end of life.

WILLS

A will determines what happens to a person's property after his or her death. Despite considerable attention to wills in the popular press, do not assume that your patients have one—half of all Americans die without one (NOLO, "Wills"). Without a will, the courts will distribute a person's assets according to state laws. Wills are particularly important for people with minor children because, without a will, the state will decide the children's guardianship (NOLO, "Estate Planning"). Wills are also important in situations in which the person is not legally married to his or her partner (e.g., common-law marriage and unmarried gay and lesbian couples) because, without a will, a survivor may inherit nothing and, worse, may lose personal property because he or she cannot prove ownership (FindLaw, "Unmarried couples and property – basics").

Many people mistakenly believe that they do not need wills because they do not have large estates. In truth, however, everyone needs a will to ensure that their wishes are followed when their assets are distributed. Handwritten, unwitnessed wills (called *holographic wills*) are valid in approximately 25 states, but more formal wills are preferable. A valid, legal will must include the following elements:

- It must be typewritten or computer generated (except holographic wills, described previously).

- The document must expressly state that it is a "Will."

- The person making the will must date and sign it.

- The will must be signed by at least two or, in some states, three witnesses who will not inherit anything under the terms of the will.

Healthcare providers should be aware that legal planning is vital for all patients but especially for HIV-infected patients. By focusing on the documents discussed previously (durable power of attorney, advance directives, POLST form, and wills) and by obtaining appropriate legal advice, the planning should not be difficult or confusing.

ARRANGING FOR CUSTODY OF MINORS

A major concern for HIV-infected parents is the welfare of their children (or grandchildren) in the event of the death of the parents. Several legal mechanisms help to address this concern, but the underlying principle is that the court will look to the best interest of the child, considering the parent's desires. A statement in a will about child custody will help inform the court of the parent's wishes. In addition, guardianships with a *springing clause for incapacity* (standby guardianship) can be used to appoint a guardian if a single parent becomes incapacitated. Adoption is a less attractive choice because it requires the parent(s) to surrender all parental rights. Because it is common for parents not to make formal legal arrangements for custody of their children in the event of the parents' death, providers can be helpful in urging patients to consider custody arrangements in advance.

ACKNOWLEDGMENTS

The author wrote or revised text from previous editions and takes responsibility for it; however, the work represents a group product including previous authors.

REFERENCES/RECOMMENDED READING

AARP. Advance directive forms. https://www.aarp.org/caregiving/financial-legal/free-printable-advance-directives/

American Bar Association. Health care advance directives. March 18, 2013. https://www.americanbar.org/groups/public_education/resources/law_issues_for_consumers/directive_review/

American Medical Association. Advance directives. Code of Medical Ethics Opinion 5.2. November 2016. https://www.ama-assn.org/delivering-care/ethics/advance-directives

Caring Connections. Advance care planning. https://caringcommunity.org/topics/advanced-care-planning/advance-directives/

Centers for Disease Control and Prevention. Factsheet. Proven HIV prevention methods. 2016. https://www.cdc.gov/nchhstp/newsroom/docs/factsheets/methods-508.pdf.

Csete J, Kaplan K, Hayashi K, et al. Compulsory drug detention center experiences among a community-based sample of injection drug users in Bangkok, Thailand. *BMC Int Health Hum Rights.* 2011;11:12.

FindLaw. State laws: living wills. http://estate.findlaw.com/estate-planning/living-wills/estate-planning-law-state-living-wills.html

FindLaw. Unmarried couples and property – basics. https://www.findlaw.com/family/living-together/unmarried-couples-and-property-basics.html

Ho VW, Thiel EC, Rubin HR, et al. The effect of advance care planning on completion of advance directives and patient satisfaction in people with HIV/AIDS. *AIDS Care.* 2000;12:97–108.

Martin DK, Thiel EC, Singer PA. A new model of advance care planning: observations from people with HIV. *Arch Intern Med.* 1999;159(1):86–92.

Massachusetts Medical Society. Health care proxies and end of life care. http://www.massmed.org/Patient-Care/Health-Topics/Health-Care-Proxies-and-End-of-Life-Care/Health-Care-Proxies-and-End-of-Life-Care/#.X16L4T-SmUk

New York State Department of Health. Choosing your health care agent. January 2020. https://www.health.ny.gov/professionals/patients/health_care_proxy/

NOLO. Estate planning: an overview. https://www.nolo.com/legal-encyclopedia/estate-planning-an-overview

NOLO. Wills. https://www.nolo.com/legal-encyclopedia/wills

Stein GL, Bonuck KA. Attitudes on end-of-life care and advance care planning in the lesbian and gay community. *J Palliat Med.* 2001;4(2):173–190.

Wenger NS, Kanouse DE, Collins RL, et al. End-of-life discussions and preferences among persons with HIV. *JAMA.* 2001;285:2880–2887.

Wolitski RJ, Rietmeijer CA, Goldbaum GM, et al. HIV serostatus disclosure among gay and bisexual men in four American cities: general patterns and relation to sexual practices. *AIDS Care.* 1998 Oct;10(5):599–610.

45.

RESEARCH DESIGN AND ANALYSIS

Sarah A. Rojas and Christian B. Ramers

INTRODUCTION

Clinical trials are used to evaluate the safety and effectiveness of drugs and devices and involve multiple phases of investigation. Each phase is governed by strict protocols, and the overall process is typically overseen by multiple regulatory bodies, including the US Food and Drug Administration (FDA) and institutional review boards. This helps ensure that drug development and approval processes are standardized.

Most early antiretroviral therapies (ARTs) entered the market via accelerated (i.e., nontraditional) approval based on changes in surrogate endpoints (i.e., plasma HIV RNA levels, CD4+ T-cell counts). However, as multiple studies subsequently demonstrated that treatment-associated decreases in HIV RNA levels were highly predictive of positive clinical outcomes, a regulatory advisory committee determined in 1997 that treatment-induced decreases in HIV RNA levels were "highly predictive of meaningful clinical benefit" and therefore HIV RNA measurements could serve as endpoints in trials designed to support *both* accelerated and traditional approvals (FDA, 2015).

Clinical trials and drug review/approval processes must be thoughtfully planned and executed, and are of critical importance to uphold patient safety and effectiveness standards. However, even if clinical research uncovers new information that is believed to hold promise in improving patient care, it often takes time for findings to be broadly adopted into practice. The process of translating research findings into clinical practice is complex, and implementation strategies are often necessary to bridge the "translation gap" and facilitate change at the individual provider, practice, and health systems levels. This may be especially relevant for HIV care, given disparities in access to treatment, HIV workforce challenges, and issues such as stigma that continue to deeply affect people with HIV (PWH) across the US and globally.

IMPLEMENTATION SCIENCE

In 2019, citing the availability of highly effective HIV treatment and prevention interventions, the US Department of Health and Human Services (DHHS) launched the *Ending the HIV Epidemic: A Plan for America* initiative, with a goal to reduce new HIV infections by 90% by 2030 (DHHS, 2019). This cross-agency collaborative involves the Centers for Disease Control and Prevention (CDC), Health Resources and Services Administration (HRSA), Indian Health Service (HIS), National Institutes of Health (NIH), and Substance Abuse and Mental Health Services Administration (SAMHSA) and focuses on 50 local jurisdictions that account for over half of new HIV diagnoses in the US. With DHHS, communities in these highly impacted areas are to tailor and implement at least one of the following key strategies: (1) Diagnose PWH as early as possible after infection; (2) Treat rapidly and effectively; (3) Prevent new HIV transmissions by using proven interventions, including preexposure prophylaxis (PrEP) and syringe service programs; and/or (4) Respond quickly to potential HIV outbreaks (https://www.hiv.gov/federal-response/ending-the-hiv-epidemic/overview). In an effort to support this work, DHHS created the America's HIV Epidemic Analysis Dashboard (AHEAD) to monitor changes in diagnosis, linkage, viral suppression, and PrEP coverage (https://ahead.hiv.gov).

Also in 2019, the NIH announced awards to participating NIH-funded Centers for AIDS Research and National Institute of Mental Health (NIMH) AIDS Research Centers that focus on implementation science. These implementation science activities will address how to translate and tailor scientific advances to priority populations at the community level (i.e., men who have sex with men, people who inject drugs, transgender persons and commercial sex workers) and further modify them to address racial, ethnic, gender, cultural, socioeconomic, and geographic parameters. Such implementation science efforts aim to address structural, legal, and societal barriers such as stigma, discrimination, criminalization, lack of access to healthcare, food insecurity, and homelessness (Eisinger et al., 2019).

EVALUATING THE STATISTICAL ANALYSIS OF CLINICAL TRIALS

LEARNING OBJECTIVES

- Differentiate between per-protocol (PP) and intent-to-treat (ITT) analyses
- Differentiate between two FDA algorithms that assess virologic response to ART regimens: time to loss of virologic response (TLOVR) and Snapshot

- Share examples of when a noninferiority analysis might be used

KEY POINTS

- Because of inherent differences in approach, the PP analysis will frequently report better outcomes than the ITT analysis due to exclusion of study dropout and loss to follow-up.

- Therapeutic responses to ART regimens may be evaluated using various approaches, such as TLOVR and Snapshot algorithms; each method may be more appropriate in certain study populations than in others.

- New ART regimens are usually compared to existing standard-of-care regimens using a type of statistical comparison called a noninferiority analysis.

- A common error in reporting and interpreting clinical trial results is not accurately distinguishing between clinical and statistical significance.

- To properly interpret and apply results of scientific studies, clinician readers should understand the difference between a statistical association and causality.

PP VERSUS ITT ANALYSIS

In randomized trials, a PP analysis (also known as "as-treated analysis," "observed analysis," or "on treatment analysis") examines outcomes in only those study participants who remain on their assigned study regimen for the duration of the trial or, in the case of an interim analysis, up to a particular time point. In contrast, an ITT analysis evaluates each patient according to the treatment group to which they were originally randomized, regardless of whether the participant received the treatment or completed the study. Both ITT and PP analyses are valuable in understanding the findings of a clinical trial.

By removing from the analysis those participants who were lost to follow-up, do not complete the study (for any reason), drop out due to side effects, or do not stay on their prescribed study regimen, a PP analysis selects for participants who tolerated study medication(s). This analysis method is therefore intrinsically biased toward a best-case scenario and may systematically bias results such that poor outcomes associated with a treatment that is not well tolerated may be hidden. The value of the ITT analysis is that it limits bias by evaluating the entire population of participants randomized to a given study regimen. ITT analyses more completely encompass efficacy, tolerability, adverse events, and the myriad other reasons why participants do not remain on or deviate from the assigned drug regimen; therefore, ITT analyses account for the influence of these factors on outcomes (Lang & Secic, 1997). The more rigorous ITT approach conveys a truer sense of a treatment's overall effectiveness and is considered to be less subject to bias.

Because of the inherent differences in these approaches, the PP analysis will frequently report better outcomes than will the ITT analysis (e.g., a higher proportion of participants achieving an undetectable HIV RNA level). PP analyses exclude participants who are noncompliant with study medications, procedures, and/or study visits and also those who drop out due to intolerance of the assigned regimen. If more participants are excluded from one treatment arm than another, the PP analysis may report a clinical difference that is quite different from the actual treatment difference obtained when all subjects are analyzed. Conversely, a PP analysis may find no difference between two treatments, whereas an ITT analysis, which better accounts for tolerability, may find a superior outcome for a treatment due to less study dropout or discontinuation.

TLOVR VERSUS SNAPSHOT ANALYSIS

Achieving an undetectable HIV RNA level (viral load) is the most widely accepted endpoint for antiretroviral clinical trials, as it is the most clinically relevant surrogate marker for outcomes that may take years to occur (e.g., progression to AIDS and death). As such, investigational ART regimens are frequently evaluated by assessing the percentage of participants achieving low (suppressed) plasma levels of HIV RNA. Because assays that detect HIV RNA have different limits of detection, it is important to know which prespecified level of HIV RNA was considered "suppressed" or "undetectable." Often, trials will allow some "forgiveness" in statistical analysis to account for small elevations or "blips" in viral load that likely do not affect ultimate clinical outcome. In addition to measuring the failure to achieve or maintain HIV RNA suppression, the TLOVR analysis also considers the introduction of a new antiretroviral drug, death, or loss to follow-up as failures (FDA, 2015). Depending on the patient population, the FDA suggests the Snapshot method of analyzing results with the goal of simplifying the evaluation of study results. Snapshot differs from TLOVR in that it primarily focuses on a virologic response at a predetermined endpoint (e.g., 24 or 48 weeks). Specifically, an outcome will be measured only if a participant is a responder with an HIV RNA of less than 50 copies/mL at week 48 (± a 1- to 2-week window) (Qaqish et al., 2010). Twenty-four weeks of follow-up data is often appropriate for drugs that have some benefit over existing options (i.e., for patients with multiple antiretroviral drug resistance, where it may not be possible to construct a fully suppressive treatment regimen; or improved efficacy, tolerability, or ease of administration), while 48 weeks is recommended for investigational therapies with comparable characteristics to existing options (FDA, 2015). Both methods of analysis have value, and clinical trials often report results in both forms, although more recent analyses have favored the Snapshot algorithm.

NONINFERIORITY ANALYSIS

In contrast to statistical analyses used to demonstrate superiority, new drug regimens may be evaluated with the aim of demonstrating equivalence or noninferior efficacy relative to a standard drug regimen. The noninferiority trial is used mainly when the added value of a new drug/regimen is related to factors such as improved convenience, better tolerability, simpler dosing schedule, lower toxicity, or lower cost (Wittkop et al., 2010). FDA industry guidance regarding procedures for new drug approval has helped to standardize the statistical methods used in clinical trials. The proportion of treatment responders at 48 weeks is often used to assess noninferiority, as this provides sufficient time for emergence of loss of tolerability, antiretroviral drug resistance, or other relevant measurable outcomes, using a specific margin of difference that is acceptable between study arms (FDA, 2015). In practical terms, a noninferiority analysis is a statistically rigorous way in which a clinical trial can demonstrate that a new therapy/regimen is at least as good as a currently available option. Often, efficacy results may appear numerically different, with one regimen achieving a slightly higher proportion of participants with undetectable viral loads at week 48, for example. In a noninferiority trial, numerical difference is less important than whether efficacy of both regimens falls within the prespecified "noninferiority margin," which then helps determine clinical equivalence. Trials are often powered differently, with larger numbers of participants if they aim to show superiority of one regimen over another rather than noninferiority. Recently, the FDA has tightened this noninferiority margin to ensure that new drugs are truly equivalent to existing therapies before coming to market.

CLINICAL VERSUS STATISTICAL SIGNIFICANCE

When evaluating research findings, clinicians should be aware of the difference between a statistically significant difference and a clinically significant difference. One of the most common errors in interpreting and reporting clinical trial results is not correctly distinguishing between clinical and statistical significance (Braitman, 1991). A clinically significant finding is one that has important implications for patient care. A statistically significant finding is a conclusion that there is evidence against the "null hypothesis"; that is, a low probability exists of getting a result as extreme or more extreme than the one observed in the study data by chance alone. Statistical significance, when applied to the terms noninferiority or superiority, indicates that the result of a clinical trial would be unlikely to occur by chance. It does not necessarily mean that the result will be important for treating patients (Braitman, 1991; Lang & Secic, 1997). Clinically significant findings typically must involve outcomes with particular relevance to clinical medicine and must have an effect size that is large enough to influence clinical decision-making.

RECOMMENDED READING

Department of Health and Human Services. Overview: what is *Ending the HIV Epidemic: A Plan for America*? February 5, 2019. https://www.hiv.gov/federal-response/ending-the-hiv-epidemic/overview
Eisinger RW, Dieffenbach CW, Fauci AS. Role of implementation science: linking fundamental discovery science and innovation science to ending the HIV epidemic at the community level. *J AIDS*. 2019;82:S171–S172. doi:10.1097/QAI.0000000000002227
Friedman LM, Furberg CD, DeMets DL. *Fundamentals of clinical trials*, 5th ed. New York: Springer; 2015.
Pocock SJ. *Clinical trials: a practical approach*. New York: Wiley; 1991.

DETERMINING CAUSE-AND-EFFECT ASSOCIATIONS

LEARNING OBJECTIVE

- Discuss the difficulties of drawing cause-and-effect conclusions about associations identified in research studies, including the limitations of observational studies and cross-study comparisons

KEY POINTS

- Randomized clinical trials (RCTs) and observational cohorts provide different but equally valuable information.

- Cohort studies frequently follow large numbers of study participants for prolonged periods and have greater representation of "real-world" populations (e.g., women and minorities) than do traditional randomized trials.

- Cohort studies lack randomization and controls but are useful in generating hypotheses and demonstrating long-term associations that can be further evaluated in randomized, prospective trials.

RCTs represent the gold standard of modern clinical research because they randomly assign equivalent groups of study participants to different treatments, thus eliminating many types of bias that might influence outcome. If randomization efforts are effectively implemented, the different arms of an RCT should be equivalent in all aspects except for the intervention/treatment administered, allowing conclusions to be drawn regarding the causality of the intervention and a given outcome. However, RCTs are expensive and time-consuming and typically must include a large number of participants in order to show results that are generalizable across patient populations. Although considered to provide a less rigorous level of evidence, observational cohort studies, cross-sectional analyses, and case–control studies have also played a major role in HIV clinical research efforts and can add value to the general scientific understanding and evidence base of a particular problem.

From the earliest findings of the Multicenter AIDS Cohort Study (MACS) to other ongoing national and international cohorts, study databases have provided crucial insights into the natural history of HIV and the efficacy and safety of various HIV treatments. Lipodystrophy, cardiovascular disease, renal and bone complications, treatment interruptions, and the timing of ART initiation are areas with recent contributions from observational studies. Compared to RCTs, cohort analyses are no more or less valuable; rather, they are simply different design methodologies designed to answer different types of questions.

Cohort studies are able to follow large numbers of participants for prolonged periods of time and often better reflect "real-world" populations, in contrast to study subjects who are able and willing to participate in randomized trials. While randomized trials will typically measure 48-, 96-, or rarely 192-week data, cohort studies run for much longer and frequently have greater representation of women, minorities, and those with comorbid conditions than do typical randomized studies (which may exclude patients with preidentified health conditions).

Cohort studies, however, do have biases. First, the quality of the results is only as good as the quality, consistency, and completeness of the data from cohort participants. Second, a lack of randomization or control of treatments administered to participants can significantly impact interpretation of the results through introduction of selection bias. For example, participants starting a particular treatment in a cohort study may be selected by investigators to avoid a perceived toxicity or selected to gain a perceived benefit, and this in turn could lead to results favoring one agent over another that may or may not be correct. Similarly, large changes in policy, availability of treatment advances, or other confounding disease states—so-called historical bias—can influence outcomes and may be more important than the specific variables being assessed. Cohort studies are useful for observing events and outcomes that only occur many years after an exposure that might be missed by a 1- to 3-year RCT. They also may find associations that can generate hypotheses, where an observation may lead to the undertaking of an RCT to confirm or refute the observations made in the cohort analysis. Cohort studies may detect associations between certain treatments or factors with an outcome that prompts a more rigorous evaluation to help determine causality. They can provide preliminary information about long-term clinical endpoints, survival, complications, and the role of comorbid conditions that may be tested later in an RCT. Thus, the observational cohort study and RCT are complementary rather than competitive.

Focused observational studies can also be valuable for evaluating factors associated with rare diseases or outcomes. In a case–control study, a set of individuals (cases) with the condition of interest is assembled (Schulz & Grimes, 2002). A corresponding set of individuals (controls) without the condition is then selected. Controls are frequently matched to be similar to the cases, and they should be selected from the same general population. Information on risk factors is then collected and analyzed to identify factors that are more (or less) common in the cases compared to the controls. For example, thresholds used to define the appropriate use of prophylaxis for opportunistic infections are largely derived from case–control studies that showed increased risk for these infections in groups of PWH with lower CD4+ counts compared to PWH with higher counts. Careful design and implementation are needed to minimize bias in case–control studies, particularly to select appropriate controls and to collect unbiased information on risk factors.

Cross-study comparisons of randomized trials—that is, trying to relate efficacy of one particular treatment to that of another when they have not been directly compared—must be undertaken with caution because patient characteristics, study protocols, and extrinsic factors may differ considerably between studies that share the same primary endpoint. A meta-analysis of related studies is more reliable than a one-to-one comparison because researchers can carefully analyze data to avoid misleading conclusions, and they can thoroughly describe what they did and why.

In summary, when attempting to determine causality between an intervention or risk factor and an outcome, RCTs provide the highest level of evidence. Observational studies such as cohort, case–control, and cross-sectional studies are useful to generate hypotheses, to show preliminary associations, and to guide the design of future clinical trials. Most of what is known about HIV's natural history, treatment response, and associated clinical risk factors for progression or virologic control is derived from these types of studies.

RECOMMENDED READING

Collins R, MacMahon S. Reliable assessment of the effects of treatment on mortality and major morbidity: I. Clinical trials. *Lancet*. 2001;357:373–380.

Ioannidis JPA, Haidich A, Pappa M, et al. Comparison of evidence of treatment effects in randomized and nonrandomized studies. *JAMA*. 2001;286:821–830.

MacMahon S, Collins R. Reliable assessment of the effects of treatment on mortality and major morbidity: II. Observational studies. *Lancet*. 2001;357:455–462.

REFERENCES

Braitman LE. Confidence intervals assess both clinical significance and statistical significance. *Ann Intern Med*. 1991;114:515–517.

Department of Health and Human Services. *Ending the HIV Epidemic: A Plan for America*. February 5, 2019. https://www.hhs.gov/blog/2019/02/05/ending-the-hiv-epidemic-a-plan-for-america.html

Eisinger RW, Dieffenbach CW, Fauci AS. Role of implementation science: linking fundamental discovery science and innovation science to ending the HIV epidemic at the community level. *J AIDS*. 2019;82:S171–S172. doi: 10.1097/QAI.0000000000002227.

Food and Drug Administration. *Guidance for industry submitting select clinical trial data sets for drugs intended to treat human immunodeficiency virus-1 infection*. Washington, DC: US Department of Health and Human Services; 2015. https://www.fda.gov/downloads/forindustry/datastandards/studydatastandards/ucm603323.pdf

Lang TA, Secic M. *How to report statistics in medicine: annotated guidelines for authors, editors, and reviewers*. Philadelphia, PA: American College of Physicians; 1997.

Qaqish R, van Wyk J, King M. A comparison of the FDA TLOVR and FDA Snapshot algorithms based on studies evaluating once-daily vs. twice daily lopinavir/ritonavir (LPV/r) regimens. *J Intl AIDS Soc*. 2010;13:P58. doi:10.1186/1758-2652-13-S4-P58

Schulz KF, Grimes DA. Case–control studies: research in reverse. *Lancet*. 2002;359:431–434.

Wittkop L, Smith C, Fox Z, et al. Methodological issues in the use of composite endpoints in clinical trials: examples from the HIV field. *Clin Trials*. 2010;7(1):19–35.

46.

ETHICAL CONDUCT OF CLINICAL TRIALS, INSTITUTIONAL REVIEW BOARDS, INFORMED CONSENT, AND FINANCIAL CONFLICTS OF INTEREST

Adam C. Bortner and Christian B. Ramers

LEARNING OBJECTIVE

- Describe the essential components of the ethical conduct of research, role of institutional review boards (IRBs), process of informed consent, potential areas of conflict of interest for clinicians participating in research, and other ethical issues related to research in HIV medicine

WHAT'S NEW

In July 2019, the US Food and Drug Administration (FDA) released draft guidance for enhancing the diversity of clinical trial populations to help further promote research enrollment practices that lead to clinical trials better reflecting the patient population(s) most likely to use a therapy/drug if it were to be approved. The guidance recommends specific approaches that sponsors of clinical trials can take to broaden eligibility criteria (as appropriate) and increase enrollment of underrepresented populations in clinical trials.

KEY POINTS

The Declaration of Helsinki and the Belmont Report remain important guides for ethical standards in research. IRBs are an essential resource for clinician investigators, beyond reviewing trial applications and monitoring study progress. However, many IRB committees and research trials continue to lack member and participant diversity; this may be an especially salient consideration for HIV-related research, given ongoing HIV-related health disparities (along racial, gender, socioeconomic, age, etc. dimensions).

INTRODUCTION

HIV prevention and treatment advances reflect decades of research initiatives involving hundreds of thousands of participants. The ethical considerations when performing research include basic ethical principles (e.g., autonomy,

confidentiality, nonmaleficence, informed consent, beneficence, justice, and utility), as well as nuances including appropriate study designs, investigator conflict of interests, and bias in all its forms. To help guide clinicians, a number of professional and governmental organizations have posted guidelines and recommendations on various aspects of clinical research (e.g., the American Medical Association, the National Institutes of Health, and the FDA).

The Declaration of Helsinki and the Belmont Report are important historical benchmarks that have laid the foundation of currently accepted ethical standards in the treatment of participants in clinical trials. The Declaration of Helsinki, first adopted in 1964 and amended multiple times (most recently updated in 2013), stresses that it is the duty of the physician to promote and safeguard the health of patients and that the well-being of the individual research participants must take precedence over all other interests (World Medical Association, 2013). Although the document does not highlight individual diseases or specific research initiatives, the following points have particular importance to people with HIV:

1. Participation in clinical trials must be completely voluntary and without undue coercion or influence.

2. It is the duty of the physician to maintain privacy and confidentiality of personal information.

3. Populations that are underrepresented in medical research should be provided appropriate access to participation in research.

Similarly, the Belmont Report (US Department of Health and Welfare, 1979) highlights three fundamental ethical principles relating specifically to the conduct of research:

1. The principle of *respect for persons* acknowledges the dignity and autonomy of individuals.

2. The principle of *beneficence* protects individuals by maximizing anticipated benefits and minimizing possible harms.

3. The principle of *justice* requires that all subjects are treated fairly.

Recognizing that certain groups remain underrepresented in clinical trials, in 2019 the FDA released draft guidance with recommendations for enhancing diversity among research participants (FDA, 2019).

Additionally, there are seven requirements for determining whether a research trial is ethical; these are discussed next.

SEVEN REQUIREMENTS FOR DETERMINING WHETHER A RESEARCH TRIAL IS ETHICAL

Emanuel et al. (2000) described the following requirements for determining whether a clinical trial is ethical:

1. *Value*: Enhancements of health or knowledge must be derived from the research.

2. *Scientific validity*: The research must be methodologically rigorous.

3. *Fair subject selection*: Scientific objective, not vulnerability or privilege, and the potential for and distribution of risks and benefits should determine the communities selected for study sites and the inclusion criteria for individual subjects.

4. *Favorable risk–benefit ratio*: Within the context of standard clinical practices and the research protocol, risk must be minimized and potential benefits enhanced, and the potential benefits to individuals and the knowledge gained for society must outweigh the risks.

5. *Independent review*: Unaffiliated individuals must review the research and approve, amend, or terminate it.

6. *Informed consent*: Individuals should be informed about the research and provide their voluntary consent.

7. *Respect for enrolled subjects*: Participants should have their privacy protected, the opportunity to withdraw from the research without penalty, and their well-being monitored.

Facing ethical dilemmas during the conduct of a clinical trial is a rather common experience. A survey of physicians engaged in clinical research found that almost all of them had recently encountered such issues (DuVal et al., 2005). Issues can arise at any stage of the research process, from trial design through execution to the final publication of the research report. Notably, this particular survey found that most ethical dilemmas occurred after IRB approval, suggesting that ethical considerations should be continuous rather than a one-time process. Approximately half of the physician respondents requested an ethical consultation before resolving the issue, and, accordingly, many institutions are beginning to offer such services outside of the IRB process.

INSTITUTIONAL REVIEW BOARDS

IRBs are charged with (1) reviewing protocols and consent documents and any modifications to them prior to their implementation and (2) monitoring approved trials on a periodic basis to ensure ethical conduct. IRBs do not have primary responsibility for trial-related safety issues; that responsibility resides with the principal investigator(s), the safety officer designated by the study sponsor, and the regulatory affairs office responsible for adverse event reporting to the FDA and other regulatory agencies (as applicable). Nonetheless, IRBs must be informed of any safety concerns as they arise because safety issues may impact the ethical conduct of the trial. Multicenter trials may utilize an independent, central IRB chosen by the trial sponsor as well as local IRBs established by participating study sites/research centers. IRB composition and responsibilities are guided by the U.S. Code of Federal Regulations (21 CFR 56.107-111), which provides minimum standards for subject safety and information. Some forms of research (e.g., retrospective chart reviews) may be considered "minimal risk" and thus eligible for an IRB exemption or waiver; however, when in doubt regarding the ethical merits of a particular research effort, an investigator or clinician should always err on the side of caution and engage a local IRB or ethics committee for guidance. In a systematic review of literature evaluating IRBs in the US, bioethicists from the National Institutes of Health (NIH) identified widespread problems, including inconsistent interpretation of federal regulations with inefficient processes as well as inadequate training and diversity of IRB members (Abbott & Grady, 2011).

RECRUITMENT AND SELECTION OF PARTICIPANTS

In addition to IRB member diversity and representation, the diversity of participants in clinical trials has gained increasing attention over the past few decades. In 1993, President Clinton signed the National Institutes of Health Revitalization Act into law, requiring "inclusion of women and minorities as subjects" as a priority in federally funded clinical research (US Congress, 1993). Twenty-six years later, the FDA put forth draft recommendations in June 2019 calling for increased enrollment in clinical research of groups underrepresented on the basis of race, ethnicity, sex, and age as well as nondemographic factors such as organ dysfunction, comorbid conditions, and extremes of weight. The guidelines specifically note that people with HIV "are often excluded from clinical trials without strong clinical or scientific justification" and advocate that participants in clinical trials better reflect the diversity of populations in which therapies may be used (FDA, 2019). Strategies to accomplish the goal of increased diversity include ensuring healthcare providers reflect this diversity and using community-based participatory research methods, where members of communities being researched are involved in research design and implementation and agenda setting. Early access for diverse populations to therapies that prolong or save lives through safe, ethical research may also benefit such communities with disproportionate disease burden and mitigate health disparities (Washington, 2006).

INFORMED CONSENT

The FDA provides a comprehensive review on the informed consent process and guidance for development of the informed consent document (FDA, 2016). The informed consent procedure involves more than simply obtaining a participant's signature; it is a process of complete and accurate information exchange that may include, in addition to reading and signing the informed consent document, participant recruitment materials, verbal instructions, a question-and-answer session, and measures of participant understanding. Researchers must provide potential participants with full disclosure of the anticipated benefits and risks of and alternatives to the study intervention. That obligation extends throughout the course of the study to include updating participants in a timely manner on emerging knowledge that might change their perception of the risks and benefits of continued participation in the trial. The informed consent document should be in a language and at a content level understandable to the subject (or the subject's representative) and provide the subject with sufficient opportunity to consider whether to participate without the possibility of coercion or undue influence. In addition, the document must state that participation is completely voluntary and that subjects can withdraw from the study at any point in time, for any reason, without loss of benefits or penalty.

CONFLICTS OF INTERESTS IN THE CONDUCT OF CLINICAL TRIALS

As research has expanded to include centers outside of academic health institutions, partnerships between pharmaceutical companies and private practice research sites have grown. As such, physicians (and other types of clinician investigators) may play dual roles of both investigator and clinician. This could lead to a conflict of interest to enroll participants in trials when financial incentives are in place. The American Medical Association (AMA) has posted recommendations to safeguard against conflicts of interest during clinical trials. Only physicians with medical expertise in the areas of the research being performed should be investigators. When financial compensation is offered from trial sponsors, it should be at "fair market value," with the rate commensurate with the efforts of the physician performing the research; additionally, compensation should not vary according to the number of participants enrolled by the physician; and any compensation must be disclosed to a potential participant as part of the informed consent process. In addition, the AMA states that it is unethical for physicians to accept payment solely for referring patients to research studies. Finally, both the AMA and the Declaration of Helsinki (2008) make specific statements about the publication of study results. The AMA states that physicians should ensure that publication of study results not be unduly delayed or otherwise obstructed by the sponsoring company, and the most recent update of the Declaration of Helsinki highlights that negative and inconclusive, as well as positive, results should be published or otherwise be made publicly available.

PERCEPTIONS AND MISPERCEPTIONS

Altruism often is a core but seldom the sole reason for volunteering to participate in a study (Kass et al., 1996). Many people participate in clinical trials for very pragmatic reasons, such as having inadequate or no health insurance, or they may have exhausted or found no relief from currently approved therapies (Kass et al., 1996; Sacristan et al., 2016). A trial may represent their only perceived access to care or hope for relief. Such a mixture of motivating factors can exacerbate the "therapeutic misconception," wherein participants believe they are receiving clinical care rather than engaging in clinical research.

With an increasing number of clinical trials being performed and the expansion of their conduct from research medical centers to private settings, the distinction between research and care can become blurred (Morin et al., 2002). It may be difficult for individual physicians to separate their roles of healthcare provider and researcher (Miller et al., 1998), both within their own minds and in communicating with patients who are potential participants in a study. This also may lead investigators to circumvent strict enrollment criteria or bypass the randomization process (Morin et al., 2002). This can heighten the potential for a participant's "therapeutic misconception." The two roles that the physician plays often then result in a tension that is ethically complex and ambiguous, and, if it cannot be avoided, it must be managed appropriately (Miller et al., 1998).

The AMA has taken the position that the physician who has treated a patient on an ongoing basis should not be responsible for obtaining informed consent. Rather, once a patient has been identified as meeting trial eligibility, a person who does not have an existing treating/therapeutic relationship should conduct the formal consent procedure (Morin et al., 2002). This is particularly important when studies are performed in institutional (or other involuntary placement) settings, including correctional facilities, in which broad supervision may impact the free will and autonomy of potential volunteers.

Clinicians must be mindful of the trust that patients place in them to guide their personal healthcare decisions, including participation in a clinical research trial, and clinicians must be clear in distinguishing between providing direct care and offering participation in a clinical trial (Kass et al., 1996). Many clinician-researchers find it helpful to separate clinical care visits temporally and geographically from research study visits in order to clearly separate the goals of each interaction.

ETHICAL CONSIDERATIONS IN INTERNATIONAL RESEARCH

Scientific advances in the treatment of HIV have produced antiretroviral medication and regimens that are highly potent, well tolerated, and convenient for most patients. As a result, the interest in patient participation in clinical trials of novel agents and regimens in high-income/industrialized countries has declined. This in turn has caused many biotechnology and pharmaceutical companies to shift a large portion of their research interests and initiatives to regions of the world that are lacking in infrastructure and/or resources to provide treatments that are considered to be "standard of care" in resource-rich settings. A 2001 editorial in the *New England Journal of Medicine* highlighted the following key issues regarding research in resource-limited settings/developing countries (Shapiro & Mesline, 2001):

1. Clinical trials conducted abroad should meet all ethical standards for trials based in the US.

2. Studies should be sensitive to the local customs, conditions, and culture of the region.

3. Careful consideration must be undertaken in areas that have high rates of illiteracy or where signing a form may be considered dangerous in countries with oppressive political regimes.

4. It is unethical to ask persons to participate in a trial in which the intervention being tested is not likely affordable in the host country or where the healthcare infrastructure cannot support its proper distribution and use.

5. The experimental intervention should, ideally, be compared with an established, effective treatment or standard of care.

6. Research participants should not be made worse off by their inability to have continued access to a successful intervention after the trial has ended.

7. A review by ethics committees in both host and sponsoring countries should be performed.

CONCLUSION

HIV-related biomedical research has resulted in a large body of preventive and therapeutic advancements and vast improvements in our scientific knowledge and clinical understanding of the biology, pathogenesis, natural history, and epidemiology of HIV infection. Foundational ethical principles such as autonomy, confidentiality, nonmaleficence, informed consent, beneficence, justice, and utility must be continually applied to the conduct of research in order to maintain ethically sound research programs that can advance health for all affected populations. IRBs and ethics consultation services can serve as important resources for researchers and clinicians. Increasing diversity among both researchers and participants may increase health equity.

REFERENCES

Abbott L, Grady C. A systematic review of the empirical literature evaluating IRBs: what we know and what we still need to learn. *J Empir Res Hum Res Ethics.* 2011;6(1):3–19. doi:10.1525/jer.2011.6.1.3

DuVal G, Gensler G, Danis M. Ethical dilemmas encountered by clinical researchers. *J Clin Ethics.* 2005;16(3):267–276.

Emanuel EJ, Wendler D, Grady C. What makes clinical research ethical? *JAMA.* 2000;283(20):2701–2711.

Kass NE, Sugarman J, Faden R, et al. Trust, the fragile foundation of contemporary biomedical research. *Hastings Cent Rep.* 1996;26(5): 25–29.

Miller FG, Rosenstein DL, DeRenzo EG. Professional integrity in clinical research. *JAMA.* 1998;280(16):1449–1454.

Morin K, Rakatansky H, Riddick FA, et al. Managing conflicts of interest in the conduct of clinical trials. *JAMA.* 2002;287:78–84.

Sacristan JA, Aguaron A, Avendano-Sola C, et al. Patient involvement in clinical research: why, when, and how. *Patient Prefer Adherence.* 2016;10:631–640.

Shapiro HT, Mesline EM. Ethical issues in the design and conduct of clinical trials in developing countries. *N Engl J Med.* 2001;345(2):139–142.

US Congress, National Institutes of Health Revitalization Act of 1993: Act to Amend the Public Health Service Act to Revise and Extend the Programs of the National Institutes of Health, and for Other Purposes. https://www.congress.gov/bill/103rd-congress/senate-bill/1

US Department of Health and Welfare, National Commission for the Protection of Human Subjects of Biomedical and Behavioral Research. The Belmont Report: ethical principles and guidelines for the protection of human subjects of research. April 18, 1979. http://www.hhs.gov/ohrp/humansubjects/guidance/belmont.html

US Food and Drug Administration. A guide to informed consent—Information sheet: Guidance for institutional review boards and clinical investigators. 2016. www.fda.gov/RegulatoryInformation/Guidances/ucm126431.htm

US Food and Drug Administration. Enhancing the diversity of clinical trial populations—Eligibility criteria, enrollment practices, and trial designs guidance for industry. June 2019. https://www.fda.gov/regulatory-information/search-fda-guidance-documents/enhancing-diversity-clinical-trial-populations-eligibility-criteria-enrollment-practices-and-trial

Washington HA. *Medical apartheid: the dark history of medical experimentation on Black Americans from colonial times to the present.* 1st ed. New York, NY: Doubleday Books; 2006.

World Medical Association. Declaration of Helsinki: ethical principles for medical research involving human subjects. *JAMA.* 2013;310(20): 2191–2194.

INDEX

Tables, figures and boxes are indicated by *t*, *f* and *b* following the page number